PERITONEAL DIALYSIS

PERITONEAL DIALYSIS

Edited by

KARL D. NOLPH

Division of Nephrology, University of Missouri Health Sciences Center,
VA Hospital, and Dalton Research Center, Columbia, Missouri, U.S.A.

Third edition

KLUWER ACADEMIC PUBLISHERS

DORDRECHT / BOSTON / LONDON

Library of Congress Cataloging in Publication Data

Peritoneal dialysis / edited by Karl D. Nolph. -- 3rd ed.
        p.   cm.
    Includes bibliographies and index.
    ISBN 0-89838-406-0 (U.S.)
    1. Peritoneal dialysis.   I. Nolph, Karl D.
    [DNLM: 1. Peritoneal Dialysis.   WJ 378 P446]
    RC901.7.P48P473 1988
    617'.461059--dc19
    DNLM/DLC
    for Library of Congress   88-23156
                                                                  CIP

Published by Kluwer Academic Publishers,
P.O. Box 17, 3300 AA Dordrecht, The Netherlands.

Kluwer Academic Publishers incorporates
the publishing programmes of
D. Reidel, Martinus Nijhoff, Dr W. Junk and MTP Press.

Sold and distributed in the U.S.A. and Canada
by Kluwer Academic Publishers,
101 Philip Drive, Norwell, MA 02061, U.S.A.

In all other countries, sold and distributed
by Kluwer Academic Publishers Group,
P.O. Box 322, 3300 AH Dordrecht, The Netherlands.

TABLE OF CONTENTS

LIST OF CONTRIBUTORS

S.R. ALEXANDER
University of Texas
Health Science Center
Department of Clinical Pediatric Nephrology
5323 Harry Hines Blvd
Dallas, TX 75235-9063, U.S.A.

J.M. BARGMAN
Division of Nephrology
Department of Medicine
Toronto Western Hospital
399 Bathurst Street
Toronto, Ontario, Canada M5T 2S8

J. BERGSTRÖM
Department of Renal Medicine
K 56, Huddinge University Hospital
Karolinska Institute
S-141 86 Huddinge, Sweden

S.T. BOEN
Department of Nephrology and Dialysis
Sint Lucas Hospital
Jan Tooropstraat 164
Amsterdam-West, The Netherlands

F.P. BRUNNER
EDTA-ERA Registration Committee
Department of Internal Medicine
University of Basel
4031 Basel, Switzerland

H.J. BURTON
Department of Psychiatry
University of Toronto
Toronto Western Hospital
399 Bathurst Street
Toronto, Ontario, Canada M5T 2S8

J.A. DIAZ-BUXO
Nall Clinic Kidney Center
928 Baxter Street
Charlotte, NC 28204, U.S.A.

P.C. FARRELL
Centre for Biomedical Engineering
P.O. Box 1
University of New South Wales
Kensington, NSW, Australia 2033

W. GEERLINGS
EDTA-ETA Registration Committee
Home Dialysis Foundation North Netherlands
Nieuwe Stationsweg 3-7
9751 CA Haren, The Netherlands

T.A. GOLPER
Division of Nephrology
Oregon Health Sciences University
Portland, OR 97201, U.S.A.

L. GOTLOIB
Department of Nephrology
Kornach Laboratory for Experimental Nephrology
Central Emek Hospital
Afula 18101, Israel

D.N. GRANGER
Department of Physiology
Louisiana State University
P.O. Box 33923
Shreveport, LA 71130, U.S.A.

M.D. HALLETT
Baxter Center for Medical Research
376 Lane Cove Road
Sydney, NSW, Australia 2113

P.A. HEIDENHEIM
Department of Medicine
Victoria Hospital
375 South Street
London, Ontario, Canada N6A 4G5

L.W. HENDERSON
VA Hospital
3350 La Jolla Village Drive
San Diego, CA 92161, U.S.A.

P. HIRSZEL
Division of Nephrology
Uniformed Services University of the Health Sciences
Bethesda, MD 20814, U.S.A.

C. JACOBS, EDTA Registry
St. Thomas' Hospital
London, England SE1 7EH

R. KHANNA
Division of Nephrology-MA436
University of Missouri Health Sciences Center
1 Hospital Drive
Columbia, MO 65212, U.S.A.

S.A. KLINE
Department of Psychiatry
Toronto Western Hospital
399 Bathurst Street
Toronto, Ontario, Canada M5T 2S8

R.J. KORTHUIS
Department of Physiology
Louisiana State Univerrsity
P.O. Box 33923
Shreveport, LA 71130, U.S.A.

P. KRAMER
EDTA Registry
St. Thomas' Hospital
London, England SE1 7EH

R.C. KUSH
247 rue de Vaugirard
Paris, 75015 France

J.K. LEYPOLDT
Departments of Medicine and AMES
University of California
San Diego and the VA Medical Center
3350 La Jolla Village
San Diego, CA 91161, U.S.A.

A.S. LINDBLAD
The EMMES Cooperation
Data Coordinating Center for the U.S.A. CAPD Registry
11325 Seven Locks Road
Suite 214
Potomac, MD 20854, U.S.A.

B. LINDHOLM
Department of Renal Medicine
Karolinska Institute
Huddinge University Hospital
Huddinge, S-141 86 Sweden

R.M. LINDSAY
The University of Western Ontario
Victoria Hospital
375 South Street
London, Ontario, Canada N6A 4G5

M.J. LYSAGHT
Baxter Center for Medical Research
376 Lane Cove Road
Sydney, NSW, Australia 2113

R.A. MACTIER
Department of Medicine
Ninewells Hospital
Dundee, DD1 9SY Scotland, United Kingdom

J.F. MAHER
Division of Nephrology
Uniformed Services University of the Health Sciences
Bethesda, MD 20814, U.S.A.

J.W. MONCRIEF
Acorn Research Laboratory and Austin Diagnostic Clinic
Austin, TX 78765, U.S.A.

R. MOORE
EDTA Registry
St. Thomas' Hospital
London, England SE1 7EH

K.D. NOLPH,
Division of Nephrology-MA436
University of Missouri Health Sciences Center
VA Hospital and Dalton Research Center
Columbia MO 65212, U.S.A.

J.W. NOVAK
The EMMES Corporation
Data Coordinating Center for the USA CAPD Registry
11325 Seven Locks Road
Suite 214
Potomac, MD 20854, U.S.A.

D.G. OREOPOULOS, Division of Nephrology
Toronto Western Hospital
399 Bathurst Street
Toronto, Ontario, Canada M5T 2S8

R.P. POPOVICH
University of Texas
Department of Chemical and Biomedical Engineering
3410 Owen
Austin, TX 78705, U.S.A.

W.K. PYLE
Acorn Research Laboratory
3410 Owen
Austin, TX 78705, U.S.A.

J. ROTTEMBOURG
Department of Nephrology, Groupe Hospitalier de la Pitié-
Salpêtrière
47-83 Blvd de l'Hôpital
75651 Paris, Cedex 13, France

J. RUBIN
Division of Nephrology
University of Mississippi Medical Center
2500 North State Street
Jackson, MS 39216, U.S.A.

B.H. SCRIBNER
University of Washington
Division of Kidney Diseases
Box Room 11
Seattle, WA 98105, U.S.A.

N.H. SELWOOD
EDTA-ERA Registration Committee
UK Transplant Service
Southmead Road, Bristol BS10 5ND, United Kingdom

A. SHUSTAK
Department of Nephrology
Central Emek Hospital
Afula 18101, Israel

Z.J. TWARDOWSKI
Division of Nephrology-MA436
University of Missouri Health Sciences Center
1 Hospital Drive
Columbia, MO 65212, U.S.A.

S.I. VAS
Department of Medical Microbiology
Toronto Western Hospital
399 Bathurst Street
Toronto, Ontario, Canada M5T 2S8

A.J. WING
EDTA-ERA Registration Committee
St. Thomas' Hospital
London SE1 7EH, United Kingdom

FOREWORD TO FIRST EDITION

A year or so after Dr. Robert Popovich arrived in Seattle in 1965 to begin working on his doctoral thesis under Dr. A.L. Babb, we had just begun work to try to prove the prediction that the peritoneum had a higher permeability to 'middle molecules' than hemodialysis membranes [1]. Several years later, when Dr. Popovich accepted a position at the University of Texas in Austin, he decided to concentrate his research efforts in the area of peritoneal dialysis and everyone knows how successful that effort has become [2]. Indeed, because of continuous ambulatory peritoneal dialysis (CAPD), long-term peritoneal dialysis after a two-decade incubation period is finally becoming an equal option to hemodialysis and transplantation in the management of chronic renal failure.

For me this development represents final vindication of a twenty-year effort to help promote peritoneal dialysis, often in the face of enormous opposition. I particularly remember a policy meeting at the NIH a few years back in which it was decided by my colleagues on the committee that long term peritoneal dialysis had no future and therefore no funds for projects in this area would be forthcoming. Based on the excellent results that Boen and later Tenckhoff had been getting in our Seattle program, I knew the committee was wrong and tried to convince them otherwise. Naturally, being the only favorable vote, I failed. I often wonder how many years this decision and others like it set back peritoneal dialysis.

Long term peritoneal dialysis was born out of necessity. After starting the first three patients on long term hemodialysis in early 1960, the program was completely shut down because the hospital administration decreed that due to lack of funding, no additional patients could be accepted until one of the first three died. Since that did not occur until 11 years later, it would have been a long wait.

Later the administrators relented – mainly on the strength of a small research grant from Dean George Aagaard that permitted us to add two more patients. The second of these, J.R., proved to be the first failure on chronic hemodialysis, who would have died had not Fred Boen arrived in Seattle about that time. J.R. was dying simply because he immediately clotted the same AV shunt that was working so well in the other 4 patients. (Imagine what might have happened if J.R. had been patient number 1 instead of number 5). The reasons for this accelerated clotting were never identified. However, recently a small subgroup of dialysis patients with an accelerated tendency to clot has been described [3] and J.R. may have belonged to that group. In any event, Dr. Boen determined to try to save J.R. by means of long term peritoneal dialysis. Figure 1

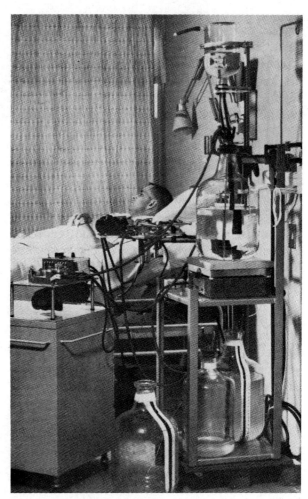

Figure 1. Patient JR on a 20-l carboy dialysis system in 1962. From 1963 onwards 40-l units were used.

shows this patient on the cycler cleverly fashioned out of equipment that had been developed five years earlier by Dr. Thomas Marr for use in gastrodialysis [4].

In 1962, when Dr. Boen started working with J.R., long term peritoneal dialysis had been abandoned because of the high incidence of peritonitis. Boen decided to eliminate the bottle change as one source of infection and developed a closed sterile system using first twenty-liter and later forty-liter carboys of dialysis fluid. This remarkable system required that a 'fluid factory' be built which could manu-

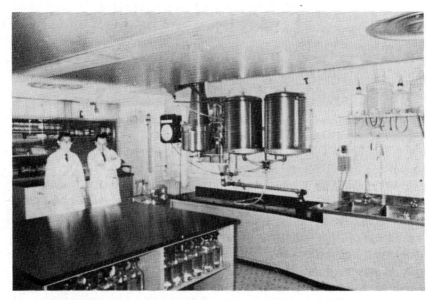

Figure 2. Dr. Fred Boen and his chief technician, Mr. George Shilipetar in the fluid factory, 1962.

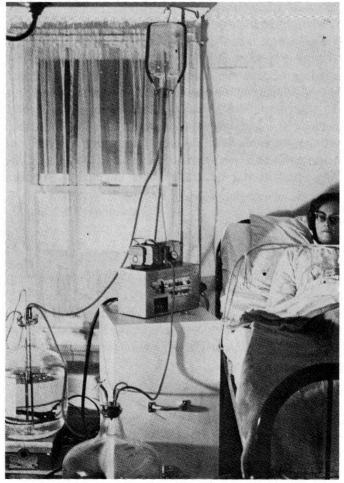

Figure 3. Patient M.O. on peritoneal dialysis at home, using a 40-l carboy cycler which remained completely closed throughout the procedure.

facture and sterilize forty-liter bottles. A remote corner in the sub-basement of the University of Washington Hospital was donated to the project and this factory, Figure 2, operated successfully until 1979, when it was finally refurbished and moved upstairs to more respectable quarters. To this day all in-hospital peritoneal dialysis still is done with forty-liter carboys. Being completely closed and sterile, it is the safest system ever devised and permitted Boen to keep J.R. going for many months until he finally became infected repeatedly through the access device and eventually died. As a result Boen decided to abandon attempts to develop a peritoneal access device and in January 1963, started a second patient, J.D., on peritoneal dialysis using a repeated puncture technique which involved inserting a catheter for each dialysis. J.D. did very well on peritoneal dialysis remaining virtually free of peritonitis for three years until she was switched to hemodialysis. Eventually she received a transplant from her sister and is alive and well today, seventeen years after starting peritoneal dialysis. Boen regards his experience with J.D. as the crucial first step in finally proving the potential feasibility of long-term peritoneal dialysis in the management of end-stage kidney disease. Boen's research fellow, Henry Tenckhoff, went one step further. He started a patient, M.O., on peritoneal dialysis and immediately moved her into the home, Figure 3. This approach required Dr. Tenckhoff to visit M.O. at home 3 times weekly to insert the peritoneal catheter.

Whereas the repeated puncture technique worked splendidly as a peritoneal access technique with very little risk of infection and thereby proved to Boen and Tenckhoff that long term peritoneal dialysis was feasible, it frustrated any wide-spread application of the technique because cannula insertion for each dialysis was so unpleasant and demanding. Some form of long term access simply had to be devised. Henry Tenckhoff finally came up with the answer after overcoming the bias against seeking a device which he inherited from his mentor, Fred Boen.

Dr. Tenckhoff received his initial encouragement from the success of the Palmer-Quinton silicone catheter which had a long subcutaneous tunnel [5]. About that time my colleague, Jack Cole, was experimenting with the bonding of dacron felt to silicone arteriovenous shunts as an anchor and infection barrier. Although this technique did not work for A.V. shunts, it permitted Tenckhoff to re-design the Palmer-Quinton catheter into a shorter device that could be inserted through a trochar and be held firmly in place by the dacron felt cuffs [6]. It is of some interest that we later modified Tenckhoff's design for use as a right atrial catheter for home parenteral nutrition [7]. This device saved that project from utter failure. Originally we had proposed to infuse through a side-arm in an A-V shunt [8]. This latter technique works well in uremia, but not in patients with chronic bowel disease who readily clot both A-V shunts and A-V fistulas.

With long term peritoneal access finally assured, there still remained the problem of a safe and practical source of peritoneal dialysis fluid. The forty-liter bottle system worked well enough, provided one had a 'fluid factory' and was willing to deliver forty-liter carboys to homes in the area. It simply was not a practical system.

Tenckhoff's first attempt to solve this problem is shown in Figure 4. This apparatus was nothing more nor less than

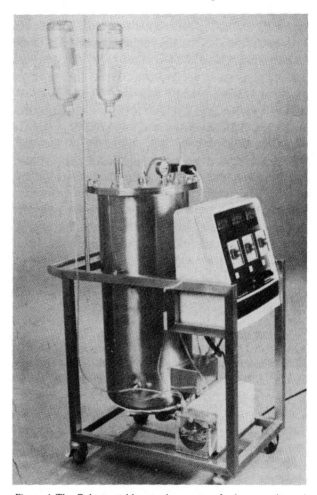

Figure 4. The Cobe portable autoclave system for home peritoneal dialysis.

a miniature fluid factory with a miniature autoclave to sterilize the fluid. Reverse osmosis replaced the still as a source of pure water. Several of these machines were built by Cobe Laboratories and used with great success locally. However, the heat of sterilization, the huge size, the weight and the complicated operational sequence precluded widespread application. The next generation of machines, developed by Curtis at the Seattle V.A. and Tenckhofff, used reverse osmosis as the method of sterilization. These machines have evolved into today's highly usuable units.

Despite the success of these reverse osmosis machines, the technique of long term peritoneal dialysis never really took hold except in a few centers. It remained for CAPD to really start things moving. I daresay that this book would not have been planned had it not been for CAPD. I believe that both CAPD and this volume will prove to be landmarks in the history of the therapy of chronic renal failure. I sincerely hope I am right – time surely will tell.

January 1981   Belding H. Scribner

REFERENCES

1. Babb AL, Johansen PJ, Strand MJ, Tenckhoff H. Scribner BH: Bidirectional permeability of the human peritoneum to middle molecules. Proc Europ Dialysis Transplant Assoc 10: 247–262, 1973.
2. Popovich RP, Moncrief JW, Nolph KD, Ghods AJ, Twardowski ZJ, Pyle WK: Continuous ambulatory peritoneal dialysis. Ann Intern Med 88: 449–456, 1978.
3. Kauffman HM, Edbom GA, Adams MB, Hussey CV: Hypercoagulability: A cause of vascular access failure. Proc Dialysis Transplant Forum 9: 28–30, 1979.
4. Marr TA, Burnell JM, Scribner BH: Gastrodialysis in the treatment of acute renal failure. J. Clin Invest 39: 653–661, 1960.
5. Palmer RA, Newell JE, Gray JE. Quinton WE: Treatment of chronic renal failure by prolonged peritoneal dialysis. N Eng J Med 274: 248–254, 1966.
6. Tenckhoff H. Schechter H: A bacteriologically safe peritoneal access device. Trans Am Soc Artif Intern Organs 14: 181–186, 1968.
7. Atkins RC, Vizzo JE, Cole JJ, Blagg CR, Scribner BH: The artificial gut in hospital and home. Technical improvements. Trans Am Soc Artif Intern Organs 16: 260–266, 1970.
8. Scribner BH, Cole JJ, Christopher TG, Vizzo JE, Atkins RC, Blagg CR: Long-term total parenteral nutrition. The concept of an artifical gut. JAMA 212: 457–463, 1970.

FOREWORD TO SECOND EDITION

When the foreword to the first edition was written the big question was whither CAPD? Many of the answers to that question will be found in the pages of this second edition.

In 1979 I predicted that a new technique of combined automated and ambulatory peritoneal dialysis might emerge as a sort of compromise between IPD and CAPD [1]. What was then rank speculation has turned out to be correct in part, at least, as CCPD has emerged as a new and apparently satisfactory approach. Now I will go one step further and predict that some form of nightly peritoneal dialysis, NPD, may evolve as the best compromise of all. It seems to me that NPD might end up as the method of choice for most patients because it has the potential to maximize the advantages of both IPD and CAPD while minimizing the disadvantages. For example, the greatest advantage of IPD was its low incidence of peritonitis, i.e. one episode every 4½ patient years in the Montpellier experience. With a properly designed reverse osmosis fluid supply system for NPD, it should be possible to reduce the number of connect-disconnect procedures to seven per week. In addition, improved connectology should make it possible to again approach this low incidence of peritonitis.

NPD would eliminate all of the mechanical disadvantages of carrying 1–2 liters of fluid in the abdomen including hernias, chronic back pain and the adverse cosmetic effect of a swollen abdomen. Also, the daily tedium and inconvenience of repeating the connect-disconnect procedure would be eliminated.

NPD probably requires lower dextrose concentrations to achieve the same amount of weekly ultrafiltration. In addition, the elimination during the day of both the dextrose load and the abdominal distension might improve protein intake and help reverse the documented trend of CAPD patients to store fat on the one hand and develop protein malnutrition on the other [2].

Finally, it should be possible to design a peritoneal fluid supply system based on modern reverse osmosis and ultrafiltration technology that would be easy to operate, virtually maintenance-free, and always ready for nightly use by the patient. Such a system would be very cost effective – the watchword of the future.

Seattle, January 1984   Belding H. Scribner

REFERENCES

1. Scribner BH: A current perspective on the role of intermittent vs continuous ambulatory peritoneal dialysis. Proc NE Regional Meeting of Renal Physicians Assoc 3: 76–81, 1979.

2. Heide B, Prenatos A et al.: Nutritional status of patients undergoing CAPD. Perit Dial Bulletin 1: 138–141, 1983.

FOREWORD TO THIRD EDITION

My former mentor, endocrinologist Dr. Robert Williams, always maintained that every new worthwhile development in medicine goes thru three phases that are visually represented by the QRS complex of an electrocardiogram. There is the initial phase of unbridled enthusiasm, the Q wave; followed by a phase of disillusionment, the R wave, and finally a leveling off above or below the baseline, depending on the long term value of the development. Currently, (early 1988), so called high flux hemodialysis is in phase one. I believe CAPD and its variations are entering phase three and I am not sure there was a really identifiable phase two. As described in the pages of this excellent volume, CAPD has come of age and found for itself an indispensable place among the dialyic options available.

Just a few months ago a lovely lady in her sixties, who had been on CAPD for over a year, was admitted to my hospital service with a peritoneal catheter tract infection. She, her husband and their personal physician all were intent on having us try to save her peritoneum, because the other options were so repugnant. This elderly couple lived in a rural area and the idea of commuting to a dialysis center, or bringing a hemodialysis machine into their modest home seemed overwhelming. The outcome was unfortunate in that we not only failed to save the peritoneal space, but almost lost the patient who remained in the hospital for over three months. A major problem was a severe depression that developed because hemodialysis was the only option left.

This anecdote encapsulates much of the 'story' of CAPD, with its strengths – weaknesses and trade-offs, all of which are beautifully detailed in this edition.

What does the future hold? Permit me to speculate with a suggested course that might be followed. Please recall that on-line manufacture of sterile peritoneal dialysis fluid at the bedside is a proven technique developed in Seattle by Tenckhoff and Curtis in the 1970's. The technique went out of favor because the complexity of the equipment and the workload were so great that it could not be adopted to a seven night per week dialysis schedule. Today modern on-line sterilizing technology for dialysis fluid has been simplified to the point where a new, fully-automatic peritoneal dialysis machine could be designed that would make nightly peritoneal dialysis simpler, safer and less expensive. This device would permit a simplified form of CCPD with only one connect/disconnect per night. I believe that such a device could be made available at an acceptable cost. Indeed the cost of the machine would be more than offset by eliminating the expensive bags of sterile dialysis fluid. Such a machine would reduce infection by eliminating the connections to the bags of dialysis fluid. The number and volume of cycles could be individualized along with the composition of dialysate. In short, such a machine undoubtedly would make home peritoneal dialysis an even more desirable option than it already has become.

January, 1988   Belding H. Scribner

PREFACE

Peritoneal dialysis represents an internal technique for blood purification. In this dialyzer the blood path, the membrane and the dialysate compartment are provided by nature. The developments of chronic peritoneal catheters, automated cycling equipment, solution preparation by reversed osmosis, manipulations of transport with drugs and the experiences with continuous ambulatory peritoneal dialysis and continuous cycling peritoneal dialysis have increased the interest in peritoneal dialysis. Publications related to peritoneal dialysis probably exceed 400 annually. *Peritoneal Dialysis International* (formally *Peritoneal Dialysis Bulletin*) the official journal of the International Society for Peritoneal Dialysis is a journal solely devoted to peritoneal dialysis experiences and developments. The Fourth International Symposium on Peritoneal Dialysis was held in Venice, Italy in 1987 and the next meeting of this new international society will be held in Kyoto, Japan in 1990. The eighth Annual CAPD Conference in Kansas City, Missouri in 1988 attracted near 1000 people from 25 countries. The USA NIH CAPD Registry has registered more than 25,000 patients on CAPD or CCPD since 1981. At this time over 35,000 patients are estimated to be maintained on CAPD worldwide. New advances in the physiology of peritoneal dialysis (such as understanding the role of peritoneal lymphatics) and in peritoneal dialysis technology (such as tidal peritoneal dialysis and new connection devices) are examples of the dynamic nature of the field.

This book is meant to provide an overview of the state of the art of peritoneal dialysis. Many clinicians are making extensive commitments to peritoneal dialysis for the first time. Nephrologists, anatomists, physiologists, pharmacologists, biomedical engineers and even physicists are involved in studies to better understand peritoneal dialysis. The complexities of peritoneal dialysis and the peritoneal membrane are becoming apparent. Studies of peritoneal dialysis increase understanding of the anatomy and physiology of biological membranes and the factors influencing the passive movement of solutes across the microcirculation and related structures. Peritoneal dialysis provides a 'window' to the visceral microcirculation in animals and humans.

Peritoneal dialysis may be useful to treat problems other than renal failure. Beneficial effects in the treatment of dysproteinemias, psoriasis, hypothermia, and many metabolic problems have been reported. The intraperitoneal administration of chemotherapeutic agents draws upon and contributes to our understanding of peritoneal dialysis.

I feel fortunate to have been involved in peritoneal dialysis research for the past 22 years. New ideas and new developments have been an almost daily occurrence. Yet, our understanding of this dialysis system is still in its infancy. The authors of the chapters in this book have been actively investigating and writing about their respective topics for many years. Most are individuals with whom I have had the good fortune to have had frequent contacts.

As in the first and second edition, each chapter is an extensive review of a given topic. I have not edited out all overlap between chapters since I feel the reader benefits by exposure to slightly different perspectives of complex material and by allowing each author to deal with all issues that relate to their respective topics.

The prefaces of the first two editions summarized the major purpose of the book with the statement 'It is hoped that this book will serve as a reference text for all those with more than a casual interest in peritoneal dialysis.'. This remains my hope for the third edition.

February, 1988   Karl D. Nolph

HISTORY OF PERITONEAL DIALYSIS

S.T. BOEN

1. FIRST PERIOD: 1923-1962

1.1. Early clinical experience

In 1923 an article by Ganter [1] was published in which he described intermittent infusion and removal of saline solution into and from the peritoneal cavity of a guinea pig made uremic by ureteral ligation. The urea-N concentration in the fluid was close to the bloodconcentration after a dwell time of 1 hr. After several instillations and removals of fluid the animal improved.

Furthermore he stated briefly that 1.5 l of saline solution was infused into the peritoneal cavity of a woman with uremia due to ureter blockage by a uterus carcinoma, and that he had the impression that there was an improvement in her condition.

Ganter was of the opinion that the peritoneal membrane would also allow passage of other kinds of toxic substances, as he observed a reversal of the unconsciousness of a patient with diabetic coma after intraperitoneal infusion of 3 l of saline solution.

Heusser and Werder [2] mentioned in 1927 that they performed peritoneal dialysis in 3 patients; they noted that there was no clinical improvement because the amount of fluid used was too small.

Prior to 1940 additional uremic patients were treated with peritoneal dyalisis by Balázs and Rosenak [3] in 3 cases, by Wear et al. [4] in 5 cases and by Rhoads [5] in 2 cases. One of Wear et al. 's patients recovered from the uremic state, and tolerated an operation for bladder stones. Rhoads used peritoneal dialysis 3 times in one patient, each session lasted 2½ hr. Although a substantial amount of urea nitrogen was removed the decline in blood urea nitrogen was small or absent.

From the many publications after 1946, we will select a few to illustrate the developments in its clinical use.

Fine et al. [6] in 1946 used peritoneal dialysis in 4 patients, in one of them for 12 days. Pulmonary edema developed in 3 cases because of too much fluid administration by

intravenous route; at the other hand using hypertonic dialysate, water could be removed by peritoneal dialysis. They mentioned also the importance of adjusting the dialysate composition in order to improve acidosis in the uremic patient. Furthermore it was calculated that using 35 l of dialysate with 2% glucose concentration in 24 hr, 200 to 300 g of glucose was absorbed in this period.

Dérot et al. [7] reported in 1949 their first successful experience in acute rental failure: 9 out of 10 patients survived compared to no survivors in 1947.

The duration of dialysis was between 5 and 240 hr, using 2.25 to 150 l of fluid. After their most recent experience it was advocated to dialyze for 24 to 36 hr, adding penicilline and sometimes streptomycine to the dialysate.

Legrain and Merrill [8] used peritoneal dialysis in 3 patients, in one of them 3 procedures were performed in a 2-week period after a renal transplant with oliguria and hyperpotassemia. In another patient a practically sodium-free hypertonic irrigating fluid with glucose was used for 7 hr. removing about 1000 mEq of sodium from a patient with marked edema due to nephrotic syndrome.

Odel et al. [9] collected 101 patients from the literature between 1923 through 1948: 63 had reversible lesions, 32 irreversible lesions and in 2 the diagnosis was undetermined. Of the 63 patients with revesible renal diseases 32 recovered. The cause of death was reported in 40 cases. Three complications accounted for the death in 88% of the cases; in 13 cases (33%) death was caused by uremia, in 16 cases (40%) it was due to pulmonary edema and in 6 cases (15%) peritonitis was the primary cause of death. It could be assumed that pulmonary edema was brought about by use of an unbalanced perfusing fluid or by injudicious and excessive use of parenteral fluid.

Grollman et al. [10] demonstrated that peritoneal dialysis can keep bilaterally nephrectomized dogs alive for periods of 30 to 70 days. Furthermore 5 patients with uremia were treated with intermittent peritoneal dialysis.

In the Netherlands peritoneal dialysis was first used by Formijne in 1946 in 2 patients with acute uremia [11].

1.2. Method and technique

1.2.1. Catheters
Usually the catheters used for peritoneal dialysis were improvised and adapted from tubings available on the ward. Wear *et al.* [4] used a regular gallbladder trocar for the inflow, and a trocar with numerous small holes in the distal third for the outflow. Fine *et al.* [6] employed a rubber catheter or a perforated small stainless steel tube as inlet tube, and a whistle-tip catheter or a large bore mushroom-tip catheter as outlet tube. Because of frequent plugging, the outlet tube later on was changed to a stainless steel sump-drain, which was similar to the metal perforated suction tube commonly used in operating rooms.

Dérot *et al.* [7] and Legrain and Merrill [8] used polyvinyl chloride tubes with small holes in the distal part of the catheter; this tube was inserted through a trocar.

Grollman *et al.* [10] used polyethylene plastic tubes. Bassett *et al.* [12] used a brass fenestrated tube as an outlet channel. Boen [13, 14] used rubber gastric tubing with side holes as a peritoneal catheter. Doolan *et al.* [15] initially used plastic gastric or nasal oxygen tubes in which additional holes were made. These proved unsatisfactory, and they developed a polyvinyl chloride catheter with transverse ridges to prevent kinking as well as to prevent blockage by the omentum.

Maxwell *et al.* described a nylon catheter, 27.5 cm in length with multiple small perforations at its distal 7.5 cm. It was slightly curved at the distal end with a rounded solid tip. It fit into a 17 F. metal trocar [16]. This catheter became commercially available and was widely used in the following years.

1.2.2. Technique
There are two techniques for peritoneal dialysis. With the continuous flow technique two catheters are used, one in the upper abdomen and a second one in the lower pelvis. Fluid is continuously infused through the upper catheter and is drained out through the lower one. This technique was used by Heusser and Werder [2] and by others [3, 6, 7, 8, 11].

With the intermittent technique only one catheter is used, which is placed with its end in the small pelvis (lowest part of the abdominal cavity) to ensure good removal of the fluid. The dialysate is run in and after a dwell time run out again through the same tube, whereafter the cycle is repeated.

Abbott and Shea [17], Grollman *et al.* [10], Boen [13, 14], Doolan *et al.* [15], Maxwell *et al.* [16] and others used this technique. It has the advantage of lesser chance for leakage, for infection and of avoiding short-cut fluid channels.

Since 1950 nearly all clinicians have been using the intermittent technique.

1.3. The dialysate

1.3.1. Composition of the fluid
In the first years of peritoneal dialysis either normal saline solution or 5% glucose solution was used as dialysate. Heusser and Werder [2] advised the use of saline solution with the addition of 2 to 5% glucose to make the dialysate hypertonic. Large shifts of water and minerals occurred during dialysis and the acidosis of uremic patients was not corrected. Later lactate was added to the fluid as a source of bicarbonate [5], and bicarbonate was part of the mineral composition when Ringer's solution (2.4 mEq bicarbonate/l) or Tyrode's solution (12 mEq bicarbonate/l) was used as dialysate. With higher bicarbonate concentrations a correction of the patient's acidosis could be achieved. Abbott and Shea [17] added 26 mEq bicarbonate per liter, Odel *et al* [9] 24 to 36 mEq/l, Grollman *et al.* [10] 35.8 mEq/l, and Boen 35 to 40 mEq/l [13, 14].

Commercial solution became available in 1959; it contains 35 to 40 mEq lactate/l. In 1962 we started to use acetate as a source of bicarbonate in a concentration of 35 mEq/l [18]; this is still being used in the Seattle area and some manufacturers are also using acetate in the dialysate.

The sodium concentration in the fluid varies from 130 to 140 mEq/l, potassium 0 to 5 mEq/l, calcium 2 to 4 mEq/l and magnesium 0 to 2 mEq/l.

Glucose concentration of the fluid is between 1.5 to 5 gm%.

Instead of glucose, 5% gelatin was added by Fine *et al.* [6] to make the fluidd hypertonic; this is not being used anymore.

In Table 1 the composition of different dialysates are seen.

1.3.2. Preparation of the fluid
Factory made fluid became available in 1959. Up till then the clinicians had to make their own dialysate. Usually mineral solutions and glucose solutions were mixed prior to dialysis, making a dialysate composition which can be adjusted to the patient's need. More glucose was added when the patient was overhydrated, and the potassium concentration was varied dependent upon the serum potassium level.

In the early nineteen-fifties we used sterile distilled water in calibrated bottles to which measured amounts of concentrated solutions of $NaCl$, $NaHCO_3$, $CaCl_2$, $MgCl_2$, KCl and glucose were added immediately before use [13, 14].

Kop [19] made dialysate by sterilizing solutions in a container consisting of 2 compartments; a smaller one of 5 l for $NaCl$, $NaHCO_3$ and KCl, and a larger one of 28 l for glucose, $CaCl_2$ and HCl. The solutions were boiled for 30 min; after cooling the solutions from the two compartments were mixed.

Caramelization of glucose had to be avoided; glucose could not be sterilized together with all the minerals. Furthermore solutions containing both calcium and bicarbonate could not be stored because of precipitation of calcium carbonate. Once calcium was added to the dialysate, the fluid had to be used soon.

Maxwell *et al.* [16] in 1959 introduced the use of factory made fluid in one liter bottles. Using a Y-connection, 2 bottles of fluid were infused simultaneously; the empty bottles were used to receive the drained out dialysate. Instead of bicarbonate, lactate was used as a source of bicarbonate. The availability of commercial fluid has enhanced the wide-spread use of peritoneal dialysis.

1.4. Quantitative data of peritoneal dialysis
In earlier publications peritoneal dialysis seemed unable

Table 1. Composition of irrigation fluid

		NaCl 0.9%	Ringer	Locke	Tyrode	Rhoads	Hartmann	Abott and Shea	Ferris	Odel
Na	mEq/l	154	156.4	156.4	166.4	276	130	131	139	143
K	mEq/l		4	3.2	2.7	5	4	5	3	3
Ca	mEq/l		4.5	7.6	3.6	4	4	4	2	2
Mg	mEq/l				2.1			1	2	2
HCO$_3$	mEq/l		2.4	2.4	12			26	36	24
Cl	mEq/l	154	162.5	164.8	162.4	257	110	114	109	109
Lactate	mEq/l					28	28			
Acetate	mEq/l									
Citrate	mEq/l									16
Glucose	Gm/l			1	1			10–20	20	20

		Grollman	Boen Amsterdam	Boen Seattle	Tenckhoff RO machine	Commercial 1	2	3 (CAPD)	4 (CAPD)
Na	mEq/l	134.5	140	135	130	130	140	132	134
K	mEq/l	2.7	0–3						0–2
Ca	mEq/l	3.6	3	3	3.5	4.0	4.0	3.0	3.5
Mg	mEq/l	1.1	0–1.5	1.5	1.0	1.5	1.5	1.5	1.0
HCO$_3$	mEq/l	35.8	40						
Cl	mEq/l	106.1	103	107.5	96.5	101	101	101.5	105.5
Lactate	mEq/l							35.0	35.0
Acetate	mEq/l			35.0	38.0	35.0	45.0		
Citrate	mEq/l		3						
Glucose	Gm/l	10–30	20 and higher	20 and higher	15 and higher	70	15	15, 42.5	5.15 42.5

to improve the blood chemistry of the uremic patient. Frequently the duration of dialysis was too short (a few hours). Furthermore although sometimes the dialysis duration was long, the amount of fluid used was too small to produce significant removal of waste products. The difference in outcome between hemodialysis and peritoneal dialysis lead Hamburger and Richet to state that only the artificial kidney can correct the abnormalities in calcium, chloride and phosphate levels, and that this can not be achieved with peritoneal dialysis [20].

Contrary to this statement, we demonstrated in 1959 that the same improvement in bloodchemistry could be achieved provided a large amount of dialysate was used and the dialysis duration is prolonged [21, 13]. Some data are seen in Figure 1.

The clearance obtained with peritoneal dialysis is far lower than the hemodialysis clearance. For instance, the peritoneal urea clearance on the average is 12ml/min when 1 l dialysate is cycled per hour and around 20ml/min with 2l/hr. 25 ml/min with 3 l/hr and around 30 ml/min, with 4 l/hr. There is a clear relationship between flow rate and clearance value. Later studies by Tenckhoff *et al.* showed a further increase of the urea clearance to 40 ml/min at a dialysate flow rate of 10l/hr [22].This value is about the limit which can be achieved by peritoneal dialysis.

Bomar *et al.* [23] and Villaroel [24] found good agreement of our data with their mathematical models.

The diffusion curves for creatinine, uric acid and phosphate are lower than the urea curves. Accordingly the peritoneal clearances of these substances are lower than the urea clearance. These differences are similar to the artificial kidney. However, the peritoneal membrane does also have areas with large pore sizes, because all fractions of serum proteins do appear in the dialysate [13]. The inverse relationship between the molecular weights of the plasma proteins and its peritoneal clearance was demonstrated in later years [25]. The permeability to molecules with a molecular weight between 1500 and 5000 daltons was investigated too [26].

Enhancement of peritoneal clearance by drugs and by osmolarity changes was demonstrated in later years, but has not been integrated in clinical practice [27–31].

2. THE PERIOD OF CHRONIC INTERMITTENT PERITONEAL DIALYSIS

2.1. Devices for access into the peritoneal cavity

When chronic peritoneal dialysis started to be used in 1962, it was felt that frequent access into the peritoneal cavity shoud be made easier. In Seattle we developed access devices made of teflon and silicone rubber tubes which were implanted in the abdominal wall [18]. The catheter was inserted through this tube, and after dialysis the tube was closed by a cap. Others also developed conduits [32–34].

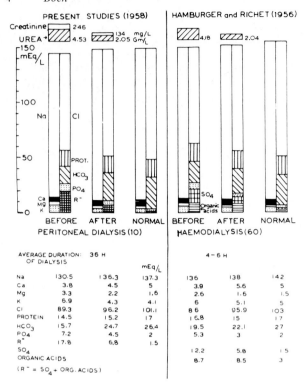

PRESENT STUDIES (1958) | HAMBURGER and RICHET (1956)

Creatinine 246
UREA+ 4.53 2.05 mg/L Gm/L   4.18   2.04

BEFORE AFTER NORMAL | BEFORE AFTER NORMAL
PERITONEAL DIALYSIS (10) | HAEMODIALYSIS (60)

AVERAGE DURATION OF DIALYSIS: 36 H   4-6 H

mEq/L

	Before	After	Normal	Before	After	Normal
Na	130.5	136.3	137.3	136	138	142
Ca	3.8	4.5	5	3.9	5.6	5
Mg	3.3	2.2	1.6	2.6	1.6	1.5
K	6.9	4.3	4.1	6	5.1	5
Cl	89.3	96.2	101.1	86	95.9	103
PROTEIN	14.5	15.2	17	16.8	15	17
HCO₃	15.7	24.7	26.4	19.5	22.1	27
PO₄	7.2	4.5	2	5.3	3	2
R⁻	17.8	6.8	1.5			
SO₄				12.2	5.8	1.5
ORGANIC ACIDS				8.7	8.5	3

(R⁻ = SO₄ + ORG. ACIDS)

Figure 1. Comparison between peritoneal dialysis and hemodialysis.

All efforts ended with failure because of peritonitis and formation of adhesions which blocked the pathway of the catheter. After a few years this approach was abandoned. An indwelling rod to provide a permanent tract for a catheter has also been developed [35]; in our experience this kind of tract between skin and the peritoneal cavity gave too easy entry of bacteria although others have used it for some period of time [36].

Subcutaneous peritoneal devices were designed and used in patients [37–39], although not extensively. More investigation seems justified as this kind of device may decrease the risk of peritonitis.

2.2. The repeated puncture technique

To prove that chronic peritoneal dialysis is possible, we had to eradicate peritonitis which was the limiting factor for long-term use of this method. In 1963 we elected to abandon indwelling devices and to use repeated puncture for each dialysis [40]. Initially a small trocar was used for insertion of a commercially available small bore nylon catheter, but by the end of 1964 we used a stylet-catheter [41]. The catheter was removed after each dialysis. Furthermore a closed sterile system during an entire dialysis run was achieved using fluid in 40l carboys and an automatic machine.

The patient had complete freedom of movement in between dialysis, and it was the first time that a patient could go on vacation-trips without any risk.

The pre-dialysis BUN concentrations varied between 100 and 150 mg%, the serum creatinine level was around 15 mg% and the uric acid concentration was 9 mg%. The post dialysis values were: BUN usually around 50 mg% (sometimes 90 mg%), serum creatinine around 9 mg% and uric acid around 5 mg%. The hematocrit was about 30% without transfusions. The serum albumin levels were in the normal range. The protein loss was between 20 and 50 g/dialysis. The blood pressure was well controlled without any hypotensive medication. Over a 2-yr period the peritoneal urea clearance was measured periodically, the values did not show a decrease. This was the first long-term successful experience with peritoneal dialysis.

Tenckhoff demonstrated, that the repeated puncture technique with the use of an automatic machine was also possible in the home-setting [42]. This method was carried out for 3½ yr at home, during which period 380 catheter punctures were performed. Later on this patient was dialyzed using the silicone rubber catheter devised by Tenckhoff. The repeated puncture technique was also successfully used in 5 patients by Lasker *et al.* [43].

2.3. Automatic machines

One of the causes of peritonitis is contamination of the dialysate when changing the bottles. Using fluid in one liter bottles during a 10-h run and a cycle volume of 4l/h, 40 bottles had to be changed with as many chances for bacterial invasion. To minimize this risk, we produced dialysate in 40-l bottles and used a closed sterile system throughout the entire dialysis. In order to minimize attendance by a nurse for clamping and opening fluid lines, timers and clamps were incorporated in the system to make the procedure automatic. The first kind of peritoneal dialysis machine was constructed in Seattle in 1962 [18]. This machine is still being used at the University Hospital in Seattle. A schematic drawing of the machine is seen in Figure 2. From the 40-l carboys the fluid is pumped into a head-tank from which it goes into the patient by gravity flow. The outflow is collected in a sterile 40-l bottle. Timers control the inflow-time, dwelltime and outflow time. In later years a camcycler was used instead of the clock-like timers [44].

To sterilize fluid in 40-l bottles special equipment was required which could not easily be installed in other places. Later commercial fluid in 2-l bottles became available; by connecting 4 bottles, a reservoir of 8 l each time was obtained and a cycler could be used for automatic dialysis [45]. Mion connected 4 to 8 plastic containers with 10 l of fluid each in series for closed circuit peritoneal dialysis [46].

Shipping large amounts of fluid to the patient's home was cumbersome, and there was a need for an apparatus which could make sterile dialysate in the home of the patient. Although cold sterilization of water has been tried using a 0.22μ filter [47, 48], small viruses and bacterial breakdown products can still pass the filter. Pyrogenic reactions and sterile peritonitis can follow (unpublished personal data and ref. [49]).In 1969 Tenckhoff *et al.* [49] described a pressure boiler tank with capacity of 160 l which was used for on the spot sterilization of either mixed dialysate or water. In the latter case the water was mixed in a 20 to 1 proportion with mineral concentrate using a proportioning roller pump. In this way the cost or dialysate could be reduced. A much refined version was used successfully both in the home and in the hospital. The weight and bulkiness of the machine

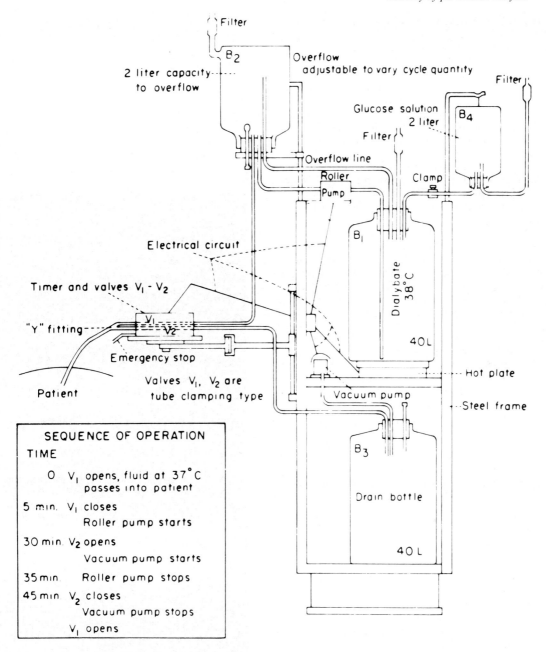

Figure 2. Schematic drawing with the sequence of operation of the first automatic peritoneal dialysis machine.

represented major disadvantages. Advances in water treatment technology permitted the development of a new system, which Tenckhoff *et al.* published in 1972 [50]. It incorporated a reverse osmosis filter to produce sterile, pyrogen free water from tap-water which is mixed by a 20:1 proportioning (roller) pump with mineral concentrate to make sterile dialysate. The machine was compact and easily movable for home or hospital use. This reverse osmosis automatic machine did increase the number of patients treated at home with peritoneal dialysis.

2.4. Indwelling catheters

Although the repeated puncture technique made long-term peritoneal dialysis a success (by preventing peritonitis), the procedure was too time-consuming for the physicians and could not be used on a larger scale. Furthermore, occasionally bleeding occurred during puncture of the abdominal wall. The stiff nylon catheter occasionally produced pain during dialysis.

Palmer *et al.* [51, 52] in 1964 devised an indwelling silicone rubber peritoneal catheter; it was 84 cm long, with a lumen of 2 mm. The intraperitoneal end of the tube was coiled and had many perforations extending 23 cm from the tip. Halfway along the tube was a triflanged step for seating the tube in the deep fascia and peritoneum. The rest of the tube was placed in a long spiral tunnel in the deep subcutaneous tissue emerging from the skin surface in the left upper quadrant of the abdomen. The catheter was sealed by a small cap if the patient was off dialysis. The long subcutaneous part was meant to prevent extension of surface infection.

Straight silicone rubber catheters were used by Gutch [53], and by McDonald *et al.* [54], the latter incorporated a teflon velour skirt in the subcutaneous tissue and a dacron-weaveknit sleeve from the skirt down to the peritoneum.

Tenckhoff's design of indwelling silicone rubber catheter [55] was accepted widely since its publication in 1968 and became the most important factor in promoting chronic peritoneal dialysis in other centers. Figure 3 shows the catheter. The silicone rubber tube had an internal diameter of 2.6 mm and an outer diameter of 4.6 mm. The intra-abdominal section of the catheter was 20 cm long and had 60 spaced perforations of 0.5 mm diameter in its terminal 15 cm; the end of the tube remained open. One dacron cuff was bonded to the catheter just outside the peritoneum; the second dacron felt cuff was immediately beneath the skin in the subcutaneous tissue. The distance between the 2 cuffs was 10 cm, and this part is placed in a curve in the subcutis. The external part of the catheter was 10 cm long. The dacron felt cuffs were designed to close the sinus tract around the catheter against bacterial intrusion. The shorter subcutaneous part compared to Palmer's catheter made it possible to implant the catheter through a specially designed trocar. Furthermore if a catheter had to removed because of infection, there was still space left for repeated puncture dialysis and reimplantation of a new catheter.

Later modification included a balloon [56] and discs in the intra-abdominal part to prevent easy dislocation of the catheter and omental wrapping [57]. A subcutaneously implanted device with 2 tubes in the peritoneal cavity has also been used [58]. With silastic catheter, the incidence of pain during dialysis is very low. Although the Tenckhoff catheter is most advantageous from the practical point of view, as an indwelling device it still carries the risk of peritoneal infection through the lumen of the catheter or alongside the catheter. Good instructions for aseptic technique remain imperative.

2.5. Clinical results

The use of the Tecnkhoff catheter and automated machines enlarged the chronic peritoneal dialysis program in the Seattle area. In 1973 Tenckhoff *et al.* reported the experience of 12 000 peritoneal dialysis sessions in 69 patients, mostly at home [59]. In 1977 in the Seattle area 161 patients had been on peritoneal dialysis, many of them for over 4 yr and one patient for 8 yr [60].

The second largest population of intermittent peritoneal dialysis patients was in Toronto, Canada. Oreopoulos reported on 150 patients in 1975 [61]. Other centers in Europe and in the USA also reported satisfactory results

(ref. [61] through [81]) and peritoneal dialysis became an alternative method for treating patients with end-stage renal disease.

However, real long-term treatment (over 4 yr) was not often achived.

Ahmad *et al.* [82] calculated the cumulative technical survival rate for the Seattle patients: 72% after 1 yr, 43% after 2 yr and 27% after 3 yr. Conversion to hemodialysis because of complications and inadequate dialysis was common. This reflects the usual experience in other centers. In contrast Diaz-Buxo reported a survival rate of 86% after 1 yr, 83% after 2 yr and 80% after 3 yr; these figures are

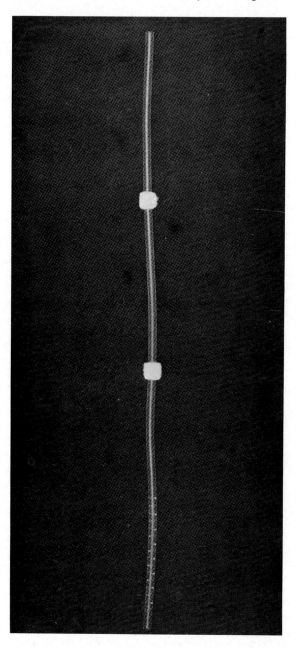

Figure 3. Tenckhoff silicone rubber catheter with two dacron cuffs.

comparable to hemodialysis survival rates [66].

Inadequate dialysis was one of the cases for conversion; it is therefore important to adjust the duration of dialysis to the declining residual renal function. Peritonitis did still occur, although the incidence was low when a closed sterile system was used with automated dialysis.

An index for adequate peritoneal dialysis using the total creatinine clearance (renal + peritoneal clearance) has been proposed [83, 84]; we observed that patients on peritoneal dialysis did as well as patients on hemodialysis although the small solutes removal was less than with hemodialysis [85]. The total creatinine clearance in peritoneal dialysis is far less than in hemodialysis, but the clearance for presumably toxic larger molecule weight substances ('middle molecules') is higher.

3. CONTINUOUS AMBULATORY PERITONEAL DIALYSIS (CAPD)

In 1976 Popovich. Moncrief *et al.* [86] submitted an abstract tot the American Society for Artificial Internal Organs describing what was called the equilibrium peritoneal dialysis technique. Two liters of dialysate were infused intraperitoneally and allowed to equilibrate 5 hr while the patient conducted his normal activities. The dialysate was then drained and fresh fluid was run in again. Five exchanges per day. 7 days per week were cartried out. In 1978 experience in more patients was reported by Popovich, Moncrief, Nolph *et al.*, and the name of the method was changed to continuous ambulatory peritoneal dialysis or CAPD [87]. The dialysate was then only available in bottles in the USA, whereas in Canada dialysate was delivered in plastic bags. Oreopoulos' modification of CAPD using bags made the technique easier to perform and decreased (but did not eliminate) the rather high incidence of peritonitis [88]. After inflow, the empty bag is folded and carried on the body allowing free movement of the patient.

The peritoneal urea clearance with 5 exchanges of 21 each per day and 21 of ultrafiltration per day is 8.4 ml/min. The clearance for larger molecules like Vit. B_{12} and inulin, however, are higher than with hemodialysis or intermittent peritoneal dialysis. For instance Vit. B_{12} clearance values are: CAPD 5 exchanges per day around 5 ml/min, intermittent peritoneal dialysis 40 hr week 1.6 ml/min. hemodialysis 15 hr/week 3.0 ml/min [89. 90].

In contrast to hemodialysis and intermittent peritoneal dialysis, the blood chemistries of patients on CAPD are steady after a few weeks of treatment because there is a constant removal of waste products from the body. This makes CAPD the most physiologic way of dialysis. Because of sufficient fluid removal each day, the fluid allowance of the patients is more liberal. The blood pressure is usually well controlled. CAPD patients show a rise in hematocrit which is not seen with other dialysis methods. The clinical condition of the patient is good provided complications like peritonitis do not occur and the patient can eat sufficient amount of protein to compensate for the protein loss with dialysis. Many more reports about CAPD have been published [91–162].

Special indications are: dialysis of diabetic patients because of easier blood sugar control (usually insulin is administered intraperitoneally) and dialysis of children.

The interest for CAPD has grown tremendously in the last few years. Many centers have started CAPD and many have expanded their program. As of December 31, 1983 there were 8532 patients on CAPD in the USA out of 71987 total dialysis patients, or 11.9% of the total [136], compared to 20 CAPD patients in 1977 and 1700 patients in 1980 [109].

On December 31, 1982 there were 1232 patients on peritoneal dialysis in Canada, which was 34% of the total dialysis population. Of the new patients accepted in 1982, 50% were on CAPD [137].

In Europe 1837 patients started CAPD in 1982 and 2141 patients in the years before 1982 [138]. In most countries a further increase of the number of CAPD patients took place after 1982. In the Netherlands 15.1% of all adult dialysis patients were on CAPD as of January 1, 1985 [139].

According to the EDTA Registry report over the year 1982, for patients aged 45–54 excluding diabetics, the patient survival was around 82% at 2 yr [138]. For the USA patient survival after 1 yr was 78.1% for diabetics and 87.8% for all others [136].

In Toronto Western Hospital the cumulative survival of diabetics at 4 yr was around 50% compared to around 70% for non-diabetics. For type I diabetics the survival at 4 yr was 62% as opposed to 27% for type II [140]. At the Vancouver General Hospital the overall patient survival at 42 months was 88.9% and the overall treatment survival was 37.5%. In the diabetic patients survival was 67.5% at 36 months compared to 92.9% for the non-diabetics [141]. In Montpellier, using intermittent peritoneal dialysis, the actuarial survival rate for type I diabetics was 83% at 4 years and around 25% for type II patients [142].

Although its real long-term success is not yet known, it is clear now that CAPD became a first choice initial treatment method for many patients. Technique survival rate is improving, but sclerosing peritonitis with loss of ultrafiltration capacity is probably an irreversible comlication. This serious problem has been seen mostly in France [143, 144]. More recently an equally serious complication was described, the progressive calcifying peritonitis, involving the visceral and parietal peritoneum which can be seen on a plain abdominal X-ray as an egg-shell calcification [145, 146].

New technical developments include the use of a bacterial filter in the fluid line [147, 148], the use of a sterile splice for connecting new dialysate bags [149, 150], the use of heat sterilization [151], or ultra violet light sterilization [152] for connections, the abandonement of carrying empty bags during dwell time [141, 153, 154, 155, 156], the introduction of new catheters like the curled Tenckhoff catheter [157], the column disc catheter [158], a new type of balloon catheter [159], a catheter with a transcutaneous segment with a cuff and a flange made from silicone elastomer and expanded polytetrafluoroethylene which allow tissue ingrowth [160] and a short catheter [161].

A modification of CAPD commonly known as continuous cyclic peritoneal dialysis, CCPD, but which also has been called prolonged dwell time peritoneal dialysis, PDPD, requires a peritoneal dialysis cycling machine [162, 163, 164]. Upon retiring at night the peritoneal catheter is connected to the cycler. The machine is usually programmed to deliver 3 exchanges of 2 l each, lasting 3 hr per exchange. After the last drainage, an additional 2 l of dialysate is infused. The equipment is then disconnected and the catheter capped. The fluid remains in the peritoneal cavity during daytime. The procedure is repeated nightly.

Another modification is the so-called semi-continuous semi-ambulatory peritoneal dialysis which can be carried out according to two schedules: (a) rapid exchange of 8 l of luid late in the evening plus equilibration of 2 l of dialysate during nighttime and daytime; (b) rapid exchange of 4 l of dialysate both in the morning and in the evening plus two equilibrations of 2 liters of dialysate at daytime and nighttime each [165].

High-volume (3 l) low-frequency CAPD gave satisfactory results in patients who can tolerate such a volume [166, 167].

As to the dialysate composition, acetate as a source of bicarbonate has been abandoned because it might have caused sclerosis of the peritoneum in some patients. Lactate is commonly used in the dialysate although there is renewed interest for the use of bicarbonate instead of lactate [168, 169]. As an osmotic agent in the dialysate, glucose is still the best. Several other substances like glycerol, amino acids, gelatin derivatives, sorbitol, xylitol and polyglucose have been tested [170].

Addition of substances in the dialysate in order to improve ultrafiltration in patients were tried; the use of phosphatidylcholine in CAPD patients with low ultrafiltration, during or outside a peritonitis episode, seems promising for increasing water removal [171].

Recent studies indicate that fluid removal during peritoneal dialysis is not only induced by osmotic pressure differences.

Net ultrafiltration equals transcapillary ultrafiltration minus lymphatic absorption. In CAPD patients it was found that lymphatic absorption was substantial and amounted to 89.5 ± 11.8 ml/hr.

Extrapolated to 4×2 l, 2.5% glucose dialysate, 6 hr exchanges per day, lymphatic drainage reduced daily ultrafiltration by $83.2 \pm 10.2\%$ [172]. Reduction of lymphatic absorption would be another way of increasing water removal during CAPD.

Peritonitis is a main complication of CAPD. Its incidence declines with better instructions and improved technology. One of the best results is reported by a group using a Y-set system which is filled with sodium hypochlorite during dwell time, and rinsed out prior to inflow of fresh dialysate [156].

That peritonitis can occur during CAPD is not unexpected. However, not to be expected and therefore of importance is the fact that some patients do not develop peritonitis at all, even after 2 to 3 yr on CAPD. Of great value would be to identify fully their strong host defense factors, and use this knowledge to boost weak factors in patients with frequent episodes of peritonitis. Investigations in this field have started and facts are accumulating. It was found, that a greater incidence of Staph. epidermidis peritonitis occurred in patients with low heat-stable opsonin in the outflow dialysate [173]. Instillation of IgG intraperitoneally increased opsonic activity and reduced the number of peritonitis episodes in patients with a high rate of peritonitis [174]. Peritoneal monocyte-macrophage populations represent an important first-line defense in patients on CAPD. Disorders in iits function could negatively affect cellular-mediated defense [175, 176]. Some defects of the peritoneal macrophage can be overcome by intraperitoneal administration of interferons [177].

The resurgence of peritoneal dialysis has been remarkable. Many have been stimulated to join the p.d. force resulting in the emergence of new develoments and better understanding of underlying patho-physiology in this field. More progress is to come.

REFERENCES

1. Ganter G: Über die Beseitigung giftiger Stoffe aus dem Blute durch Dialyse. Muench Med Wochenschr 70(2): 1478–1480, 1923.
2. Heusser H, Werder H: Untersuchungen über Peritonealdialyse. Bruns Beitr Klin Chir 141: 38–49, 1927.
3. Balazs J, Rosenak S: Zur Behandlung der Sublimatanurie durch peritoneal Dialyse Wien Klin Wochenschr 47(2): 851–854, 1934.
4. Wear JB, Sisk IR, Trinkle AJ: Peritoneal lavage in the treatment of uremia. J. Urol 39: 53–62, 1938.
5. Rhoads JE: Peritoneal lavage in the treatment of renal insufficiency. Am J Med Sci 196: 642–647, 1938.
6. Fine J, Frank H, Seligman AM: The treatment of acute renal failure by peritoneal irrigation. Ann Surg 124: 857–875, 1946.
7. Dérot M, Tanzet P, Roussillon J, Bernier JJ: La dialyse peritonéale dans le traitement de l'urémie aiguë. J Urol 55: 113–121, 1949.
8. Legrain M, Merrill JP: Short term continuous transperitoneal dialysis. N Engl J Med 248: 125–129, 1953.
9. Odel HM, Ferris DO, Power MH: Peritoneal lavage as an effective means of extrarenal excretion. Am J Med 9: 63–77, 1950.
10. Grollman A, Turner LB, Mc Lean JA: Intermittent peritoneal lavage in nephrectomized dogs and its application to the human being. Arch Intern Med 87: 379–390, 1951.
11. Formijne P: De behandeling van de acute uraemie. Ned Tijdschr voor Geneeskd 90: 1181, 1946.
12. Basset SH, Brown HR, Keutmann EH, Holler J. Van Alstine HE, Mocejunas O, Schantz H: Nitrogen and fluid balance in treatment of acute uremia by peritoneal lavage. Arch Intern Med 80: 616–636, 1947.
13. Boen ST: Kinetics of peritoneal dialysis. Medicine 40: 243–287, 1961.
14. Boen ST: Peritoneal Dialysis in Clinical Medicine. Charles C. Thomas Publ, Springfield, Illinois, 1964.
15. Doolan PD, Murphy WP, Wiggins RA, CArter NW, Cooper WC, Watten RH, Alphen EL: An evaluation of intermittent peritoneal lavage. Am J Med 26: 831–844, 1959.
16. Maxwell MH, Rockney RE, Kleeman CR, Twiss MR: Peritoneal dialysis. JAMA 170: 917–924, 1959.
17. Abbott WE, Shea P: The treatment of temporary renal insufficiency by peritoneal lavage. Am J Med Sci 211: 312–319, 1946.
18. Boen ST, Mulinari AS, Dillard DH, Scribner BH: Periodic peritoneal dialysis in the management of chronic uremia. Trans Am Soc Artif Intern Organs 8: 256–262, 1962.
19. Kop PSM: Peritoneale Dialyse (Thesis), Groningen, 1948.
20. Hamburger J, Richet G: Enseignements tirés de la pratique du rein artificiel pour l'interprétation électrolytiques de l'urémie aiguë. Rev Fr Etud Clin Biol 1: 39–54, 1956.
21. Boen ST: Peritoneal Dialysis (Thesis). Univ of Amsterdam, 1959.

22. Tenckhoff H, Ward G, Boen ST: The influence of dialysate volume and flow rate on peritoneal clearance. Proc Eur Dial Transpl Assoc 2:113–117, 1965.

23. Bomar JB, Decherd JF, Hlavinka DJ, Moncrief JW, Popovich RP: The elucidation of maximum efficiency – minimum cost peritoneal dialysis protocols. Trans Am Soc Art Intern Organs 20: 120–129, 1974.

24. Villaroel F: Kinetics of intermittent and continuous peritoneal dialysis. J Dial 1: 333–347, 1977.

25. Bonomini V, Zucchelli P, Mioli V: Selective and unselective protein loss in peritoneal dialysis. Proc Eur Dial Transpl Assoc 4: 146–149, 1967.

26. Babb AL, Johansen PJ, Strand MJ, Tenckhoff H, Scribner BH: By directional permeability of the human peritoneum to middle molecules. Proc Eur Dial Transpl Assoc 10: 247–257, 1973.

27. Henderson LW, Nolph KD: Altered permeability of the peritoneal membrane after using hypertonic peritoneal dialysis fluid. J Clin Invest 48: 992–1001, 1969.

28. Nolph KD, Rosenfeld PS, Powell JT, Danforth E: Peritoneal glucose transport and hyperglycemia during peritoneal dialysis. Am J Med Scii 259: 272–281, 1970.

29. Nolph KD, Ghods AJ, Van Stone J, Brown PA: The effects of intraperitoneal vasodilators on peritoneal clearances. Trans Am Soc Artif Intern Organs 22: 586b–591, 1976.

30. Maher JF, Shea C. Cassetta M, Hohnadel DC: Isoproterenol enhancement of peritoneal permeability. J Dial 1: 319–331, 1977.

31. Gutman RA, Nixon WP, McRae RL, Spencer HW: Effect of intraperitoneal and intravenous vasoactive amines on peritoneal dialysis. Trans Am Soc Artif Intern Organs 12: 570–573, 1976.

32. Merrill JP, Sabbaga E. Henderson L, Welzant W, Cranc C: The use of an inlying plastic conduit for chronic peritoneal irrigation. Trans Am Soc Artif Intern Organs 8: 252–255, 1962.

33. Barry KG, Shambaugh GE, Goler D, Matthews EF: A new flexible cannula and seal to provide prolonged access to the peritoneal cavity for dialysis. Trans Am Soc Artif Intern Organs 9: 105–107, 1963.

34. Henderson LW, Merrill JP, Crane C: Further experience with the inlying plastic conduit for chronic peritoneal dialysis. Trans Am Soc Artif Intern Organs 9: 108–116, 1963.

35. Jacob GB, Deane N: Repeated peritoneal dialysis by the catheter replacement method: Description of technique and a replaceable prosthesis for chronic access to the peritoneal cavity. Proc Eur Dial Transpl Assoc 4: 136–140, 1967.

36. Bigelow P, Oreopoulos DG, De Veber GA: Use of Deane prosthesis in patients on long-term peritoneal dialysis. Can Med J 109: 999–1001, 1973.

37. Malette WG, McPhaul JJ, Bledsoe F, McIntosh DA, Doegel E: A clinically successful subcutaneous peritoneal access button for repeated peritoneal dialysis. Trans Am Soc Artif Intern Organs 10: 396–398, 1964.

38. Gotloib L, Nisencorn J, Garmizo AL, Galili N, Servadio C, Sudarsky M: Subcutaneous intraperitoneal prosthesis for maintenance peritoneal dialysis. Lancet 1: 1318–1319, 1975.

39. Gotloib L. Mines M, Garmizo AL, Rodoy Y: Peritoneal dialysis using the subcutaneous intraperitoneal prosthesis. Dial Transpl 8: 217–220, 1979.

40. Boen ST, Mion CM, Curtis FK, Shilipetar G: Periodic peritoneal dialysis using the repeated puncture technique and an automatic cycling machine. Trans Am Soc Artif Intern Organs 10: 409–413, 1964.

41. Weston RE, Roberts M: Clinical use of stylet-Catheter for peritoneal dialysis. Arch Intern Med 115: 659–662, 1965.

42. Tenckhoff H, Schilipetar G, Boen ST: One year's experience with home peritoneal dialysis. Trans Am Soc Artif Intern Organs 11: 11–14, 1965.

43. Lasker N. McCauley EP, Passarotti CT: Chronic peritoneal dialysis. Trans Am Soc Artif Intern Organs 12: 94–97, 1966.

44. Curtis FK, Boen ST: Automatic peritoneal dialysis with a simple cycling machine. Lancet 2: 620, 1965.

45. Bosch E, De Vries LA, Boen ST: A simplified automatic peritoneal dialysis system. Proc Eur Dial Transpl Assoc 3: 362–365, 1966.

46. Mion C: A peritoneal dialysis program. Proc Eur Dial Transpl Assoc 12: 140–145, 1975.

47. McDonald HP: An automatic peritoneal dialysis machine: preliminary report. Trans Am Soc Artif Intern Organs 11: 83–85, 1965.

48. Vercellone A, Piccoli G, Cavalli PL, Ragni R, Alloati S: A new automatic peritoneal dialysis system. Proc Eur Dail Transpl Assoc 5:344–347, 1968.

49. Tenckhoff H, Shilipetar G, Van Paasschen WH, Swanson E: A home peritoneal dialysate delivery system. Trans Am Soc Artif Intern Organs 15: 103–107, 1969.

50. Tenckhoff H, Meston B, Shilipetar G: A simplified automatic peritoneal dialysis system. Trans Am Soc Artif Intern Organs 18: 436–439, 1972.

51. Palmer RA, Quinton WE, Gray JF: Prolonged peritoneal dialysis for chornic renal failure. Lancet 1: 700–702, 1964.

52. Palmer RA, Newell JE, Gray EJ, Quinton WE: Treatment of chronic renal failure by prolonged peritoneal dialysis. N Engl J Med 274: 248–254, 1966.

53. Gutch CF: Peritoneal dialysis. Trans Am Soc Artif Intern Organs 10: 406–407, 1964.

54. McDonald HP, Gerber N, Mishra D, Wolin L, Peng B, Waterhouse K: Subcutaneous dacron and teflon cloth adjuncts for silastic arteriovenous shunts and peritoneal dialysis catheters. Trans Am Soc Artif Intern Organs 14: 176b–180, 1968.

55. Tenckhoff H. Schechter H: A bacteriologically safe peritoneal access device. Trans Am Soc Artif Intern Organs 14: 181–186, 1968.

56. Goldberg EM, Hill W, Kabins S, Levin B: Peritoneal dialysis. Dial Transpl 4: 50–56, 1975.

57. Oreopoulos DG: Overall experience with peritoneal dialysis. Dial Transpl 7: 783–787, 1978.

58. Stephen RL, Atkin-Thor E, Kolff WJ: Recirculating peritoneal dialysis with subcutaneous catheter. Trans Am Soc Artif Intern Organs 22: 575–584, 1976.

59. Tenckhoff H, Blagg CR, Curtis KF, Hickman RO: Chronic peritoneal dialysis. Proc Eur Dial Transpl Assoc 10: 363–370, 1973.

60. Tenckhoff H: Advantages and shortcomings of peritoneal dialysis in the management of chronic renal failure. Séminar Uro-Néphrologie Hopital Pitié, pp 107–118, Paris, 1977.

61. Oreopoulos DG: Home peritoneal dialysis. Proc Eur Dial Transpl Assoc 12: 139, 1975.

62. Counts S, Hickman R, Garbaccio A, Tenckhoff H: Chronic home peritoneal dialysis in children. Trans Am Soc Artif Intern Organs 19: 157–163, 1973.

63. Black HR, Finkelstein FO, Lee RV: The treatment of peritonitis in patients with chronic indwelling catheters. Trans Am Soc Artif Intern Organs 20: 115–119, 1974.

64. Von Hartitzsch B, Medlock TR: Chronic peritoneal dialysis – a regime comparable to conventional hemodialysis. Trans Am Soc Artif Intern Organs 22: 595–597, 1976.

65. Diaz-Buxo JA, Chandler JT, Farmer CD, Smith DL: Chronic peritoneal dialysis at home – a comparison with hemodialysis. Trans Am Soc Artif Intern Organs 23: 191–193, 1977.

66. Diaz-Buxo JA, Haas VF: The influence of automated peritoneal dialysis in an established dialysis program. Dial Transpl 8: 531–533, 1979.

67. Fenton SSA, Cattran DC, Barnes NM, Waugh KJ: Home peritoneal dialysis. A major advance in promoting home dialysis. Trans Am Soc Artif Intern Organs 23: 194–200, 1977.

68. Brouhard BH, Berger M, Cunningham RJ, Petrusiek T, Allen W, Lynch RE, Travis LB: Home peritoneal dialysis in children. Trans Am Soc Artif Intern Organs 25: 90–93, 1979.

69. Roxe DM, Del Greco F, Krumlowsky F, Ghantous W, Hughes J, Ivanovich P, Quintanilla A, Salkin M, Stone N: A comparison of maintenance hemodialysis to maintenance peritoneal dialysis in the maintenance of end-stage renal disease. Trans Am Soc Artif Intern Organs 25: 81–85, 1979.

70. Dawids SG, Christensen E: Chronic home peritoneal dialysis with a simple dialysis system. Proc Eur Dial Transpl Assoc 12: 149–152, 1975.

71. Giodano C, De Santo NG, Cirillo D, Capodicasa, Rinaldi S, Cicchetti T, Di Maio F: Short daily peritoneal dialysis and protein restriction. Proc Eur Dial Transpl Assoc 12: 132–138, 1975.

72. Buoncristiani V: Clinical results of long-term peritoneal dialysis. Proc Eur Dial Transpl Assoc 12: 145–148, 1975.

73. Heal MR, England AG, Goldsmith HJ: Four year's experience with indwelling silastic cannulae for long-term peritoneal dialysis. Brit Med J 2: 596–600, 1973.

74. Lankish PG, Tonnis HJ, Fernandez-Redo E, Girndt J, Kramer P, Quellhorst E, Scheler F: Use of Tenckhoff catheter for peritoneal dialysis in terminal renal failure. Brit Med J 2: 712–713, 1973.

75. Brewer TE, Caldwell FT, Patterson RM, Flanigan WJ: Indwelling peritoneal (Tenckhoff) dialysis catheter. JAMA 219: 1011–1015, 1972.

76. Rae A, Pendray M: Advantages of peritoneal dialysis in chronic renal failure. JAMA 225: 937–941, 1973.

77. Blagg CR: Peritoneal dialysis and the Medicare ESRD program. Dial Transpl 8: 1081–1085, 1979.

78. Blumenkrantz MJ: Controlled evaluation of maintenance peritoneal dialysis. Dial Transpl 7: 797–799, 1978.

79. Mion C, Slingeneyer A, Oules R, Selam JL, Delors J, Mirouze J: Home peritoneal dialysis in diabetics with end-stage renal failure. Contrib Nephrol 1: 120–130, 1979.

80. Hood SA, Frohnert PP, Mitchell JC, Kurtz SB: Home peritoneal dialysis therapy of choice in chronic renal failure of juvenile-onset diabetes mellitus. Dial Transpl 9: 843–844, 1980.

81. Boen ST, Mion C, Slingeneyer A: The past 15 years: the role of peritoneal dialysis in the treatment of end-stage renal disease. Proc Third Capri Uremia Coufe. Publ. Wichtig Ed, Milan, 1980.

82. Ahmad S, Gallagher N, Shen F: Intermittent peritoneal dialysis: status re-assessed. Trans Am Soc Artif Intern Organs 25: 86–88, 1979.

83. Boen ST: Overview and history of peritoneal dialysis. Dial Transpl 6: 12–18, 1977.

84. Boen ST, Haagsma-Schouten WAG, Birnie RJ: Long-term peritoneal dialysis and a dialysis index. Dial Transpl 7: 377–381, 1978.

85. Scribner BH, Fergus EB, Boen ST, Thomas ED: Some therapeutic approaches to chronic renal insufficiencies. Ann Rev Med 16: 285–300, 1965.

86. Popovich RP, Moncrief JW, Decherd JF, Bomar JJB, Pyle WK: The definition of a novel portable-wearable equilibrium peritoneal technique. Abst Am Soc Artif Intern Organs 64, 1976.

87. Popovich RP, Moncrief JW, Nolph KD, Ghods AJ, Twardowski ZJ, Pyle WK: Continuous ambulatory peritoneal dialysis. Ann Intern Med 88: 449, 1978.

88. Oreopoulos DG, Robson M, Izatt G, Clayton S. De Veber GA: A simple and safe technique for continuous ambulatory peritoneal dialysis (CAPD). Trans Am Soc Artif Intern Organs 24: 481–489, 1978.

89. Popovich RP, Moncrief JW: Kinetic modeling of peritoneal transport. Contr Nephrol 17: 58–72, 1979.

90. Popovich RRP: Physiological transport parameters in patients. Dial Transpl. 7: 823–824, 842, 1978.

91. Moncrief J, Nolph KD, Rubin J, Popovich RP: Additional experience with continuous ambulatory peritoneal dialysis (CAPD). Trans Am Soc Artif Intern Organs 24: 476–483, 1978.

92. Hiatt MP, Pyle WK, Moncrief JW, Popovich RP: A comparison of the relative efficacy of CAPD and hemodialysis in the control of solute concentration. Artif Organs 4: 37–43, 1980.

93. Gill D, Morgan J, Ryan B, Gault MH, Churchill DN: Role of continuous ambulatory peritoneal dialysis in a rural population. Dial Transpl 8: 1182–1183, 1979.

94. Oreopou.os DG, Clayton S, Dombros N, Zellerman G, Katirtzoglou A: Experience with continuous ambualtory peritoneal dialysis (CAPD). Trans Am Soc Artif Intern Organs 25: 96–97, 1979.

95. Oreopoulos DG: The coming age of continuous ambulatory peritoneal dialysis. Dial Transpl 8: 460–517, 1979.

96. Rubin J, Arfania D, Nolph KD, Prowant B, Fruto L, Brown P, Moore H: Peritoneal clearances after 6–12 months on continuous ambulatory peritoneal dialysis. Trans Am Soc Artif Intern Organs 25: 104–108, 1979.

97. Fenton SSA, McCReady W, Cattran DC, Oreopoulos DG, Whiteside C: Selected clinical aspects of continuous ambulatory peritoneal dialysis. Proc Symp On CAPD, Paris, Excerpta Medica. Amsterdam, pp 107–112, 1979.

98. Price JDE, MOriarty MV: Continuous ambualtory peritoneal dialysis: selection criteria – failures and causes – deaths in diabetes mellitus. Proc Symp on CAPD, Paris. Excerpta Medica, Amsterdam, pp 113–119, 1979.

99. Gahl GM: Medical management of continuous ambulatory peritoneal dialysis. Proc Symp on CAPD, Paris. Excerpta Medica, Amsterdam, pp 181–186, 1979.

100. Lindholm B, Ahberg M, Alvestrand A. Fürst P. Karlander SG, Bergstrom J: Nutritional aspects of continuous ambulatory peritoneal dialysis. Proc Symp on CAPD, Paris. Excerpta Medica, Amsterdam, pp 199–206, 1979.

101. Lameire N, Ringoir S: An overview of peritonitis and other complications of continuous ambulatory peritoneal dialysis. Proc Symp on CAPD, Paris. Excerpta Medica, Amsterdam, pp 229–237, 1979.

102. Gokal R, Freyer R, McHugh M, Ward MK, Kerr DNS: Calcium and phosphate control in patients on CAPD. Proc Symp on CAPD, Paris. Excerpta Medica, Amsterdam, pp 283–291, 1979.

103. Mion C: Maintenance hemodialysis versus intermittent peritoneal dialysis versus continuous ambulatory peritoneal dialysis. Proc Symp on CAPD, Paris. Excerpta Medica, Amsterdam, pp 317–327, 1979.

104. Baillod RA: Continuous ambulatory peritoneal dialysis versus intermittent peritoneal dialysis at the Royal Free Hospital. Proc Symp on CAPD, Paris. Excerpta Medica, Amsterdam, pp 328–334, 1979.

105. Legrain M, Jacob C: Place of chronic ambulatory peritoneal dialysis in the treatment of end-stage renal failure. Proc Symp on CAPD, Paris, Excerpta Medica, Amsterdam, pp 347–353, 1979.

106. Nolph KD, Parker A: The composition of dialysis solutions for continuous ambulatory peritoneal dialysis. Proc Symp on CAPD, Paris. Excerpta Medica, Amsterdam, pp 341–346, 1979.

107. Thomson NM, Walker RG, Whiteside G, Scott DF, Atkins RC: Coninuous ambulatory peritoneal dialysis (CAPD) in the treatment of end-stage renal failure. Proc Eur Dial Transpl Assoc 16: 171–177, 1979.

108. Farrell PC, Randerson DH: Mass transfer kinetics in continuous ambulatory peritoneal dialysis. Proc Symp on CAPD, Paris. Excerpta Medica, Amsterdam, pp 34–41, 1979.

109. Moncrief J: CAPD Experience in USA (1980). Proc Panpacific

Symp on Peritoneal Dialysis. Churchill, Melbourne, pp 165–170, 1981.

110. Lindholm B, Bergström J, Karlander SG: Glucose metabolisms in patients on CAPD. Trans ASAIO 27: 58–60, 1981.

111. Potter DE, McDaid K, McHenry K, Mar H: Continuous ambulatory peritoneal dialysis in children. Trans ASAIO 27: 64–17, 1981.

112. Evans DH, Sorkin MI, Nolph KD, Whittier FC: Continuous ambulatory peritoneal dialysis and transplantation. Trans ASAIO 27: 320–324, 1981.

113. Chan MK, Chuah P, Raferty MJ, Baillod RM, Sweny P, Varghese Z, Moorhead JF: Three year's experience of CAPD. Lancet 1: 1409, 1981.

114. Gokal R, Ramos JM, Vertch P, Proud G, Taylor RMR, Ward MK, Wilkinson R, Kerr DNS: Renal transplantation in patients on continuous ambulatory peritoneal dialysis. Proc Eur Dial Transpl Assoc 18: 222–227, 1981.

115. Oreopoulos DG, Khanna R, Williams P et al.: Continuous ambulatory peritoneal dialysis. Nephron 30: 293–303, 1981.

116. Giangrande A, Cantie P, Limido A, de Francesco D, Malacrida V: Continuous ambulatory peritoneal dialysis and cellular immunity. Proc Eur Dial Transpl Assoc 19: 3772–379, 1982.

117. Luce E, Nakagawa D, Lovell J, Davis J, Stonebaugh BJ, Suki WN: Improvement in the bacteriologic diagnosis of peritonitis with the use of blood culture media. Trans ASAIO 28: 259–262, 1982.

118. Lindholm B, Tegner R, Tranaeus A, Bergström J: Progress of peripheral uremic neuropathy during CAPD. Trans ASAIO 28: 263–269, 1982.

119. Fabris A, Biasioli S, Chiaramonte C, Feriani M, Prisani E, Ronco C, Cantarella G, La Greca G: Buffer metabolism in CAPD: relationship with respiratory dynamics. Trans ASAIO 28: 270–275, 1982.

120. Rottembourgh J, Issad B, Gallego JL, Degoulet P, Aime F, Gueffaf B, Legrain M: Evolution of residual renal function in patients undergoing hemodialyses or CAPD. Proc Eur Dial Transpl Assoc 19: 397–403, 1982.

121. Kurtz SB, Wong VH, Anderson CF, Vogel JP, McCarthy JT, Mitchell III JC: Continuous ambulatory peritoneal dialysis. Three year's experience at the Mayo Clinic. Mayo Clin Proc 58: 633–639, 1983.

122. Prowant B. Ryan L. Nolph KD: Six years experience with peritonitis in a CAPD program. Perit Dial Bull 3: 199–200, 1983.

123. Broyer M, Niaudet P, Champion G, Jean G, Chopin N, Czernichow P: Nutritional and metabolic studies in children on continuous ambulatory peritoneal dialysis. Kidney Int 24 (Suppl) 15: 106–110, 1983.

124. Solusky JB, Kopple JD, Fine RN: Continuous ambulatory peritoneal dialysis in paediatric patients. Kidney Int 24 (Suppl) 15: 101–105, 1983.

125. Garred LJ, Canuad B, Farrell PC: A simple kinetic modelling for assessing peritoneal mass transfer in chronic ambulatory peritoneal dialysis. ASAIO 6: 131–137, 1983.

126. Blumberg A, Hanck A. Sander G: Vitamin Nutrition in patients on CAPD. Clin Nephrol 20: 244–250, 1983.

127. Lameire N, Dhaene M, Matthys E, De Paepe M, Vereerstraeten P, Dratwa M, Ringoir S: Experience with CAPD in diabetic patients. Proc Symp on Prevention and Treatment of Diabetic Nephropathy, Paris. MTP, Lancaster, pp 289–297, 1983.

128. Nolph KD, Boen ST, Farrell PC, Pyle KW: Continuous ambulatory peritoneal dialysis in Australia, Europe and the United States: 1981, Kidney Int 23: 3–8, 1983.

129. Thomson NM, Stevens BJ, Humphery TJ, Atkins RC: Comparison of trace elements in peritoneal dialyses, hemodialyses and uremia, Kidney Int 23: 9–14, 1983.

130. Gokal R, Ramos JM, Ellis HA, Parkinson I, Sweetman V,

Dewar J, Ward MK, Kerr DNS: Histological renal osteodystrophy and 25 hydroxycholecalciferol and aluminium levels in patients on CAPD. Kidney Int 23: 15–21, 1983.

131. Wideröe E, Smeby LC, Berg KJ, Jörstad S, Svartas TM: Intraperitoneal insulin absorption during intermittent and continuous peritoneal dialysis. Kidney Int 23: 22–28, 1983.

132. Von Baeyer H, Gahl GM, Riedinges H, Borowzak R, Averdunk R, Schurig R, Kessel M: Adaptation of CAPD patients to continuous peritoneal energy uptake. Kidney Int 23: 29–34, 1983.

133. Rottembourg. J, El Shahat Y, Agrafiotis A, Thuillier Y, De Groe F, Jacobs C, Legrain M: Continuous ambulatory peritoneal dialysis in insuline-dependent diabetic patients: a 40 month experience. Kidney Int 23: 40–455, 1983.

134. Zuchelli P, Chiarini C, Esposito ED, Fabbri L, Santoro A, Sturani A,: Influence of CAPD on the autonomic nervous system. Kidney Int. 23: 46–50, 1983.

135. Vas SI: Microbiologic aspects of chronic ambulatory peritoneal dialysis. Kidney Int 23: 83–92, 1983.

136. Nolph KD, Cut ler SJ, Steinberg SM, Novak JW: Continuous ambulatory peritoneal dialysis in the United States: A three year study. Kidney Int. 28: 198–205, 1985.

137. Posen G, Lam E, Rapaport A: CAPD in Canada 1982. Abstract, 4th ISAO Official Staellite Symp on CAPD. Kyoto, Japan, November 1983.

138. Wing AJ, Broyer M. Brunner FP, Brynger H, Challah S, Donckerwolcke RA, Gretz N, Jacobs C, Kramer P, Selwood NH: Combined report on regular dialysis and transplantation in Europe, XIII, 1982. Proc. Eur Dial Transpl Assoc 20: 5–67, 1983.

139. Krediet RT, Boeschoten EW, Arisz L: De kwaliteit van het buikvlies tijdens CAPD. Nederlands Tijdschrift voor Geneeskunde 1986: 110–113, 1986.

140. Khanna R, Wu G, Chrisholm L, Oreopoulos DG: Further experience with CAPD in diabetics with end-stage renal disease. Proc. Symp on Prevention and Treatment of Diabetic Nephropathy, Paris. MTP Press, Lancaster, pp 279–288, 1983.

141. Mavichak V, Moriarty MV, Cameron EC, Reeve CE, Ballon HS, Lauener RW, Price DJ: Three and a half years experience with CAPD using the beta cap technique. Trans. ASAIO 28: 253–258, 1982.

142. Mion C. Slingeneyer A, Canaud B, Oules R, Branger B, Chong G, Mourad G: Home intermittent peritoneal dialysis in the treatment of end-stage diabetic nephropathy: 1982 update. Proc.Symp on Prevention and Treatment of Diabetic Nephriopathy. Paris. MRP Press, Lancaster, pp 263–277, 1983.

143. SLingeneyer A, Mion C, Mourad G, Canaud B, Faller B, Beraud JJ: Progressive sclerosing peritonitis: a late and severe complication of maintenance peritoneal dialysis. Trans ASAIO 29: 633–640, 1983.

144. Rottembourg J, Gahl GM, Poignet JL, Mertani E, Strippoli P, Langlois P, Tranbaloc P, Legrain M: Severe abdominal complications in patients undergoing continuous peritoneal dialysis. Proc. Eur Dial Transpl Assoc 20: 236–241, 1983.

145. Canaud B, Slingeneyer A, Mourad G et al.: Peritonite sclérosante et calcifiante. In VII Gambro Symposium onc: 'La survie à long terme de l'insuffisant rénal chronique'. pp 221–225, 1986.

146. Faller B, Marichal JF, Brignon P, Benevent D, Pierre D, Ryckelyncke JP, Charra B, Verger C: Progressive calcifying peritonitis in peritoneal dialysis: Proc. 7th National Conference on CAPD, Kansas City, Febr. 1987.

147. Slingeneyer A. Mion C: Peritonitis prevention in continuous ambulatory peritoneal dialysis: long-term efficacy of a bacteriological filter. Proc Eur. Dial. Transpl. Assco. 19: 388–395, 1982.

148. Winchester JF, Ash SR, Bousquet G. Rakowski TA, Barnard WR, Heeter E, Haley S: Successful peritonitis reduction with a undirectional bacteriological CAPD filter. Trans ASAIO

29: 611–616, 1983.

149. Hamilton R. Adams P, Burkart J, Disher B, Dillingham E. Crater C: Feasibility of a sterile splice for connection in CAPD. Trans ASAIO 29: 623–628, 1983.
150. Hamilton R, Charytan C, Kurtz S *et al.*: Reduction in peritonitis frequency by the Dupont sterile connection device. Trans. ASAIO vol. XXXI: 651–654, 1985.
151. Dia Paolo N, Buoncristiani V: Automatic peritoneal dialysis. Nephron 35: 248–252, 1983.
152. Moncrief JW, Mullins-Blackson C, Le Bourglois J, Popovich RP, Pyle K: Development and testing of an ultraviolet light resterilizing procedure for CAPD. Abstract 4th ISAO Official Satellite Symposium on CAPD. Kyoto, Japan. November 1983.
153. Bazzato G, Coli U, Landini S *et al*: CAPD without wearing a bag: complete freedom of patient and significant reduction on peritonitis. Proc Eur Dial Transpl Assoc 17: 266–275, 1980.
154. Buoncristiani V. Bianchi P. Cozzari M *et al.*: A new safe simple connection system for CAPD. Int J Nephrol Urol Androl 1: 50–53, 1980.
155. Buoncristinai U. Di Paolo N: Autosterilizing CAPD connection systems. Nephron 35: 244–247, 1983.
156. Maiorca R. Cancarini GC, Brocolli R. Brasa S, Cantaluppi A. Scalamogna A, Graziani G, Ponicelli C: Prospective controlled trial of a Y-connector and disinfectant to prevent peritonitis in CAPD. Lancet 2: 642–644, 1983.
157. Rottembourg J. DE Groc F: Peritoneal access using the curled Tenckhoff catheter. Perspectives in Peritoneal Dialysis 1: 7–8, 1983.
158. Ash SR, Slingeneyer A. Schardin KE: Peritoneal access using the column-disc catheter. Perspectives in Peritoneal Dialysis 1: 9–11, 1983.
159. Valli A, Comotti C, Torelli D, Crescimanno U, Valentini A, Riegler P, Huber W, Borghi M, Gruttadauria C, Scarovanat P. Pecchini F: A new catheter for peritoneal dialysis. Trans ASAIO 29: 629–632, 1983.
160. Ehrlich LF, Powell SL: Care of the patient with a Gore-Tex peritoneal dialysis catheter. Dial Transpl 12: 572, 1983.
161. Chiaramonte S, Feriani M, Biasioli S *et al*: Clinical experience with short peritoneal catheter. Proceed. European Dialysis and Transplant Association-European Renal Association, vol. 22: 421–425, 1985.
162. Diaz-Buxo JA, Walker PJ, Farmer DF, Chandler JT, Holt KL, Cox P: Continuous cyclic peritoneal dialysis. Trans ASAIO 27: 51–53, 1981.

163. Price CG, Suki WN: Newer modification of peritoneal dialysis. Am J Nephrol 1: 97–104, 1981.
164. Nakagawa D, Price C, Stinebaugh B, Suki W: Continuous cycling peritoneal dialysis: a viable option in the treatment of chronic renal failure. Trans ASAIO 27: 55–57, 1981.
165. Buoncristiani V. Cozarri M, Carobi C, Quintaliani G. Barbarossa D, Di Paolo N: Semi-continuous semi-ambulatory peritoneal dialysis. Proc Eur Dial Transpl Assoc 17: 328–332, 1980.
166. Twardowski ZJ, Prowant BF, Nolph KD, Martinez AJ, Lampton LM: High volume low frequency CAPD. Kidney Int. 23: 64–70, 1983.
167. Twardowski ZJ, Nolph KD, Prowant BF, Moore HL: Efficiency of high volume low frequency continuous ambulatory peritoneal dialysis. Trans ASAIO 29: 53–57, 1983.
168. Ing TS, Hamayun HS, Daugirdas JF *et al.*: Preparation of bicarbonate containing dialysate for peritoneal dialysis. Int J Artif Organs 6: 217, 1983.
169. Feriani M, Basioli S, Borin D *et al.*: Bicarbonate buffer for CAPD solution. Trans ASAIO vol. XXXI: 668–672, 1985.
170. Twardowski ZJ, Khanna R, Nolph KD: Osmotic agents and ultrafiltration in peritoneal dialysis. Nephron 42: 93–101, 1986.
171. Di Paoli N, Buoncristiani V, Capotondo L *et al.*: Phosphatidylcholine and peritoneal transport during peritoneal dialysis. Nephron 44: 365–370, 1986.
172. Mactier RA, Khanna R. Twardowski Z, Moore H, Nolph KD: Contribution of lymphatic absorption to loss of ultrafiltration and solute clearances in CAPD. J Clinic Invest 80: 1311–1316, 1987.
173. Keane WF, Peterson Ph K: Host defense mechanisms of the peritoneal cavity and CAPD Peritoneal Dial Bulletin, vol. 4: 122–127, 1984.
174. Lamperi S, Carozzi S: Peritoneal defense mechanism in CAPD. Abstract ASAIO 14: 37, 1985.
175. Lamperi S, Carozzi S: Suppressor resident peritoneal macrophages and Peritonitis incidence in CAPD patients. Nephron 44: 219–225, 1986.
176. McGregor SJ, Brock JH, Briggs JD, JUnor BJR : Bactericidal activity of peritoneal macrophages from CAPD patients. Nephrol Dial Transplant 2: 104–108, 1987.
177. Lamperi S, Carozzi S : Interferons, peritoneal macrophages and peritonitis in CAPD patients. Abstract ASAIO 16: 33, 1987.

2

THE PERITONEAL DIALYSIS SYSTEM

KARL D. NOLPH and ZBYLUT J. TWARDOWSKI

1. INTRODUCTION

The peritoneal dialysis system can be considered as nature's version of a capillary kidney [1]. Peritoneal dialysis probably represents solute and fluid exchange mainly between peritoneal capillary blood and dialysis solution in the peritoneal cavity [2]. The dialysis membrane consists of the vascular wall, the interstitium, the mesothelium, and adjacent fluid films [1–2]. In this chapter, we will review the anatomy of the peritoneum and the physiology of peritoneal transport. We will also compare the peritoneal dialysis system to man-made hollow fiber dialyzers. The features of the latter have been well characterized and are very familiar to most nephrologists. Comparison of peritoneal and hollow fiber dialysis should help the reader appreciate some of the unique characteristics of the peritoneal dialysis system.

The peritoneal membrane covers visceral organs, forms the visceral mesentery that connects loops of bowel, and reflects over and covers the inner surface of the abdominal wall. This membrane is continuous and the closed space within contains small amounts of fluid (probably less than 100 ml) under normal conditions. This space can be enlarged by the instillation of fluid. Most normal-sized adults can tolerate 2 or more liters of fluid without discomfort. A thin layer of mesothelial cells covers the surface of the membrane lining the cavity. Beneath the mesothelial layer there is interstitium containing extracellular fluid, connective tissue fibers, blood vessels and lymphatics.

Visceral peritoneum courses over the surface of visceral organs. Visceral mesentery between adjacent loops of bowel is formed as the visceral peritoneum reflects over loops of bowel and consists of two layers of mesothelial cells with interstitium interspersed between these layers.

The inner surface of the abdominal wall is covered by the parietal peritoneum. The parietal peritoneum receives its blood supply from the arteries of the abdominal wall.

Visceral mesentery contains mainly large blood vessels on their way to visceral organs. Characterictics of the peritoneal microcirculation will be reviewed in the chapter by Korthuis and Granger. Many lymphatics are present in visceral mesentery but the extent of their participation in peritoneal dialysis solute and water exchange is unknown. Subdiaphragmatic and other parietal peritoneal lymphatics are thought to account for a major portion of fluid absorption from the peritoneal cavity; the effects of parietal lymphatics on the kinetics of peritoneal dialysis will be reviewed extensively in the chapter on peritoneal lymphatics by Mactier and Khanna.

The total gross surface area of the combined parietal and visceral peritoneal mesothelium is thought to approximate the surface area of the skin (1–2 m² in most adults). The exact ratio of parietal to visceral peritoneal surface area is unknown. Visceral mesentery represents a larger fraction of total peritoneal surface area because of its many folds. However, portions of the parietal peritoneum may be more vascular than some of the nearly avascular sections of mesentery. Thus, true vascular contributions of parietal and visceral peritoneum to solute transport are unknown.

2. EVIDENCE THAT PERITONEAL DIALYSIS IS PRIMARILY HEMODIALYSIS

Table 1 summarizes the indirect evidence that peritoneal capillary blood is the major source of solutes, cells, and water removed during peritoneal dialysis. It should be stressed that most of the evidence is indirect.

Table 1. Indirect evidence that peritoneal capillary blood is a major source of solutes, cells, and water removal during peritoneal dialysis.

1. Hypotension with repeated hypertonic exchanges.
2. Decreased clearances with hypotension.
3. Decreased clearances with vasoconstrictors.
4. Increased clearances with vasodilators.
5. Drugs known to increase protein leaking from venules increase protein losses during peritoneal dialysis.
6. Decreased clearances with vasculitis.
7. Decreased clearances with diabetic vascular disease.
8. Dialysate potassium concentrations approach Gibbs-Donnan equilibrium with serum, not with intracellular fluid.
9. Convective removal of potassium per liter of ultrafiltrate does not exceed extracellular concentrations.
10. Limited pools of fluid and solutes in peritoneal mesothelium and interstitium-quickly exhausted without rapid replacement.
11. Lymphatic flow presumably quite low-drainage not chylous.
12. Dialysate leukocyte counts and fibrin increase rapidly with inflammation.
13. Complement activation increases protein losses in peritoneal dialysate.
14. Early vascular changes in alloxan diabetes in rats associated with increased peritoneal clearances.
15. In peritonitis, increased protein losses are associated with increased PGE2 in dialysate-both blocked with indomethacin.

Hypertonic peritoneal dialysis solution containing 4.25% dextrose can generate net ultrafiltration in excess of 500 ml/hr [6]. Many liters per day of ultrafiltration can be tolerated with the rather rapid resolution of edema. If hypertonic exchanges are interspersed so as to avoid severe hyperglycemia or hypotension, net ultrafiltration per hypertonic exchange can remain quite consistent [6]. It seems unlikely that mesothelial cells, interstitium or lymphatics could yield net ultrafiltration of this magnitude over short periods of time. It seems more reasonable to assume that ultrafiltrate is primarily a capillary ultrafiltrate. Also, dramatic reductions in blood pressure following one or two hypertonic exchanges can sometimes be observed suggesting that net ultrafiltration without adequate mobilization of edema fluid can jeopardize blood volume.

Hypotension can result in decreased peritoneal clearances [18]. Although such reductions in clearances are often modest even in severe shock (for reasons to be discussed below) the findings do suggest that solute clearances are affected by peritoneal capillary blood flow [7-9].

Intraperitoneal or systemic vasoconstrictors have been shown to reduce peritoneal clearances [10-11]. Vasoconstrictors are known to decrease the number of peritoneal capillaries perfused as well as peritoneal capillary blood flow [12]. Decreased clearances with vasoconstrictors supports the conjecture that the status of the microcirculation influences peritoneal clearances.

Peritoneal clearances increase with intraperitoneal vasodilators [12-18]. These agents increase peritoneal capillary blood flow as well as the number of capillaries perfused [14-16]. Vasodilatation and/or direct effects of the agents used may increase capillary permeability [19]. The point to be made herein, however, is that vasoactive agents affect peritoneal clearances in the expected direction if clearances relate directly to blood flow, numbers of capillaries, and vascular permeability.

Wayland has shown that histamine applied topically to the rat peritoneum widens the intercellular gaps in small venules [19]. His techniques have included serial section studies with electron microscopy, computerized reconstruction of venular intercellular gaps, and direct observations of the movement of fluorescent tagged albumin across the walls of small vessels in the rat mesentery. The latter technique utilizes a laser beam microscope developed by

Dr. Wayland. With this device an outpouring of albumin from small venules can be seen following a topical application of histamine to rat mesentery. Miller and co-workers have reported similar findings with nitroprusside [20]. In clinical studies, the addition of nitroprusside to peritoneal dialysis solution markedly increases protein losses [13-18].

Patients with severe systemic vasculitis, presumably involving the peritoneal microcirculation have been reported to have significantly reduced peritoneal clearances [21, 23]. To date this includes reports of reduced clearances with systemic lupus erythematosus, scleroderma, and malignant hypertension.

Some patients with wide spread diabetic vascular disease have been found to have significantly reduced clearances [21]. This is not a universal finding in all diabetics but may relate to the basement membrane thickening and vascular disease as it exists in the peritoneum.

The concentration of potassium in the intracellular fluid of mesothelial cells is near 140 mEq/1 [24-26]. Nevertheless, dialysis solution in the peritoneal cavity approaches Gibbs-Donnan equilibrium with the potassium concentration in serum water [27-28]. Since dialysis solution is similar in composition to extracellular fluid it is not surprising that the mesothelial cells would maintain their normal internal milieu even though bathed with dialysis solution. However, the fact that intracellular electrolytes do not participate in peritoneal dialysis exchange to any great extent does not rule out the possibility that some creatinine and urea are removed from intracellular fluid.

Using hypertonic solutions and thus generating net ultrafiltration, solutes can be removed by convection in the absence of a concentration gradient for net diffusion [29-32]. The net removal of potassium by convection per liter of ultrafiltrate does not appear to exceed amounts of potassium in extracellular fluid [27, 33-34].

Certainly it is likely that diffusible solutes are removed from peritoneal interstitium and perhaps to some extent from mesothelial intracellular fluid [1-4, 19, 35]. Ultrafiltrate would, of course, involve water movement through the interstitium and perhaps to some extent through or from mesothelial cells [31]. However, mesothelial cells could only tolerate a modest degree of dehydration and interstitial pools of water and solute would quickly be exhausted without rapid replacement from peritoneal capillaries. The point is that most of the water and solutes removed during peritoneal dialysis must represent water and solute movement from peritoneal capillaries into the peritoneal cavity by way of pathways through the interstitium and the mesothelial layer.

Solutes and water could move into the peritoneal interstitium from visceral peritoneal lymphatics [35]. It is unknown what portion of net removal of solutes or water comes from peritoneal lymphatics. This has been assumed to be of minor importance since lymphatic flow rates are presumably low and drainage is not usually chylous. We have followed one patient on continuous ambulatory peritoneal dialysis whose drainage after an episode of streptococcal peritonitis obviously contained lymph for nearly three years. Drainage was milky, particularly after meals, and contained high triglyceride concentrations. There was no evidence of inflammation (dialysate white counts were low and there were no symptoms). This particular finding however is extremely unusual.

Additional evidence that peritoneal capillary blood can contribute rapidly and significantly to what is removed in peritoneal dialysis solution is the finding that with infection dialysate leukocyte counts can increase over several hours from less than 100 to many thousands of white cells/mm^3 [36–37]. Also it would appear that an outpouring of fibrinogen and the formation of fibrin in dialysate can occur quite quickly in the presence of inflammation.

Activation of the alternate pathway of complement may cause changes in protein losses during peritoneal dialysis [38]. In rats, the movement of intra-arterial injected rat serum albumin conjugated to a fluorescent dye into the peritoneal cavity can be monitored. Zymosine activated rat serum and endotoxin injections (both intraperitoneal and intra-arterial), each of which may activate the alternate pathway of complement, produce dramatic increases in dialysate protein concentrations.

Early diabetes mellitus can cause increases in glomerular permeability [39]. In rats, alloxan induced diabetes mellitus can result in increased peritoneal clearances of urea, inulin and albumin. These changes are associated with findings of small adipose cells in the capillary basement membranes and neovascularization in the peritoneums of the diabetic rats. Whether diabetes mellitus decreases transport or increases transport may depend on the duration of the disease and the extent of the vascular alterations. Vasoactive prostoglandins are involved in the pathophysiology of increased peritoneal protein losses in the early phases of CAPD associated peritonitis [40]. Indomethacin administration can diminish the amount of PGE2 in dialysate and prevent increased protein losses.

Thus, indirect evidence supports the hypothesis that peritoneal dialysis represents fluid and solute exchange between peritoneal capillary blood and dialysis solution in the peritoneal cavity. The capillary endothelium, peritoneal interstitium, and mesothelium represent the resistance sites which must be crossed by fluid and solutes and result in a net exchange.

3. PERITONEAL CAPILLARY BLOOD FLOW

The absolute peritoneal capillary blood flow which participates in peritoneal dialysis exchange is unknown. In adult humans, total splanchnic blood flow may exceed 1200/ml/min [41]. However, most of this blood is on its way to visceral organs and not to the small vessels of the peritoneum. In fact our observations of the rat peritoneum would suggest that the mesentery is not particularly vascular and that most of the small vessels capable of participating in exchange may be located at those sites where the peritoneum reflects over loops of bowel [42–43].

In adult humans maximum urea clearances usually do not exceed 40 ml/min even with the most rapid cycling [44–46]. One possible explanation has been that effective peritoneal capillary blood flow may not exceed 30 to 40 ml/min and maximum urea clearances are approaching effective peritoneal capillary flow. There is abundant indirect evidence to suggest that this is not the case. Table 2 summarizes indirect evidence that maximum peritoneal urea clearances are not primarily blood flow limited.

First in animal studies it has been shown that urea clearances remain above 70% of control even with severe shock and 38% reductions in splanchnic blood flow [7]. Although the magnitude of change in the effective peritoneal capillary flow from control to shock conditions is unknown, this observation would suggest that effective peritoneal capillary flow is well above urea clearance in the control state and only falls into a modest flow limiting range with severe hypotension.

Secondly, urea clearances increase only modestly (usually less than 20%) with intraperitoneal vasodilators [13–18]. Vasodilators are also known to influence the number of capillaries perfused, induce venodilation and in some instances directly alter vascular permeability [12, 42–43]. Since these latter effects might also account for the modest increases in small solute clearances these findings suggest that any increases in effective capillary flow with vasodilators have little or no effects on urea clearances and that there is not a major blood flow limitation on urea clearances.

In fact vasodilators primarily increase clearances of larger solutes [14–15]. Such increases may exceed 100% for solutes of molecular weight 5200 daltons or above. These obser-

Table 2. Indirect evidence that maximum peritoneal urea clearances[a] are not primarily blood flow limited.

1. Urea clearances remain 70% of control even in shock.
2. Urea clearances increase <20% with vasodilators.
3. Vasodilators increase clearances of larger solutes more than urea clearances.
4. Clearances of CO_2 and H_2 gases nearly three times maximum urea clearances.
5. Urea clearances, if only $1/3$ of effective capillary blood flow (as gas clearances suggest), would be minimally flow limited according to kinetic modeling analysis and in vitro simulations.
6. Increasing evidence that fluid films can readily explain low urea clearances.

[a] Very high dialysate flow, >4 l/hr yields urea clearances in man <40 ml/min.

vations would support the contention that vasodilator effects may be more related to venodilation and alterations in permeability rather than effects on blood flow per se [19, 43, 47]. This is not to deny the possibility that vasodilators may increase effective peritoneal capillary flow. However, if this were the main effect of the drugs and if urea clearances were flow limited, proportionally greater increases in urea clearances should occur as compared to increases in clearance of larger solutes.

Peritoneal clearances of CO_2 gas in humans and hydrogen gas in rabbits are two to three times maximum urea clearances [2, 8]. Gas clearances should also be limited by effective peritoneal capillary flow and should not exceed urea clearance to any great extent if effective capillary flow were the main determinant of urea clearance. On the other hand gases should be able to diffuse across all membrane resistances more rapidly. Gases might also utilize trans-cellular routes while evidence to be discussed later suggests that nongaseous solutes pass primarily via vesicles or through intercellular gaps and extracellular pathways [48–50]. The fact that gas clearances can be two to three times urea clearances suggests that urea clearances are limited by total membrane resistances, including fluid films rather than effective peritoneal capillary flow.

If it is true that urea clearances are only one third to one half of the effective capillary blood flow, kinetic modeling analyses and in vitro simulations of peritoneal dialysis suggest that under such conditions effective capillary flow would exert only modest limitations on peritoneal urea clearances and that the relationship of urea clearance to effective capillary flow would be in the 'plateau' portion of the clearance to blood flow relationship [2]. Figure 1 shows a hypothetical relationship of urea clearance to blood flow at high dialysis solution flow rates for peritoneal dialysis compared to typical findings with a hollow fiber artificial kidney. For the hollow fiber, dialysate flow would be near 500 ml/min and, for peritoneal dialysis, flow rates would exceed 4 l/hr. If effective peritoneal capillary flow rate in adult humans is near 70 ml/min (as CO_2 gas diffusion studies suggest) then urea clearances would show a nearly 'plateau' relationship with effective blood flow. This plateau presumably represents effects of membrane and fluid film resistances. On the other hand, the hollow fiber dialyzer fluid film and membrane resistances to urea transport are so low the system is primarily blood flow limited. Urea clearances remain at a high fraction of blood flow up to very high blood flows.

Finally, there is increasing evidence that fluid films can

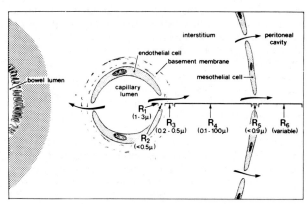

Figure 2. Resistance to solute movement during peritoneal dialysis. See text for definitions of R_1 thru R_6. Reprinted with permission from Nolph and Sorkin: CAPD in *Chronic Renal Failure* edited by Brenner and Stein. Churchill Livingstone, New York, 1981, p. 197.

readily account for the low urea clearance [2, 48]. Figure 2 shows the hypothetical resistance sites which solutes must cross in moving from peritoneal capillaries into the peritoneal dialysis solution. The dimensions listed in Figure 2 are based on rat studies. R_1 would represent stagnant fluid films in the peritoneal capillary and R_2 the endothelium. The work of Karnovsky and others suggest that the major path for solute movement across the endothelium may be through intercellular gaps [48, 50]. R_3 would represent the basement membrane of the capillary endothelium, R_4 the peritoneal interstitium, and R_5 the mesothelial layer. Intercellular gaps may be important pathways for solute and water movement across the mesothelium during peritoneal dialysis [48, 50]. Finally, R_6 represents the stagnant fluid films in the peritoneal cavity. There is increasing evidence that the interstitium and the fluid films in the peritoneal cavity may account for the major limitations on urea clearance [19, 51]. The number of capillaries

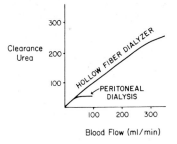

Figure 1. Urea clearance is related to blood flow in hollow fiber and peritoneal dialysis. Dialysate flow is assumed non-limiting.

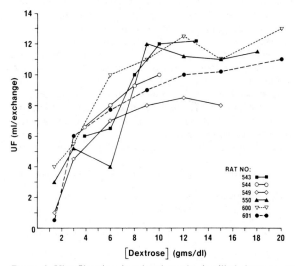

Figure 3. Ultrafiltration is related to the instilled dextrose concentration in series of 16 ml exchanges in 6 rats. A plateau of ultrafiltration per exchange is seen above 10 gms/dl.

involved may also limit total pore area even though mean pore size may be relatively high.

Although we have just summarized evidence that capillary blood flow may not limit urea clearance under normal circumstances it is possible that capillary blood flow limits maximum ultrafiltration rate [52–53]. Figure 3 shows net ultrafiltration (ml/exchange) in rats receiving series of exchanges (16 ml instillations) with progressive increases in dialysis solution dextrose concentration. The total cycle time for each exchange was 30 min. Net UF per exchange appears to reach a plateau. Based on previous estimates of effective capillary blood flow rate, filtration fractions at maximum rates of ultrafiltration may be approaching 50%. One hypothetical explanation for the limitation on ultrafiltration rate is depicted in Figure 4. As blood flows along peritoneal capillaries, oncotic pressure increases while net hydrostatic and osmotic pressure gradients favoring ultrafiltration decrease. The shaded areas between the lines represent an index of total net ultrafiltration. At instillation dextrose concentrations of 10 gm% or more, the rise in oncotic pressure in capillary plasma is so steep as to reach equilibrium with the sum of opposing hydrostatic and osmotic pressures. The area representing net ultrafiltration does not increase with higher dextrose concentrations because of the earlier filtration pressure equilibrium and the constancy of the shaded area as an index of net ultrafiltration. Theoretical aspects of ultrafiltration will be discussed in more detail in the chapter by Henderson.

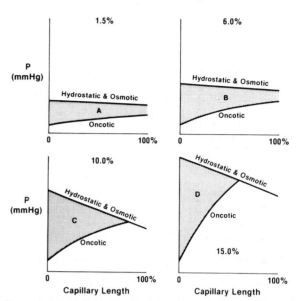

Figure 4. A hypothetical explanation of the findings in Figure 3 postulating steep increases in oncotic pressure and filtration pressure equilibrium at high filtration fractions.

4. INDIRECT EVIDENCE THAT FLUID FILMS AND/OR INTERSTITIAL RESISTANCE LIMIT UREA CLEARANCE DURING PERITONEAL DIALYSIS

Table 3 summarizes the indirect evidence that fluid films and/or the interstitial resistance are important in limiting urea clearances during peritoneal dialysis. First, as mentioned above, maximum urea clearance do not appear to exceed 40 ml/min in most humans even with rapid cycling or the use of intraperitoneal vasodilators [44–46]. The rapid cycling should minimize limitations due to dialysis solution flow rate. Vasodilators which presumably increase the number of capillaries perfused and alter capillary permeability should minimize endothelial resistance. Studies in isolated mesentery suggest that some mesothelial intercellular gaps are greater than 500 Å in width and offer very little resistance [54–56]. Thus, under the conditions of rapid cycling and the use of intraperitoneal vasodilators (and assuming that effective peritoneal capillary flow is not limiting) major resistance sites that explain the limits on urea clearances should be the interstitium and the stagnant

fluid films in the peritoneal cavity.

Secondly, dialysate is always relatively stagnant in the peritoneal cavity within the many folds of the mesentery even with rapid cycling [44–46].

Thirdly, dialysate channels are probably relatively wide [46]. Figure 5 shows a comparison of dialysate channel dimensions during peritoneal dialysis with those in a man-made hollow fiber kidney. Note that in the hollow fiber kidney much of the cross section of the dialyzer represents blood path. In small dialysate channels there is rapid counter-current flow with minimal fluid film resistance [57–58]. In contrast, in the peritoneal system the interstitium and stagnant pools of fluid between folds of mesentery represent substantial fluid film resistances.

The interstitial solute path probably represents a usually relatively long distance [4]. In Figure 2 we see that it may represent 100 μ or more. Figure 6 shows that the situation may be even more complex. The work of Wayland suggests that the interstitium may represent a network of aqueous channels through mucopolysaccharide and collagenous gels [19]. Hypertonic peritoneal dialysis solutions may dehydrate the interstitium and, although the total distance may be

Table 3. Indirect evidence that fluid films and/or interstitial resistance limit urea clearances during peritoneal dialysis.

1. Maximum urea clearances near 40 ml/min even with rapid cycling or vasodilators.
2. Dialysate relatively stagnant.
3. Probably very wide dialysate channels.
4. Interstitial solute path-potentially long distance.
5. In vitro simulations of peritoneal dialysis demonstrate high fluid film resistance.
6. Little evidence to support blood flow limitation.
7. Vascular resistance appears low for small solutes.
8. Recent theoretical models of peritoneal transport emphasize interstitial diffusivity.

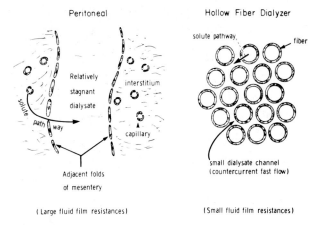

Peritoneal   Hollow Fiber Dialyzer

(Large fluid film resistances)   (Small fluid film resistances)

Figure 5. Dialysate channel features for peritoneal and hollow fiber dialysis are compared.

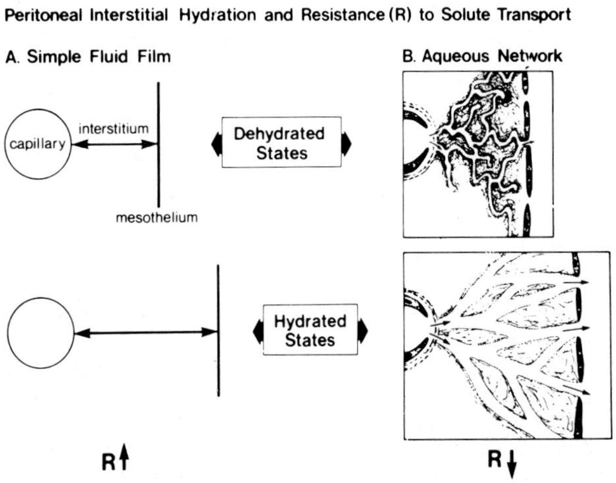

Peritoneal Interstitial Hydration and Resistance (R) to Solute Transport

A. Simple Fluid Film   **B. Aqueous Network**

R↑   R↓

Figure 6. The interstitium is hypothetically shown as a simple film (A) or network of water channels (B) dehydrated by hypertonic solutions in the peritoneal cavity. If it were a simple fluid film (A), going from dehydration to hydration should increase resistance (R) by increasing distance. In B., hydration decreases R by widening channels.

shortened, the aqueous network of channels could become more torturous and the resistance to solute movement actually increase [43, 59].

In vitro simulations of peritoneal dialysis, using hollow fiber dialyzers placed in stagnant pools of fluid with the outer shell of the dialyzer removed, demonstrate rapid deterioration in urea clearances attributable to high fluid film resistances [2, 51]. Even with the most rapid cycling techniques in and out of the simulated peritoneal cavity, clearances cannot be restored. Vigorous shaking of the cavity and improved mixing will diminish the effects of fluid film resistance to some extent but never approach the performance that can be achieved with rapid counter current flow of dialysate in the usual manner [51].

As mentioned above, there is little evidence to support a blood flow limitation and, therefore, the importance of the fluid films is implied.

Studies by Wayland suggest that endothelium offers very little resistance to small solute movement from peritoneal capillary blood into peritoneal dialysis solution [19]. If rats are injected with fluorescent tagged small solutes, extensive migration of the solute into the interstitium can be observed. This is in contrast to what is seen following injection of fluorescent tagged albumin; movement of albumin across vascular walls is not obvious over many minutes unless agents which increase vascular permeability are administered in solutions bathing the peritoneum [19].

Recently published distributed models of peritoneal-plasma transport have stressed the importance of tissue diffusivity [60]. Key parameters of the model include peritoneal surface area, tissue diffusivity, capillary permeability, tissue void fraction and hydrostatic in osmostic pressures in the capillaries and interstitium.

5. EVIDENCE THAT VASCULAR PERMEABILITY IS A MAJOR RESISTANCE FOR LARGER SOLUTES

In contrast to the situation for small solutes where interstitial and fluid films appear to be major determinants of removal efficiency, the permeability of the microcirculation appears to be a major influence of the clearances of larger solutes [13–20, 47]. The evidence for this is summarized in Table 4.

First, we have already mentioned that increased protein losses occur with the topical application to the mesentery of agents known to increase venular permeability [19]. Intraperitoneal nitroprusside, for example, markedly increases protein losses.

Secondly, there are proportionally larger increases in inulin clearances as compared to urea clearances with vasoactive drugs [13, 18]. There is evidence to suggest that vasoactive drugs alter vascular permeability [19–20]. This would explain the greater proportional effects on larger solutes where vascular permeability has a major effect on clearances.

Thirdly, it is well known that protein losses increase with peritoneal inflammation [5, 61–63]. Peritoneal inflammation from any cause stimulates an outpouring of white cells into the peritoneal dialysis solution [37]. Inflammation in other tissues of the body is usually associated with vasodilation and it seems reasonable to assume that this would also occur in the peritoneum. Thus the protein losses with inflammation may simply reflect endogenous mechanisms that induce vasodilation. Vasodilation per se may result in the perfusion of more permeable capillaries [64]. Local release of histamine may increase vascular permeability. Evidence for a close association between peritoneal prostaglandin production [40] and compliment activation [38] has been cited and supports the concept that microcirculatory permeability is a major determinant of protein losses and large molecular transport across the peritoneum.

Finally, studies with fluorescent tagged albumin already have been mentioned [19]. Following an injection of this material into the rat, the albumin remains within the microcirculation over many minutes of observation without obvious leaking into the interstitium. With topical peritoneal application of agents that alter vascular permeability, there is an almost explosive outpouring of albumin from the microcirculation into the interstitium over a matter of seconds.

Table 4. Evidence that vascular permeability is a major resistance for large solutes.

1. Increased protein losses with agents known to increase venular permeability.
2. Proportionately larger increases in inulin clearances (as compared to urea clearances) with vasoactive drugs.
3. Increased protein losses with peritoneal inflammation.
4. Laser studies with fluorescent tagged albumin in the rat microcirculation.

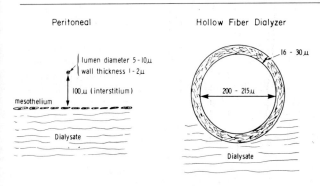

Figure 7. The intercellular gaps of the peritoneal endothelium are relatively wide but few. In hollow fibers, 'pores' are smaller but many.

6. A COMPARISON OF CAPILLARY DIMENSIONS OF THE PERITONEAL DIALYSIS SYSTEM WITH THE HOLLOW FIBER DIALYZER

Figure 7 shows cross sections of a peritoneal capillary and a synthetic fiber in a hollow fiber dialyzer. The dimensions are drawn to scale as indicated. Although the synthetic fiber wall is much thicker, a high fraction of the wall luminal surface may represent 'pore' area. The fiber wall is a mesh of synthetic material with many spaces between interstices. In contrast, the peritoneal capillary may not only have a very small relative total luminal surface but only a small fraction (less than 0.2% according to Pappenheimer [65]) of that luminal surface may represent 'pore' area. This is only true, of course, if indeed intercellular gaps are the major pathways for solute and water movement from the capillary.

Figure 8 shows lateral views of the fiber walls. This demonstrates even more readily the great distance that may be between intercellular slits in capillary endothelium and, in contrast, the high fraction of synthetic fiber walls representing space available for solute exchange between the molecules composing the wall.

Figure 9 shows lateral views of the course of capillaries in the peritoneal membrane and synthetic fibers in a hollow fiber dialyzer. Notice that the capillary network in the peritoneal system would be quite complex with many interconnections. The total number of capillaries participating in exchange is unknown. In contrast, in the hollow fiber dialyzers each fiber is a separate entity. There are no interconnections and the numbers are well known depending on the brand of hollow fiber dialyzer. In the peritoneal system only a portion of capillaries may be perfused at any one time as others may be essentially closed down by pre-capillary sphincter tone [4]. In contrast, in the hollow fiber dialyzer most of the fibers are perfused at any one time in the absence of fiber plugging [66].

7. DIALYSATE FLOW

Figure 10 compares typical flow rates in ml per minute and in liters per week for dialysis with a hollow fiber dialyzer (12 hr per week), intermittent peritoneal dialysis (40 hr per week), and continuous ambulatory peritoneal dialysis (four 2–1 exchanges per day). The figure does not include ultrafiltration rates which have little impact on the figures for hollow fiber dialysis and intermittent peritoneal dialysis but add substantially to total flow for continuous ambulatory peritoneal dialysis.

For hollow fiber dialysis, urea clearances are primarily blood flow limited. For intermittent peritoneal dialysis urea clearances during treatment are probably limited primarily by fluid film resistances for the reasons discussed above. For continuous ambulatory peritoneal dialysis, the urea

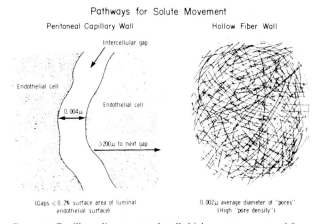

Figure 8. Capillary diameters and wall thickness are compared for peritoneal and hollow fiber dialyzers. Note that hollow fiber dialyzers are in direct contact with dialysate while peritoneal capillaries are not.

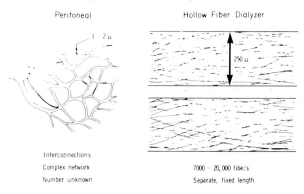

Figure 9. Capillary arrangements in peritoneal and hollow fiber dialysis.

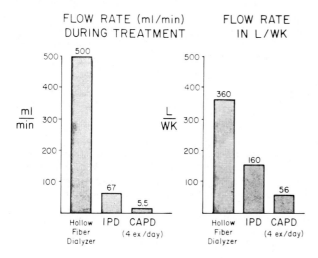

Figure 10. Comparison of typical dialysate flow rates in hollow fiber, intermittent peritoneal (IPD), and continuous ambulatory peritoneal dialysis (CAPD); ml/min and 1 week.

clearances are limited by dialysis solution flow rate and are nearly identical to dialysis solution flow rate.

Figure 11 shows that urea clearances typically are nearly one third of dialysis solution rate for both hollow fiber dialysis and intermittent peritoneal dialysis during the treatment seesions. For continuous ambulatory peritoneal dialysis, the ratio of urea clearance to flow rate of dialysis solution approaches 1.0 [67–72].

8. A SUMMARY OF THE IMPORTANCE OF DIFFERENT RESISTANCES FOR LARGE AND SMALL SOLUTES DURING HOLLOW FIBER DIALYSIS AND PERITONEAL DIALYSIS

Figure 12 shows a summary of the important resistance sites during peritoneal dialysis and during hollow fiber dialysis. The height of each bar is a hypothetical value since the actual numbers are for the most part unknown.

The upper figures show a summary of the important resistance sites on an absolute scale. In peritoneal dialysis, the vascular wall probably offers substantial resistance only for the much larger solutes above 1000 daltons in molecular weight [19]. For smaller solutes this is a short distance to traverse with a relatively large mean pore size (perhaps greater than 40 Å in width at the venular end of the capillary) [48–50]. The interstitial resistance is substantial for both small and large solutes. This would again be an even greater resistance for large solutes since they must diffuse across this distance and greater hindrance by the dimensions of the aqueous channels (if such truly exist) would be expected. The fluid films in the peritoneal cavity offer substantial resistance to both small and large solutes. The resistance to the latter would again be greater because of the distances involved and their poorer diffusibility. Mesothelial resistance is not shown since intercellular gaps may be 500 Å or more in diameter and there is little evidence to suggest that mesothelium is a major resistance site [54–56]. Very recent findings, to be reviewed below, are challenging the concept of a very 'open' mesothelium, however, and argue for greater mesothelial resistance in some areas of the peritoneum. Intracapillary stagnant fluid films and capillary basement membranes are not shown since they are also not known to be major resistance sites.

Below these hypothetical absolute resistance values for peritoneal dialysis is a figure showing relative resistances. In the case of urea clearance, the interstitium and the fluid films are proportionately greater resistances. Because the vascular wall is a major resistance site for large solutes, interstitial and dialysis solution fluid films are proportionally shown as less important.

In the hollow fiber dialyzer are only two major resistance sites, the fiber wall and fluid films. The mean pore size of the fiber wall may be 20 Å or less [73]. For very large

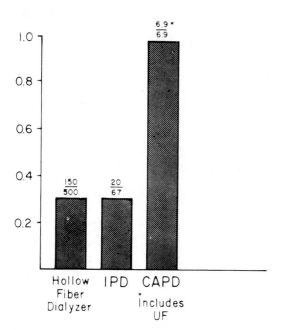

Figure 11. Ratios of typical urea clearances to dialysate flow rates in different dialysis techniques as in Figure 10.

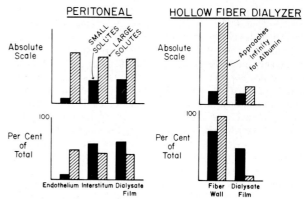

Figure 12. Hypothetical absolute and relative resistance values in peritoneal and hollow fiber dialysis.

solutes, like albumin, synthetic fiber resistance approaches infinity since fibers are impermeable to albumin. The thickness of the fiber wall makes the fiber an important resistance site for urea, perhaps primarily because of the distance involved. Dialysis solution fluid film resistances are much smaller than in peritoneal dialysis for reasons discussed. Thus on a relative scale the fiber wall would offer a high proportion of the total resistance to the movement of both small and large solutes.

9. POSSIBLE MECHANISMS FOR THE NET ELECTROLYTE SIEVING EFFECTS WITH PERITONEAL ULTRAFILTRATION

There are numerous studies to suggest that ultrafiltration induced with osmotic pressure removes water primarily from peritoneal capillaries. The net removals of sodium and potassium by convection per liter of ultrafiltrate are usually well below respective extracellular fluid concentrations [31–33]. The net convective component of sodium and potassium removal can be calculated by subtracting net removal accountable to diffusion from the net total removal [33]. Another way to estimate convective transport is to instill solutions with sodium and potassium concentrations in Gibbs-Donnan equilibrium with serum water [31–33, 74–75]. Although a net sieving effect creates a concentration gradient for some net diffusion, net electrolyte removal per liter of ultrafiltrate still remains far below that in extracellular fluid. Severe hypernatremia has been observed as a result of overzealous peritoneal ultrafiltration and removal of extracellular water without amounts of sodium equal to extracellular fluid concentrations [32].

In contrast, it is well known that ultrafiltration by hydrostatic pressure in a hollow fiber dialyzer results in the net removal of an ultrafiltrate with electrolytes in proportions comparable to those in extracellular fluid [76–77]. Isolated ultrafiltration in hollow fibers yields an essentially protein free ultrafiltrate of serum containing electrolytes in amounts near those predicted by Gibbs-Donnan equilibrium.

How is it possible that a membrane as permeable as the peritoneum (more permeable than hollow fibers in terms of protein losses) can hinder the convective movement of electrolytes with ultrafiltration? The answer to this question is not available. Table 5 summarizes possible mechanisms for the net electrolyte sieving effect with peritoneal ultrafiltration.

First, there is substantial evidence to suggest that the width of intercellular gaps progressively increases from proximal to distal portions of the capillaries with the most permeable portions being in the small venules [19]. The

capillaries of the peritoneum may differ from man-made fibers in having a progressive increase in pore width along the capillary while man-made fibers are more homogenous. At the proximal end of the capillaries hydrostatic pressure should be higher [64]. Glucose should be more osmotically effective across this tighter portion of the capillary whereas in the distal portion of the capillary glucose may be readily absorbed and exert little osmotic pressure. Thus combined hydrostatic and osmotic pressure could induce maximum ultrafiltration rates across portions of the capillary that are least permeable.

If most of the water flows through the intercellular gap where junctions are rather narrow, then endothelial cell surfaces in close proximity and their repective charges could impede the movement of electrolytes through the gap.

If transmembrane hydrostatic and osmotic pressures are high enough, perhaps some transendothelial cell water movement does occur [31]. Such net movement of water across the cell may occur without proportional movement of electrolytes through the very complex internal cell milieu.

Surface charges on the capillary basement membrane or on the surfaces of interstitial gels may impede the movement of charged solutes. This could be akin to the charge interference offered by polar molecules in the glomerulus [78]. The work of Glassock and others suggest that albumin is held back more by charge than by pore dimensions [78].

Mesothelial cell surface charges in intercellular gaps could influence electrolyte movements. However, if it is true that the permeability of the mesothelium is much greater than that of the endothelium, then this could be less important than the same phenomenon in the endothelium.

The movement of ultrafiltrate from the interstitium into the peritoneal cavity could occur by hydrostatic pressure with the build up of fluid in the interstitium and with some osmotic pressure induced by glucose gradients across the mesothelium. If it is true that the mesothelium is more permeable than the endothelium then the major glucose gradient could be across the vessel wall with only a modest glucose gradient maintained across the mesothelium. Nevertheless, if water did move through mesothelial cells this again could interfere with the convective transport of electrolytes.

Finally, we have published studies to show that even neutral molecules may not accompany ultrafiltration induced by glucose osmotic pressure in the same proportions as when the ultrafiltration is induced across the same membrane with hydraulic pressure [79]. This is not an effect of osmotic pressure per se as perhaps due to the use of a solute such as glucose which can enter the membrane and move up stream against the flow of ultrafiltrate [80]. We have proposed a hypothesis that molecular interaction within the membrane may alter the net sieving effects [74].

Table 5. Possible mechanisms for the net electrolyte sieving effect with peritoneal ultrafiltration.

1. Ultrafiltration through narrow intercellular gaps in proximal capillaries.
2. Endothelial cell surface charges in interrcellular gaps.
3. Trans-endothelial cell water movement.
4. Interstitial gel surface charges along aqueous channels.
5. Mesothelial cell surface charges in intercellular gaps.
6. Trans-mesothelial cell water movement.
7. Glucose interaction with cations in intercellular gaps or interstitial channels.

Rubin et al. have measured net sieving coefficients in clinical studies where solutes were added to dialysis solutions prior to instillation at concentrations near those of body fluid [81]. A concentration gradient for net diffusion was thus absent at the beginning of the exchange. Net sieving coefficients of multiple solutes (for 4.25% dextrose exchanges with a 30-min dwell time) were calculated as mass transfer/ultrafiltration volume/plasma water concentration. Progressively lower net sieving coefficients were found as molecular weight increased (see Table 6). Charged ions such as sodium and potassium yielded net sieving coefficients lower than that of neutral solutes at comparable molecular weight.

10. COMPARISONS IN ANIMALS AND HUMANS

Techniques to assess dialysis efficiency will be reviewed in the chapter by Popovich. The mass transfer area coefficient represents the maximum clearance possible by diffusion at rapid dialysis solution flow rates. It is limited by the permeability and effective pore area of the membrane. Dedrick has compared peritoneal mass transfer area coefficients for urea and inulin in several species as a function of body weight (Figure 13) [82]. Some of the values represent clearance measurements at high flow rates but presumably approach the mass transfer area coefficients. Several values for gas clearance (hydrogen in rabbit and carbon dioxide in humans) are shown. Gas clearances provide minimum estimates of effective capillary blood flow. Lower urea and inulin mass transfer area coefficients support the contention that mass transfer area coefficients for urea and inulin are not limited by blood flow but by membrane resistances and area. Nearly linear relationships with body weight suggest that the peritoneal dialysis system behaves quite similarly from species to species in proportion to the dimensions represented therein. These studies suggest that there are not striking differences in membrane properties between species.

11. VESICLES VS INTERCELLULAR GAPS

In recent years interest has focused on the relative importance of vesicles and intercellular gaps in regard to the passive movement of solutes across peritoneal endothelium and mesothelium [77–85].

Table 6. Net sieving coefficients per exchange[a]

Solute	Mean ± SEM net sieving coefficient	Number of exchanges
Sodium	0.56 ± 0.04	14
Potassium	0.40 ± 0.04	11
Urea	0.63 ± 0.06	10
Creatinine	0.57 ± 0.09	8
Inulin	0.41 ± 0.08	6

[a]Mass transfer/ultrafiltration volume/plasma water concentration for 4.25% dextrose exchanges with a 30-min dwell (from Rubin et al. [81]; reproduced with permission).

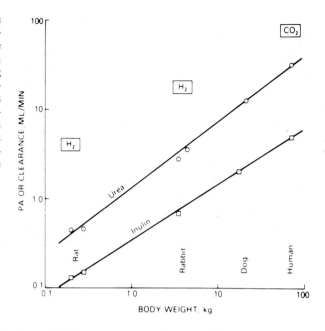

Figure 13. Peritoneal mass transfer area coefficients are compared for urea and inulin in several species as a function of body weight. Some values are clearances at high flow rates thought to be approaching the mass transfer area coefficients, clearances of hydrogen gas in the rat and rabbit and of carbon dioxide in humans are also shown (from Dedrick *et al.* [82]; published with permission).

Wide intercellular gaps have been noted in certain species particularly in the sub-diaphragmatic area [89–90]. In addition, earlier reports suggested that the movement if tracers up to 30 000 daltons molecular weight occurs mainly between cells rather than through cells via vesicles [48–50]. Conversely, recent studies in rabbits have noted very tight intercellular mesothelial cell junctions and numerous intra-cytoplasmic vesicles [91]. Capillaries were of the continuous type and endothelial cells were also noted to contain many vesicles. Following intravenous injection of iron dextran, an electron dense tracer, the iron dextran was found mainly in vesicles in the peritoneum of the rabbit. Scanning electron microscopy of rat mesentery has also revealed very tight intercellular junctions between mesothelial cells [92].

More work is needed to determine the relative role of intercellular gaps and vesicles in passive solute transport across the peritoneum. This may vary from species to species, in different areas of the peritoneum and for solutes of different molecular weight. Although the peritoneal microvascular bed is formed mainly by capillaries of the continuous type, occasional fenestrated capillaries have been reported in rabbits and in humans [93]. In human biopsies fenestrated capillaries have been noted in 1.7% of capillaries studied; in contrast, the incidence of fenestrated capillaries in rabbits approaches 29% in the diaphragmatic peritoneum [93]. It is not clear as to how peritoneal morphology and solute transport in animals relate to humans. Also, it is not clear how tissue processing may artifactually misrepresent the number of vesicles and/or the dimensions of intercellular gaps in vivo. Finally, in vivo, inflammation such as with peritonitis, may widen intercellular gaps resulting in misrepresentation of the situation under non-infected conditions [86].

12. CHANGES WITH PERITONITIS

In humans and animals peritonitis has been associated with changes in peritoneal transport [92, 94–95]. Clearances, glucose absorption rate and protein losses tend to increase suggesting increases in permeability. Rapid glucose absorption is associated with an earlier osmotic equilibrium, early loss of the osmotic pressure gradient for ultrafiltration and less net ultrafiltration with long dwell exchanges (greater than 3 hrs of dwell).

Verger and his colleagues have shown a marked widening of intercellular gaps in visceral mesentery in rats with peritonitis (see Figures 14–16) [92]. There is also loss of mesothelial microvilli and the appearance of round forms (presumably white cells) that seem to be moving through the wide intercellular gaps. With peritonitis there are also changes in the interstitium and microcirculation; interstitial cellular infiltration and vasodilatation are seen. Thus, it is impossible to determine whether changes are primarily the result of mesothelial interstitial or vascular alterations.

13. THE IMPORTANCE OF MESOTHELIAL RESISTANCE

Verger and colleagues produced morphological changes in the mesothelium of the rat peritoneum with a laparotomy,

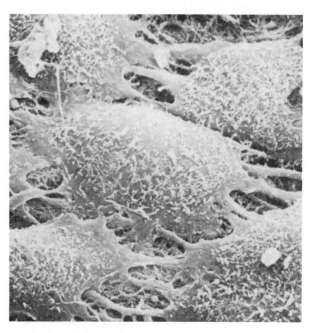

Figure 15. Scanning electron microscopy of mesentery with peritonitis. Note intercellular spaces bridged by cytoplasmic processes (from Verger *et al.* [92]; reproduced with permission).

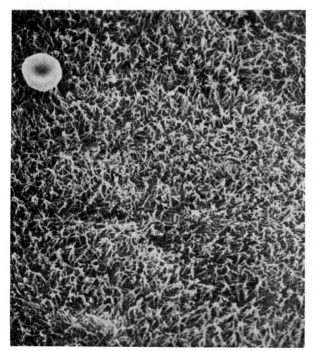

Figure 14. Normal rat mesentery by SEM. There are many microvilli; ×2000 (from Verger *et al.* [92]; reproduced with permission).

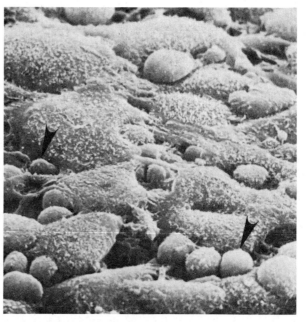

Figure 16. Scanning electron microscopy of infected mesentery. Round forms appear to be moving through the intercellular spaces. Arrows point to several round cells; × 1500 (from Verger *et al.* [92]; reproduced with permission).

heat drying technique and subsequent closure. One to two days post-operatively, increases in clearances, protein loss and glucose absorption were similar to increases with peritonitis [92]. Histological studies at the same time showed mesothelial changes similar to peritonitis in visceral mesentery except for the absence of inflammatory cells. However, there were no interstitial or microcirculatory alterations.

These studies suggest that mesothelial resistance may be much greater than previously believed, at least in some species and some areas of the peritoneum. Mesothelial injury with or without vasodilatation may alter the passive transport characteristics of the membrane. Further work is necessary to clarify these issues.

Intraperitoneal coitochalasin B increases the permeability in the rat to inulin, urea and albumin [96]. Mesothelial cells exposed to coitochalasin B develop membrane protuberances (zeiotic knobs). Coitochalasin D has been noted to increase peritoneal transport in rabbits [97]. Verapamil and bupivacaine increase transmesothelial flux of calcium in rabbits [98]. The authors of these studies with calcium channel blockers suggest the permeability of the mesothelium may be dependent on intracellular calcium ion concentration and that drugs that affect transperitoneal transport of solute may achieve their effects by changes in the state of intracellular calcium. The local anaesthetic, procaine, added to peritoneal dialysis solutions increases peritoneal clearances in rabbits [99]. In vitro studies on rabbit mesentery show influences of procaine on transmesothelial transfer of urea and inulin. Recent in vitro studies have explored the permeability of mesothelium to rubidium and albumin [100]. Only 0.03% of mesothelial surface appeared available for free diffusion of rubidium and results suggested that mesothelium was 10 times less permeable than that described in earlier reports. In vivo studies in rabbits and in vitro studies with isolated rabbit mesentery show that phosphatidylcholine increases the permeability of the mesothelium to water, urea, and glucose [101]. Following exposure of the peritoneal membrane to Alcian blue, a positively charged dye, phosphatidylcholine has no effect on mesothelial permeability. The authors suggest that the action of phosphatidylcholine depends on attachment to the anionic sites of the mesothelium and this in turn diminishes the thickness of stagnant fluid layers trapped between microvilli. We have mentioned above that peritoneal injuries due to peritonitis or heat drying result in increased peritoneal transport associated with mesothelial alterations. All of these studies raise questions about the relative importance of the mesothelium as a resistance site. Perhaps previous impressions that the mesothelium offered little resistance need to be reconsidered. On the other hand many of the inferences about the mesothelium from the studies are highly speculative.

The mesothelial microvilli are 1.5–3.0 microns long and 400–900 Å wide in mice [85]. Microvilli markedly increase gross surface area. Surface charges may trap water between microvilli and prevent friction of adjacent surfaces [86]. At the base of microvilli, the open ends of surface vesicles can be seen [87]. There is much to be learned about the effects of cellular structures on mesothelial passive transport properties during peritoneal dialysis.

14. CAPACITIES AND PRESSURES IN THE DIALYSIS SOLUTION CHAMBER OF THE PERITONEAL DIALYSIS SYSTEM

Twardowski and co-workers [102] have related intra-abdominal pressure to intraperitoneal volume in normal sized adults. The mean results from his studies are summarized in Figure 17. Note an almost linear increase in intra-abdominal pressure in each position studied. The hydrostatic pressures shown relate to the umbilicus in the supine position and the xiphoid process in the upright position. Filling the peritoneal cavity is somewhat like inflating a collapsed balloon. In upright positions the muscle tone of the abdominal wall is greater and higher pressures are required to inflate the less compliant wall. Many normal-sized adults tolerated up to 4 l of intraperitoneal volume without discomfort. Those who develop dyspnea at intraperitoneal volumes between 2.5 to 4 l have had an associated decrease in forced vital capacity. This occurred even though their intra-abdominal pressure at the higher volumes was the same as those who did not develop dyspnea or a decrease in forced vital capacity. Therefore, it would appear that the major difference between patients who tolerate and patients who do not tolerate large volumes has to do with diaphragmatic strength rather than the workload. Obviously at the extremes of patient size variation, the relationship of intra-abdominal pressure to intraperitoneal volume may be different.

In patients who tolerate larger volumes, daily clearances may be increased by the use of larger volumes at the same

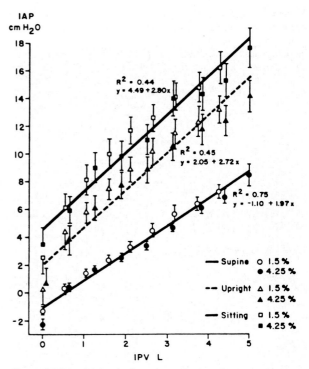

Figure 17. Intra-abdominal pressure (IAP) related to calculated intraperitoneal volume (IPV) of 1.5 and 4.25% glucose solutions. Means ± SEM and linear regressions are shown (from Twardowski *et al.* [102]; reproduced with permission).

frequency or maintained with larger volumes and fewer daily exchanges. Clearance increases with 3-l volumes as compared to 2-l volumes at fixed cycle times are mainly a function of the increased dialysis solution flow rate [103]. Small solute clearances increase most; larger solute clearances and protein losses remain stable, as they tend to do with increases in dialysis solution flow rate by any technique. Studies in adult patients by Goldschmidt and co-workers [104] showed similar clearances of small solutes with 1-l and 2-l volumes provided the dialysis solution flow rates remained unchanged. This suggests that solution membrane contact is near maximum with 1-l volumes and that larger volumes mainly increase the width of the dialysis solution channels with little effect on membrane contact. Thus, in most adults, all or most finger-like projections of the peritoneal cavity must be filled with fluid with 1-l intraperitoneal volumes. Three-liter volumes may stretch them more but do not open new projections. There must be some point below 1-l volumes, however, where solution membrane contact would decrease and area losses would reduce large solute clearances.

15. THE ROLE OF LYMPHATIC OUTFLOW FROM THE PERITONEAL CAVITY

It has become apparent that there is a convective back leak of intraperitoneal fluid into subdiaphragmatic lymphatics and/or abdominal wall tissues [105–108]. The back leak in the tissues could reflect hydraulic pressure effects. The role of lymphatics in peritoneal dialysis will be reviewed in detail in the chapter by Mactier and Khanna. In brief accumulating studies suggest that there is a back flux of fluid from the peritoneal cavity during peritoneal dialysis in adult humans of approximately 90–100 ml/hr. The absorption of substances of a molecular weight greater than 20,000 daltons from the peritoneal cavity to plasma is probably primarily in association with this convective back leak and eventually into peritoneal lymphatics. Large openings (stomata) between mesothelial cells on the undersurfaces of the diaphragm lead to lymphatic lacunae. Endothelial cell extensions called microfilaments prevent back flux of fluid from lymphatic into the peritoneum during diaphragmatic contraction. With diaphramatic relaxation fluid moves between mesothelial cells into the low pressure lacunae which have been emptied of their fluid contents by diaphragmatic contraction pushing the fluid into more cephalad lymphatics. The stomata seem highly permeable permitting the movement of large molecules, particles and even cells from the peritoneal cavity into this system.

This brief summary is included in the chapter only to remind the reader that any understanding of net peritoneal clearances and net ultrafiltration are dependent on net drainage volume. Net drainage volume in return is influenced not only by instillation volume and true transcapillary ultrafiltration induced by ostomic pressure, but also by the convective back movement of fluid into the abdominal wall-lymphatic systems.

ACKNOWLEDGEMENT

Supported in part by Veterans Administration Merit Review Funds, NIH Division of Research Resources, General Clinical Research Center, Grant N05-M01RR00287 and NIH contracts USPH N01-AM5-2216, USPH N01-AM 7-2217, and USPH N01-AM9-2208 USPH N01-AM-3-2244 and N01-AM-3-2245.

REFERENCES

1. Nolph KD: CAPD – A logical approach to peritoneal dialysis limitations (A comparison of the peritoneal dialysis system and hollow fiber kidneys). NUA 1:5–8, 1980.
2. Nolph KD, Popovich RP, Ghods AJ, Twardowski Z: Determinants of low clearances of small solutes during peritoneal dialysis. Kidney Int 13: 117–123, 1978.
3. Nolph KD: The peritoneal dialysis system. In: Today's Art of peritoneal dialysis. Contrib Nephrol 17: 44–49, 1979.
4. Nolph KD, Miller FN, Rubin J. Popovich R: New directions in peritoneal dialysis concepts and applications. Kidney Int 18 (Suppl 10): S111, 1980.
5. Nolph KD: Peritoneal dialysis. In: Drukker W, Parsons FM, Maher JF (eds), Replacement of Renal Function by Dialysis. Martinus Nijhoff Medical Division, The Hague, pp 277–321, 1978.
6. Rubin J, Nolph KD, Popovich RP, Moncrief J, Prowant B: Drainage volumes during CAPD. ASAIO 2: 2, 1979.
7. Erbe RW, Greene JA Jr, Weller JM: Peritoneal dialysis during hemorrhagic shock., J Appl Physiol 22: 131–135, 1967.
8. Aune S: Transperitoneal exchange 2. Peritoneal blood flow estimated by hydrogen gas clearance. Scand J Gastroenterol 5: 99, 1970.
9. Texter E, Clinton JR: Small intestinal blood flow. Am J Digest Dis 8: 587, 1963.
10. Hare HG, Valtin H, Gosslin RE: Effects of drugs on peritoneal dialysis in the dog. J Pharmacol Exp Ther 145: 122–129, 1964.
11. Henderson LW, Kintzel JE: Influence of antidiuretic hormone on peritoneal membrane area and permeability. J Clin Invest 50: 2437–2443, 1971.
12. Nolph KD, Ghods AJ, Brown O, Van Stone JC, Miller FN, Wiegmann DL, Harris PD: Factors affecting peritoneal dialysis efficiency. Dial Transpl 6: 52–90, 1977.
13. Nolph KD, Ghods AJ, Van Stone J, Brown PA: The effects of intraperitoneal vasodilators on peritoneal clearances. Trans Am Soc Artif Intern Organs 22: 586–594, 1976.
14. Miller FN, Nolph KD, Harris PD, Rubin J, Wiegman DL, Joshua IG, Twardowski ZJ, Ghods AJ: Microvascular and clinical effects of altered peritoneal dialysis solutions. Kidney Int 15: 630–639, 1979.
15. Miller FN, Nolph KD, Harris PD, Rubin J, Wiegman DL, Joshua IG: Effects of peritoneal dialysis solutions on human clearances and rat arterioles. Trans Am Soc Artif Intern Organs 24: 131–132, 1978.
16. Nolph KD: Effects of intraperitoneal vasodilators on peritoneal clearances. Dial Transpl 7: 812–817, 1978.
17. Nolph KD, Rubin J, Wiegman DL, Harris PD, Miller FN: Peritoneal clearances with three types of commercially available peritoneal dialysis solutions: Effects of pH adjustment and intraperitoneal nitroprusside. Nephron 24: 35–40, 1979.
18. Nolph KD, Ghods AJ, Brown PA, Twardowski ZJ: Effects of intraperitoneal nitroprusside in peritoneal clearances with variation in dose, frequency of administration, and dwell times. Nephron 24: 114, 1979.
19. Wayland H: Action of histamine on the microvasculature. Proc Ist CAPD Int Symp. Excerpta Medica, Amsterdam, 1980, 18–27.
20. Miller FN, Joshua IG, Harris PD *et al.*: Peritoneal dialysis

solutions and the microcirculation. (Vol 17 of Contributions to Nephrology). Trevino-Becerra A, Boen F(eds), In: Today's Art of Peritoneal Dialysis. S. Karger, Basel, pp 51–58, 1979.

21. Nolph KD, Stoltz M, Maher JF: Altered peritoneal permeability in patients with systemic vasculitis. Ann Intern Med 78: 891–984, 1973.

22. Nolph KD, Miller L, Husted FC, Hirszel P: Effects of intraperitoneal isoproterenol on reduced peritoneal clearances in patients with systemic vascular disease. J Int Urol Nephrol 8: 161–169, 1976.

23. Brown ST, Ahearn DJ, Nolph KD: Reduced peritoneal clearances in scleroderma increased by intraperitoneal isoproterenol. Ann Intern Med 78: 891–894, 1973.

24. Manery JF: Water and electrolyte metabolism. Physiol Rev 34: 334–417, 1954.

25. Tarail R, Hacker ES, Tavmor R: The ultrafiltrability of potassium and sodium in human serum. J Clin Invest 31: 23–26, 1952.

26. Folk BP, Zierler KL, Lilienthal JL: Distribution of potassium and sodium between serum and certain extracellular fluids in man. Am J Physiol 153: 381–385, 1948.

27. Brown ST, Ahearn DJ, Nolph KD: Potassium removal with peritoneal dialysis. Kidney Int 4: 67–69, 1973.

28. Kelton JG, Vlan R, Stiller C, Holmes E: Comparison of chemical composition of peritoneal fluid and serum. Ann Intern Med 89: 67–70, 1978.

29. Henderson LW: Peritoneal ultrafiltration dialysis: Enhanced urea transfer using hypertonic peritoneal dialysis fluid. J Clin Invest 45: 950, 1966.

30. Henderson LW, Nolph KD: Altered permeability of the peritoneal membrane after using hypertonic peritoneal dialysis fluid. J Clin Invest 48: 992–1001, 1969.

31. Ahearn DJ, Nolph KD: Controlled sodium removal with peritoneal dialysis. Trans Am Soc Artif Intern Organs 28: 423–428, 1972.

32. Nolph KD, Hano JE, Teschan PE: Peritoneal sodium transport during hypertonic peritoneal dialysis: Physiologic mechanisms and clinical implications. Ann Intern Med 70: 931–941, 1969.

33. Nolph KD, Sorkin MI, Moore H: Autoregulation of sodium and potassium removal during continuous ambulatory peritoneal dialysis. Trans Am Soc Artif Intern Organs 26, 1980.

34. Maher JF, Chokrabarti E: Ultrafiltration by hyperosmotic peritoneal dialysis fluid excludes intracellular solutes. Am J Nephrol 4: 169–172, 1984.

35. Wayland H, Silberberg A: Blood to lymph transport. Microvasc Res 15: 367, 1978.

36. Nolph KD, Prowant B: Complications during contionuous ambulatory peritoneal dialysis. Proc 1st Int Symp on CAPD. Excerpta Medica, Amsterdam, pp 258–262, 1980.

37. Rubin J, Roger WA, Taylor HM, Everett ED, Prowant BP, Fruto LV, Nolph KD: Peritonitis during continuous ambulatory peritoneal dialysis. Ann Intern Med 92: 7–13, 1980.

38. Miller FN, Hammerschmidt DE, Anderson GL et al: Protein loss induced by complement activation during peritoneal dialysis. Kidney Int 25: 480–485, 1984.

39. Zimmerman AL, Sablay LB, Aynedjian HS et al: Increased peritoneal permeability in rats with alloxan-induced diabetes mellitus. J Lab Clin Med 103: 720–730, 1984.

40. Steinhauer HB, Schollmeyer P: Prostaglandin-mediated loss of proteins during peritonitis in continuous ambulatory peritoneal dialysis. Kidney Int 29: 584–590, 1986.

41. Rubin R, Roger WA, Taylor HM, Everett ED, Prowant BP, Fruto LV, Nolph KD: Peritonitis during continuous ambulatory peritoneal dialysis. Ann Intern Med 92: 7–13, 1980.

42. Miller FN, Nolph KD, Joshua IG: The osmolality component of peritoneal dialysis solutions. Proc 1st Int Symp on CAPD. Excerpta Medica, Amsterdam, pp 12–17, 1980.

43. Nolph KD: Anatomy, physiology and kinetics of peritoneal transport during peritoneal dialysis. Proc 1st Int Symp on CAPD. Excerpta Medica, Amsterdam, pp 7–11, 1980.

44. Tenckhoff H, Ward G, Boen ST: The influence of dialysate volume and flow rate on peritoneal clearance. Proc Eur Dial Transpl Assoc 2: 113–117, 1965.

45. Stephen RL, Atkin-Thor E, Kolff WJ: Recirculating peritoneal dialysis with subcutaneous catheter. Trans Am Soc Artif Intern Organs 22: 575–585, 1976.

46. Goldschmidt ZH, Pote HH, Katz MA, Shear L: Effect of dialysate volume on peritoneal dialysis kinetics. Kidney Int 5: 240–245, 1975.

47. Miller FN, Wiegman DL, Joshua IG, Nolph KD, Rubin J: Effects of vasodilators and peritoneal dialysis solution on the microcirculation of the rat cecum. Proc Soc Exp Biol Med 161: 605–608, 1979.

48. Karnovsky MJ: The ultrastructural basis of capillary permeability studies with peroxides as a tracer. J Cell Biol 35: 213–235, 1967.

49. Cotran RS: The fine structure of the microvasculature in relation to normal and altered permeability. In: Reeve EB, Guyton AC (eds), Physical Bases of Circulatory Transport: Regulation and Exchange. WB Saunders, Philadelphia, pp 249–275, 1967.

50. Karnovsky MJ: The ultrastructural basis of transcapillary exchanges. In: Biological Interfaces: Flows and Exchanges. Little Brown, Boston, pp 64–95, 1968.

51. McGary TJ, Nolph KD, Rubin J: In vitro simulations of peritoneal dialysis: A technique for demonstrating limitations on solute clearances due to stagnant fluid films and poor mixing. J Lab Clin Med 96: 1, 148–157, 1980.

52. Levin TN, Rigden LB, Nielsen LH, Moore HL, Twardowski ZJ, Khanna R, Nolph KD: Maximum ultrafiltration rates during peritoneal dialysis in rats. Kidney Int 31: 731–735, 1987.

53. Ronco C, Brendolan A, Bragantini L, Chioramonte S, Feriani M, Fabris A, Dell Aquila R, Milan M, La Greca G: Flusso ematico capillare effettivo nel sistema dialitico peritoneale. In: Lamperi S, Capelli G, Milano CS (eds), Dialysi Peritoneale. Wichtig Editore, pp 21–28, 1985.

54. Nagel W, Kuschinsky W: Study of the permeability of isolated dog mesentery. Eur J Clin Invest 1: 149–154, 1970.

55. Gosslin RE, Berndt WO: Diffusional transport of solutes through mesentery and peritoneum. J Theor Biol 3: 487–495, 1962.

56. Rasio EA: Metabolic control of permeability in isolated mesentery. Am J Physiol 276: 962–968, 1974.

57. Maher JF, Nolph KD: Factors effecting optimal performance of coil dialyzers. Proc Int Congr Nephrol, Florence Italy, 1975, p 657.

58. Maher JF, Nolph KD: Resistance to diffusion in dialyzers. Clin Nephrol 1: 333–335.

59. Rubin J, Nolph KD, Arfania D, Miller FM, Wiegman DL, Josua IG, Harris PD: Studies on non-vasoactive periotoneal dialysis solutions. J Lab Clin med 93: 910–915, 1979.

60. Flessner MF, Dedrick RL, Schultz JS: A distributed model of peritoneal-plasma transport: Theoretical considerations. Am J Physiol 246: R597–R607, 1984.

61. Blumenkrantz MJ, Roberts CE, Card B et al: Nutritional management of the adult patient undergoing peritoneal dialysis.. J Am Diet Assoc 73(3): 251–256, 1978.

62. Giordano C, De Santo NG: Dietary management of patients on peritoneal dialysis. In: Trevino-Beccerra A, Boen F (eds), Today's Art of Peritoneal Dialysis. S Karger, Basel, pp 77–92, 1979.

63. Kobayashi K, Manji T, Hiramatsu S et al: Nitrogen metabolism in patients on peritoneal dialysis. (Vol 17 of Contriv Nephrol). In Trevino-Beccerra A, Boen F (eds), Today's Art of Peritoneal Dialysis. S Karger, Basel, pp 93–100, 1979.

64. Renkin EM: Exchange of substances through capillary walls:

circulatory and respiratory mass transport. In: GEW Wolstenholme (eds), Ciba Foundation Symp. Little Brown & Company, Boston, pp 55–60, 1969.
65. Pappenheimer JR: Passage of molecules through capillary walls. Physiol Rev 33: 387, 1953.
66. Nolph KD, Ahearn DJ, Esterly JA, Maher JF: Irreversible morphological and functional changes in hollow fiber kidneys with a single dialysis. Trans Am Soc Artif Intern Organs 20: 4604–612, 1974.
67. Nolph KD: Peritoneal clearances. (Invited Editorial). J Lab Clin Med 94: 519–525, 1979.
68. Nolph KD, Popovich RP, Moncrief JW: Theoretical and practical implications of continuous ambulatory peritoneal dialysis. (Invited Editorial). Nephron 21: 117–122, 1978.
69. Popovich RP, Moncrief JW: Kinetic modeling of peritoneal transport. In: Trevino-Becerra A, Boen F (eds), Today's Art of Peritoneal Dialysis. S Karger, Basel, p. 59, 1979.
70. Popovich RP, Pyle WK, Moncrief JW et al: Peritoneal dialysis. AIChE Symp Series 75: 31.
71. Popovich RP: Metabolic transport, kinetics in peritoneal dialysis. Proc Ist Int Symp on CAPD. Excerpta Medica, Amsterdam, pp 28–33, Amsterdam, 1980.
72. Popovich R, Moncrief JW, Nolph KD, Ghods AJ, Twardowski ZJ, Pyle WK: Continuous ambulatory peritoneal dialysis. Ann Intern Med 88: 449–456, 1978.
73. Green DM, Antwiler GD, Moncrief JW, Decherd JF, Popovich RP: Measurement of the transmittance coefficient spectrum of cuprophan. Trans Am Soc Artif Intern Organs 22: 627–636, 1976.
74. Donnan FG: The theory of membrane equilibrium. Chem Rev 1: 73, 1924–1925.
75. Loeb J: Donnan equilibrium and physical properties of proteins. J Gen Physiol 3: 691, 1920–1921.
76. Nolph KD, New DL: Effects of ultrafiltration on solute clearances in hollow fiber artificial kidneys. J Lab Clin Med 88: 593–600, 1976.
77. Nolph KD, Stolz ML, Maher JF: Electrolyte transport during ultrafiltration of protein solutions,. Nephron 8: 473–487, 1971.
78. Glassock RJ: The nephrotic syndrome. Hosp Prac 14: 105–129, 1979.
79. Nolph KD, Hopkins CA, New D, Antwiler GD, Popovich RP: Differences in solute sieving with osmotic vs hydrostatic ultrafiltration. Trans Am Soc Artif Intern Organs 22: 618–626, 1976.
80. Twardowski ZJ, Nolph KD, Popovich RP, Hopkins CA: Comparison of polymer, glucose and hydrostatic pressure induced ultrafiltration in a hollow fiber dialyzer: Effects on convective solute transport. J Lab Clin Med 92: 619–633, 1978.
81. Rubin J, Klein E, Bower JD: Investigation of the net sieving coefficient of the peritoneal membrane during peritoneal dialysis. ASAIO J 5: 9–15, 1982.
82. Dedrick RL, Flessner MF, Collins JM et al: Is the peritoneum a membrane? ASAIO J 5: 1–8, 1982.
83. Feriani M, Biasioli S, Chiaramonte S et al: Anatomical bases of peritoneal permeability: A reappraisal. Anatomy of peritoneum. Int J Artif Organs 5: 345, 1982.
84. Odor DL: Observations of the rat mesothelium with the electron and phase microscopes. Am J Anat 95: 433, 1954.
85. Baradi AF, Rao SN: A scanning electron microscope study of mouse peritoneal mesothelium. Tissue Cell 8: 159, 1976.
86. Andrews PM, Porter KR: The ultrastructure morphology and possible functional significance of mesothelial microvilli. Anat Res 177: 409, 1973.
87. Baradi AF, Rayns DJ: Mesothelial intercellular junctions and pathways. Cell Tissue Res 173: 133, 1976.
88. Simioescu M, Simionescu N: Organization of cell junctions in the peritoneal mesothelium. J Cell Biol 74: 98, 1977.
89. Tsilibray EC, Wissig SL: Absorption from the peritoneal cavity; SEM study of the mesothelium covering the peritoneal surface of the muscular portion fo the diaphragm. Am J Anat 199: 127, 1977.
90. Dumont AE, Robbins E, Martelli A, Iliescu H: Platelet blockade of particle absorption from the peritoneal surface of the diaphragm (41138). Proc Soc Exp Biol Med 167: 137, 1981.
91. Goitloib L, Digenis GE, Rabinovich S, Medline A, Oreopoulos DG: Ultrastructure of normal rabbit mesentery. Nephron 34: 248, 1983.
92. Verger C, Luger A, Moore HL, Nolph KD: Acute changes in peritoneal morphology and transport properties with infectious peritonitis and mechanical injury. Kidney Int 23: 823, 1983.
93. Gotloib L, Shustak A, Bar-Sella P et al: Fenestrated capillaries in human parietal and rabbit diaphragmatic peritoneum. Nephron 41: 200–202, 1985.
94. Rubin J, McFaraland S, Hellems EW et al: Peritoneal dialysis during peritonitis. Kidney Int 19: 460, 1981.
95. Smeby LC, Wideroe THE, Svartas TM et al: Changes in water removal due to peritonitis during continuous peritoneal dialysis. In: KD Nolph (eds), Advances in Peritoneal Dialysis. Gahl GM, Kessel M. Excerpta Medica, Amsterdam, p 287, 1981.
96. Alavi N, Lianos E, Van Liew JB et al: Peritoneal permeability in the rat: Modulation by microfilament-active agents. Kidney Int 27: 411–419, 1985.
97. Hirszel P, Didge K, Maher JF: Acceleration of peritoneal solute transport by cytochalasin D. Uremia Invest 8: 85–88, 1984–1985.
98. Breborowicz A, Knapowski J, Breborowicz G: Intracellular calcium ions modulate permeability of the peritoneal mesothelium in vivo. Perit Dial Bull 5(2): 105–108, 1985.
99. Breborowicz A, Knapowski J: Augmentation of peritoneal dialysis clearance with procaine. Kidney Int 26: 392–396, 1984.
100. Breborowicz A, Knapowski J: Studies on the resistance of the peritoneal mesothelium to solute transport. Perit Dial Bull 4: 37–40, 1984.
101. Breboroiwicz A, Sombolos K, Rodela H, Ogilvie R, Bargman J, Oreopoulos D: Mechanism of phosphatidylcholine action during peritoneal dialysis. Perit Dial Bull 7(1): 6–9, 1987.
102. Twardowski ZJ, Prowant BF, Nolph KD et al: High volume, low frequency continuous ambulatory peritoneal dialysis. Kidney Int 23: 64–70, 1983.
103. Twardowski ZJ, Nolph KD, Prowant B, Moore HL: Efficiency of high volume, low frequency CAPD. Trans ASAIO 29: 53–57, 1983.
104. Goldschmidt ZH, Pote HH, Katz MD, Shear L: Effects of dialysate volume on peritoneal dialysis kinetics. Kidney Int 5: 240–245, 1974.
105. Flessner MF, Dedrick RL, Schultz JS: Exchange of macromolecules between peritoneal cavity and plasma. Am J Physiol 248: H15–H25, 1985.
106. Flessner MF, Fenstermacher JD, Blasberg RG et al: Peritoneal absorption of macromolecules studies by quantitative autoradiography. Am J Physiol 248: H26–H32, 1985.
107. Nolph KD, Mactier R, Khanna R, Twardowski ZJ, Moore H, McGary T: The kinetics of ultrafiltration during peritoneal dialysis: the role of lymphatics. Kidney Int 32: 1987.
108. Mactier R, Khanna R, Twardowski Z, Nolph K: Role of peritoneal cavity lymphatic absorption in peritoneal dialysis. Kidney Int 32: 1987.

3

ROLE OF THE PERITONEAL MICROCIRCULATION IN PERITONEAL DIALYSIS

RONALD J. KORTHUIS and D. NEIL GRANGER

1. INTRODUCTION

Peritoneal dialysis represents a feasible and increasingly popular alternative to maintenance hemodialysis for the patient with end-stage renal disease. The continued preference for extracorporeal dialyzers results primarily from the greater efficiency of this mode of therapy in removing low molecular weight toxins from blood than peritoneal dialysis. Transperitoneal clearances of large molecular weight solutes such as insulin generally equal or exceed plasma clearances of such solutes produced by hemodialysis. In contrast, the clearance of solutes the size of urea during peritoneal dialysis is usually one-sixth the value obtained with hemodialysis. However, the results of numerous recent studies indicate that transperitoneal clearances of both small and large solutes can be augmented by pharmocologic and physiologic manipulation of microcirculatory function. This information, coupled to a better understanding of peritoneal transport characteristics, has led to the design of therapeutic manipulations which enhance the efficiency of peritoneal dialysis to an extent where it may become an even more popular alternative treatment for renal failure [1–9].

Rational use of drugs and other manipulations to increase the efficiency of peritoneal dialysis requires a firm understanding of the physiology of the peritoneal microcirculation as well as knowledge of the effects of such pertubations on that circulation. Thus, a major aim of this treatise is to review the available information regarding peritoneal microcirculatory function. In addition, those factors which may allow for controlled manipulation of peritoneal transport via modification of microcirculatory function will be discussed relative to mechanisms of action and ability to optimize the clearance of solutes.

2. PERITONEAL MEMBRANE ANATOMY

The peritoneum is a thin, coninuous, and transluscent membrane which covers the visceral organs (visceral pe-ritoneum) and lines the inner surface of the abdominal wall (parietal peritoneum). The surface of the peritoneal membrane is lined by a single layer of mesothelial cells which encloses a space that normally contains less than 100 ml of fluid (which serves a lubricating function) but can accomodate a 20 fold increase in volume without patient discomfort [10]. Specialized regions, the omenta and mesenteries, are double-layered folds of peritoneum which connect certain viscera to the posterior abdominal wall or to each other. For example, the greater omentum hangs as a large fold from the greater curvature of the stomach to attach to the inferior border of the transverse colon. In other areas, short double-layered folds of peritoneum called ligaments (e.g., falciform ligament of the liver) attach solid viscera to the abdominal wall. The peritoneal ligaments and mesenteries such as the greater omentum are capable of storing large amounts of fat. Lying between the liver and diaphragm are the subphrenic spaces bounded by two layers of peritoneum. These compartments of the peritoneal cavity are of particular importance in view of the generous and specialized lymphatic drainage associated with the undersurface of the diaphragm (see below).

The vascular and lymphatic systems supplying the peritoneal membrane and the underlying organs constitute a complex and efficient system for solute delivery to and removal from the peritoneal cavity. This exchange system is composed of three essentially separate but interdependent components: 1) the blood circulation of the visceral peritoneum, 2) the blood circulation of the parietal peritoneum, and 3) the lymphatic circulations of the parietal and visceral peritoneum. Physiologic, pharmacologic, and pathologic modification of the transport properties of these components can dramatically alter the efficiency of peritoneal dialysis.

2.1. Circulation in the visceral and parietal peritoneum

The visceral mesentery contains primarily large vessels arising from the celiac and mesenteric arteries. These large vessels function primarily as conduits to supply blood to the visceral organs. Although mesenteric capillaries are relatively sparse, the large vessels coursing through the mesentery divide as they reflect over the bowel surface, forming capillary beds which presumably participate in transperitoneal fluid and solute exchange [10, 11]. The venous vessels draining the visceral organs and peritoneum empty into the portal vein.

The arterial blood supply to the parietal peritoneum and to the underlying abdominal wall musculature arises from the circumflex, iliac, lumbar, intercostal, and epigastric arteries. In contrast to the visceral peritoneum, the venous vessels of the parietal peritoneum empty into the systemic veins rather than the hepatic portal system. A potentially important consequence of this vascular arrangement is that drugs and other solutes that are absorbed from peritoneal dialysis solutions primarily across the visceral peritoneum are immediately vulnerable to metabolism by the liver. In contrast, solutes absorbed primarily across the parietal peritoneum bypass first-pass hepatic metabolism. Thus, compounds such as atropine, caffeine, glucose, glycine, and progesterone, which are absorbed primarily via the visceral peritoneum [12], may undergo first pass metabolism by the liver and thereby exert minimal systemic effects when administered with dialysis solutions. In contrast, substances absorbed primarily via the parietal peritoneum bypass first-pass hepatic metabolism and may exert profound systemic effects when administered by intraperitoneal injection. In addition, the fact that the blood supply of the visceral peritoneum empties into the portal vein while that of the parietal peritoneum drains into systemic veins suggests that fluid movement and solute clearances in the visceral vasculature may be altered by portal hypertension associated with cirrhosis or obstruction (e.g., carcinoma). However, portal hypertension should exert little or no influence on fluid and solute exchange across the parietal peritoneum since the vasculature supplying these structures drains into systemic veins.

The total surface area of the peritoneum in adults appears to approximate the surface area of the skin (1–2 m^2, ref. 13). Of the total peritoneal membrane area, parietal peritoneum accounts for 10% while visceral peritoneum accounts for the remaining 90% [14]. Although the entire peritoneal membrane is presumably available for peritoneal exchange during dialysis, functional estimates of the surface area available for exchange indicate that effective peritoneal membrane surface area is much lower [15]. In addition, the effective surface area may be further reduced in some patients as a result of adhesion formation secondary to prior abdominal surgery or infections [16]. Given that the visceral peritoneum comprises 90% of the total peritoneal membrane surface area, one might suspect that the contribution of the visceral peritoneum to total peritoneal membrane exchange would predominate over that portion contributed by the partietal membranes. However, the relative contributions of the parietal and visceral peritoneum to peritoneal exchange during dialysis are unknown since some sections of the parietal peritoneum are more vascular than the relatively avascular visceral mesentery [17–19]. Rubin and coworkers [20] have attempted to determine the relative importance of the visceral peritoneum in dialysis exchange by performing dialysis rates studies

in eviscerated rats and comparing these rates to those obtained in control animals with intact visceral peritoneum. Surprisingly, these investigators found that peritoneal absorption rates for urea, creatinine, glucose, and inulin were only slightly reduced in eviscerated rats relative to control animals. Since evisceration did not alter blood flow or diffusive properties of the parietal membranes, the results may be interpreted to suggest that the contribution of the visceral peritoneum to peritoneal dialysis exchange is slight despite the fact that it comprises 90% of the total peritoneal membrane area. However, an equally plausible interpretation is that evisceration resulted in improved contact between thee dialysate and the peritoneal membranes.

2.2. Peritoneal lymphatics

In addition to the vascular systems associated with the visceral and parietal peritoneum, there is the potential for mass transport via the elaborate and extensive lymphatic system in the abdominal cavity. For example, there is a generous and specialized lymphatic drainage located on the undersuface of the diaphragm which is thought to play an important role in the drainage of fluid and solutes from the peritoneal cavity [21]. An even more important function ascribed to these lymphatics is that they serve as the primary route for the uptake of macromolecules and particles such as cells from the abdominal cavity to the bloodstream [22–28].

In addition to the diaphragmatic lymphatics, other subserosal lymphatic vessels can be recognized in the small intestine of species such as mice and bats but cannot be demonstrated in normal human jejunum [29]. Despite the apparent lack of these lymphatics in normal jejunum, lymphatics are clearly visible in the serosal-muscular layer of the jejunum of patients with cirrhosis and ascites [30]. While the role that these vessels play in peritoneal drainage in cirrhotic patients is uncertain, it has been suggested that they represent a specific adaptation to longstanding edemagenic stress [31, 32].

Although the subject of great debate for many years, it now appears established that a fine network of lymphatic vessels, which anastomose with gastric lymphatics, also exists in the greater omentum, at least in the dog [33]. However, the flow of lymph in this omental-gasric system appears to be slow. Moreover, it is generally accepted that the uptake of particulate matter from the peritoneal cavity by omental lymphatics is relatively minor compared to diaphragmatic lymphatic vessels.

Finally, hepatic subcapsular lymphatic vessels do not appear to play any significant role in the uptake of fluid, solutes, or particulate matter from the peritoneal cavity. It is thought that the fibrous tissue of the capsule of the liver forms a significant barrier that prevents access of peritoneal fluid and solutes to the hepatic subcapsular lymphatic network [34].

3. BARRIERS TO PERITONEAL DIALYSIS TRANSPORT

The transport of solutes and water from the blood to the peritoneal cavity occurs across several anatomic structures that act as resistance barriers to peritoneal exchange. These barriers are arranged in series and include the microvascular wall, the interstitium, and the mesothelium. In addition, unstirred water layers at the capillary blood-endothelial cell interface and at the mesothelial cell-dialysate interface offer resistance to solute transfer across the peritoneal membrane.

In moving from the blood to the peritoneal cavity, the first barrier a solute encounters is the unstirred water layer at the capillary blood-endothelial cell interface. The effective resistance to solute diffusion offered by this layer is influenced by turbulence and concentration polarization [35]. It is likely that the resistance to solute diffusion offered by the unstirred layer is relatively small since the high capillary blood flow effectively reduces the thickness of this layer [35].

The microvascular wall provides the second important resistance to solute transfer across the peritoneum and consists of an endothelial cell lining and the underlying basement membrane. Although terminal arterioles have a discontinuous muscle layer, and consequently only endothelium and basement membrane to act as barriers to solute transfer in portioins of their walls, most solute transfer across the peritoneal microvasculature occurs across capillaries and postcapillary venules [36–38]. The capillaries of the peritoneum are generally lined by a continuous layer of endothelial cells that form a very effective barrier against solute transfer [37, 39–41]. Solute transport across the endothelium appears to occur via intracellular junctions or vesicular transport [39, 41–45]. Intravital fluorescence microscopy studies of mesenteric capillaries indicate that rapid passage of small molecules (MW, 389–3400) occurs along the entire length of most capillaries although most leakage occurs in venous capillaries and venules [46]. For solutes (dextrans) with molecular weights in excess of 19000 daltons (>30 Å radius), leakage is localized to the venular ends of the microcirculation [46]. Dextrans as large as 393000 Daltons (150 Å radius) are observed to enter the perivascular space surrounding postcapillary venules [46]. These findings suggest that peritoneal capillaries are perforated by small pores of approximately 30 Å radius and large pores which are larger than 150 Å radius. Furthermore, these results suggest that the large pore system resides solely in the venular segments of the microcirculation.

Estimates of the capillary osmotic reflection coefficient (σ_d) for sodium chloride, urea, sucrose, raffinose, and vitamin B*12* range between 0.02–0.20 in rabbit, cat and human peritoneum and frog mesentery [47–53]. Moreover, these studies generally indicate there is a strong correlation between σ_d and molecular size. For myoglobin (21 Å radius), albumin (36 Å radius), and sulphate-substituted dextrans (Dextran 118, 61 Å radius; Dextran 242, 90 Å radius), the reflection coefficient is 0.35, 0.82, 0.99, and 1.00 respectively [50]. The σ_d values are comparable to those reported for continuous capillary beds of other organs such as skeletal muscle [38, 54–56]. Furthermore, the σ_d values are consistent with cylindrical pores of 55–70 Å radius, which is also comparable to the small pore dimension predicted for various organs using lymph protein flux data [38]. The aforementioned studies indicate that the peritoneal membrane is a highly selective barrier with restrictive properties comparable to those reported for continuous capillary beds [38, 54–56].

The basement membrane underlying the endothelium is thought to be permeable to most solutes. However, the transport of larger molecules, such as plasma proteins, appears to be impeded by this structure [57–62]. This notion is supported by the work of Granger and Taylor [63] who have demonstrated that the restrictive properties of intestinal capillaries to endogenous macromolecules are similar to those of mesenteric, skin, or skeletal muscle capillaries despite the fact intestinal capillaries are perforated by numerous large fenestrations [38, 63]. Thus it would appear that the actual barrier to macromolecular movement resides beyond the endothelium, perhaps at the basement membrane or interstitium. In support of this notion, colloidal carbon penetrates the intercellular clefts of continuous capillaries exposed to histamine but their transport into the interstitial space is retarded at the basement membrane [64–65].

The peritoneal interstitial space represents the fourth important barrier to peritoneal exchange. The interstitium is composed largely of glycosaminoglycan fibers enmeshed in a network or lattice of collagen fibers which are mechanically entangled and cross-linked to produce an elastic, three dimensional reticulum or gel-like structure which behaves as if it is perforated by pores of approximately 200–250 Å radius [46, 66–70]. Interspersed in the gel-like matrix is a free fluid phase through which substances can be transported by both convection and restricted diffusion, while transport through the gel phase is limited to the process of restricted diffusion [71]. For dextrans with molecular weights ranging from 3400 to 41200 daltons, the calculated diffusion coefficients in mesenteric tissue are essentially the same as for free diffusion in water. However, restricted diffusion by the mesenteric interstitium is observed for larger dextrans (MW>150000) [46]. Finally, it is likely that the path solutes must traverse in crossing the interstitium can be quite long since some capillaries lie 100 microns or more from the mesothelial cells [44, 72, 73].

The major physicochemical properties of the interstitium apparently derive in large part from the behavior of the glycosaminoglycan molecules [66–70]. For example, these mucopolysaccharides aid in the maintenance of an optimal diffusion distance for blood-tissue (peritoneal cavity) exchange by immobilizing tissue fluid. Another important property, of great functional significance, is the ability of the gel reticulum to exclude solutes from portions of the available gel water [66–70]. That is, large molecules, such as plasma proteins, normally distribute only in a fraction of the interstitial volume because large solute molecules cannot gain access to certain regions of the matrix. Therefore, the solute distributes itself into the matrix spaces which have dimensions larger than the solute (the accessible volume) and conversely are excluded from microdomains with smaller dimensions (the excluded volume). The functional significance of the exclusion phenomenon relates, in part, to the fact that the excluded volume and consequently the effective surface area for diffusion varies inversely with matrix hydration which, in turn, may be affected by the dialysate composition [40, 42, 69, 70, 74, 75]. For example, a hypertonic dialysate may dehydrate the peritoneal interstitium which compacts the peritoneal interstitium and increases the excluded volume. Conversely, a hypotonic dialysate may decrease the density of matrix fibers and the fraction of tissue fluid from which the solute is excluded and thereby increase matrix porosity. Thus, hydration of the peritoneal interstitium may be an important determinant of the rate of solute diffusion during peritoneal dialysis.

The fifth barrier a solute must cross before entering the peritoneal cavity from blood is a layer of mesothelial cells and its basement membrane. Most morphometric evidence suggests this barrier is a negligible resistance to solute movement across the peritoneum [76–80]. Mesothelial cells are covered by numerous microvilli which may function to increase the mesothelial surface area available for exchange between these cells and the peritoneal cavity [13, 77, 81, 92]. In addition, it has been proposed that the microvilli protect the mesothelial surface from frictional injury by entrapping water and a serous exudate [82]. Ultrastructural studies indicate that clefts between mesothelial cells in mesentery are 35–50 Å in radius [76]. In diaphragmatic mesothelium two types of intercellular gaps are present [77], one being formed by interlacing filamentous processes from adjacent mesothelial cells. The other type consists of a circular pore formed between several mesothelial cells resulting in a well-defined channel (4–10 μ diameter) or 'stomata' which opens directly into the peritoneal cavity [77, 80]. Colloidal particles and red blood cells readily traverse these channels through gaps between diaphragmatic mesothelium that widen with respiration [83]. It has been predicted that the pores in the mesothelium occupy 0.2% of the total area of the peritoneum [76]. These studies suggest that intercellular channels or pores provide the major path for solute transfer across the peritoneum. Transport via transcellular pathways is negligible. However, the visceral mesentery of rabbits and rats contains primarily tight junctions and large solute transport may occur across transcellular paths [84, 85]. Physiologic studies suggest that the mesothelium significantly limits the diffusion of ions (Na, K, Rb) across the peritoneum [14, 41, 76]. The K^+ permeability of the mesothelium, estimated using K^+-sensitive electrodes, is approximately 25 times less than that reported for mesenteric capillaries [86], suggesting greater restriction to ion movement across the mesothelial layer. Measurements of sodium and potassium fluxes across in vivo preparations of the parietal and visceral peritoneum indicate that the mesothelium of the latter membrane is more permeable [76, 87]. This notion is supported by the observation that the absorption of drugs after intraperitoneal injection occurs largely across blood vessels of the visceral peritoneum [12].

The final resistance barrier the solute must cross in moving from the blood to the peritoneal cavity is the unstirred layers at the mesothelial cell-dialysate interface. Although the resistance provided by the unstirred layer at the capillary blood-endothelial cell interface is thought to be relatively small, the resistance contributed at the mesothelial cell-dialysate interface may be substantial since dialysis flow rate is considerably less than blood flow in capillaries and diffusion distances are much longer [10]. In addition, even with the most rapid dialysate cycling, the many folds of the mesentery assures that dialysate remains relatively stagnant in the peritoneal cavity. The notion that unstirred layers at the mesothelial cell-dialysate

interface represent an important barrier to transperitoneal solute transport is supported by in vitro simulations of peritoneal dialysis using hollow fiber dialyzers with the outer shell removed [9, 88]. In these studies, urea clearances across the dialyzer are markedly reduced after placement of the dialyzer in stagnant pools of fluid. Furthermore, vigorous shaking of the dialyzer or rapid cycling of dialysate fluid to improve mixing and decrease the thickness of the unstirred layers increased urea clearance although not to levels achieved by normal use of the dialyzer (i.e., with rapid countercurrent flow of dialysate in an intact dialyzer). These findings suggest that the unstirred layers may represent an important barrier to solute exchange across the peritoneum.

Although the available morphologic and physiologic data on permeability of the aforementioned barriers to transperitoneal transfer do not allow for a clear delineation of which barrier is rate-limiting regarding small solute fluxes, the microvascular wall appears to provide the major resistance to large solute transport under normal conditions. This notion is based largely on the observation that fluorescien-labelled albumin and dextrans remain in the vasculature several minutes after injection with no obvious leakage into the interstitial space [46, 89]. However, application of agents known to increase microvascular permeability (e.g., histamine) cause extensive leakage of the tagged macromolecules into the interstitium within seconds of application [89]. The rate-limiting barrier to small solute transperitoneal exchange is less well defined.

4. RESTRICTIVE PROPERTIES OF THE PERITONEUM

The most popular index of the rate at which solutes move from blood into the peritoneal cavity is peritoneal clearance since it provides a means to assess dialysis efficiency [7, 8]. Peritoneal clearances (C) are determined using the plasma (P) and dialysate (D) concentrations of intravenously administered (inulin, creatinine) or endogenous solutes (urea), the drainage volume (V_D), and the time of exchange (dwell time) during dialysis:

$$C \text{ (ml/min)} = (D/P) \times (V_D/T). \qquad [1]$$

Thus, peritoneal clearance represents the volume of plasma cleared of a substance per unit time. While equation 1 represents the most popular method for calculating peritoneal clearances, modifications of this method have been employed [7, 8]. Numerous studies in patients and experimental animals consistently reveal a reduction in peritoneal clearance as molecular size increases from urea to large molecular weight dextrans and albumin [1, 90, 91]. In order to assess whether the reduction in clearance with increasing solute size is due to restricted diffusion, clearance ratios (urea clearance/inulin clearance) are often used. For solutes between the size of urea and inulin, clearance ratios generally predict that the reduction in clearance with increasing solute size are proportional or less than the predicted fall of the free diffusion coefficients [1, 90, 91]. Thus, for solutes in this size range one cannot predict restricted diffusion across the peritoneal membrane, suggesting the existence of large pores in the limiting barrier of the peritoneum. Restricted diffusion is frequently predicted using clearance ratios of large solutes (e.g., dextrans, albumin). From the relative clearances of inulin to albumin, Aune [90] proposed that the degree of restricted diffusion is consistent with pores of 130 Å radius. However, according to newer hydrodynamic formulations, the predicted pore radius would be 65 Å.

One of the most elaborate analyses of peritoneal membrane permeability using clearance ratios was performed by Arturson [82]. Transperitoneal clearances of urea, ^{131}I-albumin and dextrans of different sizes (20–60 Å radius) were measured in the rat. The clearance of dextrans (referenced to urea) displayed a steep fall in permeation in the dextran size range below 30 Å radius. Above 30 Å there was an extension of residual permeability with little decrement in clearances for molecules as large as 60 Å radius. Arturson [82] applied the dextran clearance data to pore theory and suggested that the data was best explained by a heteroporous membrane with a small pore population of 15–20 Å radius and a large pore system of approximately 70 Å radius, with one large pore per 10 000 small pores. Although the dextran clearance data clearly demonstrates selective restriction of solute on the basis of molecular size, the pore distribution predicted by Arturson's analysis is inconsistent with the degree of solute restriction generally predicted by both small and large solutes in the peritoneum. For a relatively isoporous membrane consisting of 17 Å pores, one would expect significant restricted diffusion of molecules the size of urea and inulin. Furthermore, an osmotic reflection coefficient of essentially one would be predicted for molecules the size of albumin for such a barrier. This notion is supported by the recent study of Leypoldt and colleages [93] who reported that reflection coefficients for neutral dextrans with radii ranging between 13 and 35 Å exceed 0.9.

There is some evidence that the peritoneal membrane behaves as a negatively charged barrier. For example, the clearance of albumin is lower than that measured for dextrans of similar molecular radii [82]. In addition, phosphate transport rates across the peritoneum are much lower that predicted from its size [1].

Although much of what is known about peritoneal membrane permeability is based on clearance rate or clearance ratio data, there are several assumptions inherent in these approaches which may limit their usefulness in describing the transport characteristics of the peritoneum. Use of clearance ratios to estimate whether restricted diffusion exists across the peritoneum assumes that: 1) the clearance of a molecule is not limited by how rapidly the blood flow can deliver the tracer to the tissue, 2) the surface area available for exchange is the same for the various solutes, and 3) diffusion is the sole mechanism for transperitoneal transport of the solutes studied. The frequent finding that the clearance ratio of urea to a larger solute (e.g., inulin, albumin) is much lower than the ratio of the free diffusion coefficients may be explained by inaccuracies in all of the aforementioned assumptions. Due to its relatively small size and partial lipid solubility, one may expect blood flow limitation (this possibility will be discussed in greater detail in a subsequent section) and a greater surface area for exchange of urea (due to transcellular movement). Since the contribution of convection to solute

exchange increases with solute size during filtration across semipermeable membranes, one would predict greater restricted diffusion using urea-to-albumin or inulin-to-albumin clearance ratios if compensation for convective exchange of the larger solute is allowed.

A novel approach for studying the selectivity of the peritoneum was described by Aune [90]. By measuring the ^{131}I-albumin activity in peritoneal fluid (D) and plasma (P) at different transperitoneal filtration rates, a value for the osmotic reflection coefficient (σ_d) was obtained. At high ultrafiltration rates, the contribution of diffusion to establishing the filtrate concentration is negligible and the D:P ratio under such conditions defines the sieving or separative capacity of the peritoneum [38, 94, 95] such that:

$$\sigma_d = 1 - D/P. \qquad [2]$$

Using this approach, a σ_d value of 0.70 was obtained for albumin. This value is in reasonable agreement with values reported for mesenteric capillaries [50]. According to current hydrodynamic theory, a σ_d of 0.70 for albumin is consistent with a membrane perforated by 65 Å radius pores. The prediction of a homoporous barrier is due to the fact that only one solute (albumin) was applied successfully to this analysis. Nonetheless, application of the same approach to other organs yields similar values for σ_d and pore size [38]. A more thorough description of the restrictive properties and pore distributions of the peritoneum can be obtained using this approach if macromolecules of different size are studied. Indeed, analysis of transperitoneal clearances of solutes with graded molecular radii using a nonlinear flux equation indicates that the selective properties of peritoneal capillaries can be described in terms of a two pore system: a small pore system with a radius of 63 Å and a large pore system with a radius of 221 Å (ref. 53, Figure 1). In addition, this analysis indicates that the ratio of small to large pores is 6158:1.

It appears likely that the morphologic equivalent of the small pore predicted by hydrodynamic theory is the intercellular junction [38]. This structure probably represents the major path for small solute transport across peritoneal capillaries. The morphologic equivalent of the large pores is less well defined. Peritoneal capillary dimensions have been obtained in the mouse and indicate that capillary thickness decreases in the venular end of capillaries while the number of micropinocytotic vesicles (400–800 Å diameter) per cubic micron increases [73]. The vesicles may form confluent chains across the endothelial cells [38, 73]. These transendothelial channels are more numerous in the venular segments of the microcirculation and may represent important pathways for solute movements across the endothelial barrier [38, 46]. In addition, postcapillary venular endothelium contains many large vesicles (2000 Å diameter) in addition to the micropinocytotic vesicles found in capillaries [73]. These large vesicles may also fuse to form patent transendothelial channels to provide a direct pathway for macromolecule transport. Finally, large gaps may exist between endothelial cells lining postcapillary venules thereby providing an additional route for protein transport [38, 46].

Taken as a whole, the available information on peritoneal mass transport does not support the prevailing concept of a high permeability. Although there are inconsistencies

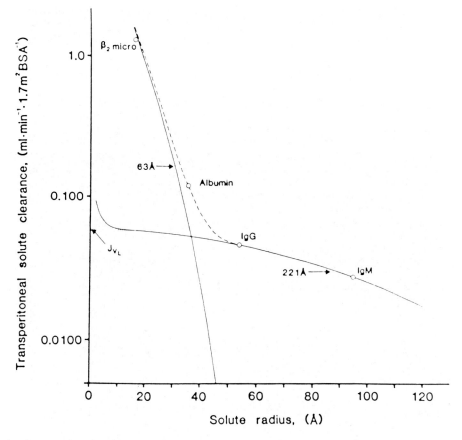

Figure 1. Analysis of transperitoneal solute clearances as a function of solute radius. Application of a pore stripping technique (38) predicts two equivalent pore populations for the peritoneal membrane; a large pore system (221 Å radius) and a small pore system (63 Å radius). This analysis also predicts a ratio of small: large pore numbers of 6158:1. Analysis performed by B. Rippe (unpublished observations).

regarding the degree of restriction offered to various solutes by the peritoneum, the transport characteristics of the peritoneum are generally similar to that reported in mesentery and other organs. This similarity suggests that the capillary wall may be the limiting barrier to solute movement across the peritoneum as a whole. One conclusion which may be drawn from the available information on peritoneal mass transport is that changes in the clearance ratio for small solutes (e.g., urea, creatinine, inulin) are difficult to interpret relative to peritoneal membrane permeability since the relative transport rates of these solutes are normally less than predicted for free diffusion in water.

5. ROLE OF LYMPHATIC VESSELS IN PERITONEAL MASS TRANSPORT

When fluid is introduced into the peritoneal cavity, small, readily diffusible molecules rapidly equilibrate between the injected fluid and plasma in the blood capillaries. The contribution of peritoneal lymphatics in the clearance of these small solutes is negligible. However, larger, poorly diffusible solutes require more time for equilibration to occur when placed in the peritoneal cavity. Protein uptake by peritoneal capillaries would primarily involve convective transport that is coupled to fluid absorption inasmuch as an uphill protein concentration gradient normally exists. However, available evidence indicates that the contribution of this route for large solute absorption is negligible. Rather, the results of several studies indicate that absorption of colloids and particles (up to the size of red blood cells or larger) from the peritoneal cavity occur almost exclusively via subdiaphragmatic lymphatics [22–28, 83, 96–101, 105]. For example, whole blood injected into the peritoneal cavity (20 ml/kg) is completely removed by peritoneal lymphatics within 24 hr, 48 hr, and 72 hr in the rat, rabbit, and guinea pig, respectively [101]. In dogs, 20–100% of injected red cells are removed by peritoneal lymphatics within 24 hr [102]. In all species studied, the plasma was absorbed more rapidly than the red cells. It is interesting to note that nearly all red cells escape macrophage ingestion while in the peritoneal cavity and lymph nodes, yet bacteria are readily ingested by phagocytes, especially in the omentum [97].

Several anatomic features of the peritoneal lymphatic vessels support the notion that these vessels may participate in the uptake of macromolecules and large particles from the peritoneal cavity. For example, mesenteric lymphatics

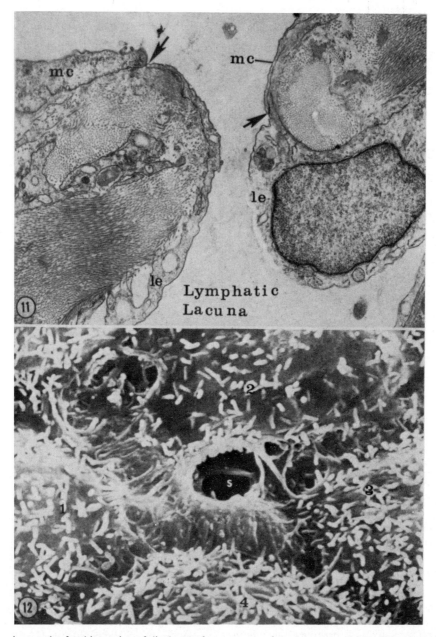

Figure 2. Electron micrograph of a thin section of diaphragm from an area of the lacunar roof. Note that the lymphatic endothelial cells (le) extend onto the peritoneal surface to form intercellular junctions (arrows) with the surface mesothelial cells (mc). This intimate contact between mc and le cells provides a direct pathway ('stomata' or 'pore', see lower panel) between the peritoneal cavity and the lymphatic lacuna. Magnification × 17 800. From ref. 77.

may provide a large surface area for water and solute exchange since approximately 4% of the mesenteric mesothelial surface covers adjacent lymphatics [84]. In addition, while lymphatic endothelium is similar in structure to the endothelial cells lining blood capillaries, tight junctions are not observed [84]. Furthermore, the underlying basement membrane is discontinuous [84]. These observations suggest that the numerous mesenteric lymphatics may be very permeable and thus may play an important role in solute exchange across the peritoneum.

Macromolecules and particles gain access to peritoneal lymph by first passing through the small openings (stomata) formed by intercellular junctions at the cell margins of peritoneal mesothelial cells of the diaphragm [2]. Similar stomata are formed by the intercellular junctions of lymphatic endothelial cells. For example, Leak and Rahil [77] have shown that the peritoneal mesothelium, which normally exists in a flattened cell form, takes on a cuboidal appearance when overlying submesothelial lymphatic lacunae. These investigators described two forms of inter-

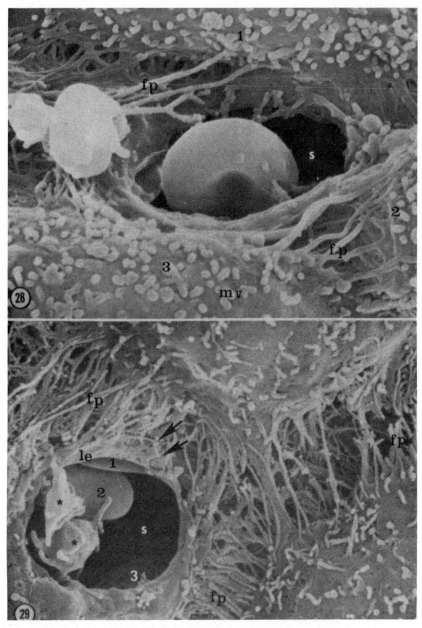

Figure 3. Electron micrograph depicting red blood cells in diaphragmatic stomata. From ref. 77.

cellular gaps between these cuboidal cells. One type has interlacing filamentous processes from adjacent mesothelial cells which overly a thin layer of connective tissue [77]. The second type of gap is a circular pore formed among several mesothelial cells whose membranes form adhesions with the cell membranes of underlying lymphatic endothelial cells (Figure 2). It is through such well defined channels that particles and cells can readily pass, as illustrated in Figure 3.

The contribution of lymphatics to the clearance of macromolecules from the peritoneal cavity should be largely determined by solute size. This notion is supported by the work of Flessner and coworkers [103] who noted that solutes

of molecular weight greater than 39 000 are transported from the peritoneal cavity to plasma almost exclusively via peritoneal lymphatics. However, small macromolecules are removed from the peritoneal cavity by both lymphatics and blood capillaries.

A number of investigators have attempted to define the maximum size of particles that can be removed by peritoneal lymphatics. The largest spherical particle that can be removed by peritoneal lymphatics is 16.8 μm (diameter) in the mouse and 24 μm in the rat and cat [99].

Although size is an important determinant of the accessibility of intraperitoneal particles to diaphragmatic lymph vessels, the net electrical charge on solutes and particles may also be important. For example, Leak [104] has demonstrated that there is a high density of anionic sites along the intercellular clefts of both mesothelial and lymphatic endothelial cells. This finding suggests that negatively charged solutes and particles may encounter more resistance in gaining access to peritoneal lymph than neutral or positively charged solutes of the same size and conformation.

While it is thought that peritoneal lymphatics play an important role in the removal of the fluid that normally accumulates in the peritoneal cavity [21, 106, 107], the contribution of these vessels in removing fluid during peritoneal dialysis remains largely undefined. Studies performed in rats indicate that total peritoneal lymph flow ranges between 10 and 35 ml/(min · kg body weight)([98]. Simultaneous estimates of peritoneal absorption rate range between 100 and 450 ml/(min · kg body weight). Based on this information, one would predict that peritoneal lymphatics may account for 2–30% of the fluid absorbed during peritoneal dialysis. Furthermore, Flesner and coworkers [98] have observed that thoracic duct lumph flow

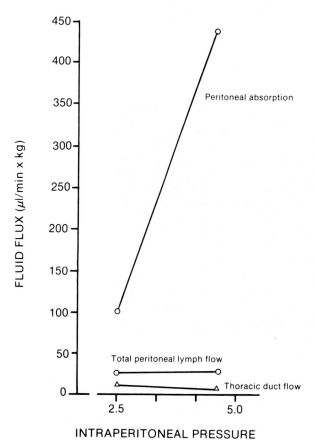

Figure 4. Effect of elevated intraperitoneal pressure on peritoneal fluid absorption rate, total peritoneal lymph flow and thoracic duct flow in the rat after injection of 5% albumin in Krebs-Ringer solution. Note that neither total peritoneal lymph flow or thoracic duct lymph flow was affected although peritoneal fluid absorption rate was markedly elevated. Modified from reference 96. Data from ref. 98.

is elevated by approximately 40% during peritoneal dialysis. This rise in thoracic duct lymph flow during dialysis suggests that the contribution of peritoneal lymphatics to fluid absorption may be larger than predicted above.

Over 60 yr ago, Florey [25] suggested that increments in intra-abdominal pressure should facilitate the absorption of peritoneal fluid and particles. A number of subsequent studies have substantiated this suggestion [99, 108–110]. Moreover, Zink and Greenway [110] have demonstrated that the rate of peritoneal fluid absorption is directly proportional to intraperitoneal pressure over a range of 0 to 22 mm Hg in the cat. As a consequence, it is generally held that peritoneal lymph flow is also positively correlated with intraperitoneal pressure. However, attempts to demonstrate a correlation between thoracic duct (or right lymphatic trunk) lymph flow and intraperitoneal pressure have largely failed. For example, although total peritoneal absorption rate is increased 4.5 fold by an increase in intraperitoneal pressure from 2.5 to 4.4 mm Hg, neither total peritoneal lymph flow nor thoracic duct flow is affected (Figure 4) [98]. Thus, it appears that the relative contribution of peritoneal lymphatics to total fluid absorption is reduced at elevated intraperitoneal pressures [98].

A wide variety of disease states are associated with pathological changes in diaphragmatic lymphatics that may interfere with peritoneal lymphatic drainage and alter the efficiency of peritoneal dialysis exchange. For example, fibrous thickening of the peritoneum is a feature of chronic ascites. Buhac and Jarmolych [30] have noted that the thickness of the peritoneum increases six-fold in patients dying of cirrhosis with ascites. Histopathologic evidence suggests a chronic nonspecific peritonitis with an increase in small blood vessels and lymphatics in the thickened peritoneum [30, 96]. Similar results have been noted in the peritoneum of the hemidiaphragm in patients with shistosomal hepatic fibrosis [111]. It has been suggested that obliteration of diaphragmatic stomata may be a major factor contributing to ascites in these patients [111]. Obviously, absorption of proteins and particles from the peritoneal cavity would be severely hindered in these patients. Nephrogenic ascites also results in impaired fluid drainage from the peritoneal cavity [112].

6. FACTORS AFFECTING PERITONEAL TRANSPORT RATES

The recent increase in clinical use of peritoneal dialysis has been accompanied by considerable expansion in the knowledge of factors which augment or impair peritoneal mass transport and the role that the peritoneal microcirculation plays in these responses. Table 1 lists some of the factors which have been shown to alter peritoneal clearances through effects on microcirculatory function. Although this

Table 1. Factors which influence peritoneal clearance via modulation of peritoneal microcirculatory function

Procedural variables	Ultrafiltration
Blood flow	Composition of dialysate
Drugs and hormones	Peritonitis

list is not all inclusive, it does present those factors which have been afforded clinical and/or experimental attention. An understanding of the role of the circulation in the effects and mechanisms of action of these factors is fundamental for developing rational methods of enhancing the efficiency of peritoneal dialysis. This latter point is of critical importance in view of the fact that inefficient peritoneal transport necessitates more frequent changes of dialysis solutions thereby contributing to the danger of peritonitis, the major complication of chronic peritoneal dialysis.

6.1. Variables of procedure

There are several procedural variables in routine peritoneal dialysis which may alter peritoneal clearance rates. These include: volume of dialysis fluid, dwell time, and the rate of flow of dialysis fluid. The general tendency has been to use a volume of dialysis fluid of 2 l without question, presumably because this is convenient (due to commercial availability) and not large enough to cause patient discomfort. One would expect that increasing dialysis volumes should augment peritoneal clearances since this would maintain a larger concentration gradient for diffusion between the blood and dialysate at any given dwell time. However, since dialysis volumes between 1 and 3 l cause a doubling of inferior vena cava pressure [113], it might be expected that stroke volume, cardiac output, and arterial pressure would decrease. As a consequence, it is possible that large dialysis volumes could decrease peritoneal clearances as a result of decreased peritoneal blood flow secondary to a fall in arterial pressure. However, experimental evidence does not support this notion since dialysis volumes between 1 and 3 l do not alter central hemodynamic parameters (cardiac output, stroke volume, arterial pressure) in patients despite the doubling of inferior vena caval pressure [113]. Moreover, evidence obtained in experimental animals and patients indicate that increments in dialysis volume increase the clearance of urea [9, 114. 115]. However, the volumes required to produce a reasonable increment in clearance (50%) appear impractical for clinical use [9, 114, 115].

Considerable attention has been given to the effects of dwell time (time dialysis solution is in the abdomen) on peritoneal clearances. Presumably this interest is related to the notion that increased dwell time should decrease peritoneal clearance rates since sufficient time is allowed for equilibration of the solute between blood and dialysis fluid, thereby reducing the diffusive gradient for peritoneal exchange. This is an important consideration since there is a substantial variation in the time dialysis fluid is allowed to remain in the abdomen (30 min to 8 hr, depending on the physician and type of dialysis, e.g., intermittent vs continuous ambulatory). Experimental evidence suggests that alterations in dwell time between 10 and 60 min significantly influence urea clearance rates. For example, in rabbits a 30 min dwell time produces clearance values for urea which are 50% greater than that obtained with 60 min dwell times [114]. With the development of continuous ambulatory peritoneal dialysis (CAPD), dialysis solutions may be left in the peritoneal cavity for 4–8 hr prior to drainage. Studies in humans show that with either 1.5% or 4.25% glucose dialysis solutions, urea approaches

diffusion equilibrium at approximately 4 hr [116]. Although larger solutes (creatinine, inulin) are not at equilibrium at 4 hr, the clearance rates fall dramatically with dwell times beyond 3 hr. Even though net solute removal by diffusion is expected beyond 3–4 hr, the efficiency of dialysis is so markedly reduced by the extended dwell time as to question the practicality of dwell times > 4 hr with CAPD.

A major determinant of diffusive solute transfer across the peritoneum is the magnitude of the concentration gradient for the solute. This gradient dissipates as solute leaves the circulation and accumulates in the dialysate. One way to maintain optimal concentration gradients is to increase the rate of dialysis solution exchange. Several investigators have attempted to identify the dialysis solution flow rate which produces maximal peritoneal clearance rates [9, 117, 118]. A typical value for dialysis flow rate in many clinical settings is approximately 30 ml/min representing 2100 ml drainage volume/70 min exchange. A reduction in dialysis flow rate to 15 ml/min typically results in a 35% reduction in urea clearance, while an increase in flow rate to 50 ml/min produces a 50% increase in urea clearance. Increasing dialysis flow rate above 50 ml/min does not significantly alter urea clearance. The clearance of larger, poorly diffusible solutes (inulin, albumin) are virtually unaffected by increases in dialysis flow rate above 10 ml/min [9].

The temperature of dialysis solutions is routinely allowed to equilibrate with that of room air prior to use. It has been shown that the exchange of urea between blood and peritoneal fluid in patients can be accelerated by heating the dialysis solutions to 37 °C [118]. Dialysis solutions warmed from 20 °C to 37 °C result in a 35% increase in urea clearance [118]. This increase is considered to result from temperature effects on peritoneal blood flow. However, more recent studies indicate that instillation of dialysate at room temperature does not significantly alter peritoneal clearances when compared to dialysate instillation at body temperature, apparently because heat exchange between dialysate and the body fluids occurs very rapidly [119].

6.2. Blood flow

There is considerable evidence indicating that alterations in peritoneal blood flow significantly influence the clearance of small solutes [8, 40]. Several mechanisms may be responsible for the effects of blood flow on peritoneal solute transport. These include: blood flow-limited delivery of the solute, passive (or active) recruitment (or derecruitment) of perfused peritoneal capillaries, and enhanced capillary filtration (and convective exchange) due to increased capillary hydrostatic pressure. Although the latter possibility may alter the clearance of large solutes, it is unlikely that ultrafiltration will significantly alter the clearance of solutes the size of urea. Recruitment of previously nonperfused (or poorly perfused) capillaries should increase the clearance of small and large solutes due to an effective increase in the surface area available for exchange. Estimates of peritoneal capillary exchange capacity at various blood flows are lacking due to technical difficulties. Therefore, an assessment of the role of capillary recruitment in the blood flow-induced increases in urea clearance is not possible at present.

The results of several studies show that some splanchnic vasodilators produce a greater increase in the clearance of urea than that of larger solutes (e.g., inulin) [120–122]. This observation, coupled to the common finding that the ratio of urea clearance to inulin clearance (approx. 2.5–3.0) is significantly less than the urea/inulin free diffusion coefficient ratio (8.6), suggests that urea clearance may be blood flow-limited. The possibility that the clearance of urea across the peritoneum is blood flow limited is usually dismissed based on indirect evidence [9]. A systematic analysis of the relationship between urea clearance and peritoneal blood flow is necessary to resolve this issue. Total blood flow to the peritoneum cannot be measured directly due to the diffuse nature of this tissue and its vasculature. However, effective peritoneal perfusion rates have been derived using the inert gas (H_2, Xe) washout technique. Estimates of peritoneal blood flow range between 2.5 and 6.2 ml/min per kg body weight in rabbits [123] to 7.5 ml/min × 100 g body weight in rats [124]. In rats, 91% of the effective peritoneal perfusion is due to splanchnic blood flow and superior mesenteric flow alone accounts for 89% of peritoneal perfusion [124]. Analysis of carbon dioxide diffusion into the peritoneal cavity of man yield estimates of peritoneal blood flow ranging between 68 and 82 ml/min (approximately 1–2 ml/min per kg body weight). From the ratio of urea clearance to peritoneal blood flow (assuming diffusion alone accounts for urea transport across the peritoneum), Aune [123] predicted minimal blood flow limitation of urea clearance, i.e., a doubling of peritoneal blood flow would produce less than a 10% increase in urea

clearance. However, vasodilation increases the clearances of large solutes (>5200 Daltons) by 100% or more, presumably by increasing convective flux [8]. Considering the emphasis now being placed on the use of vasodilators to augment peritoneal clearance, future studies should be designed to directly assess the possibility that the clearance of urea is limited by how rapidly the blood flow can deliver urea to the peritoneum.

6.3. Drugs and hormones

The demonstration that the impaired peritoneal mass transport accompanying systematic vascular disease can be restored to normal by vasoactive agents [3], such as isoproterenol, has led to a proliferation of studies designed to assess the effect of drugs and hormones on peritoneal mass transport in the absence of vascular disease (Table 2). These studies have shown that peritoneal clearances can be manipulated by a large number of drugs. The drugs and hormones which have been reported to modify peritoneal clearances are listed in Table 2. In general, agents which enhance peritoneal clearances are vasodilators in splanchnic organs [3, 134, 166, 179, 180, 182, 184, 185, 200], while splanchnic vasoconstrictors generally tend to decrease peritoneal clearances [3, 122, 149–151, 179, 185]. A notable exception to this general rule is aminophylline which increases intestinal blood flow [156, 181] but does not alter peritoneal clearances [178]. Of the agents that alter peritoneal clearances, most generally produce changes which range between 15–65%. However, there is much

Table 2. Effects of drugs and hormones on peritoneal transport

Agents that increase clearance

Albumin [125–128]	Insulin [79]
Aminoproprionate [129]	Isoproterenol [141, 159–162]
Anthranilic acid [130, 131]	Lipid in dialysate [163]
Arachidonic acid [132]	Methylprednisolone [164]
Bradykinin [121]	Nitroprusside [141, 157, 165–167]
Cetyl trimethyl NH_4Cl [133]	N-myristyl alanine [130]
Cholecystokinin [134]	Procaine hydrochloride [172]
Desferrioxamine [135–137]	Prostaglandin A_1 [168, 169]
Dialysate alkalinization [138, 139]	Prostaglandin E_1 [168, 169]
Diazoxide [140, 141]	Prostaglandin E_2 [168, 169]
Dioctyl sodium sulfosuccinate [133, 142]	Phenazine methosulfate [170]
Dipyridamole [143–148, 164]	Phentolamine [171]
Dopamine [122, 149–151, 177]	Protamine [173]
Edetate calcium disodium [152]	Puromycin [174]
Ethacrynic acid [153]	Salicylate [127, 156]
Furosemide [153, 154]	Secretin [134, 145]
Glucagon [134, 155, 180, 185]	Serotonin [149]
Histamine [79, 89, 121]	Streptokinase [149]
Hydralazine [156]	Tolazoline [4]
Hypertonic glucose [72, 157, 158]	Tris hydroxymethyl aminomethane (THAM) [138, 151, 176]
Indomethacin [156]	

Agents that decrease clearance

Calcium [151]	Prostaglandin F_2 [168]
Dopamine [182]	Vasopressin [149–151]
Norepinephrine [122, 177]	

References in [ ]
Modified from ref. 8.

evidence indicating that the route of administration (intravenous vs intraperitoneal) determines the magnitude of the effect of the drug on peritoneal mass transport [134, 180, 182]. Generally, the drugs that augment peritoneal clearances when administered i.p. are small solutes which rapidly cross the peritoneum. The high molecular weight agents, such as glucagon and secretin, must be administered intravenously to augment peritoneal mass transport.

Nitroprusside and isoproterenol appear to be the most effective agents which augment peritoneal clearances [141, 157, 159–162, 165–167, 183, 186]. Both are potent splanchnic vasodilators [156, 181] and produce increments in creatinine clearance of 50–60% when administered i.p.. Nitroprusside increases the clearance of urea, creatinine, inulin, and protein in a dose-dependent manner, with small solute clearance being most affected at lower doses and the large solute clearances increasing more dramatically at higher doses [187]. The effects of nitroprusside on peritoneal clearances are promptly reversed after removal of the vasodilator from the dialysis fluid. A major disadvantage to the clinical use of nitroprusside is its peripheral vasodilatory effect. Nonetheless, preliminary trials with this drug in patients appear promising and suggest that the hypotensive effects are minimal with i.p. administration [3]. Isoproterenol accelerates peritoneal transport when administered i.p. in experimental animals and man, yet is considered to offer greater potential danger to patients due to its cardiac actions [160].

Most of the evidence that vasodilator-induced increments in peritoneal clearance is due to concomitant increments in splanchnic blood flow is inferential since splanchnic blood flow is not monitored in a majority of the studies. In a recent study [180], the effects of isoproterenol and glucagon on peritoneal clearances of creatinine and inulin were determined while monitoring superior mesenteric blood flow (SMBF). Intravenous isoproterenol increases SMBF by 88%, yet did not alter peritoneal clearances. Intraperitoneally administered isoproterenol increased the clearance of both solutes and produced a rise in SMBF comparable to that observed after i.v. injection. When blood flow was returned to normal during i.p. isoproterenol by partially occluding the aorta, the clearance returned to control values. Glucagon given i.v. increased SMBF by 80% and caused clearances to rise. Reducing SMBF with the aortic clamp returned the clearance values to control levels. The results of this study indicates that peritoneal clearance changes induced by vasoactive agents can be dissociated from blood flow responses. It is difficult to further interpret the results of this study without some knowledge of the changes in peritoneal blood flow produced by the experimental pertubations. Nonetheless, it does point to the need for more studies on the relationship between vasodilator-induced changes in splanchnic and peritoneal blood flows, and peritoneal clearances.

In the clinical setting, patients suffering from acute renal failure secondary to shock may require peritoneal dialysis and vasoconstrictor therapy. The finding that most vasopressor agents decrease peritoneal mass transport [3, 122, 149–151, 155, 179] suggests that application of certain pressor agents may not be advantageous in this situation. However, in contrast to the effects of most vasoconstrictor agents, some studies indicate that dopamine may produce a significant increase in peritoneal mass transport. This result is most likely explained by fact that although dopamine increases cardiac output and total peripheral resistance, the splanchnic vasculature demonstrates only a transient vasoconstriction followed by dilation [188]. Thus, it has been suggested that in patients undergoing peritoneal dialysis who also require vasoconstrictor therapy, the pressor agent dopamine may be the drug of choice [122]. However, other studies suggest that peritoneal clearances may decrease with dopamine administration [182].

The mechanism(s) involved in the drug or hormone-induced changes in peritoneal clearance may include: blood flow-limited delivery of the solute, recruitment of capillaries, increased capillary and/or mesothelial permeability, and enhanced ultrafiltration. While blood flow-limited delivery could account for acceleration of urea clearance, other mechanisms must be invoked to explain the enhanced clearance of larger solutes. Vasoactive agents which are known to increase capillary permeability (histamine, bradykinin) in the mesentery and other tissues exert only moderate effects on small solute clearances relative to isoproterenol [121]. The disproportionately greater increase in protein clearance observed with high doses of nitroprusside is compatible with enhanced permeability [40]. The latter possibility is supported by reports of enhanced leakage of fluorescein-tagged albumin across mesenteric microvessels after exposure to nitroprusside [189].

The most likely mechanism involved in the augmented peritoneal clearances induced by most drugs is capillary recruitment. There is evidence that most of the agents which augment peritoneal clearance also increase the capillary exchange area of many splanchnic organs, including mesentery [181]. Since many vasoactive agents do not produce proportional increments in the clearance of small and large solutes, either the newly recruited capillaries are more permeable than those continuously perfused or mechanisms other than recruitment are also involved in the augmented transport. It is difficult to assess the role of mesothelial permeability in drug-induced increases in peritoneal clearance since the mesothelium is not generally considered to be a limiting barrier to the exchange of solutes across the peritoneum. However, the fact that furosemide, nitroprusside, procaine hydrochloride and other agents have been shown to increase the permeability of the mesothelium to small solutes [141, 172], indicates that mesothelial permeability changes could play a role in drug-induced augmentation of peritoneal transport.

6.4. Ultrafiltration

Most commercially available dialysis solutions are hypertonic due to the presence of glucose in concentrations equal to or exceeding 1.5 gm%. Glucose is added to match or exceed the osmolarity of the uremic extracellular fluid. As a result of the osmotic imbalance between blood and peritoneal fluid, net fluid filtration into the peritoneum occurs thereby increasing peritoneal volume [190, 191]. Peak intraperitoneal volume has been assumed to occur at or near osmotic equilibrium [190]. However, recent evidence, discussed later in this section, suggests this may not be the case.

With a 1.5 gm% glucose dialysis solution, net ultrafiltration occurs at a rate of 3.0 ml/min/m² body surface area (0.17 ml/min for a 4 kg rabbit) and increases by approximately 1.7 ml/min/m² for each gm% increment in dialysis glucose concentration [4, 115]. Because of the inward diffusion of glucose, the blood-peritoneal osmotic pressure gradient dissipates rapidly resulting in a concomitant reduction in ultrafiltration rate. In patients undergoing 8–10 hr of dialysis with hyperosmolar dialysis fluid (2–4 gm%), an average weight loss of 1.6 kg occurs due to ultrafiltration [113].

Significant augmentation of peritoneal clearances frequently accompanies the use of hypertonic dialysis solutions. These higher rates of solute clearance are often explained by enhanced convective transport of solutes across the peritoneum due to ultrafiltration [115]. The convective flux of urea produced by hypertonic dialysis solutions in rabbits is approximately 0.8 ml/min for each ml/min of net ultrafiltration [158]. Using this approximation, convection should account for less than 15% of the total urea flux observed with commercially available dialysis solutions. Other evidence also suggests that ultrafiltration is not primarily responsible for the augmented peritoneal transport produced by hypertonic dialysis solutions. In some studies, use of hypertonic dialysis solutions produces a greater increase in the clearance of urea than that of larger solutes (e.g., inulin) [120]. With ultrafiltration one would predict a proportionally greater rise in the clearance of larger solutes if convection were the sole mechanism enhancing transport. Hypertonic dialysis solutions enhance peritoneal clearances even when ultrafiltration does not occur [121]. Furthermore, enhanced peritoneal mass transport persists when hypertonic and isotonic solutions are interchanged [192]. Finally, secretin, a hormone known to enhance peritoneal ultrafiltration, does not alter peritoneal solute clearances [134].

Alternative explanations for the augmented peritoneal transport produced by hypertonic solutions have been presented. For example, it has been suggested that hypertonic solutions increase peritoneal capillary permeability. Support for this hypothesis is provided by the frequent observation that large solute clearances are increased by a greater extent than that of small solutes [158] and that intestinal capillary permeability is increased following 20 mM increments in blood glucose concentration [193]. As discussed in greater detail in the following section, hypertonic dialysis solutions increase blood flow and number of perfused capillaries in the mesentery. Thus, vasodilation and capillary recruitment could account for the augmented peritoneal transport. Another possibility is that the fluid entering the peritoneal cavity with hypertonic solutions is withdrawn from cells or across pores which are too small to let solutes through. Since this fluid would be devoid of solutes, it would decrease the concentration of solutes in the peritoneal cavity by dilution. The steeper concentration gradient would then increase the rate of clearance of solutes, such as urea or inulin.

Absorption of peritoneal fluid into blood capillaries after dialysate crytalloids have attained an osmotic equilibrium with plasma is described by the Starling equation as:

$$J_v = L_pA \, (\Delta P - \sigma \Delta \pi) - J_L, \qquad [3]$$

where J_v represents fluid flow from peritoneum to plasma,

L_pA represents the peritoneal membrane filtration coefficient which in turn represents a product of peritoneal membrane hydraulic conductivity (L_p) and surface area (A), ΔP represents the effective hydrostatic pressure gradient between the capillaries and peritoneal cavity, $\Delta \pi$ represents the effective colloid osmotic pressure gradient between the capillaries and peritoneal cavity, and J_L represents the lymph flow from the peritoneal cavity. The rate of absorption across the peritoneal membrane after crystalliod equilibration is −0.9 to −1.1 ml/min in human patients [51, 194]. The peritoneal membrane filtration coefficient has been estimated [195] from equation 1 by inserting this value for J_v, ΔP = 10 mm Hg, σ = 0.90, $\Delta \pi$ = 20 mm Hg, and J_L = 0.2 ml/min. Such a calculation yields a value for L_pA of 0.1 ml min⁻¹ mm Hg⁻¹ [195] which is in close agreement with that obtained by Rippe *et al.* [52] for cat peritoneum (0.12 ml min⁻¹ mm Hg⁻² body surface). Comparisons of the ratios of hydraulic conductivity and potassium permeability in skeletal muscle and mesentery are similar suggesting that the molecular structures responsible for the resistance to water and small solute movements across capillaries in these tissues are similar [196].

From equation 3, it is apparent that lymphatic fluid absorption can influence net ultrafiltration rate. In a recent study, Nolph and co-workers [197] have demonstrated that net ultrafiltration is substantially reduced by lymphatic absorption (Figure 5). Thus, the net ultrafiltration rate induced by instillation of hypertonic dialysis solutions into the peritoneal cavity is well below true transcapillary filtration rate. Another important finding presented in this study is that peak intraperitoneal volume does not occur at osmotic equilibrium. Rather, the peak volume occurs when transcapillary ultrafiltration rate equals lymphatic absorption rate (Figure 6) [197].

Ronco and co-workers [198, cited in 199] have suggested

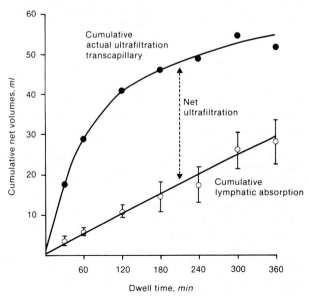

Figure 5. Simultaneous estimates cumulative transcapillary ultrafiltration, net ultrafiltration, and cumulative lymphatic absorption induced by instillation of hypertonic dialysis solutions into the peritoneal cavity. Note that net ultrafiltration is substantialy reduced by lymphatic absorption. From ref. 197.

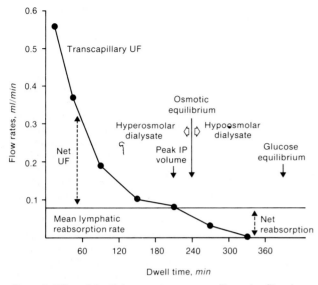

Figure 6. Effect of dwell time on mean transcapillary ultrafiltration rate and lymphatic absorption rate. Note that peak intraperitoneal volume occurs before osmotic equilibrium is attained. From ref. 197.

that filtration pressure equilibrium may occur in peritoneal capillaries during peritoneal dialysis with very hypertonic exchange solutions. This notion is based on the fact that steep increases in plasma osmotic pressure should occur when the filtration fraction (peritoneal ultrafiltration rate divided by peritoneal plasma flow) approaches 50%. Further increments in filtration fraction should produce little or no increase in ultrafiltration rate since plasma osmotic pressure increases markedly with only slight increases in filtration fraction above this level. Attainment of such an ultrafiltration maximum with very hypertonic dialysate exchanges has recently been demonstrated in the rat [199].

6.5. Composition of the dialysis solution

Peritoneal dialysis solutions differ from non-vascoactive bicarbonate-buffered Krebs solution by having a high osmolality (335–350 mOsm) due to glucose, an acetate or lactate buffer system, and a lower pH (5.5 vs 7.4). Nolph and co-workers [185] have hypothesized that the acidic nature of most commercial peritoneal dialysis solutiuons could alter dialysis efficiency by causing arteriolar relaxation and increased capillary blood flow. Subsequent work by this group [40, 75, 184, 189, 200] had indicated that commercial peritoneal dialysis solutions produce a transient vasoconstriction (1–4 min) which is followed by sustained vasodilation when they are topically applied to arterioles of the rat cremaster (a model for parietal peritoneum) or on the mesothelial surface of the rat cecum (a model for visceral peritoneum). However, it is unlikely that the low pH (5.3–5.8) of the commercial dialysis solutions accounts for their vasoactive properties since adjustment of pH to 7.0–7.4 does not alter the vasodilatory response in the rat cremaster [200] and does not alter peritoneal urea, creatinine, inulin or protein clearances in patients [187]. Moreover, Granger and co-workers [201] have reported that

Tyrode's solution (pH 7.4) and Tyrode's lactate (pH 5.3) had similar effects on blood flow in the peritoneal cavity.

Although dialysate pH adjustments do not affect clearances of a variety of substances [187], these results cannot be extrapolated to all solutes since alkalinization of dialysate fluid enhances the clearance of weak acids such as urate or barbiturates [138, 139, 151, 176]. This result is most likely explained by the phenomenon of ionic trapping. That is, elevation of dialysate pH promotes the conversion of non-charged weak acids to ionized salts. The charged salts are less diffusible than the weak acid forms and are thus trapped in the dialysis solution. This may represent an important mechanism whereby tris hydroxymethyl amino-methane (THAM) increases peritoneal urea clearance [138, 151, 176]. Moreover, pH adjustments can have marked effects on the proportion of drugs and other solutes bound to proteins. Obviously, clearance of a solute that binds to protein will increase when pH adjustments increase the bound (non-difusible) form in the peritoneal cavity since this maintains a steeper concentration gradient for the free form and also minimizes back diffusion. A similar line of reasoning has been applied as a rationale for the addition of sorbents (zirconium phosphate) [202], chelators (EDTA and desferrioxamine) [135-137, 152], and proteins (albumin) [125-128] to dialysate fluid to enhance clearances of certain solutes.

Hyperosmolality produced by glucose does produce submaximal vasodilation. Normal osmolality acetate or lactate solutions also produce submaximal dilation of cremaster arterioles. However, the combination of hyperosmolality and either acetate or lactate produced maximal vasodilation [75]. Although hyperosmotic dialysis solutions are known to augment peritoneal solute clearances [203], it is uncertain whether lactate or acetate alters peritoneal mass transport. It has been shown, however, that peritoneal clearances of urea, creatinine and inulin are not significantly different between hyperosmotic dialysis solutions containing lactate or acetate [204]. Clinical studies with nonvasoactive dialysis solutions show a reduction in the clearances of urea and creatinine but not inulin when compared to commercial solutions [192].

The results of the *in vivo* microscopy studies on the peritoneal microcirculation are of importance for they suggest that the commercially available dialysis solutions are vasoactive. Furthermore, they define some of the factors in peritoneal dialysis solutions that could be altered to produce predictable changes in small solute clearances via changes in peritoneal blood flow in conscious animals or patients. The observation in whole organ studies that the intestinal vasculature is more sensitive to changes in blood osmolality than other organs [193] supports the possibility that commercial dialysis solutions will dilate the vasculature of the visceral peritoneum in conscious animals or man. To directly assess this possibility, Granger and co-workers [201] monitored superior mesenteric blood flow and peritoneal blood flow in anesthetized cats during intraperitoneal administration of commercial dialysis solutions (Dianeal). Their results indicate that commercial peritoneal dialysis solutions dramatically increase blood flow to mesentery, omentum, intestinal serosa, and parietal peritoneum (Figure 7). However, these changes were not accompanied by significant alterations in blood flow in the major

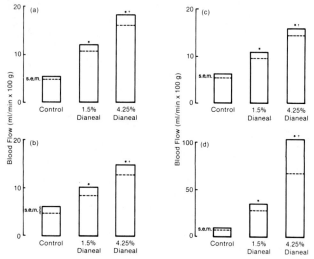

Figure 7. Effects of 1.5% and 4.25% dextrose-Dianeal solutions on blood flow in mesentery (Panel A), parietal peritoneum (Panel B), omentum (Panel C), and intestinal serosa (Panel D). Control values were obtained with Tyrode's solution in the abdomen. * denotes P<0.05 compared to control; t denotes P<0.01 compared to 1.5% Dianeal. (Modified from ref. 201).

abdominal organs (liver, stomach, intestine, pancreas, and spleen). The selective vasodilation of the 'thin' tissues (mesentery, omentum, parietal peritoneum, and intestinal serosa) presumably results from a greater access (shorter diffusion distance) of the vasoactive constituent(s) to resistance vessels [201]. Although this study only assessed the effects of Dianeal solutions on splanchnic blood flow, the similarity in chemical compositions of most commercial peritoneal dialysis solutions would suggest that other commercial peritoneal dialysis solutions (e.g., Inpersol and McGaw) exert similar effects on blood flow to tissues in the abdominal cavity [201]. Extrapolation of this data to conscious man indicates total peritoneal blood flow in man exceeds 100 ml/min during dialysis (50). However, it should be kept in mind that the applicability of this data obtained in the cat to conscious man on peritoneal dialysis depends on the assumption that blood flows per unit mass of tissue are similar in cat and man and on extent to which peritoneal blood flow is influenced by anesthesia or by the hypertension and uremia observed in peritoneal dialysis patients.

6.6. Peritonitis and prolonged CAPD

Peritonitis is the most frequent complication associated with peritoneal dialysis. During episodes of peritonitis in patients undergoing intermittent or continuous ambulatory peritoneal dialysis (CAPD), there is either an increase or no change in the clearance of small solutes (urea, creatinine) yet there is usually an increased protein loss into the peritoneal cavity [13, 85, 205, 206]. These changes are consistent with the increased capillary permeability and blood flow usually associated with inflammation. The enhanced protein loss is considered to account, at least in part, for the general catabolic state associated with peritonitis. Other diseases have been shown to depress

peritoneal mass transport. These include malignant hypertension, scleroderma, collagen vascular disease with severe vasculitis, and advanced diabetic vasculitis [7].

There is some difference of opinion as to whether peritoneal clearances are altered by long-term peritoneal dialysis. In some studies the clearance of urea, creatinine, inulin, and protein are not significantly altered after 6 months to 1 yr of CAPD [205]. This stability of clearances with time is also observed after numerous episodes of peritonitis. Furthermore, the ability of nitroprusside to enhance peritoneal clearances is not altered by one year of CAPD. Therefore, according to these studies, the integrity of the peritoneal membrane and the responsiveness of peritoneal microvessels is not adversely affected by one year of CAPD. The results of other studies [207], however, suggest that the peritoneum is more permeable in patients undergoing CAPD than IPD. A corresponding difference is observed in patients transferred from IPD to CAPD. The reasons for the discrepancy in results of the above studies are not readily apparent. However, different severities and frequencies of peritonitis between the two patient populations may account for these differences. Irrespective of the reasons for these discrepancies, all of the information obtained indicates that peritoneal clearances are not reduced after prolonged CAPD.

ACKNOWLEDGEMENTS

Ronald J. Korthuis is the recipient of an Established Investigatorship from the American Heart Association and is supported by a grant (HL-36069) from the National Heart, Lung, and Blood Institute. D. Neil Granger's work is supported by HL-26441 from the National Heart, Lung, and Blood Institute.

REFERENCES

1. Hirszel P, Larisch M, Maher JM, Maher JF: Prediction of solute transport during peritoneal dialysis. Artific Org 3: 228–229, 1979.
2. Maher JF: Principles of dialysis and dialysis of drugs. Am J Med 62: 475–481, 1977.
3. Maher JF: Acceleration of peritoneal mass transport by drugs and hormones. Artific Org 3: 224–227, 1977.
4. Maher JF, Hirszel P, Lasrich M: An experimental model for study of pharmacologic and hormonal influences on peritoneal dialysis. Contr Nephrol 17: 131–138, 1979.
5. Mattocks AM, El-Bassiouni EA: Peritoneal dialysis: A review. J Pharm Sci 60: 1767–1782, 1971.
6. Nolph KD: Short dialysis, middle molecules, and uremia. Ann Int Med 86: 93–97, 1977.
7. Nolph KD: Peritoneal clearances. J Lab Clin Med 94: 519–525, 1979.
8. Nolph KD: Peritoneal dialysis. In: The Kidney, vol. 2, BM Brenner FC Rector, Jr. (eds), WB Saunders, Philadelphia, pp 1847–1906.
9. Nolph KD, Popovich RP, Ghods AJ, Twardowski Z: Determinants of low clearances of small solutes during peritoneal dialysis. Kid Int 13: 117–123, 1978.
10. Nolph KD, Twardowski Z: The peritoneal dialysis system. In: KD Nolph (ed), Peritoneal Dialysis. Martinus Nijhoff, Boston, pp 23–50, 1985.
11. Crafts RC: A Textbook of Human Anatomy, New York, The Ronald Press Company, 1966.

12. Lukas G, Brindle SD, Greengard P: The route of absorption of intraperitoneally administered compounds. J Pharmacol Exp Ther 178: 562–566, 1966.
13. Verger C: Peritoneal ultrastructure. In: KD Nolph (ed) Peritoneal Dialysis, Martinus Nijhoff, Boston pp 95–113, 1985.
14. Knapowski J, Feder E, Simon M, Zabel M: Evaluation of the participation of parietal peritoneum in dialysis: physiological, morphological, and pharmacological data. Proc Eur Dial Trans Assoc 16: 155–164, 1979.
15. Henderson LW: The problem of peritoneal membrane and permeability. Kid Int 3: 409–410, 1973.
16. Mion CM, Boen ST: Analysis of factors responsible for the formation of adhesions during chronic peritoneal dialysis. Am J Med Sci 250: 675–679, 1965.
17. Miller FN, Nolph KD, Joshua IJ: The osmotic component of peritoneal dialysis solutions. Proc 1st Int Symp on CAPD. Amsterdam, Excerpta Medica, pp 12–17, 1980.
18. Nolph KD: Anatomy, physiology and kinetics of peritoneal transport during peritoneal dialysis. Proc 1st Int Symp on CAPD Amsterdam, Excerpta Medica, pp 7–11, 1980.
19. Popovich RP, Pyle WK, Bomar JB, Moncrief JW: Peritoneal dialysis. American Institute of Chemical Engineering Symposium, series 75: 31–45, 1978.
20. Rubin J, Jones Q, Planch A, Stanek K: Systems of membranes involved in peritoneal dialysis. J Lab Clin Invest 110: 448–453, 1987.
21. Allen L, Vogt E: A mechanism of lymphatic absorption from serous cavities. Am J Physiol 119: 776–782, 1937.
22. Von Rechlinghausen FT: Zur fettre sorption. Arch Pathol Anat Physiol 26: 172 (abstract). Cited in ref. 109, 1863.
23. Allen L: The peritoneal stomata. Anat Rec 67: 89–93, 1936.
24. Casley-Smith JR: Endothelial permeability. The passage of particles into and out of diaphragmatic lymphatics. Quart J Exp Physiol 49: 365–383, 1964.
25. Florey HW: Reactions of, and absorption by lymphatics, with special reference to those of the diaphragm. Br J Exp Path 8: 479–490, 1927.
26. French JE, Florey HW, Morris B: The absorption of particles by the lymphatics of the diaphragm. *Quart J Exp Physiol 45: 88*–203, 1960.
27. Higgens GM, Graham AS: Lymphatic drainage from the peritoneal cavity in the dog. Arch Surg Chicago 19: 453–465, 1929.
28. Morris B: The absorption of fatty chyle and artificial fat emulsions from the peritoneal cavity. Aust J Exp Biol Med Sci 34: 173–180, 1956.
29. Azzali G: Ultrastructure of small intestine, submucosal and serosal-muscular lymphatic vessels. Lymphology 15: 106–111, 1982.
30. Buhac I, Jarmolych J: Histology of the intestinal peritoneum in patients with cirrhosis of the liver and ascites. Dig Dis 23: 417–422, 1978.
31. Korthuis RJ, Kinden DA, Brimer GE, Slattery KA, Stogsdill P, Granger DN: Intestinal capillary filtration in acute and chronic portal hypertension. Am J Physiol *254*: G339–G345, 1988.
32. Witte CL, Witte MH: The circulation in portal hypertension. Yale J Biol Med 48: 141–155, 1975.
33. Nylander G, Tjernberg B: The lymphatics of the greater omentum. An experimental study in the dog. Lymphology 2: 3–7, 1969.
34. Barrowman JA: Physiology of the Gastrointestinal Lymphatic System. Monographs of the Physiology Society, Cambridge University Press, Cambridge, 1978.
35. Sorkin MI, Nolph KD: Dynamics of peritoneal transfer. In: Atkins RC, Thompson NM, Farrell PC (eds), Peritoneal Dialysis, Edinburgh, UK, Churchill, Livingstone, pp 12–21, 1981.
36. Chambers R, Zwiefach BW: Functional activity of the blood capillary bed, with special reference to visceral tissue. Ann NY Acad Sci 46: 683–694, 1946.
37. Rhodin JAG: Histology: A Text and Atlas. New York, Oxford University Press, 1974.
38. Taylor AE, Granger DN: Exchange of macromolecules across the circulation. In: Renkin EM, Michel CC (eds) Handbook of Physiology, Microcirculation section, Chapter 11, Baltimore, American Physiological Society, pp 467–520.
39. Renkin EM: Relation of capillary morphology to transport of fluid and large molecules: A review. Acta Physiol Scand Suppl 463: 81–91, 1979.
40. Miller FN: The peritoneal microcirculation. In: Nolph KD (ed), Peritoneal Dialysis. Martinus Nijhoff, Boston, pp 51–93, 1985.
41. Karnovsky MJ: The ultrastructural basis of capillary permeability. J Cell Biol 35: 213–236, 1967.
42. Bruns RR, Palade GE: Studies on blood capillaries. II. Transport of ferritin molecules across the wall of muscle capillaries. J Cell Biol 37: 277–299, 1968.
42. Bruns RR, Palade GE: Studies on blood capillaries. II. Transport of ferritin molecules across the wall of muscle capillaries. J Cell Biol 37: 277–299, 1968.
43. Johansson BR: Permeability of muscle capillaries to interstitially microinjected horseradish peroxidase. Microvasc Res 16: 340–361, 1978.
44. Nolph KD, Miller FN, Rubin J, Popovich R: New directions in peritoneal dialysis concepts and applications. Kid Int 18: S111–S116, 1980.
45. Westergaard E, Brightman MW: Transport of proteins across normal cerebral arterioles. J Comp Neurol 152: 17–44, 1973.
46. Nakamura Y, Wayland H: Macromolecular transport in the cat mesentery. Microvasc Res 9: 1–21, 1975.
47. Aune S: Transperitoneal Exchange. IV. The effect of transperitoneal fluid transport on the transfer of solutes. Scand J Gastroent 5: 241–252, 1970.
48. Curry FE, Mason JC, Michel CC: Osmotic reflection coefficients of capillary walls to low molecular weight hydrophilic solutes measured in single perfused capillaries of the frog mesentery. J Physiol 261: 319–336, 1976.
49. Michel CC: Reflection coefficients in single capillaries compared with results from whole organs. Bibl Anat 15: 172–176, 1977.
50. Michel CC: Filtration coefficients and osmotic reflection coefficients of the walls of single frog mesenteric capillaries. J Physiol 309: 341–355, 1980.
51. Pyle WK, Moncrief JW, Popovich RP: Peritoneal transport evaluation in CAPD. In: Moncrief JW, Popovich RP (eds), Proc 2nd Int Symp on CAPD, New York, Masson, pp 35–39, 1981.
52. Rippe B, Perry MA and Granger DN: Permselectivity of the peritoneal membrane. Microvasc Res 29: 89–102, 1985.
53. Rippe B, Stelin G, Ahlmen J: Basal permeability of the peritoneal membrane during continuous ambulatory peritoneal dialysis (CAPD). In: Advances in Peritoneal Dialysis. Proc. of the 2nd International Symposium in Peritoneal Dialysis, Excerpta Medica, Amsterdam, pp 5–9, 1981.
54. Diana JN, Laughlin MH: Effect of ischemia on capillary pressure and equivalent pore radius in capillaries of the isolated dog hind limb. Circ Res 35: 77–101, 1974.
55. Korthuis RJ, Granger DN: Peritoneal dialysis: An analysis of factors which influence peritoneal mass transport. In Stigmark B (ed) Peritoneum and Peritoneal Access. London, John Wiley and Sons, (in press), 1988.
56. Rippe B, Haraldson B: Capillary permeability in rat hindquarters as determined by estimations of capillary reflection coefficients. Acta Physiol Scand 127: 289–303, 1986.
57. Clementi F, Palade GE: Intestinal capillaries. I. Permeability to peroxidase and ferritin. J Cell Biol 41: 33–58, 1969.
58. Fox JR, Wayland H: Interstitial diffusion of macro-molecules

in the rat mesentery. Microvasc Res 18: 255–274, 1979.

59. Johansson BR: Permeability of muscle capillaries to interstitially microinjected ferritin. Microvasc Res 16: 362–368, 1978.

60. Laurent TC: Interaction between proteins and glycosaminoglycans. Fed Proc 36: 24–27, 1977.

61. Watson PD, Grodins FS: An analysis of the effects of the interstitial matrix on plasma-lymph transport. Microvasc Res 16: 19–41, 1978.

62. Wiederheim CA: The interstitial space. In: Fung YC, Perrone N, Anliker M (eds), Biomechanics, its Foundations and Objectives, Prentice Hall, Englewood Cliffs, New Jersey, pp 273–286, 1972.

63. Granger DN, Taylor AE: Permeability of intestinal capillaries to endogenous macromolecules. Am J Physiol 238: H457–H464, 1980.

64. Majno G: Ultrastructure of the vascular membrane. In: Handbook of Physiology-Circulation, section 2, vol. 3, Baltimore, Williams and Wilkins, pp. 2293–2376, 1965.

65. Majno G, Palade GE: Studies on inflammation. I. The effect of histamine and serotonin on vascular permeability: an electron microscopic study. J Biophys Biochem Cytol 11: 571–606, 1961.

66. Barrowman JA, Perry MA, Kvietys PR, Granger DN: Exclusion phenomena in the liver interstitium. Am J Physiol 234: G410–G414, 1982.

67. Bert JL, Pearce RH: The interstitium and microvascular exchange. In: Handbook of Physiology: The Cardiovascular System, Sect. 2, Vol. IV, The Microcirculation, Part 1, Renkin EM and Michel CC (eds), Bethesda, Williams and Wilkins, p 521–548, 1982.

68. Comper WD, Laurent TC: Physiological functions of connective tissue polysaccharides. Physiol Rev 58: 255–315, 1978.

69. Granger HJ: Physicochemical properties of the extracellular matrix. In: Tissue Fluid Pressure and Composition, AR Hargens (ed), Baltimore, Williams and Wilkins, pp 43–62, 1981.

70. Granger HJ, Shepherd AP: Dynamics and control of the microcirculation. Adv Biomed Eng 7: 1–63, 1979.

71. Guyton AC, Taylor AE, Granger HJ: Circulatory Physiology. II. Dynamics and Control of the Body Fluids. Philadephia, Saunders, 1975.

72. Nolph KD: The first hemodialyzer. ASAIO J 1: 273. Simionescu N, Simionescu M, Palade GE. (1978). Structural basis of permeability in sequential segments of the microvasculature of the diaphragm. II. Pathways followed by microperoxidase across the endothelium. Microvasc. Res. 15: 17–36, 1978.

74. Granger HJ, Taylor AE: Permeability of connective tissue linings isolated from implanted capsules. Implications for interstitial fluid pressure measurements. Circ Res 36: 222–228, 1975.

75. Miller FN, Nolph KD, Joshua IG, Weigman DL, Harris PD, Andersen DB: Hyperosmolality, acetate and lactate: Dilatory factors during peritoneal dialysis. Kid Int 20: 397–402, 1981.

76. Gosselin RE, Berndt WO: Diffusional transport of solutes through mesentery and peritoneum. J Theoret Biol 3: 487–499, 1962.

77. Leak LV, Rahil K: Permeability of the diaphragmatic mesothelium: The ultrastructural basis for stomata. Am J Anat 151: 557–579, 1978.

78. Nagel W, Kuschinsky W: Study of the permeability of the isolated dog mesentery. Eur J Clin Invest 1: 149–154, 1970.

79. Rasio EA: Metabolic control of permeability in isolated mesentery. Am J Physiol 226: 962–968, 1974.

80. Tsilibray EC, Wissig SL: Absorbtion from the peritoneal cavity; SEM study of the mesothelium covering the peritoneal surface of the muscular portion of the diaphragm. Am J Anat 149: 127–133, 1977.

81. Odor L: Observations of the rat mesothelium with the electron and phase microscopes. Am J Anat 95: 433–465, 1954.

82. Arturson G: Permeability of the peritoneal membrane. In: Proceedings of the 6th European Conf. Microcirculation, pp 197–202, 1970.

83. Dumont AE, Robbins E, Martelli A, Iliescu H: Platelet blockade of particle absorption from the peritoneal surface of the diaphragm. Proc Soc Exp Biol Med 167: 137–142, 1981.

84. Gotloib L, Digenis GE, Rabinovich S, Medline A, Oreopoulos DM: Ultrastructure of Normal Rabbit Mesentery. Nephron 34: 248–255, 1983.

85. Verger C, Luger A, Moore HL, Nolph KD: Acute changes in peritoneal morphology and transport properties with infectious peritonitis and mechanical injury. Kid. Int. 23: 823–831, 1983.

86. Frokjaer-Jensen J, Christensen O: Potassium permeability of the mesothelium of the frog mesentery. J Physiol 102: 2A, 1978.

87. Knapowski JM, Simon MP, Feder EM: Preparation of parietal peritoneum for measurements of in vitro permeability. Artific Org 3: 219–223, 1979.

88. McGary TJ, Nolph KD, Rubin J: In vitro simulations of peritoneal dialysis. A technique for demonstrating limitations on solute clearances due to stagnant fluid films and poor mixing. J Lab Clin Med 96: 148–157, 1980.

89. Wayland H: Action of histamine on the microvasculature. In: Legrain M (ed), Proc 1st CAPD Int Symp, Amsterdam, Excerpta Medica, pp 18–27, 1980.

90. Aune S: Transperitoneal exchange. I. Peritoneal permeability studied by transperitoneal plasma clearance of urea, PAH, inulin and serum albumin in rabbits. Scand J Gastroent 5: 86–97, 1970.

91. Hirszel P, Chakrabati EK, Bennett RA, Maher JF: Permselectivity of the peritoneum to neutral dextrans. Trans Am Soc Artif Intern Organs 30: 625–627, 1984.

92. Andrews PM, Porter KR: The ultrastructural morphology and possible functional significance of mesothelial microvilli. Anat Rec 177: 409–426, 1973.

93. Leypoldt JK, Parker HR, Frigon RP, Henderson LW: Molecular size dependence on peritoneal transport. J Lab Clin Invest 110: 207–216, 1987.

94. Bresler EH, Groome LJ: On equations for combined convective and diffusive transport of neutral solute across porous membranes. Am J Physiol 241: F469–F476, 1981.

95. Granger DN, Granger JP, Brace RA, Parker RE, Taylor AE: Analysis of the permeability characteristics of intestinal capillaries. Circ Res 44: 335–344, 1979.

96. Barrowman JA, Granger DN: Lymphatic drainage in the peritoneal cavity. In: B Stigmark (ed), Peritoneum and Peritoneal Access. London, John Wiley and Sons, (in press), 1988.

97. Bettendorf U: Lymph flow mechanism of the subperitoneal diaphragmatic lymphatics. Lymphology 11: 111–116, 1978.

98. Flessner MF, Parker RJ, Sieber SM: Peritoneal lymphatic uptake of fibrinogen and erythrocytes in the rat. Am J Physiol 244: H89–H96, 1983.

99. Yoffrey JM, Courtice FC: Lymphatics, Lymph and the Lymphomyeloid Complex. London, Academic Press, p 295, 1979.

100. Mactier RA, Khanna R, Twardowski ZJ, Nolph KD: Role of peritoneal cavity lymphatic absorption in peritoneal dialysis. Kid Int 32: 165–172, 1987.

101. Courtice FC, Harding J, Steinbeck AW: The removal of free red blood cells from the peritoneal cavity of animals. Aust J Exp Biol Med 31: 215–226, 1953.

102. Hahn PF, Miller LL, Robscheit-Robbins FS, Bale FS, Whipple G: Peritoneal absorption. Red cells labelled by radio-iron hemoglobin move promptly from the peritoneal cavity into the circulation. J Exp Med 80: 77–82, 1944.

103. Flessner MF, Dedrick RL, Schultz JS: Exchange of macro-

molecules between peritoneal cavity and plasma. Am J Physiol 248: H15–H25, 1985.

104. Leak LV: Distribution of cell surface changes on mesothelium and lymphatic endothelium. Microvasc Res 31: 18–30, 1986.

105. Leak LV: Permeability of peritoneal mesothelium. A T.E.M. and S.E.M. study. J Cell Biol 19: 423A, 1976.

106. Szabo G, Magyar Z, Serenyi P: Lymphatic drainage of the peritoneal cavity in experimental ascites. Acta Med Acad Sci Hung 32: 337–348, 1975.

107. Lill SR, Parsons RH, Buhac I: Permeability of the diaphragm and fluid resorption from the peritoneal cavity in the rat. Gastroenterology 76: 997–1001, 1979.

108. McKay T, Zink J, Greenway CF: Relative rates of absorption of fluid and protein from the peritoneal cavity in cats. Lymphology 11: 106–110, 1978.

109. Ruszniak I, Foldi M, Szabo G: Lymphatics and Lymph Circulation. Pergamon Press, Oxford, 1967.

110. Zink J, Greenway CV: Intraperitoneal pressure in formation and resorption of ascites in cats. Am J Physiol 233: H185–H190, 1977.

111. Ismail AH, Mohamed FS: Structural changes of the diaphragmatic peritoneum in patients with shistosomal hepatic fibrosis: its relation to ascites. Lymphology 19: 82–87, 1986.

112. Morgan AG, Terry SI: Impaired peritoneal fluid drainage in nephrogenic ascites. Clin Nephrol 15: 61–65, 1981.

113. Schurig R, Gahl GM, Becker H, Schiller R, Kessel M, Paeprer H: Hemodynamic studies in long-term peritoneal dialysis patients. Artific Organs 3: 215–218, 1979.

114. Penzotti SC, Mattocks AM: Effects of dwell time, volume of dialysis fluid, and added accelerators on peritoneal dialysis of urea. J Pharm Sci 60: 1520–1522, 1971.

115. Maher JF: Peritoneal transport rates: Mechanisms, limitation and methods for augmentation. Kid Int 18: S117–S121, 1980.

116. Nolph KD, Twardowski ZJ, Popovich RP, Rubin J: Equilibration of peritoneal dialysis solutions during long dwell exchanges. J Lab Clin Med 93: 246–256, 1979.

117. Boen ST: Peritoneal dialysis in clinical medicine. Springfied, Ill: Charles C. Thomas, 1964.

118. Gross M, McDonald HP Jr: Effects of dialysate temperature and flow rate on peritoneal clearance. JAMA 202: 363–365, 1967.

119. Indraprasit S, Namwongprom A, Sooksriwongse CO: Effects of dialysate temperature on peritoneal clearances. Nephron 34: 45–47, 1983.

120. Aune S: Transperitoneal exchange. III. The influence of transperitoneal fluid flux on the peritoneal plasma clearance of serum albumin in rabbits. Scand J Gastroent 5: 105–113, 1970.

121. Brown EA, Kliger AS, Goffinet J, Finkelstein FO: Effect of hypertonic dialysate and vasodilators on peritoneal dialysis clearances in rats. Kid Int 13: 271–277, 1978.

122. Hirszel P, Larisch M, Maher JF: Divergent effects of catecholamines on peritoneal mass transport. Trans Am Soc Artif Intern Organs 25: 110–113, 1979.

123. Aune S: Transperitoneal exchange. II. Peritoneal blood flow estimated by hydrogen gas clearance. Scand J Gastroent 5: 99–104, 1970.

124. Bulkley GB: Washout of intraperitoneal Xenon: effective peritoneal perfusion as an estimation of splanchnic blood flow. In: Measurements of Blood Flow: Applications to the Splanchnic Circulation, Granger DN, Bulkley GB (eds), Baltimore, Williams and Wilkins, pp 441–453, 1981.

125. Campion DS, North JDK: Effect of protein binding of barbiturates on their rate of removal during peritoneal dialysis. J Lab Clin Med 66: 549–563, 1965.

126. Cole DEC, Lirenman DS: Role of albumin enriched peritoneal dialysate in acute copper poisoning. J Pediatr 92: 955–977, 1978.

127. Etteldorf JN, Dobbins WT, Summit RL, Rainwater WT, Fischer RL: Intermittent peritoneal dialysis using 5% albumin in the treatment of salicylate intoxication in children. J Pediatr 58: 226–236, 1961.

128. Schultz JC, Crouder DG, Medart WS: Excretion studies in ethylchlorovynol (placidil) intoxication. Arch Intern Med 117: 409–411, 1966.

129. El-Bassiouni EA, Mattocks AM: Acceleration of peritoneal dialysis with minimal N-myristyl-B-aminoproprionate. J Pharm Sci 62: 1314–1316, 1973.

130. Kudla RM, El-Bassiouni EA, Mattocks AM: Accelerated peritoneal dialysis of barbiturates, diphenylhydantion and salicylate. J Pharm Sci 60: 1065–1067, 1971.

131. Mattocks AM: Accelerated removal of salicylate by additives in peritoneal dialysis fluid. J Pharm Sci 58: 595–598, 1969.

132. Hirszel P, Lasrich M, Maher JF: Arachidonic acid increases peritoneal clearances. Trans Am Soc Artif Intern Organs 27: 61–63, 1981.

133. Penzotti SC, Mattocks AM: Acceleration of peritoneal dialysis by surface-acting agents. J Pharm Sci 57: 1192–1195, 1968.

134. Maher JF, Hirszel P, Lasrich M: Effects of gastrointestinal hormones on transport by peritoneal dialysis. Kid Int 16: 130–136, 1979.

135. Covey TJ: Ferrous sulfate poisoning: a review, case summaries and therapeutic regimen. J Pediatr 64: 218–226, 1964.

136. Stanbaugh GH Jr, Homes AW, Gillit D: Iron chelation therapy in CAPD: A new effective treatment for iron overload disease in ESRD patients. Perit Dial Bull 3: 99–103, 1983.

137. Williams P, Khanna R, Crapper McLachlan DR: Enhancement of aluminium removal by desferrioxamine in a patient on continuous ambulatory peritoneal dialysis with dementia. Perit Dial Bull 1: 73–77, 1981.

138. Knochel JP, Clayton E, Smith WL, Barry KG: Intraperitoneal THAM: An effective method to enhance phenobarbital removal during peritoneal dialysis. J Lab Clin Med 64: 257–268, 1964.

139. Knochel JP, Mason AD: Effect of alkalinization on peritoneal diffusion of uric acid. Am J Physiol 210: 1160–1164, 1966.

140. Limido A, Cantu P, Allaria P et al: Velocita di flusso ed efectto dei farmaci nella valutazione dell'efficienza della dialisi peritoneale. Minerva Nephrol 26: 161. Cited in ref. 8, 1979.

141. Nolph KD, Ghods AJ, Van Stone J, Brown PA: The effects of intraperitoneal vasodilators on peritoneal clearances. Trans Am Soc Artif Intern Organs 22: 586–594, 1976.

142. Mattocks AM, Penzotti SC: Acceleration of peritoneal dialysis with minimum amounts of dioctyl sodium sulfosuccinate. J Pharm Sci 61: 475–476, 1972.

143. Diaz-Buxo JA, Farmer CD, Walker PJ: Effects of hyperparathyroidism on peritoneal clearances. Trans Am Soc Artific Intern Organs 28: 276–279, 1982.

144. Maher JF, Hirszel P: Augmenting peritoneal mass transport. Int J Artif Organs 2: 59–63, 1979.

145. Maher JF, Hohnadel DC: Peritoneal permeability and drugg enhancement in uremia. Proc 9th Annual Contractors Conf Artif Kidney Chronic Uremia Program NIH NIAMDD DHEW publication No. (NIH)77:1167, 9: 116–120, 1976.

146. Maher JF, Hirszel P, LeGrow W: Enhanced peritoneal permeability with methyl prednisolone. Clin Res 26: 64A, 1978.

147. Rubin J, Adair C, Barnes T, Bower JD: Augmentation of peritoneal clearance by dipyridamole. Kid Int 22: 658–661, 1982.

148. Ryckelynck JP, Pierre D, DeMartin A, Rottenbourg J: Amelioration des clairances peritoneales par le dipyridamole. Nouv Presse Med 7:472. Cited in ref. 8, 1978.

149. Hare HG, Valtin H, Gosselin RE: Effects of drugs on peritoneal dialysis in the dog. J Pharmacol Exp Ther 145: 122–129, 1964.

150. Henderson LW, Kintzel JE: Influence of antidiuretic hormone on peritoneal membrane area and permeability. J Clin Invest 50: 2437–2443, 1971.

151. Shear L, Harvey JD, Barry KG: Peritoneal sodium transport: enhancement by pharmacologic and physical agents. J Lab Clin Med 67: 181–188, 1966.

152. Mehbod H: Treatment of lead intoxication. Combined use of peritoneal dialysis and edetate calcium disodium. Jama 201: 972–974, 1967.

153. Maher JF, Hohnadel DC, Shea C, SiSanzo F, Cassetts M: Effects of intraperitoneal diuretics on solute transport during hypertonic dialysis. Clin Nephrol 7: 96–100, 1977.

154. Grzegorzewska A, Baczyk K: Furosemide-induced increase in urinary and peritoneal excretion of uric acid during peritoneal dialysis in patients with chronic uremia. Artific Organs 6: 220–224, 1982.

155. Nolph KD, Ghods AJ, Brown P, Van Stone JC: Factors affecting peritoneal dialysis efficiency. Dial Transpl 6: 52–56, 1977.

156. Granger DN, Richardson PDI, Kvietys PR, Mortillaro NA: Intestinal blood flow. Gastroenterology 78: 837–863, 1980.

157. DeSanto NG, Capodicasa G, Capasso G: Development of means to augment peritoneal urea clearances: the synergic effects of combining high dialysate temperature and high dialysate flow rates with dextrose and nitroprusside. Artif Organs 5: 409–414, 1981.

158. Henderson LW, Nolph KD: Altered permeability of the peritoneal membrane after using hypertonic peritoneal dialysis fluid. J Clin Invest 48: 992–1001, 1969.

159. Brown ST, Aheran DJ, Nolph KD: Reduced peritoneal clearances in scleroderma increased by intraperitoneal isoproterenol. Ann Intern Med 78: 891–897, 1973.

160. Maher JF, Shea C, Cassetta M, Hohnadel DC: Isoproterenol enhancement of peritoneal permeability. J Dial 1: 319–331, 1977.

161. Nolph KD, Miller L, Husted FC, Hirszel P: Peritoneal clearances in scleroderma and diabetes mellitus. Effects of intraperitoneal isoproterenol. Int Urol Nephrol 8: 161–154, 1976.

162. Vanichayakornkul S, Nimmanit S, Chirawong P: Accelerated peritoneal dialysis with intraperitoneal isoproterenol. J Med Assoc Thailand 61 Suppl. 1: 127–128, 1978.

163. Shinaberger JH, Shear L, Clayton LE: Dialysis for intoxication with lipid soluble drugs: enhancement of glutethimide extraction with lipid dialysate. Trans Am Soc Artif Organs 11: 173–177, 1965.

164. Maher JF, Hirszel P, Abraham JE: The effect of dipyridamole on peritoneal mass transport. Trans Am Soc Artif Intern Organs 23: 219–223, 1977.

165. Miller FN, Nolph KD, Harris PD: Effects of peritoneal dialysis solutions on human clearances and rat arterioles. Trans Am Soc Artif Intern Organs 24: 131–132, 1978.

166. Nolph KD: Effects of intraperitoneal vasodilators on peritoneal clearances. DIal Transpl 7: 812, 1978.

167. Nolph KD, Ghods AJ, Brown PA, Twardowski ZJ: Effects of intraperitoneal nitroprusside on peritoneal clearances with variations in dose, frequency of administration, and dwell times. Nephron 24: 114–120, 1979.

168. Maher JF, Hirszel P, Lasrich M: Modulation of peritoneal transport rates by prostaglandins. Adv Prostaglandin Thromboxame Res 7: 695–700, 1980.

169. Hirszel P, Larisch M, Maher JF: Peritoneal transport rates and inhibition of prostaglandin synthetase by mefenamic acid. Abstr Am Soc Artif Intern Organs 9: 48, 1980.

170. Cascarano J, Rubin AD, Chick WL, Zweifach BW: Metabolically induced permeability changes across mesothelium and endothelium. Am J Physiol 206: 373–382, 1964.

171. Parker HR, Schroeder JP, Henderson LW: Influence of dopamine and Regitine on peritoneal dialysis in unanesthetized dogs. Abstracts Am Soc Artif Int Organs 7: 43, 1978.

172. Breborowicz A, Knapowski J: Augmentation of peritoneal dialysis clearances with procaine. Kid Int 26: 392–396, 1984.

173. Alavi N, Lianos E, Andres G: Effect of protamine on the permeability and structure of rat peritoneum. Kidney Int 21: 44–53, 1982.

174. Avasthi PS: Effects of aminonucleoside on rat blood-peritoneal barrier permeability. J Lab Clin Med 94: 295–302, 1979.

175. Richardson PDI: The actions of natural secretin on the small interstinal vasculature of the anesthetized cat. Br J Pharm 58: 127–135, 1976.

176. McLean WM, Poland DM, Cohon MS, Penzotti SC, Mattocks AM: Effect of Tris (hydroxymethyl) aminomethane on removal of urea by peritoneal dialysis. J Pharm Sci 56: 1614–1621, 1967.

177. Hirszel P, Larisch M, Maher JF: Augmentation of peritoneal mass transport by dopamine. Comparison with norepinephrine and evaluation of pharmacologic mechanisms. J Lab Clin Med 94: 747–754, 1979.

178. Maher JF, Cassetts M, Shea C, Hohnadel DC: Peritoneal dialysis in rabbits. A study of transperitoneal theophylline flux and peritoneal permeability. Nephron 20: 18–23, 1978.

179. Maher JF: Pharmacologic manipulation of peritoneal transport. In: KD Nolph (ed) Peritoneal Dialysis, The Hague, Martinus Nijhoff, p. 213, 1981.

180. Felt J, Richard C, McCaffrey C, Levy M: Peritoneal clearance of creatinine and inulin during dialysis in dogs: Effect of splanchnic vasodilators. Kid Int 16: 459–469, 1979.

181. Chou CC, Kvietys PR: Physiological and pharmacological alternations in gastrointestinal blood flow. In: Granger DN, Bulkley GB (eds), Measurement of Blood Flow: Applications to the Splanchnic Circulation. Williams and Wilkins, Baltimore, pp 477–509, 1981.

182. Gutman RA, Nixon WP, McRae RL, Spencer HW: Effect of intraperitoneal and intravenous vasoactive amines on peritoneal dialysis: study in anephric dogs. Trans Am Soc Artif Intern Organs 22: 570–573, 1976.

183. Hirszel P, Maher JF, Chamberlin M: Augmented peritoneal mass transport with intraperitoneal nitroprusside. J Dial 2: 131, 1978.

184. Miller FN, Nolph KD, Joshua IG, Nolph KD, Rubin J: Effects of vasodilators and peritoneal dialysis solution on the microcirculation of the rat cecum. Proc Soc Expt Biol Med 161: 605–608, 1979.

185. Hirszel P, Maher JF, LeGrow W: Increased peritoneal mass transport with glucagon acting at the vascular surface. Trans Am Soc Artific Organs 24: 136–138, 1978.

186. Raja RM, Kramer MS, Rosenbaum JL: Enhanced clearance with intraperitoneal nitroprusside in high flow recirculation peritoneal dialysis. Trans Am Soc Artif Int Organs 24: 133–135, 1978.

187. Nolph KD, Rubin J, Wiegman DL, Harris PD, Miller FN: Peritoneal clearances with three types of commercially available peritoneal dialysis solutions. Nephron 24: 35–40, 1979.

188. Goldberg LI: Cardiovascular and renal actions of dopamine: Potential clinical implications. Pharmacol Rev 24: 1–30, 1972.

189. Miller FN, Joshua JG, Harris PD, Wiegman DL, Jauchem JR: Peritoneal dialysis solutions and the microcirculation. Contr Nephrol 17: 51–58, 1977.

190. Rubin J, Nolph KD, Popovich RP, Moncrief JW, Prowant B: Drainage volumes during continuous ambulatory peritoneal dialysis. Am Soc Artif Int Org 22: 54–60, 1979.

191. Twardowski ZJ, Khanna R, Nolph KD: Osmotic agents and ultrafiltration in peritoneal dialysis. Nephron 42: 93–101, 1986.

192. Rubin J, Nolph KD, Arfania D, Joshua IG, Miller FN, Wiegman DL, Harris PD: Clinical studies with a nonvasoactive peritoneal dialysis solution. J Lab Clin Med 93: 910–915, 1979.

193. Levine SE, Granger DN, Brace RA, Taylor AE: Effect of hyperosmolality on vascular resistance and lymph flow in the cat ileum. Am J Physiol 234: H14–H20, 1978.

194. Pyle WK, Popovich RP, Moncrief JW: Mass transfer in peritoneal dialysis. In: Advances in peritoneal dialysis: Proceedings of the 2nd international symposium on peritoneal dialysis. Amsterdam, Excerpta Medica, pp 41–49, 1981.

195. Rippe B, Stelin G, Ahlmen J: Lymph flow from the peritoneal cavity in CAPD patients. In: Frontiers in Peritoneal Dialysis, New York, Field, Rich & Associates, pp 24–30, 1986.

196. Curry FE, Frokjaer-Jensen J: Water flow across the walls of single muscle capillaries in the frog, rana pipiens. J Physiol 350: 293–307, 1984.

197. Nolph KD, Mactier R, Khanna R, Twardowski ZJ, Moore H, McGary T: The kinetics of ultrafiltration during peritoneal dialysis: The role of lymphatics. Kid Int 32: 219–226, 1987.

198. Ronco C, Brendolan A, Bragantini L, Chiramonte S, Feriani M, Fabris A, Dell Aquila A, Milan R, La Greca G: Flusso ematico capillare effettivo nel sistema dialitico peritoneale. In Lamperi S, Capelli G, Carozzi S (eds) Dialsysi Peritoneale, Milano, Italy, Wichtig Editore, pp 21–28. Cited in ref. 199, 1985.

199. Levin TN, Rigden LB, Nielsen LH, Moore HL, Twardowski ZJ, Khanna R, Nolph KD: Maximum ultrafiltration rates during peritoneal dialysis in rats. Kid Int 31: 731–735, 1987.

200. Miller FN, Nolph KD, Harris PD, Rubin J, Wiegman DL, Joshua JG, Twardowski ZJ, Ghods AJ: Microvascular and clinical effects of altered peritoneal dialysis solution. Kid Int 15: 630–639, 1979.

201. Granger DN, Ulrich M, Perry MA, Kvietys PR: Peritoneal dialysis solutions and feline splanchnic blood flow. Clin Exp Pharmacol Physiol 11: 473–483, 1984.

202. Blumenkrantz MJ, Gordon A, Roberts M, Lewin AJ, Pecker EA, Moran JK, Coburn JW, Maxwell MH: Applications of the Redy sorbent system to hemodialysis and peritoneal dialysis. Artific Org 3: 230–236, 1979.

203. Zelman A, Giser D, Whittam PJ, Parsons RH, Schuyler R: Augmentation of peritoneal dialysis efficiency with programmed hyper/hypoosmotic dialysate. Trans Am Soc Artif Intern Organs 23: 203–209, 1977.

204. Rubin J, Nolph KD, Arfania D, Wiegman DL, Miller FN, Harris PD: Comparison of the effects of lactate and acetate on clinical peritoneal clearances. Clin Nephrol 12: 145–147, 1979.

205. Rubin J, Arfania D, Nolph KD, Prowant B, Fruto L, Brown P, More H: Peritoneal clearances after 6–12 months of CAPD. Trans Am Soc Artif Intern Organs 25: 104–109, 1979.

206. Rubin J, McFarland S, Hellems EW, Bower JD: Peritoneal dialysis during peritonitis. Kid Int 19: 460–464, 1981.

207. Farrell PC, Randerson DH: Membrane permeability changes in long-term CAPD. Trans Am Soc Artif Intern Organ 26: 197–200, 1980.

4

PERITONEAL CAVITY LYMPHATICS

ROBERT A. MACTIER and RAMESH KHANNA

1. INTRODUCTION

Intraperitoneal fluid is absorbed continuously by convective flow into the peritoneal cavity lymphatics [1, 2]. The importance of lymphatic absorption from the peritoneal cavity in the pathophysiology of ascites is well established [3–16] and the considerable absorptive capacity of the peritoneal cavity lymphatics has been exploited clinically to perform intraperitoneal blood transfusions in the fetus and in children [17–21]. Nevertheless, until recently, studies of the kinetics of peritoneal dialysis 'ascites' have neglected the role of the peritoneal cavity lymphatics and have focused only on fluid and solute exchange between the peritoneal microcirculation and the hypertonic dialysis solution instilled into the peritoneal cavity [22–34]. Recent investigations, however, have demonstrated a significant contribution of lymphatic absorption to loss of ultrafiltration and solute clearances after long-dwell peritoneal dialysis exchanges [35–39]. Accordingly, the major objectives of this review are to summarize current knowledge of the anatomy and physiology of the peritoneal cavity lymphatics, to provide a reappraisal of peritoneal dialysis kinetics which includes the role of the peritoneal cavity lymphatics and finally, to discuss the theoretical and practical implications of lymphatic absorption during peritoneal dialysis.

2. ANATOMY AND PHYSIOLOGY OF THE PERITONEAL LYMPHATICS

2.1. Lymphatic pathways of the peritoneal lymphatics

Lymphatic drainage from the peritoneal cavity is primarily via specialized end lymphatic openings (stomata) located in the subdiaphragmatic peritoneum [40–43]. Moreover, absorption of intraperitoneal fluid is greatest from the right side overlying the liver [42]. In contrast, absorption by the lymphatic capillaries within the interstitium of the mesentery, omentum and parietal peritoneum only contributes a relatively minor proportion of total peritoneal lymphatic drainage [2, 43, 44].

The lymphatic capillaries leading from the subdiaphragmatic stomata coalesce to form a plexus of collecting lymphatics within the muscular portion of the diaphragm. This subperitoneal plexus also communicates with the lymphatics from the pleural surface. From the diaphragm and the diaphragmatic lymph nodes, most of the lymphatic trunks accompany the internal mammary vessels to the anterior mediastinal lymph nodes around the thymus and thereafter return almost 80% of the peritoneal lymphatic drainage to the venous circulation via the right lymph duct [2, 45]. Some of the efferent lymphatics from the anterior mediastinal nodes may, however, occasionally drain to the central veins on the left side either in association with or separate from the thoracic duct. The lymphatic drainage from the remainder of the peritoneum, including part of the subdiaphragmatic peritoneum, returns to the systemic circulation through the thoracic duct [2]. Consequently cannulation of the thoracic duct during peritoneal dialysis in the rat collected less than 30% of total estimated lymphatic absorption [46]. The major substernal and other minor lymphatic pathways from the peritoneal cavity are summarized in Figure 1.

2.2. The subdiaphragmatic stomata

Von Recklinghausen in 1863 was the first to suggest that carbon particles, red blood cells, proteins and fluid were transported directly from the peritoneal cavity into the lymphatics of the diaphragm via openings in the subdiaphragmatic peritoneum, which he called stomata [47]. Other investigators subsequently claimed that the stomata were artifacts [48–50] but the presence of these specialized terminal lymphatics in animals and man has since been confirmed by light and electron microscopy [51–56].

The lacunae of the terminal lymphatics of the subdiaphragmatic peritoneum are only separated from the peritoneal cavity by a thin triple-layer, consisting of small, rounded, and interdigitating mesothelium, a loose network of connective tissue and lymphatic endothelium [52, 54]. Scanning and transmission electron microscopy have shown that the stomata permit absorption of intraperitoneal particles, cells, colloids and fluid into the underlying lymphatic lacunae via extracellular pathways [52, 57] (Figure 2). The mesothelial cells which overlie the lymphatic lacunae are

smaller and separate from each other more readily than the cells in the surrounding mesothelium [52, 58]. Internally the lacunar mesothelial cells have bands of actin filaments arranged along their base [54]. The stomata are formed by the separation of adjacent mesothelial cells and, in the rat, can accommodate spherical particles up to 22.5 μ in diameter [59]. At the stomata the submesothelial basement membrane and the underlying lattice of connective tissue become fenestrated [60] and so allow the mesothelial cells to adjoin the lymphatic endothelial cells to form a channel from the peritoneal cavity to the lumen of the underlying lacuna [61, 62].

2.3. Mechanism of lymphatic absorption

The rate at which intraperitoneal fluid is absorbed by the peritoneal cavity lymphatics depends on the excursions of the diaphragm during respiration [63–65]. As the diaphragm relaxes during expiration, the adjacent mesothelial and endothelial cells in the roofs of the lymphatic lacunae separate from each other and intraperitoneal fluid is absorbed as suction is created by the distension of the lacunae. In inspiration the contraction of the diaphragm closes the gaps between the overlying mesothelial and endothelial cells and the contents of the lacunae are emptied into the efferent lymphatics. The presence of abundant actin filaments in the cytoplasm of both the mesothelial and endothelial cells, however, suggests that there may be an active as well as a passive mechanism for maintaining the patency of the stomata [63, 64]. Backflow of the absorbed fluid into the peritoneal cavity is prevented during inspiration by the overlapping of the endothelial cells in the roofs of the lacunae [53, 54] (Figure 3). Forward flow, induced by lymphatic contractility and changes in intrathoracic pressure, is maintained by the presence of valves in the efferent lymphatics [53, 54, 65]. The higher lymphatic absorption rate from the right hemidiaphragm is probably due to compression of the liver against the subdiaphragmatic stomata during respiration [58]. The ultrastructure and the mechanism of absorption of the peritoneal cavity lymphatics may be reviewed in greater detail elsewhere [66].

2.4. Function of peritoneal cavity lymphatics

The lymphatics draining the peritoneal cavity act as a one-way system returning excess intraperitoneal fluid and protein to the systemic circulation. The sum of hydrostatic and osmotic pressure gradients across the peritoneum normally favors a minor net inflow of fluid into the peritoneal cavity [31]. Bidirectional transperitoneal transfer of small solutes occurs by diffusion and by solvent drag. However, macromolecules (molecular weight greater than 20 000) exhibit minimal direct reabsorption into the peritoneal capillaries [67] and consequently, after unidirectional transport from the peritoneal microcirculation into the peritoneal cavity, are returned to the venous circulation by convective flow into the lymphatics. Normally peritoneal lymphatic drainage of serous fluid equals its rate of formation and only a small volume of isosmotic fluid is maintained within the peritoneal cavity.

The second major function of the lymphatics is their contribution to the host defenses of the peritoneal cavity.

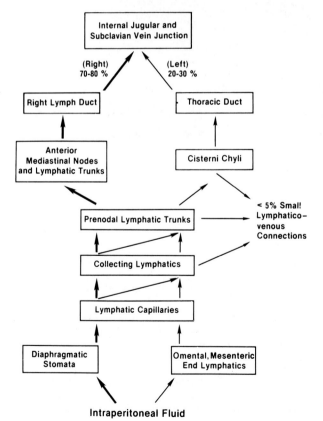

Figure 1. Anatomical pathways of lymphatic absorption of intra peritoneal fluid. (Reproduced with permission from ref. 36).

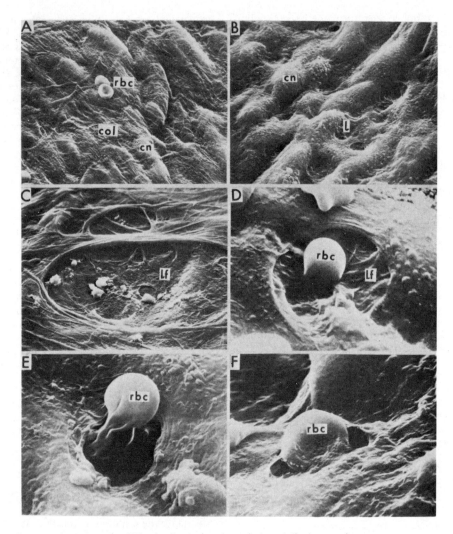

Figure 2. Scanning electron microscopy of red blood cells passing through the subdiaphragmatic stomata.
A.   Non-absorbing surface in the rat diaphragm; rbc, red blood cell; col, collagen fibers; cn, mesothelial cell nucleus. × 780.
B.   Absorbing surface overlying lymphatic lacunae (L) in the rat diaphragm. × 1200.
C.   Rabbit diaphragm showing the roof of a lacuna (Lf).
D.   Red blood cell passing through a slit in the roof of lacuna in the rabbit diaphragm. × 3120.
E.   Red blood cell passing between mesothelial cells in the rat diaphragm. × 4200.
F.   As for E. × 3780.
(Reproduced with permission from ref. 57).

Absorption by the peritoneal cavity lymphatics and phagocytosis by the resident intraperitoneal and omental macrophages are the first lines of defense after an inoculum of bacteria gains entry to the peritoneal cavity [68, 69]. The macrophages in the omentum provide an effective defense against bacteria but the omental lymphatics play only a minor role in the absorption of fluid from the peritoneal cavity [44]. Likewise, it is important to emphasize that although the lymphatics carrying fluid and solutes from the intestinal mucosa traverse the mesentery before draining into the cisterna chyli and the thoracic duct, they are not significantly involved in absorption of isosmotic fluid from the peritoneal cavity per se [2, 43].

2.5. Absorptive capacity of the peritoneal lymphatics

The lymphatics draining the peritoneal cavity, therefore, are virtually the only pathway for absorption of intraperitoneal isosmotic fluid, biologically inert particles, colloids and cells [2, 58, 65, 70]. Consequently the absorptive capacity of the peritoneal cavity lymphatics has been evaluated in normal animals from the rate of uptake of isosmotic fluid (plasma, whole blood, crystalloid solutions) infused into the peritoneal cavity [41–43, 71–80]. Representative values from these studies indicate that lymphatic absorption rates from the peritoneal cavity in animals and man are considerable (Table 1). Furthermore, obliteration

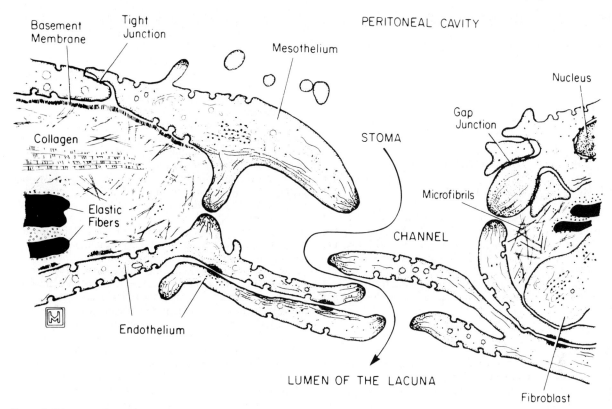

Figure 3. Diagram of a typical stoma and underlying channel linking the peritoneal cavity with the lumen of a lymphatic lacuna. (Reproduced with permission of ref. 54).

Table 1. Rates of isosmotic fluid absorption from the peritoneal cavity in different species

Species	Infusion volumes	Infused solution	Absorption rate	Ref.
Rat	20 ml (per kg)	Homologous plasma	6 ml/kg/hr	74
Rabbit	20 ml (per kg)	Homologous plasma	3.5 ml/kg/hr	74
Cat	50 ml (2.4-2.7 kg)	Homologous serum	4.2–6.0 ml/hr	43
Dog	1000 ml (13–18 kg)	0.9% Saline	16.8 ml/hr*	75
Man	1000 ml (45–86 kg)	0.9% Saline	33 ml/hr*	76

* After serum and intraperitoneal fluid reached osmolar equilibrium (ref. 75 and 76)

of the subdiaphragmatic peritoneum [43, 73] or ligation of the parasternal lymphatic trunks [74] greatly reduces the rate of intraperitoneal fluid absorption.

2.6. Factors controlling peritoneal lymphatic absorption

From studies performed mainly in animals, several physiological factors have been shown to alter the rate of lymphatic absorption from the peritoneal cavity. Hyperventilation, which was induced by breathing carbon dioxide, increased whereas anesthesia and acute phrenic neurectomy reduced lymphatic absorption [79, 80]. Lymphatic and peritoneal transcapillary absorption were both enhanced by increasing intraperitoneal hydrostatic pressure [78] and decreased after paracentesis [81]. Upright posture with small intraperitoneal volumes reduced the rate of lymphatic flow, although absorption still occurred due to propulsion of the intraperitoneal fluid towards the diaphragm by intestinal peristalsis [74]. Indeed, the circulation of intraperitoneal fluid towards the diaphragm is the most likely explanation for the relative frequency of abscess formation in the right subphrenic space following entry of bacteria into the peritoneal cavity [82]. Fowler successfully localized infection in the pelvis of patients with diffuse peritonitis by elevating the head of their beds by twelve to fifteen inches [83]. Even though obstruction of the peritoneal cavity lymphatics by fibrin or fibrosis may decrease lymphatic absorption after infectious peritonitis, chemical peritonitis induced by sodium hypochlorite was observed to increase the rate of lymphatic absorption in the recovery period [84]. This rise in lymphatic flow may be related to rapid regeneration of end lymphatics after injury [85]. The factors known to influence peritoneal lymphatic drainage are summarized in Table 2.

Table 2. Factors influencing lymphatic absorption from the peritoneal cavity

---

1. Intraperitoneal fluid volume.
2. Intraperitoneal hydrostatic pressure.
3. Rate and depth of respiration.
4. Posture.
5. Intestinal peristalsis.
6. Patency of the diaphragmatic and mediastinal lymphatics.

---

3. LYMPHATIC ABSORPTION IN ASCITES

3.1. Role in the pathophysiology of ascites

Ascites develops when the net transperitoneal inflow of fluid into peritoneal cavity exceeds the rate of fluid efflux via the peritoneal cavity lymphatics [3–8]. The fluid flux rate across the peritoneum (Jw) is determined by the product of peritoneal hydraulic permeability (Lp), the effective membrane area (A) and the sum of osmotic ($\Delta\pi$) and hydrostatic (ΔP) transmembrane pressure gradients. That is:

$$Jw = Lp.A \, (\Delta\pi + \Delta P). \qquad [1]$$

Accordingly, net inflow of fluid into the peritoneal cavity is observed in conditions where there is a rise in hepatic sinusoidal and portal venous hydrostatic pressure, a reduction in serum albumin concentration and/or an increase in peritoneal permeability. The accumulation of intraperitoneal fluid is countered by its continuous reabsorption by the peritoneal cavity lymphatics at a rate influenced by the volume of ascites, the intraperitoneal hydrostatic pressure and the patency of the lymphatic pathways (Table 2). This continuous bidirectional transport of fluid in ascites, however, precludes direct estimation of lymphatic drainage from the rate of absorption of isosmotic fluid as in normal animals (Table 1).

3.2. Lymphatic absorption rates in ascites

The peritoneal lymphatic absorption rate in ascites has been estimated indirectly from the rate of mass transfer of labelled colloids from the peritoneal cavity to the systemic circulation. This formulation is dependent on prior observations that intraperitoneal macromolecules (molecular weight greater than 20000) are returned to the venous circulation almost exclusively by the peritoneal lymphatics [2, 67, 86, 87] and that isosmotic intraperitoneal fluid is drained by the peritoneal lymphatics without change in the concentration of index macromolecules [77, 78, 88–90]. This methodology underestimates lymphatic absorption from the peritoneal cavity for several reasons. A significant proportion of the tracer colloid, absorbed by the peritoneal lymphatics, does not reach the systemic circulation during the study time due to delayed transit or permanent entrapment in the diaphragmatic and mediastinal lymph nodes. Indeed, this physiological function of the draining lymph nodes is utilized in mediastinal lymphoscintigraphy [10–13, 91]. Secondly, the rise in blood concentration of the tracer colloid must be corrected for redistribution of the tracer out of the blood volume during the study interval

[46, 67, 90]. Nevertheless, peritoneal to plasma mass transfer rates of radio-iodinated serum albumin [9, 10, 90] and other radio-colloids [10–13] have provided a valid comparison of the relative peritoneal lymphatic flow rates in patients with hepatic [9, 10, 90], malignant [10–13] and dialysis associated ascites [9]. Estimations of peritoneal lymphatic absorption by this method in 10 patients with hepatic ascites ranged from 24 to 223 ml per hour and averaged 80 ml per hour [9, 10, 90]. Presumably the large intraperitoneal fluid volume ensures constant contact of fluid with the undersurface of the diaphragm and the concurrent rise in intraperitoneal pressure enhances convective movement of fluid into the diaphragmatic lymphatics. In contrast, metastatic invasion of the subdiaphragmatic peritoneum is not uncommon in patients with intra-abdominal malignancy [92, 93] and may at least partially obstruct lymphatic drainage from the peritoneal cavity [14, 15]. Subdiaphragmatic lymphatic capillaries filled with malignant cells are shown in Figure 4. Peritoneal lymphatic absorption in 22 patients with malignant ascites ranged from 1 to 63 ml per hour and averaged only 11 ml per hour [10]. Mediastinal lymphoscintigraphy in patients with malignant ascites often failed to demonstrate patent diaphragmatic lymphatics or identify mediastinal lymph nodes [10–13]. Moreover, the calculated lymphatic absorption rate correlated with the concurrently performed lymphoscintigram [10]. Likewise, patients with schistosomal hepatic fibrosis and ascites have significant fibrous thickening of the subdiaphragmatic peritoneum, which most likely limits flow into the diaphragmatic lymphatics [16]. In support of this mechanism, obliteration of the diaphragm with fibrous tissue significantly increased the incidence and severity of ascites in animals with infrahepatic portal hypertension [94]. The role of lymphatic absorption in the pathophysiology of these different forms of ascites is summarized in Table 3.

4. ROLE OF LYMPHATIC ABSORPTION IN PERITONEAL DIALYSIS

4.1. Rationale

Several theoretical considerations and clinical observations support the concept that peritoneal cavity lymphatic absorption plays an important role in the kinetics of peritoneal dialysis 'ascites' and thereby significantly reduces potential net ultrafiltration and solute mass transfer after long-dwell exchanges:

1) Review of the anatomy and physiology of the peri-

Table 3. Transcapillary fluid influx and lymphatic absorption rates in ascites

Form of ascites	Net transcapillary fluid influx rate	Lymphatic absorption rate
Hepatic	++++	++
Malignant	+	−
Nephrogenic	+	−
Peritoneal Dialysis	+++	+?

Abbreviations: + increase; − decrease.

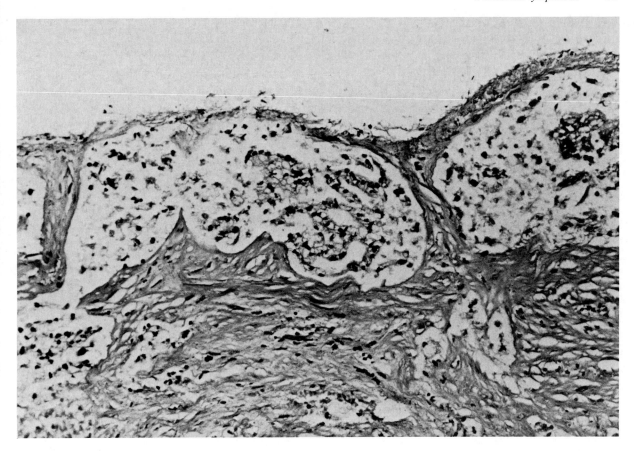

Figure 4. High power photomicrograph showing malignant cells partially occluding the subdiaphragmatic lymphatic capillaries in a patient with malignant ascites secondary to adenocarcinoma of the pancreas.

toneal cavity lymphatics has already shown that the absorptive capacity of the lymphatics is considerable (Tables 1 and 3).

2) In patients with ascites lymphatic drainage exceeds 50 ml per hour unless the diaphragmatic or mediastinal lymphatics are obstructed by tumor of fibrosis [10]. Intraperitoneal fluid volumes during peritoneal dialysis are routinely greater than 2 l and should also ensure continuous contact of fluid with the undersurface of the diaphragm. Furthermore, the patency of the peritoneal cavity lymphatics should be preserved in peritoneal dialysis if the subdiaphragmatic parietal peritoneum only undergoes the same minor histological changes as have been observed in the parietal peritoneum lining the anterior abdominal wall [95–97].

3) The ultrafiltrate from the peritoneal capillaries reaches the peritoneal cavity via pathways through the interstitium and consequently must bypass absorption by the lymphatics within the interstitium. Small increments in interstitial hydrostatic pressure are known to increase the lymphatic flow rate until a maximum is reached when tissue hydrostatic pressure is 2 mmHg above normal [98]. Even though the hydrostatic pressure within the peritoneal interstitium during peritoneal dialysis is unknown, submesothelial edema which is frequently observed in specimens of peritoneum from patients on CAPD [95, 96] may enhance fluid absorption by the interstitial lymphatics.

4) Isosmotic intraperitoneal fluid is absorbed primarily by the lymphatics [41–43, 74–80]. In nine uremic patients, an average of 546 ml of fluid was absorbed over seven hours after infusion of almost 2 l of 0.9% saline (308 mOsm/l) into the peritoneal cavity [99]. The average absorption rate of 78 ml per hour, however, may include net transcapillary absorption of fluid early in dwell time due to an initial osmotic gradient between infused isotonic saline and uremic plasma [100].

5) In hypertonic peritoneal dialysis the intraperitoneal fluid volume begins to decrease before isosmolality of the dialysis solution and plasma is observed [29, 32], indicating that net fluid absorption occurs before net transcapillary ultrafiltration is complete (Figure 5). In addition, osmolar equilibrium is reached before osmotic pressure and glucose equilibrium [29]. The dialysis solution becomes isosmolar with the plasma before glucose equilibrium because of solute sieving with transcapillary ultrafiltration [24, 25, 101]. The total transperitoneal osmotic pressure gradient is the sum of the products of the concentration gradient and the peritoneal reflection coefficient of each solute. Accordingly, the higher peritoneal reflection coefficient of glucose than other small molecular weight solutes [102] tends to maintain an osmotic pressure gradient into the dialysis solution after isosmolality is reached and thereby allows net transcapillary

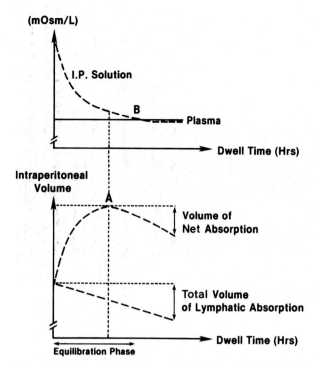

Figure 5. Changes in osmolality and intraperitoneal fluid volume following infusion of a hypertonic dextrose dialysis solution. The peak intraperitoneal volume (point A) precedes osmolar equilibrium (point B). Thereafter net fluid absorption represents lymphatic absorption in excess of net transcapillary ultrafiltration. (Reproduced with permission from ref. 36).

ultrafiltration to continue at a slow rate until osmotic pressure equilibrium is approached later in the dwell time. This mechanism has also been invoked to explain the net ultrafiltration observed following intraperitoneal infusion of electrolyte-free 5% dextrose solution (252 mOsm/l) [102]. Since the dialysis solution becomes hypoosmolar to the plasma towards the end of the dwell time [37, 38], this further suggests that net transcapillary ultrafiltration continues after osmolar equilibrium is first observed. Consequently the reduction in intraperitoneal volume (ΔV) after peak ultrafiltration really represents the lymphatic absorption rate (L) in excess of the concurrent net transcapillary ultrafiltration rate (Jw in equation 1). Thus,

$$\Delta V = Lp.A\,(\Delta \pi + \Delta P) - L. \qquad [2]$$

Direct measurements of drain volumes after sequential dwell times in 29 CAPD patients showed that the rate of decrease in the intraperitoneal volume ranged from 8 to 89 ml per hour and averaged 39 ml per hour [28, 29]. The net absorption rate was not significantly different, irrespective of whether 2 l volumes of 1.5%, 2.5% or 4.25% dextrose dialysis solution were instilled [28, 29]. Moreover, net absorption rates during dialysis with 2.5 l infusion volumes also averaged 37 ml per hour in 16 CAPD patients [26].

In conclusion, by analogy with ascites and by extrapolation from previous studies of drain volumes after infusion of isotonic and hypertonic solutions, the average daily lymphatic absorption rate during CAPD may be predicted to be at least 1 l per day.

4.2. Definitions

The existing terminology used to describe the kinetics of peritoneal dialysis has been modified to incorporate the role of the peritoneal cavity lymphatics [36–39]. The measurable net ultrafiltration volume represents the net change in the intraperitoneal fluid volume at the end of the dwell time and, assuming that the residual volume remains constant, equals the dialysate drain volume minus the infusion volume. However, as discussed above (equation 2), the net ultrafiltration volume is, in effect, the difference between cumulative net transcapillary ultrafiltration *into* the peritoneal cavity and total lymphatic absorption *out* of the peritoneal cavity during the dwell time (Figure 6). These two formulations of net ultrafiltration may be designated directly measured and calculated net ultrafiltration (UF), respectively. That is:

> Measured net UF = drain volume – infusion volume
> Calculated net UF = cumulative net transcapillary UF
>   – lymphatic absorption

Cumulative net transcapillary ultrafiltration defines the total net influx of fluid from the peritoneal microcirculation into the peritoneal cavity during the dwell time in response to the osmotic pressure of the dialysis solution. This definition allows for bidirectional transcapillary water movement during the dwell time but acknowledges that inflow into the peritoneal cavity dominates and that only the *net* fluid flux can be measured. The resultant net inflow of fluid would equal measured net ultrafiltration if it was not for cumulative drainage via the lymphatics during the dwell time (Figure 6).

4.3. Methods of estimating lymphatic absorption

Peritoneal lymphatic flow rates in hypertonic peritoneal dialysis can only be estimated indirectly since the changes in intraperitoneal volume after any given dwell time reflect the balance of cumulative net transcapillary ultrafiltration and lymphatic absorption. Two methods have been described for measuring lymphatic drainage during peritoneal dialysis [35–39, 46]. Both apply the same physiological functions of the peritoneal cavity lymphatics. By assuming that intraperitoneal marker colloids are returned to the systemic circulation exclusively by the lymphatics and that intraperitoneal fluid is drained by the peritoneal lymphatics

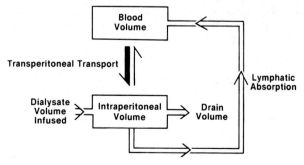

Figure 6. Schematic representation of the role of lymphatic absorption in the kinetics of peritoneal dialysis. (Reproduced with permission from ref. 36).

without increase or decrease in concentration of index colloids [2, 67, 77, 86–90], the lymphatic absorption rate may be estimated either from the mass transfer rate of marker colloids from the peritoneal cavity to the blood [35, 46] or from their rate of disappearance from the peritoneal cavity [36–39].

4.3.1. Mass transfer rates of intraperitoneal colloids to the blood

The first method essentially represents the peritoneal to blood clearance of a radio-labelled colloid. That is:

$$L = \frac{V_D \times \Delta C_D}{C_p} \qquad [3]$$

where

L = total lymphatic flow during the time of the study
V_D = volume of distribution of the tracer colloid (plasma volume)
ΔC_D = rise in plasma concentration of the tracer colloid
C_p = time averaged mean intraperitoneal concentration of the tracer colloid.

Using this approach, the average lymphatic absorption rate in 10 CAPD patients was only 11 ml per hour [35], compared with the aforementioned predicted rate from serial drain volumes of at least 39 ml per hour [28, 29]. The absolute lymphatic absorption rate during CAPD was underestimated in this study since the plasma volume of the CAPD patients was extrapolated from their body weight, the elimination rate of the radio-colloid from the plasma was not included in the initial calculations and, most importantly, the plasma appearance rate of radio-iodinated serum albumin, as in similar studies in patients with ascites [90, 103], was only 20% of the peritoneal disappearance rate. As well as confirming that there is an initial lag phase before the plasma concentration of the radio-colloid begins to increase linearly [9, 10, 46, 90], Spencer and Farrell have recently shown that the mass transfer of intraperitoneal radio-iodinated albumin to the blood in CAPD patients was significantly greater after 24 hours than after the end of a four hour study exchange [33]. Thus, lymphatic transfer of radio-colloids continues after the washout exchange at the end of the study time and cannot be accurately timed to the duration of the exchange. These factors also explain why lymphatic flow rates calculated by this method are much lower than direct observations of absorption of intraperitoneal plasma or whole blood in the same animal model [41, 46].

4.3.2. Mass transfer rates of colloids from the peritoneal cavity

Alternatively the lymphatic absorption rate (L) may be estimated from the mass transfer rate of intraperitoneal macromolecules from the peritoneal cavity. That is:

$$L = \frac{(V_0 \times C_0) - (V_t \times C_t)}{C_p} \qquad [4]$$

where

V_0 and V_t = intraperitoneal fluid volumes at time 0 and t
C_0 and C_t = intraperitoneal concentration of marker colloid at times 0 and t

C_p = time averaged mean intraperitoneal concentration of marker colloid.

This mass balance equation avoids the error in calculating lymphatic flow in the previous method due to delayed transfer of radio-labelled colloids from the diaphragm and interstitial lymphatics to the blood. This formulation, however, not only depends on the assumption that intraperitoneal macromolecules are absorbed exclusively from the peritoneal cavity by convective flow via the lymphatics, but further assumes that all of the intraperitoneal marker colloid lost from the peritoneal cavity is absorbed by the non-restrictive pathways of the lymphatics. In connective tissue spaces, back diffusion of colloids into capillaries is negligible [104], the osmolality and the concentration of protein in the tissue fluid and end lymphatic lymph are equal [98, 105] and absorption of tissue protein is fully accounted for by lymphatic flow [104, 106]. Several observations indicate that these findings also pertain to intraperitoneal fluid and colloid kinetics and that intraperitoneal fluid absorption may be estimated from the rate of loss of an intraperitoneal marker colloid.

a) The concentration of marker colloids remains unchanged during absorption of intraperitoneal isosmotic fluid [41, 46, 47], suggesting that colloids are absorbed with fluid by convective transport presumably through lymphatic pathways.

b) Fractional peritoneal absorption of albumin and IgG [90] and gelatins of different molecular weight [107] are similar, further suggesting that absorption of macromolecules is by convective flow.

c) The intraperitoneal content of radio-iodinated serum albumin during hypertonic peritoneal dialysis decreases at a linear rate averaging 3% per hour [35] and, late in the dwell time, correlates with net fluid absorption [32, 35].

However, with microquantities of radio-colloid, a significant proportion of the administered dosage may be absorbed to the peritoneal mesothelium, dialysis bag and administration set or be absorbed by the adjacent subperitoneal tissues [35, 46, 108]. The addition of a large quantity of unlabelled colloid, such as albumin, instead of microamounts of radio-labelled colloid should obviate this potential error. Thus, lymphatic absorption during peritoneal dialysis may theoretically be estimated most accurately from the net rate of removal of high intraperitoneal concentration of a colloid from the peritoneal cavity. Cumulative net transcapillary ultrafiltration can be estimated concurrently from the dilution of the initial dialysate marker colloid concentration [38, 39] since the intraperitoneal colloid concentration is unchanged by lymphatic absorption of intraperitoneal fluid [86, 87] and thus any decrease in the dialysate colloid concentration during the dwell time results from net influx of fluid from the peritoneal microcirculation.

4.4. Rates of lymphatic absorption during peritoneal dialysis

The above method has been utilized to study lymphatic drainage during peritoneal dialysis in a rat model [37] and in CAPD patients [38, 109].

4.4.1. Peritoneal dialysis in rats

Serial direct measurements of net ultrafiltration and calculated concurrent lymphatic absorption rates during six

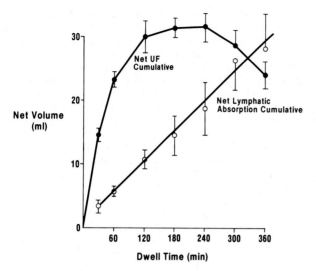

Figure 7. Cumulative lymphatic absorption and cumulative net ultrafiltration (mean ± SEM) during six hour exchanges with 15% dextrose dialysis solution in rats. (Reproduced with permission from ref. 37).

hour exchanges in rats using 17 ± 0.3 (SEM) ml of 15% dextrose dialysis solution are depicted in Figure 7. Cumulative net ultrafiltration began to decrease after the four hour dwell time whereas cumulative lymphatic absorption increased almost linearly throughout the exchange [37]. Consequently in this study lymphatic drainage proceeded at a nearly constant rate and at the end of the six hour dwell time reabsorbed greater than half of the total cumulative transcapillary ultrafiltration during the exchange. Further analysis of the temporal relationships of key events during these exchanges showed that the peak intraperitoneal volume was observed before osmolar equilibrium between

the dialysis solution and plasma was reached (Figure 8). Transperitoneal osmolar equilibrium in turn preceded glucose equilibrium (Figure 8). Therefore the peak intraperitoneal volume occurs when the net transcapillary ultrafiltration rate has fallen exponentially to equal the lymphatic absorption rate. At this point the overall net ultrafiltration rate is zero. Thereafter, the intraperitoneal volume decreases even though net transcapillary ultrafiltration continues at a slow rate and osmolar equilibrium is not reached until later in the dwell time.

During similar exchanges using near isosmotic Ringer's lactate solution instead of hypertonic dextrose dialysis solution, lymphatic absorption also continued at a relatively constant rate and correlated closely (r = 0.98) with directly measured net fluid absorption (Figure 9). Moreover, as in previous studies [46, 67], the concentration of the intraperitoneal marker colloid remained constant during the absorption of the isosmotic intraperitoneal fluid. These observations suggest that absorption of isosmotic intraperitoneal fluid is primarily by convective flow via the peritoneal cavity lymphatics. The calculated lymphatic absorption rates during these studies are comparable to direct measurements of absorption rates following intraperitoneal infusion of homologous plasma in the rat [74] and provide further support for utilizing the above method to estimate lymphatic absorption rates during peritoneal dialysis.

4.4.2. Peritoneal dialysis in man
Cumulative lymphatic absorption during standardized four hour peritoneal dialysis exchanges using 2 l of 2.5% dextrose dialysis solution (Dianeal[R] PD-2) with 30 g added human serum albumin averaged 343 ± 39 (SEM) ml in 18 stable CAPD patients [109]. These lymphatic absorption rates are consistent with prior observations in patients with ascites who have no fibrosis or tumor invasion of the diaphrag-

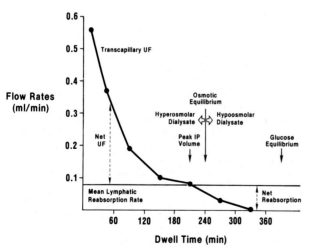

Figure 8. The net transcapillary ultrafiltration rate (mean ± SEM) and mean lymphatic absorption rate are related to dwell time and key events during exchanges with 15% dextrose dialysis solution in rats. The peak intraperitoneal volume precedes osmotic equilibrium which in turn preceses glucose equilibrium. (Reproduced with permission from ref. 37).

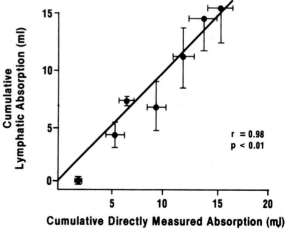

Figure 9. Cumulative lymphatic absorption (mean ± SEM), calculated by the albumin absorption method, is related to directly measured fluid absorption (mean ± SEM) during six hour exchanges with Ringer's lactate solution in rats. The identity line is shown. (Reproduced with permission from ref. 37).

matic and mediastinal lymphatics [10–13, 90] and have a major influence on ultrafiltration kinetics in long-dwell peritoneal dialysis exchanges (Figure 10). Due to cumulative lymphatic absorption, peak net ultrafiltration occurred near the two hour dwell time and calculated net ultrafiltration at the end of the exchanges averaged only 44 ± 6% of the total net transcapillary ultrafiltration volume during the four hour dwell time (Figure 10). As in hypertonic peritoneal dialysis in the rat [37], the maximum intraperitoneal volume during CAPD exchanges preceded osmolar equilibrium which in turn preceded glucose equilibrium between serum and the dialysis solution (Figure 11). If lymphatic absorption during CAPD is assumed to be constant [37], the maximum intraperitoneal volume, and hence the peak ultrafiltration volume, is observed when the net transcapillary rate has decreased to equal the lymphatic absorption rate (Figure 12). Since net transcapillary ultrafiltration is not yet complete at this point, the net absorption rate represents the lymphatic absorption rate minus the concurrent net transcapillary ultrafiltration rate (Figure 12). These calculated net fluid absorption rates after peak ultrafiltration are in agreement with absorption rates derived from sequential direct measurements of dialysate drain volumes in CAPD patients [28, 29] and infer that net fluid absorption in CAPD is mainly due to the peritoneal cavity lymphatics.

Lymphatic absorption rates in these studies may be higher than in active CAPD patients since the exchanges were all performed with the patient supine and fluid contact with the diaphragm may have been more extensive than if the patient was in the upright posture [74]. Alternatively, the increase in intraperitoneal pressure with upright posture [110, 111] may tend to increase lymphatic absorption in active CAPD patients [78]. None of the patients were studied within three months of peritonitis since acute peritonitis may alter lymphatic absorption rates [84]. Even though seven of the 18 CAPD patients in this study had 20 prior episodes of peritonitis, the lymphatic absorption rates were unrelated to the frequency of peritonitis. This observation suggests that CAPD associated peritonitis has no significant long-term effect on the patency or function of the peritoneal cavity lymphatics. However, the influence of posture and peritonitis on lymphatic absorption rates during CAPD has still to be evaluated.

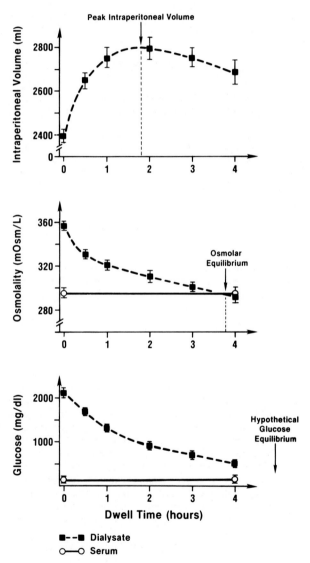

Figure 11. Intraperitoneal volume, serum and dialysate osmolality and glucose concentrations (mean ± SEM) during four hour exchanges in 18 CAPD patients using 2 l of 2.5% dextrose dialysis solution. Arrows indicate peak intraperitoneal volume, osmolar equilibrium and hypothetical glucose equilibrium. (Reproduced with permission from ref. 109).

Figure 10. Cumulative lymphatic absorption, net ultrafiltration and cumulative net transcapillary ultrafiltration (mean ± SEM) during four hour exchanges in 18 CAPD patients using 2 l of 2.5% dextrose dialysis solution. (Reproduced with permission from ref. 109).

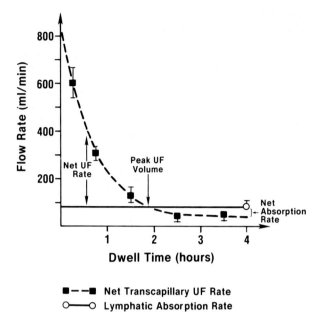

Figure 12. Net transcapillary ultrafiltration and lymphatic absorption rates (mean ± SEM) during four hour exchanges in 18 CAPD patients using 2 l of 2.5% dextrose dialysis solution. Peak ultrafiltration volume (arrowed) occurs when the net transcapillary ultrafiltration rate equals the lymphatic absorption rate. (Reproduced with permission from ref. 109).

4.5. Consequences of lymphatic absorption during peritoneal dialysis

The physiological roles of the peritoneal cavity lymphatics in the absorption of intraperitoneal isosmotic fluid, macromolecules, particles and bacteria are normally beneficial. However, lymphatic absorption has mainly adverse effects on the clinical application of long-dwell peritoneal dialysis as an effective form of renal replacement therapy.

4.5.1. Loss of ultrafiltration
Lymphatic drainage of intraperitoneal fluid throughoiut the dwell time significantly reduces the potential drain volume and, thus net ultrafiltration, in all CAPD patients [38]. Since net transcapillary ultrafiltration occurs mainly during the first hours of each exchange whereas lymphatic absorption is continuous (Figure 12), fluid absorption via the lymphatics has a greater influence on ultrafiltration kinetics in CAPD than in intermittent peritoneal dialysis with rapid exchanges. In short-dwell exchanges cumulative net transcapillary ultrafiltration greatly exceeds lymphatic drainage and consequently the reduction in the dialysate drain volume resulting from lymphatic absorption is relatively minor.

Wide interindividual [112–116] and intraindividual [117–120] variation in net ultrafiltration has been observed in CAPD patients even if the dwell time, osmolality and volume of exchanges are standardized. Poor peritoneal ultrafiltration capacity has usually been ascribed to high peritoneal permeability × area, rapid absorption of glucose from the dialysate, early dissipation of the transperitoneal

osmolar gradient and thus reduced cumulative net transcapillary ultrafiltration [115–120]. In addition, since transperitoneal osmotic pressure is equivalent to the sum of the products of the osmolar gradient and the peritoneal reflection coefficient of each solute, the lower peritoneal reflection coefficient for glucose in patients with high peritoneal permeability × area will further reduce transcapillary ultrafiltration (Jw) by generating reduced osmotic pressure ($\Delta\pi$) at any given glucose concentration gradient (equation 1). Interpatient differences in peritoneal ultrafiltration capacity after long-dwell exchanges may, however, depend on lymphatic absorption as well as peritoneal permeability × area (equation 2).

The influence of lymphatic drainage in ultrafiltration kinetics was compared in adult CAPD patients with normal and high peritoneal permeability × area [38, 109]. The patients were divided into two groups using peritoneal transport rates (dialysate/serum urea and creatinine and effluent/initial dialysate glucose ratios) during the standardized study exchanges as indices of peritoneal permeability × area [116, 121]. All patients remained supine during the four hour exchanges using 2 l of 2.5% dextrose dialysis solution with 30 g added albumin. Ten patients (group 1) had urea, creatinine and glucose ratios within the normal range (± 1 SD) and eight patients (group 2) had dialysate/serum urea and creatinine ratios greater than 1 SD above the mean (Figures 13 and 14) and effluent/initial dialysate glucose more than 1 SD below the mean of the CAPD population at the University of Missouri-Columbia (Figure 15). The mean age, duration of CAPD and number of

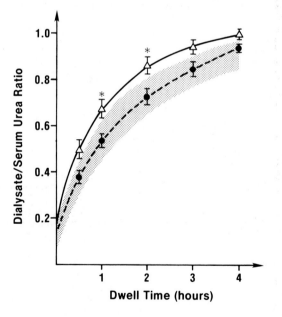

Figure 13. Dialysate/serum urea ratios (mean ± SEM) during four hour exchanges using 2 l of 2.5% dextrose dialysis solution in groups 1 and 2 with average and high peritoneal permeability × area, respectively. The reference range (mean ± 1 SD) is shaded. (Reproduced with permission from ref. 109.) (*p<0.05.)

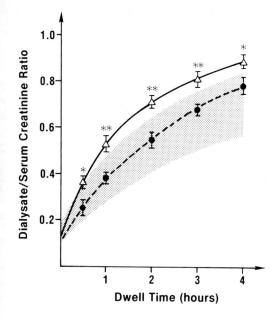

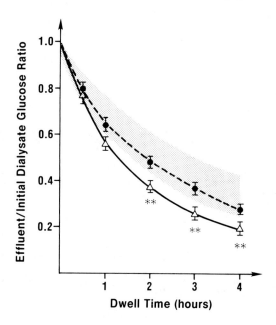

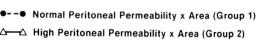

●--● Normal Peritoneal Permeability x Area (Group 1)

△—△ High Peritoneal Permeability x Area (Group 2)

●--● Average Peritoneal Glucose Transport (Group 1)

△—△ High Peritoneal Glucose Transport (Group 2)

Figure 14. Dialysate/serum creatinine ratios (mean ± SEM) during four hour exchanges using 2 l of 2.5% dextrose dialysis solution in groups 1 and 2 with average and high peritoneal permeability × area, respectively. (Reproduced with permission from ref. 109). (**p<0.01; *p<0.05.)

Figure 15. Effluent/initial dialysate glucose ratios (mean ± SEM) during four hour exchanges using 2 l of 2.5% dextrose dialysis solution in groups 1 and 2 with average and high peritoneal permeability × area, respectively. (Reproduced with permission from ref. 109). (**p<0.01.)

previous episodes of peritonitis did not differ between the two groups. None of the patients had peritonitis within three months of study [119], none had clinical or biochemical features of chronic liver disease, none had evidence of extraperitoneal dialysate leaks and all of the patients had only used lactate containing dialysis solution. Ultrafiltration kinetics in each group are shown in Figure 16. Cumulative net transcapillary ultrafiltration at the end of the exchanges in patients with normal peritoneal permeability × area (group 1) averaged 806 ± 77 ml and in patients with high peritoneal permeability × area (group 2) averaged 536 ± 92 (p < 0.05), whereas cumulative lymphatic absorption over the four hour dwell time did not differ between the two groups (332 ± 65 ml in group 1 and 356 ± 36 ml in group 2). As expected, peak intraperitoneal volume and transperitoneal osmolar equilibrium were observed earlier in the dwell time during the exchanges in group 2 (Figure 17). Thus, even though lymphatic absorption rates were similar in both groups, lymphatic drainage caused a proportionately greater reduction in net ultrafiltration in patients with high peritoneal permeability × area since these patients had more rapid absorption of glucose from the dialysis solution (Figure 15), earlier loss of the transperitoneal osmolar gradient (Figure 17) and lower cumulative net transcapillary ultrafiltration (Figure 16). Extrapolated to four exchanges with 2 l of 2.5% dextrose dialysis solution per day, the group 2 patients with high peritoneal permeability × area had negative daily ultrafiltration even though daily net transcapillary ultrafiltration averaged 2.1

± 0.4 l per day (Figure 18). Consequently, in the absence of a dialysate leak, failure of peritoneal ultrafiltration occurs in CAPD patients when daily lymphatic absorption equals or exceeds daily net transcapillary ultrafiltration.

The contribution of lymphatic absorption to loss of ultrafiltration has also been evaluated during similar exchanges in six children on peritoneal dialysis [122]. Dialysis mechanics in children of differing body size were standardized by performing four hour exchanges using 40 ml/kg of 1.5% albumin, 2.5% dextrose dialysis solution in each child. To enable analysis of group data from exchanges with variable infusion volumes, lymphatic absorption, cumulative net transcapillary ultrafiltration and net ultrafiltration were expressed either as a percentage of the intraperitoneal volume at the beginning of each exchange (Figure 19) or in relation to body surface area (Table 4). Calculated net ultrafiltration at the end of the exchanges represented only 27 ± 10% of total net transcapillary ultrafiltration during the dwell time (Figure 19). When compared to adult CAPD patients with average peritoneal permeability × area (group 1), maximum intraperitoneal volume was observed earlier in the dwell time at around 90 minutes (Figure 19) and glucose was absorbed more rapidly from the dialysate (Figure 20). Indeed, the kinetics of ultrafiltration in children (Figures 19 and 20) simulate adults with high peritoneal permeability × area (Figures 15 and 16). Moreover, net ultrafiltration, scaled for body weight, was confirmed to be lower in children than in adults [123–125] and is most likely due to a combination of

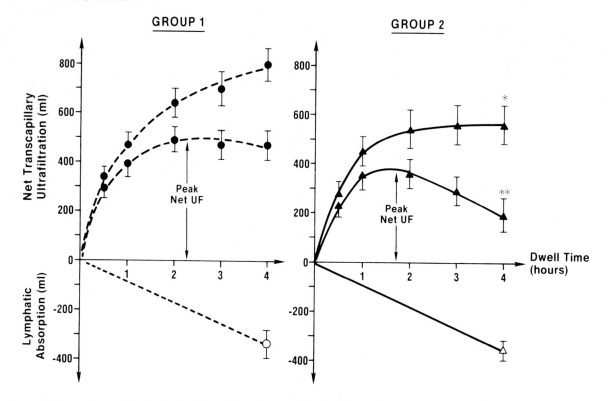

Figure 16. Comparison of cumulative lymphatic absorption, net ultrafiltration and cumulative net transcapillary ultrafiltration (mean ± SEM) during four hour exchanges using 2 l of 2.5% dextrose dialysis solution in CAPD patients with average (group 1) and high (group 2) peritoneal permeability × area. (Reproduced with permission from ref. 109). (**p<0.01; *p<0.05.)

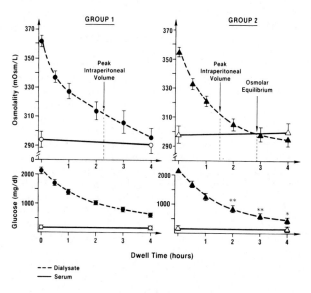

Figure 17. Comparison of serum and dialysate osmolality and glucose concentrations (mean ± SEM) during four hour exchanges using 2 l of 2.5% dextrose dialysis solution in CAPD patients with average (group 1) and high (group 2) peritoneal permeability × area. Arrows indicate peak intraperitoneal volume and osmolar equilibrium. (Reproduced with permission from ref. 109). (**p<0.01; *p<0.05.)

relatively lower net transcapillary ultrafiltration and higher lymphatic absorption (Table 4).

These findings indicate that net ultrafiltration volumes are significantly decreased by cumulative lymphatic absorption after long-dwell exchanges in all CAPD patients. Nevertheless lymphatic drainage produces a relatively greater reduction in net ultrafiltration in adults with high peritoneal permeability × area and in children. This observation explains why these two groups of patients often require shorter dwell times to capture maximum ultrafiltration, to avoid fluid absorption later in the dwell time and thereby to achieve desired daily net ultrafiltration. Ultrafiltration failure is observed in patients with high peritoneal permeability × area (Type 1 membrane failure) when, despite reducing the dwell time and/or increasing the osmolality of exchanges, daily net transcapillary ultrafiltration is less than daily lymphatic absorption.

4.5.2. Loss of solute mass transfer

The continuous absorption of dialysate solutes by convective flow via the peritoneal cavity lymphatics significantly decreases solute mass transfer during CAPD [38, 109]. Peritoneal solute clearances were calculated as the product of daily drain volume and drain dialysate solute concentration divided by the mean serum solute concentration while reverse solute clearances (via the lymphatics) were estimated from the product of daily lymphatic drainage and mean dialysate solute concentration divided by the

Table 4. Comparison of ultrafiltration kinetics in children and in adults with average peritoneal permeability × area

	Children (N = 6)	*Adults (N = 10)*
Infusion volume	1333 + 156	1254 ± 63
Total transcapillary UF	406 ± 61	430 ± 42
Lymphatic flow	271 ± 48	180 ± 36
Measured net UF	111 ± 52	237 ± 26*

Results (mean ± SEM) after a four hour exchange using 2.5% dextrose dialysis solution were expressed as ml/m² estimated body surface area.
*p < 0.05 by Student's t-test.

mean serum solute concentration. Extrapolated to four exchanges using 2 l of 2.5% dextrose dialysis solution per day, lymphatic drainage in 18 CAPD patients reduced the potential daily drain volume by 18 ± 2%, potential daily urea clearance by 14 ± 1.4% and potential daily creatinine clearance by 13.3 ± 1.5% (Figure 21). Similar calculations in children using four exchanges of 40 ml/kg of 2.5% dextrose dialysis solution per day found that the reduction in daily potential urea and creatinine clearances due to lymphatic absorption (Figure 22) was even greater than in adults (p < 0.05) [126]. These findings indicate that estimates of transperitoneal solute transport, which are based on the dialysate drain volume and solute concentration, are erroneously low since no allowance has been

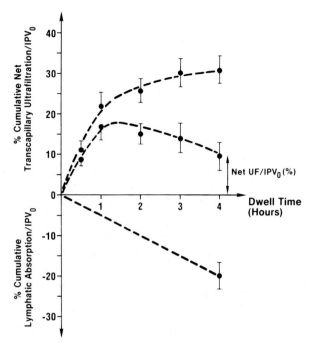

Figure 19. Cumulative net transcapillary ultrafiltration, lymphatic absorption and net ultrafiltration (mean ± SEM) during four hour exchanges in children using 40 ml/kg of 2.5% dextrose dialysis solution. All values are expressed as a percentage of the intra-peritoneal volume at the beginning of the exchange (IPV_0).

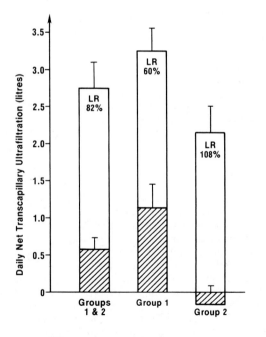

LR Daily Lymphatic Reabsorption

/// Daily Net Ultrafiltration/Absorption

Figure 18. Daily net transcapillary ultrafiltration, lymphatic absorption and net ultrafiltration (mean ± SEM) in CAPD patients with average (group 1) and high (group 2) peritoneal permeability × area using four exchanges of 2 l, 2.5% dextrose dialysis solution per day. (Reproduced with permission from ref. 109).

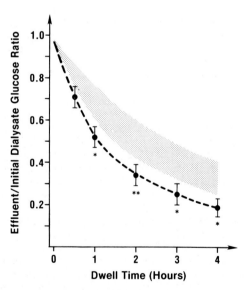

Figure 20. Effluent/initial dialysate glucose ratios (mean ± SEM) during exchanges with 2.5% dextrose dialysis solution in children. The reference range (mean ± 1 SD) in adults is shaded. Glucose ratios in children and adults with average peritoneal permeability × area (group 1, Figure 14) were compared by Student's t-test. (**p<0.01; *p<0.05.)

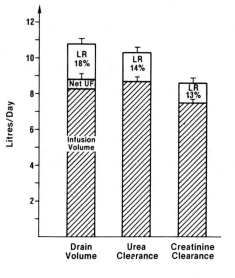

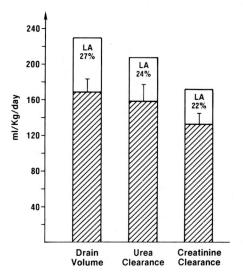

Figure 21. Contribution of lymphatic absorption to loss of potential daily drain volume, urea clearance and creatinine clearance (mean ± SEM) in adult CAPD patients (n = 18) using four exchanges of 2 l of 2.5% dextrose dialysis solution per day.

Figure 22. Contribution of lymphatic absorption to loss of daily drain volumes and solute clearances in children using four exchanges with 40 ml/kg of 2.5% dextrose dialysis solution per day. Observed drain volumes and solute clearances (mean ± SEM) are expressed as ml/kg/day.

made for translymphatic absorption throughout the dwell time. Accordingly the efficiency of the peritoneum as a dialyzing membrane is greater than previously recognized [27, 33, 34, 127–130] and a reduction in lymphatic absorption may therefore provide an alternative means of increasing net ultrafiltration and solute mass transfer without requiring enhanced transperitoneal transport of water and solutes into the peritoneal cavity. Preliminary studies in a rat model of peritoneal dialysis suggest that drug manipulation of lymphatic drainage can augment the efficiency of long-dwell peritoneal dialysis [131, 132].

4.5.3. Absorption of intraperitoneal bacteria

The uptake of intraperitoneal bacteria by the peritoneal cavity lymphatics is well established [133, 134]. Nevertheless, blood cultures are infrequently positive during CAPD associated peritonitis [135] and secondary pulmonary infections or right sided endocarditis are very rare complications of peritonitis [69, 135]. The bacteria are presumably filtered and effectively trapped by the mediastinal lymph nodes.

Transient loss of peritoneal ultrafiltration capacity is observed during episodes of CAPD associated peritonitis and results, at least in part, from a temporary rise in peritoneal permeability, increase in glucose absorption from the dialysate and subsequent reduction in transcapillary ultrafiltration [119, 136, 137]. The lymphatic trunks have inherent contractility as well as innervation by non-myelinated autonomic fibers [138, 139]. Since the contractility of the lymphatic trunks is increased by prostaglandins and leukotrienes [140] and these mediators of inflammation are transiently elevated in the dialysis solution of CAPD

patients with peritonitis [141], loss of ultrafiltration during episodes of CAPD peritonitis may be related to an increase in lymphatic absorption as well as reduced transcapillary ultrafiltration. However, the role of lymphatic absorption in ultrafiltration kinetics during CAPD associated peritonitis has yet to be evaluated.

4.5.4. Absorption of intraperitoneal polymers and particles

The uptake of large solutes and particles by convective flow into the peritoneal cavity lymphatics has several implications for peritoneal dialysis. Alternative, less absorbable osmotic agents than glucose have been sought to reduce the undesired metabolic sequelae of dialysate glucose absorption and, most importantly, to induce sustained net transcapillary ultrafiltration [31, 142–146]. However, lymphatic drainage results in significant systemic absorption of all polymer osmotic agents [146, 147], regardless of their molecular weight, and has hindered the development of safe and effective alternative osmotic agents to glucose. Consequently, despite initial promising results, the routine clinical use of glucose polymer as an osmotic agent has been limited by its systemic absorption and potential toxicity [143–146].

Particulate material entering the peritoneal cavity in the dialysis solution will also be absorbed by the peritoneal cavity lymphatics. Thus contaminants in commerical dialysis solutions should be avoided to prevent their systemic accumulation and toxicity as well as their potentially adverse effects on the peritoneal membrane [114, 148]. Human recombinant erythropoietin (molecular weight = 34 000) has been shown to correct anemia in chronic hemodialysis patients [149, 150] and, absorption via the peritoneal lymphatics following intraperitoneal infusion in the dialysis solution may provide a convenient and adequate route of administration in CAPD patients, especially if instilled in the long-dwell exchange overnight.

5. CONCLUSION

Lymphatic absorption rates during peritoneal dialysis are considerable and have a major influence on the kinetics of ultrafiltration in long-dwell exchanges. The currently available range of glucose containing dialysis solutions has been developed to induce sufficient net transcapillary ultrafiltration to offset lymphatic drainage and therefore achieve adequate daily peritoneal ultrafiltration in most CAPD patients. Nevertheless, a reduction in lymphatic drainage during peritoneal dialysis would allow either an increase in the efficiency of long-dwell peritoneal dialysis by augmenting ultrafiltration and solute removal or alternatively, decreases in the osmolality of currently used dialysis solutions. The pharmacological manipulationn of lymphatic absorption therefore merits further investigation.

REFERENCES

1. Allen L: Lymphatics and lymphoid tissues. Ann Rev Physiol 29: 197, 1967.
2. Courtice FC, Steinbeck AW: The lymphatic drainage of plasma from the peritoneal cavity of the cat. Austral J Exp Biol Med Sci 28: 161, 1950.
3. Hyatt RE, Smith JR: The mechanisms of ascites: physiological appraisal. Am J Med 16: 434, 1954.
4. Courtice FC: Ascites: the role of the lymphatics in the accumulation of ascitic fluid. Med J Aust 26: 945, 1959.
5. Witte MH, Witte CL, Dumont AE: Progress in liver disease: physiological factors involved in the causation of cirrhotic ascites. Gastroenterology 61: 742, 1971.
6. Levy M: Pathophysiology of ascites formation. In: Epstein M (ed), The Kidney in Liver Disease (2nd edition). New York, Elsevier Biomedical, p. 245, 1983.
7. Barrowman JA: Liver lymph. In: Barrowman JA (ed), Physiology of the Gastrointestinal Lymphatic System. Cambridge, Cambridge University Press, p. 229, 1978.
8. Witte CL, Witte MH, Dumont AE: Lymph imbalance in the genesis and perpetuation of the ascites syndrome in hepatic cirrhosis. Gastroenterology 78: 1059, 1980.
9. Morgan AG, Terry SI: Impaired peritoneal fluid drainage in nephrogenic ascites. Clin Nephrol 15: 61, 1981.
10. Bronskill MJ, Bush RS, Ege GN: A quantitative measurement of peritoneal drainage in malignant ascites. Cancer 40: 2375, 1977.
11. Coates G, Bush RS, Aspin N: A study of ascites using lymphoscintigraphy with 99m Tc sulfur colloid. Radiology 107: 577, 1973.
12. Atkins HL, Hauser W, Richards P: Visualization of mediastinal lymph nodes after intraperitoneal administrations of 99m Tc sulfur colloid. Nuclear-medizin 9: 275, 1970.
13. Kroon BBR: Over het ontstaan en de chirurgische behandeling van maligne ascites. M.D. Thesis, University of Amsterdam, 1986.
14. Feldman GB, Knapp RC: Lymphatic drainage of the peritoneal cavity and its significance in ovarian cancer.
15. Feldman GB: Lymphatic obstruction in carcinomatous ascites. Cancer Res 35: 325, 1975.
16. Ismail AH, Mohamed FS: Structural changes of the diaphragmatic peritoneum in patients with schistosomal hepatic fibrosis in relation to ascites. Lymphology 19: 82, 1986.
17. Clausen J: Studies on the effect of intraperitoneal blood transfusion. Acta Paediat 27: 24, 1940.
18. Cole WC, Montgomery JC: Intraperitoneal blood transfusion. Report of 237 transfusions in 117 patients in private practice. Am J Dis Child 37: 497, 1929.
19. Siperstein DM, Sansby JM: Intraperitoneal transfusion with citrated blood. Am J Dis Child 25: 107, 1923.
20. Scopes JW: Intraperitoneal transfusion of blood in newborn babies. Lancet i: 1027, 1963.
21. Liley AW: Intrauterine transfusion of the foetus in haemolytic disease. Br Med J ii: 1107, 1963.
22. Nolph KD, Popovich RP, Ghods AJ, Twardowski Z: Determinants of low clearances of small solutes during peritoneal dialysis. Kidney Int 13: 117, 1978.
23. Nolph KD, Miller F, Rubin J, Popovich R: New directions in peritoneal dialysis concepts and applications. Kidney Int. 18: S111, 1980.
24. Nolph KD: Solute and water transport during peritoneal dialysis. Perspect Perit Dial 1: 4, 1983.
25. Nolph KD, Miller FN, Pyle WK, Popovich RP, Sorkin MI: An hypothesis to explain the ultrafiltration characteristics of peritoneal dialysis. Kidney Int 20: 543, 1981.
26. Twardowski Z, Janicka L: Three exchanges with a 2.5 liter volume for continuous ambulatory peritoneal dialysis. Kidney Int. 20: 281, 1981.
27. Pyle WK, Popovich RP, Moncrief JW: Mass transfer evaluation in peritoneal dialysis. In: Moncrief JW, Popovich RP (eds), CAPD Update. New York, Masson Publishing USA, Inc. p. 35, 1981.
28. Twardowski Z, Ksiazek A, Majdan M, et al.: Kinetics of continuous ambulatory peritoneal dialysis (CAPD) with four exchanges per day. Clin Nephrol 15: 119, 1981.
29. Rubin J, Nolph KD, Popovich RP, Moncrief JW, Prowant B: Drainage volumes during continuous ambulatory peritoneal dialysis. ASAIO J 2: 54, 1979.
30. Krediet RT, Boeschoten EW, Zuyderhoudt FMJ, Arisz L: The relationship between peritoneal glucose absorption and body fluid loss by ultrafiltration during continuous ambulatory peritoneal dialysis. Clin Nephrol 27: 51, 1987.
31. Twardowski ZJ, Khanna R, Nolph KD: Osmotic agents and ultrafiltration in peritoneal dialysis. Nephron 42: 93, 1986.
32. Lindholm B, Werynski A, Bergstrom J: Kinetics of peritoneal dialysis with glycerol and glucose osmotic agents. ASAIO Trans 33: 19, 1987.
33. Spencer PC, Farrell PC: Solute and water kinetics in CAPD. In: Gokal R (ed), Continuous Ambulatory Peritoneal Dialysis. Edinburgh, Churchill Livingstone, p. 38, 1986.
34. Krediet RT, Boeschoten EW, Zuyderhoudt FMJ, Arisz L: Peritoneal transport characteristics of water, low-molecular weight solutes and proteins during long-term continuous ambulatory peritoneal dialysis. Perit Dial Bull 6: 61, 1986.
35. Rippe B, Stelin G, Ahlmen J: Lymph flow from the peritoneal cavity in CAPD patients. In: Maher JF, Winchester JF (eds), Frontiers in Peritoneal Dialysis. New York, Field, Rich and Associates, Inc., p. 24, 1986.
36. Mactier RA, Khanna R, Twardowski Z, Nolph KD: Role of peritoneal cavity lymphatic absorption in peritoneal dialysis. Kidney Int. 32: 165, 1987.
37. Nolph KD, Mactier RA, Khanna R, Twardowski ZJ, Moore H, McGary T: The kinetics of ultrafiltration during peritoneal dialysis: the role of lymphatics. Kidney Int 32: 219, 1987.
38. Mactier RA, Khanna R, Twardowski ZJ, Moore H, Nolph

KD: Contribution of lymphatic absorption to loss of ultra-filtration and solute clearances in CAPD. J Clin Invest 80: 1311, 1987.

39. Mactier RA, Khanna R, Twardowski ZJ, Nolph KD: Failure of ultrafiltration in CAPD due to excessive lymphatic absorption. Am J Kidney Dis 10: 461, 1987.

40. Olin T, Saldeen T: The lymphatic pathways from the peritoneal cavity: a lymphangiographic study in the rat. Cancer Res 24: 1700, 1964.

41. Courtice FC, Simmonds WJ: Physiological significance of lymph drainage of the serous cavities and lungs. Physiol Rev 34: 419, 1954.

42. Higgins GM, Graham AS: Lymphatic drainage from the peritoneal cavity in the dog. Arch Surg 19: 452, 1929.

43. Raybuck HE, Allen L, Harms WS: Absorption of serum from the peritoneal cavity. Am J Physiol 199: 1021, 1960.

44. Simer PH: The drainage of particulate matter from the peritoneal cavity by lymphatics. Anat Rec 88: 175, 1944.

45. Courtice FC, Harding J, Steinbeck AW: The removal of free red blood cells from the peritoneal cavity of animals. Aust J Exp Biol Med Sci 31: 215, 1953.

46. Flessner MF, Parker RJ, Sieber SM: Peritoneal lymphatic uptake of fibrinogen and erythrocytes in the rat. Am J Physiol 244: H89, 1983.

47. Von Recklinghausen F: Zur Fettresorption. Archiv fur Pathologische Anatomie und Physiologie und fur Klinische Medicin. 26: 172, 1863.

48. MacCallum WG: On the mechanism of absorption of granular material from the peritoneum. Bull John Hopkins Hosp 14: 105, 1903.

49. Cunningham RS: Studies in absorption from serous cavities IV. On the passage of blood cells and particles of different size through the walls of the lymphatics in the diaphragm. Am J Physiol 62: 248, 1922.

50. Hertzler AE: The morphogenesis of the stigmata and stomata occurring in peritoneal and vascular endothelium. Trans Am Micro Soc 22: 63, 1901.

51. Allen, L.: The peritoneal stomata. Anat Rec 67: 89, 1937.

52. French JE, Florey HW, Morris B: The absorption of particles by the lymphatic of the diaphragm. Q J Exp Physiol 45: 88, 1960.

53. Casley-Smith JR: Endothelial permeability – the passage of particles into and out of diaphragmatic lymphatics. Q J Exp Physiol 49: 365, 1964.

54. Tsilibary EC, Wissig SL: Light and electron microscope observations of the lymphatic drainage units of the peritoneal cavity of rodents. Am J Anat 180: 195, 1987.

55. Tsilibary EC, Wissig SL: Absorption from the peritoneal cavity: SEM study of mesothelium covering the peritoneal surface of the muscular portion of the diaphragm. Am J Anat 149: 127, 1977.

56. Hedenstedt S.: Elliptocyte transfusions as a method in studies on blood destruction, blood volume and peritoneal resorption. Acta Chir Scandinav 95(Suppl 128): 105, 1947.

57. Morris B, Murphy MJ, Bessis M: The passage of red blood cells from the peritoneal cavity. In: Yoffey JM, Courtice FC (eds), Lymphatics, Lymph and Lymphoid Tissue. London, Academic Press, p. 303, 1970.

58. Florey HW: Reactions of, and absorption by, lymphatics with special reference to those of the diaphragm. Br J Exp Path 8: 479, 1927.

59. Allen L: On the penetrability of the lymphatics of the diaphragm. Anat Rec 124: 639, 1956.

60. Allen L, Weatherwood T: Role of fenestrated basement membrane in lymphatic absorption from the peritoneal cavity. Am J Physiol 197: 551, 1959.

61. Leak LV, Rahil K: Permeability to the diaphragmatic mesothelium: the ultrastructural basis for stomata. Am J Anat 151: 557, 1978.

62. Tsilibary EC, Wissig SL: Structural plasticity in the pathway for lymphatic drainage from the peritoneal cavity. Microvasc Res 17: S144, 1979.

63. Bettendorf U: Lymph flow mechanism of the subperitoneal diaphragmatic lymphatics. Lymphology 11: 111, 1978.

64. Tsilibary EC, Wissig SL: Lymphatic absorption from the peritoneal cavity: regulation of patency of mesothelial stomata. Microvasc Res 25: 225, 1983.

65. Allen L, Vogt E: A mechanism of lymphatic absorption from serous cavities. Am J Physiol 119: 776, 1937.

66. Khanna R, Mactier R, Twardowski ZJ, Nolph KD: Peritoneal cavity lymphatics. Perit Dial Bull 6: 113, 1986.

67. Flessner MF, Dedrick RL, Schultz JS: Exchange of macromolecules between peritoneal cavity and plasma. Am J Physiol 248: H15, 1985.

68. Dunn DL, Barke RA, Knight NB, Humphrey EW, Simmons RL: Role of resident macrophages, peripheral neutrophils and translymphatic absorption in bacterial clearance from the peritoneal cavity. Infect Immun 49: 257, 1985.

69. Keane WF, Peterson PK: Host defence mechanisms of the peritoneal cavity and continuous ambulatory peritoneal dialysis. Perit Dial Bull 4: 122, 1984.

70. Simer PH: The passage of particulate matter from peritoneal cavity into the lymph vessels of the diaphragm. Anat Rec 101: 333, 1948.

71. Clark AJ: Absorption from the peritoneal cavity. J Pharmacol Exp Ther 16: 415, 1920.

72. Courtice FC, Steinbeck AW: The rate of absorption of heparinized plasma and of 0.9% Na Cl from the peritoneal cavity of the rabbit and guinea-pig. Austral J Exp Biol Med Sci 28: 171, 1950.

73. Allen L, Raybuck HE: The effects of obliteration of the diaphragmatic lymphatic plexus on serous fluid. Anat Rec 137: 25, 1960.

74. Courtice FC, Steinbeck AW: The effects of lymphatic obstruction and of posture on the absorption of protein from the peritoneal cavity. Austral J Exp Biol Med Sci 29: 451, 1951.

75. Shear L, Castellot J, Barry KG: Peritoneal fluid absorption: effect of dehydration on kinetics. J Lab Clin Med 66: 232, 1965.

76. Shear L, Swartz C, Shinaberger JA, Barry KG: Kinetics of peritoneal fluid absorption in adult man. New Engl J Med 272: 123, 1965.

77. Bolton C: Absorption from the peritoneal cavity. J Path Bact 24: 429, 1921.

78. Zink J, Greenway CV: Control of ascites absorption in anesthetized cats: effects of intraperitoneal pressure, protein and furosemide diuresis. Gastroenterology 73: 1119, 1977.

79. Morris B: The effect of diaphragmatic movement on the absorption of red cells and protein from the peritoneal cavity. Aust J Exp Biol Med Sci 31: 239, 1953.

80. Higgins GM, Beaver MG, Lemon WS: Phrenic neurectomy and peritoneal absorption. Am J Anat 45: 137, 1930.

81. Shear L, Ching S, Gabuzda GJ: Compartmentalisation of ascites and oedema in patients with hepatic cirrhosis. New Engl J Med 282: 1391, 1970.

82. Hau T, Ahrenholz DH, Simmons RL: Secondary bacterial peritonitis: the biologic basis of treatment. Curr Probl Surg 16:1, 1979.

83. Fowler GR: Diffuse septic peritonitis, with special reference to a new method of treatment, namely, the elevated head and trunk posture, to facilitate drainage into the pelvis. With a report of nine consecutive cases of recovery. Medical Rec 57: 617, 1900.

84. Levine S: Post-inflammatory increase of absorption from peritoneal cavity into lymph nodes: particulate and oily inocula. Exp Mol Path 43: 124, 1985.

85. Casley-Smith JR: The lymphatic system in inflammation. In:

Zweibach BW, Grant L, McCluskey RT (eds), The Inflammatory Process. New York: Academic Press, 2: 161, 1973.
86. Lill SR, Parsons RH, Bohac I: Permeability of the diaphragm and fluid resorption from the peritoneal cavity in the rat. Gastroenterology 76: 997, 1979.
87. Aune S: Transperitoneal exchange IV. The effect of transperitoneal fluid transport on the transfer of solutes. Scand J Gastroenterol 5: 241, 1970.
88. Courtice FC, Steinbeck AW: Absorption of protein from the peritoneal cavity. J Physiol 1951, 114: 336, 1951.
89. Nicoll PA, Taylor AE: Lymph formation and flow. Ann Rev Physiol 39: 73, 1977.
90. Henriksen JH, Lassen NA, Parving H, Winkler K: Filtration as the main transport mechanism of protein exchange between plasma and the peritoneal cavity in hepatic cirrhosis. Scand J Clin Invest 40: 503, 1980.
91. Goranson LR, Jonsson K, Olin T: Parasternal scintigraphy with technetium – 99m sulfide colloid in human subjects: a comparison between two techniques. Acta Radiol Diagnosis 15: 639, 1974.
92. Bergman F: Carcinoma of the ovary: a clinicopathological study of 86 autopsied cases with special reference to mode of spread. Acta Obstet Gynecol Scand 45: 211, 1966.
93. Baglley CM, Young RC, Schein PS, Chabner BA, DeVita VT: Ovarian carcinoma metastatic to the diaphragm – frequently undiagnosed at laparotomy. Am J Obstet Gynecol 116: 397, 1973.
94. Raybuck HE, Weatherwood T, Allen L: Lymphatics in the rat. Am J Physiol 198: 1207, 1960.
95. Dobbie JW, Zaki M, Wilson L: Ultrastructural studies on the peritoneum with special reference to chronic ambulatory peritoneal dialysis. Scott Med J 26: 213, 1981.
96. Di Paolo N, Sacchi G, De Mia M, et al.: Morphology of the peritoneal membrane during peritoneal dialysis. Nephron 44: 204, 1986.
97. Verger C, Brunschvigg O, Le Carpentier Y, Laverone A: Structural and ultrastructural peritoneal membrane changes and permeability alterations during CAPD. Proc EDTA 18: 199, 1981.
98. Taylor AE, Gibson WH, Granger HJ, Guyton AC: The interaction between intercapillary and tissue forces in the overall regulation of interstitial fluid volume. Lymphology 6: 192, 1973.
99. Daugirdas JR, Ing TS, Gandhi VC, Hano JE, Chen WT, Yuan L: Kinetics of peritoneal fluid absorption (from the peritoneal cavity) in patients with chronic renal failure. J Lab Clin Med 95: 351, 1980.
100. Starling EH, Tubby AH: On absorption from and secretion into the serous cavities. J Physiol 16: 140, 1894.
101. Nolph KD, Hano JE, Teschan PE: Peritoneal sodium transport during hypertonic peritoneal dialysis: Physiologic mechanisms and clinical implications. Ann Intern Med 70: 931, 1969.
102. Knochel JP: Formation of peritoneal fluid hypertonicity during dialysis with isotonic glucose solutions. J Appl Physiol 27: 233, 1969.
103. Dykes PW, Jones JH: Albumin exchange between plasma and ascitic fluid. Clin Sci 34: 185, 1968.
104. Arfors KE, Rutili G, Svensjo E: Microvascular transport of macromolecules in normal and inflammatory conditions. Acta Physiol Scand 463: S90, 1979.
105. Rutili G, Arfors KE: Interstitial fluid and lymph protein concentration in the subcutaneous tissue. Bibl Anat 13: 70, 1975.
106. Noer I, Lassen NA: Evidence of active transport (filtration?) of plasma proteins across the capillary walls in muscle and subcutis. Lymphology 11: 133, 1978.
107. Cheek TR, Twardowski ZJ, Moore HL, Nolph KD: Absorption of inulin and high molecular weight gelatin isocyanate

solution from peritoneal cavity of rats. Proceedings of IVth International Symposium on Peritoneal Dialysis (in press).
108. Flessner MF, Fentschermacher JD, Blasberg RG, Dedrick RL: Peritoneal absorption of macromolecules studied by quantitative autoradiography. Am J Physiol 248: H26, 1985.
109. Mactier RA: The role of lymphatic absorption in peritoneal dialysis. M.D. Thesis, University of Glasgow, 1988.
110. Twardowski ZJ, Prowant B, Nolph KD, Martinez AJ, Lampton LM: High volume, low frequency continuous ambulatory peritoneal dialysis. Kidney Int 23: 64, 1983.
111. Twardowski ZJ, Khanna R, Nolph KD et al.: Intra-abdominal pressures during natural activities in patients treated with continuous ambulatory peritoneal dialysis. Nephron 44: 129, 1986.
112. Nikolakakis N, Rodger RSC, Goodship THJ et al.: The assessment of peritoneal function using a single hypertonic exchange. Perit Dial Bull 5: 186, 1985.
113. Smeby LC, Wideroe TE, Jorstad S: Individual differences in water transport during continuous peritoneal dialysis. ASAIO J 4: 17, 1981.
114. An International Co-operative Study. A survey of ultrafiltration in continuous ambulatory peritoneal dialysis. Perit Dial Bull 4: 137, 1984.
115. Khanna R, Nolph KD: Ultrafiltration failure and sclerosing peritonitis in peritoneal dialysis patients. In: Nissenson AR, Fine RN (eds), Dialysis Therapy. Philadephia, Hanley and Belfus, Inc., p. 122, 1986.
116. Verger C, Larpent L, Dumontet M: Prognostic value of peritoneal equilibration curves in CAPD patients. In: Maher JF, Winchester JF (eds), Frontiers in Peritoneal Dialysis. New York, Rich and Associates, Inc., p. 88, 1986.
117. Slingeneyer A, Canaud B, Mion C: Permanent loss of ultrafiltration capacity of the peritoneum in long-term peritoneal dialysis: an epidemiological study. Nephron 33: 133, 1983.
118. Faller B, Marichal JF: Loss of ultrafiltration in continuous ambulatory peritoneal dialysis: a role for acetate. Perit Dial Bull 4: 10, 1984.
119. Raja RM, Khanna MS, Barber K: Solute transport and ultrafiltration during peritonitis in CAPD patients. ASAIO J 7: 8, 1984.
120. Wideroe TE, Smeby LC, Mjaaland S, Dahl K, Berg KJ, Aas TW: Long-term changes in transperitoneal water transport during continuous ambulatory peritoneal; dialysis. Nephron 38: 238, 1984.
121. Twardowski ZJ, Nolph KD, Khanna R et al.: Peritoneal equilibration test. Perit Dial Bull 7: 138, 1987.
122. Khanna R, Mactier RA, Nolph KD, Groshong T: Why is ultrafiltration lower in children on CAPD? Kidney Int 33: 247A, 1988.
123. Popovich RP, Pyle WK, Rosenthal DA, Alexander SR, Balfe JW, Moncrief JW: Kinetics of peritoneal dialysis in children. In: Moncrief JW, Popovich RP (eds), CAPD Update. New York, Masson Publishing USA, Inc., p. 227, 1981.
124. Kohaut EC, Alexander SR: Ultrafiltration in the young patient on CAPD. In: Moncrief JW, Popovich RP (eds), CAPD Update. New York, Masson Publishing USA, Inc., p. 221, 1981.
125. Balfe JW, Vigneux A, Willumsen J, Hardy BE: The use of CAPD in children with end-stage renal disease. Perit Dail Bull 1: 35, 1981.
126. Mactier RA, Khanna R, Moore H, Russ J, Nolph KD, Groshong T: Kinetics of peritoneal dialysis in children: Role of lymphatics. Kidney Int 34: 82, 1988.
127. Randerson DH, Farrell PC: Mass transfer properties of the human peritoneum. ASAIO J 3: 140, 1980.
128. Popovich RP, Moncrief JW: Transport kinetics. In: Nolph KD (ed), Peritoneal Dialysis (2nd edition). Boston, Martinus Nijhoff, p. 115, 1985.

129. Garred LJ, Canaud B, Farrell PC: A simple kinetic model for assessing peritoneal mass transfer in chronic ambulatory peritoneal dialysis. ASAIO J 6: 131, 1983.
130. Selgas R, Rodriguez-Carmona A, Martinez ME *et al.*: Peritoneal mass transfer in patients on long-term CAPD. Perit Dial Bull 4: 153, 1984.
131. Mactier RA, Khanna R, Nolph KD, Twardowski Z, Moore H: Neostigmine increases ultrafiltration and solute clearances in peritoneal dialysis by reducing lymphatic drainage. Perit Dial Bull 7: S50, 1987.
132. Mactier RA, Khanna R, Moore H, Twardowski Z, Nolph K: Phosphatidylcholine enhances the efficiency of peritoneal dialysis by reducing lymphatic reabsorption. Kidney Int 33: 247A, 1988.
133. Steinberg B: Infections of the peritoneum. New York, Paul Hoeber, Inc., 1984.
134. Durham HE: The mechanism of reaction to peritoneal infection. J Path Bact 4: 338, 1897.
135. Vas SI: Peritonitis. In: Nolph KD (ed), Peritoneal Dialysis (2nd edition). Boston, Marinus Nijhoff Publishers, p. 403, 1985.
136. Krediet RT, Zuyderhoudt FMJ, Boeschoten EW, Arisz L: Alterations in peritoneal transport of water and solutes during peritonitis in continuous ambulatory peritoneal dialysis patients. Eur J Clin Invest 17: 43, 1987.
137. Rubin J, Ray R, Barnes T, Bower T: Peritoneal abnormalities during infectious episodes of continuous ambulatory peritoneal dialysis. Nephron 29: 124, 1981.
138. Olsewski WL, Engeset A: Intrinsic contractility of prenodal lymph vessels and lymph flow in human leg. Am J Physiol 239: H775, 1980.
139. McHale NG: Innervation of the lymphatic circulation. In: Johnston MG (ed), Experimental Biology of the Lymphatic Circulation. Amsterdam: Elsevier Science Publishers, p. 121, 1985.
140. Johnston MG: Involvement of lymphatic collecting ducts in the physiology and pathophysiology of lymph flow. In: Johnston MG (ed), Experimental Biology of the Lymphatic Circulation. Amsterdam, Elsevier Science Publishers, p. 81, 1985.
141. Steinhauer HB, Schollmeyer P: Prostaglandin-mediated loss of proteins during peritonitis in continuous ambulatory peritoneal dialysis. Kidney Int 29: 584, 1986.
142. Wu G: Osmotic agents for peritoneal dialysis solutions. Perit Dial Bull 2: 151, 1982.
143. Mistry CD, Mallick NP, Gokal R: The advantage of glucose polymer as an osmotic agent in continuous ambulatory peritoneal dialysis. Proc EDTA 22: 415, 1985.
144. Winchester JF, Stegink LD, Ahmad S *et al.*: A comparison of glucose polymer and dextrose as osmotic agents in CAPD. In: Maher JF, Winchester JF (eds), Frontiers in Peritoneal Dialysis. New York, Field, Rich and Associates, Inc., p. 231, 1986.
145. Higgins JT, Gross ML, Somani P: Patient tolerance and dialysis effectiveness of a glucose polymer containing peritoneal dialysis solution. Perit Dial Bull 4: S131, 1984.
146. Mistry CD, Mallick NP, Gokal R: Ultrafiltration with an isosmotic solution during long peritoneal dialysis exchanges. Lancet ii: 178, 1987.
147. Twardowski ZJ, Nolph KD, Khanna R, Hain H, Moore H, McGary TJ: Charged polymers as osmotic agents for peritoneal dialysis. Materials Research Society Symposium Proceedings, 55: 319, 1986.
148. Junor BJR, Briggs JD, Forwell MA, Dobbie JW, Henderson IS: Sclerosing peritonitis: role of chlorhexidine in alcohol. Perit Dial Bull 5: 101, 1985.
149. Winearls CG, Pippard MJ, Downing MR, Oliver DO, Reid C, Cotes PM: Effect of human erythropoietin derived from recombinant DNA on the anaemia of patients maintained by chronic haemodialysis. Lancet ii: 1175, 1986.
150. Eschbach JW, Egrie JC, Downing MR, Browne JK, Adamson JW: Correction of the anemia of end stage renal disease with recombinant human erythropoietin. N Engl J Med 316: 73, 1987.

5

PERITONEAL ULTRASTRUCTURE

L. GOTLOIB and A. SHOSTAK

'In this life, every living thing has its own life'.

BHAGAVAD GITA

1. INTRODUCTION

Ninety years ago, Robinson [1], after summarizing more than two centuries of research, defined the diverse natural functions of the peritoneum as follows: a) to regulate fluid for nutrient and mechanical purposes; b) to facilitate motion; c) to minimize friction, and d) to conduct vessels and nerves to the viscera.

Several medical and scientific developments which occurred during the twentieh century originated a new approach at the peritoneum being used as a dialyzing membrane for long term life support [2, 3, 4, 5, 6]. These same developments created the need for a deeper understanding of periotoneal ultrastructure.

The peritoneum is a serous membrane embryologically derived from mesenchyma and composed of thin layers of loose connective tissues covered by a sheet of mesothelium [7]. When the membrane is folded, forming the omentum and the mesentery, both luminal surfaces are coevred by mesothelium.

The peritoneal surface area for the human adult is considered to range between 2.08 [8] and 1.72 m^2 [9], with a ratio of area/body weight of 0.284. The intestinal mesothelium together with that of mesentery make up 49% of the total mesothelial area [10]. For infants having a body weight of 2.700–2.900 g, the total peritoneal surface was found to oscillate between 0.106 [10] and 0.151 m^2 [8], with an area to body weight ratio that fluctuates between 0.383 [10] and 0.522. In infants, the contribution of intestine and mesentery to the total surface area is of 67.5% [10].

Peritoneal thickness is not uniform and varies according to the area examined. Measurements are quite problematic in parietal and diaphragmatic peritoneum due to the considerable amount of connective tissue and at times fat, intervening between the peritoneum itself and the underlying tissue. The submesothelial connective tissue layer of visceral peritoneum is firmly bound to the fibrous tissue of the viscus. Therefore the mesentery, having mesothelial lining on both surfaces and including its trabecular con-

nective framework, appears to be the most appropriate peritoneal portion for estimation of membrane thickness which, in the rabbit, ranges between 30 and 38 μ [11, 12,] (Figure 1).

2. NORMAL MESOTHELIUM

Electron microscopic studies done on mouse embryo disclosed that the mesothelium is derived from mesenchymal cells which become flattened; form their own basement membrane; and develop intercellular junctions, mostly desmosomes [13] (Figure 4 – inset). These cells show an oval nucleus with an even distribution of chromatin and a prominent nucleolus. Both pinocytotic vesicles and rough endoplasmic reticulum were present. Yolk sac of human embryos at the 5th to 7th week of gestation also exhibit flattened mesothelial cells lying on a hyaline, homogeneous basement membrane [14].

The resting normal mesothelium generally appears as a continuous layer formed by flattened, elongated cells; the thickness of which ranges, in the rabbit, between 0.6 and 2 μ [11, 12] (Figure 2). The number of mesothelial cells per unit area seems higher on the visceral than on the parietal peritoneal surface [15].

The cell plasmalemma shows, when stained specifically, the typical trilaminar structure observed in all biological cell membranes [16]. The normal mesothelium occasionally shows macrophages implanted on the luminal peritoneal surface instead of mesothelial cells (Figure 4).

The luminal aspect of the mesothelial cell plasmalemma has numerous cytoplasmic extensions: the microvilli (Figure 1, 2, 3), whose existence was originally reported by Kolossov [17] and many years later confirmed by electron-microscopy done on the serosa covering the rat oviduct [18, 19]. Even though microvilli are more frequently observed in visceral than in parietal peritoneum [20, 21], their distribution is variable and fluctuates from very numerous to completely absent [21, 22]. The human omentum has not yet been

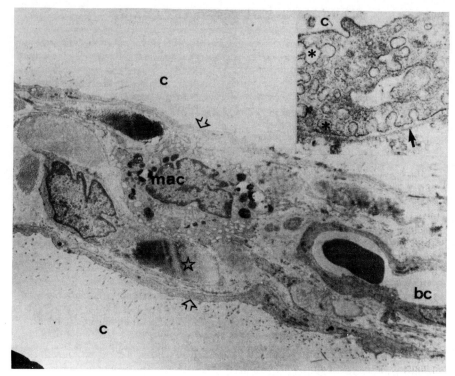

Figure 1. Section of normal rabbit mesentery showing the mesothelial layer (open arrows) covering both aspects of the mesenteric surface area facing the abdominal cavity (c). The interstitium contains as continuous blood capillary (bc), bundles of collagen (open star), as well as a macrophage (mac). Numerous microvilli can be seen at the lower mesothelial surface. (Original magnification: × 4750).

Inset. (Upper right). Parietal peritoneum of normal mice. Note the presence of numerous pinocytotic vesicles (*) which, on the left side of the electron micrograph, form a chain between the luminal aspect of the mesothelial cell facing the abdominal cavity (c) and the abluminal one, lying on the continuous basement membrane (arrow). (× 41 500).

studied in great depth. However, some ultrastructural investigations performed in mice and rats [19, 23] seem to indicate that there is little variation between species [24] and that in mice, omental mesothelial cells can transiently increase their population of microvilli up to seven-fold, suggesting that their concentration in any given area could reflect functional adaptation rather than static structural variation [25].

The presence of pinocytotic vesicles in microvilli has been both reported [18, 20, 26] and denied [25].

Experimental studies done in mice and rats [26, 27, 28] using cationic tracers like ruthenium-red (MW 551 d) and cationized ferritin (MW 445000 d) revealed the existence of anionic fixed charges on the luminal surface of the microvilli cytoplasmic membrane (Figure 5 – inset). This cell membrane coating or glycocalyx, composed of fine fibers that are continuous with the membrane itself [29], furnish the microvilli's surface with electronegative charge which most likely plays a significant role in the transperitoneal transfer of anionic macromolecules like plasma proteins [27, 30]; as well as in that of charged small molecules, as suggested by Curry and Michel [31] in their fiber matrix model of capillary permeability.

Length of microvilli in rodents ranges between 0.42 and 2,7 μ and their average diameter is of 0.1 μ (11, 18, 20, 23). We have observed a similar range in adult humans.

However, mesothelial cells of human embryos 5th to 7th week of gestation) showed microvilli up to 3,5 μ long [14].

It has been estimated that microvilli present in the striated border of intestinal epithelium increase the surface area of the intestine by a factor of 20 [32]. Consequently, it has been speculated that mesothelial microvilli could increase the actual peritoneal surfaces are up to 40 m^2 [33].

Plasmalemma of mesothelial cells shows, like that of microvilli, electronegatively charged glycocalyx [26, 27, 28, 34] (Figure 5).

Pinocytotic vesicles, originally described by Lewis [35] in macrophages of rat omentum, are conspicuously present in mesothelial cells at both the basal and the luminal borders, as well as in the paranuclear cytoplasm [18, 19, 20, 23, 36, 37, 38] (Figure 1 – inset). Their average diameter is approximately 0.717 μ [11]. At times, pinocytotic vesicles appear clustered together and communicating with each other (Figure 1 – inset). Occasionally, they appear forming transcellular channels similar to those described in endothelial cells of blood capillaries [39, 40], apparently communicating both aspects, luminal and abluminal, of the mesothelial cell. These channels can be formed by a chain of several vesicles (Figure 1 – inset) or just by two adjoining vesicles (Figure 6 – inset). Often pinocytotic vesicles appear to open through the plasma membrane into the luminal or abluminal aspect of the cell (Figure 1 – inset, Figure

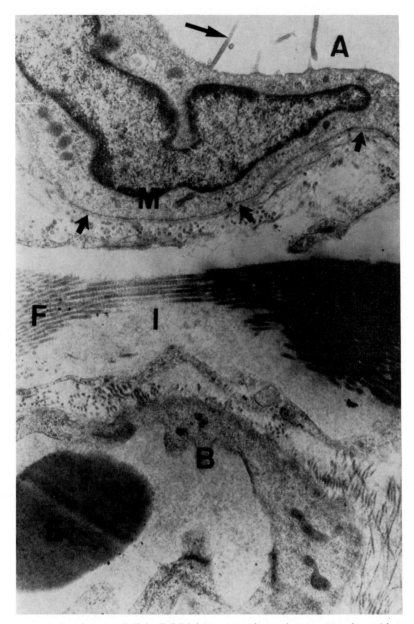

Figure 2. Rabbit mesentery: normal resting mesothelial cell (M) lying on a continuous basement membrane (short arrows). (A: abdominal cavity; long arrow: microvilli; I: interstitium; F: collagen fibers; B: blood capillary; E: erythrocyte). (Original magnification: × 27 500).

5), as well as into the intercellular space (Figure 5); exhibiting a neck and a mouth whose respective average diameters are 0.176 and 0.028 μ [11]. With respect to the density distribution of pinocytotic vesicles, it has been suggested that the parietal mesothelium is less well endowed than the visceral [38].

Palade [41] first proposed that a large part of the macromolecular transport across capillary walls could be attributed to exchange of pinocytotic vesicles between the internal and external surfaces of endothelial cells. This concept was repeatedly applied to the mesothelium. Several electron-dense tracers like native ferritin [38], iron dextran [11, 23] and melanin [19] were found randomly distributed within pinocytotic vesicles of mesothelial cells after being injected intraperitoneally. Casley-Smith [37] calculated that the median transit time of vesicles through mesothelial cells ranges between 3 and 5 sec, and that approximately 40% of the released vesicles reach the cytoplasmic membrane on the opposite side of the cell. It was even observed that metabolic inhibitors like dinitrophenol, poisons (cyanide) or slow cooling to 0 °C did not completely preclude the uptake of electron-dense macromolecules by pinocytosis [38, 42]. This information, supporting Palade's prediction [41] that pinocytotic vesicles could be the structural equivalent of the large pore theory [43] was challenged by stereological analysis of plasmalemmal vesicles. This study

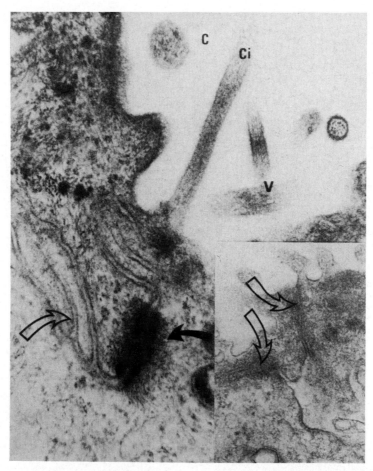

Figure 3. Biopsy of parietal peritoneum taken from a chronic uremic patient on maintenance peritoneal dialysis. Note the presence of an oligocilium (Ci) showing the deviated axial microtubule (open arrow) and the attached basal body (black arrow). Their function is unknown. (C: abdominal cavity; V: microvilli). (× 42 900).
Inset. (Lower right). Rabbit mesentery: the open arrows show tight junctions between adjoining mesothelial cells. (× 62 500).

apparently showed that vesicles represent just invaginations of the plasmalemma from both sides of the capillary wall of frog mesentery [44]. It was suggested that this organization of the vesicular system is incompatible with the concept that macromolecules could be transferred across cells by vesicular transport. The methodology followed in this study has been reviewed and criticized, and its conclusions have been refuted [45]. Therefore, it is generally accepted that pinocytotic vesicles and transcellular channels function as a continuous operating conveyor belt for macromolecules, fusing with each other and moving through the cell [39, 40, 46, 47]. The source of energy fueling vescicular movement still remains one of the many open questions [38, 42, 48, 49, 50, 51, 52].

Simionescu *et al.* [53] showed the existence of differentiated microdomains on the luminal surface of capillary endothelium, where they found a distinct and preferential distribution of anionic sites. Cationic tracers, which did not bind to plasmalemmal vesicles nor to transcellular channels, decorated the luminal glycocalyx, coated pits and coated vesicles [46; 51, 53]. Recent studies done by applying cationic tracers like ruthenium-red and cationized ferritin

in rat and mouse peritoneum also showed a preferential distribution of anionic charges at the level of the mesothelial cells'luminal surface [27, 28, 34] (Figure 5).

The existence of differentiated microdomains in the mesothelial cell plasmalemma is an example of biochemical heterogeneity within a continuous membrane bilayer [47]. Coated pits and vesicles, whose coating consists primarily of clathrin [54], are thought to be cell membrane specializations involved in receptor mediated endocytosis from the extracellular phase to intracellular organelles [51, 55]. The significance of this process is stressed by estimations that cultured cells may form as many as 3000 vesicles per minute [56]. Furthermore, a cultured cell cann internalize up to 50% of the cell membrane in one hour [55]. Uncoated pinocytotic vesicles and transcellular channels are most likely involved in fluid phase pinocytotis [57], as suggested by the random distribution of electron dense tracers within the vesicular contents [11, 23], and also in receptor mediated transcytosis of albumin [57]. It seems, therefore, that Henle's prediction that the essential anatomy and physiology of the peritoneum are located in its 'endothelia' has been, at least in part, confirmed [58].

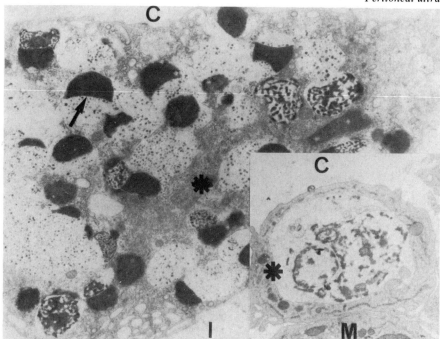

Figure 4. Mesentery of normal rabbit: A macrophage (*) is covering a denuded area of peritoneum. (C: abdominal cavity; black arrow: lysosome; I: interstitium). (Original magnification: × 27 500).

Inset. (Lower right). Mouse mesenteric mesothelium: a signet ring macrophage (*) is covering a recently implanted mesothelial cell (M). (Original magnification: × 15 400).

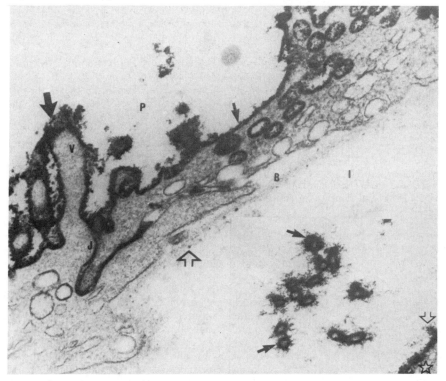

Figure 5. Section of rat mesentery showing microvilli (V) with heavily ruthenium red decorated glycocalyx (large arrow) also evident on the mesothelial cell plasmalemma (small arrow). The cationic dye also stains a long portion of the intercellular junction (J). The basement membrane (B) shows quite regularly distributed anionic sites (open arrow). (P̂: abdominal cavity); I: interstitium). (Original magnification: × 50 720).

Inset. Rat mesentery: transversal section of microvilli showing the fibrilar ruthenium red stained glycocalyx (arrows). (× 50 720).

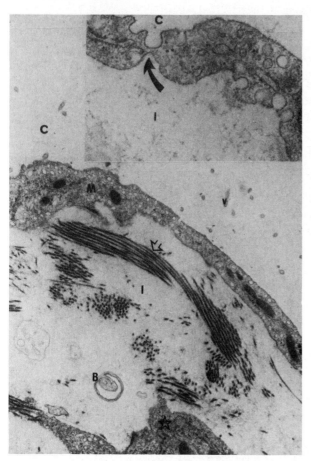

Figure 6. Sample of rat mesentery obtained after 33 intraperitoneal injections of 0.2% furfural, performed on a daily basis. Microvilli (V) are present. The elongated mesothelial cell (M) is lying directly on the connective tissue. The basement membrane is absent. Note the intensity of interstitial edema (I), which is evident even between the collagen fibers (open arrow). (B: myelinoid body; C: abdominal space). (Original magnification: × 15 400).

  Inset. (Upper right). A different area of the same sample showing a transmesothelial channel (black arrow) formed by vesicles. Notice the lack of submesothelial basement membrane. (I: edematous interstitium; C: abdominal cavity). (Original magnification: × 41 500).

Mesothelial cell boundaries are tortuous, with adjacent cells often tending to overlap (Figure 3 – inset, Figure 5). Tight junctions close the luminal side of the intercellular boundaries [11, 18, 23] (Figure 7 – inset). When studied in the horizontal plane by using the freeze-fracture technique, these junctional contact areas were defined as cell extensions and finger-like processes, overlapping into the adjacent cell body. Cell processes were wedge-shaped and numerous, and the cell periphery appeared serrated [59]. Desmosomes have also been observed near the cellular luminal front [11, 20, 22, 23] (Figure 7 – inset, Figure 8) and so have gap junctions [22]. The abluminal portions of cell interfaces usually show an open intercellular channel (Figure 5). Completely open intercellular interphases have not been observed in normal, resting mesothelium [11, 18, 23]. Even desquamated mesothelial cells showing severe

degenerative changes can keep their junctional system almost intact (Figure 8). These junctional morphological features are, however, different from those observed between mesothelial cells covering the diaphragmatic lymphatic lacunae, which are more cuboidal and prominent than mesothelial cells observed in other areas of the peritoneal surface. The existence of stomata (open inter-mesothelial communications between the abdominal cavity and the submesothelial diaphragmatic lymphatics), predicted by William Hewson [1] 100 yr before being discovered by Von Recklinghausen [60], have been the subject of a long and rich controversy along the years. Accepted by some [61, 62, 63] and denied by others [64, 65, 66], it was not until the advent of electron microscopy that their existence was demonstrated [34, 67, 68]. Scanning electron microscopy disclosed the patent intermesothelial junctions forming gaps whose average diameter ranged between 4 and 12 μ +67, 68] and circumscribed by cuboidal mesothelial cells. These gaps open into submesothelial lympathics [34] and have not been observed in diaphragmatic mesothelium covering non-lacunar areas [68].

Stomata have been ascribed the role of a preferential pathway for the output of fluids, cells, particles and bacteria from the abdominal cavity [69]. However, the luminal surface of mesothelial cells (which limits the gaps) displayed, after staining with cationized ferritin, dense labelling of their cytoplasmic plasmalemma as well as coated pits and coated vesicles. The same cationic tracer also decorated the lymphatic endothelial plasmalemma which circumscribed the stomatal openings [34]. If so, the passage of solutes through stomata is most likely dependent not only on molecular weight, size and shape, but also on electric charge [34].

Studies done in rat and mouse perfused with ruthenium-red revealed that intermesothelial cell junctions were, in general, stained just at the level of their infundibulum, even though the dye decorated now and then the junctional complex, staining approximately 50% of its length [28] (Figure 5).

Nuclei are generally located in the central region of mesothelial cells, showing an elongated, oval or reniform appearance with occasional irregularities in their outlines and sometimes protrusions and indentations (Figure 2). The chromatin is fine, evenly distributed and forms a dense rim around the nuclear membrane (Figure 2). Nucleoli have been reported both als present [18, 23]. Rough endoplasmic reticulum and ribosomes are dispersed in the cytoplasm. Mitochondria and the Golgi complex are evident mainly in perinuclear areas (Figure 2). Although seldem observed, isolated cilia may emerge from the luminal aspect of mesothelial cells, showing in their cytoplasmic part the axial microtubule as well as the attached basal body (Figure 3). More frequently observed in splenic mesothelium [70], their functional significance is still unknown [71].

The submesothelial basement membrane (which was originally described bij Todd and Bowman [72] and later on reported as hyaline, homogeneous, one layered and continuous [61, 73], with an average thickness of approximately 40 nm for mouse and rabbit peritoneum [11, 19] normally appears lying under the mesothelial layer of visceral, parietal and diaphragmatic peritoneum [74] (Figure 2, Figure 7). As an exception, the functional signi-

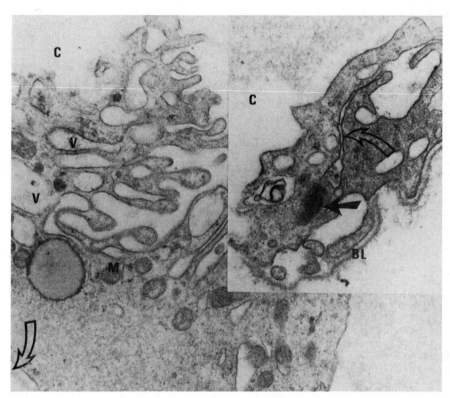

Figure 7. Biopsy of parietal peritoneum taken from a 67 year old chronic uremic patient who was on IPD for a period of almost two years. A young mesothelial cell shows numerous vacuoles (V) giving a worm-like appearance, which is why this structure is called micropinocytosis vermiformis. The abluminal aspect of the mesothelial cell is lying on a hyaline basement membrane (open arrow). (C: abdominal cavity; M: mitochondrion). ($\times$ 26 000).

Inset. (Upper right). Another area of the same biopsy. This electron micrograph shows the vacuolized cytoplasm of two adjacent mesothelial cells developing a new intercellular junction (open arrow). Note the presence of a typical desmosome (black arrow). The basement membrane (BL) is still discontinuous. (Original magnification: $\times$ 30 740).

ficance of which is still unknown, the omental mesothelium of mice and humans lacks basement membrane [19, 75].

Submesothelial basement membrane of visceral, parietal and diaphragmatic peritoneum of rat and mouse, perfused with the cationic tracer ruthenium-red, consistently shows anionic fixed charges periodically distributed along the lamina rara externa and/or the lamina rara interna, and forming double rows at times [27, 28] (Figure 5).

The reported average diameter of ruthenium-red stained particles in the basement membrane was 2.7 nm whereas the average distance measured between the one-row oriented basal lamina dye particles was 90 nm [11].

Reduplicated submesothelial basement membrane has been observed in non-diabetic chronic uremic patients treated by maintenance peritoneal dialysis [76] (Figure 9). It has been shown that perivascular basement membrane thickness increases with age [77, 78] as well as in the direction of head to foot [78, 79]. This same ultrastructural alteration has been observed in diabetics [78, 80]. It has been suggested that diabetes alone is not responsible for excessive accumulation of basement membrane associated with aging [82]. Therefore, it seems likely that the reduplication of basement membrane observed in human mesothelium is al by-product of cell renewal regardless of the cause of cell death that triggers the process of repopulation [76, 81].

3. INTERSTITIUM

Connective tissue which originates from mesenchyma is composed of cells and fibers embedded in an amorphous substance. The main connective tissue cell is the fibroblast and the main fiber is collagen [83].

The submesothelial connective tissue normally has a low cell population surrounded by high molecular weight intercellular material. Fibroblasts, mast cells in the proximity of blood microvessels (Figure 10), occasional monocytes and macrophages (Figure 1) are frequently observed.

Substantial amounts of quite compact bundles of collagen are usually interposed between the blood microvessels and the mesothelial layer (Figures 1, 2). The collagen density distribution in the different regions of visceral peritoneum is quite variable [74].

The macromolecular common denomination of connective tissues is a broad molecular class of polyanions: the tissue polyaccharides. The form a gel-like structure with the collagen fibers [84] which, when stained with ruthenium-red, shows the presence of anionic fixed charges [28].

4. BLOOD MICROVESSELS

Capillaries of human and rodent parietal [85] and visceral

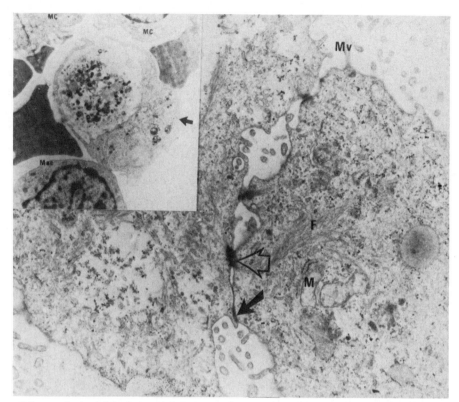

Figure 8. Effluent dialysate obtained from a non infected patient on peritoneal dialysis. Two desquamated mesothelial cells show severe degenerative changes: swollen mitochondria (M) with broken membranes, sheaves of filaments (F) and swollen cytoplasm. Part of the tight junction is still present (black arrow), as well as a desmosome (open arrow). (Mv: microvilli). (Original magnification: × 15 400).

Inset. (Upper left). Effluent dialysate obtained from the same patient. Note the presence of a signet-ring macrophage (arrow), as well as part of two floating mesothelial cells (Mc). (Mac: macrophage). (Original magnification: × 8600).

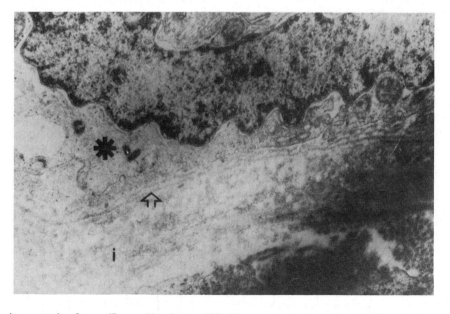

Figure 9. Parietal peritoneum taken from a 67 year old patient on IPD. The open arrow shows the reduplicated submesothelial basement membrane. (*: mesothelial cell; i: submesothelial interstitium). (Original magnification: × 24 600).

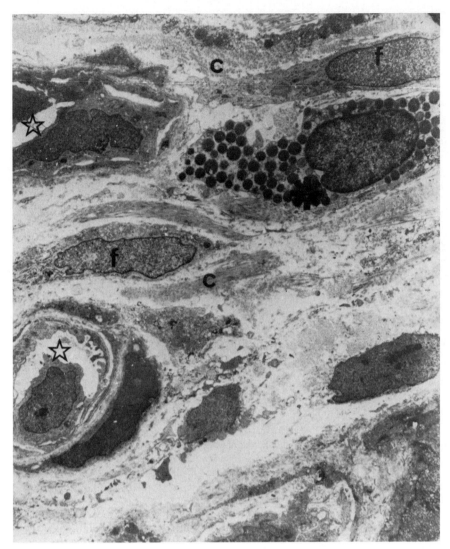

Figure 10. Interstitial tissue of human parietal peritoneum. Bundles of collagen (C) and fibroblasts (f) are interposed between the blood microvessels (open stars) and the mesothelial cells (not included in this electron micrograph). Mast cells (*) are frequently observed near blood microvessels. (Original magnification: × 42 900).

peritoneum [33, 86] have been reported to be of the continuous type (Figures 1, 2, 11, 12, 13, 14), according to the classification of Majno [87]. However, the existence of fenestrated capillaries in human parietal and rabbit diaphragmatic peritoneum [89] (Figure 11), as well as in mouse mesentery [89], has been reported. The incidence of fenestrated capillaries in human parietal peritoneum appears to be low (1.7% of the total number of capillaries) [88]. The density distribution of submesothelial microvessels along the different portions of the peritoneum is variable. In the rabbit, the mesentery appears to be the most vascularized peritoneal segment (contributing 71.1% of the total number of observed capillaries). The reported diaphragmatic and parietal contributions to the total microvascular bed examined were of 17.9% and 10.9% respectively [90]). Distances between the microvessels and the mesothelial layer are variable, ranging between a few microns

(Figure 1) and, at times, as much as 100 μ [91].

In rabbit mesentery the main population of continuous blood microvessels is represented by:

a) true capillaries (without perithelial cells), the mean luminal diameter of which is 7.2 μ and whose mean wall thickness is 0.4 μ (Figures 1, 2, 11, 13, 14);

b) venous capillaries, usually formed by the confluence of two of three capillaries. These show a thin endothelial layer, occasional peripheral perithelial cells, and have a mean luminal diameter of 9.2 μ;

c) post-capillary venules whose luminal diameter ranges between 9.4 and 20.6 μ, whereas their reported mean wall thickness is 1.6 μ [33]. With increasing luminal diameter there is a proportional increase in wall thickness due to the presence of more perithelial cells encircling the endothelial layer [92] (Figure 12). The average ration of luminal diameter to wall thickness is approximately 10/1 [92]. All

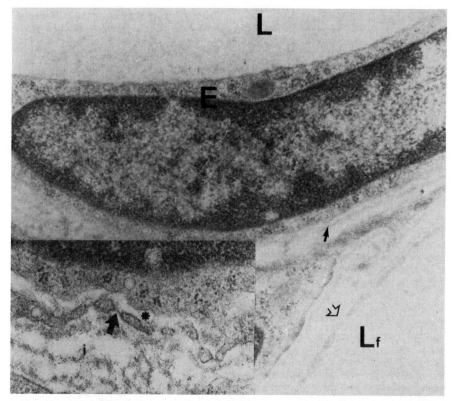

Figure 11. Continuous capillary of a blood mesenteric rabbit capillary whose endothelial layer (E) is lying on the basement membrane (black arrow). The lower right part of this electron micrograph shows a fenestrated capillary (open arrow). (L: lumen of continuous capillary; Lf: lumen of fenestrated capillary). (Original magnification: × 47 400).

   Inset. (Lower left). Fenestrated capillary of human parietal peritoneum. (The arrow points to a fenestral diaphragm. (i: interstitium; *: lumen of fenestrated capillary). (Original magnification: × 42 900).

aforementioned exchange vessels present at their luminal aspect a limiting area that separates the endothelial cell from the circulating blood and is formed by the plasmalemma with its trilaminar structure [16] (Figure 13) and the glycocalyx (Figure 13). The latter, originally described by Luft [29] in other vascular beds, has also been observed at the luminal aspect of peritoneal microvessels [93]. The presence of sialoconjugates, proteoglycans and acidic glycoproteins organized as a fibrous network provides the plasmalemmal glycocalyx with electronegative charge [94].

   There is evidence tha anionic plasma proteins (albumin and IgG) are adsorbed to the glycocalyx of microvascular endothelial cells [95]. The fiber-matrix model of capillary permeability envisages the glycocalyx as a meshwork of glycoprotein fibers which, after adsorbing circulating proteins, would tighten its mesh, thereby rendering the underlying endothelium less accessible to water and other water-soluble molecules [31]. Furthermore, it has been shown that the adsorption of circulating anionic plasma proteins to the glycocalyx renders the underlying endothelium relatively impermeable to large, electron dense, anionic tracers like native ferritin (MW ̃ 450 000 d) [95].

   The mean endothelial cell-width of rabbit mesenteric capillaries is 0.4 μ unless the cytoplasm bulges up to more than 1 μ at the site of the nucleus (Compare Figures 2 and 13). The cytoplasm includes the usual cell organelles:

mitochondria, rough endoplasmic reticulum and free ribosomes [11, 87].

   The mitochondrial content of vascular endothelial cells in frog mesentery decreases gradually from arterioles toward venous capillaries and subsequently increases toward venules [96].

   The Golgi complex displays variable degrees of development in biopsies taken from different patients. This same variability was observed when comparing different peritoneal microvascular endothelial cells present in a single sample.

   The cytoplasmic matrix of endothelial cells shows long filaments parallel to the longitudinal cellular axis. Their diameter ranges between 20 and 100 A [87], and at times they appear in bundles. These intermediate size filaments seem to be a common component of the cytoplasmic matrix of vascular endothelial cells showing, however, a lower density distribution than that observed in other cell types [71].

   Nuclei are generally oval, elongated (Figure 11) or occasionally kidney-shaped with focal surface irregularities (Figures 2 and 9). Their mean short-axis width in rabbit mesentery is 0.957 ± 0.417 μ [11].

Pinocytotic vesicles, which can be found in most cell types, are particularly common in capillary endothelia [97], where theu occupy approximately 7% of the cell volume [49]

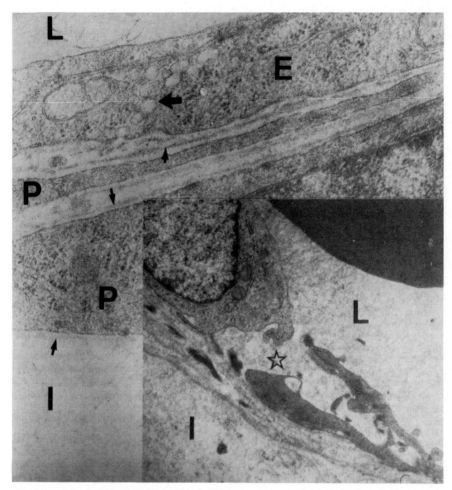

Figure 12. Postcapillary venule of rabbit mesentery. The large arrow shows a transcellular channel (L: microvascular lumen; E: endothelial cell; short arrow: subendothelial basement membrane; P: pericyte; longer arrows: subperithelial basement membrane; I: interstitium). (× 62 500).

Inset. (Lower right). Human parietal peritoneum taken from a 21 year old patient with *E. coli* peritonitis. The star shows an open interendothelial junction of a blood capillary. Note part of an erythrocyte in the upper right quadrant. (L: capillary lumen; I: interstitium). (Original magnification: × 41 500).

(Figures 12, 13). Their outer diameter is approximately 700 A (it ranges between 500 and 900 A) [11, 36, 40] and they have a round or oval shape surrounded by a three-layered membrane of 80 A thickness (Figure 13 – inset).

According to their location in the cytoplasmic matrix, vesicles can be classified into three groups: a) vesicles attached to the plasmalemma limiting the blood front of the endothelial cell; b) free vesicles within the cytoplasmic matrix; c) attached vesicles, but this time, to the tissue front of the endothelial cell plasmalemma [40] (Figure 13). The density population of pinocytotic vesicles varies considerably from one vascular segment to another, even within the same microvascular territory [39, 40]. In the mouse diaphragm, arterioles show 200 vesicles/μ^2, true capillaries 900/μ^2, venular segments of capillaries 1200/μ^2 and postcapillary venules 600/μ^2 [39].

Most vesicles that open to the extracellular medium have necks whose diameter can be as small as 100 A [40]. Transendothelial channels formed by a chain of vesicles

opening simultaneously on both fronts of the endothelium have been described in capillaries of mouse diaphragmatic muscle [39] as well as in post-capillary venules of rabbit mesentery (Figure 12) [11]. The relative frequency of transendothelial channels has been found to be higher in true capillaries than in arterioles and venules, with the highest density in the venular segment of capillaries [51]. Microvessels of frog mesentery showed a density distribution of 3 transendothelial channels for every 400 vascular profiles examined [96]. Just as in observations made on mesothelial cells, pinocytotic vesicles and transendothelial channels do not bind cationic electron-dense tracers which, on the other hand, decorate the luminal aspect of coated pits and coated vesicles [46, 53] in the peritoneal microvasculature [28].

The functional significance of pinocytotic vesicles, transendothelial channels, coated pits and coated vesicles was discussed in paragraph 2.

In fenestrated capillaries, endothelial cells are pierced by

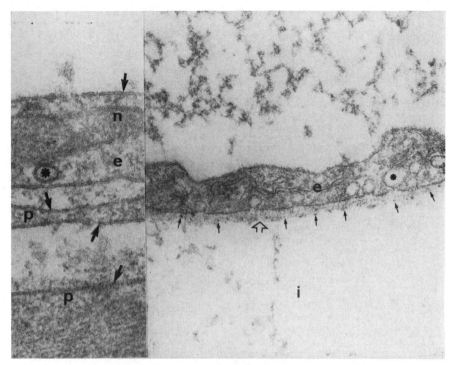

Figure 13. The right part of the figure shows part of a blood capillary wall observed in a sample of diaphragmatic peritoneum obtained from a normal rat. The luminal aspect (upper cell border) of the endothelial cell (e) shows a fine reticular glycocalyx stained by ruthenium red which, on the other hand, does not decorate pynocytotic vesicles (*). The subendothelial basement membrane (open arrow) is continuous and shows quite regularly distributed ruthenium red stained anionic sites (small arrows) along both the lamina rara externa and the lamina rara interna. (Original magnification: × 50 720).

Inset. (Left part of the figure). Part of a post-capillary venule observed in mesentery of a rat, 5 days after induction of peritonitis. The trilaminar structure of the endothelial (e) and perithelial cell plasmalemma is clearly observed (arrows), as well as that of the limiting membrane of the pinocytotic vesicle (*). Glycocalyx, basement membrane and anionic sites are absent. (n: nucleus of endothelial cell). (Original magnification: × 84 530).

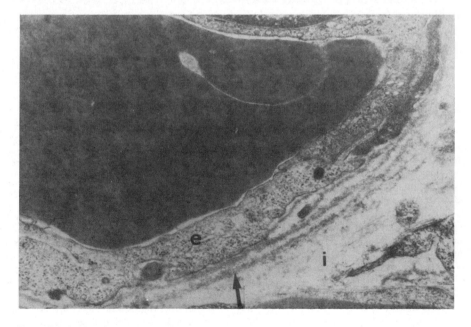

Figure 14. Blood capillary of parietal peritoneum taken from a 69 year old uremic patient on IPD for almost three years. The endothelial cell (e) is lying on a reduplicated basement membrane (arrow). (i: interstitium) (× 24 600).

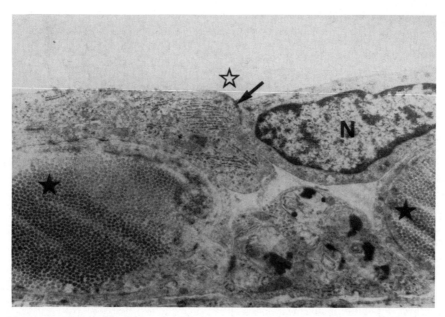

Figure 15. Blood capillary of rabbit mesentery. The black arrows points to a tight junction formed by two adjoining endothelial cells. A macrophage can be observed lying under the endothelial cells and separating two bundles of collagen (black stars). (Open star: capillary lumen; N: nucleus of endothelial cell). (Original magnification: × 85 000).

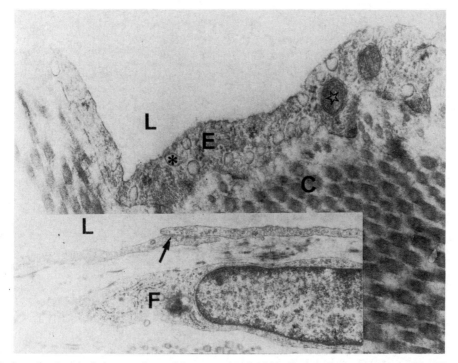

Figure 16. Partial view of a lymphatic lacuna observed in a sample of rabbit diaphragmatic peritoneum. The thin endothelial cell (E) shows numerous pinocytotic vesicles (*) and occasional mitochondria (star). Note the absence of subendothelial basement membrane. (L: lacunar lumen; C: collagen fibers). (Original magnification: × 85 0000).
  Inset. (Lower left). Lymphatic capillary of rabbit diaphragmatic peritoneum. Two adjoining endothelial cells forming a tight junction (arrow) appear lying on the interstitial tissue. Basement membrane as well as anchoring filaments are not observed. (L: capillary lumen; F: fibroblast). (Original magnification: × 62 500).

fenestrae whose diameter ranges between 20 and 120 nm and may either be open or closed by a diaphragm [98] (Figure 11). Fenestrae are not static structures. It has been shown that they can increase during acute inflammation and under the influence of sexual hormones [86].

High concentrations of negative fixed charges (heparin and heparan sulphate) have been found on the blood front of fenestral diaphragms in several microvascular beds [46, 53, 98, 99, 100, 101, 102]. They are expected to discriminate against anionic macromolecules, essentially anionic plasma protein. The possible presence of anionic fixed charges on fenestral diaphragms of human parietal and rabbit diaphragmatic peritoneum remains to be demonstrated.

Capillary endothelial cells are linked to each other by tight junctions (zonula occludens), originally described by Farquhar and Palade [103, 104, 105] (Figure 15). Communicating or gap junctions have been observed in arteriolar endothelium [104]. Post-capillary venules have loosely organized junctions with discontinuous ridges and grooves of which 25 to 30% appear to be open with a gap of 20 to 60 A [40]. They also sometimes show gap junctions [11].

Even though it has been argued that the identification of the small pore pathway for lipid-insoluble molecules with the intercellular junctions still remains questionable [106], some studies suggest that intercellular junctions of continuous capillaries are permeable to molecules of approximately 10-17 A diameter [40, 91].

Cytoplasmic plasmalemma bordering both sides of junctions also shows anionic fixed charges [28]. Their functional significance in relation to the passage of charged molecules remains to be established.

The basement membrane of true capillaries is normally a thin sheet at the interface between the abluminal aspect of the endothelial cell and the connective tissue (Figures 2, 11). In post-capillary venules it is interposed between the endothelial and the perithelial cell (Figure 12). Generally uniform for a given structure, its thickness varies among the different parts of the body. True capillaries of normal rabbit mesentery have a mean basal membrane thickness of 0.234 ± 0.095 μ [11]. As was described for the submesothelial basement membrane, that of human capillaries also exhibits a significantly increasing thickness in the direction of head to foot [78]. It has been suggested that these regional variations are secondary to difference in venous hydrostatic pressure effective on the capillary bed [78]. Chronic uremic patients that showed reduplicated submesothelial basement had similar alterations on the capillary basement membrane of parietal peritoneum [76]. Peritoneal capillaries of rats and mice perfused with ruthenium-red presented regularly distributed, anionic fixed charges along the subendothelial basement membrane [27, 28].

Summarizing the information obtained from ultrastructural and physiological studies, it can be stated that the microvascular endothelial cell should be considered a highly active structure serving not only as a permeability barrier and an effective thrombo-resistant surface, but also as the location of important synthetic and other metabolic activities [96, 105].

Continuous capillaries are more permeable to larger molecules than fenestrated capillaries [107]. Coated pits and coated vesicles are involved in receptor-mediated endocy-

tosis, whereas the uncharged pinocytotic vesicles and transcellular channels may be involved in the transfer of proteins and fluid-phase pinocytosis. Additionally, all the resistances described by Nolph [107] along the pathway leading from the microvascular lumen to the abdominal cavity, are negatively charged [28, 30].

5. LYMPHATICS

The role of lymphatic absorption during peritoneal dialysis has been recently focused on by Mactier et al. [109]. The lymphatic system of the peritoneum consists of: a) pre-initial and initial lymphatics [110, 111, 112, 113, 114, 115]; b) lymphatic capillaries; c) lymphatic lacunae whose significance has been a matter of debate since Van Recklinghausen [60]; d) precollecting and collecting lymphatics [1].

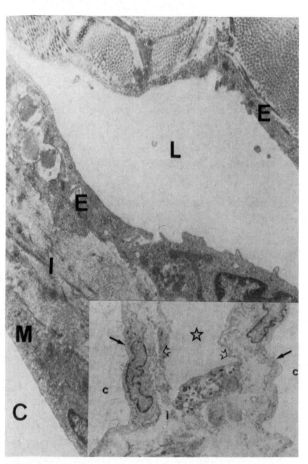

Figure 17. Lymphatic lacuna of rabbit diaphragmatic peritoneum. The wide lacunar lumen (L) is surrounded by the lymphatic endothelium (E). Connective tissue (I) is interposed between the lacuna and the mesothelial cell layer (M). (C: abdominal cavity). (Original magnification: × 17 750).

Inset. (Lower right). Lymphatic lacuna of rabbit mesentery. The open star shows the lacunar lumen surrounded by a thin endothelial layer (open arrows). Mesothelial cells (black arrows) are covering both aspects of the mesenteric peritoneal surface. (i: interstitium; c: abdominal cavity). (Original magnification: × 4750).

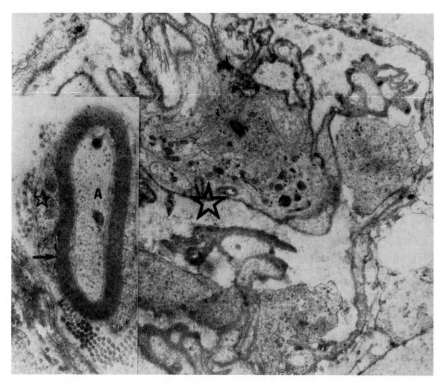

Figure 18. Parietal peritoneum taken from a 67 year old chronic uremic patient on IPD, showing a transversal cut of an unmyelinated nerve (star) (× 12 600).

Inset. Rabbit mesentery showing a myelinated nerve fiber (star: Schwann cell cytoplasma; arrow: myelin; A: axon). (Original magnification: × 47 400).

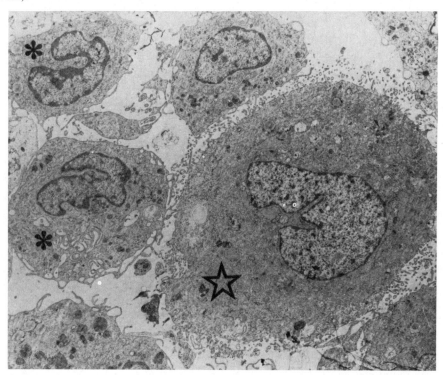

Figure 19. Effluent dialysate obtained from a non-infected chronic uremic patient, showing a floating mesothelial cell (star), as well as macrophages (*) (× 6900).

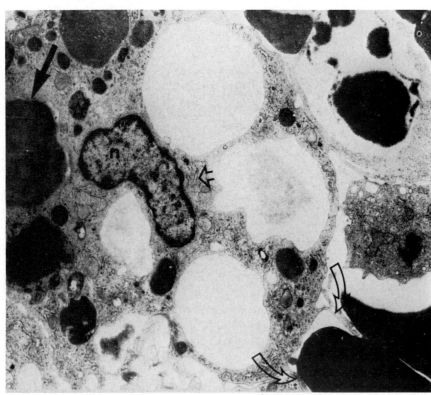

82   *Gotloib, Shostak*

5.1. Pre-initial and initial lymphatics

Prelymphatic tissue channels (or low resistance pathways along the surface of elastic fibers) observed in rabbit and cat mesentery do not show a microcopically recognizable wall structure [115]. They are usually located in the perivascular space of venules and small collecting venules [112, 113]. According to Hauck [115] this most peripheral part of the lymph vessel system is a completely open net of tissue channels which would eventually drain, at least in cat mesentery, into a network of fine, irregularly countoured endothelial tubes of approximately 20–30 μ width [111] (which are considered to be the initial lymphatics) [115]. However, other studies done in cat and rat mesentery showed the additional presence of blind, saccular formations with a wall made up of a simple layer of thin endothelial cells [111, 114].

5.2. Lymphatic capillaries

Approximately 4% of the mesenteric mesothelial surface area of the rabbit covers underlying lymphatic vessels [11]. Lymphatic capillaries are generally wider and more irregular than blood capillaries. Their diameter ranges between 15 and 40 μ [115]. The luminal aspect is covered by a continuous layer of thin endothelial cells which, in non nuclear areas, show an average thickness of approximately 0.3 μ (Figure 16) [36]. Nuclei are flattened and elongated,

with an irregular outline and have a thin peripheral rim of dense chromatin (Figure 17 - inset).

The cytoplasm is made up of an abundant, clear matrix which contains rough endoplasmic reticulum, a vesiculated Golgi complex, mitochondria (Figure 16), and free ribosomes. Pinocytotic vesicles similar to those described in blood microvessels are commonly observed [36, 116, 117, 118] (Figure 16).

Several types of junctions have been described: approximately 2% of the whole junctional system consists of open junctions showing gaps of up to 100 nm [63, 67]; 10% of the junctions are zonula adherens; whereas the rest are tight junctions [118] (Figure 16 - inset). This frequency distribution of the several types of intercellular junctions varies between different lymphatic territories. However, gap or communicating junctions have not been observed [105].

The subendothelial basement membrane may appear but shows numerous interruptions. There are, however, many places in which it completely vanishes [116] (Figure 16 - inset). In these areas, anchoring filaments are inserted on the tissue front of the endothelial plasma membrane and, on the other side, bind the lymphatic endothelial cells to the adjoining interstitial structures [116, 120, 121].

5.3. Lymphatic lacunae

One of the characteristic features of diaphragmatic lymphatics is the presence of flattened, elongated cisternae of

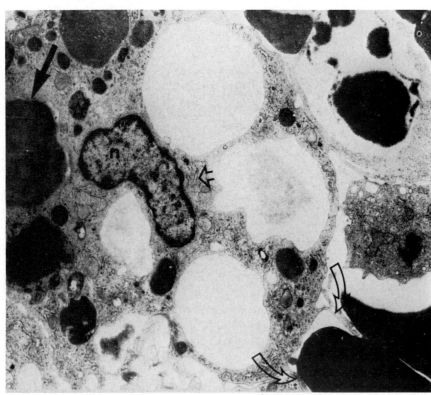

Figure 20. Peritoneal effluent obtained from a chronic uremic patient on peritoneal dialysis. The macrophages depicted in the figure shows phagolysosomes digesting erythrocytes (black arrow). Note the presence of rough endoplasmic reticulum (short open arrow) near the nucleus (n). The former normally appears in macrophages when the cells are involved in phagocytic activity. The curved open arrows are pointing to cell processes engulfing red blood cells. (Star: mitochondrion) (× 8600).

about 0.3–0.6 cm. length with a long axis that runs parallel with the long axis of the muscle fibers [68] (Figures 16, 17).

The endothelial cell lining of lymphatic lacunae is thin and shows no tight junctions. Adjacent cells usually overlap leaving an open basal interface which at times can be as wide as 12 μ in diameter [68]. The cytoplasm of endothelial cells shares the characteristics described for lymphatic capillaries. The same can be said of the subendothelial basement membrane and anchoring filaments (Figure 16).

It is not yet known whether the stomata, which have been discussed previously, represent a portal or a direct pathway to the lacunar lumen [68].

Recent studies done using cationized ferritin as an electron dense tracer showed large clumps of ferritin particles accumulated within the portals of mesothelial stomata as well as adhering to the mesothelial and lymphatic endothelial surfaces that form the boundary of the stomatal openings. The clefts of intercellular junctions between mesothelial and lymphathic endothelial cells were also heavily decorated by cationic ferritin, indicating the presence of a high density of anionic fixed charges [34]. Furthermore, another study done using several electron-dense charged tracers provided evidence for assymetry of both charge sign and charge density between abluminal and luminal aspects of the lacunar lymphathic endothelium. The luminal plasma membrane showed both cationic and anionic fixed charges, although the latter outnumbered the former. The abluminal plasma membrane prsented few anionic fixed charges [122].

Lymphathic lacunae which do not show morphological evidence of inflow sites for initial lympathics usually join together to form a wide channel which, in turn, becomes a one-way valve vessel as described by Rusch in the 18th century [1], with muscle cells around the endothelial tube. This arrangement is more frequently observed towards the down-stream end of the segment [123, 124].

6. PERITONEAL INNERVATION

The first report announcing the presence of nerves in the peritoneal instertitium was made by Haller in 1751 [125] and confirmed during the 19th century by Ranvier and Robin who, using osmic acid and silver nitrate, described nerve trunks, branches and nerve endings accompanying arteries and veins. Robinson [1] described the peritoneum as being richly supplied with myelinated and non-myelinated nerves (Figure 18). More recently [126] silver stain was used to study the innervation of large lymph vessels and lymph capillaries in the mesentery of dogs and cats. This research proved that these large vessels are supplied with myelinated nerves that reach only the adventitial surface and with non-myelinated nerve fibers that penetrate into the region of valve attachment. The latter are supposed to conduct the motor stimuli for the peristalsis of lymphatic vessels. Contraction is mediated by activation of α-adrenoreceptors via post-ganglionic sympathetic nerves, whereas relaxation is mainly mediated by β-adrenoreceptors [127].

In rat mesentery, networks of adrenergic axons innervate the principal and small arteries and arterioles. Precapillary arterioles, collecting venules and small veins are not innervated, and are most likely under the influence of humoral vasoactive substances [128].

In 1741, Vater observed that the submesothelial connective tissue of cat mesentery contained oval corpuscles with a diameter of approximately 1–2 mm. In 1830, Paccini rediscovered and gave a systemic description of this corpuscle which is known as the Vater-Paccini corpuscle [1]. It takes the form of a non-myelinated nerve ending which in transverse section appears as a sliced onion. In humans, it has been observed in the peritoneum of mesentery and in visceral ligaments, functioning as the main receptor for perception of pressure.

7. CYTOLOGY OF THE PERITONEAL FLUID

The peritoneal fluid of laboratory animals has classically been a favored site for experiments dealing with the inflammatory response [129] as well as for those designed

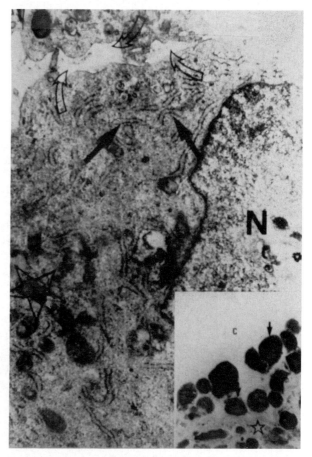

Figure 21. Parietal peritoneum of a patient on IPD. The biopsy was taken 13 hours after peritoneal dialysis was interrupted. This electron micrograph shows two recently implanted new mesothelial cells, still separated by a wide intercellular space (open arrows). The cytoplasm is rich in rough endoplasmic reticulum (black arrows) and mitochrondria (open star). (N: nucleus). (× 19 200).

Inset. (Lower right). Wandering mesothelial cells (arrows) coming from the peritoneal space (c) are repopulating the denuded peritoneal surface. The smaller round cells are macrophages. (Original magnification: × 400).

to analyze the biological reaction to infection [130].

More than 50 yr ago, Josey and Webb realized that fluid shifts into and out of the peritoneal cavity could change the concentration of cells without affecting their absolute number [131, 132, 133, 134]. The methodological answer to this question was given by Seeley and coll. who weighed peritoneal fluid and measured the cellular concentrations, and so were able to estimate the absolute number of cells [135]. Padawer and Gordon [133], after analyzing the cellular elements present in peritoneal fluid of eight different normal mammals, concluded that the most frequently observed cells were eosinophils, mast cells and mononuclears (including lymphocytic and macrophagic elements). Total cell numbers, as well as percentages of the different cells varied greatly among the species examined. Neutrophils were never observed in normal animals. Total absolute counts were higher for females than for males, as well as for older animals compared with younger ones. In the individual animal under normal conditions, the number of cells present within the abdominal cavity was constant [133].

Observation of peritoneal fluid obtained from healthy women showed that macrophages and mesothelial cells contributed more than 70% of the whole cell population, whereas lymphocytes and polymorphonuclears contributed to a lesser extent (18% and 7% respectively) [137]. Other investigators observed that at the midphase of the menstrual cycle, macrophages, which comprised 82% to 98% of the peritoneal cells, showed morphological as well as biochemical heterogeneity and were seen to be involved in phagocytosis of erythrocytes [138] (Figure 20). However, other studies showed up to four different types of cytologic patterns in peritoneal fluid of women during the course of the menstrual cycle, in all of which mesothelial cells contributed substantially to the total cell counts. The paramenstrual type was in most cases hemorrhagic and highly cellular [139].

The apparently puzzling effect of intraperitoneal saline inducing substantial influx of neutrophils into the abdominal cavity, which was observed long ago [130], was not confirmed when the experiments were carried out using sterile techniques. Bacterial lipopolysaccharides proved to be very effective in producing intraperitoneal exudate rich in cells [134]. This phenomenon was inhibited by previous intraperitoneal injection of cortisone [140].

In humans, sterile inflammatory effusions are characterized by a rich cellular content including neutrophils, lymphocytes, macrophages, mesothelial cells, eosinophils and basophils; usually in that order of frequency [141]. The presence of macrophages, mesothelial cells, lymphocytes, eosinophils and even plasma cells has been confirmed by electron microscope studies [142, 143, 144].

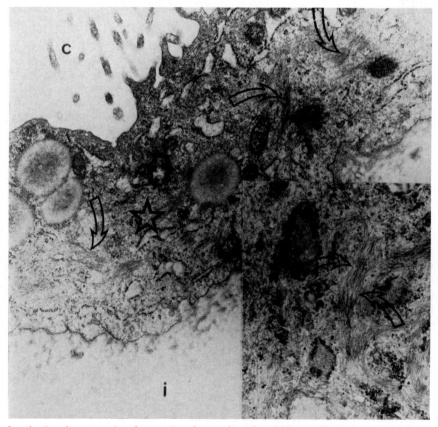

Figure 22. Biopsy of parietal peritoneum taken from a chronic uremic patient 16 hours after interruption of peritoneal dialysis. This recently implanted (˜4–5 days) mesothelial cell (star) shows microvilli on its luminal aspect facing the abdominal cavity (C). The open arrows point to intermediate size filaments. The basement membrane is still lacking. (i: interstitium). (× 15 400).

Inset. (Lower right). Intermediate size filaments at higher magnification (open arrows) (× 24 600).

Peritoneal eosinophilia (eosinophils > 10–50%) has been experimentally induced by intraperitoneal injection of iodine, chalk, nucleic acid, pilocarpine, hemoglobin or red blood cells, egg albumin, gold salts, mineral and vegetable oils, hydatidic fluid, and saline [141, 145]. On the other hand, intraperitoneal injection of bacteria and/or bacterial endotoxins induce a massive migration of neutrophils and monocytes into the peritoneal cavity [133, 146, 147].

The information presented above suggests that the cell content of effluent peritoneal dialysate is likely to be modified by so many factors that a concise description of a standardized cytologic pattern becomes extremely difficult. There are, however, a few aspects of peritoneal effluent dialysate which have been defined: a) patients on IPD have total cell counts up to 1200 cells/ml in the first exchange volume [148]; b) the cell population tends to decrease significantly with further exchanges [149]; c) during infectious peritonitis there is a substantial increase in total cell number [148], as well as in the number of neutrophils [5]; d) peritoneal fluid eosinophilia has been observed occacionally [150, 151].

7.1. Ultrastructure of peritoneal fluid cells

Free floating mesothelial cells are round or oval in shape and show a central, round nucleus (Figure 19, Figure 20 –l inset). Nuclear chromatin is quite evenly distributed and a small nucleolus may be observed. Numerous slender and sometimes branching microvilli emerge from the cytoplas-mic membrane [142, 144, 152, 153, 154]. Branching microvilli, similar to those observed in human embryos [14], can be quite crowded in some cells, whereas in others they are scarce [144]. Mitochondria, numerous cisternae of rough reticulum and free ribosomes are mainly located in the outer part of the cytoplasm, and so are pinocytotic vesicles [142, 154]. The presence of intermediate size filaments, perinuclear or irregularly scattered along the cytoplasm has been documented in young free-floating mesothelial cells [141, 143], as well as in those recently implanted on the peritoneal surface (Figure 22). These free-floating mesothelial cells should be distinguished from desquamated, degenerating mesothelial cells wandering in the peritoneal fluid (Figure 8) [152]. Free floating mesothelial cells in culture undergo mitotic activity [155].

Macrophages, which can be observed in large numbers, usually show an irregular and, at times, kidney-shaped nucleus with distorted masses of chromatin concentrated along the nuclear membrane (Figures 19, 20). The cytoplasmic outline of macrophages is irregular, with thin processes of variable length which, at times, engulf degenerated cells (Figure 20) or take the form of signet ring macrophages (Figure 8 – inset). Mitochondria, a small Golgi complex and phagolysosomes are more evident when the cell is involved in phagocytic activity (Figure 20).

The ultrastructural aspect of inflammatory cells that eventually appear in the peritoneal fluid is similar to that classically described for other tissues.

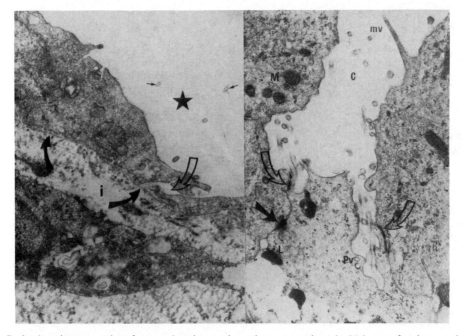

Figure 23. Left: Parietal peritoneum taken from a chronic uremic patient, approximately 14 hours after interruption of peritoneal dialysis. A few transversally sectioned microvilli (small arrows) can be seen in the peritoneal cavity (star). Two young adjacent mesothelial cells are separated by an open intercellular junction (open arrow). The basement membrane (black arrows) is, at times, interrupted. (i: interstitium). (Original magnification: × 16 250).
Right. Another area of the same biopsy. The general appearance of the tissue is quite close to that observed in normals and to that reported by Ryan-Majno in rats, seven days after injury. Note the presence of microvilli (mv), tight junctions (open arrows) and a desmosome (black arrow). (Pv: pinocytotic vesicles; M: mitochondria; L: lysosome; C: abdominal cavity). (Original magnification: × 16 250).

8. PERITONEAL ULTRASTRUCTURAL CHANGES DURING LONG TERM PERITONEAL DIALYSIS

Mesothelial cells ar extremely sensitive to minor injury. Mild drying or wetting of rat caecal peritoneum for five minutes induced mesothelial cell degeneration and detachment, and severe interstitial edema [156, 157]. Biopsies taken from CAPD patients also showed detachment of mesothelial cells (Figure 8) and similar severe degenerative changes: lack or scarcity of microvilli (Figures 23, 24 – inset); widened intercellular spaces (Figure 23) between mesothelial cells [158] and variable degrees of interstitial edema (Figures 24, 25, 26) [158, 159, 160].

Increased thickness of the submesothelial collagenous layer, apparently leading to a decreased peritoneal ultrafiltration potential, has also been reported [160].

An extreme degree of fibrosis has been observed in IPD as well as in CAPD patient developing sclerosing peritonitis [161, 162, 163, 164]. This severe complication was first described by Battle after ovariotomy [165], and later was associated with the use of β-blockers [166] and intraperitoneally administered substances [164, 167]. Even though the pathophysiology of this complication is still unclear, experimental studies suggest that a substantial decrease in the mesothelial fibrinolytic activity could be the most likely initiating mechanism [168, 169, 170].

Some researchers have reported small plastic particles [158, 160] as well as cytoplasmic inclusions of crystals

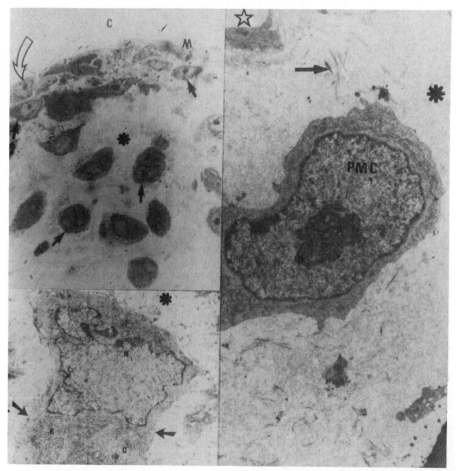

Figure 24. Biopsy taken from a chronic uremic patient 14 hours after interruption of peritoneal dialysis. *Upper left:* Mesothelial cell precursors (black arrows) appear to be progressing towards the peritoneal surface facing the abdominal cavity (C). One of these cells (open arrows) is already implanted on the luminal surface of the peritoneum. The elongated mesothelial cell (M) shows a nucleus quite similar to that of the precursors. The interstitium (*) is edematous. This situation is similar to that observed by Ryan and Majno 3 days after experimentally induced severe mesothelial injury. (Original magnification: × 400). *Lower left.* This submesothelial interstitial cell (arrows) is interpreted as a mesothelial cell precursor. The cytoplasm shows protrusions and indentations. The irregularly shaped nucleus (N) shows fine and evenly distributed chromatin with a dense rim along the nuclear membrane. The presence of numerous cisternae of rough endoplasmic reticulum (R) indicate the high metabolic activity of this cell. The Golgi complex (G) is poorly developed as is usually observed in stem cells and fast growing cells. (*: interstitium). (Original magnification: × 10450). *Right:* This cell is interpreted as a primitive mesenchymal cell (PMC). The nucleus (N) is oval, with some irregularities and shows a granular and even distribution of chromatin. A fine chromatin rim underlines the nuclear membrane. The nucleolus is prominent. These cells are usually arranged along interstitial blood capillaries (star). Note collagen fibers (arrow) between the cell and the blood capillary. (*: interstitium) (× 4400).

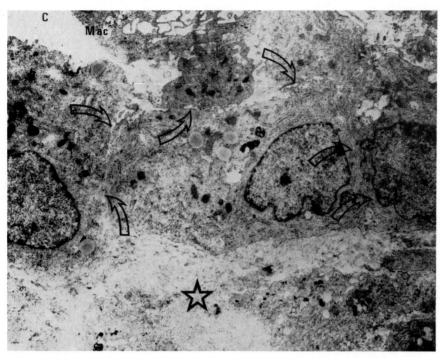

Figure 25. Biopsy of parietal peritoneum taken from a chronic uremic patient 13 hr after interruption of peritoneal dialysis. Note adjacent recently implanted mesothelial cells touching one another (open arrows), forming new intercellular junctions. There is no evidence of basement membrane. This situation is similar to that experimentally observed by Ryan-Majno 3 to 4 days after severe mesothelial injury. (C: abdominal cavity; Mac: macrophage; star: interstitium). (Original magnification: × 5600).

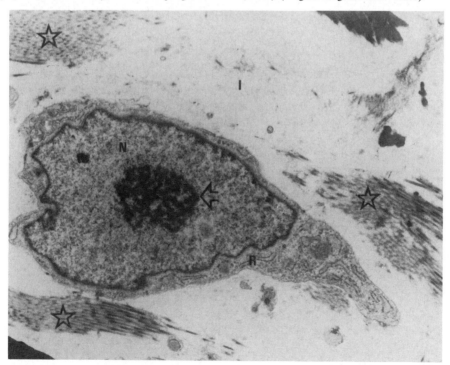

Figure 26. Biopsy of parietal peritoneum taken from an IPD patient (14 months on IPD). The young fibroblast depicted in the figure shows irregular cytoplasmic outline. The nucleus (N) is large, irregular with faint, widely distributed chromatin which is concentrated at the nuclear periphery, forming a thin rim. Note a large, granular and central nucleolus (open arrow). The interstitium shows bundles of collagen fibers (open stars) as well as large areas of edema (I). (R: rough endoplasmic reticulum) (× 8600).

(Figure 27), both resulting, most likely, from the use of contaminated dialysis solutions or defective lines and/or bags. The idea that most of the previously mentioned ultrastructural mesothelial changes are due to cell injury is not accepted by all the investigators. It has been stated that ultrastructural deviations from normality found in mesothelium exposed to dialysate may not in fact denote damage, and that separation between mesothelial cells result from cell shrinkage induced by the hyperosmolar dialysate [171].

It has been shown that the mesothelium has powerful regenerative capabilities [156, 157]. Comparison of experimental observations with those obtained from patients on maintenance peritoneal dialysis suggests that most of the observed peritoneal ultrastructural changes are the end results of two processes occurring simultaneously: mesothelial injury and regeneration [172].

Biopsies taken from IPD patients approximately 14 to 16 hr after completion of peritoneal dialysis showed peritoneal areas denuded of mesothelium and covered just by smooth muscle cells. Round, mononuclear, wandering mesothelial cells coming up from the peritoneum and, at times, macrophages were observed settling at the injured areas (Figure 21 – inset, Figure 24 – inset, Figure 25). These findings resemble those made by Ryan [156] 24 hours after experimental mesothelial injury. Other areas of the same

biopsies showed recently implanted young mesothelial cells (Figure 23 – Left, Figure 25 – Left, upper inset). Both the mesothelial basement membrane and microvilli were absent. Adjoining mesothelial cells occassionally appeared forming new intercellular junctions which were still more or less open (Figure 23 – left, Figure 25). The submesothelial interstitium was grossly edematous (Figure 24 – upper left, Figures 25, 26). Similar ultrastructural features were observed experimentally 3 days after mesothelial injury [156, 157]. Other specimens, taken from patients approximately 14–16 hr after peritoneal dialysis, showed young mesothelial cells building a new basement membrane (Figures 7, 23) as well as new microvilli which sometimes took the worm-like appearance of micropinocytosis vermiformis (Figure 7). These were reminiscent of the branching microvilli observed in mesothelial cells of human embryos in the 5th–8th week of gestation [14]. This sequence of mesothelial regeneration is compatible with that observed 4–5 days after experimental mesothelial injury [156]. Biopsies taken 10 or more days after the last peritoneal dialysis had a normal mesothelial lining which, in one case, showed intracytoplasmic crystalline inclusions (Figure 27).

In summary, studies done on IPD patients disclosed that different blocks taken from one biopsy of parietal peritoneum showed each of the above mentioned steps of mesothelial reegeneration taking place simultaneously in

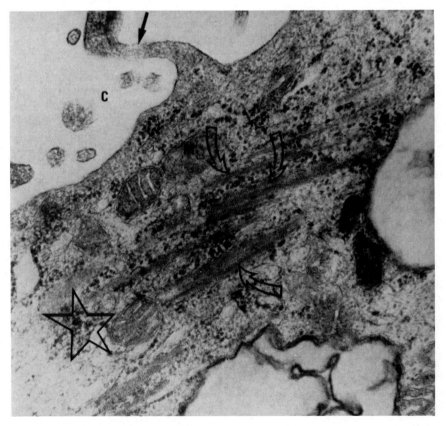

Figure 27. Biopsy of partietal peritoneum taken from a chronic uremic 10 days after interruption of peritoneal dialysis. This patient was on peritoneal dialysis for 7 months. The mesothelial cell (star) depicted in the figure shows crystalline inclusions (open arrows), mitochondria (M), smooth endoplasmic reticulum (framed by the open star), as well as microvilli (black arrow). (C: abdominal cavity) ($\times 50\,720$).

different areas of the peritoneal surface [172]. From these observations it can be inferred that the currently used peritoneal dialysis solutions induce a situation of continuous mesothelial injury, which is restored by a continuous process of repair. Similar ultrastructural changes were experimentally induced by intraperitoneal injections of furfural, one of the many substances resulting from the non-enzymatic degradation of glucose [173].

Interstitial edema (Figures 22, 24) results from the inflammatory reaction after injury. The presence of wide-open intercellular channels (Figures 21, 23, 24, 26) occurring after mesothelial injury would reflect a specific stage in the process of building new junctions by the new mesothelial cells [153, 157, 174, 175] (Figures 21, 23, 25). Ultrastructural studies done on mouse embryo [13] revealed that mesothelial cells directly derived from mesenchymal cells showed increasing numbers of microvilli according to the extent of their differentiation. Therefore, the aforementioned lack or scarcity of microvilli could just denote the presence of less mature, regenerating mesothelial cells at the peritoneal luminal surface [22].

8.1. The origin of the new mesothelial cells

It has been shown experimentally that small and large mesothelial wounds heal at the same rate within 7 to 10 days after injury [176]. The basal, normally observed mitotic rate of mesothelial cells, as measured in the rat by H^3-thymidine incorporation, is of approximately 1%/day. This rate is significantly increased during peritonitis, reaching maximal values of up to 19% between 1 and 3 days after injury, and returning to the basal activity on the 4th or 5th day [177]. It should be noted, however, that proliferation of fibroblasts as well as mesothelial cell repair are substantially inhibited in experimental uremic animals [177, 178, 179].

The origin of the new mesothelial cells repopulating denuded areas of injury is still controversial. Four different hypotheses haven been proposed:

a) The repopulating cells originate from the bone marrow [50]. Other experimental studies showed, however, that whole-body irradiation sufficient to depress peripheral white blood cell count as well as cell replacement by the bone marrow did not prevent mesothelial healing [180]. Therefore, the existence of a circulating mesothelial precursor originating from the bone marrow seems to be unlikely.

b) Mature mesothelial cells from adjacent and/or opposed areas proliferate, exfoliate and migrate to repopulate the affected surface [175, 175, 181]. This hypothesis has neither been accepted by other investigators [178, 182, 183], nor supported by our own observations. In fact, we have not observed mature mesothelial cells covering areas with evidence of recent mesothelial injury.

c) Other studies [152, 178, 1874] suggested the sequence of a two stage process; during the first 24 hr, macrophages forming the first line of defence [185] and coming from the peritoneal fluid repopulate the wound surface (Figure 21 – inset, Figure 25). Later on, during the second stage, new mesothelial cells, arising from metaplasia of mesenchymal precursors located in the interstitial tissue well below the site of injury, migrate to the surface and differentiate into mature mesothelial cells (Figure 24). This hypothesis

has not been universally accepted [22, 156, 157, 174, 176], It has also been suggested that the early implanted macrophages are gradually transformed into mesothelial cells [174]. However, Raftery [186], after labelling peritoneal macrophages with polystyrene spheres presented strong evidence against the hypothesis that peritoneal macrophages could be transformed into mesothelial cells.

Primitive mesenchymal cells which have been observed deep in the interstitial tissue [187] (Figure 24 – right) are multipotential and can give rise to a wide variety of cells, including mesothelium [182]. Mesothelial cell precursors coming up from the submesothelial connective tissue were also observed under the damaged areas. The nuclear and cytoplasmic aspect of these cells were identical to that showed by new mesothelial cells already implanted on the peritoneal surface (Figure 24 – upper left).

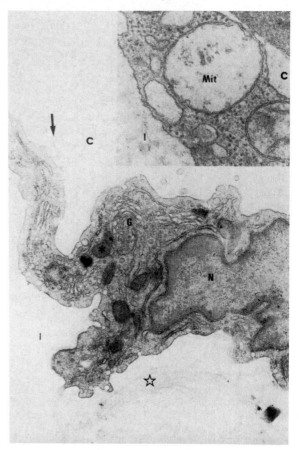

Figure 28. **Mesentery of rat. The animal was sacrified after 14** consecutive intraperitoneal injections of 0.2% furfural, on a daily basis. The young mesothelial cell appearing in this electron micrograph shows some microvilli (black arrow), an irregularly shaped nucleus (n), hypertrophic Golgi complex (G), and mitochondria (*). The normally observed submesothelial membrane is absent. The interstitial space (I) is grossly edematous. A few collagen fibers (star) can be seen at the bottom. (Original magnification: × 24 600).

Inset. (Upper right). A different mesothelial cell of the same sample showing marked mitochondrial swelling (Mit) as well as absence of basement membrane. (C: abdominal cavity; I: interstitium). (Original magnification: × 50 720).

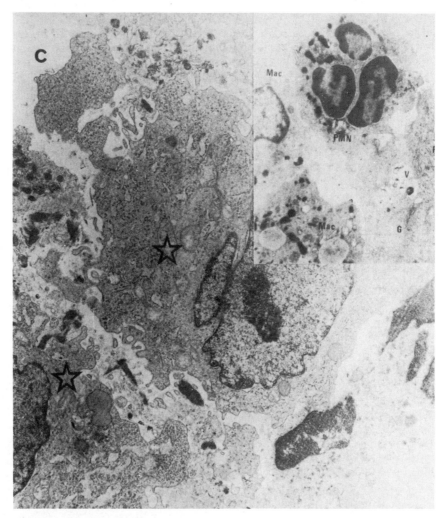

90   *Gotloib, Shostak*

Figure 29. Biopsy of parietal peritoneum taken, during an episode of peritonitis, from a chronic uremic patient on peritoneal dialysis. Recently implanted (1–2 days) mesothelial cells (stars), apparently coming from the abdominal cavity (C), are repopulating the denuded peritoneal surface. (Original magnification: × 8400).

Inset. (Upper right). A different area of the same biopsy showing a recently implanted mesothelial cell with vacuoles (V), rough endoplasmic reticulum (R) and hyperthrophic Golgi complex (G). Notice the presence of macrophages (Mac) and polymorphonuclears (PMN). (Original magnification: × 12 600).

d) Free-floating cells of the serosal cavity settle on the injured areas and gradually differentiate into new mesothelial cells [156, 157, 172, 182] (Figure 21 – inset). It should be noticed that desquamated, mature mesothelial cells show degenerative changes ((Figure 8) which, as was previously stated, are absent in the young, free floating mesothelial cells (Figure 19).

All this evidence suggests that, most likely, mesothelial cell regeneration takes place through two different processes occurring simultaneously: implantation of young wandering mesothelial cells, and migration of mesothelial cell precursors coming from the underlying connective tissue.

8.2. Ultrastructural changes during septic peritonitis

This condition results in acute inflammatory changes affecting all the peritoneal structures. Mesothelial cells, ne-

crotic or showing severe degenerative changes, exfoliate. The submesothelial basement membrane disappears (Figure 29), together with the normally present anionic fixed charges (Figure 30).

Experimental studies have shown that the anionic fixed charges of mesothelial glycocalyx and microvilli, which were still present 24 hr after induction of peritonitis, were not observed 5 days later, and partially reappeared 13 days after the onset of the experiment [93].

The interstitium becomes grossly edematous (Figure 30) as well as infiltrated by acute inflammatory cells. The microvessels occasionally show wide-open intercellular junctions (Figure 12 – inset), as well as a sharp decrease in the subendothelial density distribution of anionic fixed charges (Figure 13 – left) [93].

Almost simultaneously, macrophages and young mesothelial cells start to repopulate the denuded luminal pe-

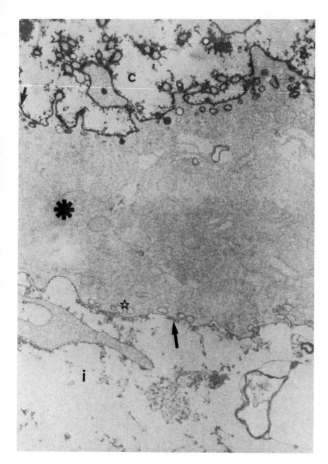

Figure 30. Section of rat mesentery taken 24 hours after induction of *E. coli* peritonitis. The glycocalyx of mesothelial cell plasmalemma (short black arrow), as well as that of microvilli (open arrow) are still present. The mesothelial cell (*) is lying on an interrupted and disorganized basement membrane (long black arrow). Note the absence of submesothelial anionic sites as well as the intensity of the interstitial edema (i). (Star: uncoated pinocytotic vesicles; C: abdominal cavity). (Original magnification: × 24 600).

ritoneal surface (Figure 29). Polymorphonuclears (Figure 29 – inset) and monocytes are usually present at the luminal surface, as well as in the submesothelial connective tissue.

Complete morphological and functional return to normality may be expected to occur approximately 2 weeks after recovery from the infectious episode.

9. CONCLUSION

There is no doubt that today we know much more about the ultrastructure and cell biology of the peritoneal constituents than 10 years ago. A different picture of ...'the living peritoneum as a dialyzing membrane' [188] is emerging. Perhaps, the most significant contribution of the numerous research studies included in our long list of references is that we are starting to know how much we still do not know. In essence, as stated by Nagel [189] ...'The

mark of scientific progress becomes the discovery of new problems rather than the solution of old ones'.

REFERENCES

1. Robinson B: The peritoneum. WT Keener Co., Chicago, p. 13, 1897.
2. Ganter, G: Uber die Beseitigung giftiger Stoffe aus dem Blute durch dialyse. Munchen Med Wchnschr 70: 1478–1480, 1923.
3. Boen ST: Peritoneal dialysis in clinical medicine. Charles C. Thomas. Springfield, 1964.
4. Tenckhoff H, Schechter H: A bacteriologically safe peritoneal access device for repeated dialysis. Trans Am Soc Artif Inter Organs 14: 181–187, 1968.
5. Popovich RP, Moncrief JW, Decherd JF, Bomar JB, Pyle WK: Preliminary verification of the low dialysis clearance hypothesis via a novel equilibrium peritoneal dialysis technique. Abst Am Soc Artif Intern Organs 5: 64, 1976.
6. Nolph KD, Sorkin M, Rubin, J, Arfania D, Prowant B, Fruto L, Kennedy D: Continuous ambulatory peritoneal dialysis: three-year experience at one center. Annals Int Med 92: 609–613, 1980.
7. Luschka H: Die Structure der serosen haute des menschen. Tubingen, 1851.
8. Putiloff PV: Materials for the study of the laws of growth of the human body in relation to the surface areas of different systems: the trial on Russian subjects of planigraphic anatomy as a mean of exact antropometry. Presented at the Siberian branch of the Russian Geographic Society. Omsk, 1886.
9. Wegner G: Chirurgische bemerkingen uber die peritoneal Hole, mit Besonderer Berucksichtigung der ovariotomie. Arch Klin Chir 20: 51–59, 1877.
10. Esperanca MJ, Collins DL: Peritoneal dialysis efficiency in relation to body weight. J Pediatric Surg 1: 162–169, 1966.
11. Gotloib L, Digenis GE, Rabinovich S, Medline A, Oreopolous DG: Ultrastructure of normal rabbit mesentery. Nephron 34: 248–255, 1983.
12. Gosselin RE, Berndt WO: Diffusional transport of solutes through mesentery and peritoneum. J Theor Biol 3: 487, 1962.
13. Haar JL, Ackerman GA: A phase and electron microscopic study of vasculogenesis and erythropoiesis in the yolk sac of the mous. Anatom Record 170: 199–224, 1971.
14. Ukeshima A, Hayashi Y, Fujimore T: Surface morphology of the human yolk sac: endoderm and mesothelium. 49: 483–494, 1986.
15. Puulmala RM: Morphologic comparison of parietal and visceral peritoneal epithelium in fetus and adult. Anatom Record 68: 327–330, 1937.
16. Robertson JD: Molecular structure of biological membranes. In: A. Lima de Faria (ed), Handbook of Molecular Cytology. North Holland Publ Amsterdam and London, p. 1404, 1969.
17. Kolossow A: Weber die struktur des endothels der pleuroperitoneal hole der blut und lymphgefasse. Biol Centralbl Bd 12: S87–94, 1892.
18. Odor L: Obervations of the rat mesothelium with the electron and phase microscopes. Am J Anat 95: 433–465, 1954.
19. Felix DM, Dalton AJ: A comparison of mesothelial cells and macrophages in mice after the intraperitoneal inoculation of melanine granules. J Biophys and Biochem Cyt 2, Suppl part 2: 109–117, 1956.
20. Baradi AF, Hope J: Obervations on ultrastructure of rabbit mesothelium. Exper Cell Res 34: 33–44, 1964.
21. Baradi AF, Crae SN: A scanning electron microscope study of mouse peritoneal mesothelium. Tissue Cell 8: 159, 1976.
22. Whitaker D, Papadimitriou JM, Walters MNI: The mesothelium and its reactions: a review. CRC Critical reviews in Toxicology 10: 81–144, 1982.

23. Fukata H: Electron microscopic study on normal rat peritoneal mesothelium and its changes in adsorption of particulate iron dextran complex. Acta Pathol Japonica 13: 309–325, 1963.
24. Lieberman-Meffet D, White H: The greater omentum: anatomy, physiology, pathology, surgery with an historical survery. Springer-Verlag, Berlin. p 6.
25. Madison LD, Bergstrom MU, Porter B, Torres R, Shelton E: Regulation of surface topography of mouse peritoneal cells. J Cell Biol 82: 783, 1979.
26. Gotloib L, Shostak A: Ultrastructural morphology of the peritoneum: new findings and speculations on transfer of solutes and water during peritoneal dialysis. Perit Dial Bull (in press).
27. Gotloib L: Anatomical basis for peritoneal permeability. In: La Greca G, Chiaramonte S, Fabris A, Feriani M, Ronco C (eds), Peritoneal Dialysis. Wichtig Ed, Milano, pp 3–10.
28. Gotloib L, Shostak A, Jaichenko J: Ruthenium red stained anionic charges of rat and mice mesothelial cells and basal lamina: the peritoneum is a negatively charged dialyzing membrane. Nephron (in press).
29. Luft JH: Fine structure of capillary and endocapillary layer as revealed by ruthenium ed. Fed Proc 25: 1173–1183, 1966.
30. Gotloib L, Bar-Sella P, Jaichenko J, Shostak A: Ruthenium red stained polyanionic fixed charges in peritoneal microvessels. Nephron 47: 22–28, 1987.
31. Curry FE, Michel CC: A fiber matrix model of capillary permeability. Microvasc Res 20: 96–99, 1980.
32. Moog F: The lining of the small intestine. Scientific American 2455: 116–125, 1981.
33. Gotloib L: Anatomy of the peritoneal membrane. In: La Greca G, Biasoli G, Ronco C (eds), Wichtig Ed, Milan, pp 17–30, 1982.
34. Leak LV: Distribution of cell surface charges on mesothelium and lymphatic endothelium. Microvasc Res 31: 18–30, 1986..
35. Lewis WH: Pinocutosis. Bull Johns Hopkins Hosp 49: 17–23, 1931.
36. Casley-Smith JR: The dimensions and numbers of small vesicles in cells, endothelial and mesothelial and the significance of these for endothelial permeability. J Microscopy 90: 251–269, 1969.
37. Casley-Smith JR, Chin JC: The passage of cytoplasmic vesicles across endothelial and mesothelial cells. J Microscopy 93: 167–189, 1971.
38. Fedorko ME, Hirsch JG, Fried B: Studies on transport of macromolecules and small particles across mesothelial cells of the mouse omentum. Exp Cell Res 63: 313–323, 1971.
39. Simionescu N, Simionescu M, Palade GE: Structural basis of permeability in sequential segments of the microvasculature. II. Pathways followed by microperoxidase across the endothelium. Microvasc Res 15: 17–36, 1978.
40. Palade GE, Simionescu M, Simionescu N: Structural aspects of the permeability of the microvascular endothelium. Acta Physiol Scand Suppl 463: 11–32, 1979.
41. Palade GE: Fine structure of blood capillaries. J Appl Phys 24: 1424, 1953.
42. Florey HW: The transport of materials across the capillary wall. Quart J Exper Physiol 49: 117–128, 1964.
43. Pappenheimer JR, Renkin EM, Borrero LM: Filtration, diffusion and molecular sieving through peripheral capillary membranes. A contribution to the pore theory of capillary permeability. Am J Physiol 167: 13–46, 1951.
44. Frokjaer-Jensen J: The plasmalemmal vesicular system in capillary endothelium. Prog Appl Microcirc 1: 17–34, 1983.
45. Wagner RC, Robinson CS: High voltage electron microscsopy of capillary endothelial vesicles. Microvascc Res 28: 197–205, 1984.
46. Simionescu N, Simionescu M, Palade GE: Differentiated microdomains on the luminal surface of capillary endothelium. I. Preferential distribution of anionic sites. J Cell Biol 90: 605–613, 1981.
47. Steinman RM, Mellman IS, Muller WA, Cohn ZA: Endocytosis and the recycling of plasma membrane. J Cell Biol 96: 1–27, 1983.
48. Shea SM, Karnovesky MJ: Brownian motion: a theoretical explanation for the movement of vesicles across the endothelium. Nature, London 212: 353–354, 1966.
49. Simionescu M, Simionescu N, Palade GE: Morphometric data on the endothelium of blood capillaries. J Cell Biol 60: 128–152, 1974.
50. Wagner JC, Johnson NF, Brown DG, Wagner MMF: Histology and ultrastructure of serially transplanted rat mesotheliomas. Brit J Cancer 46: 294–299, 1982.
51. Petersen OW, Van Deurs B: Serial section analysis of coated pits and vesicles involved in adsorptive pinocytosis in cultered fibroblasts. J Cell Biol 96: 277–281, 1983.
52. Peters KR, Carley WW, Palade GE: Endothelial plasmalemmal vesicles have a characteristic striped bipolar surface structure. J Cell Biol 101: 2233–2238, 1985.
53. Simionescu M, Simionescu N, Silbert J, Palade G: Differentiated microdomains on the luminal surface of the capillary endothelium. II. Partial characterization of their anionic sites. J Cell Biol 90: 614–621, 1981.
54. Pearse BMF: Clathrin: a unique protein associated with intracellular transfer of membrane by coated vesicles. Proc Natl Acad Sci USA 73: 1255–1259, 1976.
55. Goldstein JL, Brown MS, Anderson RGW, Russell, DW, Schneider WJ: Receptor mediated endocytosis: concepts emerging from the LDL receptor system. Ann Rev Cell Biol 1: 1–39, 1985.
56. Pastan I, Willingham MC: The pathway of endocytosis. In: Pastan I, Willingham MC (eds), Endocytosis. Plenum Press, New York. pp 1–44, 1985.
57. Ghitescu L, Fixman A, Simionescu M, Simionescu N: Specific binding sites for albumin restricted to plasmalemmal vesicles of continuous capillary endothelium: receptor mediated transcytosis. J Cell Biol 102: 1304–1311, 1986.
58. Henle FGJ: Splacnologie. Vol II, p 175, 1875.
59. Simionescu M, Simionescu N: Organization of cell junctions in the peritoneal mesothelium. J Cell Biol 74: 98, 1977.
60. Von Recklinghausen FD: Zur Fettresorption. Arch of Path Anat u Physiol, Bd 26: S172–208, 1863.
61. Bizzozero G, Salvioli G: Sulla suttura della membrane sierosa e particolarmente del peritoneo diaphragmatico. Giornale della R Acad di Medicina di Torino. 19: 466–470, 1876.
62. Allen L: The peritoneal stomata. The Anat Record 67: 89–103, 1937.
63. French JE, Florey HW, Morris B: The adsorption of particles by the lymphatics of the diaphragm. Quarterly J Exper Physiol 45: 88–102, 1959.
64. Tourneux F, Herrman G: Recherches sur quelques epitheliums plats dans la serie animale (Deuxieme partie). J de L'Anat et de la Physiol. 12: 386–424, 1876.
65. Kolossow A: Uber die struktur des pleuroperitoneal und gefassepithels (endothels). Arch f Mikr Anat 42: 318–383, 1893.
66. Simer PM: The passage of particulate matter from the peritoneal cavity into the lymph vessels of the diaphragm. The Anatom Record 101: 333–351, 1948.
67. Leak LW, Just EE: Permeability of peritoneal mesothelium. J Cell Biol 70: 423a, 1976.
68. Tsilibarry EC, Wissig SL: Absorption from the peritoneal cavity: SEM study of the mesothelium covering the peritoneal surface of the muscular portion of the diaphragm. Am J Anat 149: 127–133, 1977.
69. Yoffey JM, Courtice FC: Lymphatics, lymph and lymphoid tissue. Edward Arnold Ltd, London. p 176, 1956.
70. Andrews PM, Porter KR: The ultrastructural morphology

and possible functional significance of mesothelial microvilli. Anat Rec 177: 409–414, 1973.

71. Ghadially FN: Ultrastructural pathology of the cell. Butterworths, London and Boston. p 403, 1978.

72. Todd RB, Bowman W: The physiological anatomy and physiology of man. Vols I and II. London. 1845 and 1846.

73. Muscatello G: Uber den Bau und das Aufsaugunsvermogen des Peritanaums. Virchows Archiv f Path Anat, Bd 142: 327–359, 1895.

74. Baron MA: Structure of the intestinal peritoneum in man. Am J Anat 69: 439–496, 1941.

75. Maximow A: Bindgewebe und blutbildende gcwebe. Handbuch der mikroskopischen Anatomie des menschen. Bd 2 T 1: S232–583. v. Mollendorf. 1927.

76. Gotloib L, Shostak A, Bar-Sella P, Eiali V: Reduplicated skin and peritoneal blood capillaries and mesothelical basement membrane in aged non-diabetic chronic uremic patients. Perit Dial Bulletin 4: S28, 1984.

77. Gersh I, Catchpole HR: The organization of ground substances and basement membrane and its significance in tissue injury, disease and growth. Am J Anat 85: 457–522, 1949.

78. Williamson JR, Vogler NJ, Kilo Ch: Regional variations in the width of the basement membrane of muscle capillaries in man and giraffe. Am J Path 63: 359–367, 1971.

79. Vracko R: Skeletal muscle capillaries in nondiabetics. A quantitative analysis. Circulation 16: 285–297, 1970.

80. Parthasarathy N, Spire RG: Effect of diabetes on the glycosaminoglycan component of the human glomerular basement membrane. Diabetes 31: 738–741, 1982.

81. Vracko R, Pecoraro RE, Carter WB: Overview article: Basal lamina of epidermis, muscle fibers, muscle capillaries, and renal tubules; changes with aging and in diabetes mellitus. Ultrast Pathol 1, 559–574, 1980.

82. Vracko R: Basal lamina scaffold-anatomy and significance for maintenance of orderly tissue structure. A review. Am J Pathol 77: 313–346, 1974.

83. Hruza Z: Connective tissue. In: Kaley G, Altura BM (eds), Microcirculation. Univ Park Press, Baltimore. Vol 1, pp 167–183, 1977.

84. Comper WD, Laurent TC: Physiological function of connective tissue polysaccharides. Physiol Reviews 58: 255–315, 1978.

85. Simionescu N: Cellular aspects of transcapillary exchange. Physiol Reviews 63: 1536–1579, 1983.

86. Wolff JR: Ultrastructure of the terminal vascular bed as related to function. In: Kaley G, Altura BM (eds), Microcirculation. University Park Press, Baltimore. Vol I, pp 95–130, 1977.

87. Majno G: Ultrastructure of the vascular membrane. Handbook of Physiology. Section II - Circulation. Vol III. Am Physiol Soc Washington DC, pp 2293–2375, 1965.

88. Gotloib L, Shostak A, Bar-Sella P, Eiali V: Fenestrated capillaries in human parietal and rabbit diaphragmatic peritoneum. Nephron 41: 200–202, 1985.

89. Gotloib L, Shostak A, Jaichenko J. Unpublished observations.

90. Gotloib L, Shostak A, Bar-Sella P, Eiali V: Heterogeneous density and ultrastructure of rabbit's microvasculature. Int J Artif Organs 7: 123–125, 1984.

91. Nolph KD, Miller F, Rubin J, Popovich R: New directions in peritoneal dialysis concepts and applications. Kidney Int 18, Suppl 10: S111–S116, 1980.

92. Rhodin YAG: Ultrastructure of mammalian venous capillaries, venules and small collecting veins. J Ultrast Research 25: 452–500, 1968.

93. Gotloib L, Shostak A, Jaichenko J: Loss of mesothelial and microvascular fixed anionic charges during murine experimentally induced septic peritonitis. Presented at the IV Int Symposium on Peritoneal Dialysis, Venice, 1987. 1987.

94. Simionescu M, Simionescu N, Palade GE: Differentiated microdomains on the luminal surface of capillary endothelium: distribution of lectin receptors. J Cell Biol 94: 406–413, 1982.

95. Schneeberger EE, Hamelin M: Interactions of serum proteins with lung endothelial glycocalyx: its effect on endothelial permeability. Am J Physiol 247: H206–H217, 1984.

96. Bundgaard M, Frokjaer-Jensen J: Functional aspects of the ultrastructure of terminal blood vessels: a quantitative study on consecutive segments of the frog mesenteric microvasculature. Microvasc Res 23: 1–30, 1982.

97. Palade GE: Transport in quanta across the endothelium of blood capillaries. Anat Rec 116: 254, 1960.

98. Milici AJ, L'hernault N, Palade GE: Surface densities of diaphragmed fenestrae and transendothelial channels in different murine capillary beds. Circ Res 56, 709–717, 1985.

99. Simionescu M, Simionescu N, Palade GE: Sulfated glycosaminoglycans are major components of the anionic sites of fenestral diaphragms in capillary endothelium. J Cell Biol 83: 78a, 1979.

100. Milici AJ, L'Hernault N: Variation in the number of fenestrations and channels between fenestrated capillary bed. J Cell Biol 97: No. 5, 336, 1983.

101. Peters KR, Milici AJ: High resolution scanning electron microscopy of the luminal surface of a fenestrated capillary endothelium. J Cell Biol 97: 336a, 1983.

102. Bankston PW, Milici AJ: A Survey of the binding of polycationic ferritin in several fenestrated capillary beds: indication of heterogeneity in the luminal glycocalyx of fenestral diaphragms. Microvasc Res 26: 36–48, 1983.

103. Farquhar MG, Palade GE: Junctional complexes in various epithelia. J Cell Biol 17: 375–442, 1963.

104. Simionescu M, Simionescu N, Palade G: Segmental differentiations of cell junctions in the vascular endothelium. J Cell Biol 67: 863–885, 1975.

105. Thorgeirsson G, Robertson AL Jr: The vascular endothelium. Pathobiologic significance. Am J Pathol 95: 801–848, 1978.

106. Renkin EM: Multiple ways of capillary permeability. Circ Research 41: 735–743, 1977.

107. Bearer EL, Orci L: Endothelial fenestral diaphragms: a quick-freeze deep-etch study. J Cell Biol 100: 418–428, 1985.

108. Nolph KD: The peritoneal dialysis system. Contr Nephrol 17: 44–50, 1979.

109. Mactier RA, Khanna R, Twardowski ZJ, Nolph KD: Role of peritoneal lymphatic absorption in peritoneal dialysis. Kidney Int 32: 165–172, 1987.

110. Casley-Smith JR: The role of the endothelial intercellular junctions in the functioning of the initial lymphatics. Angiologica 9: 106, 131, 1972.

111. Crone Ch: Exchange of molecules between plasma, interstitial tissue and lymphatics. Pflugers Arch 336: S65–S79, 1972.

112. Hauck G: Functional aspects of the topical relationship between blood capillaries and lymphatics of the mesentery. Pflugers Arch 339: 251–256, 1973.

113. Hauck G: Permeability of the mesenteric vasculature. Bibl Anat 13: 9–12, 1975.

114. Rhodin JAG, Sue SL: Combined intravital microscopy and electron microscopy of the blind beginnings of the mesenteric lymphatic capilalries of the rat mesentery. Acta Physiol Scand 463: 51–58, 1979.

115. Hauck G: The connective tissue space in view of lymphology. Experientia 38: 1121–1122, 1982.

116. Leak LV: Electron microscopic observations on lymphatic capillaries and the structural components of the connective tissue-lymph interface. Microvasc Res 2, 361–391, 1970.

117. Leak LV: Studies on the permeability of lymphatic capillaries. J Cell Biol 50: 300–323, 1971

118. Jones WR, O'Morchoe PJ, O'Morchoe CCC: The organization of endocytotic vesicles in lymphatic endothelium.

Microvasc Res 25: 286–299, 1983.

119. Casley-Smith JR: The functioning and interrelationships of blood capillaries and lymphatics. Experientia 32: 1–12, 1976.

120. Leak LV, Burke JF: Fine structure of lymphatic capillaries and the adjoining connective tissue area. Am J Anat 118: 785–809, 1966.

121. Leak LV, Burke JF: Ultrastructural studies on the lymphatic anchoring filaments. J Cell Biol 36: 129–149, 1968.

122. Jones WR, O'Morchoe CCC, Jarosz HM, O'Morchoe PJ: Distribution of charged sites on lymphatic endothelium. Lymphology 19: 5–14, 1986.

123. Hortsmann E: Anatomie and physiologie des lymphgefab-systems in Bauchraum. In: H Bartelheimer und N Hesig. Actuelle Gastroenterologie Verh Stuttgart. Thieme 1968, 1967.

124. Wayland H, Silbergberg A: Meeting report: blood to lymph transport. Microvasc Res 15, 367–374, 1978.

125. Haller A: Primae linae physiologiae in usum Praelectionum Academicarum avetae et emendato. Gottingae, Capit 25: p 421, 1751.

126. Vajda J: Innervation of lymph vessels. Acta Morphol Acad Sci Hung 14: 197–208, 1966.

127. Ohkashi T, Kobayashi S, Tsukahara S, Azuma T: Innervation of bovine mesenteric lymphatics from the histochemical point of view. Microvasc Res 24: 377–385, 1982.

128. Furness JB: Arrangement of blood vessels and their relation with adrenergic nerves in the rat mesentery. J Anat 115: 347–364, 1973.

129. Beattie JM: The cells of inflammatory exudations: an experimental research as to their function and density, and also as to the origin of the mononucleated cells. J Path Bacteriol 8: 130–177, 1903.

130. Durham HE: The mechanism of reaction to peritoneal infection. J Path Bacteriol 4: 338–382, 1897.

131. Josey AL: Studies in the physiology if the eosinophil. V. The role of the eosinophil in inflammation. Folia Haematol 51: 80–95, 1934.

132. Webb RL: Changes in the number of cells within the peritoneal fluid of the white rat, between birth and sexual maturity. Folia Haematol 51: 445–451, 1934.

133. Padawer J, Gordon AS: Cellular elements in the peritoneal fluid of some mammals. The Anatom Record 124: 209–222, 1956.

134. Fruhman GJ: Neutrophil mobilization into peritoneal fluid. Blood 16: 1753–1761, 1960.

135. Seeley SF, Higgins GM, Mann FC: The cytologic response of the peritoneal fluid to certain substances. Surgery 2: 862–876, 1937.

136. Montgomery LG: Preliminary studies of the cells of the peritoneal fluid in certain laboratory animals. Proc Staff Meetings of the Mayo CLinic 7: 589–591, 1932.

137. Bercovici B, Gallily R: The cytology of the human peritoneal fluid. Cytol 22, 124–127, 1978.

138. Becker S, Halme J, Haskill S: Heterogeneity of human peritoneal macrophages: cytochemical and flow cytometric studies. J Reticuloendothelial Soc (RES) 33: 127–138, 1983.

139. De Brux JA, Dupre-Froment J, Mintz M: Cytology of the peritoneal fluids sampled by coelioscopy or by cul de sac puncture. Its value in gynecology. Acta Cytol 12: 395–403, 1968.

140. Fruhmann GJ: Adrenal steroids and neutrophil mobilization. Blood 20: 355–363, 1962.

141. Spriggs AI, Boddington MM: The cytology of effusions. Grune-Straton, Inc New York. Second Edition. pp 5–17, 1968.

142. Domagala W, Woyke S: Transmission and scanning electron microscopic studies of cells in effusions. Acta Cytol 19: 214–224, 1975.

143. Efrati P, Nir E: Morphological and cytochemical investigation of human mesothelial cells from pleural and peritoneal effusions. A light and electron microscopy study. Israel J Med Sciences 12: 662–673, 1976.

144. Bewtra Ch, Greer KP: Ultrastructural studies of cells in body cavity effusions. Acta Cytol 29: 226–238, 1985.

145. Chapman JS, Reynolds RC: Eosinophilic response to intra-peritoneal blood. J Lab Clin Med 51: 516–520, 1958.

146. Northover BJ: The effect of various anti-inflammatory drugs on the accumulation of leucocytes in the peritoneal cavity of mice. J Pathol and Bacteriol 88: No. 1, 332–335, 1964.

147. Hurley JV, Ryan GB, Friedman A: The mononuclear response to intrapleural injection in the rat. J Path Bact 91: 575–587, 1966.

148. Gotloib L, Mines M, Garmizo AL, Rodoy, Y: Peritoneal dialysis using the subcutaneous intraperitoneal prosthesis. Dial and Transp 8: No. 3, 217–220, 1979.

149. Cichoki T, Hanicki Z, Sulowicz W, Smolensky O, Kopec J, Zembala M: Output of peritoneal cells into peritoneal di-alysate. Nephron 35, 175–182, 1983.

150. Nolph KD, Sorkin MI, Prowant BF, Kennedy JM, Everett ED: Asymptomatic eosinophilic peritonitis in continuous ambulatory peritoneal dialysis. Dial and Trans 11: 309–313, 1982.

151. Humayun HM, Todd SS, Daugisrdas JT, Ghandi VC, Popli S, Robinson JA, Hano JE, Zayas I: Peritoneal fluid eosin-ophilia in patients undergoing maintenance peritoneal dialy-sis. Arch Int Med 141: 1172, 1981.

152. Leak LV: Interaction of mesothelium to intraperitoneal sti-mulation. Lab Invest 48: 479–490, 1983.

153. Raftery AT: Regeneration of parietal and visceral peritoneum: an electron microscopical study. J Anat 115: 375–392, 1973.

154. Raftery AT: Mesothelial cells in peritoneal fluid. J Anat 115: 237–253, 1973.

155. Koss LG: Diagnostic cytology and its histopathologic bases. Third Edition. Lippincot, Philadelphia. Chapters 16–25, 1979.

156. Ryan GB, Grobety J, Majno G: Postoperative peritoneal adhesions: a study of the mechanisms. Am J Pathol 65: 117–148, 1971.

157. Ryan GB, Grobety J, Majno G: Mesothelial injury and recovery. Am J Pathol 71: 93–112, 1973.

158. Di Paolo N, Sacchi G, De Mia M, Gaggiotti E, Capotoude L, Rossi P, Bernini M, Pucci AM, Ibba L, Sabatelli P, Alessandrini C: Does Dialysis modify the peritoneal struc-ture?' In: La Greca G, Chiaramonte S, Fabris A, Feriani M, Ronco C (eds), Peritoneal Dialysis. Wichtig Ed, Milano. Pages 11–24.

159. Dobbie JW, Zaki M, Wilson L: Ultrastructural studies on the peritoneum with special reference to chronic ambulatory peritoneal dyalisis. Scott Med J 26: 213–223, 1981.

160. Verger C, Brunschvicg O, Le Charpentier Y, Lavergne A, Vantelon J: Structural and ultrastructural peritoneal mem-brane changes and permeability alterations during continuous ambulatory peritoneal dialysis. Proc EDTA 18: 199–205, 1981.

161. Tenckhoff H: Chronic peritoneal dialysis manual. Univ Was-hington School of Medicine. Seattle. pp 5, 634, 79, 1974.

162. Gandhi VC, Humayun HM, Todd S, Daugirdas JT, Jablokow VR, Shunzaburo I, Geis P, Hano JE: Sclerotic thickening of the peritoneal membrane in maintenance peritoneal dialysis patients. Arch Int Med 140: 1201–1203, 1980.

163. Slingeneyer A, Canaud B, Mourad G, Beraud JJ, Balmes M, Mion C: Sclerosing peritonitis (SP): late and severe complications of long term home peritoneal dialysis (HPD). Abstr 29th Ann Meet Am Soc Artif Intern Organs, p 66, 1982.

164. Ing TS, Daugirdas JT, Gandh VC: Peritoneal sclerosis in peritoneal dialysis patients. Am J Nephrol 4: 173–176, 1984.

165. Battle W: Intestinal obstruction coming on four years after the operation of ovariotomy. Lancet 1: 818–820, 1883.

166. Brown P, Baddeley H, Read AE, Davies JD, Mc Garry J: Sclerosing peritonitis, an unusual complication of an adre-

nergic blocking drug (practolol). Lancet II: 1477–1481, 1974.

167. Junor BJR, Briggs JD, Forwell MA, Dobbie JW, Henderson I: Sclerosing peritonitis. The contribution of chlorhexidine in alcohol. Pert Dial Bulletin 5: 101–104, 1985.

168. Myhre-Jensen O, Bergmann Larsen S, Astrup T: Fibrinolytic activity in serosal and synovial membranes. Rats, guinea pigs and rabbits. Arch Pathol 88: 623–630, 1969

169. Gervin AS, Puckett ChL, Silver D: Serosal hypofibrinolysis. A cause of postoperative adhesions. Am J Surg 1225: 80–88, 1973.

170. Buckman RF, Woods M, Sargent L, Gervin AS: A unifying pathogenetic mechanism in the etiology of intraperitoneal adhesions. J Surg Res 20, 1–5, 1976.

171. Dobbie JW, Zaki MA: The ultrastructure of the parietal peritoneum in normal and uremic man and in patients on CAPD. In: Maher JF, Winchester JF (eds), Frontiers on Peritoneal Dialysis. Field, Richh and assoc. New York, p 3, 1986.

172. Gotloib L, Shostak A, Bar-Sella P, Cohen R: Continuous mesothelial injury and regeneration during long term peritoneal dialysis. Perit Dial Bulletin (in press).

173. Gotloib L, Shostak A, Jaichenko J: Continuous mesothelial injury and regeneration. A possible role of the non enzymatic degradation of glucose. Presented at the IV Congress of the Int Soc of Peritoneal Dialysis, Venice.

174. Eskeland G, Kjaerheim A: Regeneration of parietal peritoneum in rats. 2. An electron microscopical study. Acta Pathol Microbiol Scand 68, 379–395, 1966.

175. Watters WB, Buck RC: Scanning electron microscopy of mesothelial regeneration in the rat. Lab Invest 26, 604–609, 1972.

176. Whitaker D, Padadimitriou J: Mesothelial healing: morphological and kinetic investigations. J Pathol Bact 73, 1–10, 1957.

177. Renvall SY: Peritoneal metabolism and intrabdominal adhesion formation during experimental peritonitis. Acta Chirurg Scanb Suppl 503, 1–48, 1980.

178. Ellis H, Harrison W, Hugh TB: The healing of peritoneum under normal and pathological conditions. Brit J Surg 52, 471–476, 1965.

179. Ellis H: The cause and prevention of postoperative intraperitoneal adhesions. Surg Gynecol Obstet 133, 497–511, 1971.

180. Whitaker D, Papadimitriou J: Mesothelial healing: morphological and kinetic investigations. J Pathol 145, 159–175.

181. Cameron GR, Hassan SM, De SN: Repair of Glisson's capsule after tangential wounds of the liver. J Pathol Bacteriol 73, 1–10, 1957.

182. Johnson FR, Whitting HW: Repair of parietal peritoneum. Brit J Surg 49, 653–660, 1962.

183. Eskeland G: Regeneration of parietal peritoneum in rats. A light microscopical study. Acta Path Microbiol Scandina 68, 355–378, 1966.

184. Williams DC: The peritoneum. A plea for a change in attitude towards this membrane. Brit J Surg 42, 401–405, 1955.

185. Shaldon S: Peritoneal dialysis: the first line of defense. In: La Greca G, Chiaramonte S, Fabris A, Feriani M, Ronco C (eds), Peritoneal Dialysis. Milano, p 201, 1986.

186. Raftery AT: Regeneration of parietal and visceral peritoneum. A light microscopical study. Brit J Surgery 60, 293–299, 1973.

187. Maximow AA, Bloom W: A textbook of histology. WB Saunders Comp. Philadelphia, pp 63–66, 1942.

188. Patnam TJ: The living peritoneum as a dialyzing membrane. Am J Physiol 63, 548–565, 1923.

189. Nagel E: Teleology revisited and other essays on the phylosophy and history of science. Columbia Univ Press. New York, p 75, 197.

6

TRANSPORT KINETICS

ROBERT P. POPOVICH, JACK W. MONCRIEF and W. KEITH PYLE

1. INTRODUCTION

Comprehensive mathematical models of the patient-peritoneal dialysis system are fundamental to the analysis and understanding of metabolite and fluid transport in peritoneal dialysis. Theoretical models serve to: (1) illustrate the system parameters which are most significant, (2) define how these parameters relate to each other, (3) predict the behavior of the system, allowing manipulation of the variables to produce optimized clinical results, (4) aid in the design of clinical protocols to measure the parameters, and (5) suggest areas requiring additional investigation. In short, a great deal of information can be acquired from modeling of the peritoneal dialysis system in general with multiple applications to the diagnosis and treatment of individual patients.

2. HISTORICAL PERSPECTIVE

Ganter [1] is credited as being the first to use peritoneal dialysis in the treatment of uremia in 1923. Following experimentation with animals, he dialyzed a patient who demonstrated some clinical improvement. Other investigators, reviewed by Cunningham [2], studied the absorption of a wide range of particulate and soluble substances from the peritoneal cavity. As early as 1921, Clark [3] demonstrated that intraperitoneal fluid tended to equilibrate both chemically and osmotically with blood. This was later confirmed by Schechter et al. [4] who further demonstrated that hypertonic glucose solutions infused into the peritoneal cavity increased in volume before being absorbed. The effectiveness of peritoneal lavage in resolving uremic symptoms in nephrectomized dogs was demonstrated by Bliss [5] in 1931. In 1950, Odel et al. [6] published an extensive literature review in which they noted over 100 reported cases of peritoneal dialysis. They concluded that peritoneal dialysis had earned a definite place in the treatment of acute renal failure.

Grollman et al. [7] resolved many of the technical problems and complications of chronic peritoneal dialysis. The development of the Tenckhoff catheter [8], coupled to subsequent refinements in techniques and the availability of commercial dialysis supplies and solutions, has made peritoneal dialysis a simple, safe, and commonly employed technique in the treatment of renal failure [9–17].

3. PHYSIOLOGICAL PRINCIPLES

The peritoneum is the largest serous membrane of the body. It lines the inside of the abdominal wall (the parietal peritoneum) and is reflected over the viscera (the visceral peritoneum). The space between the parietal and visceral portions of the membrane is called the peritoneal cavity. This is normally a potential space lubricated by serous fluid secreted by mesothelial cells which cover its free surface [18–21].

The detailed microscopic anatomy of the peritoneum has been described by Baron [21]. It consists of five layers of fibrous and elastic connective tissue covered by mesothelial cells. Blood and lymphatic capillaries are located in the deepest layers in adults. Thus, for a substance to pass from the bloodstream into the peritoneal cavity, it must pass the capillary endothelium, the interstitium, the mesothelium and any fluid film resistances. This is illustrated schematically in Figure 2 of Chapter 2. Six resistances to the diffusion of metabolites from blood are shown. R^1 represents the mass transfer resistance of the blood fluid film where the diffusion distance in the capillary is illustrated

96

between 1 and 3 μ (the capillary radius). R^2 and R^3 represent the resistances to diffusing past the endothelial intercellular channel and the basement membrane, respectively. R^4 represents the resistance of the interstitial fluid. The interstitium may be a dense matrix of collagenous fibers and mucopolysaccharide gels with channels or pores through which the metabolites must diffuse. The nature of the pores may depend on the degree of hydration [22] of the matrix. Note that the interstitial diffusion path can approach 100 μ which would represent an appreciable resistance to diffusion. R_5 represents the resistance of the mesothelial cells and R_6 is the dialysate fluid film resistance. The total resistance is the sum of all the individual resistances.

The precise nature of absorption from the peritoneal cavity varies in relation to the physical and chemical properties of the substance in question. Neutral, noncolloidal substances such as urea will be transported primarily by passive diffusion. On the other hand, it is postulated that plasma proteins, red blood cells, and other particulate matter may be absorbed through the lymphatics because of the greater permeability of the lymph capillaries to large molecules or particles [2, 23–25]. Allen and Weatherford [23] have demonstrated that spherical particles up to 24 μ are absorbed through the peritoneum in the cat and rat. From this they have postulated that there is a porous basement membrane through which particles pass into the lymphatics.

The movement of fluid and solutes across the peritoneum in response to osmotic agents is well-documented [3, 26–31]. Henderson [28] demonstrated the transfer of inulin and urea across the peritoneal membrane in the absence of a concentration gradient. This led Nolph [26] to conclude that solute transport across the peritoneum occurs to some extent by convection or ultrafiltration.

The area of the peritoneal membrane available for mass transfer is uncertain. The total peritoneal area was directly measured and found to be 20 718 cm² with an area-to-body weight ratio of 284 cm²/kg in an adult male [32, 33]. The authors calculated an area-to-body weight ratio of 522 cm²/kg in infants [33]. Esperanca and Collins [33] also obtained a ratio of approximately 2 for infant peritoneal area to adult peritoneal area per kilogram of body weight. Kallen [32] has suggested a scaling approximation of:

$$S = 1000 \ W^{0.7}, \qquad [1]$$

where S is the peritoneal surface area in square centimeters and W is the body weight in kilograms.

These measurements may provide an estimate of the total anatomical peritoneal surface area. However, the precise pore area of the adult peritoneum is unknown. Gosselin and Berndt [34] computed a 0.6% open pore area for the mesentery and a 0.2% open pore area for the intestinal peritoneum in rabbits. The average thickness of the rabbit visceral peritoneum was 38.1 ± 1.7 μ.

The area of the peritoneum available for transfer may also depend on the volume of dialysate infused. The precise peritoneal surface area-to-dialysate volume relationship is also unknown. The data of Miller *et al.* [15] indicate that a linear volume/area relationship and a constant area relationship are unsatisfactory to explain observed equilibration data. Goldschmidt *et al.* [35] have demonstrated that the relationship does not conform to that expected

for a sphere unless the dialysate volume is large (approximately 3 l).

4. CLINICAL PROTOCOLS

Modeling of the patient-peritoneal dialysis system will to some extent be dependent upon the details of the clinical protocol employed. Miller *et al.* [15] have classified six intermittent methods:

Technique I – standard peritoneal dialysis (PD)
Technique II – recirculation PD
Technique III – continuous flow PD
Technique IV – continuous flow recirculation PD
Technique V – rapid intermittent PD
Technique VI – continuous flow compound dialysis

Several recent additions since the publication of Miller's paper are reciprocating PD and Continuous Ambulatory Peritoneal Dialysis (CAPD) and Continuous Cyclic Peritoneal Dialysis (CCPD).

Technique I, standard intermittent peritoneal dialysis, was the usual clinical procedure prior to the introduction of CAPD. In Technique I, two liters of dialysate solution at 37 °C are rapidly infused into the peritoneal cavity and allowed to equilibrate for approximately 30 min. The dialysate fluid is then drained by gravity flow and two liters of fresh dialysate are infused. The exchanges are repeated until the desired clinical result is obtained. The bulk of the theoretical models in the literature are aimed at understanding and optimizing this standard clinical procedure.

Intermittent recirculation PD (Technique II) is similar to Technique I except that the dialysate is recirculated through the abdomen during the equilibration phase. It was thought that this would greatly improve solute transport by preventing stagnation of the dialysate. Unfortunately, Miller *et al.* [15] demonstrated a slight decrease in clearance using Technique II relative to Technique I controls.

Continuous flow PD (Technique III) employs two widely spaced catheters with continuous infusion and drainage of dialysate. It has been used succesfully by early clinicians [6, 17, 36, 37] but, again, Miller *et al.* [15] have demonstrated that no significant improvements in clearance are obtained. Indeed, the addition of a recirculation loop to achieve higher flow rates through the peritoneal cavity (Technique IV – continuous recirculation PD) by Miller and colleagues [15] did not yield results up to expectations. They suggested that this may have resulted from channeling of dialysate at the higher flow rates. As will be demonstrated, this may instead be a result of the peritoneal transport being limited by membrane resistances (R_1 to R_5).

Rapid intermittent peritoneal dialysis (Technique V) has also been applied by many investigators [15, 17, 38–40]. Drainage is started as soon as an infusion is completed in this technique, in an attempt to achieve maximum dialysate flow rates (4 to 5 l/h).

Continuous compound dialysis (Technique VI) is a continuous flow procedure in which the peritoneal dialysis fluid is recirculated through a hemodialyzer. Shinaberger *et al.* [41, 42] reported reduced protein losses using this method. Rosenbalm and Mandanas [43] used this technique and recirculated the dialysate through ion exchange columns to obtain enhanced phenobarbital removal.

A slight modification of this basic procedure termed reciprocating peritoneal dialysis [7, 18–21, 23–24] has also been attempted. In this case, a preset volume of dialysate is removed from the peritoneal cavity and pumped through a hollow fiber artificial kidney. This is schematically illustrated in Figure 1. Recent advances involve the addition of a dialysate regeneration circuit to the basic reciprocating system [44].

A novel approach to continuous peritoneal dialysis (developed by Popovich and Moncrief) has recently been described [45–47] and termed Continuous Ambulatory Peritoneal Dialysis. This technique and the analogous CCPD procedure employs the continuous presence (24 hr a day, 7 days a week) of peritoneal dialysis solution in the peritoneal cavity. Dialysate fluid is drained and immediately replaced 3 to 5 times per day. Additional procedural details of these methods of dialysis are available in Chapters 7–9.

5. THEORETICAL ANALYSIS OF THE PATIENT-PERITONEAL DIALYSIS SYSTEM

A complete exposition of the kinetic models associated with each of the various peritoneal dialysis techniques is beyond the scope of this publication. Therefore, only those models associated with techniques currently utilized in general clinical practice will be examined. These include the various forms of standard intermittent dialysis, CAPD and CCPD. For models of the less frequently employed procedures, the literature should be consulted. For example, Villarroel [48] has presented an excellent characterization of continuous models of peritoneal dialysis. Kablitz *et al.* [44] have described a model of reciprocating peritoneal dialysis. Naturally, the general principles of peritoneal transport apply to all the techniques.

5.1. Diffuse mass transfer models

In 1966, Kallen [32] suggested the use of a simple exponential model for approximating the decrease in blood urea concentration as a function of total dialysis time. No provisions were included for the effects of infusion and

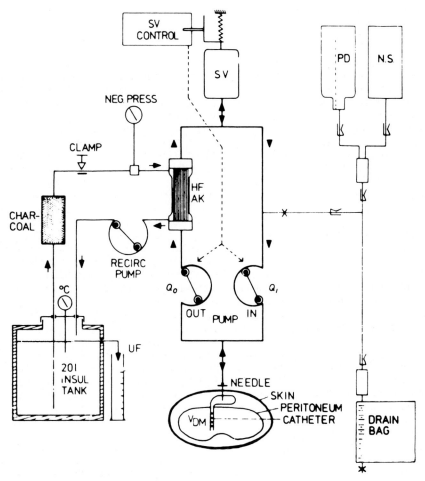

Figure 1. Schematic of reciprocating peritoneal dialysis (reprinted with permission of Dialysis & Transplantation (ref 44)).

drainage, or for fluid transfer. This model tended to over-predict the urea removal in clinical trials. The basic parameter of his model was the mean urea clearance which, as will be subsequently demonstrated, is highly dependent upon the dialysis conditions.

Miller et al. [15] also suggested a simple model for the decay of the concentration gradient between the body fluid and the dialysate during a single exchange. On the basis of this model, they concluded that there are three primary factors affecting mass transport. These are: (1) the general permeability characteristics of the peritoneum, including its underlying interstitial space and the capillary walls (resistances R_4 and R_2, respectively); (2) the volumes of distribution of the metabolite present on either side of the peritoneum; and (3) the transperitoneal metabolite concentration gradient. Clearance measurements using the techniques (I–III) outlined previously suggested that the dialysate side of the dialysate fluid film diffusion resistance (R_6) is of less importance.

Henderson and Nolph [30] employed the classic two-pool (body fluid and dialysate) compartmental model utilized in pharmacodynamic studies [49] to characterize diffusive mass transfer during a single exchange. They clearly demonstrated that the dialyse clearance changes during the residence period and that the mass transfer rate is relatively insensitive to large errors in estimating the metabolite space. Mattocks [50] employed a similar two-pool model to characterize salicylate transfer in the presence of transfer accelerators. Popovich et al. [51] expanded the two-pool model to include the effects of metabolite generation (an important parameter), protein binding, and nonequilibrium distribution. They simplified the mathematical analysis considerably by replacing the infusion and drainage times with an equivalent residence time. Many important relationships between the mass transfer parameters were demonstrated. They defined an overall peritoneum mass transfer coefficient by

$$\dot{m} = KA\ (C_B - C_D), \qquad [2]$$

where $\dot{m}$ is the mass transfer rate, K is the overall mass transfer coefficient, A is the effective peritoneal transfer area, and C_B and C_D are instantaneous blood and dialysate metabolite concentration levels. They demonstrated the important fact that, unlike the dialysis clearance, the overall mass transfer coefficient is independent of the dialysis schedule.

Equation 2 can be compared to the more familiair form of mass transfer – Ficks' Law of Diffusion:

$$\frac{\dot{m}}{A} = D_{AM}\ \frac{dC_A}{dx} \qquad [3]$$

where D_{AM} is the diffusivity of solute A in the peritoneum and C_A is the solute concentration of A as a function of distance across the peritoneum, X. Assuming steady-state transport across a well-defined membrane film of thickness δ, this can be simplified to:

$$\frac{\dot{m}}{A} = D_{AM}\ \frac{(C_B - C_D)}{\delta} = \frac{(C_B - C_D)}{R_M} \qquad [4]$$

where R_M is the resistance to transport across the membrane. A comparison of equations 2 and 4 illustrates that

for a single well-defined film resistance the mass transfer coefficient (K) is equal to the membrane diffusivity (D_{AM}) divided by the membrane thickness (δ). It is also equal to the reciprocal of the membrane resistance.

In actual practice metabolites diffusing from the blood to the dialysate encounter an entire series of resistances, not a particularly well-defined one such as would be described by equation 4.

A total of six potential resistances have been identified as noted in Figure 2, Chapter 2. Under these more complex circumstances the mass transport coefficient is related to these resistances by the reciprocal relationship:

$$K = \frac{1}{R_1 + R_2 + R_3 + R_4 + R_5 + R_6}. \qquad [5]$$

The relative magnitudes of the individual resistances and the effective mass transfer area have not been clearly defined. Therefore, Popovich et al. [51] suggested that the product of the mass transfer coefficient (K) times the area (A), known as the mass transfer-area coefficient (KA), is the transport parameter to be utilized to characterize mass transfer in peritoneal dialysis. They also demonstrated that the metabolite generation rate must be included in the analysis.

5.2. Peritoneal dialysis optimizations

Bomar et al. [52] presented the first comprehensive analytical optimizations of standard intermittent peritoneal dialysis. They also employed a two-pool model and accounted for metabolite transfer during the infusion and drainage periods. In addition, metabolite generation and residual renal clearance were included to allow simulation of the interdialytic period. The model was employed to determine optimum peritoneal dialysis protocols for urea removal.

As would be expected, this model predicts that the maximum urea clearance is obtained if the residence time is reduced to near zero, as in continuous flow intermittent peritoneal dialysis (Technique III). Villaroel [48] confirmed these findings in a comparison of intermittent and continuous peritoneal dialysis. He concluded that 'continuous flow peritoneal dialysis is more efficient than the intermittent mode, particularly at higher flow rates'. However, Bomar found that only a very slight decrease in urea removal rates occurs if the residence time is increased from 0 to 10 min. Slightly increasing the residence time greatly reduces the total volume of dialysate used. Thus, it was concluded that short-residence-time standard intermittent peritoneal dialysis was economically superior to continuous flow dialysis with minimal effect on efficiency.

Bomar et al. [52] also determined the residence time which yielded the maximum urea removal per liter of dialysate (the 'dialysate utilization optimum') for various degrees of reduction of serum blood urea nitrogen. They found the optimum residence time to range from 40 to 50 min for reductions in serum BUN ranging from 20% to 60%.

Finally, a cost function was generated to reflect both the fixed and variable costs associated with peritoneal dialysis [52] . The model was used in conjunction with this cost function to determine the dialysate residence time which yielded the minimum cost. For the cost parameters selected, it was determined that a minimum in cost would be obtained using a 29 min residence phase for a 60% reduction in blood urea nitrogen.

5.3. Combined diffusive and convective mass transfer models

The pure diffusive models outlined above all assume no significant ultrafiltration occurs during an exchange. However, osmotic agents are routinely added to dialysate [12] to remove excess fluid. As will subsequently be demonstrated, this gives rise to significant ultrafiltration rates (up to 26 ml/min) [53]. This fluid movement has been shown to carry solute with it as it traverses the peritoneum [26, 30]. Neglecting this important mass transfer mechanism results in the computation of higher mass transfer-area coefficients than if it was included in the models because of the model's attempt to 'best fit' the clinical data without the convective term. For small molecular weight, rapidly-transferring solutes like urea, ultrafiltration effects are small compared to diffusion [54] such that forcing a fit with a pure diffusion model yields reasonable agreement between model predictions and urea clearance. This will not hold true if high ultrafiltration rates are obtained. Pyle [54] and Popovich *et al.* [53] have also demonstrated that the convective mass transfer mechanism becomes increasingly important as the molecular weight of a solute increases. Thus, models which account for the transport effects of ultrafiltration are required to properly analyze most metabolites in peritoneral dialysis.

In 1973, Babb *et al.* [56] utilized a simplified transport model which included convective transport. The authors assumed that convective mass transport operated as a parallel mechanism with diffusion and included a term to describe its effect. This model was also employed by Popovich *et al.* [45, 57] who included provisions for variable blood concentration and metabolite generation. These models utilized a sieving coefficient, S, as measured by Henderson and Nolph [30] in the ultrafiltration term. In the mathematical terms, the mass transfer rate is expressed in the form (compare with equation 2):

$$\dot{m} = KA\,(C_B - C_D) + SQ_u C_B, \qquad [6]$$

where Q_u is the ultrafiltration rate.

Garred *et al.* [58] simplified this approach to provide for routine analysis of patient kinetics in the clinical setting. They assumed: (i) a non-selective membrane (S = 1.0 in equation 6); (ii) constant blood concentration, $\bar{C}_B$; (iii) $KA/\overline{V}_D$ = constant; (iv) positive Q_u; and (v) negligible lymphatic involvement. The mass transfer area coefficient is computed from the simple equation:

$$KA = \frac{\overline{V}_D}{t}\,\ln\left[\frac{V_D^0\,(\bar{C}_B - \bar{C}_D^0)}{V_D^t\,(\bar{C}_B - \bar{C}_D^t)}\right] \qquad [7]$$

where $\overline{V}_D$ is the mean dialysate volume, V_D^0 and V_D^t are initial and final dialysate volumes, C_D^0 and C_D^t are intial and final dialysate concentrations over a dwell period t.

If blood and dialysate concentrations are measured at various timed intervals during the dwell period, equation 7 can be rewriten as:

$$\ln\left[V_D^t\,(\bar{C}_B - \bar{C}_D^t)\right] = \ln\left[V_D^0\,(\bar{C}_B - \bar{C}_D^0)\right] - \frac{KA\cdot t}{\overline{V}_D} \cdot \qquad [8]$$

A graph can be prepared in which the ordinate is the logarithm term on the left hand side of equation 8, and the abscissa is time. The slope of the line obtained by regression analysis equals KA/V_D from which KA may be computed. As demonstrated by Lindholm [59], this model yields a straight forward way to compute KA if it is applied during the time of treatment when isovolemia occurs (near the top of the volume curves illustrated in Figures 4 and 5). Leypoldt *et al.* [60] and Villarroel *et al.* [61] also derived analytical expressions for the case where S was less than unity (selective membrane) and for a constant ultrafiltration rate.

Bomar [62] presented a comprehensive mathematical model based upon a non-equilibrium thermodynamics approach [63, 64]. It is a generalized, open, three-pool model in which the dialysis volume and metabolite distribution volumes vary as a function of time. Provision is made for solute generation, G, in either pool and for residual renal clearance. The model is extremely complex, requiring the simultaneous solution of over eight non-linear differential equations for fluid and mass transfer. Excellent fits were obtained for blood and dialysate concentration levels for urea, creatinine and vitamin B-12 over multiple exchanges. The results are summarized by Popovich *et al.* [65].

6. DEFINITION OF A MODEL OF PERITONEAL DIALYSIS

The most desirable mathematical model is one which closely duplicates the natural events which occur during peritoneal dialysis but is an acceptable compromise of utility and theoretical accuracy. Numerous models have been proposed as outlined above with varying degrees of complexity. We believe that in order for a model to accurately represent the patient-peritoneal dialysis system, it must at a minimum account for fluid transport with resulting variable ultrafiltration rates and dialysate volumes, both diffusive and selective convective transport, metabolite generation, and residual renal and/or metabolic clearance. While early models neglected some of these factors, later models, such as Bomar's, were extremely complex and difficult to apply to the clinical situation.

Figure 2 presents a schematic of a model which conforms to all the criteria outline above [53]. The peritoneum separates a dialysate compartment from a body compart-

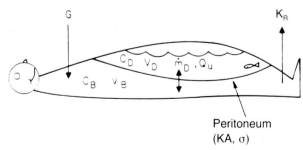

Figure 2. Schematic of the patient undergoing peritoneal dialysis.

ment. Both pools are assumed to be well-mixed with concentrations designated by C_B and C_D, and volumes by V_B and V_D for blood and dialysate, respectively. Metabolite generation is assumed to occur at a constant rate, G. Removal by remaining renal function or metabolism is at the constant clearance, K_R. Ultrafiltration occurs under the influence of hydrostatic and osmotic forces at a variable rate denoted by Q_u. The peritoneal membrane is characterized by two membrane phenomenological coefficients: the mass transfer area coefficient for diffusion and the reflection coefficient for convective transport. The reflection coefficient is a constant employed to determine the fraction of metabolite transferred by entrainment in ultrafiltration from one compartment to another. These coefficients are assumed to be time invariant and independent of osmotic and metabolite concentration gradients for a particular solute.

Mathematically, the metabolite mass balance for the dialysate compartment and peritoneal membrane is given by:

$$\frac{d\,(V_D C_D)}{dt} = KA\,(C_B - C_D) \qquad + (1-\sigma)\,Q_u\,C \qquad [9]$$

Rate of accumulation   Transfer by diffusion   Transfer by convection

where

$$C = C_B - f\,(C_B - C_D) \qquad [10]$$

KA = mass transfer-area coefficient
σ = reflection coefficient
Q_u = ultrafiltration rate

$$f = \frac{1}{\beta} - \frac{1}{\exp(\beta) - 1} \qquad [11]$$

$$\beta = \frac{Q_u\,(1 - \sigma)}{KA} \qquad [12]$$

The form of the convective term conforms to homogeneous membrane theory [66] and pore theory [67, 68]. It is equal to the product of the complement of the reflection coefficient, the instantaneous ultrafiltration rate, and the weighted average transmembrane concentration. The function, f, is dependent on the ratio of convective to diffusive transport, characterized by the Peclet Number, β [69]. An overall metabolite balance for the system is:

$$C_B V_B + C_D V_D = C_B^0 V_B + C_D^0 V_D^0 + Gt - K_R \!\int\! C_B dt, \qquad [13]$$

where the superscript, 0, refers to an initial state. Pyle *et al.* [53, 54] have demonstrated that the ultrafiltration rate can be characterized by the exponential function:

$$Q_u = a_1 \exp\,(a_2 t) + a_3 . \qquad [14]$$

The dialysate volume is determined by intergrating this equation over time to yield:

$$V_D = \frac{a_1}{a_2}\,[\exp\,(a_2 t) - 1] + a_3 t + V_D^0 . \qquad [15]$$

Combining equations 9–15 and solving yields characteristic expressions for the dialysate and blood concentrations as functions of the model parameters and time. Details of the solution are presented elsewhere [54].

7. CLINICAL MEASUREMENT OF MODEL PARAMETERS

In order to measure the membrane parameters using the model outlined above, concurrent evaluations of fluid and solute transport are required [53, 54]. The rate of fluid transfer was determined by the degree of dilution obtained with a large molecular weight substance added to the dialysate. Prior to dialysate infusion, a known quantity of sterile, pyrogen-free radioisotopically tagged dextran (70 000 mol. wt.) was infused into the dialysate. In order to investigate a wide range of osmotic effects, three dialysate solutions with varying osmolalities were employed. These were Ringer's lactate (244 mOsm/l), and two commercially-used Dianeal® dialysis fluids with 1.5% dextrose (332 mOsm/l), and 4.25% dextrose 477 mOsm/l). Following the completion of infusion, dialysate samples were obtained at frequent time intervals. Blood samples were obtained immediately at post-infusion and at the mid-point and end of dwell to determine the degree of transport of the tagged dextran. By employing the dilution principle, corrected for such dextran transfer, intraperitoneal dialysate volumes were calculated at each sample time. A computer program [54] was employed to fit equation 11 to the calculated volumes using Gauss' non-linear least squares algorithm [70, 71]. The resulting coefficients were then utilized to compute the instantaneous ultrafiltration rate using equation 14.

Transport parameters can be determined for any desired solute once the intraperitoneal volume profile is known. Concentration-time data have been generated for a variety of solutes by appropriate analyses of samples selected from simultaneous fluid transfer evaluations [53, 54]. Since the solution of equation 9 specifies the dialysate concentration profile for a given set of transport parameters, a least squares fit to the solute data gives the mass transfer-area and reflection coefficients characteristic of the patient's peritoneum.

8. FLUID TRANSFER PARAMETERS

Typical intraperitoneal volume profiles for Ringer's lactate, 1.5 and 4.25 dextrose dialysis solution (Dianeal, Baxter-Travenol), are illustrated in Figures 3–5 [53, 54]. In each figure, the asterisks indicate the actual volume data while the solid line is the least squares fit of equation 15 to this data. The coefficients which gave these fits are shown in Table 1. Due to the initial hypotonicity of Ringer's lactate, the curve in Figure 3 shows an initial rapid drop in volume. As the osmolality of the dialysate rises due to solute transfer, the rate of volume decline asymptotically approaches a constant rate. That is, ultrafiltration is initially high from dialysate to blood (negative ultrafiltration), decreasing to a small negative value. When a hypertonic solution such as 1.5 g/dl dextrose dialysis solution is employed, the intraperitoneal volume will increase before reabsorption begins, as shown in Figure 4. In this case, ultrafiltration is positive (from blood to dialysate) for the first 136 min resulting in a maximum volume of 2408 ml. Since the volume at the end of infusion was 2130 ml (t = 0), approximately 278 ml were unfiltered during the residence phase. After

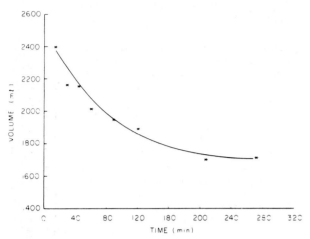

Figure 3. Intraperitoneal volume profile – Ringer's lactate (reprinted with permission of Pyle WK (ref 54.))

the maximum was reached, the volume begins to decrease and subsequently approaches a constant rate of reabsorption. Since the 4.25 dialysis solution is also hypertonic but to a greater degree than the 1.5 g/dl dialysis solution, the 4.25 intraperitoneal volume profile shown in Figure 5 is similar to that of Figure 4 but with a higher ultrafiltered volume and greater initial slope. The peak volume for this exchange was 3325 ml at 177 min. The 1337 ml of ultrafiltration represents at 67% increase over the post-infusion volume of 1988 ml. As in each of the other cases, fluid reabsorption eventually begins and approaches a constant rate.

Table 1. Volume profile equation coefficients.

Solution	$V_D t = 0$	a_1	a_3	a_3
Isotonic	2841.0	−21.4	−0.0195	−0.231
1.5	2130.0	7.48	−0.0207	−0.452
4.25	1988.0	28.4	−0.0170	−1.40

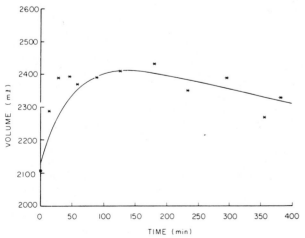

Figure 4. Intraperitoneal volume profile – 1.5 g/dl dextrose dialysis solution (reprinted with permission of Pyle WK (ref. 54)).

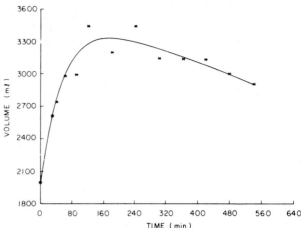

Figure 5. Intraperitoneal volume profile – 4.25 g/dl dextrose dialysis solution (reprinted with permission of Pyle WK (ref. 54)).

The volume profile coefficients of Table I also specify the ultrafiltration profile through equation 14. The ultrafiltration profile corresponding to the 1.5 g/dl dialysis solution volume profile of Figure 4 is shown in Figure 6 [53, 54]. The ultrafiltration rate is approximately 7 ml/min immediately post-infusion. The ultrafiltration rate decreases to 0 at 136 min, and levels off at about −0.45 ml/min. As indicated above, the higher tonicity of the 4.25 dialysis solution increases the magnitude of the initial ultrafiltration. The profile shown in Figure 7 is derived from the volume curve of Figure 5. The initial rate exceeds 26 ml/min dropping to −1.4 ml/min after 4 to 5 hr.

Pyle *et al.* [53] have reported the fluid transfer results in four studies each with 1.5 g/dl and 4.25 g/dl dextrose dialysate. The average results are summarized in Table 2. From these studies, the 1028 ml ultrafiltration induced by the 4.25 solution is approximately three times that removed with the average 1.5 solution. Since the concentration of the osmotic agent is higher in the 4.25 dialysis solution, the osmotic gradient will be maintained longer. Thus, ultrafiltration is positive for a longer period when the 4.25 solution is employed. On the average, ultrafiltration is positive for 140 and 247 min with the 1.5 and 4.25 solutions, respectively. Since fluid reabsorption begins after these respective times, these times mark the point of maximum fluid removal and maximum intraperitoneal volume. The initial or maximum ultrafiltration rate which will occur is also dependent on the magnitude of the initial osmotic gradient. These studies have shown the average post-infusion ultrafiltration rate to be 11.7 ml/min for the 1.5 and 16.6 ml/min for the 4.25 solution. The reabsorption rates reported by Pyle *et al.* [53] were −0.68 and −0.87 ml/min for 1.5 and 4.25 dialysis solution, respectively, which may be related to lymphatic interaction. Since both of these values, shown in Table 2, were subject to relatively large variations, they may represent a single value (p > 0.65). Reabsorption may be utilized clinically to introduce fluids into the vascular space of a hypovolemic patient by leaving the fluid in the peritoneal cavity.

Considerable variations in ultrafiltration characteristics between patients have been noted [53, 72]. Some of the

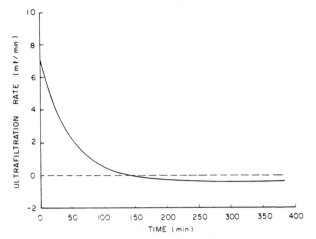

Figure 6. Transperitoneal ultrafiltration profile – 1.5 g/dl dextrose solution (reprinted with permission of Pyle WK (ref. 54)).

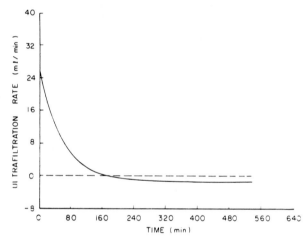

Figure 7. Transperitoneal ultrafiltration profile – 4.25 g/dl Dextrose solution (reprinted with permission of Pyle WK (ref. 54)).

variations may be attributed to differences in mass transfer characteristics and the relative degree of drainage. Dilution of fresh solutions by residual dialysate can reduce fluid transfer. Nolph has hypothesized that ultrafiltration is actually the result of two different fluid transfer mechanisms: high proximal capillary ultrafiltration and lower negative distal ultrafiltration [73]. This suggests that a patient's ultrafiltration characteristics can be affected by permeability changes at either the proximal or distal portions of the capillary or both. Undoubtedly, fluid transfer is influenced by hydrostatic and osmotic pressures in both the capillaries and in the dialysate, the interstitial water path dimensions, and molecular surface charges in the interstitium [73]. Detailed studies will be required to identify the importance of the various factors and the sources of the reported interpatient variations.

9. SOLUTE TRANSFER PARAMETERS

Popovich *et al.* [74] have reported peritoneal mass transfer area coefficients (MTAC) resulting from 34 studies in 8 patients on Intermittent Peritoneal Dialysis and CAPD. These early studies predated the concurrent evaluations of fluid and solute transfer. As a consequence, they assumed constant ultrafiltration rates. Also, the convective term was assumed to be equal for all solutes in the studies using hypertonic solutions after the results of Henderson and Nolph [30]. From the mean mass-transfer area coefficients, they produced the first empirical correlation of MTAC to solute molecular weight, shown in Figure 8. While the MTAC's for the different solutes exhibited considerable interpatient variations, a trend given by:

$$KA = 333.6 \, (MW)^{-0.561} \qquad [16]$$

was evident over six orders of magnitude of molecular weight.

Pyle *et al.* [53] later performed sixteen comprehensive transport studies in five CAPD patients, measuring fluid transfer rates and diffusive and convective solute transfer parameters. Figures 9–12 present representative dialysate concentration profiles for BUN, creatinine, inulin, and total protein, respectively, from these studies. Dialysate concentrations are shown by the asterisks with the solid line indicating their model's predictions. Blood levels are shown by circles and the dashed lines. From this sequence of figures, the effect of molecular size on transport rates becomes apparent. Due to its small molecular size (60 daltons), urea has a relatively high MTAC of 15.3 ml/min and low reflection coefficient of 0.126. These membrane properties lead to a rapid rise in the dialysate urea level and a slight drop in the blood concentration during the first 90 min of the exchange as seen in Figure 9. Creatinine (113 daltons) is larger than urea and transfers more slowly, as shown by Figure 10. In this case, the parameters are

Table 2. Average fluid transfer results.

	Mean ± S.D.: (n = 4)	
	1.5 Dianeal®	4.25 Dianeal®
Maximum ultrafiltered volume (ml)	331 ± 187	1028 ± 258
Time of maximum volume (min)	140 ± 48	247 ± 61
Maximum ultrafiltration rate (ml/min)	11.7 ± 13.0	16.6 ± 7.7
Reabsorption rate (ml/min)	−0.68 ± 0.61	−0.87 ± 0.55

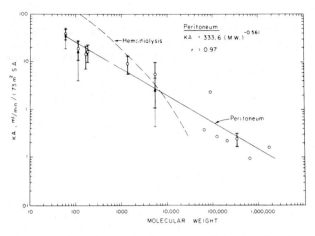

Figure 8. Peritoneal mass transfer – area coefficient as a function of solute molecular weight (reprinted with permission of the American Institute of Chemical Engineers (ref. 61)).

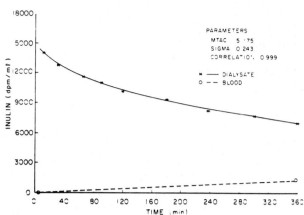

Figure 11. Inulin concentration profiles in CAPD (reprinted with permission of Pyle WK (ref. 54)).

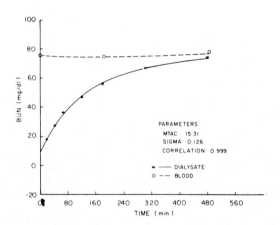

Figure 2. Blood urea nitrogen concentration profiles in CAPD (reprinted with permission of Pyle WK (ref. 54)).

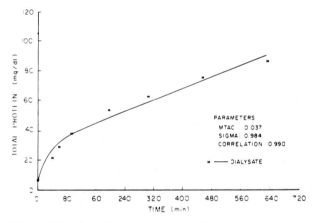

Figure 12. Total protein concentration profile in CAPD (reprinted with permission of Pyle WK (ref. 54)).

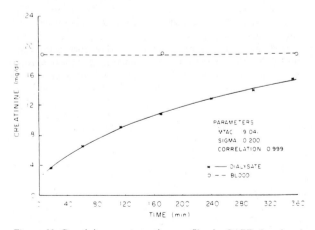

Figure 10. Creatinine concentration profiles in CAPD (reprinted with permission of Pyle WK (ref. 54)).

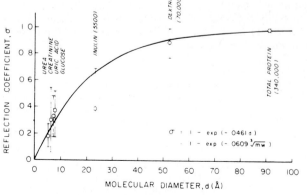

Figure 13. Peritoneal membrane reflection coefficients as a function of molecular size (reprinted with permission of Pyle WK (ref. 54)).

an MTAC of 9.0 ml/min and a reflection coefficient of 0.200. Since the transfer rate is slower, the creatinine dialysate concentration profile does not show the high initial slope or strong curvature of the BUN profile. Also, the difference between blood and dialysate levels is greater at any given residence time for the larger metabolite. This effect is even more prominent for inulin (5500 daltons) and total protein (340 000 daltons, weighted mean) shown in Figures 11 and 12, respectively. In Figure 12, the plasma protein level of 7900 mg/dl is so much greater than in the dialysate that it is not practical to show it on the graph.

The protein concentration profile of Figure 12 also illustrates the effect of high fluid transfer rates on solute transfer. For about the first 80 min of the residence phase of this exchange, the ultrafiltration was positive and relative high, similar to the situation shown in Figure 7. The high fluid transfer rate resulted in the convection of protein across the peritoneum by entrainment and a rapid initial rise in the dialysate protein level of about 30 mg/dl. As the ultrafiltration rate declines, solute convection becomes relatively less important than diffusion and the concentration profile assumes a nearly linear trend. At the lower diffusion induced transfer rate, about 320 min is required to obtain another 30 mg/dl rise in the protein level. Thus, even a small period of convective transport can be quite important in the dialysis of large solutes.

An important aspect of the studies by Pyle *et al.* [53] was the first determination of peritoneal membrane reflection coefficients for a variety of solutes. Mean reflection coefficients for urea (60 daltons), creatinine (113), uric acid (158), glucose (180), inulin (5500), dextran (70 000 mean) and total protein (340 000 weighted mean) are presented in Figure 13 with an empirical correlation function to molecular size. Prior to these studies, the most frequently referenced work [30] on convective coefficients indicated that both urea and inulin had peritoneal reflection coefficients of about 0.2. While these values fall within the range of variation reported by Pyle, the mistaken conclusion that peritoneal sieving is equivalent for all solutes could be drawn from the earlier work. Figure 13 indicates that this is clearly not the case as confirmed by Morgenstein *et al.* [75] and Rubin *et al.* [76]. In these studies, the reflection coefficient ranged from a mean of 0.18 for urea to 0.992 for total protein and was well-correlated to the expression

$$\sigma = 1 - \exp[-0.0609(\text{MW})^{(1/3)}]. \qquad [17]$$

This function indicates that the majority of smaller solutes, such as urea, entrained in the ultrafiltrate are convected through the membrane. Conversely, less than one percent of the protein in the same ultrafiltrate passes through due to the higher degree of reflection. As indicated above, the convective transfer rate of large solutes can still be appreciable if the fluid transfer rate is significant.

Yamashita *et al.* [77] extended this approach to include intracellular and extracellular body fluid compartments for small solutes, and interstitial and extracelular compartments for albumin. Other numerical models include diffusion with non-selective convective transport by Randeron and Farrell [78], and diffusion with selective convective transport by Smeby *et al.* [79], and Jaffrin *et al.* [80].

Dedrick, Flessner *et al.* [81–83] took a different approach. The homogenous membrane outlined above is replaced with a section of tissue in which a series of capillaries are uniformly distributed with access to dialysate on one side only. Their modeling work stemmed from an interest in antineoplastic drug transport during intraperitoneal chemotherapy protocols. Solute transport occurred by movement into the capillaries via blood flow, diffusion across the endothelium, and transit through a hydrogel barrier before reaching the dialysate pool. Solute transport via lymph flow from the peritoneal cavity was included. A characteristic exponential concentration profile in the interstitial region was predicted and experimentally confirmed.

10. CONTINUOUS AMBULATORY PERITONEAL DIALYSIS

Prior to 1975, chronic peritoneal dialysis techniques were generally performed intermittently, two or three times per week. The high efficiency of hemodialysis clearances allowed for short treatment times; a total of approximately 15 h/week. The less efficient standard intermitttent peritoneal dialysis required 30–40 h of treatment per week. This difference in treatment times is one factor resulting in the vast majority of patients being treated with hemodialysis at that time.

During a typical 5 h hemodialysis treatment, the concentration of blood urea nitrogen is reduced from approximately 100 mg/dl to about 40 mg/dl concomitant with the removal of approximately 2–3 l of water. For the next 43 to 67 h, no dialysis is performed, and urea, other metabolites, and fluids accumulate. The cycle is repeated by subsequent periods of dialysis and reaccumulation. Kjellstrand *et al.* [84] have hypoethesized that these fluctuations may be detrimental to the patients' health. In fact, the application of very high efficiency hemodialysis results in a 'disequilirbium syndrome' characterized by headache, nausea, vomiting and severe blood pressure declines. Arieff *et al.* [85] have suggested that this syndrome is a result of large intracellular-to-extracellular concentration gradients with concomitant fluid movement under the resulting osmotic gradients, particularly across the blood-brain barrier. This hypothesis is supported by the results of Popovich *et al.* [86] who have shown that resistance to mass transfer across the cellular membranes can result in significant transcellular concentration disequilibrium during hemodialysis.

The clinical symptoms associated with short-term intensive dialysis treatments can be eliminated by performing the treatment continuously at a modest efficiency analogous to normal kidney function but at a reduced clearance. A clinical technique which accomplishes this using peritoneal dialysis was developed by Popovich and Moncrief in 1975 [46]. This procedure is termed Continuous Ambulatory Peritoneal Dialysis (CAPD).

11. THEORETICAL BASIS OF CAPD

The clinical protocol which will yield desired blood metabolite concentrations levels employing CAPD can be specified by the use of a simple mathematical model for the patient-peritoneal dialysis system. Popovich *et al.* [86]

have demonstrated that a single body pool assumption, such as the one schematically outlined in Figure 2, is valid for low dialysis clearance systems such as CAPD. The verbal statement which applies to metabolites in the body is that accumulation is equal to the rate of generation, G, minus the rate by residual renal clearance, K_R, or dialysis clearance, K_D. This verbal statement is illustrated in equation 18.

$$\frac{d}{dt}(V_B C_B) = \quad G \quad - \quad K_R C_B \quad - \quad K_D C_B. \quad [18]$$

| Rate of accumulation | Rate of generation | Renal removal rate | Dialysis removal rate |

As noted, the accumulation term is the time derivative of the total mass of metabolite in the system (the blood concentration, C_B, times the volume of distribution, V_B). This term will equal zero if the dialysis treatment is continuous, i.e. the concentrations and volumes are constant. Setting the accumulation term equal to zero and solving the resulting algebraic equation for the steady state body metabolite concentration level in term of the system parameters yields:

$$C_B = \frac{G}{K_d + K_d} = \frac{G}{K}. \quad [19]$$

where K is the total metabolite clearance or the sum of dialysis, renal and, if present, metabolic clearance. Note that these clearances are additive.

A typical blood area nitrogen generation rate for dialysis patients is 5.7 mg/min [87]. If one desires to maintain a patient at a continuous BUN level of 80 mg/dl, equation 19 predicts that a total clearance of 7.1 ml/min is required as illustrated.

$$K = \frac{G}{C_B} = \frac{5.7 \text{ mg/min}}{0.8 \text{ mg/ml}} = 7.1 \text{ ml/min.} \quad [20]$$

Multiplying this by 1440, the number of minutes per day, yields the daily clearance requirement:

$$K = (7.1 \text{ ml/min}) (1440 \text{ min/day}) = 10\,200 \text{ ml/day.} \quad [21]$$

Thus, a total clearance of about 10 l/day is required to maintain a patient with a BUN of about 80 mg/dl.

This clearance can be obtained using any dialysis technique. Peritoneal dialysis clearance is defined by:

$$K_D = \frac{V_D C_D}{T C_B}. \quad [22]$$

where V_D is the drained dialysate volume at a mean concentration of C_D over a total time T.

As noted in Figure 9, the dialysate BUN concentration asymptotically approaches the blood concentration level following infusion of fresh dialysis fluid. If the residence phase is sufficiently long, equilibration will occur such that $C_B = C_D$. Under these circumstances equation 18 reduces to:

$$K_D = \frac{V_D}{T} = Q_D = \text{dialysate flow rate.} \quad [23]$$

This model leads directly to the clinical protocol of CAPD. The theory predicts that a patient will maintain

a steady BUN level of 80 mg/dl if 10 l dialysate are allowed to equilibrate with body fluids on a daily basis. Since the normal infusion volume is 2.0 l, four infusions per day will result in a total of 8.0 l. Approximately 2 l/day are ultrafiltered yielding a total drained volume of 10 l/day as predicted. Four exchanges per day will require a mean residence time of approximately 6 hr per exchange for continuous treatment. This is more than adequate to achieve equilibration for BUN. Equilibration will not be achieved for higher molecular weight substances such as inulin (5500 MW) and proteins.

12. CAPD EXCHANGE RATE CRITERIA

Table 3 presents a list of the major factors which affect CAPD exchange rate criteria. Under ordinary conditions, two liter infusions are employed. Mean peritoneum transport characteristics and ultrafiltration volumes have been determined as outlined above. Using this data, Popovich *et al.* [88] have computed the number of two liter exchanges per day which will be required to maintain a BUN of less than 80 mg/dl in a typical CAPD patient. The results are presented in Figure 14. The results demonstrate that the typical patient with low residual renal clearances (0 to 1.0 ml/min) will generally require 4 exchanges per day. Patients with zero residual renal clearance will have a steady state

Table 3. Factors affecting exchange rate.

Major factors	Influenced by
Generation rate	Diet, weight, metabolic rate
Residual renal clearances	
Ultrafiltration rate	Fluid intake, dialysate tonicity
Mass transfer-area coefficient	Peritonitis, vascular disease, vasodilation

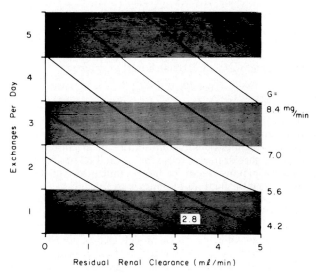

Figure 14. CAPD exchange rate determined by residual renal clearance and BUN generation rate (reprinted with permission of Excerpta Medica (ref. 88)).

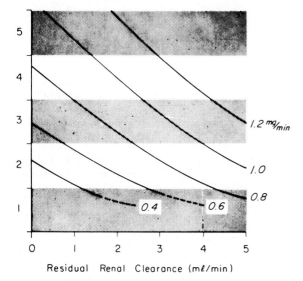

Figure 15. CAPD exchange rate determined by residual renal clearance and creatinine generation rate.

BUN near 80 mg/dl. Patients with renal clearances near 1.0 ml/min will obtain an additional 1.4 l/day clearance resulting in a BUN level of about 67 mg/dl. At a renal clearance of approximately 1.5 ml/min, only three exchanges per day are predicted to maintain the patients at a BUN of 80 mg/dl. Two exchanges per day are predicted for a residual renal clearance function of approximately 3.0 ml/min. Of course, the generation rate is also an important parameter which can be related to protein intake [74]. Figure 15 presents identical information but is based on maintaining a steady creatinine level below 12 mg/dl.

13. MEMBRANE TRANSPORT LIMITATIONS

The authors caution that the above results are based on patients with average ultrafiltration rates and peritoneal transport characteristics [88]. Indeed, Popovich *et al.* [89] have recently presented a documented case of a patient who developed uremic symptoms on 4 exchanges per day as a consequence of drastically reduced peritoneum mass transfer ability. The patient developed nausea, vomiting anorexia, and lethargy while undergoing CAPD with four exchanges per day. The patient became asymptomatic when placed on five exchanges per day. Detailed transport studies were obtained at this time. The exchange schedule was again altered from 5 to 4 to 5 exchanges per day with the development and abatement of symptoms. Symptoms did not reappear following a final shift to 4 exchanges per day. Again, transport studies were obtained. The resulting mass transfer-area coefficients are presented in Table 4.

The authors found that the patient had a creatinine mass transfer-area coefficient of only 5.1 ml/min (22% of normal) during the period he developed uremic symptoms on four exchanges per day. His BUN and creatinine levels were 97 and 21.5 mg/dl, respectively. The creatinine MTAC had increased to 12.8 ml/min (54% of normal) when he was asymptomatic on four exchanges per day. This led the authors to conclude that decreased mass transport can result in insufficient metabolite removal and the development of uremic symptoms on CAPD [89]. Also, because of high MTAC's for middle molecules in the patient and the known large removal rates of middle molecules for CAPD, relative to other dialysis techniques [88], the authors suggested that it is the smaller metabolites which were responsible for the uremic symptoms noted.

A simple clinical protocol to evaluate the mass transport capabilities of a patient based on the degree of equilibration of creatinine during a test exchange has been presented [89]. The clinical protocol is outlined in Table 5. This can be performed using a needle for dialysate infusion if a nephrologist wishes to test a patient's ability to perform CAPD prior to insertion of an indwelling catheter.

Table 4. Mass transfer-area coefficients (ml/min).

Solute (mol. wt)	Study 1 5 ex/day	Study 2 4 ex/day	Controls (averaged results)
BUN (60.1)	12.6	17.0	33.5
Creatinine (113)	5.1	12.8	23.5
Glucose (180)	5.2	6.6	18.1
Inulin (5500)	3.7	4.0	2.7
Dextran (70000)	1.2	1.9	0.6

Table 5. Transfer evaluation protocol.

1. Infuse 2.01 1.5 gm% dextrose dialysis solution intraperitoneally
2. Let solution dwell for 4 hours post-infusion
3. Sample dialysate and plasma for creatinine concentration.
4. Calculate D/P creatinine concentration ratio.
5. Find D/P ration on 4 hour creatinine equilibration curve.
6. Read corresponding MTAC from abscissa.

The degree of creatinine equilibration in a four-hour period is determined using 2.0 l of standard 1.5% dextrose Dianeal®. The four-hour period indicated refers to the period between the end of infusion and sampling of the blood and dialysate. The MTAC can be estimated from the degree of equilibration using Figure 16 which is based on the authors' theoretical correlations [89].

The average creatinine MTAC is about 23.5 ml/min [74] corresponding to 92% of equilibration for creatinine after a four-hour dwell period. The authors suggest that patients with MTAC's less than one-fourth of average (less than 50% equilibration) may develop symptoms of under-dialysis and require additional exchanges [89]. Patients with greater than one-half average MTAC should be considered suitable candidates for CAPD from the standpoint of mass transport ability.

Another factor which can influence CAPD exchange rate criteria is the necessity to maintain proper fluid balance. Generally, CAPD provides excellent control of fluids [72]. However, there may be difficulties in achieving adequate ultrafiltration during episodes of peritonitis [90]. This may result from increased glucose transport with resulting rapid loss of osmotic gradients. Randerson and Farrell [91] have demonstrated substantial increases in the MTAC in two patients during bouts of peritonitis. This may necessitate more frequent exchanges employing more hypertonic solutions.

Occasionally, patients under routine treatment exhibit hypotension [90]. This can be alleviated by using less of the higher tonicity dialysate. During hypotensive episodes, it may also be helpful to skip the next scheduled exchange. By leaving the fluid in for a period of two exchanges, the body reabsorbs dialysate fluid at approximately 1 ml/min during the second four to six hour period. This will help any acute situations with little noticeable increase in BUN levels.

14. CAPD IN CHILDREN

CAPD is currently enjoying rapid expansion in the treat-ment of adult patients with end stage renal disease. This is due in part to the advantages that CAPD exhibits over hemodialysis [92–94]. These include: (1) continuous bio-chemical and fluid control, (2) patient mobility and freedom from a machine, (3) greatly reduced dietary restrictions, (4) simplicity of operation, and (5) elimination of the need for routine blood access. Because of these advantages, preliminary clinical studies suggest that CAPD may be an attractive alternative to hemodialysis in the treatment of infants and children. Promising clinical results have been reported in limited clinical trials [95–96].

It is known that metabolite transport in children differs from that in adults [32, 33, 84]. However, only recently have detailed transport studies been conducted by Popovich *et al.* [98] to characterize their differences. Peritoneal mass transfer characteristics were measured in seven studies in four children with an age range of 17 months to 6 years. The clinical protocol of Pyle [54] outlined above was employed using radioiodated human serum albumin (RISA) in place of the tagged dextran [98]. The volume of the dialysate fluid present in the peritoneal cavity was computed using the degree of dilution of the RISA. Mass transfer-area coefficients were computed from an analysis of the concentration-time profiles and known ultrafiltration rates.

Typical concentration-time results are presented in Figure 17. The BUN dialysate to plasma concentration ratio versus time in three patients is illustrated. Note that results similar to the adult reference are obtained. The same held true for creatinine, uric acid and glucose [98].

The actual intraperitoneal dialysate volumes as a function of dwell time for 1.5% and 4.25% dextrose solutions in a typical patient are illustrated in Figure 18. Again, the results are similar to that in adults. A rapid increase in dialysate volume is obtained shortly after infusion. This occurs as a result of high glucose concentration gradients with concomitant osmotic driving forces. The glucose is rapidly absorbed causing the volume to reach a maximum and then decline as dialysate is reabsorbed under the influence of the oncotic force of the blood. Dwell times corresponding to maximum ultrafiltration were approxi-mately 3 to 4 h.

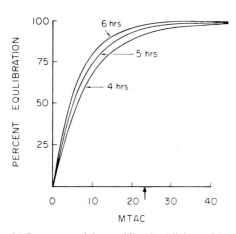

Figure 16. Percent creatinine equilibration (dialysate/plasma ratio) as a function of mass transfer coefficient and dwell time (reprinted with permission of Artificial Organs (ref. 93)).

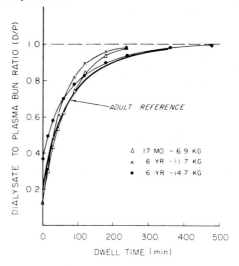

Figure 17. BUN dialysate/plasma ratio in children on CAPD.

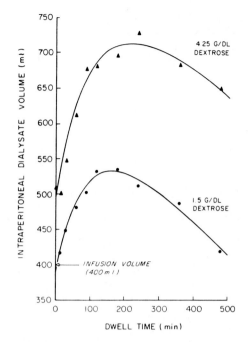

Figure 18. Intraperitoneal volume profiles for a 14.7 kg child on CAPD.

Mean mass transfer-area coefficients, determined by Popovich *et al.* [98], are presented in Table 6 with an adult reference. Clearly, the MTAC's are quite different from the adults. Some relationship between the MTAC and child size is evident. The reader will recall the MTAC is a measure of the maximum possible dialysis clearance which would occur if the dialysate metabolite concentration level was somehow maintained at zero at all times. It is also equal to the area available for mass transport divided by the sum of all resistances to transport (see equation 5). If the anatomical and physiological characteristics of the peritoneum in the child per unit area are simular to that in adults, the sum of the resistances would also be similar. This suggests that the decrease in the MTAC's might be related to a decrease in the area for transport which could be correlated for adult values by some scaling factor.

Table 7 shows how the mean solute MTAC's are scaled by body surface area and weight. Scaling by weight gives a much better correlation with adult values in the children studied [98].

Scaling by weight rather than body surface area is also supported by an ultrafiltration comparison. The mean rate of ultrafiltration immediately following dialysate infusion (the maximum ultrafiltration rate) was determined to be 2.5 to 3.0 ml/min compared to 11.7 to 16.6 ml/min in adults [98]. Table 8 illustrates that the mean maximum ultrafiltration rates give better correlation to adult values if scaled by weight.

Popovich *et al.* [98] noted the apparent contradiction of metabolite concentration equilibration data similar to adults in the face of drastically reduced mass transfer-area coefficients. They resolved this by rearranging the basic mass transport relationship (equation 9) for the change of dialysate concentration versus time to obtain:

$$\frac{dC_D}{dt} = \frac{KA}{V_d}(C_B - C_D) + \frac{Q_u}{V_d}[(1-\sigma)C - C_D]. \qquad [24]$$

The parameters which determine the rate of dialysate equilibration are KA/V_D and Q_u/V_D. The authors had demonstrated that both KA and Q_u appear to correlate in direct proportion to body weight. Therefore, if the infused

Table 6. Mean mass transfer area coefficients.

Patient/wt (kg)	in ml/min				
	1 7.0	2 8.2	3 11.7	4 14.7	Adult reference
Solute					
Urea	2.69	6.14	7.50	7.71	33.6
Creatinine	1.49	1.51	3.36	4.15	23.5
Uric acid	0.88	2.59	4.34	4.40	19.5
Glucose	1.67	3.35	4.15	3.52	18.1

Table 7. Mean BUN mass transfer-area coefficients scaled by body surface area and weight.

Patient	KA ml/min	Surface area M²	WT kg	KA scaled by surface area	KA scaled by wt	Adult reference
1	2.69	0.34	7.0	13.7	26.9	33.6
2	6.14	0.38	8.2	28.0	52.4	33.6
3	7.50	0.51	11.7	25.4	44.9	33.6
4	7.71	0.65	14.7	20.5	36.7	33.6
Mean				21.9 ± 5.4	40.2 ± 9.5	33.6

Table 8. Maximum ultrafiltration rates scaled by body surface area and weight.

% Dextrose	Measured ml/min	Scaled by surface area	Scaled by weight	Adult mean
1.5	2.5	5.3	9.5	11.7
4.25	3.0	9.6	17.8	16.6

dialysate volume, V_D, is also decreased proportionally to decreasing weight, the parameter will have constant values. For this case, mass transfer solutions of equation 24 will yield similar dialysate concentration profiles regardless of patient size. In fact, clinicians treating children have typically scaled infusion volumes by body weight, which explains the rather consistent D/P curves obtained for the different children.

Finally, the authors predicted daily infusion volumes necessary to obtain specified creatinine concentration levels for adults and children using four CAPD exchanges per day. Creatinine was selected because of the wealth of generation rate data for children and adults [100–102]. The mass transfer-area coefficients and ultrafiltration rates were assumed to scale by weight. Residual renal clearance was assumed to be negligible as a worst case basis.

The results of the computations are illustrated in Figures 19 and 20. Also shown are data points corresponding to actual infused volumes and weights of children treated with CAPD. Excellent agreement was obtained between the predicted and clinical results. However, the authors caution that 'their curves are based on average data and should only be utilized to obtain an initial estimate. Considerable individual variations in peritoneal transport characteristics are common. Generation rates also vary' [98]. Nevertheless, the curves provide a basis for a first estimate of infusion volume which can be adjusted depending on the particular circumstances involved.

KINETIC STUDIES OF DIALYSIS

15.1. Effects of convective transport

It has long been recognized that fluid transfer occurs in peritoneal dialysis and that some entrainment or convection of solutes must result. Until the studies of Pyle *et al.* [53, 54], however, definitive data on solute convection was not available and the contribution of convection to total solute transport could only be estimated [103]. From comprehensive transport studies in CAPD patients, Pyle [54] has determined the individual diffusive and convective mass transfer rates as a function of time. Figure 21 illustrates the fraction of total solute transfer resulting from convection for the solute concentration profiles shown in Figures 9 to 12 [54]. This data shows that convection is a small but significant mechanism in urea transport. At the maximum, the contribution is about 12%. As solute size increases, the importance of convective transport increases dramatically. Immediately post-infusion (t = 0), convection accounts for about 86% of the total protein transfer. Thus, it is apparent that convection cannot be neglected as a transport mechanism, especially for large solutes. If this

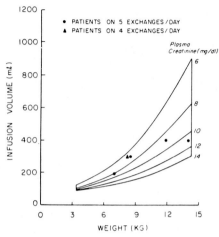

Figure 19. Predicted infusion volume required for CAPD patients as a function of weight (3 to 14 kg).

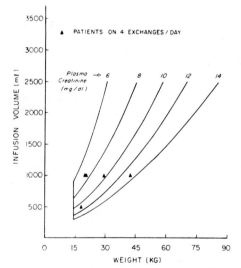

Figure 20. Predicted infusion volume required for CAPD patients as a function of weight (greater than 14 kg).

mechanism is not included in models employed in the evaluation of transport parameters, the remaining parameters may be seriously over-estimated.

15.2. Technique comparisons

The two classic treatments of uremia via dialysis are hemodialysis and peritoneal dialysis, with many technical variations on each. The evaluation of these various pro-

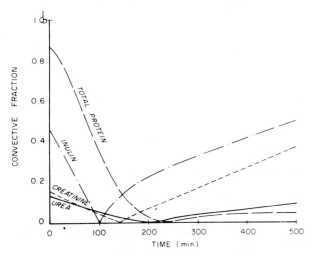

Figure 21. Fraction of solute transport due to convection in peritoneal dialysis (reprinted with permission of Pyle WK (ref. 54)).

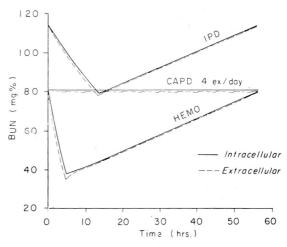

Figure 22. BUN concentration profiles for stable, average patient on IPD, CAPD, and hemodialysis.

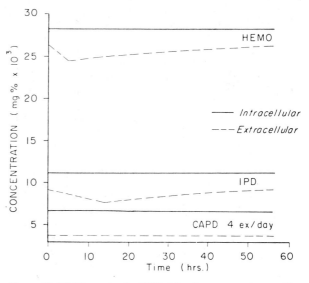

Figure 23. Middle molecule (5500 dalton) concentration profiles for stable, average patient on IPD, CAPD, and hemodialysis.

cedures is complicated by the lack of a clear understanding of uremia itself, i.e. what the toxins involved are, and which are the most important. However, more recent comparative studies have employed mathematical models of the dialysis techniques to identify the important variables and their effects. Through the ability of these models to stimulate a variety of therapeutic conditions, it is possible to draw comparisons of techniques as dissimilar as hemodialysis and peritoneal dialysis.

Popovich *et al.* [88, 105, 106] have employed a two-pool patient model to compare these techniques and CAPD for the ability to remove urea, creatinine, vitamin B-12 (1355 daltons) and inulin (5500 daltons). Their model generated concentration profiles for intra- and extracellular body compartments as shown for urea and the 5500 dalton solute in Figures 22 and 23, respectively. This data confirms that 40 hour/week intermittent peritoneal dialysis is a less efficient method of dialyzing urea than 15 hour/week hemodialysis. However, CAPD with 4 exchanges/day results in lower metabolite levels than IPD. In this case, the minimum IPD levels and the CAPD levels (which are nearly constant) are both approximately equal. The predialysis IPD levels are approximately 40% higher than the CAPD levels. Also note the nearly constant BUN levels with CAPD patients relative to the saw-tooth concentration pattern for both of the intermittent procedures.

As outlined in Figure 23, the results are significantly different for a 5500 dalton 'middle' molecule. While CAPD is still more efficient than IPD (i.e. CAPD results in lower concentration levels), both are substantially better than hemodialysis. This is because of the rapid decrease in hemodialysis clearance with increasing molecular weight relative to peritoneal dialysis [89]. Again, the CAPD levels are relatively constant, due to the continuous application of the procedure.

It is interesting to note that in CAPD there is very little transcellular difference in the urea levels compared to the conditions during hemodialysis. As absolute size increases, the transcellular concentration gradient increases in magnitude, but the gradient is never as great as with hemo-

dialysis. Hiatt *et al.* [93] have shown that the CAPD transcellular disequilibrium is virtually the same as would be found in individuals with normal renal function. They have illustrated this by performing mathematical simulations of concentration levels in subjects with normal renal function and in those undergoing dialysis. The maximum disequilibrium was then determined and a ratio of the dialysis to normal values was calculated. The ratios, shown in Table 9, indicate that the disequilibrium experienced by CAPD is never more than four percent greater than that in normals while it may exceed 900% in hemodialysis patients. It has been hypothesized [85, 107] that this abnormal degree of disequilibrium is detrimental to the patients' health.

It is apparent from the concentration profiles in Figures 22 and 23 that there is some solute size for which hemodialysis and CAPD are equivalent at steady state. Figure

Table 9. Maximum intracellular to extracellular metabolite disequilibrium ratio.

Solute	Mol. wt.	CAPD/normal	IPD/normal	HD/normal
Urea	60	1.04	3.5	9.6
Vit. B-12	1.355	1.02	2.7	4.6
Inulin	5.500	1.00	1.3	1.5

24 shows the ratio of the predialysis hemodialysis to CAPD concentration levels as a function of solute molecular weight. For urea, this ratio indicates that four CAPD exchanges per day are roughly equivalent to three 5-hr hemodialyses per week. As solute size increases, the hemodialyzer is relatively less efficient and the concentration ratio increases. The increase is largely due to three factors: the rapid decrease in membrane permeability with increasing molecular weight for hemodialyzer membranes, the relatively high permeability of the peritoneum to large solutes, and the longer treatment time with CAPD. Thus, for metabolites which behave similar to inulin, four daily CAPD exchanges results in a metabolite level one-seventh of that found in hemodialysis.

Another method with which to compare the various treatment modalities is to quantitate them on the basis of solute clearances [89]. Representative clearance values on a weekly basis are presented in Table 10 along with normal kidney clearances. From this data, the superiority of hemodialysis in the removal of small solutes is apparent. For urea or a similar-sized solute, hemodialysis can clear 107 l of body fluids in a week while CAPD (4 exchanges per day) and IPD clear only 70 and 60 l/week, respectively. However, none of these procedures can duplicate the removal rate of two kidneys, 756 l/week. As solute size increases, there is a drastic drop in the hemodialyzer clearance. The peritoneal dialysis procedures are less strongly affected for the reasons noted above. For a solute of 5500 daltons, the hemodialyzer clearance declines to 5 l/week, only 4.6% of the urea clearance. In contrast, the 5500 dalton clearances for CAPD (4 exchanges per day) and IPD of 26 and 12 l/week represent 37 and 20%, respectively, of the urea clearance. Thus, either of the peritoneal dialysis procedures will provide better large solute removal ability, with CAPD being the clearly superior technique. There can be little doubt that CAPD would be the treatment of choice if the object of the treatment is the removal of large molecular weight toxins.

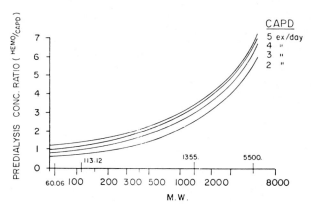

Figure 24. Hemodialysis to CAPD predialysis concentration ratio as a function of molecular weight (reprinted with permission of Artificial Organs (ref. 93)).

16. TRANSPORT LIMITATIONS: THE DIFFERENCE BETWEEN CAPD AND IPD

The BUN clearance of peritoneal dialysis is a complex function of three dominant parameters [89]: the peritoneal blood flow rate, Q_B, the dialysate flow rate, Q_D, and the mass transfer-area coefficient, MTAC. The clearance can never exceed the lowest value of these three parameters. Also, the clearance will be approximately equal to the value of one of the parameters if it is very much less than the other two. For example, the clearance will be approximately equal to the MTAC if the value of the blood and dialysate flow rates are very much larger than the value of the MTAC. In this case the clearance is said to be *mass transfer limited*, and increasing either the blood or dialysate flow rates will not significantly increase the clearance. The clearance of a solute is said to be *dialysate flow rate limited* if the value of the dialysate flow rate is much lower than the blood flow rate and the MTAC. In this case the clearance will essentially equal the value of dialysate flow rate.

These concepts are illustrated in Figure 25. The urea clearance is presented as a function of dialysate flow rate for peritoneal dialysis. Intermittent peritoneal dialysis is generally performed with dialysate flow rates of 30–40 ml/min, with a urea clearance near 20 ml/min. Note that the urea clearance levels off at approximately 35 ml/min (a value equal to the average MTAC) at high dialysate flow rates. This demonstrates that the clearance of intermittent peritoneal dialysis is limited to a considerable extent by a low mass transfer-area coefficient. This assumes that under

Table 10. Weekly solute clearances

Solute	Normal kidneys	Hemodyalisis (15 hr/week)	IPD (40 hr/wk)	CAPD exchanges day		
				3	4	5
Urea	756	107	60	57	70	83
1355 dalton	1260	15	19	39	42	45
5500 dalton	1260	4	12	25	26	27

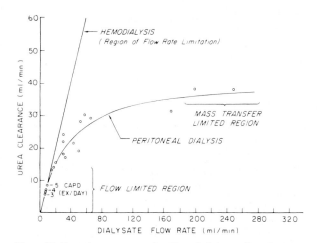

Figure 25. Urea clearances as a function of dialysate flow rate.

ordinary circumstances the peritoneum capillary blood flow rate is sufficiently high to preclude it becoming a limiting parameter. This assumption is supported by inferential evidence presented by Nolph *et al.* [96].

With the typical IPD dialysate flow rates of 30 to 40 ml/min, the urea clearance is approximately 55% of the maximum possible clearance for a patient with average peritoneal mass transfer ability. If a patient has impaired transport ability, the maximum clearance will be decreased proportionately. This effect can have serious consequences in an intermittent technique such as IPD where efficiency must be maximized to provide adequate therapy. As shown in Figure 22, IPD is the least effective technique in terms of urea removal for the average patient. Any loss or intrinsic lack of peritoneal transport capability will make IPD less efficient, and will result in higher metabolite concentration.

There is known to be substantial interpatient variability in peritoneal mass transfer-area coefficients. Some patients' MTAC's have been found to be about 20% of the average value [105]. Due to the low clearances found even under the best circumstances, these patients are poor candidates for IPD. If treated with IPD, they may well exhibit symptoms of under-dialysis or develop other serious complications. Indeed, this may explain the poor survivability of some IPD patients [108]. These problems can generally be overcome by performing longer treatments to compensate for any transport limitations. However, long IPD treatments present practical difficulties. CAPD overcomes the problem of low efficiency inherent in peritoneal dialysis by making continuous operation an integral part of the procedure.

Since CAPD operates at much lower dialysate flow rates (7 to 9 ml/min) than IPD, CAPD becomes a flow rate limited system with a maximum clearance of no more than 9 ml/min. Thus, on first examination, it would seem that CAPD might be an even poorer therapy than IPD. However, CAPD is performed continuously (168 h/week) as opposed to only about 40 h/week for IPD. CAPD provides a much higher weekly solute clearance for all solutes because of this longer treatment time, as shown in Table 10. This shows that CAPD is, in fact, a much more efficacious means of maintaining solute concentration control than IPD.

There is also a hidden benefit in the low clearance of CAPD. Since the dialysate flow rate is much less than the average mass transfer-area coefficient, the flow rate is the dominant factor in determining solute clearances. That is, the mass transfer-area coefficient would have to drop to less than half of the average value before membrane properties could exert a significant effect on clearances. Thus, only those patients with severe loss or lack of transport ability will have decreased CAPD clearances with the concomitant problems. In many of these cases, adding another CAPD exchange each day can compensate for the decrease in clearance in these patients. With IPD, even a slight decrease in transport ability may significantly affect clearances.

These results suggest that IPD should be employed with caution due to the possible consequences of under-dialysis. Probably those patients with known membrane-transport problems should not be considered for chronic IPD unless there is a significant amount of residual function to assist in solute clearance. Most patients thus excluded from IPD can be successfully maintained by CAPD with or without residual renal function.

Patients being considered as peritoneal dialysis candidates may be tested for peritoneal membrane transport properties before being placed on either IPD or CAPD by employing the simple clinical protocol of Popovich [89] outlined above. Those patients with average or greater than average transport ability will probably be acceptable candidates for either IPD or CAPD. For those in which any significant impairment is noted, CAPD may prove generally preferable to IPD.

Finally, these results demonstrate that IPD and CAPD are fundamentally different procedures in terms of transport limitations with resulting dissimilarities in their abilities to maintain biochemical control. These differences suggest that IPD clinical results should not be employed in attempting to make comparison between CAPD and hemodialysis.

Numerous recent publications concerning the kinetics of peritoneal transport may be consulted for additional information [110–129].

REFERENCES

1. Ganter G: Uber die Beseitigung giftiger Stoffe aus dem Blut durch Dialyse. Munch Med Wochschr 70: 1478–1480, 1923. (from Boen ST) Kinetics of Peritoneal Dialysis. Medicine 40: 243–287, 1961.
2. Cunningham RS: The physiology of the serous membranes. Physiol Rev 6: 242–280, 1926.
3. Clark AJ: Absorption from the peritoneal cavity. J Pharm Exp Ther 16: 415–433, 1921.
4. Schlechter AJ, Cary MK, Carpentier AL, Darrow DC: Changes in composition of fluids injected into the peritoneal cavity. Am J Dis Child, 46: 1015–1026, 1933.
5. Bliss S, Kastler AO, Nadler SB: Peritoneal lavage. Effective elimination of nitrogenous wastes in the absence of kidney function. Proc Soc Exp Biol Med 29: 1078–1079, 1932.
6. Odel HM, Ferris DO, Power MH: Peritoneal lavage as an effective means of extrarenal excretion. Am J Med 9: 63–77, 1950.
7. Grollman A, Turner LB, McLean JA: Intermittent peritoneal lavage in nephrectomized dogs and its application to the human being. Arch Intern Med 87: 379–389, 1951.

8. Tenckhoff HA, Schechter H: A bacteriologically safe peritoneal access device. Trans Am Soc Artif Intern Organs 14: 181–187, 1968.

9. Feldman W, Beliah T, Drummond KN: Intermittent peritoneal dialysis in the management of chronic renal failure in children. Am J Dis Child 116: 30–36, 1968.

10. Tenckhoff HA, Blagg CR, Curtis KF, Hickman RO: Chronic peritoneal dialysis. Eur Dial Transpl Assoc 10: 363–370, 1973.

11. Flanigan WJ, Henderson LW, Merrill JP: The clinical application and tecvhnique of peritoneal dialysis. Gen Pract 28: 98–109.

12. Mattocks AM, El-Bassiouni EA: Peritoneal dialysis. A review. J Pharm Sci 60: 1767–1782, 1971.

13. Jones JH: Peritoneal dialysis. Br Med Bull 27: 165–169, 1971.

14. Vidt DG: Intermittent peritoneal dialysis. Ohio State Med J 64: 1149–1153, 1968.

15. Miller JH, Gipstein R, Margules R, Swartz M, Rubin ME: Automated peritoneal dialysis: analysis of several methods of peritoneal dialysis. Trans Am Soc Artif Intern Organs 12: 98–105, 1966.

16. Maxwell MW, Rockney RE, Kleeman CR, Twiss MR: Peritoneal dialysis. 1. Technique and application, JAMA 170: 917–924, 1959.

17. Boen ST: Kinetics of peritoneal dialysis: a comparison with the artificial kidney, Medicine 40: 243–287, 1961.

18. Gray H: Anatomy of the Human Body, 27th ed. C. Mayo (ed), Lea and Febiger, Philadelphia, pp 1253–1272, 1959.

19. Copenhauer WM, Johnson DD (1958) Bailey's Textbook of Histology, 14th ed. Williams and Wilkins, Baltimore, 1958.

20. Grant JCB: An atlas of anatomy, 4th eds. Williams and Wilkins, Baltimore, 1956.

21. Baron MA: Structure of the Intestinal Peritoneum in Man. Am J Anat 69: 439–496, 1941.

22. Wayland H: Transmural and interstitial molecular transport. Proc Int'l. CAPD Symp. Paris, 1979. Excerpta Medica, pp 18–27, 1980.

23. Allen L, Weatherford T: Role of fenestrated basement membrane in lymphatic absorption from peritoneal cavity. Am J Physiol 197: 551–554, 1959.

24. Karnovsky MJ: The ultrastructural basis of capillary permeability studied with perioxides as a tracer. J Cell Biol 35: 213–235, 1967.

25. Lieb WR, Stein WD: Biological membranes behave as nonporous polymeric sheets with respect to the diffusion of nonelectrolytes. Nature 224: 240–243, 1969.

26. Nolph KD, Hano JE, teschan PE: Peritoneal sodium transport during hypertonic peritoneal dialysis: physiologic mechanisms and clinical implications. Ann Intern Med 70: 931–941, 1969.

27. Stolz ML, Nolph KD, Maher JF: Factors affecting calcium removal with calcium free peritoneal dialysis. J Lab Clin Med 78: 389–398, 1971.

28. Henderson LW: Peritoneal ultrafiltration dialysis: enhanced urea transfer using hypertonic peritoneal dialysis fluid. J Clin Invest 45: 950–955, 1966.

29. Nolph KD, Rosenfeld PS, Powell JT, Danforth E: Peritoneal glucose transport and hyperglycemia during peritoneal dialysis. Am J Med Sci 259: 272–281, 1970.

30. Henderson LW, Nolph KD: Altered permeability of peritoneal membrane after using hypertonic peritoneal dialysis fluid. J Clin Invest 48: 992–1001, 1976.

31. Raja RM, Cantor RE, Boreyko C, Busheri H, Kramer MS, Rosenbaum JL: Sodium transport during ultrafiltration peritoneal dialysis. Trans Am Soc Artif Intern Organs 18: 429–435, 1972.

32. Kallen RJ: A method for approximating the efficacy of peritoneal dialysis for uremia. Am J Dis Child III: 156–160, 1966.

33. Esperanca MJ, Collins DL: Peritoneal dialysis efficiency in relation to body weight. J Pediat Surg O: 162–169, 1966.

34. Gosselin RE, Berndt WO: Diffusional transport of solutes through mesentery and peritoneum. J Theor Biol 3: 487–495, 1962.

35. Goldschmidtt ZH, Pote HH, Katz MA, Shear L: Effect of dialysate volume on peritoneal dialysis kinetics. Kidney Int, 5: 240–245, 1974.

36. Frank HA, Seligman AM, Fine JJ: Treatment of uremia after acute renal failure by peritoneal irrigation. J Am Med Assoc 130: 703–705.

37. Seligman AM, Frank HA, Fine JJ: Treatment of experimental uremia by means of peritoneal irrigation. J Clin Invest 25: 211–219, 1946.

38. Penzotti SC, Mattocks AM: Effects of dwell time, volume of dialysis fluid, and added accelerators on peritoneal dialysis of urea. J Pharm Sci 60: 1520–1522, 1971.

39. Pirpasopoulos M, Lindsay RM, Rahman M, Kennedy AC: A cost-effectiveness study of dwell times in peritoneal dialysis. Lancet 2: 1135–1136, 1972.

40. Gross M, McDonals HP: Effect of dialysate temperature and flow rate on peritoneal clearance. JAM A 202: 363–365, 1967.

41. Shinaberger JH, Shear L, Clayton LE, Barry FG, Knowlton M, Goldbaum LR: Dialysis for intoxications with lipid soluble drugs: enhancement of glutathimide extraction with lipid dialysate. Trans Am Soc Artif Intern Organs 11: 173–177, 1965.

42. Shinaberger JH, Shear L, Barry KG: Pertitoneal-extracorporeal recirculation dialysis: a technique for improving efficiency of peritoneal dialysis. Invest Urol 2: 555–560, 1965.

43. Rosenbaum JI, Mandanas R: Treatment of phenobarbitol intoxication in dogs with anion-recirculation peritoneal dialysis technique. Trans Soc Artif Intern Organs 13: 183–189, 1967.

44. Kablitz C, Stephen RL, Duffy DP, Jacobsen SC, Zelman A, Kolff WJ: Technological augmantation of peritoneal urea clearance: past, present, and future. Dial & Transpl 9(8): 741–744, 1980.

45. Popovich RP, Pyle WK, Moncrief JW, Decherd JF, Brooks S: Preliminary verification of the low dialysis clearance hypothesis via a novel equilibrium peritoneal dialysis technique. Proc 2nd Austral Conf Heat Mass Transfer 2: 217–223, 1977.

46. Popovich RP, Moncrief JW, Decherd JF, Bomar JB, Pyle WK: The definition of a novel portable/wearable equilibrium peritoneal dialysis technique. Abst Am Soc Artif Interm Organs 5: 64, 1976.

47. Popovich RP, Moncrief JW, Nolph KD, Ghods AJ, Twardowski ZJ, Pyle WK: Continuous ambulatory peritoneal dialysis. Ann Intern Med 88: 449–456, 1978.

48. Villarroel F: Kinetics of intermittent and continuous peritoneal dialysis. J Dial (4): 333–347, 1977.

49. Rescigno A, Segre G: Drug and tracer kinetics, Blaisdell, Waltham, Mass, 1966.

50. Mattocks AM: Accelerated removal of salicylate by additive in peritoneal dialysis fluid. J Pharm Sci 58: 595–598, 1969.

51. Popovich RP, Moncrief JW, Okutan M, Decherd JF: A model of the peritoneal dialysis system. Proc 25th Ann Conf on Engr in Med And Biol 14: 172, 1966.

52. Bomar JB, Decherd JF, Hlavinka DJ, Moncrief JW, Popovich RP: The elucidation of maximum efficiency minimum cost peritoneal dialysis protocols. Trans Am Soc Artif Intern Organs 20: 120–129, 1974.

53. Pyle WK, Popovich RP, Moncrief JW: In: Moncrief JW, Popovich RP (eds), Mass transfer evaluation in peritoneal dialysis. Masson NY, pp 32–52, 1981.

54. Pyle WK: Mass transfer in peritoneal dialysis. Ph.D. Dissertation, Univ. of Texas, 1981.

55. Popovich RP, Cristopher TG, Babb AL: The effects of membrane diffusion and ultrafiltration properties on hemodialyzer design and performance. Chem Eng Prog Symp Ser

67(114): 105–115, 1971.

56. Babb AL, Johansen PJ, Strand MJ, Tenckhoff H, Scribner BH: Bi-directional permeability of the human peritoneum to middle molecules. Proc 10th Cong Europ Dial Transpl Assoc, Vienna 10: 247–262, 1973.

57. Popovich RP, Moncrief JW: Clinical development of the low dialysis clearance hypothesis via equilibrium peritoneal dialysis. 1ste Ann Rep No. NO1-AM-6-2211, AK-CUP, NIAMDD, NIH, Bethesda, MD, 1977.

58. Garred LJ, Canand B, Farrell PC: A simple kinetic model for assessing peritoneal mass transfer in chronic ambulatory peritoneal dialysis. Am Soc Artif Intern Organs J, 6(3): 131–137, 1983.

59. Lindholm B, Werynsky A, Bergstrom J: Kinetics of peritoneal dialysis with glycerol and glucose as osmotic agents. Trans Am Soc Artif Intern Organs, 33: 19–27, 1987.

60. Leypoldt JK, Parken HR, Frigon RPP, Henderson LW: Molecular size dependence of peritoneal transport, 110(2): 207–216, 1987.

61. Villarroel F, Popovich RP, Nolph KD: Evaluation of permeance in peritoneal dialysis. J Dial 2(4): 361–378, 1978.

62. Bomar JB: The transport of uremic metabolites in peritoneal dialysis. Ph.D. Dissertation, Univ of Texas.

63. Kedem, O, Katchalsky A: Thermodynamic analysis of the permeability of biological membranes to non-electrolytes. Biochem Biophys Acta 27: 229–246, 1958.

64. Katchalsky A, Curran PF: Nonequilibrium thermodynamics in biophysics. Harvard University Press, Cambridge, Mass, 1967.

65. Popovich RP, Pyle WK, Moncrief JW, Bomar JB: Peritoneal dialysis. Chronic replacement of kidney function. AIChE Symp Series, 75(187): 31–45, 1979.

66. Villarroel F, Klein E, Holland F: Solute flux in hemodialysis and hemofiltration membranes. Trans Am Soc Artif Intern Organs 23: 225–233, 1977.

67. Anderson JL, Quinn JA: Restricted transport in small pores: a model for steric exclusion and hindered particle motion. Biophys J 14: 130–150, 1974.

68. Brenner J, Gaydos LJ: The contrained brownian movement of spherical particles in cylindrical pores of comparable radius: models of the diffusive and convective transport of solute molecules in membranes and porous media. J Colloid Interface Sci 58: 312–356, 1977.

69. Bird RB, Steward WE, Lightfoot EN: Transport phenomena, John Wiley and Sons, New York, 1960.

70. Conte SD, de Boor C: Elementary numerical analysis, 2nd ed., McGraw-Hill, New York, 1965.

71. Brown KM: Computer-oriented methods for fitting tabular data in the least squares sense. Fall Joint Computer Conf., Natl Center for Atmospheric Res., Boulder, Colo, 1972.

72. Rubin J, Nolph KD, Popovich RP, Moncrief JW, Prowart B: Drainage volumes during continuous ambulatory peritoneal dialysis. J Am Soc Artif Intern Organs 2(2): 54–60, 1979.

73. Nolph KD, Sorkin MJ: A hypothesis to explain the ultrafiltration characteristics of peritoneal dialysis. Kidney Int (in press).

74. Popovich RP, Moncrief JW, Nolph KD, Pyle WK, Sawyer JW: Physiological Transport Parameters in Peritoneal and Hemodialysis. 3rd Ann Rep No NO1-AM-3-2205, AK-CUP, N1AMDD, N1H, Bethesda, Md, 1977.

75. Morgenstern BZ, Pyle WK, Gruskin AB, Kaiser BA, Perlman SA, Polinsky MS, Baluarte HJ: Convective characteristics of pediatric peritoneal dialysis. Perit Dialysis Bull 4: S155–S158, 1984.

76. Rubin J, Klein E, Bower JD: Investigation of net sieving coefficient of the peritoneal membrane during peritoneal dialysis. Am Soc Artif Intern Organs J 5: 9–15, 1982.

77. Yamashita A, Nagumo H, Hidai H, Kumano K, Iidaka K, Sakai T: Efficiency of diffusion and convective transport for solute removal in CAPD. Japan J Artif Organs 14: 111, 1985.

78. Randerson DH, Farrell PC: Mass transfer properties of the human peritoneum. Am Soc Artif Intern Organs J 3: 140–146, 1981.

79. Smeby LC, Wideroe TE, Jorstad S: Individual differences in water transport during continuous peritoneal dialysis. Am Soc Artif Intern Organs J 4: 17–27, 1981.

80. Jaffrin MY, Odell RA, Farrell PC: A model of ultrafiltration and glucose mass transfer kinetics in peritoneal dialysis. Artif Organs 11(3): 198–207, 1987.

81. Dedrik RL, Flessner MF, Collins JM, Schulz JS: Is the peritoneum a membrane? Am Soc Artif Intern Organs 5: 1–8, 1982.

82. Flessner MF, Dedrik RL, Schulz JS: A distributed model of peritoneal-plasma transport: theoretical considerations. Am J Physiol 246: 597–607, 1984.

83. Flessner MF, Dedrik RL, Schulz JS: A distributed model of peritoneal-plasma transport: analysis of experimental data in the rat. Am J Physiol 248: 413–424, 1985.

84. Kjellstrand CM, Rosa AA, Shideman JR, Rodrigo F, Davin T, Lynch RE: Optimal dialysis frequency and duration: the 'unphysiology hypothesis'. Kidney Int 13 (suppl. 8): S-120-S-124, 1978.

85. Arieff AJ, Guisado R, Massry SG: Uremic encephalopathy: studies on biochemical alterations in the brian. Kidney Int 7 (Suppl): S-194-S-200, 1975.

86. Popovich RP, Hlavinka DJ, Bomar JB, Moncrief JW, Decherd JF: The consequences of physiological resistances on metabolite removal from the patient-artificial kidney system. Trans Am Soc Artif Intern Organs 21: 108–115, 1975.

87. Gotch FA, Sargent JA, Keen M, Lam M, Prowitt M, Grady M: Solute kinetics in intermittent dialysis therapy. 9th Ann Rep – Contractors Conf, pp 98–101, 1976.

88. Popovich RP, Pyle WK, Hiatt MP, McCullough WS, Moncrief JW: Metabolite transport kinetics in peritoneal dialysis. Proc Int CAPD Symp, Paris, Nov 2–3, 1979. Excerpta Medica, pp 28–33, 1980.

89. Popovich RP, Hiatt MP, Moncrief JW, Pyle WK: Mathematical in modeling and minimum treatment requirements peritoneal dialysis. Proc 3rd Capri Conf on chronic Uremia, 1980 (in press).

90. Moncrief JW: Personal communication, Aug. 28, 1980.

91. Randerson DH, Farell PC: Assessment of mass transfer properties of the peritoneal membrane during peritoneal dialysis. J Am Soc Artif Intern Organs, 1980 (in press).

92. Moncrief JW, Popovich RP, Nolph KD, Rubin J, Robson M, Dombros N, de Veber G, Oreopoulous DG: Clinical experience with continuous ambulatory peritoneal dialysis. J Am Soc Artif Intern Organs 2(3): 114–118, 1979.

93. Moncrief JW, Popovich RP: Peritoneal dialysis for a greater number of patients. Chap. In: Controversies in Nephrology, Schreiner GE, ed, Georgetown Universitv Press, Washington D.C., 1979.

94. Moncrief JW, Popovich RP: Continuous ambulatory peritoneal dialysis. Contrib Nephrol 17: 139–145, 1979 (Karger, Basel).

95. Balfe JW, Irwin MA, Oreopolous DG: An assessment of continuous ambulatory peritonean dialysis in children. Proc CAPD Int Symp II, May 9–10, 1980, Austin, Tx (in press).

96. Shmerling J, Kohaut E, Perry S: Cost and social benefits of CAPD in a pediatric population. Proc. CAPD Int Symp II, May 9–10, Austin, Tx (in press).

97. Kohaut EC, Alexander S: Ultrafiltration in the young patient on CAPD. Proc CAPD Int Symp II, May 9–10, 1980, Austin, Tx (in press).

98. Popovich RP, Pyle WK, Rosenthal DA, Alexander S, Balfe JW, Moncrief JW: Kinetics of Peritoneal dialysis in children. Proc CAPD Int Symp II, May 9–10, 1980, Austun, Tx (in

press).

99. Moncrief JW, Pyle WK, Simon P, Popovich RP: Hypertriglycerdemia, Diabetes Mellitus, and Insulin administration in patients undergoing continuous ambulatory peritoneal dialysis. Proc CAPD Int Symp II, May 9–10, Austin, Tx (in press).
100. Arant BS, Edelman CM, Spitzer A: The congruence of creatinine and inulin clearances in children – use of the technicion auto analyzer. J Pediat 81(3): 559–561, 1972.
101. Clark LC, Thompson HL, Beek EI, Jacobson W: Excretion of creatine and creatinine by children. Am J Dis Child 81: 774–783, 1951.
102. Shull BC, Haughey D, Koup J, Baliah T, Li PK: A useful method for predicting creatinine clearance in children. Clin Chem 24(7): 1167–1169, 1979.
103. Popovich RP, Moncrief JW: Kinetic modeling of peritoneal transport. Contrib Nephrol 17: 59–72. (Karger, Basel).
104. Babb AL, Popovich RP, Christopher TG, Scribner BH: The genesis of the square meter-hour hypothesis. Trans Am Soc Artif Intern Organs 17: 81–91, 1971.
105. Popovich RP, Pyle WK, Hiatt MP, Moncrief JW: Comparative Kinetic Studies of Dialysis. Proc Northeastern Physicians Conf., New York, Oct 20, 1979 (in press).
106. Hiatt MP, Pyle WK, Moncrief JW, Popovich RP: A comparison of the relative efficacy of CAPD and hemodialysis in the control of solute concentration. Artif Organs 4(1): 37–43, 1980.
107. Kjellstrand CM, Evans RL, Peterson RJ, Shideman JR, von Hartitzsch B, Buselman TJ: The 'Unphysiology' of dialysis: a major cause of dialysis side effects? Kidney Int 7: 530–534, 1975.
108. Kjellstrand CM et al.: Proc 3rd Capri Conf on Uremia, 1980 (in press).
109. Nolph KD, Miller F, Rubin J, Popovich RP: New directions in peritoneal dialysis concepts and applications. Kidney Int 18(S-10): S-111-S-116.
110. Feriani M, Biasioli S, Chiaramonte A et al.: Anatomical bases of peritoneal permeability: a reappraisal. Int J Artif Organs 5: 345-348, 1982.
111. Nolph KD: Solute and water transport during peritoneal dialysis. Perspec Perit Dial 1: 4–8, 1983.
112. Garini G, Tagliavini D, Occhialini L: Mechanisms of transport and kinetics of the solutes in peritoneal dialysis. Recent Prog Med 73: 569–580, 1982.
113. Rubin J, Klein E, Bower JD: Investigation of the net sieving coefficient of the peritoneal membrane during peritoneal dialysis. ASAI0 J 5: 9–15, 1982.
114. Indraprasit S, Namwongprom A, Sookriwongse C et al.: Effect of dialysate temperature on peritoneal clearances. Nephron 34: 45–47, 1983.
115. Maher J: Transport kinetics in peritoneal dialysis. Perit Dial Bull 3 (suppl): 4–6, 1983.
116. Nath IV, Sehgal S, Chugh KS et al.: Loss of immunoglobulins during peritoneal dialysis. J Assoc Physicians India 29: 927–929, 1982.
117. Ku K, Anderson R, Shoenfeld P: Kinetic modeling of urea in peritoneal dialysis. Dial Transpl 12: 374–381, 1983.
118. Oreopoulos DG: Criteria for adequacy of peritoneal dialysis. Perit Dial Bull 3: 1–2, 1983.
119. Diaz-Buxo JA, Farmer CD, Walker PJ et al.: Effects of hyperparathyroidism on peritoneal clearances. Trans Am Soc Artif Intern Organs 28: 276–279, 1982.
120. Grzegorzewska A, Baczyk K: Furosemide-induced increase in urinary and peritoneal excretion of uric acid during peritoneal dialysis in patients with chronic uremia. Artif Organs 6: 220–224, 1982.
121. Hall K, Meatherall B, Krahn J et al.: Clearance of quinidine during peritoneal dialysis. Am Heart J 104: 646-647, 1982.
122. Rubin J, Adair C, Barnes T et al.: Augmentation of peritoneal clearance by dipyridamole. Kidney Int 22: 658–661, 1982.
123. Lang HL, Nolph KD, McGary TJ: Enhancement of clearances by activated charcoal in an *in vitro* model of peritoneal dialysis. Clin Exp Dial Apheresis 6: 85–95, 1982.
124. Ratnu KS, Haldia KR, Panicker S et al.: A new technique – semicontinuous rapid flow, high volume exchange – for effective peritoneal dialysis in shorter periods. Nephron 31: 159–164, 1982.
125. Twardowski ZJ, Prowant BF, Nolph KD et al.: High volume, low frequency continuous ambulatory peritoneal dialysis. Kidney Int 23: 64–70, 1983.
126. Lopot F: Ultrafiltration characteristics of peritoneal dialysis. Vnitr Lek 29: 230–237, 1983.
127. Manuel A: Failure of ultrafiltration in patients on CAPD. Perit Dial Bull 3 (Suppl): 38–k41, 1983.
128. Slingeneyer A, Canaud B, Mion C: Permanent loss of ultrafiltration capacity of the peritoneum in long-term peritoneal dialysis: an epidemiological study. Nephron 33: 133–138, 1983.
129. Kraus MA, Shasha SM, Nemas M et al.: Ultrafiltration peritoneal dialysis and recirculating peritoneal dialysis with a portable kidney. Dial Transpl 12: 385–388, 1983.

7

ULTRAFILTRATION WITH PERITONEAL DIALYSIS

LEE W. HENDERSON and JOHN K. LEYPOLDT

1. INTRODUCTION

There is a clinical requirement to remove excess body water and electrolytes on a regular basis from patients with end-stage renal failure. The removal of fluid during peritoneal dialysis requires a different approach from that employed during extracorporeal artificial kidney treatment such as hemodialysis or hemofiltration. Whereas fluid can be easily ultrafiltered across a hemodialysis or hemofiltration membrane by applying a difference in hydrostatic or hydraulic pressure, fluid is removed from the patient during peritoneal dialysis by creating a difference in osmotic pressure between dialysis solution and blood. Fluid removal during peritoneal dialysis is therefore more similar to the classical membrane process of osmosis rather than ultrafiltration [1, 2]. The term ultrafiltration, however, has come to be more broadly understood to mean fluid movement induced by either hydrostatic or osmotic pressure driving forces, and we will use the term ultrafiltration to mean fluid movement in this broader sense. We will make a distinction then between ultrafiltration and the movement of fluid out of the peritoneal cavity via the lymphatics and/or into the tissues surrounding the peritoneal cavity. The following discussion will focus primarily on the use of glucose as the osmotic agent driving ultrafiltration across the peritoneum.

1.1. The model

The route taken by water and solute molecules from blood to the dialysis solution across the peritoneum is complex and is described in detail in Chapter 2. It is not possible to quantitatively represent all such details in a simple model of the peritoneum and still retain clinical utility. In the present discussion we will cast the peritoneum in terms of a homogeneous membrane. Such a peritoneal membrane is simply defined functionally as the resistance to mass transport that separates the bulk phase of plasma water from the bulk phase of well-mixed dialysis fluid. With this definition, the peritoneal membrane will comprise both anatomical structures such as the capillary endothelium,

interstitium, and mesothelium and the unstirred layers of solution both within the capillary and the peritoneal cavity. Any heterogeneities between tissues investing different peritoneal regions, such as possible differences between parietal and visceral peritoneum, are ignored.

The practice of referring to the peritoneum as a membrane is very old [3]. At least as far back as the 19th century the terms peritoneum and peritoneal membrane were used synonymously. This historical concept of a peritoneal membrane originated from the structure of the peritoneum as was observed in surgical procedures within the abdominal cavity. It is important to note that this historical concept of a membrane is not necessarily that which is employed in describing peritoneal transport. For this latter purpose, the peritoneal membrane is defined functionally and is a theoretical construct that simplifies the description of water and solute transport to and from the peritoneal cavity.

The primary reason for invoking a membrane model is that it is the simplest model that explains the relevant kinetic data on water and solute transport. As reviewed by Cunningham, in 1926 [3], studies performed around the turn of the century showed that alterations in either dialysate or blood osmolality influenced the rate of absorption of solutions from the peritoneal cavity as expected based upon the known laws of osmosis and diffusion. Additional studies of both water and solute movement by others [4, 5] confirmed that the diffusion of solutes as well as the absorption of fluids out of the peritoneal cavity occurred as expected based upon simple physical laws acting qacross a peritoneal membrane. Moreover, the concept of enhancement of solute movement by solvent drag [6] and the application of nonequilibrium thermodynamics [7] have been incorporated more recently into a modern description of the peritoneal membrane. As well shall see, recent work demonstrates that the assembled clinical and laboratory data on solute and water transport cannot be adequately explained by describing the peritoneum as a simple membrane containing pores of a uniform size. Nevertheless, the point to be made here is that virtually every element of the data taken separately can be quite adequately explained in terms of such a membrane. Thus, the response to adding glucose to the dialysis fluid may be fully conceptualized in terms of a membrane and an osmotic driving force. Similarly, solute movement in response to either a concentration gradient or solvent drag may satisfactorily be explained as if the peritoneum was a membrane. As described below, it is only when approaching the problem in totality that paradoxes arise when employing a simple membrane model.

It should be emphasized that the membrane model is not unique; thus, other models that exhibit identical transport kinetics may also apply. In particular, the model of peritoneal transport described by Dedrick *et al.* [8] presents a formidable alternative. There are two major differences between this new model of the peritoneum and the membrane model. First, the barrier separating blood from dialysate is envisioned to consist of not a single homogeneous phase but rather to include two distinct elements: capillary wall and interstitium (mesothelium is ignored). The second difference is that the blood phase is not lumped together on one side of a hypothetical membrane but is instead distributed or smeared homogeneously within the peritoneal interstitium. Dedrick *et al.* [8] have shown that the kinetics of solute diffusion predicted by this distributed model are identical to those predicted by the membrane model. The advantages of this distributed model of peritoneal transport are that: 1) it relates peritoneal transport parameters to the properties of the capillary microcirculation; and 2) it permits a prediction of solute concentration profiles within the tissues surrounding the peritoneal cavity. The model has only recently been extended to include elements of convective transport to and from the peritoneal cavity [9]. Because of the additional complexities, however, it is difficult to compare the kinetics of water and solute transport predicted by this distributed model with those predicted by the membrane model when dealing with ultrafiltration during peritoneal dialysis. We will therefore confine our discussion of this new transport model to conceptual differences between it and the membrane model. Our discussion will focus on the membrane model because of its simplicity and its familiarity to nephrologists who frequently employ hemodialysis.

2. ULTRAFILTRATION OF WATER ACROSS THE PERITONEUM

2.1. The driving force

The driving force for water movement across an ideal semipermeable membrane, i.e. one that does not permit solute movement, is simply the transmembrane difference in hydrostatic and osmotic pressures. A pressure difference will be designated here in either millimeters of mercury (mm Hg) or osmolal concentration. An osmole (Osm) is by definition 6.023×10^{23} osmotically active solute particles, and osmolal concentration is usually defined as the number of osmoles per kg H_2O. For easy comparison between units, a 1 milliosmole (mOsm) per kg H_2O transmembrane concentration difference will exert enough force at physiological temperature to support a 19 mm column of mercury. For a substance that does not dissociate in aqueous solution,

e.g. glucose, 1 osmole is equivalkent to 1 mole of solute. For a dissociable solute such as NaCl there is the potential of 2 osmoles for each mole of solute as NaCl will dissociate into its constituent ions, each of which is an osmotically active particle. Empirically measured osmotic pressures are lower than those calculated based upon the number of solute particles because of incomplete dissociation of salts and other solution nonidealities. For typical peritoneal dialysis solutions, the measured osmotic pressure is approximately 93% of that calculated.

Osmotic pressure is a colligative property of the solution and is independent of the membrane under consideration. It is well known, however, that the driving force for transmembrane ultrafiltration also depends upon the properties of the membrane. For a given solution osmotic pressure, the driving force for ultrafiltration is greatest across an ideal semipermeable membrane and decreases as the membrane becomes more leaky to solute movement. This phenomenon is important when dealing with the peritoneal membrane as it is not ideally semipermeable; however, it also makes the task of quantifying the driving force for ultrafiltration across the peritoneum quite complicated. If the peritoneal membrane was completely impermeable to all solutes yet permeable to water, then one would need only to determine the concentration difference across the peritoneum for each of the solutes present and convert each concentration term into an osmotic pressure term $\Delta\pi$. Their sum would be the computed osmotic transmembrane pressure difference that would drive ultrafiltration. Furthermore, if the hydraulic conductivity or permeability L_p and area A of the peritoneal membrane were known, it would be possible to compute the ultrafiltration rate Q_f for the clinical circumstance.

As the peritoneal membrane is not ideally semipermeable to the solutes present in dialysis fluid, a correction factor is required for each solute concentration difference to adjust for the degree of membrane leakiness. This correction factor is called the osmotic or Staverman reflection coefficient σ [10], and it depends on the properties of both the solute and the membrane. Values of σ vary between 0 and 1. Written more formally, these concepts could be set down as follows

$$Q_f = -L_pA\,(\sigma_1\Delta\pi_1 + \sigma_2\Delta\pi_2 + ... \text{etc.})^1 \qquad [1]$$

where for example $\sigma_1\Delta\pi_1$ would equal the osmotic driving force for sodium, $\sigma_2\Delta\pi_2$ would equal that for potassium, etc. until each of the solutes present in plasma and dialysis solution are represented. The negative sign is required by convention since water movement flows from the low osmotic pressure solution to the high osmotic pressure solution. This equation illustrates that solutes that are nearly equal in concentration on both sides of the membrane would, of course, contribute little or no driving force for ultrafiltration. On the other hand, solutes such as glucose, urea and albumin, which by therapeutic intent or biological circumstance will have a large concentration difference across the peritoneal membrane, may contribute significant osmotic driving force. This equation, moreover, indicates that it is not possible to estimate the ultrafiltration flow rate in the clinical setting without knowledge of σ values for each solute present as well as the parameter L_pA. Further inspection of equation 1 suggests that only the product of L_pA and σ, the osmotic conductance or permeability $L_pA\sigma$ for each solute, is all that is necessary to predict ultrafiltration flow rate. Yet, the measurement of this product for each solute of interest remains a challenging and unaccomplished task.

An understanding of the relative importance of concentration differences for glucose, urea and albumin as driving forces for ultrafiltration requires further exploration of the term σ and an appreciation of the fact that the larger the size of the solute the less likely it is to be present in biological solutions at a concentration that contributes significantly to the total osmolality. Albumin, for example, probably has a σ value near unity. Assuming a plasma albumin concentration of 3.4 g/dl, a molecular weight of 68 000 and σ equal to 1, the osmotic pressure contributed by albumin to resisting movement of plasma water into the peritoneal space is:

$$\frac{34 \text{ g/kg } H_2O}{68000 \text{ g/Osm}} = 0.5 \text{ mOsm/kg } H_2O = 9 \text{ mm Hg}.$$

There is an additional, possible 3–4 mm Hg contributed by the unequal distribution of electrolytes in an ionized colloidal system such as plasma (Gibbs-Donnan phenomenon). The total contribution of 12–13 mmHg is on the order of the capillary hydrostatic pressure and must be considered small.*

Meanwhile, glucose is added to dialysis fluid at concentrations that greatly exceed the 100 mg/dl plasma level, and therefore this solute contributes a large potential driving force for ultrafiltration. For example, the net osmotic pressure difference across the peritoneum contributed by glucose when using dialysis fluid containing 1.5% or 4.25% dextrose** is 71 mOsm/kg H_2O (1350 mm Hg) or 210 mOsm/kg H_2O (3990 mm Hg), respectively. This potential is never manifest, however, because of the relatively low value of σ for glucose across the peritoneal membrane. Even if the value of σ for glucose is as small as 0.1, the driving force for ultrafiltration that is contributed by glucose is still an order of magnitude greater than that for albumin with its value of σ near unity.

The osmotic force contributed by urea may be arrived at in a similar indirect manner. A plasma urea concentration of 300 mg/dl (BUN of approximately 120 mg/dl) offers a 50 mOsm/kg H_2O (950 mm Hg) potential osmotic driving force for ultrafiltration. The value of σ for urea to be used in equation 1 has never been directly measured, but measured values of sieving coefficient (see below) suggest that the value should be approximately 0.2. A relationship between σ values for urea and glucose can then be derived approximately as follows. Clinical wisdom identifies that a 1.5% dextrose containing dialysis solution when used in patients with a BUN concentration of approximately 120 mg/dl usually results in little or no net removal of excess total body water. By using this empirical observation, neglecting solute concentration changes during the dwell period, assuming urea and glucose are the only important osmotic solutes, and assuming osmotic pressures for urea and glucose of 950 and 1350 mm Hg, respectively, we can obtain a ballpark estimate for the ratio of solute reflection coefficients for urea σ_u and glucose σ_g. We conclude from this ballpark calculation that $\sigma_u < \sigma_g$, $\sigma_u/\sigma_g = 0,7$, and $\sigma_g = 0.3$.

Besides calculations such as this, there is very limited information regarding osmotic reflection coefficients of the human peritoneal membrane for the various solutes that are present in the peritoneal dialysis system, i.e. soluble constituents of uremic plasma water and of dialysis fluid. The direct measurement in man of σ values for these solutes using only ultrafiltration flow rates is not presently possible. Rippe *et al.*[11] have recently determined information about osmotic reflection coefficients in the cat by measuring water flow rates out of the peritoneal cavity during a 20 min period using different test solutes as osmotic agents. The osmotic conductance of the peritoneal membrane $L_pA\sigma$ for a variety of solutes was calculated from the difference in rate of fluid absorption from the peritoneal cavity for a 0.9% NaCl solution and that for a 0.9% NaCl solution containing the test solute. By assuming a σ value of unity for large molecular weight solutes, they calculated osmotic reflection coefficients for NaCl, glucose, raffinose and inulin of 0.011, 0.019, 0.025, and 0.110, respectively. These values of σ are low when compared with those determined using solute transport measurements (see below) but are comparable to those previously reported for the mammalian capillary wall by others [11].

An additional factor that makes the direct calculation of ultrafiltration flow rates complicated during continuious ambulatory peritoneal dialysis (CAPD) is the long dwell time. As the peritoneum is rather leaky, solute concentrations in the dialysis fluid, and therefore the driving force for ultrafiltration, changes with time because of diffusion down concentration gradients. Figures 1 and 2 show the decrease in the total solution osmolality and glucose concentration in the dialysis solution as a function of dwell time during CAPD that are typical [12, 13] for 1.5% and 4.25% dextrose containing solutions, respectively. Dialysate osmolality equilibrates with serum osmolality more rapidly with 1.5% than with 4.25% dextrose containing solution.

---

* This equation is usually written for ultrafiltering capillaries with an additonal term to express the hydrostatic driving force resulting from the blood to interstitional pressure gradient ΔP, i.e.,

$$Q_f = L_pA \left(\Delta P - \overset{n}{\underset{j=1}{\sigma}} \sigma_j \Delta \pi_j\right).$$

Because the peritoneal space under normal circumstances is free of significant quantities of fluid, we may reasonably assume that the hydrostatic driving forces at play across the capillary wall are in balance with lymphatic run off. In order to effect net accumulation of ultrafiltrate in the peritoneal space, these forces must be unbalanced by the osmotic force contributed by the presence of glucose in the dialysis fluid. For a 2 l exchange added to the peritoneal space, the hysdrostatic force contributed would result either from the elastic recoil of the abdominal wall and/or the hydrostatic head of pressure generated by the column of water above the dependent portion of the peritoneal membrane. As such, it would be expected to be small and in a direction favoring net uptake across the peritoneal membrane from dialysate to blood. To be precise, therefore, this hydrostatic driving force should be added to equation 1 as ΔP.

** As it is encountered in peritoneal dialysis solutions in the United States, dextrose refers to glucose monohydrate. In this chapter we will refer to dextrose in this manner. As used herein, therefore, differentitaion between dextrose and glucose is only important when calculating glucose concentrations.

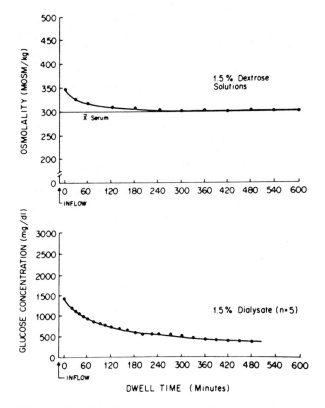

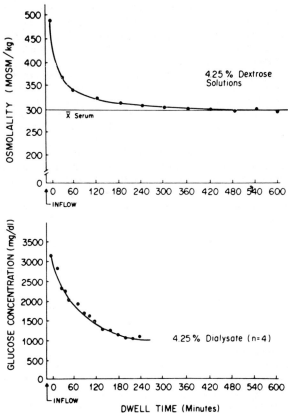

Figure 1. Changes in dialysate osmolality and glucose concentration when using 1.5% dextrose containing dialysis solution plotted as a function of dwell time. Mean plasma osmolality of 300 mOsm/kg H₂O would be expected for a patients with comparatively good control of BUN as occures during CAPD. Note that osmolal equilibrium is achieved before the glucose concentration reaches a value comparable to a normal plasma. This reflects both the dilution of other osmotically active constituents of dialysis fluid by ultrafiltered plasma water as well as the elevation of the plasma glucose levels and dialysis fluid urea concentration. Adapted from ref. 12 and 13.

Note that when using either solution, osmolal equilibriium is achieved before the glucose concentration reaches a value typical for normal plasma. Thus, quantitative predictions of ultrafiltration rates across the peritoneal membrane from first principles requires a simultaneous assessment of transperitoneal solute diffusion rates. This aspect is of clinical importance since the fall off of ultrafiltration with time on CAPD treatment could be due to the loss of either the driving force for ultrafiltration (high diffusive permeability of the osmotic solute) or alternatively the ultrafiltration capacity (low peritoneal hydraulic or water permeability).

Based upon an inverse correlation between the ultrafiltration rate and plasma protein concentration in clinical studies, Ronco *et al.* [14] have suggested that the blood flow rate to peritoneal tissues is an important additional factor determining the ultrafiltration flow rate. In analogy with the dynamics of ultrafiltration in the glomerular capillary and that during extracorporeal treatment with continuous arteriovenous hemofiltration, a low blood flow rate might limit the ultrafiltration rate by an increase in the effective oncotic force within the capillary. Levin *et al.*

Figure 2. Changes in dialysate osmolality and glucose concentration when using 4.25% dextrose containing dialysis solution plotted as a function of dwell time. Adapted from ref. 12 and 13.

[15] have tested this hypothesis in a rat model of peritoneal dialysis by determining the ultrafiltration rate as a function of glucose concentration in the dialysis fluid. These workers reported a plateau in the ultrafiltration rate at very high glucose concentration (approximately 9 g/dl), a result that is compatible with the suggestion of Ronco *et al.* Levin *et al.* found, however, that there was no enhancement of the ultrafiltration rate when drugs believed to increase peritoneal blood flow rates were added to these animals. Furthermore, the plateau in the ultrafiltration rate is not apparent until glucose concentrations are much above those in common clinical use. Based upon these studies in the rat, it seems unlikely that peritoneal blood flow significantly limits the ultrafiltration rate under typical clinical conditions.

2.2. Determining the ultrafiltration rate

Because of the number of complexities involved, only a few attempts have been made to calculate ultrafiltration flow rates using the above described principles. To keep the calculations reasonable, liberal assumptions are required concerning the relative importance of the osmotic solutes. For example, Jaffrin *et al.* [16] have described a mathematical model of ultrafiltration during peritoneal dialysis that assumes that glucose (or glycerol) is the only osmotic solute whose concentration changes with dwell time. By using peritoneal transport parameters that were determined previously by others, Jaffrin *et al.* demonstrated that their model was able to simulate the empirical dependence of dialysate volume on dwell time. Nakanishi *et al* [17] have described a similar model but have considered the importance of three osmotic solutes in determining the transperitoneal ultrafiltration rate: urea, sodium and glucose. By comparing the measured volume of dialysis solution as a function of time with the model predictions, they estimated optimal values of the osmotic conductance for the peritoneal membrane $L_pA\sigma$ for each of the osmotically active solutes. The determined parameters for urea in this three solute model were not physically realistic; therefore, they concluded that urea was not an important osmotic solute determining transperitoneal ultrafiltration. A simpler two solute model employing only sodium and glucose was equally able to simulate the dialysate volume data, and the optimal osmotic conductance value for sodium was approximately 2 times greater on average than that for glucose. If the hydraulic permeability L_pA is assumed to be a constant value, then this result suggests that the osmotic reflection coefficient for sodium is twice as large as that for glucose. This result contrasts with that of Rippe *et al* [11] described above but is consistent with reflection coefficients estimated by solute transport measurements (see below). Although these models are new and stimulating, they are limited because of the large number of unknown parameter.

Predictive calculations of the ultrafiltration rate from the distributed model of peritoneal transport [9] is more complex and requires even more assumptions. In this model the capillary wall is assumed to be the major osmotic barrier, and therefore the osmotic driving force for ultrafiltration is the difference in solute concentration across the capillary wall. The additional complication arises here because there are significant solute concentration gradients within the tissues surrounding the peritoneal cavity [18]; therefore, the solute concentration in dialysis fluid is not equal to that just outside the capillary wall. Flessner *et al.* [19] have predicted the ultrafiltration flow rate assuming paramters based on existing microcirculatory data and compared their predictions with experimental measurements in the rat during peritoneal dialysis with hypertonic solutions using mannitol as the ostomic agent. Agreement between the model predictions and the measured water flow rates required an assumed interstitial tissue thickness that was so large as to be anatomically unreasonable. Accurate predictions of ultrafiltration rates during peritoneal dialysis using the distributed model will first require a better understanding of the relative importance of the different transport barriers (capillary wall, interstitium and mesothelium) in determining rates of solute diffusion and ultrafiltration.

Instead of predicting ultrafiltration rates from first principles, most workers have been content with the emperical assessment of ultrafiltration by determining the change in dialysate volume with time under the few conditions of clinical interest. The accurate measurement of dialysate volume has not proven to be as simple as one might expect, but it is of utmost importance when empirically determining ultrafiltration during peritoneal dialysis.

The method used for assessing dialysate volume depends to a large degree on the study objective. Some studies have simply measured the volume of solution drained from the peritoneal cavity. The drained volume is the clinically relevant measure of dialysate volume since it is important in assessing the total amount of fluid and solute removed from the patient. Drained volumes suffer however from several disadvantages for physiological studies. First, they are subject to variable errors due to a residual volume of fluid remaining in the peritoneal cavity. The residual volume depends on several technical considerations such as catheter design, catheter placement and time permitted for drainage. Second, the determination of dialysate volume by drainage is inconvenient when it is necessary to have measurements at several different times throughout the dwell period. Such serial measurements are important when assessing peritoneal solute transport rates. The last reason that drained volumes are disadvantageous is that they only indicate the net change in the volume of dialysis solution. If there are two different, competing mechanisms for fluid movement from the peritoneal cavity such as across the peritoneal membrane as well as through an alternative route such as the lymphatics, then measurement of drained volume can only assess the resultant change; it does not provide information on the comparative contribution of each of the competing pathways to the net result.

The majority of investigators have therefore used the indicator dilution principle for assessing changes in the volume of dialysis solution. In the conventional application of this technique a large molecular weight indicator or index solute is added to the dialysis solution before infusion into the peritoneal cavity. The change in the volume of the dialysis fluid is then calculated based on the change in the concentration of the index solute. One of the requirements of this technique is that there is no loss of the index solute from the peritoneal cavity. It is well known however that large molecules, even red blood cells, that are added to the peritoneal cavity find their way into the blood stream. Until recently, most peritoneal dialysis studies using the indicator dilution method accounted for index solute loss by correcting for the amount appearing in plasma [20, 21].

Based upon this approach Pyle *et al.* [21] showed that the dependence of dialysate volume V and the ultrafiltration rate on time could be described respectively by the following equations:

$$V = a_1/a_2 (\exp [a_2t] - 1) + a_3t + V_0 \qquad [2]$$

$$Q_f = a_1 \exp [a_2t] + a_3 \qquad [3]$$

where a_1, a_2, and a_3 are empirically determined constants, and V_0 is the starting volume of dialysis solution. The resultant equations obtained using data from 5 patients are shown graphically in Figures 3 and 4 for 1.5% and a 4.25% dextrose contaning dialysis solutions, respectively. In either case dialysate volume reaches a maximum value, after which volume decreases slowly with dwell time. The nadir for Q_f is reached earlier with the 1.5% dextrose containing solution. As expected, the ultrafiltration rate is greater with the 4.25% dextrose containing solution. It should be noted that these are averaged results, and there exists cinsederable interpatient variability [22, 23].

In clinical studies of dialysis patients Daugirdas *et al.*

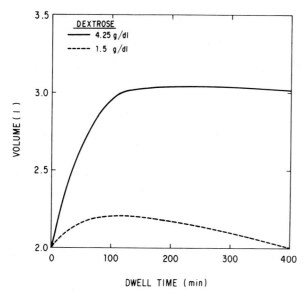

Figure 3. Dialysate volume plotted as a function of time for both 4.25% and 1.5% dextrose containing dialysis solutions. Equation 3 was used here using the empirical results of Pyle and co-workers [21, 22]. The initial volume was assumed to be 2 l.

[24] have shown, however, that this approach may be systematically in error. These investigators used radio-labeled albumin as the index solute and measured simultaneously the amount of albumin lost from the peritoneal cavity as well as that in plasma. Over a 7 hr dwell period they found that 17% of the albumin that was initially infused into the peritoneal cavity was lost, but only 24% of the albumin lost from the peritoneal cavity appeared in plasma. Flessner *et al.* [25] have confirmed these findings in the

rat and have suggested that the index solute is lost primarily into the tissues surrounding the peritoneal cavity, especially in the diaphragm and in anterior abdominal muscle tissue. The clinical studies of Daugirdas *et al.* have recently been confirmed by others [26, 27].

Our recent work in a rabbit model [28] has quantified the magnitude of the errors incurred when determining dialysate volume using the conventional indicator dilution techniques as described above. For this purpose we compared the measurements of dialysate volume by the conventional indicator dilution technique with those using a modified, short-dwell indicator dilution technique. The latter method assessed dialysate volume by determining the distribution volume of an index solute 2 min after its injection into the peritoneal cavity. This method gives a reasonable estimate of the true volume of fluid in the rabbit peritoneal cavity [28]. By using multiple injections, it was possible to determine dialysate volume as a function of dwell time during peritoneal dialysis using this modified indicator dilution technique. These latter measurements are less susceptible to index solute loss since the dwell period of newly injected index solute was limited to only 2 min.

Figure 5 shows the difference in dialysate volume when measured by either the conventional indicator dilution method (SIIS) or the modified, short-dwell indicator dilution method (MIIS) [28]. Results are shown in this figure using both isotonic and hypertonic (7% glucose containing) solutions in an awake rabbit model of peritoneal dialysis. Dialysate volume is overestimated by using the conventional indicator dilution technique and the error becomes greater the longer the duration of the exchange. Moreover, the use of a hypertonic solution exaggerates the overestimation of dialysate volume by the conventional indicator dilution

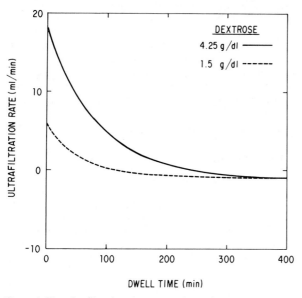

Figure 4. The ultrafiltration rate across the peritoneum plotted as a function of time for both 4.25% and 1.5% dextrose containing dialysis solutions. Equation 4 was used here using the empirical results of Pyle and co-workers [21, 22].

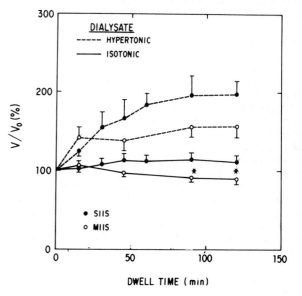

Figure 5. Dialysate volume relative to the initial volume V/V_0 plottewd as a function of dwell time when using isotonic and hypertonic dialysis solutions in a rabbit model of peritoneal dialysis. Dialysate volume was measure by either the conventional indicator dilution technique (SIIS) or by a shortdwell indicator dilution technique (MIIS). Adapted from ref. 28. The asterisk indicates a statistically significant difference.

method. We concluded from this study that dialysate volume determined by the conventional indicator dilution technique is larger than the true volume of dialysis solution within the peritoneal cavity; it indicates the distribution volume of the index solute which includes that contributed by presence of the index solute in the lymphatics and adjacent tissue spaces [24–27].

To facilitate interpretation of these different measures of dialysate volume, we also developed a mathematical model for fluid transport to and from the peritoneal cavity that accounts for loss of fluid into the lymphatics and into adjacent tissues surrounding the peritoneal cavity [28]. With simultaneous measures of the conventional indicator dilution volume and the true dialysate volume, this model permitted the calculation of fluid transport rates both across the peritoneal membrane as well as that through the lymphatics and into adjacent tissue spaces. We calculated fluid transport rates through the lymphatics and into adjacent tissue spaces that were comparable to those reported by others when the difference in animal size was taken into account. Moreover, we demonstrated that the ultrafiltration rate calculated simply by the rate of change of the conventional indicator dilution volumes was not different from the more rigorously calculated value using both volume measures. Thus, although the conventional indicator dilution technique overestimates dialysate volume, the rate of change of the conventional indicator dilution volume still proves to be a good estimate of the ultrafiltration rate across the peritoneum. With respect to the previous work of Pyle *et al.* [21], this result suggests that equation 2 above may be in error; however, equation 3 above remains approximately correct. The difference between equation 2 and true dialysate volumes is due to index solute loss into the lymphatics and the adjacent tissue spaces.

Because of the simplicity of employing the conventional indicator dilution technique, several groups have attempt to correct for the total loss of the index solute from the peritoneal cavity by back calculation [29–31]. Although the calculations from each investigator are likely somewhat different, the main approach appears similar. For example, one method [29] first determines the total amount of index solute lost from the peritoneal cavity during the entire exchange by the difference between that infused and that recovered after drainage (including that remaining within the residual volume after drainage). By assuming a mechanism for index solute loss that is the same throughout the exchange, the instantaneous rate of index solute loss can then be back calculated and corrections to the conventional indicator dilution volume can be made. While this approach appears sound and produces reasonable results, the assumption of a mechanism for index solute loss that is constant throughout the exchange remains yet to be demonstrated.

2.3. Alternative osmotic agents

The problem of overloading the patient with carbohydrate calories in the form of glucose is significant. As a result, other osmotically active agents are presently being tested. The principles described above are general and apply also to these alternative osmotic agents. We will confine our comments to differences in the effectiveness of these agents

to produce ultrafiltration. A more complete discussion regarding the advantages and disadvantages of the osmotic agents presently under consideration is given elsewhere [32].

Solutes that are both smaller and larger than glucose are potentially useful as osmotic agents. Agents smaller than glucose, such as glycerol, have been successfully employed to induce significant ultrafiltration rates both in the rat [33] and in man [34]. Small solutes have the advantage that less mass of solute is required to produce an equivalent dialysis solution osmotic pressure. Small solutes, however, will likely have low osmotic reflection coefficients as well as high diffusive permeabilities. Both of these factors will limit their osmotic effectiveness. The recent report by Lindholm *et al.* [34] demonstrates that the osmotic effect per molecule for glycerol is similar to that for glucose initially, but the effective period of ultrafiltration is shorter because of a more rapid dissipation of the driving concentration gradient. Small solutes as osmotic agents will, in general, only be effective during short exchanges.

The majority of alternative osmotic agents that have been tested are larger than glucose. Large solutes will have high osmotic reflection coefficients as well as low diffusive permeability and will therefore be more osmotically effective. The amount of solute mass required to produce a given ultrafiltration rate, however, is large and creates other problems, such as high solution viscosity, potential toxicity, and cost. A polymer of glucose has recently been shown to have comparable osmotic effectiveness to glucose only over a long, 12 hr dwell period [35]. The long term concerns of systemic toxicity and high cost still need to be adressed. Large solutes as osmotic agents will, in general, only be effective during long exchanges.

3. CONVECTIVE SOLUTE TRANSPORT ACROSS THE PERITONEUM

Solute removal from the patient is enhanced when using hypertonic compared with isotonic dialysis solutions. Ultrafiltration of water across the peritoneum not only dilutes the dialysis fluid resulting in an increased solute concentration gradient but also directly entrains solute in the solvent stream and transports it by convection. The relative importance of these two mechanisms depends on the size of the solute; we will concern ourselves with the latter mechanism only.

Based upon the observation in rabbits that intravascularly administered glucose also increased peritoneal mass transport rates, Maher *et al.* [36] have recently challenged the above mentioned conventional views regarding the mechanisms governing the increase in transperitoneal solute transport rates when employing hypertonic dialysis solutions. They speculated that hypertonic dialysis solutions increase peritoneal solute transport rates because the absorbed glucose causes extracellular volume expansion and presumably enhanced splanchnic blood flow rate. Further study of this interesting speculation seems warranted.

There are two common measures of convective solute transport: the sieving coefficient and the solute or solvent drag reflection coefficient. We will examine each separately below.

3.1. Measuring the sieving coefficient

The convective solute transport parameter that is easiest to determine clinically is the sieving coefficient for the peritoneal membrane. In analogy with that for synthetic membranes, the sieving coefficient S is defined here as the ratio of the solute concentration in the ultrafiltrate C_f to that in plasma water C_w

$$S = \frac{C_f}{C_w}.$$

To measure S clinically, previous experiments involved the use of a hypertonic dialysis solution to produce a large volume of ultrafiltrate. The test solute of interest was also added to the dialysis solution at a concentration equal to that in plasma water to minimize solute transport across the peritoneal membrane by diffusion. The rate of solute transport by convection across the peritoneal membrane $\overline{Q}_s$ was then computed by the difference in total mass between outflowing and inflowing dialysis solutions, factored for the time of the exchange. In like manner the volume of dialysis fluid drained in excess of that infused provided the ultrafiltration volume which was also factored for the exchange time $\overline{Q}_f$. The average concentration of the test solute in the ultrafiltrate $\overline{C}_f$ is then given by

$$\overline{C}_f = \frac{\overline{Q}_s}{\overline{Q}_f}.$$

The concentration of the test solute in peripheral plasma water is then determined. This concentration value is measured in plasma C_p, but a correction factor for the displaced volume occupied by plasma proteins can convert the measured value to plasma water concentration. The equation employed here is $C_w = C_p/(1 - \theta)$, where θ is the volume fraction of hydrated proteins and is taken as 0.0107 times the concentration of total plasma proteins (7.4 g/dl in normal plasma) [37]. The sieving coefficient can then be calculated from these measured values as described above.

Sieving coefficients for the human peritoneal membrane have been determined for various solutes [38–41]; the reported values are shown in Table 1. The measured sieving coefficients are scattered, are not equal to unity even for the smallest solutes, and do not depend appreciably on molecular size over the range from urea (3 Å) to inulin (14 Å). An additional observation of note from these data is that the values of S for the cations, sodium and potassium, are consistently lower than might be anticipated on the basis of their atomic weight.

3.2. Measuring the solute reflection coefficient

An alternative approach to determining a convective solute transport property of the peritoneum requires the use of kinetic or mathematical modeling techniques. A more detailed description of the mathematical models commonly employed is given in Chapter 6. In this approach the peritoneal membrane is characterized by two different mass transport parameters: PA (or KA), the diffusive permeability-area product (or mass transfer-area coefficient) and σ the solute reflection coefficient. It should be noted that the reflection coefficient determined from solute transport studies is not necessarily equal to the osmotic reflection coefficient described above. The theory of nonequilibrium thermodynamics asserts that they should be identical [1], but there is little empirical evidence in support of this contention. The mathematical models of solute transport determine optimal values of PA and σ for the peritoneal membrane by comparing their predictions with the measu-

Table 1. Sieving coefficient S and one minus the solute reflection coefficient 1-σ measured for the human peritoneal membrane

Solute	Molecular weight	Molecular radius $\mathring{A}$	S ± SEM	1-σ ± SD	Ref.
Urea	60	2.7	0.81±0.0003		38
			0.63±0.06[a]		41
				0.73±0.10	22
				0.83±0.10[c]	42
Creatinine	113	–	0.57±0.09[a]		44
				0.70±0.26	22
				0.71±0.01[c]	42
Uric Acid	168	–		0.67±0.15	22
				0.54±0.14[c]	42
Chloride	35	3.9	0.78±0.21		39
Potassium	37	4.0	0.36±0.05		40
			0.40±0.04		41
Glucose	180	4.4		0.54±0.28[b]	22
				0.56±0.03[bc]	42
Sodium	23	5.1	0.54±0.18		39
			0.56±0.04[a]		41
Inulin	5200	14.0	0.83±0.05		38
			0.41±0.08[a]		41
Protein				0.42±0.33[b]	22
				0.01±0.01	22

[a] Values measured in this study were obtained using 4.25% dextrose containing solutions, a 30 min dwell and a 20 min drain time. The other values were measured using a 7% dextrose containing, a 30 min dwell and a 30 min drain time.
[b] Values were determined when net solute transport was in the dialysate to blood direction.
[c] Values measured in children.

red solute transport rates; the latter are determined from the dependence of the dialysate volume and the solute concentrations in plasma and dialysate on time during an exchange.

The determination of optimal values of PA and σ from the dependence of the solute transport rate on time is complicated and needs to be done with careful attention to experimental and mathematical detail. This estimation procedure is best performed under certain specific conditions. The type of conditions that are optimal will be illustrated here by simulating the dependence of the solute concentration in the dialysis solution on time for some specific cases. The present examples were calculated assuming that the volume of dialysis solution varied with time in a manner identical to that shown in either Figure 3 or 4. Moreover, the test solute concentration in blood was assumed constant so that its volume of distribution within the body and its generation rate are not important factors. The simulations will be illustrated by calculating the predicted dependence of the dialysate solute concentration on time for σ values equal to both 0 and 1. The greater the difference between these two extreme cases, the more reliable is the estimate of σ. The photographic analog of this circumstance identifies that the greater the number of shades of gray between black and white the more precise will be the rendering of the shadow details in the final print.

Figure 6 shows the dependence of the relative dialysate concentration C_d/C_b on time for two different values of PA during an exchange with a 4.25% dextrose containing dialysis solution. The PA values of 20 ml/min and 4 ml/

min were chosen as representative for urea and inulin, respectively [21, 22]. These simulations illustrate that the lower the value of PA, the easier it is to determine unique values of the solute reflection coefficient. Figure 7 shows the same simulations for an exchange with a 1.5% dextrose containing solution. It is clear that it is virtually impossible to estimate unique values for σ during an isotonic exchange even when the PA value is low.

For solutes initially present in the dialysis solution such as the added osmotic agents (glucose), a similar procedure for estimating σ values has been previously employed but now with net solute transport in the dialysate to blood direction. Figure 8 illustrates the decrease in the solute concentration in the dialysis fluid relative to its initial value $C_d/C_d(0)$ as a function of time during an exchange with a 4.25% dextrose containing dialysis solution for the same assumed membrane parameters as employed in Figure 6. The differences between the simulated concentration curves when assuming σ equal to either 0 or 1 are considered small when compared with Figure 6. We feel it is questionable whether unique values of solute reflection coefficients for glucose may be computed from such an experiment. At best, such computed σ values are only approximate. We conclude from these simulations that solute reflection coefficients estimated by kinetic modeling techniques are most reliable then determined using hypertonic dialysis solutions and for large solutes with low diffusive permeability across the peritoneal membrane. Solute reflection coefficients determined during an isotonic exchange are unreliable. Moreover, solute reflection coefficients determined when net solute transport is in the

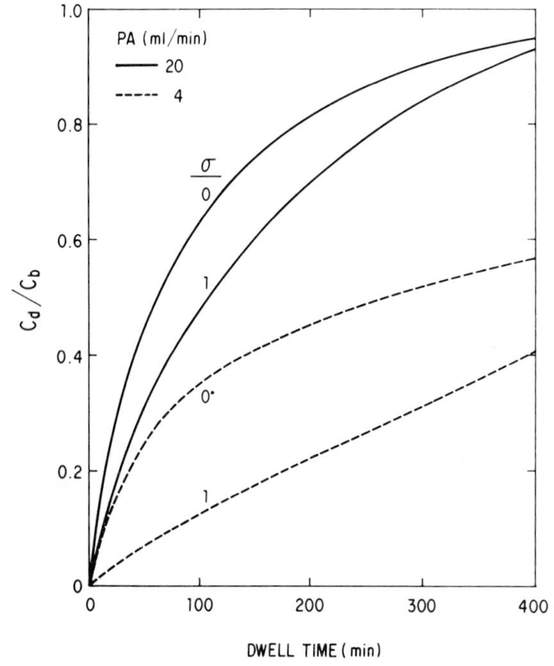

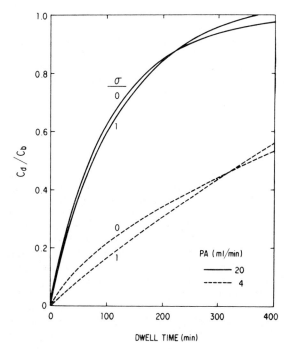

Figure 6. The dependence of the dialysis solution concentration divided by the blood concentration C_d/C_b on dwell time during a hypertonic exchange (4.25% dextrose) for solutes with PA values of 20 and 4 ml/min, respectively. Simulated results are shown for both σ equal to 0 and 1.

Figure 7. The dependence of the dialysis solution concentration divided by the blood concentration C_d/C_b on dwell time during an isotonic exchange (1.5% dextrose) for solutes with PA values of 20 and 4 ml/min, respectively. Simulated results are shown for both σ equal to 0 and 1.

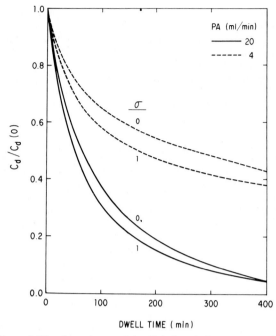

Figure 8. The dependence of the dialysis solution concentration relative to its initial value $C_d/C_d(0)$ on dwell time during a hypertonic exchange (4.25% dextrose) for solutes with PA values of 20 and 4 ml/min, respectively. Simulated results are shwon for both σ equal to 0 and 1. The blood concentration was assumed constant and equal to 5% of the initial dialysis solution concentration.

Table 2. Values of one minus reflection measured for the peritoneal membrane in animal models

Solute	Animal	$1-\sigma \pm SEM$	Ref.
glycerol	rat	0.72[a]	33
glucose	rat	0.63[a]	33
creatinine	rabbit	0.82±0.20	43
p-amminohippurate	rabbit	0.86±0.14	43

[a] Values were determined when net solute transport was in the dialysate to blood direction. No error estimates were reported.

There is a considerable body of theoretical information about σ for synthetic and biological membranes in the literature of nonequilibrium thermodynamics that will not be included in the present chapter; however, an understanding of the relationship between these convective solute transport parameters S, R and σ will provide a satisfactory theoretical background to understand the forces at work when ultrafiltration occurs.

In simple systems where a solution is ultrafiltered across a membrane, we define the rejection coefficient as

$$C_f = S\ C_w = (1 - R)\ C_w .$$

The rejection coefficient is given in this case by the following relationship [44]

$$R = \frac{\sigma\ (\ 1 - \exp[-\beta]\ )}{1 - \sigma \exp\ [-\beta]}$$

where the parameter coefficient β is defined by the following equation

$$\beta = Q_f\ \frac{(1 - \sigma)}{PA}$$

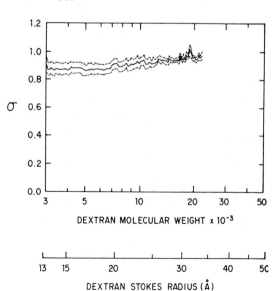

Figure 9. Dextran reflection coefficient σ determined in the rabbit during a hypertonic (7% glucose containing) exchange plotted as a function of molecular weight and Stokes radius. The mean value is shown as the solid line, and the dashed lines indicate the mean values ± 1 SEM. Taken from ref. 43.

dialysate to blood direction must be viewed cautiously. This latter result is important as it is often the manner whereby the effectiveness of a new osmotic agent is evaluated.

One minus solute reflection coefficients that have been determined in adult man [22] and in children [42] using the above described methods are shown in Table 1. One minus solute reflection coefficients for small solutes that have been determined in animal models of peritoneal dialysis are illustrated in Table 2 [33, 43]. Figure 9 shows solute reflection coefficients for larger solutes determined in the rabbit using neutral dextran as test solutes [43]. The molecular size range shown in this figure covers that from inulin (14 Å) to proteins the size of IgG (54 Å).

A comparison between these two measures of convective solute transport is helpful. The value of the sieving coefficient, like that of the solute reflection coefficient, varies between 0 and 1. The sieving coefficient will have a value of 1 and the reflection coefficient a value of 0 when there is no membrane rejection of solute. The sieving coefficient will have a value of 0 and the reflection coefficient a value of 1 when there is complete solute rejection by the membrane. Thus, the solute sieving coefficient is closely related to the reflection coefficient. Indeed, one might intuitively expect that

$$S = 1 - R \approx 1 - \sigma$$

where the above equation may be thought of as defining a third parameter R which is called the rejection coefficient.

When ß is large, then R → σ. When ß is small, then R → 0.

In order to provide an estimate or typical ß values during peritoneal dialysis, one needs estimates of both the ultrafiltration rate and the solute diffusive permeability-area product. With references to Figure 4, the maximum ultrafiltration rate is observed at the onset of an exchange containing 4.25% dextrose when the glucose gradient is greatest, and it ranges from 12–16 ml/min [22]. It is not possible to use a single value of the diffusive permeability-area product as this parameter depends on molecular size. As described above, typical values range from 20 ml/min for urea to 4 ml/min for inulin. Thus, both Q_f and PA are the same order of magnitude. We would therefore expect that for most solutes moving convectively across the peritoneum that R would be less than σ. This analogy with synthetic membranes implies that although the sieving coefficient is primarily a measure of convective solute transport, it may be augmented significantly by diffusive solute transport. As such, R (and S) are phenomenologic coefficients that should be altered by such parameters as the ultrafiltration flow rate. The similarity between S and 1−σ values for the solutes shown in Table 1 suggests, however, that the present analogy between the peritoneal and synthetic membranes may not apply directly, at least quantitatively.

3.3. Interaction between convective and diffusive transport – unstirred layers

The impact of convection on overall solute transport across the peritoneal membrane has been previously addressed theoretically by different workers [6, 22, 43, 45]. These treatments are based upon those previously developed for synthetic membranes [44, 46, 47]. Therefore, these previous works consider the peritoneum as a simple, homogeneous membrane whose transport properties are not altered by the addition of significant transmembrane fluid movement. These models may not apply directly to the peritoneum however. For example, there is evidence that the diffusive permeability of the peritoneum is increased upon exposure to hypertonic dialysis solutions that is unrelated to the increase in solute transport induced by fluid movement [38]. This effect is not explicitly taken into account in previous theoretical treatments of diffusive and convective solute transport across the peritoneum as described above. Other factors particular to the peritoneum may therefore complicate the interpretation of solute transport measurements during ultrafiltration. We will discuss one such complication in detail below, that of the presence of significant unstirred layers of solution.

Peritoneal dialysis fluid is unstirred, and it is likely that unstirred layers of solution may be as important as anatomical structures in determining the overall convective and diffusive transport properties of the peritoneal membrane. Indeed, there is evidence suggesting that unstirred layers of solution have a major impact on diffusive solute transport, as described in greater detail in Chapter 2. In this section we will confine our comments as to how fluid movement across the peritoneal membrane may impact on simultaneously occurring diffusive solute transport.

Let us now examine heuristically the possible impact of

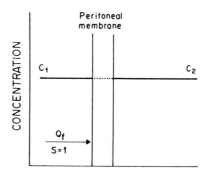

Figure 10. Concentration profile for a solute with S=1 during ultrafiltration across the peritoneal membrane. The dialysis fluid has been made to contain a concentration of solute C_2 that is equal to that in plasma water C_1.

fluid movement on diffusive solute transport across the peritoneum. Take first the case of a solute of small weight for which S is equal to 1. Figure 10 depicts the concentration profile for such a solute across a stylized peritoneal membrane that separates plasma water from dialysis fluid. The concentration in the dialysis solution has been adjusted to be equal to that in plasma water as would occur during experiments to determine solute sieving coefficients. The concentration profile is drawn for the conditions existing a few moments after the onset of ultrafiltration and is constant. That is, there is no change in solute concentration of the ultrafiltered plasma water as it crosses the membrane and the attendant unstirred layers.

In the usual clinical situation, however, there is no test solute initially present in the dialysis fluid and a solute concentration difference across the peritoneal membrane exists. Diffusion and convection then occur simultaneously during the exchange. Reasoning from analogy with transport theory developed for synthetic membranes, a qualitative understanding of the interaction between these two

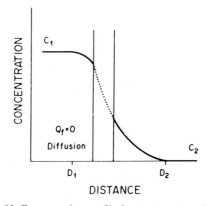

Figure 11. Concentration profile for a solute that diffuses across the peritoneal membrane in the absence of ultrafiltration. The steepness of the driving gradient for diffusion is depicted by the difference in concentration between the bulk phase of plasma water C_1 and that of the dialysis fluid C_2 acting over a distance D_1 to D_2, i.e. the diffusion rate is proportional to $(C_1-C_2)/(D_2-D_1)$.

modes of solute transport may be achieved. First, let us examine the case where no ultrafiltration occurs as is illustrated in Figure 11. The decrease in concentration from the bulk phase of plasma water to the surface of the membrane represents the unstirred layer on the blood side that is partially depleted of solute by diffusion across the membrane into the dialysis fluid. Similarly, the unstirred layer on the dialysate side is depicted as a continuing reduction in concentration with distance into the dialysis fluid before achieving the dialysate bulk phase concentration (which at the start of the exchange will be zero).

Imposing a transmembrane driving force for ultrafiltration on the conditions shown in Figure 11 in the changes shown in Figure 12 for a solute with a sieving coefficient equal to 1. The blood side unstirred layer of solution could be dramatically reduced by the fluid movement; indeed, the blood side fluid film might be reduced to zero. Such conditions would enhance solute diffusion by shortening the path length over which the gradient for diffusion is acting between the bulk phase of plasma water and that of dialysate (D_1 to D_2). In addition, the drop in concentration within the membrane might be completely obliterated, again shortening the path over which the concentration gradient is exercised. Finally, there will likely be an increase in the thickness of the dialysate side fluid film because of the presence of ultrafiltration from blood to dialysate. This effect would be to decrease the rate of solute diffusion. Alternatively, it is also possible that the presence of ultrafiltration might increase mixing of the dialysis solution, a result that would decrease the dialysate side fluid film thickness and enhance the rate of solute diffusion. Note that this formulation assumes no change to intrinsic membrane properties such as diffusive permeability as a result of adding an osmotic agent to the bath. Nevertheless, the net effect here of fluid movement would likely be to increase the apparent diffusive permeability.

Figure 13 shows the circumstances for a larger molecule where there is significant membrane restraint of solute ($S < 1$). The solute is convected to the membrane surface where because of rejection by the membrane the concentration increases significantly near the membrane surface

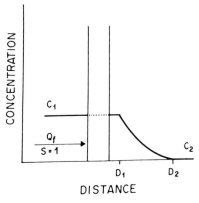

Figure 12. Concentration profile for a solute with S=1 moments after ultrafiltration has begun. Note the steeper driving concentration gradient for diffusion created by the obliteration of the unstirred layer on the blood side, i.e. $D_2 - D_1$ for diffusion compared with that shown in Figure 11.

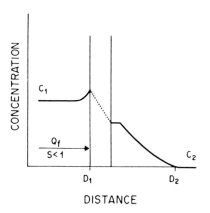

Figure 13. Concentration profile for a solute that is partially rejected by the membrane (S<1) moments after the onset of ultrafiltration. The concentration gradient is made steeper by the increase of solute at the membrane surface and acts over a shorter distance than for simple diffusion (Figure 11).

(solute or concentration polarization) [48]. The concentration within the membrane falls with distance and the dialysate side fluid film is displaced in a manner analogous to the situation in Figure 12. Here, the overall effect is likely to steepen the concentration gradient enhancing the diffusive component of transport. Precise quantitation of this enhancement for the solutes routinely dealt with in uremic plasma, is not presently available for the peritoneal membrane and would be technically difficult to obtain. This qualitative understanding of the interaction between convention and diffusion suggests, however, that fluid movement may alter the apparent diffusive permeability even though the intrinsic transport properties of the peritoneum are not altered.

4. THE EMERGING PARADOX

Studies of solute diffusion across the human peritoneum have previously demonstrated that the peritoneal membrane is more open or permeable than the hemodialysis membrane made from cuprophane [45]. A more open or more permeable membrane, in this respect, is one where PA or dialysance decreases less rapidly with increasing molecular size. For example, the peritoneal membrane is considered more permeable than a cuprophane hemodialysis membrane because the ratio of inulin to urea PA values during peritoneal dialysis is approximately 0.3, whereas the dialysance ratio for the cuprophane membrane is 0.06 [49]. This conclusion about diffusive permeability also holds for animal models of peritoneal dialysis such as the rabbit where the clearance ratio of inulin to urea was reported to be 0.25 [50]. Therefore, all previous work on solute diffusion supports the contention that the peritoneum is an open or permeable transport barrier or membrane.

Examination of the data on sieving and reflection coefficients in Tables 1 and 2, however, provides a contrasting view of the peritoneal membrane. These data suggest that the peritoneal membrane significantly restricts the passage of uncharged solutes even as small as urea ($S \approx 0.8$). This paradox of membrane openness to diffusion yet tightness to convection has been bothersome to us who have worked on peritoneal transport over the years. Several explanations for the paradox have been put forward. Certain workers have dismissed it as experimental artifact [51]. It has also brought forth the suggestion that hypertonic dialysis solution draws water from sources that are presumably free of the solute for which sieving coefficient is being measured, e.g. intracellular water might be expected to be free of the administered test solute inulin. This dilutional event then would account for S values for inulin below unity even though the permeability of the membrane as assessed by PA values is high. This rationale would not, however, explain the data for urea which has a space of distribution equal to total body water. Moreover, the low sieving coefficients for the cations, sodium and potassium, could be related to a combined effect of molecular charge and active transport mechanisms that reduce their ability to move freely across cell membranes. Thus, heterogeneity of structure and physical properties found in the test solutes has clouded the interpretation of these data.

To resolve this concern about a heterogeneity in test solute properties we have examined transport across the peritoneum using neutral dextrans ranging in molecular size from 13 to 50 Å as test solutes [43]. All of the dextrans used in these studies would likely equilibrate only in extracellular fluid and with time would have equal distribution volumes. Using an awake rabbit model, we performed peritoneal dialysis using isotonic and hypertonic (7% glucose containing) solutions and measured the transport of neutral dextran from plasma to dialysis fluid. Values of PA were determined during the isotonic exchange for each molecular size of dextran from the dependence of the dialysis solution concentration on time using the modeling techniques described above and in Chapter 6. In order to assess the degree of hindrance to solute diffusion provided by the peritoneum we divided the PA value by the solute diffusivity (D) in water. As solute diffusivity in free solution decreases with molecular size, this manipulation isolates the effect of the peritoneum on solute diffusion. The computed PA/D values are plotted versus dextran molecular weight and size in Figure 14. The PA/D values are relatively constant and do not decrease significantly with increasing molecular size. Said another way, the peritoneal membrane does not result in a significant increase in hindrance to solute diffusion with increasing molecular size and is therefore an open diffusional transport barrier. These observations confirm the above mentioned previous work on solute diffusion across the peritoneal membrane. It is interesting to note the high degree of membrane openness to solute diffusion observed in these studies. Indeed, if one was to assign a pore size to the peritoneum based on these data, it would be in excess of 500 Å.

During the hypertonic exchange we computed values of σ for dextran using the modeling techniques described above. Figure 9 plots the computed σ values versus dextran molecular weight and size. Note that the values of σ are approximately equal to unity and independent of molecular size. The results are again in agreement with a conclusion drawn from the clinical data in Table 1. Therefore, the peritoneal membrane is both open to diffusion yet tight to convection, observations that are independent of such variables as test solute charge or space of distribution and

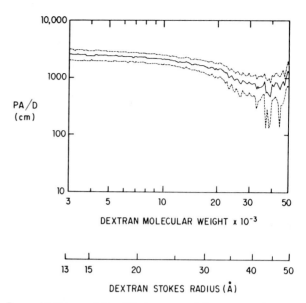

Figure 14. Values of the diffusive permeability-area product for dextran determined in the rabbit during an isotonic exchange divided by the solute diffusivity in free solution PA/D plotted as a function of molecular weight and Stokes radius. The mean value is shown as the solid line, and the dashed lines indicate the mean value ± 1 SEM. Taken from ref. 43.

special cell membrane transport mechanisms.

The hypothesis by which this paradox is commonly resolved is by postulating a heteroporous peritoneal membrane [52]. Heteroporosity of the peritoneal membrane is justified by assuming that the capillary wall, a structure widely believed to contain two distinct pore sizes [53], is the primary transport barrier. Diffusion is postulated to take place through a different set of pores than does convection [52]. For example, the large pores are located primarily at the venular end of the capillary and are postulated as the primary location for diffusional solute transport. The small pores are located primarily at the arteriolar end of the capillary and are postulated as the primary location for convective solute transport. An important element of this hypothesis is the mechanism that confines convection to the small pores. It is hypothesized that the venular pores are so large that they are exempted from water flow because glucose can only exert an osmotic driving force across the small arteriolar pores. Therefore, the peritoneal membrane appears open to diffusion because solute diffusion occurs primarily through large, venular pores. On the other hand, the peritoneal membrane appears tight to convection because solute convection occurs primarily through small, arteriolar pores.

Although this hypothesis appears reasonable, it has never been experimentally tested. An alternative hypothesis that could explain this paradox is to postulate that there are two functional membranes in series between blood and dialysis fluid, each with different properties. The barrier proximal to blood is postulated to be thin and have a small mean pore size. It is not necessary for this barrier to consist of only a single pore size; the only requirement is that the mean pore size be small. A likely anatomical candidate for this barrier is the capillary wall or endothelium. The barrier distal to blood is postulated to be thick yet be very open in structure and offer little additional hindrance to solute diffusion than would a simple water layer of comparable thickness. A likely anatomical candidate for this barrier is the interstitium. An unstirred layer of peritoneal dialysis fluid could also be a candidate for this transport barrier. Now, the overall transport properties of such a dual barrier membrane is complex, but it has been studied theoretically by others [54, 55]. For describing peritoneal transport, however, this theory may be employed as follows. The overall resistance to solute diffusion across such a dual barrier membrane is simply the sum of the diffusional resistances of each element since they are arranged in series. It should be noted that the permeability of each barrier is proportional to solute diffusivity within that barrier but also is inversely proportional to the barrier thickness. We postulate that the thickness of the distal barrier is so large that this barrier dominates the overall diffusive permeability. Therefore, solute diffusion across the peritoneum would be dominated by the open second series barrier, i.e. interstitium. On the other hand, convection across such a dual barrier membrane is dominated by the properties of the proximal barrier. The transport properties of the distal barrier are not important to overall convective solute transport. Thus, the overall solute sieving or reflection coefficient would simply be that of the capillary wall. Reflection coefficients for the capillary wall have been determined previously, and the values that have been reported are comparable to reflection coefficients across the peritoneal membrane. Thus, such a dual barrier membrane could explain a peritoneal membrane that appeared open to solute diffusion yet tight to solute convection and is also compatible with the clinical and experimental data on diffusion and convection across the peritoneal membrane.

It is instructive to note the relationship between the hypothesized models. It is of interest that the dual barrier membrane model can be considered an extension of the heteroporous membrane model. Both models require a heteroporous capillary wall as the major transport barrier to solute convection. The primary difference between the two models is that openness of the peritoneal membrane to solute diffusion cannot be fully explained by postulating only a heteroporous membrane (see below). It is also of interest to note the relationship between the dual barrier membrane model to the distributed model of peritoneal transport described by Dedrick, Flessner and co-workers [8, 9]. Both the dual barrier membrane model and the distributed model contain two different transport resistances that would need to be traversed in series by solute when in transit from blood to dialysis solution. Therefore, one might expect them to predict similar overall transport properties. Indeed, a preliminary study by us [56] has shown that when predicting solute diffusion and convection across the peritoneum, the distributed model is equivalent to the dual barrier membrane model.

4.1. Preliminary testing of models

Recent work by ourselves [57] suggests indeed that a model that includes only a heteroporous peritoneal membrane does not withstand a rigorous test. In these experiments we measured sieving coefficients across the rabbit peritoneal membrane when employing a hydrostatic driving pressure for ultrafiltration (vacuum in the peritoneal space) [57]. The test solutes employed in these studies were again neutral dextran, and sieving coefficients were calculated as the concentration in the ultrafiltrate divided by that in plasma. For technical reasons surgical removal of the bowel and the omentum was necessary. The rationale here was to measure sieving coefficients using a driving force that would be exerted across both large and small pores during the ultrafiltration process. If the heteroporous membrane model was adequate, one would expect that the peritoneal membrane would appear open to hydrostatically driven convection. Stated in other words, the heteroporosity membrane model would predict no hindrance to convective solute transport; sieving coefficients would be equal to unity for all solutes tested. This result should contrast nicely with that observed during osmotically-driven ultrafiltration where substantial hindrance to solute convection occurs. Interestingly, we observed S values that were larger than obtained during osmotically-driven ultrafiltration, but the values of S did not increase to unity (Figure 15). These observations, while in support of a heteroporous peritoneal membrane, do not suggest that a heteroporous membrane alone explains the paradoxical diffusive and convective solute transport properties of the peritoneum.

Additional recent work by us has tested the dual barrier membrane model in our rabbit model of peritoneal dialysis [58]. A unique property of a dual barrier membrane that has been predicted theoretically is that such a membrane

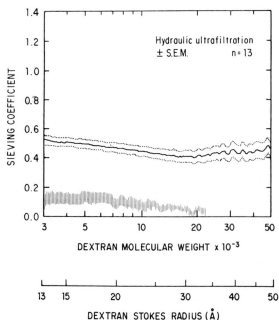

Figure 15. Dextran sieving coefficients determined in the eviscerated rabbit during hydraulically-driven convective solute transport plotted as a function of molecular weight and Stokes radius, The mean value is shown as the solid line, and the dashed lines indicate the mean value ± 1 SEM. The hatched area shows the range of sieving coefficients that were previously determined [43] during osmotically-driven ultrafiltration. Taken from ref. 57.

would exhibit the property of rectification of solute transport [54, 55]. Rectification in this case indicates that solute transport by convection would be asymmetric. Being specific to the peritoneal membrane, the dual barrier membrane model would predict that convective solute transport from blood to dialysate would appear tight, but convective solute transport from dialysate to blood transport would appear open. Previous studies by others had demonstrated that the peritoneum indeed appears open when protein transport in the peritoneal space to blood direction is considered in response to a hydrostatic pressure driving force [59, 60]. Our studies measured reflection coefficients using modeling techniques described above during ultrafiltration in the dialysate to blood direction that was induced by using a hypotonic dialysis solution. The test solutes employed in these experiments were again neutral dextran. Contrary to expectations based upon prediction of the dual barrier membrane model and previous data, we observed that the peritoneal membrane appears tight to solute convection when determined in the dialysate to blood direction under these conditions. This result argues powerfully against the dual barrier membrane model alone as fully explanatory of the paradoxical convective and diffusive solute transport properties of the peritoneum. As a corollary, the equivalency of the dual barrier membrane and distributed models in describing peritoneal transport [56] suggests that the distributed model also is not sufficient to fully explain all known peritoneal solute transport properties.

4.2. What position remains to us?

It is apparent from all of the studies performed so far that the peritoneal mass transport barrier is complex and cannot be adequately modeled as a simple semipermeable membrane even though selected observations may fit this model very nicely. Second, it is clear that reconciliation of the paradox by simply hypothesizing a heteroporous peritoneal membrane has *not* withstood the test of recent experimentation. Lastly, our recent experiments suggest that neither a dual barrier membrane nor a distributed model of peritoneal transport is likely sufficient to explain the paradoxical properties of the peritoneum.

These observations leave us with an unsatisfactory and unsatisfying position with regard to undersatanding the nature of the peritoneum. There are, however, certain empirical realities that any transport model of the peritoneum will have to explain. They are:

1) A mass transport barrier that appears very open to solute diffusion.

2) A mass transport barrier that appears very tight to solute convection when ultrafiltration is induced by small osmotic solutes.

3) A mass transport barrier that appears open to solute convection when ultrafiltration is induced by hydraulic pressure [25, 57, 59, 60].

In speculating about a new model that would contain these three experimentally demonstrated elements, we would postulate a triple barrier or membrane (functionally) consisting of a thin but convectively tight barrier on the blood side (capillary wall), a thick open middle barrier (interstitium), and a thin and convectively tight barrier on the dialysate side (mesothelium). Solute transport across such a triple barrier would be similar to that across a dual barrier membrane where net transport is in the blood to dialysate direction. An important feature of this speculative model is that the mesothelial barrier would contain certain regions such as those covering the diaphragm and the anterior abdominal wall [25] that would be convectively open but regions covering other tissues that would be convectively tight. The open sites would permit the hydrostatically driven egress of macromolecules such as reported by McKay et al. [59] and Flessner *et al.* [25] but would still be consonant with the observation of an osmotically tight mesothelial membrane – reasoning in a manner analogous to that of Nolph *et al.* [52] with respect to the dual pore membrane. Time and experimentation will be needed to confirm or deny these speculations.

REFERENCES

1. Katchalsky A, Curran PF: Nonequilibrium Thermodynamics in Biophyscs, Harvard University Press, Cambridge, MA, 1965.
2. Schultz SG: Basic Principles of Membrane Transport, Cambridge University Press, Cambridge, England, 1980.
3. Cunningham RS: The physiology of the serous membranes. PhysiolRev 6: 242–280, 1926.
4. Clark AJ: Absorption from the peritoneal cavity. J Pharmacol & Exp Ther 16: 415–433, 1921.
5. Putnam TJ: The living peritoneum as a dialyzing membrane. Am J Physiol 63: 548–565, 1922–23.
6. Henderson LW: Peritoneal ultrafiltration dialysis: enhanced urea transfer using hypertonic peritoneal dialysis fluid. J Clin Invest 45: 950–955, 1966.
7. Knochel JP: Formation of peritoneal fluid hypertonicity during dialysis with isotonic glucose solutions. J Appl Physiol 27: 233–236, 1969.
8. Dedrick RL, Flessner MF, Collins JM, Schultz JS. Is the peritoneum a membrane? asaio J 5: 1–8, 1982.
9. Flessner MF, Dedrick RL, Schultz JS: A distributed model of peritoneal-plasma transport: theoretical considerations. Am J Physiol 2487: H15–H25., 1984.
10. Staverman AJ: The theory of measurement of osmotic pressure. Rec trav chim 70: 344–352, 1951.
11. Rippe B, Perry MA, Granger DN: Permselectivity of the peritoneal membrane. Microvasc Res 29: 89–102, 1985.
12. Rubin J, Nolph KD, Popovich RP, Moncrief JW: Drainage volumes during continuous ambulatory peritoneal dialysis. asaio J 2: 54–60, 1979.
13. Nolph KD, Twardowski ZJ, Popovich RP, Rubin J: Equilibration of peritoneal dialysis solutions during long-dwell exchanges. J Lab Clin Med 93: 246–256, 1979.
14. Ronco C, Borin D, Brendalon A, Bragantini L, Chiaramonte S, Feriani M, Fabris A, La Greca G: Influence of blood flow and plasma protein on UF rate in peritoneal dialysis. In: Frontiers in Pertitoneal Dialysis, Maher JF, Winchester JF (eds), Field, Rich and Associates, Inc., New York, NY, pp 82–87, 1986.
15. Levin TN, Rigden LB, Nielsen LH, Morre HL,m Twardowski ZJ, Khanna R, Nolph KD: Maximum ultrafiltration rates during peritoneal dialysis in rats. Kidney Int 31: 731–735, 1987.
16. Jaffrin MY, Odell RA, Farrell PC: A model of ultrafiltration and glucose mass transfer kinetics in peritoneal dialysis. Artif Organs 11: 198–207, 1987.
17. Nakanishi TY, Tanaka Y, Fuyjii M, Fukuhara Y, Orita Y:

Nonequilibrium thermoidynamics of glucose transport in continuous ambulatory peritoneal dialysis. In: Maekawa M, Nolph KD, Kishimoto T, Moncrief JW (eds), Machine Free Dialysis for Patient Convenience, ISAO Press, Cleveland, OH, pp 39–44.

18. Flessner MF, Fenstermacher JD, Dedrick RL, Blasberg RG: A distributed model of peritoneal-plasma transport: tissue concentration gradients. Am J Physiol 248: F425–F435, 1985.

19. Flessner MF, Dedrick RL, Schultz JS: A distributed model of peritoneal-plasma transport: analysis of experimental data in the rat. Am J Physiol 248: F413–F424, 1985.

20. Shear L, Swartz C, Shinaberger JA, Berry KG: Kinetics of peritoneal abosorption in adult man. NM Engl J Med 272: 123–127, 1965.

21. Pyle WK, Popovich RP, Moncrief JW: Peritoneal transport evaluation in CAPD. In: Moncrief JW, Popovich RP (eds), CAPD Update, Masson, New York, NY, pp 35–52, 1981.

22. Pyle WK: Mass Transfer in Peritoneal Dialysis, Ph.D. Dissertation Univ of Texas, Austin, 1981.

23. Smeby LC, Wideroe T-E, Jorstad S: Individual differences in water transport during continuous peritoneal dialysis. asaio J 4: 17–27, 1981.

24. Daugirdas JT, Ing TS, Gandhi VC, Hano JE, Chen W-T, Yuan L: Kinetics of peritoneal fluid absorption in patients with chronic renal failure. J Lab Clin Med 95: 351–361, 1980.

25. Flessner MF, Parker RJ, Sieber SM: Peritoneal lymphatic uptake of fibrinogen and erythrocytes in the rat. Am J Physiol 244: H89–H96, 1983.

26. Rippe B, Stelin G, Ahlem J: Lymph flow from the peritoneal cavity in CAPD patients. In: Maher JF, Winchester JF (eds), Frontiers in Pertitoneal Dialysis, Field, Rich and Associates, Inc., New York, NY, pp 24–30, 1986.

27. Spencer PC, Farrell PC: Solute and water transfer kinetics in CAPD. In: Gokel R (ed), Continuous Ambulatory Peritoneal Dialysis, Churchill Livingstone, Edinburgh, UK, pp 38–55, 1986.

28. Pust AH, Leypoldt JK, Frigon RP, Henderson LW: Peritoneal dialysate volume determined by indicator dilution measurements. Kidney Int 33: 64–70, 1988.

29. Lindholm B, Werynski A, Tranaeus A, Österberg T, Bergström J: Kinetics of peritoneal dialysis with animo acids as osmotic agents. In: Nosé Y, Kjellstrand C, Ivanovich P, (eds), Progress in Artifical Organs – 1985, ISAO Press, Cleveland, OH, pp 284–288, 1986.

30. DePaepe M, Kips J, Belpaire F, Lamaire N: Comparison of different volume markers in peritoneal dialysis. In: Maher JF, Winchester JF (eds), Frontiers in Peritoneal Dialysis, Field, Rich and Associates, Inc., New York, NY, pp 279–282, 1986.

31. Krediet RT, Zuyderhoudt FMJ, Boeschoten EW, Arisz L: Alterations in the peritoneal transport of water and solutes during peritonitis in continuous ambulatory peritoneal dialysis patients. Eur J Clin Invest 17: 43–52, 1987.

32. Twardowski ZJ, Khanna R, Nolph KD: Osmotic agents and ultrafiltration in peritoneal dialysis. Nephron 42: 93–101, 1986.

33. Daniels FH, Leonard EF, Cortell S: Glucose and glycerol compared as osmotic agents for peritoneal dialysis. Kidney Int 25: 20–125, 1984.

34. Lindholm B, Werynski A, Bergström J: Kinetics of peritoneal dialysis with glycerol and glucose as osmotic agents. Trans Am Soc Artif Intern Organs 33: 19–27, 1987.

35. Mistry CD, Mallick NP, Gokal R: Ultrafiltration with an isosmotic solution during long peritoneal dialysis exchanges. Lancet ii: 178–182, 1987.

36. Maher JF, Bennett RR, Hirszel P, Chakrabarti E: The mechanism of dextrose-enhanced peritoneal mass transport rates. Kidney Int 28: 16–20, 1985.

37. Colton CK, Smith KA, Merrill EW, Friedman S: Diffusion of urea in flowing blood. AIChE J 17: 800–808, 1971.

38. Henderson KW, Nolph KD: Altered permeability of the peritoneal membrane after using hypertonic peritoneal dialysis fluid. J Clin Invest 48: 992–1001, 1969.

39. Nolph KD, Hano JE, Teschan PE: Peritoneal sodium transport during hypertonic peritoneal dialysis. Ann Intern Med 70: 931–941, 1969.

40. Brown ST, Ahearn DJ, Nolph KD: Potassium removal with peritoneal dialysis. Kidney Int 4: 67–69, 1973.

41. Rubin J, Klein E, Bower JD: Investigation of the net sieving coefficient of the peritoneal membrane during peritoneal dialysis. asaio J 5: 9–15, 1982.

42. Morgenstern B, Pyle WK, Gruskin A, Baluarte HJ,. Perlman S, Polinsky M, Kaiser B: Transport characteristics of the pediatric peritoneum. Kidney Int 25: 259 (Abstract), 1984.

43. Leypoldt JK, Parker HR, Frigon RP, Henderson LW: Molecular size dependence of peritoneal transport. J Lab Clin Med 110: 207–216, 1987.

44. Spiegler KS, Kedem O: Thermodynamics of hyperfiltration (reverse osmosis): criteria for efficient membranes. deaslination 1: 311–326, 1966.

45. Babb Al, Johansen PJ, Stand MJ, Tenckhoff H, Scribner BH: Bidirectional permeability of the human peritoneum to middle molecules. Proc Eur Dial Transpl Assoc 10: 247–261, 1973.

46. Villarroel F, Klein E, Holland F: Solute flux in hemodialysis and hemofiltration membranes. Trans Am Soc Artif Intern Organs 23: 225–233, 1977.

47. Green DM, Antwiller GD, Moncrief JW, Decherd JF, Popovich R: Measurements of the transmittance coefficient spectrum of Cuprophan and RP69 membranes: applications to middle molecule removal via ultrafiltration. Trans Am Soc Artif Intern Organs 22: 627–636, 1976.

48. Blatt WF, Dravid A, Michael AS, Nelson L: Solute polarization and cake formation in membrane ultrafiltration: causes, consequences and control techniques. In: Flinn JE (eds), Plenum, New York, NY, pp 47–97, 1970.

49. Henderson LW: The problem of peritoneal membrane area and permeability. Kidney Int 3: 409–410, 1973.

50. Aune S: Transperitoneal Exchange. I. Peritoneal permeability studies by transperitoneal plasma clearance of urea, PAH, inulin, and serum albumin in rabbits. Scand J Gastroent 5: 85–97, 1970.

51. Randerson DH, Farrell PC: Mass transfer properties of the human peritoneum. asaio J 3: 140–146, 1980.

52. Nolph KD, Miller FN, Pyle WK, Sorkin MI: An hypothesis to explain the ultrafiltration characteristics of peritoneal dialysis. Kidney Int 20: 543–548, 1981.

53. Taylor AE, Granger DN: Exchange of macromolecules across the microcirculation. In: Renkin EM, Michel CC, (eds), Handbook of Physiology. Section 2: The Cardiocavular System. Volume IV. Microcirculation, American Physiological Society, bethesda, MD, pp. 467–520, 1984.

54. Patlak CS, Goldstein DA, Hoffman JF: The flow of solute and solvent across a two-membrane system. J theor Biol 5: 426–442.

55. Wendt RP, Mason EA, Bresler EH: Effect of heteroporosity on flux equations for membranes. Biophys Chem 4: 237–247, 1976.

56. Leypoldt JK, Henderson LW: The effect of convection on bidirectional peritoneal solute transport: predictions from a distributed model. J theor Biol (in review), 1988.

57. Bell JL, Leypoldt JK, Frigon RP, Henderson LW: Heteroporosity model of peritoneal transport is not supported by hydraulically-driven convective transport. Kidney Int 33: 243 (Abstract), 1988.

58. Chiu AS, Leopoldt JK, Frigon RP, Henderson LW: Peritoneal dialysis to blood transport. Kidney Int 31: 249 (Abstract), 1987.

59. McKay T, Zink J, Greenway CV: 1978, Relative rates of absorption of fluid and protein from the peritoneal cavity in cats. Lymphology 11: 106–110, 1978.

60. Lill SR, Parsons RH, Buhac I: Permeability of the diaphragm and fluid resorption from the peritoneal cavity in the rat. Gastroent 76: 997–1001, 1979.

8

NEW APPROACHES TO INTERMITTENT PERITONEAL DIALYSIS THERAPIES

ZBYLUT J. TWARDOWSKI

1. HISTORICAL PERSPECTIVE

In 1923, Ganter [1] reported what probably was the first clinical application of peritoneal dialysis. He infused 1.5 l of normal saline in one patient and 3 l in another. Only single exchanges were used. In later years, two techniques of peritoneal dialysis were developed: a) continuous flow and b) intermittent flow. In continuous flow peritoneal dialysis, dialysis solution was infused through a trocar or tubing into the upper abdomen and drained simultaneously through another trocar or tubing introduced into the lower abdomen. This technique dominated in the 1920s and 1930s [2–5]. In intermittent flow peritoneal dialysis only a single trocar or rubber catheter was used. Fluid was infused into the peritoneal cavity, equilibrated for a short time, and drained through the same trocar or catheter. This method was studied in laboratory animals in the early 1930s [6, 7]. The first intermittent flow peritoneal dialysis in a patient was probably performed by Rhoads on June 17, 1936 [8]. Abbott and Shea [9] made further improvements in the intermittent flow technique. In 1948, Frank et al. [10] reported their experience in 18 patients treated with peritoneal dialysis; twelve were treated with the continuous flow technique, five with the intermittent flow technique, and one patient was treated with both techniques. The authors slightly favored the continuous flow technique as technically simpler and somewhat more efficient. Odel et al. [11] reviewed 101 cases reported in the literature from 1923 to 1948. Seventy three patients were treated with the continuous and twenty two with the intermittent technique. The mortality was slightly lower in patients treated with the continuous technique but the authors did not draw definitive conclusions regarding the inferiority of the intermittent technique. The continuous technique was frequently used up to the late 1950s [12, 13]. During the same period the intermittent technique was markedly improved [14]. Two papers published in the late 1950s established superiority of the intermittent technique [15, 16]. In the 1960s continuous flow peritoneal dialysis was mostly abandoned and the intermittent flow technique was commonly employed for treatment of acute and chronic renal failure [17–20].

2. TERMINOLOGY

2.1. Intermittent flow peritoneal dialaysis technique

This is a technique where dialysis solution is infused and dialysate is drained through a single catheter. During a fluid exchange three distinctive periods occur – inflow, dwell, and outflow. After the outflow and before the next inflow and during the dwell the flow of fluid is interrupted, hence the term intermittent. In the early 1960s Boen *et al.* [18] introduced peritoneal dialysis for the treatment of chronic renal failure. The dialysis sessions were performed periodically, several times per week, consequently the term 'periodic peritoneal dialysis' was applied to this regimen. Single dialysis sessions were performed with the intermittent flow technique and gradually the term 'intermittent' became synonymous with 'periodic' and the latter term was abandoned. In the late 1970s, after the introduction of continuous ambulatory peritoneal dialysis, the term 'continuous' meant that the dialysis was performed around the clock with only brief, insignificant interruptions for infrequent exchanges. Thus, yet another terminology was established. In this chapter when describing regimens performed periodically the term intermittent peritoneal dialysis will be used. However, when describing techniques the term *intermittent flow* peritoneal dialysis will be used in its original meaning.

3. ADVANTAGES AND DISADVANTAGES OF INTERMITTENT PERITONEAL DIALYSIS (IPD)

3.1. Advantages of IPD compared to hemodialysis

IPD for chronic renal failure was introduced by Boen *et al.* in 1962 [18], but the method gained popularity after two crucial developments: a safe and permanent chronic peritoneal access [21] and an automated delivery system of dialysis solution that allowed therapy at home [22, 23]. Compared to hemodialysis, IPD did not require blood access, extracorporeal circulation or systemic anticoagulation, and appeared to be simpler and safer. Because of less rapid changes in body chemistries and hydration state, IPD was considered superior to hemodialysis in patients with unstable cardiovascular systems, elderly, diabetics with active retinopathy, blood access failures, bleeding tendencies, and those living alone but willing to perform home dialysis [24]. A possibility of maintaining hematocrit above 20% without blood transfusion constituted an incentive to peritoneal dialysis in Jehovah Witnesses [24].

3.2. Disadvantages of IPD compared to hemodialysis

The main disadvantage of IPD is a shorter technique survival than on other forms of renal replacement therapy. This unsatisfactory outcome stems from two major deficiencies of IPD, especially in patients who lost residual renal function: 1) inadequate dialysis clearances and 2) inadequate sodium balance resulting in poor blood pressure control. Dropouts to hemodialysis, or CAPD, from IPD were the rule rather than an exception in the early 1980's.

3.2.1. Long term survival

Despite the apparent enthusiasm for IPD in the 1970's [24–29], and Tenckhoff's experience indicating that 20 to 25% of end-stage renal disease patients would be best treated by peritoneal dialysis, the total population of renal failure patients in the United States treated with IPD did not exceed 3% [30] in the late 1970s and dropped further in the early 1980's. At the end of 1986 only 700 out of 90,886 end stage renal disease patients (0.77%) were treated with IPD [31]. Although survival rates were comparable to those on hemodialysis during the initial one year of therapy, there was a sudden increase in mortality after the first or the second year [32–34]. Ahmad *et al.* in a retrospective study, reported only 26% of patients remaining on IPD after three years [32].

3.2.2. Adequacy of dialysis

Since the early years of chronic hemodialysis, adequate dialysis was considered as treatment by which the symptoms and signs of uremia were eradicated and the patient was fully rehabilitated [35, 36]. Adequate peritoneal dialysis must fulfill the same criteria. In our peritoneal dialysis program the patients are considered as adequately dialyzed if they feel well, have no clinical symptoms or signs of uremia, maintain hematocrit above 25% (without anabolic steroids or erythropoietin), have stable or increasing nerve conduction velocity (if not diabetic), and well controlled blood pressure. Manifestations of inadequate dialysis may be subtle and often develop insidiously. Most commonly, inadequate dialysis results in such symptoms as insomnia, weakness, dysgeusia, nausea and anorexia leading to poor nutrition with wasting and loss of lean body weight. Blood urea nitrogen may be low because of poor protein intake, but creatinine level is usually high. Unfortunately there is no particular creatinine level at which all patients develop symptoms of underdialysis. According to our personal experience, serum creatinine levels above 20 mg% are associated with subtle to obvious underdialysis symptoms in the majority of peritoneal dialysis patients; however, serum creatinine levels above 15 mg% may be associated with inadequate dialysis, especially in nonmuscular persons. Per contra, most muscular hemodialysis patients with a serum creatinine above 20 mg% have clinically adequate dialysis.

A controversial issue is whether other symptoms and signs of uremia should indicate inadequate dialysis. Control of serum phosphorus to prevent secondary hyperthyroidism by dialysis alone without phosphate binders is unrealistic, thus, hyperphosphatemia and hyperparathyroidism are not considered as indicating inadequate dialysis. Serositis may occur in otherwise adequately dialyzed patients and generally is not considered as indicating inadequate dialysis.

3.2.3. Minimum adequate clearances

Even after several decades of research, there is no general agreement on adequate body clearances of uremic toxins. Advocates of middle molecules as the most important uremic toxins propose that the combined clearances (dialysis and renal) of these molecules should exceed 3.0 ml/min (4.32 l/day or 30.24 l/week) as a minimum adequate clearance [37]. For hemodialysis, a urea fractional index of 2000–2900 ml/week per liter of body water is considered as providing sufficient dialysis [38, 39]. For adequate peritoneal dialysis, a combined creatinine clearance of 5.5 ml/min (7.92 l/day, or 55.44 l/week) has been postulated in a standard patient with body surface area (BSA) of 1.73 m^2 [40]. My personal experience indicates that patients fulfilling criteria of adequate dialysis have at least a combined creatinine clearance of 4.0–5.0 ml/min/1.73 m^2 (5.8–7.2 l/day; 40–50 l/week).

A combined creatinine clearance (K) is composed of average weekly dialysis (K_d) and renal (K_r) clearances according to the formula

$$K = K_D + K_r. \qquad [1]$$

In a continuous peritoneal dialysis regimen a direct measurement of renal and peritoneal clearances is sufficient.

In an intermittent (periodic) peritoneal dialysis (IPD) regimen

$$K_d = \frac{K_{di} \times T_d}{168} \qquad [2]$$

where:

K_{di} = IPD clearance in ml/min
T_d = IPD time in hours/week
168 = total hours in one week.

An anuric patient with a K_{di} of 12.0–15.0 ml/min/1.73 m^2 may have adequate dialysis with 56 hr of IPD per week.

3.2.4. Thirst, sodium and water balance, blood pressure control

Thirst is common in IPD patients, occurs usually after several hours of a dialysis session or immediately thereafter and may lead to excessive water intake and weight gain before the next dialysis. This is due to the low sodium concentration in ultrafiltrate resulting in hypernatremia.

The problem may be overcome by lowering sodium concentration in dialysis solution to increase the diffusion gradient. Throughout the decades the sodiuum concentrations in dialysis solutions have been gradually lowered. In the 1920's and 1930's the solutions contained more than 150 mEq/l of sodium [1–4, 5]. Rhoads used solution containing a sodium concentration of 276 mEq/l [8]. In the 1940's and 1950's sodium concentrations between 140 and 145 mEq/l were generally used [10, 11, 16] and only a few authors recommended sodium concentrations of 130–131 mEq/l [9, 12]. Boen used 140 mEq/l of sodium when he worked in Amsterdam[17] and later used 135 mEq/l when working in Seattle [18]. The use of solutions with sodium concentrations close to 140 resulted in severe thirst and poor blood pressure control [41]. Hypernatremia over 160 mEq/l has been reported [42, 44]. Many patients did not develop hypernatremia because of high water intake during dialysis due to severe thirst [41]. In the late 1960's and early 1970's, when hypernatremia was explained by molecular sieving [45], the concentration of sodium in the dialysis solutions was decreased. Ahearn and Nolph[46] recommended a sodium concentration of 110 mEq/l for 7% glucose solutions. Tenckhoff recommended 130 mEq/l for solutions with a lower glucose content [47]. In 1973, a special workshop recommended a sodium concentration of 132 mEq/l and a maximum glucose concentration of 4.5% [48]. Since that time, most commercial solutions contain such a concentration of sodium. Notwithstanding

this lower sodium concentration, many patients continue to have thirst, hypernatremia, and poor blood pressure control on IPD. In 1978 Shen *et al.* [49] proposed a sodium concentration of 118 for 2.5% glucose solutions and 109 mEq/l for 4.5% glucose solutions. At that time, continuous ambulatory peritoneal dialysis was introduced and the disappearance of thirst and spectacular improvement in blood pressure control was noted within a few days after conversion from IPD to CAPD [50]. Dialysis solution sodium concentration of 132 mEq/l seems appropriate for CAPD. Solutions with the lower sodium concentrations have never been commercially available.

Recently, with the introduction of nightly intermittent peritoneal dialysis (NIPD) and using dialysis solution containing 132 mEq/l of sodium we have observed tendencies to thirst and more difficult blood pressure control in two types of patients [51, 52]. Type one patients have chronically low serum sodium concentration, probably because of reset osmostat, and the sodium concentration gradient between dialysate and serum is so low that the sodium diffusion cannot compensate even for moderate sieving. After NIPD a relative hypernatremia develops and, due to severe thirst, the patient increases water intake to bring down serum sodium concentration to the level congruous with the osmostat set. Type two patients have low peritoneal permeability and/or area, and very low ultrafiltrate sodium concentration due to sieving. Diffusion cannot compensate for sieving and an absolute hypernatremia develops after NIPD. Blood pressure control is difficult in both types of patients.

4. FEATURES OF CAPD COMPARED TO IPD

4.1. Advantages of CAPD

4.1.1. Clearances

The main advantages of CAPD over IPD are higher dialysis clearances for solutes in all molecular weight ranges. A mean creatinine clearance is about 6.3 l/day (4.4 ml/min.) [51], a value providing adequate dialysis. There are other advantages, as listed in Table 1, but there is no question in my mind that adequate dialysis is the main reason why CAPD is so successful as a therapy.

4.1.2. Thirst, sodium balance, and blood pressure control

One of the striking features after switching the patient from IPD to CAPD were the disappearance of thirst within a few days and an excellent control of blood presure [50]. Dialysis solutions containing sodium of 132 mEq/l have been generally used in CAPD patients. Sodium sieving occurs early during the dwell time when the ultrafiltration rate is high; however, the ultrafiltration rate diminishes rapidly with glucose absorption and a dissipation of osmotic gradient. The lower the ultrafiltration rate, the less sieving. Simultaneously, due to a high sodium concentration gradient between plasma and dialysate, the sodium diffusion rate increases. After a several hour dwell time, ultrafiltration ceases and continuing diffusion increases the dialysate sodium concentration [53]. Ultimately, when the dialysate is drained, its sodium concentration is still below, but closer to that of serum. Usually, water and sodium losses are

Table 1. Advantages of CAPD compared to home IPD

	CAPD *4 daily 2l exchanges*	Home IPD *30-40 hr per week*
Medical		
Weekly clearances	Adequate	Inadequate
Sodium removal	Sufficient	Insufficient
Thirst	Absent	Present
Blood pressure	Usually well controlled	Frequently poorly controlled
Blood chemistries	Steady	Fluctuating
Psychosocial		
Equipment	Simple	Machines
Travel	Easy	Difficult
Bed confinement	None	Prolonged

nearly proportionate to water and sodium intakes, serum sodium does not increase, no thirst is present, and sodium removal is sufficient to control blood pressure. Dialysis solution sodium concentration of 132 mEq/l seems to be appropriate for CAPD.

4.1.3. Psycho-social
CAPD is a very simple procedure. It does not require machines; a suitable environment can be relatively easily created to perform dialysis exchanges, thus there are essentially no restrictions for travel. The interruption of daily activities to perform exchanges is short. Dialysis is carried out when the patient is ambulatory or asleep. Intermittent peritoneal dialysis requires a bed confinement for prolonged periods, although most dialysis may be performed during the night. Machines for IPD require running water and/or electricity, thus travel is difficult.

4.2. Disadvantages of CAPD relative to IPD

Table 2 presents undesirable features of CAPD compared to IPD. Although the continuous presence of dialysis fluid in the peritoneal cavity is favorable for the dialysis clearances, sodium balance, and steady state chemistries in CAPD patients, it is disadvantageous in several aspects.

4.2.1. Peritonitis
Peritoneal defense mechanisms against infections are compromised with the presence of an nonphysiologic fluid in the peritoneal cavity. Immunoglobulin concentrations in the high volume dialysate are lower than in the few milliliters of fluid which are normally present in the peritoneal cavity; bacterial opsonization is thus decreased. The phagocytes are also diluted in the fluid, and their contact with bacteria, essential for effective phagocytosis, is hampered. Moreover, the efficiency of phagocytic cells decrease at low pH and high osmolality of dialysis solution [54]. Patients on intermittent peritoneal dialysis have long periods when the peritoneum is without solutions and normal defense mechanisms may contain and eradicate a small bacterial inoculum. Although hypothetical, it is an attractive explanation of the higher peritonitis rates in CAPD than in IPD patients. Another reason for lower infection rates could be the lower number of peritoneal dialysis system openings

per week. Using automated reverse osmosis systems, the number of connection-disconnections in IPD have been three to four per week (156–208 per year), whereas CAPD requires 28 connection-disconnections per week (1460 per year). However, when IPD has been performed on cyclers, the number of connection-disconnections was 50 per week (2600 per year), even higher than on CAPD, yet the peritonitis rate on IPD was 0.14 per year and for CAPD 0.63 per year [55]. Certainly, the lower number of system openings cannot fully explain lower peritonitis rates on IPD.

4.2.2. Relative malnutrition
Another disadvantage of CAPD is high glucose absorption from the solution. An initial high glucose concentration in dialysis solution is needed for adequate ultrafiltration. The higher the glucose load, the longer ultrafiltration lasts [56], but during the second half of a long dwell, the fluid is absorbed and glucose continues to be absorbed. Net ultrafiltration volume per mass of absorbed glucose is lower on CAPD than on IPD. Glucose absorption in CAPD patients may reach 300 grams per day [57]. This constant and high glucose absorption probably contributes to obesity and lipid disturbances [58]. This dextrose load, coupled with abdominal distension, decreases appetite leading to the documented trend of CAPD patients to store fat and develop relative malnutrition [59].

4.2.3. Fluid leaks, hernias, and hemorrhoids
Abdominal hernias are relatively common complications of CAPD. Several authors have reported 9–28% incidence

Table 2. Disadvantages of CAPD relative to home IPD

Medical

More frequent peritonitis episodes
Higher glucose absorption, obesity, relative malnutrition
Higher rates of abdominal fluid leaks, hernias and hemorrhoids
Lower back pain is a more frequent complication

Psychosocial

Distorted body image
Inconvenient exchange schedule in school-attending and employed patients or their helpers
Worse compliance with number of exchanges

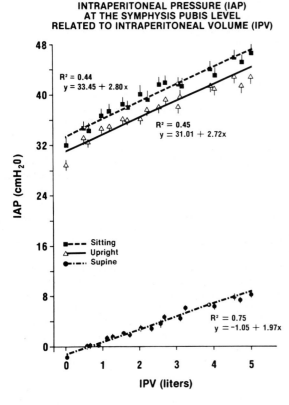

INTRAPERITONEAL PRESSURE (IAP)
AT THE SYMPHYSIS PUBIS LEVEL
RELATED TO INTRAPERITONEAL VOLUME (IPV)

of hernias in CAPD patients [60–65], whereas only 2% of IPD patients develop hernias [66]. Also, hemorrhoids and abdominal and pericatheter leaks are frequent on CAPD [65, 67–69]. Undoubtedly, it is related to the constant presence of fluid in the peritoneal cavity. This contention is supported by increased rates of hernias and even spontaneous hernia ruptures in patients with ascites [70]. Several investigators have recently demonstrated a linear relationship between the intra-abdominal pressure and intraperitoneal fluid volume in relaxed patients [71–73]. This linear relationship (Figure 1) is observed regardless of the patient position, but the curves are shifted upwards in vertical positions [71–72]. Natural activities have a profound effect on intra-abdominal pressure (Figure 2) [74]. Whereas the relaxed patients in the supine position have pressures close to 0 mm Hg at the umbilicus level, in the vertical positions the pressures are markedly higher. The position has greater influence on intra-abdominal pressures than has intraperitoneal volume. Because an elevated intra-abdominal pressure is a risk factor for the development of fluid leaks, hernias and hemorrhoids, this may explain higher rates of these complications in CAPD than in IPD patients.

Figure 1. Intraabdominal pressure (IAP) at the symphysis pubis level related to intraperitoneal volume (IPV) in 18 relaxed patients in the supine, upright and sitting positions. Means ± SEM. Linear regressions are also shown. Results obtained in the study previously reported [71] but recalculated for the symphysis pubis as a reference level.

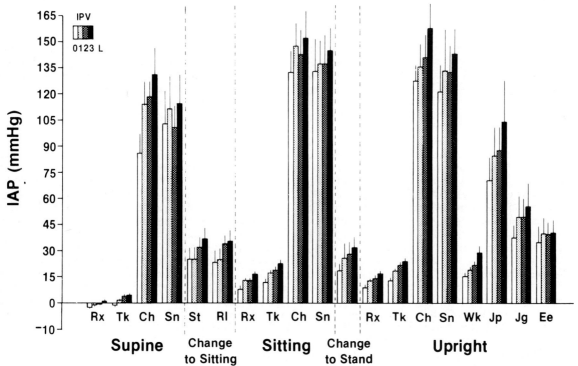

Figure 2. Intraabdominal pressures (IAP) at the umbilicus level during natural activities with 0, 1, 2, and 3 l intraperitoneal volumes (IPV). Means ± SEM in 6 patients. Rx = Relax; Tk = Talk; Ch = Cough; Sn = Strain; St = Straight; Rl = Roll; Wk = Walk; Jp = Jump; Jg = Jog; Ee = Exercycle. (Reprinted from ref. 74 with permission.)

4.2.4. Chronic back pain

Back pain is a frequent complication of CAPD, probably related to the change in body posture with the presence of fluid in the peritoneal cavity [75].

4.2.5. Psycho-social

A protruding abdomen due to the chronic artificial ascites distorts the body image in some CAPD patients. An empty abdomen during the day in IPD patients is not associated with this adverse cosmetic effect.

Frequent CAPD exchanges during the daytime are tedious and inconvenient, especially for the employed and school-attending patients. Dialysis exchanges require creation of a proper environment and are less easily performed outside the home or dialysis facility. If exchanges are performed in inappropriate conditions, the risk of peritoneal system contamination is increased. This inconvenience predisposes to noncompliance in performing all prescribed exchanges. The less exchanges per day, the better the compliance. IPD does not require daytime exchanges. Patient compliance relative to the number of exchanges is better on IPD; however, the compliance relative to the time of dialysis may be worse.

CAPD is not convenient for patients who require a helper because of age and/or disability. Since much less of the aid's time is needed for IPD compared with CAPD, the former is a preferred mode of therapy in patients requiring a helper.

5. NIGHTLY PERITONEAL DIALYSIS (NPD)

NPD is a peritoneal dialysis performed every night or may be considered as CCPD without long dwell daytime exchanges. NPD performed with an intermittent flow technique is called nightly intermittent peritoneal dialysis (NIPD). Since 1982 we have used NIPD in patients with recurrent abdominal leaks and hernias, bladder prolapse, rapid glucose absorption resulting in poor ultrafiltration on CAPD, abdominal discomfort, chronic hypotension, and patient preference [51, 76, 77]. In 1985, Scribner postulated that 'Some form of Nightly Peritoneal Dialysis, NPD, may prove as the best compromise of all [forms of peritoneal dialysis]' [78]. Because of reduced dialysis time compared to CAPD and CCPD, the main problem of NIPD is to achieve adequate clearances. The efficiency of peritoneal dialysis is dependent on peritoneal transport characteristics in individual patients. Therefore, I will first discuss a variation in the peritoneal mass transfer and its measurement pertinent to the NIPD prescription.

5.1. Peritoneal mass transfer

5.1.1. Mass transfer area coefficient

Dialysate to plasma ratios of solute concentrations change at different rates in different patients on peritoneal dialysis [10, 11, 16]. Peritoneal clearances measured during standard intermittent peritoneal dialysis vary from patient to patient [17, 79–81]. The mass transfer area coefficient (MTAC) was introduced to separate influences of dialysate flow rate and convective transport on solute transfer. This coefficient, based on kinetic models of the solute mass transfer process,

is the inverse of peritoneal diffusion resistance and represents the clearance rate which would be realized in the absence of both ultrafiltration and solute accumulation in the dialysate. The MTAC concept is described in detail elsewhere in this book. To determine MTAC, a test exchange is performed with at least two measurements of dialysate and plasma solute concentrations at different dwell times. The MTAC is expressed in ml/min. Results show a very wide variation of MTAC among patients and among studies. Garred *et al.* reported a mean creatinine MTAC of 10 and range from 2.6 to 21.4 ml/min [82]. Popovich *et al.* [83] reported an average value of 23.5 ml/min and the lowest of 5.1 ml/min. It is worth noting the discrepancy in mean values by the two groups. This reflects, probably, the difference in measurement techniques and laboratory methods.

The MTAC measurement is seldom ulitized in routine clinical practice as a guide in selection of the optimal dialysis regimen. There are at least 3 reasons for this failure: 1) the reproducibility of the results is unsatisfactory, 2) different solutes show conflicting results in individuals, and 3) the method of presentation as MTAC is not readily accepted because of the complexity of calculations. To overcome the last problem, a nomogram was published [84] to calculate MTAC from a single measurement of solute dialysate to plasma ratio at 4, 5, or 6 hr dwell time. Such a recalculation is not necessary if values of dialysate to plasma ratios obtained during peritoneal equilibration test in a large patient population are correlated with the clinical results of treatment with various peritoneal dialysis regimens.

5.1.2. Equilibration test procedure

The full details of our technique and its complete usefulness for diagnostic and prognostic purposes are beyond the scope of this chapter and are reported elsewhere [85]. Below is described a simplified peritoneal equilibration test as currently routinely performed in our institution. To achieve a satisfactory reproducibility of results, the procedure must be standardized including the exchange preceding the equilibration test. According to our protocol the preceding exchange must dwell for 8–12 hr. This pretest exchange is completely drained over 20 min in the sitting position and 2 l of 2.5% dialysis solution (Dianeal^R 2.5%) is infused at a rate of 400 ml per 2 min over a total of 10 min. The patient is in the supine position during infusion and rolls from side to side after each 400 ml is infused for better mixing of residual volume and infused solution. Exactly 10 min after the start of infusioin, at the completion of infusion (0 dwell time), 200 ml of solution is drained into the bag, mixed well, a 10 ml sample of dialysate is taken and the remaining 190 ml reinfused. The patient is ambulatory during the dwell period. After 120 min of dwell time a sample of dialysate is taken with the same technique as at 0 dwell time and a blood sample is obtained. After a 4 hr dwell time, the dialysate is drained over 20 min with the patient in the sitting position, total volume is measured and a sample taken. The total time of the equilibration exchange is 270 min.

5.1.3. Laboratory assays

Concentrations of creatinine and glucose are measured in

the dialysate and blood samples. Handling of samples is extremely important. Chemistries should be best run immediately after samples are taken. If dialysate is frozen the samples have to be thoroughly thawed, preferably at 37 °C for at least 2 hr and very well mixed before runs. Although, it should be common knowledge that sample problems arise during freezing and thawing, many analysts are not aware of this. Omong and Vellar [86] found the highest concentration of solutes at the bottom of tubes after thawing. This phenomenon is produced during thawing, when more concentrated solution thaws first and runs down to the bottom along the tube walls. Simple inversion of tubes is not sufficient. The sample should be additionally mixed on a vortex. The error due to incomplete mixing is more likely in dialysate than in the serum because of high osmolality of the former.

Glucose interferes with the Jaffe reagent for creatinine, thus creatinine values in dialysate are overestimated. In our laboratory the relationship between glucose concentrations and creatinine readings are linear within the range of 0–2500 mg/dl (r=0.98). Each mg% of glucose overestimates creatinine concentration by 0.000531415 mg/dl. Creatinine values are corrected for glucose interference before further calculations.

The correction of creatinine concentration for glucose interference is usually small after long dwell time, but it is significant after short dwell time and a substantial error arises when creatinine clearance is calculated, particularly in short dwell exchanges. For example, in the above mentioned study [52, 85] the mean dialysate to plasma ratio of uncorrected creatinine at 0.5 hr dwell time was 0.32, whereas the mean of corrected creatinine was 0.23. Creatinine clearance without correction would be overestimated by 0.32/0.23, i.e. 1.39 or 39%. Similar calculations for 4 hr dwell times reveal only a moderate error of 0.69/0.65, i.e. 1.06 or 6%. Because many reports have not provided detailed descriptions of laboratory methods, it is difficult to compare clearance values and mass transfer area coefficients reported in the literature, and it is not surprising that mean IPD creatinine clearances in one report were 18 ml/min [87] and in the other, 12 ml/min [88]. For this reason, it is so difficult to establish minimal clearance requirements acceptable for all peritoneal dialysis centers.

5.1.4. Equilibration test results and interpretation

Dialysate to plasma ratios (D/P) of creatinine at the times specified above and the ratios of dialysate glucose at 2 and 4 hr dwell time to dialysate glucose at 0 dwell time (D/DO) are calculated. Based on the results of 103 peritoneal equilibration tests the transport rate is categorized as low, low average, high average, and high [85] (Figure 3). A low transport rate is defined as a D/P ratio < mean − 1SD or a D/DO > mean + 1SD. Low average transport is defined as a D/P between the mean − 1SD and the mean, or a D/DO between the mean and the mean + 1SD. High average transport is a D/P between the mean and the mean + 1SD or a D/DO between the mean − 1SD and the mean. A high transport rate is present if D/P is > the mean + 1SD or D/DO is lower than the mean − 1SD. Drain volumes are categorized using the same principle as for dialysate to plasma ratios (Figure 4).

The curve of an individual test is categorized according to the position of 2 points at 2 and 4 hr dwell time and the results are superimposed on standard curves. The visual presentation of the results is simple to understand. Table 3 summarizes the prognostic usefulness of the baseline peritoneal equilibration test. The patients with high peritoneal transport rates have poor ultrafiltration on standard CAPD, sometimes even with mostly hypertonic dialysis solutions. These patients, even after losing residual renal function have adequate dialysis and ultrafiltration with less than 24 hr of dialysis per day; such as NIPD or daytime ambulatory peritoneal dialysis (DAPD).

The best candidates for standard dose CAPD (total dialysis solution infusion volume below 9 l) are patients with high average peritoneal transport rates. They can achieve adequate dialysis even after losing residual renal function and obtain adequate ultrafiltration with moderate dialysis solution glucose concentrations.

Most patients with low average peritoneal transport can be maintained on the standard dose CAPD; however, many of them may require a modified prescription (CAPD with total dose of dialysis solution > 9 l per day, high dose CCPD) when residual renal function becomes negligible, particularly if they have high body surface area. These patients have excellent ultrafiltration with moderate dialysis solution glucose concentrations.

Finally, patients with low peritoneal transport rates usually have excellent ultrafiltration with low dialysis solution glucose concentration and are very likely to develop symptoms of inadequate dialysis on standard CAPD when their residual renal function becomes negligible [79, 87, 89, 90].

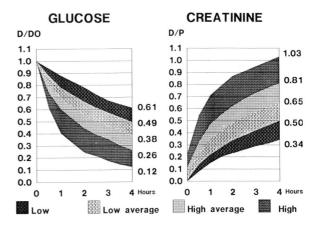

Figure 3. The equilibration test results in the study population. Areas shaded in different patterns portray results representing high, high average, low average, and low peritoneal transport rates. For creatinine the higher dialysate to plasma ratio (D/P) the higher the transfer rate; because glucose transport direction is opposite to that of creatinine the higher the concentration ratio of dialysate glucose at particular dwell time to dialysate glucose at 0 dwell time (D/DO) the lower the transfer rate. The numbers at the borders of the four categories designate maximal, mean + 1SD, mean, mean − 1SD, and minimal values at four hour dwell time. (Based on data from ref. 52 and 85).

DRAIN VOLUME

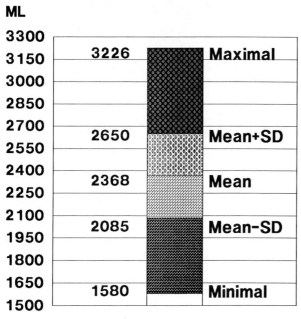

Figure 4. Drain volumes after four hour dwell time in the study population. Because patients with high solute transport rates have usually low drain volumes and vice versa the stack bar areas are shaded in the patterns corresponding to categories portrayed in Figure 3. (Based on data from ref. 52 and 85).

5.2. NIPD technique

All NIPD treatments are performed overnight on a PD cycler with 1.5 to 2 l fill volumes of commercial peritoneal dialysis solutions. Total dialysis time ranges from 8 to 12 hr per night (56–84 hr per week). A total volume of used dialysis solution per dialysis ranges from 8–20 l (56–140 l per week). The time of dialysis and dialysis dose are adjusted according to the patient's peritoneal membrane permeability area. In our patients, with the assays used in our laboratory, we found the combined corrected creatinine clearance (dialysis + renal) of 4.0–5.0 ml/min/1.73 m^2 (5.8–7.2 l/day; 40–50 l/week) as sufficient to achieve adequate dialysis.

Drain time is restricted to 12–15 min (maximum 1 min for 150 ml) to minimize the period when the peritoneal cavity is almost empty and dialysis efficiency is markedly reduced. If a low drain alarm is triggered during the initial one or two exchanges, the patients are instructed not to prolong drain time but to bypass cycles and thus create some sump volume in the peritoneal cavity. Low drain alarms usually do not occur during third or later cycles, unless the extension tubing is occluded.

Table 4 shows treatment time, exchange volume, dialysis solution sodium concentration, and the amount of dialysis solution prescribed at the time of this writing for 12 patients treated with NIPD as well as the patients' peritoneal transport rates. NIPD time is 10 hr or more per night for adequate clearances in 11 patients; one patient with high peritoneal transport characteristics can be dialyzed for 9 hr. At present only one patient requires a lower dialysis sodium concentration to achieve appropriate negative sodium balance and blood pressure control. In the past we

Table 3. Prognostic value of the baseline peritoneal equilibration test results in patients with well functioning catheter after break-in

Peritoneal solute transport	Drain volume	Predicted long term response to standard dose CAPD or CCPD[a] after loss of residual renal functions		Preferred dialysis prescription after loss of residual renal functions
		Ultrafiltration	Dialysis	
High	Low	Poor	Adequate	NIPD, DAPD[b]
High average	Low average	Adequate	Adequate	Standard, dose PD[a]
Low average	High average	Good	Adequate or inadequate[c]	Standard, dose PD[a] High dose PD[d]
Low	High	Excellent	Inadequate	High dose PD[d] Hemodialysis[e]

[a] – Standard dose PD = standard dose CAPD or CCPD.
 – Standard dose CAPD = CAPD with 7.5–9.0 l of dialysis solution used per 24 hr.
 – Standard dose CCPD = CCPD with 6–8 l of dialysis solution used overnight and 2 l daytime.
[b] – NIPD = Nightly Intermittent Peritoneal Dialysis;
 DAPD = Daytime Ambulatory Peritoneal Dialysis.
[c] – Inadequate dialysis likely in patients with body surface area >2.00 m^2.
[d] – High dose PD = high dose CAPD or CCPD.
 – High dose CAPD = CAPD with >9.0 l of dialysis solution used per 24 hr.
 – High dose CCPD = CCPD with >8 l of dialysis solution used overnight and/or >2 l daytime.
[e] – Hemodialysis may be needed in patients with body surface area >2.00 m^2.

used custom-made solutions with lower sodium concentration, but the solutions were too expensive for routine use. Recently we add 5% glucose solution (D5W) to peritoneal dialysis solution in an appropriate proportion to achieve the desired sodium concentration. For instance, 2 l of D5W added to 20 l of dialysis solution lowers the sodium concentration from 132 mEq/l to 120 mEq/l. Dilution of other electrolytes is of little significance. The use of additional, little (1 l) bags increases a demand of the procedure and risk of contamination. Certainly it would be safer and more convenient to have premixed dialysis solutions with lower sodium concentrations for some NIPD patients.

5.3. Clinical results

NIPD is in an early developmental stage with only 23 patients treated in our institution. The method is being used in other institutions (it is frequently called CCPD with dry daytime), but no reports on the results have been published yet. Table 5 portrays the results in our NIPD program.

5.3.1. Incentives to NIPD
The most common incentives for NIPD are complications related to high intraabdominal pressure and poor ultrafiltration due to high peritoneal transport rates. One patient with peritoneo-pleural leak on CAPD was successfully treated with NIPD for 2 yr before receiving a cadaveric kidney transplant. This experience confirms a previous similar observation [91] and indicates that a peritoneo-pleural leak occurring on CAPD is not an absolute contraindication to peritoneal dialysis in the supine position.

5.3.2. Outcome of NIPD
Among our 23 patients, three were transplanted, three died, two were switched back to CAPD, two were switched to CCPD (one CAPD and one CCPD patient returned to NIPD due to deterioration of hernias) and three were transferred to hemodialysis; twelve patients coninue on NIPD, the longest survivor being 4.5 yr. It is worth stressing that for 19 of these patients, NIPD was the only viable peritoneal dialysis option and six of them failed previous hemodialysis. The major reason of transfer from NIPD was a requirement of long dialysis duration because of low peritoneal transport rates. No patient with low peritoneal transport (D/P creatinine >0.50) is currently treated on our NIPD program.

Table 5. Incentives for and outcomes of nightly intermittent peritoneal dialysis (NIPD) in 23 patients at the University of Missouri

Main incentive for NIPD	Number of patients
Abdominal leaks, hemorrhoids and/or hernias	8
Peritoneo-pleural leak	1
Bladder prolapse	2
Abdominal discomfort, poor appetite	3
High glucose absorption, poor ultrafiltration	4
Convenient dialysis schedule	3
Chronic hypotension	1
Body image	1
Total	23
Outcome	
Continue on NIPD	12
Transplanted	3
Died	3
High dose CAPD[a]	1 (a)
High dose CCPD[b]	1 (a)
Hemodialysis	3 (a = 2, b = 1)
Total	23

[a] – High dose CAPD = CAPD with >9.0 l of dialysis solution used per 24 hr.

[b] – High dose CCPD = CCPD with >8 l of dialysis solution used overnight and/or >2 l daytime.
(a) – low peritoneal transport rate, long NIPD time required;
(b) – insufficient ultrafiltration due to excessive lymphatic absorption.

Table 4. Current NIPD prescriptions at the University of Missouri

Patient	Treatment time hr/night	Exchange volume l	Solution dose l/night	Dialysis solution concentration of sodium (mEq/l)	Peritoneal transport rate
1	9	1.6	10	132	High
2	10	1.5	15	132	High average
3	10	1.5	15	132	High average
4	10	1.4	11	132	High average
5	10	1.5	15	132	High average
6	10	1.9	10	132	High average
7	10	2.0	22	120	High average
8	10	1.8	15	132	Low average
9	11	1.5	15	132	Low average
10	11	1.4	15	132	Low average
11	11	1.5	20	132	Low average
12	12	1.5	15	132	Low average

5.3.3. Peritonitis

The rates of peritonitis both in NIPD and CAPD patients have been one episode per 16 patient-months for the last 12 months. Since the number of connections has been higher on NIPD than on CAPD, it seems to support the hypothesis of Vas [54, 55] as discussed earlier.

5.3.4. Advantages of NIPD

The main medical advantages of NIPD relative to CAPD and CCPD are an empty abdomen during the daytime and lower glucose absorption per volume of ultrafiltration (Table 6). An empty abdomen during the daytime is associated with lower inclination to hernias, leaks and hemorrhoids, back pain, less abdominal distension, low glucose loads during daytime with consequent better appetite and higher protein intakes.

Psycho-social advantages are similar to or even better than those for CCPD: better body image, convenient dialysis time for employed patients and for helpers if they are needed.

5.3.5. Disadvantages of NIPD

Because of reduced dialysis time compared to CAPD and CCPD, the greatest disadvantage of NIPD is a lower efficiency of dialysis. (Table 7) In most patients, the time of NIPD had to be increased to greatly exceed a normal bedtime of eight hours. To increase efficiency, the number of exchanges has to be increased, and the cost of dialysis has substantially exceeded the cost of CAPD or CCPD.

To assess the possibility of performing only eight hours NIPD we measured clearances of urea, creatinine, phosphorus, potassium, glucose absorption, sodium balance, and ultrafiltration in nine patients using up to 26 l of dialysis solution per treatment [51]. In patients with supranormal transport (peritoneal permeability and/or area), the clearances of urea, creatinine, and potassium were higher than those on standard CAPD. In patients with close to average peritoneal transport, only urea and potassium clearances matched those of CAPD. In subnormal transport patients, all clearances were lower on NIPD than on CAPD. Protein losses were similar on NIPD and CAPD, and glucose absorption was lower in NIPD with adequate ultrafiltration. Sodium balance was inadequate on eight hour NIPD, especially in patients with low peritoneal transport.

5.3.6. Current status of NIPD

Because of higher cost and lower efficiency of dialysis compared to CCPD and CAPD, NIPD is not a viable alternative to CAPD or CCPD at present. Only for patients who cannot be on ambulatory peritoneal dialysis because

Table 6. Advantages of NIPD relative to CAPD and CCPD

1. Empty abdomen during daytime.
   a. Less inclinations to hernias, leaks and hemorrhoids.
   b. Better body image.
   c. Less abdominal distention, no glucose load during daytime – better appetite – higher protein intake.
   d. Lower incidence of peritonitis?
2. Lower glucose absorption/ultrafiltration.

Table 7. Disadvantages of NIPD relative to CAPD and CCPD

1. Lower daily peritoneal creatinine clearances in most patients with 8 hr dialysis.
2. Insufficient sodium removal relative to ultrafiltration in patients with low peritoneal solute transport rates and/or chronically low serum sodium concentration.
3. Inconvenient long bed stay in patients requiring more than 8 hr dialysis.
4. Higher cost.
5. Requires a cycler, electricity – Travel difficult (relative to CAPD).

of complications related to elevated intraabdominal pressure and cannot be on hemodialysis or for patients with supranormal peritoneal transport rates does NIPD remain the best dialysis choice [52].

6. CHOICE OF PERITONEAL DIALYSIS THERAPY

Standard CAPD is the most prevalent prescription in our institution. More than 50% of patients are on standard dose (7.5–9.0 l of dialysis solution used per 24 hr) CAPD, but less than 35% are on standard dose CAPD with 2 l exchanges. Table 8 shows a cross section of peritoneal dialysis prescriptions used in our patients at the time of this writing. High dose prescriptions are used in patients with low average or low peritoneal transport rates. Low dose prescriptions are used in patients with well preserved residual renal function, standard dose DAPD or NIPD in patients with high peritoneal transport rates. NIPD is also used in patients with inclinations to complications related to high intraabdominal pressure or in patients who want to have an empty abdomen during daytime.

7. FUTURE OF NPD

I believe that NPD is a promising dialysis regimen as predicted by Scribner [78], but its future depends on three improvements: 1) the cost of dialysis must be decreased, 2) dialysis solution compositions, particularly sodium concentration, must be modified, and 3) the efficiency of dialysis has to be increased.

7.1. Cost of dialysis

Cost of dialysis has to match that of CAPD. Machines for peritoneal dialysis have to be redesigned. Automated production of dialysis solution from pretreated water and concentrate would be needed to decrease the cost of dialysis.

7.2. Dialysis solution

Sodium concentration in dialysis solution for NPD should be lower than that for CAPD or CCPD, especially for patients with normal or below normal peritoneal glucose absorption rates and those with chronically low serum sodium concentrations. The concentrations between 120 and 132 mEq/l seem to be appropriate. It would be desirable

Table 8. Current peritoneal prescriptions in adults at the University of Missouri

Prescription[a]	Number of patients		Percent	
Standard dose CAPD	28		52.8	
Standard volume		18		34.0
High volume		8		15.1
Low volume		2		3.8
High dose CAPD	4		7.5	
High volume		3		5.7
Standard volume		1		1.9
Low dose CAPD	2		3.8	
High dose CCPD	2		3.8	
Standard dose DAPD	1		1.9	
Low dose DAPD	1		1.9	
NIPD	12		22.6	
Chronic TPD study	3		5.7	
Total	53		100.0	

[a]
- Standard dose CAPD = CAPD with 7.5–9.0 l of dialysis solution used per 24 hr.
- High dose CAPD = CAPD with >9.0 l of dialysis solution used per 24 hr.
- Low dose CAPD = CAPD with <7.5 l of dialysis solution used per 24 hr.
- Standard volume CAPD = CAPD with 2.0 l exchange volume.
- High volume CAPD = CAPD with >2.0 l exchange volume.
- Low volume CAPD = CAPD with <2.0 l exchange volume.
- Standard dose CCPD = CCPD with 6–8 l of dialysis solution used overnight and 2 l daytime.
- High dose CCPD = CCPD with >8 l of dialysis solution used overnight and/or >2 l daytime.
- Standard dose DAPD = DAPD with 6.0–9.0 l of dialysis solution used per day.
- Low dose DAPD = DAPD with <6.0 l of dialysis solution used per day.
- NIPD = Nightly intermittent peritoneal dialysis – nightly peritoneal dialysis performed with intermittent flow technique.
- TPD = Tidal peritoneal dialysis.

to design peritoneal dialysis machines with a possibility of setting various sodium concentrations (eg. 120, 123, 126, 129, 132 mEq/l). Also concentrations of other electrolytes may need adjustment.

7.3. Manipulations to increase the efficiency of dialysis

7.3.1. High flow peritoneal dialysis techniques

During the IPD era, many dialysis techniques were tried to increase dialysis efficiency. The techniques are portrayed in Figures 5, 6, 7 and in Table 9.

Technique Ia, standard intermittent flow peritoneal dialysis was the usual clinical procedure prior to introduction of CAPD. In this technique, 2 l of dialysis solution at 37°C are infused by gravity over 10 min into the peritoneal cavity and allowed to equilibrate for approximately 30 min. The dialysate is then drained by gravity flow over 20 min and 2 l of fresh dialysis solution is infused immediately after previous drainage is completed. Because during infusion and drainage the peritoneal cavity is not completely filled, the average intraperitoneal fluid volume over 1 hr is approximately 1.5 l (Figure 5) and the efficiency of dialysis is not optimal during the whole cycle. It may be assumed that during an initial 5 min of inflow time and last 15 min of outflow time the average efficiency is only 50% of that during the dwell because dialysis solution is not in

contact with the whole peritoneal membrane area. Consequently, approximately 10 min (17%) out of 60 min total exchange time is lost for dialysis (Figure 5). The bulk of the theoretical models in the literature are aimed at understanding and optimizing this standard procedure. The urea and creatinine clearances reported in the literature vary widely; therefore, in Table 9 the values are presented as 100% of efficiency. Most authors (with few exceptions) compared the results of other techniques with this standard technique and the relative efficiencies of other techniques are presented as percentages of the standard technique.

In rapid intermittent peritoneal dialysis with no dwell time (Technique Ib) the drainage starts immediately after infusion, dialysate flow is doubled markedly increasing the concentration gradient between plasma and dialysate, but, with a 2 l infusion volume an average intraperitoneal volume is only 0.9 l over 1 hr. Assuming again that the full efficiency of dialysis exists only with the intraperitoneal volume exceeding 1 l, the efficient dialysis time is decreased by 20 min (34%) per hour (Figure 5). Most authors report clearances higher than those with the standard technique [17, 19, 80].

Technique Ic, rapid intermittent peritoneal dialysis with short dwell exchanges utilizes lower dialysate flows, but an efficient dialysis time is higher than in Technique Ib. Clearances are even better than with Technique Ib [17, 80]

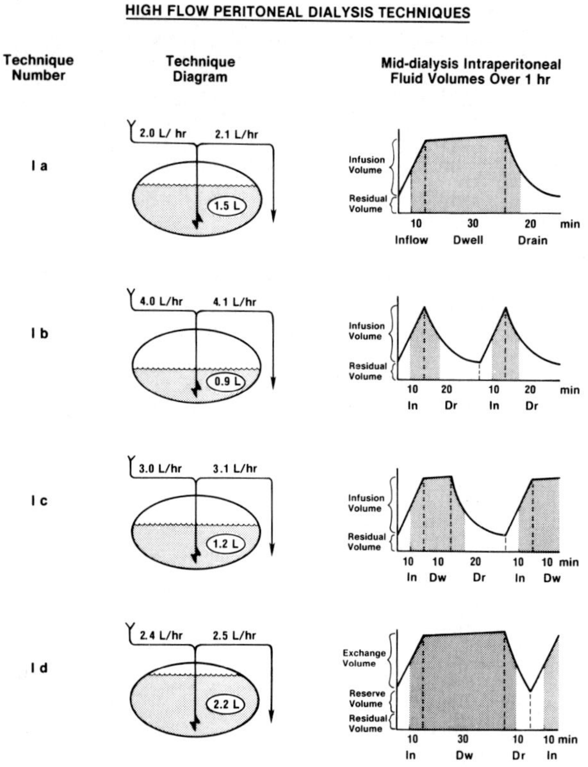

Figure 5. Intermittent peritoneal dialysis techniques with a single catheter. Technique numbers correspond to those in Table 9. Inflow and outflow rates and average intraperitoneal dialysate volumes (◯) over one hour are shown in diagrams (left). Mid-dialysis intraperitoneal fluid volumes over one hour are shown to the right. Unshaded areas under volume lines portray periods of diminished dialysis efficiency due to incompletely filled peritoneal cavity. Out of 60 min total exchange time, approximately 10 min (17%) in Technique Ia, 20 min (34%) in Technique Ib, 12 min (20%) in Technique Ic, and 5 min (8%) in Technique Id are lost for dialysis. Due to limited outflow time with Technique Id, some amount of reserve (sump) volume is created and drained only at the completion of dialysis.

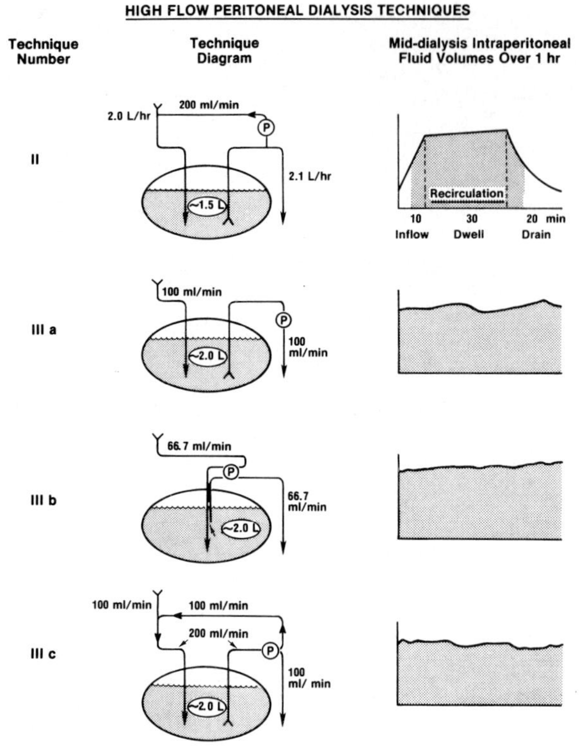

Figure 6. High flow peritoneal dialysis techniques with two catheters (Techniques II, IIIa or IIIc) or double lumen catheter (Technique IIIb). Recirculation loop added in Technique IIIc. Technique II is intermittent, others are continuous. Due to irregularities in inflow and outflow rates the intraperitoneal volumes are shown as fluctuating (right-Techniques IIIa, IIIb, and IIIc). High flows achieved with pumps (P). See Table 9, Figure 5, and text for further explanations.

which indicates that the longer full contact between the peritoneal membrane and dialysate may have substantial influence on the dialysis efficiency.

Tenckhoff [92] recommended to limit drainage times to reduce the period when the peritoneal cavity is almost empty, drainage is very slow, and no dialysis occurs. Some amount of sump volume also prevents catheter occlusiuon by the bowels and/or omentum and facilitates faster drainage. Our own unpublished observations indicate that this intermittent peritoneal dialysis with restricted outflow time (Technique Id) slightly increases the efficiency of dialysis. Indraprasit *et al.* [93] showed about 30% increases in clearances; however, they also increased dialysate flow by 25%. It is worth reiterating that unnecessarily prolonged drain time (a technique sometimes inadvertently used), markedly decreases efficiency of dialysis.

Intermittent recirculation peritoneal dialysis (Technique II) is similar to Ia except that the dialysate is recirculated during the dwell phase through two widely spaced catheters.

It was thought that this would improve solute transport by preventing stagnation of dialysate. However, Miller *et al.* [79], demonstrated a slight decrease in clearances compared to Technique Ia, the reason of which is unclear.

Continuous flow peritoneal dialysis (Technique III) employs two widely spaced catheters (Technique IIIa) [2–5, 10–12, 79, 94] or a double lumen catheter (Technique IIIb) [95]. It has been successfully used by early clinicians [2–5, 10–12, 94] until it was gradually replaced by intermittent peritoneal dialysis. To evaluate the efficiency of Technique III, Miller *et al.* [79] used two catheters and a pump for drainage (Technique IIIa), Lange *et al.* [95] used a double lumen catheter and a double pump for the inflow and drainage (Technique IIIb). In Technique IIIc, to increase mixing, the recirculation loop was added, but clearances were not higher than with Technique IIIa, probably due to fluid channeling; however, clearances were generally 30–85% better than those with Technique Ia.

Technique IV is similar to Technique III with the exception that the dialysate is regenerated in the dialyzer added into the circuit. The regeneration of fluid was expected to decrease protein losses and cost of dialysis. Shinaberger [96, 97] reported 3 times higher clearances than with the standard intermittent technique. Other authors [79, 98] did

HIGH FLOW PERITONEAL DIALYSIS TECHNIQUES

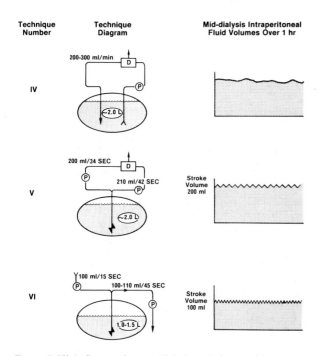

Technique Number	Technique Diagram	Mid-dialysis Intraperitoneal Fluid Volumes Over 1 hr

Figure 7. High flow peritoneal dialysis techniques with two ca-theters and dialyzer (D) for dialysate regeneration (Technique IV), single catheter and dialyzer (Technique V), and single catheter without dialyzer (Technique VI). Fluid flow rates shown in diagrams. Stroke (exchange) volume in Technique V – 200 ml; in Technique VI – 100 ml. Reserve volume drained at the completion of dialysis. See also Table 9, Figure 5, and text for explanations.

not confirm these results.

Techniques III and IV have not gained popularity because of technical difficulties. Catheters holes were frequently occluded by the bowel and/or omentum due to the suction; patients suffered pain with rapid inflows, sometimes fluid channeling actually decreased efficiency [98].

Because of these technical difficulties, the Utah group [83] introduced reciprocating peritoneal dialysis (Technique V) with a single catheter and fluid alternately infused and drained in approximately 200 ml strokes. A regeneration of fluid in a dialyzer was similar to that in Technique IV. This system also has not been accepted in clinical practice because of complexity, high cost, and a small gain in efficiency.

In studies of semi-continuous peritoneal dialysis (Technique VI) Di Paolo [99] used a single catheter, assisted inflow and outflow with pumps, and a high dialysate flow up to 50 l per 8 hr. After an initial fill with 1000–1500 ml of solution, a 100 to 110 ml portion of fluid was drained and replaced with 100 ml of fresh solution during frequent cycles. No regeneration system was used. The efficiency of the dialysis was about 50% higher than with Technique Ia. Di Paolo reported his technique in 1978 when CAPD attracted the attention of researchers and clinicians and his results have not been reevaluated. This technique can accommodate net flow rates of 6 l/hr or more with better patient tolerance and without the manipulations of patient position often required for complete drainage.

Studies in rats also showed that maintaining a fluid reservoir in the peritoneal cavity and exchanging only a portion of the fluid yields urea clearances more than 30% higher compared to the complete drainage technique at the same dialysate flows [100].

With the return of nightly peritoneal dialysis and the

Table 9. High flow peritoneal dialysis techniques in humans

	Technique	Author (ref.)	Relative clearance (%)	
			Urea	Creatinine
Ia	Standard intermittent		100	100
Ib	Rapid intermittent with no dwell	Boen [17]	125[a]	130[a]
		Miller *et al.* [79]	114	118
		Pirpasopoulos *et al.* [80]	104	107
Ic	Rapid Intermittent with short dwell	Boen [17]	130[a]	135[a]
		Pirpasopoulos *et al.* [80]	110	115
Id	Intermittent with restricted outflow time	Own unpublished	114	109
		Indraprasit *et al.* [93]	138[b]	129[b]
II	Intermittent recirculating	Miller *et al.* [79]	96	87
IIIa	Continuous	Miller *et al.* [79]	146	144
IIIb	Automatic continuous	Lange *et al.* [95]	185[c]	
IIIc	Continuous recirculating	Miller *et al.* [79]	135	155
IV	Peritoneal-extracorporeal recirculation	Shinaberger *et al.* [96, 97]	331	303
	Continuous compound	Miller *et al.* [79]	100	87
	Recirculating	Stephen *et al.* [98]	130	101
V	Reciprocating	Kablitz *et al.* [81]	129[d]	
VI	Semicontinuous	Di Paoblo [99]	145[a]	160[a]

[a] – Clearance calculated from data in figure.
[b] – One liter exchanges; dialysate flow in technique Id higher by 25% compared to Technique Ia.
[c] – Calculated from indirect data.
[d] – Compared to Technique Ib.

need of increasing dialysis efficiency, some of the techniques studied in the 1960's and 1970's may become again attractive and reevaluated.

7.3.2. Pharmacologic agents

Many drugs, given systemically or intraperitoneally, have been tried with the expectation of increasing dialysis efficiency. An extensive review of pharmacologic agents influencing peritoneal transport has recently been published [101]. Unfortunately, most agents augmenting transport of uremic toxins also increase protein losses. Further studies in this field are warranted.

8. TIDAL PERITONEAL DIALYSIS (TPD)

8.1. Theoretical background

The results of our study on NIPD efficiency [51] where we used techniques similar to Ia and Ic showed that eight hours of nightly dialysis yield creatinine clearances higher than those of 24 hr CAPD in patients with high peritoneal transport rates but lower in the remaining patients. The lower the peritoneal transport rate the lower the 8 hr NIPD creatinine clearance compared to that of 24 hr CAPD. Consequently, to match CAPD clearances, NIPD has to be prolonged by 10–40% over a usual resting time of 8 hr. Thus, the efficiency of NPD needs to be improved by 10 to 40% to make it attractive for anuric patients with high average, low average, or even low peritoneal transport characteristics.

Assuming that automatic peritoneal dialysis machines will be available in the future and the cost of dialysis will not be a limiting factor in improving its efficiency, we decided to re-evaluate some of the techniques described in Section 7.3.1. Techniques Ib, Id, and II are not promising from the efficiency point of view. Techniques III, IV and V are too complicated and technically difficult to be considered as viable options for routine home dialysis. The most promising seems to be the technique of Di Paolo.

Because of problems with high inflow and particularly outflow rates encountered by earlier investigators, as discussed in Section 7.3.1., the method has to rely on moderate flow rates. Inflow rates close to 200 ml/min and outflow rates close to 170 ml/min can be easily achieved by gravity on the PAC–X 2 cycler. With such flows and no dwell time more than 40 l of fluid may be delivered into and drained from the peritoneal cavity in eight hours.

Assuming high and constant dialysate flow, there are at least two factors determining the efficiency of dialysis with this technique: 1) the minimal volume of fluid in the peritoneal cavity assuring constant and full contact between the peritoneal membrane and dialysate (reserve volume), and 2) proper mixing of fluid in the peritoneal cavity by sufficiently high exchange or stroke or tidal volume.

Spencer and Farrel [102] found higher mass transfer area coefficients with 2 l volumes than with 1 l intraperitoneal volumes, indicating that 1 l of intraperitoneal fluid is not in full contact with the whole peritoneal surface area. Studies with 2 versus 3 l intraperitoneal volumes did not show differences in fluid-membrane contact [103, 104]. Thus, the minimal volume of fluid in the peritoneal cavity should

be higher than 1 l but need not be higher than 2 l.

Mixing is better with higher volume delivered into the peritoneal cavity with each exchange, but the maximal exchange volume is determined by the minimal reserve volume and maximum tolerable intraperitoneal fluid volume, which should not exceed 3 l.

8.2. TPD terminology

Tidal peritoneal dialysis: a technique where after an initial fill of the peritoneal cavity only a portion of dialysate is drained and replaced by fresh dialysis fluid with each cycle, leaving the majority of dialysate in constant contact with the peritoneal membrane until the end of dialysis session when the fluid is drained as completely as possible. The term tidal peritoneal dialysis was adopted from respiratory physiology. Figure 8 compares respiratory physiology and TPD glossary. Figure 9 portrays in detail volume and time terms used in TPD.

Residual volume: The volume of fluid remaining in the peritoneal cavity after the drainage is apparently complete on clinical grounds.

Reserve volume (RV): The volume of fluid above the residual volume which remains in the peritoneal cavity throughout the tidal peritoneal dialysis session.

Reservoir volume: The sum of residual and reserve volumes.

Total functional peritoneal capacity: the total intraperitoneal volume of fluid which may be accommodated by the patient without discomfort.

Tidal exchange: Inflow, dwell, and outflow during tidal peritoneal dialysis with the exception of initial fill and last drain. These terms relate to times and volumes.

Tidal inflow (fill) volume: The volume of fluid instilled into the peritoneal cavity with each cycle.

Tidal outflow (drain) volume: The volume of fluid drained from the peritoneal cavity with each cycle. Tidal drain volume equals the sum of tidal fill volume and expected volume of generated ultrafiltration per cycle.

Tidal volume (TV): the mean of tidal fill and tidal drain volumes.

Initial fill volume: The sum of reserve and tidal fill volumes

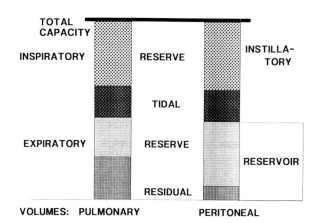

Figure 8. TPD terminology compared to that of respiratory physiology.

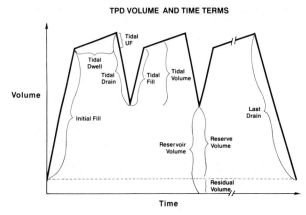

TPD VOLUME AND TIME TERMS

Figure 9. Details of volume and time terminology in TPD.

instilled at the beginning of tidal peritoneal dialysis session.

Dwell volume: The sum of tidal and reserve volumes.

Last drain volume: The volume of fluid drained at the end of TPD session. Last drain volume equals the sum of reserve volume and tidal drain volume. If residual volume remains unchanged during TPD and generated ultrafiltration equals expected ultrafiltration then last drain volume equals initial fill volume plus expected ultrafiltration volume per cycle.

Instillatory reserve volume: the difference between the total peritoneal capacity and the sum of the reservoir volume and the tidal volume.

Tidal inflow time: Time required to deliver tidal inflow volume.

Tidal outflow time: Time required to drain tidal outflow volume.

Tidal dwell time: Time from the end of tidal inflow to the beginning of tidal outflow.

Tidal exchange (cycle) time: Time from the beginning of tidal inflow to the end of tidal outflow.

NOTE: The intermittent flow peritoneal dialysis technique may be considered as a particular kind of tidal peritoneal dialysis where reserve volume equals zero.

8.3. Cycler

In collaboration with Travenol Laboratories [105] a pro-

tocol has been developed to evaluate tidal peritoneal dialysis efficiency. A PAC-X 2 cycler was redesigned but a main feature of gravity propelled flow into and from the peritoneal cavity was retained. A dual-flow peristaltic pump was used only to transfer fluid from the supply bag to the heater bag and from the drain bag to the disposal bag. The volumes were measured gravimetrically. Inflow, outflow, and dwell times could be adjusted from 1 to 9.9 min, tidal inflow volume could be adjusted from 300–1490 ml, the drain phase was regulated by a target volume.

8.4. Dialysis schedules

The study was performed in three phases: NIPD, TPD 1, and TPD 2. Each phase lasted 5 days and was performed several months apart in our dialysis clinic. One study day of CAPD was performed prior to each phase. All NIPD treatments lasted approximately 8 hr with 1.9–2.0 l exchanges of Dianeal[R] 137 solutions. A different total dialysis solution dose (TDSD) was used on each day and varied from 14–26 l. Five schedules with different TV, RV, and total dialysis solution dose (TDSD) were used in TPD 1 and TPD 2 phases as shown in Table 10. The number of exchanges varied according to tidal volumes, dwell times were adjusted according to the patients' inflow and outflow rates to keep a constant total dialysis time of 8 hr. A study group in each phase consisted of six patients; three of them had above mean (AA) and three had below mean (BA) peritoneal transport characteristics. Categorization of patients according to the peritoneal transport characteristics was based on the results of the peritoneal equilibration test, as described in Section 5.1.4. Patients with high and high average dialysate to plasma ratio for creatinine (Figure 3–D/P>0.65) were categorized as above mean (AA) in peritoneal transport characteristics, the remaining patients were categorized as below mean (BA) in peritoneal transport characteristics.

8.5. TPD efficiency

Similar to our previous study with NIPD [51], dialysis solution inflows of 17 and 26 l yielded significantly higher clearances than 14, 20, and 23 l schedules. TPD 1 schedules A and D clearances were significantly lower than those of schedules B, C, and E. TPD 2 schedule E clearances

Table 10. Tidal peritoneal dialysis (TPD) schedules

	TPD 1				TPD 2		
Schedule	TV (L)	RV (L)	TDSD (L)	Schedule	TV (L)	RV (L)	TDSD (L)
A	0.3	2.1	23.0	E	0.9	1.1	23.0
B	0.6	1.9	23.0	F	0.6	2.1	27.0
C	0.9	1.7	23.0	G	0.9	1.9	27.0
D	0.3	1.6	23.0	H	1.2	1.7	27.0
E	0.9	1.1	23.0	I	1.5	1.5	27.0

TV   – Tidal volume.
RV   – Reserve volume.
TDSD   – Total dialysis solution dose.

were significantly lower than those of other schedules. schedule I yielded the highest clearances, although not significantly different than schedules F, G, and H.

In figures, only one NIPD (261) and one TPD (1) schedule yielding the highest clearances are compared to CAPD. Urea clearances are presented in Figure 10. TPD yields 16–27% higher clearances than CAPD and 24% higher than NIPD. The gain in TPD clearances compared to CAPD is higher in AA than in BA patients. Figure 11 portrays creatinine clearances. Compared to CAPD, TPD creatinine clearances tend to be higher in AA patients, and lower in BA patients. Compared to NIPD, the TPD clearances are 10–26% higher, significantly in AA patients. Figure 12 presents ultrafiltration per glucose absorption. Ultrafiltration volume per mass of glucose absorption is markedly higher in TPD and NIPD than in CAPD, particularly in BA patients.

This preliminary study on a small group of patients indicates that TPD is approximately 20% more efficient than NIPD at similar dialysis solution inflows. Although the highest clearances in TPD were achieved with 1.5 l of both RV and TV at 27 l dialysis solution inflow, the clearances were not significantly different from those achieved with schedules F, G, and H. Tidal volumes of 300 with both reserve volumes of 2.1 and 1.6 l yielded lower clearances than those with higher tidal volumes. Thus, high tidal and reserve volumes are important for optimal efficiency. The best possible schedule has not been identified yet [105].

The difference in clearances between AA and BA patients is generally higher in TPD than in CAPD. This is not unexpected because solute gradient in the latter is dissipated early during dwell in AA patients. BA patients have the solute gradient well maintained in CAPD, thus, time of dialysis plays a more important role in efficiency than dialysate flow. BA patients have lower protein losses [105] than AA patients and these patients need higher efficiency of dialysis, thus, pharmacologic agents increasing dialysis clearances might be particularly beneficial in these patients.

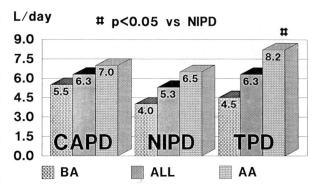

Figure 11. Mean creatinine clearances in the same patients as in Figure 10. (Based on data from ref. 105).

8.6. Technical problems

Because of the constant presence of intraperitoneal reservoir volume there are minimal difficulties with fluid outflow. With constant height of the heater and drainage bags the inflow and outflow rates depend on the height of the bed. The best flow conditions are when the height of the patient is in the middle between the heater and drainage bags (approximately 80 cm in both directions). The drainage problems occurred almost exclusively when the extension tube was obstructed (e.g. by kinking), and may occur more frequently during home dialysis at night than it was observed during the study.

Prediction of ultrafiltration is important to assure that the reserve volume remains unchanged during dialysis. If ultrafiltration volume were overestimated the reserve volume would become gradually depleted. If ultrafiltration volume were underestimated the reserve volume would gradually increase leading to decreased instillatory reserve volume and abdominal discomfort. During our study ul-

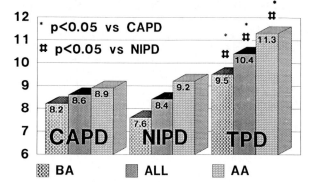

Figure 10. Mean urea clearances in 24 hr CAPD, 8 hr NIPD, and 8 hr TPD in 3 patients with below mean (BA), 3 patients with aboven mean (AA) peritoneal transport characteristics and in all (ALL) 6 patients. (Based on data from ref. 105).

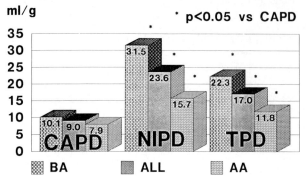

Figure 12. Mean ultrafiltration volume per mass of absorbed glucose. See legend to Figure 10 for further explanations. (Based on data from ref. 105).

trafiltration predictions were relatively precise. The highest deviations did not exceed 700 ml in either direction. The predictions were much better if the patient had at least one previous TPD session. With repeated TPD schedules for chronic dialysis, the precise ultrafiltration prediction should not be difficult.

8.7. Future of TPD

Our study indicates that TPD is approximately 20% more efficient than NIPD at dialysate flow of 3.25–3.5 l/hr.

Compared to 24 hr of CAPD, 8 hr NTPD generates sufficient ultrafiltration with a lower glucose load, renders similar protein losses, but provides inferior phosphate clearance [105]. Eight hour nightly TPD (NTPD) may provide adequate dialysis in anuric patients with above average peritoneal transport characteristics. Other anuric patients may require 9–10 hr of NTPD for adequate dialysis.

Eight hour NTPD creatinine clearances augmented by 5–20%, using pharmacologic agents or higher dialysate flows, may match those of 24 hr CAPD even in patients with low peritoneal transport rates.

REFERENCES

1. Ganter G: Ueber die Beseitigung giftiger Stoffe aus dem Blute durch Dialyse. Münch Med Wchnschr: 70: 1478–1480, 1923.
2. Rosenak S, Siwon P: Experimentelle Untersuchungen über die Peritoneale Ausscheidung harnpflichtiger Substanzen aus dem Blute. Mitt a d Grenzgeb d Med u Chir 39: 391–408, 1926.
3. Heusser H, Werder H: Untersuchungen über Peritonealdialyse. Bruns Beiträge z klin Chir 141: 38–49, 1927.
4. Balázs J, Rosenak S: Zur Behandlung der Sublimatanurie durch peritoneale Dialyse. Wien Med Wchnschr 47: 851–854, 1934.
5. Wear JB, Sisk IR, Trinkle AJ: Peritoneal lavage in the treatment of uremia. J Urol 39: 53–62, 1938.
6. Bliss S, Kastler AO, Nadler SB: Peritoneal lavage. Effective elimination of nitrogenous wastes in the absence of kidney function. Proc Soc Exp Biol Med 29: 1078–1079, 1932.
7. Haam v E, Fine A: Effect of peritoneal lavage in acute uremia. Proc Soc Exp Biol Med 30: 396–398, 1932.
8. Rhoads JE: Peritoneal lavage in the treatment of renal insufficiency. Am J Med Sci 196: 642–647, 1938.
9. Abbott WE, Shea P: The treatment of temporary renal insufficiency by peritoneal lavage. Am J Med Sci 211: 312–319, 1946.
10. Frank HA, Seligman AM, Fine J: Further experiences with peritoneal irrigation for acute renal failure. Ann Surg 128: 561–608, 1948.
11. Odel HM, Ferris DO, Power MH: Peritoneal lavage as an effective means of extrarenal excretion. A clinical appraisal. Am J Med 9: 63–77, 1950.
12. Legrain M, Merrill JP: Short-term continuous transperitoneal dialysis: A simplified technique. N Engl J Med 248: 125–129, 1953.
13. Ascari S, Morales P, Hotchkiss RS: Peritoneal dialysis. NY State J Med 59: 1981–1985, 1959.
14. Grollman A, Turner LB, McLean JA: Intermittent peritoneal lavage in nephrectomized dogs and its application to the human being. Arch Int Med 87: 379–390, 1951.
15. Doolan PD, Murphy WP, Wiggins RA, Carter NW, Cooper WC, Watten RH, Alpen EL: An evaluation of intermittent peritoneal lavage. Amer J Med 26: 831–844, 1959.
16. Maxwell MH, Rockney RE, Kleeman CR, Twiss MR: Peritoneal dialysis. I. Technique and applications. JAMA 170: 917–924, 1959.
17. Boen ST: Kinetics of peritoneal dialysis. Medicine, Balt. 40: 243–287, 1961.
18. Boen ST, Mulinari AS, Dillard DH, Scribner BH: Periodic peritoneal dialysis in the management of chronic uremia. Trans Am Soc Artif Intern Organs 8: 256–262, 1962.
19. Tenckhoff H, Ward G, Boen ST: The influence of dialysate volume and flow rate on peritoneal clearance. Proc Eur Dial Transpl Assoc 2: 113–117, 1965.
20. Tenckhoff H, Schilipetar G, Boen ST: One year experience

with home peritoneal dialysis. Trans Am Soc Artif Intern Organs 11: 11–14, 1965.
21. Tenckhoff H, Schechter H: A bateriologically safe peritoneal access device. Trans Am Soc Artif Intern Organs 14: 181–186, 1968.
22. Tenckhoff H, Schilipetar G, Van Paasschen WH, Swanson E: A home peritoneal dilaysate delivery system. Trans Am Soc Artif Intern Organs 15: 103–107, 1969.
23. Tenckhoff H, Meston B, Shilipetar G: A simplified automatic peritoneal dialysis system. Trans Am Soc Artif Intern Organs 18: 436–439, 1972.
24. Tenckhoff H: Peritoneal dialysis today: A new look. Nephron 12: 420–436, 1974.
25. Von Hartitzsch B, Medlock TR: Chronic peritoneal dialysis – a regime comparable to conventional hemodialysis. Trans Am Soc Artif Intern Organs 22: 595–597, 1976.
26. Diaz-Buxo JA, Chandler JT, Farmer CD, Smith DL: Chronic peritoneal dialysis at home – a comparison with hemodialysis. Trans Am Soc Artif Intern Organs 23: 191–193, 1977.
27. Diaz-Buxo JA, Haas VF: The influence of automated peritoneal dialysis in an established dialysis program. Dial Transpl 8: 531–533, 1979.
28. Fenton SSA, Cattran DC, Barnes NM, Waugh KJ: Home peritoneal dialysis. A major advance in promoting home dialysis. Trans Am Soc Artif Intern Organs 23: 194–200, 1977.
29. Gutman RA: Automated peritoneal dialysis for home use. Q J Med 47: 261–280, 1978.
30. Annual Report to Congress-End Stage Renal Disease Program, Health Care Financing Administration, Department of Health, Education and Welfare. Baltimore, Maryland, 1979.
31. End Stage Renal Disease Program Highlights, 1986. Data Summary distributed by Health Care Financing Administration, Washington, DC, 1987.
32. Ahmad S, Gallagher N, Shen FH: Intermittent peritoneal dialysis: Status reassessed. Trans Am Soc Artif Intern Organs 25: 86–88, 1979.
33. Schmidt RW, Blumenkrantz MJ: IPD, CAPD, CCPD, CRPD-Peritoneal dialysis: Past, present and future. Int J Artif Organs 4: 124–129, 1981.
34. Ghantous WN, Salkin MS, Adelson BN, Ghantous S, McGinnis K, Valenziano A, Cronin M: Limitations of peritoneal dialysis (PD) in the treatment of ESRD patients. Trans Am Soc Artif Intern Organs 25: 100–103, 1979.
35. Pendras JP, Erickson RV: Hemodialysis: a successful therapy for chronic uremia. Ann Intern Med, 64: 293–311, 1966.
36. Twardowski Z: The adequacy of haemodialysis in treatment of chronic renal failure. Acta Med Pol, 15: 227–243, 1974.
37. Babb AL, Strand MJ, Uvelli DA, Milutinovic J, Scribner BH: Quantitative description of dialysis treatment: a dialysis index. Kidney Int 7(Suppl 2): S-23–S-29, 1975.
38. Johnson WJ, Schniepp BJ: Comparison of urea kinetic modeling with other approaches to dialysis prescription. Dial Transplant 10: 280–284, 1981.
39. Teschan PE, Ginn HE, Bourne JR, Ward JW, Schaffer JD:

A prospective study of reduced dialysis. ASAIO J, 6: 108–122, 1983.

40. Boen ST, Haagsma-Schouten WAG, Birnie RJ: Long-term peritoneal dialysis and a peritoneal dialysis-index. Dial Transplant 7: 377–380, 1978.

41. Twardowski Z, Lebek R, Hakuba A, Klosowski B, Nowak H, Orawski L: Treatment of chronic irreversible renal insufficiency by means of repeated peritoneal dialysis. Acta Med Pol 11: 343–362, 1970.

42. Boyer J, Gill GN, Epstein FH: Hyperglycemia and hyperosmolality complicating peritoneal dialysis. Ann Intern Med 67: 568–572, 1967.

43. Miller RB, Tassistro CR: Peritoneal dialysis. New Engl J Med 281: 945–949, 1969.

44. Gault MH, Ferguson EL, Sidhu JS, Corbin RP: Fluid and electrolyte complications of peritoneal dialysis. Choice of dialysis solutions. Ann Intern Med 75: 253–262, 1971.

45. Nolph KD, Hano JE, Teschan PE: Peritoneal sodium transport during hypertonic peritoneal dialysis: Physiologic mechanisms and clinical implications. Ann Intern Med 70: 931–941, 1969.

46. Ahearn DJ, Nolph KD: Controlled sodium removal with peritoneal glucose transport during peritoneal dialysis. Trans Am Soc Artif Int Organs 17: 423–428, 1972.

47. Tenckhoff H: Choice of peritoneal dialysis solutions. Ann Intern Med 75: 313–314, 1971.

48. Vidt DG: Recommendations on choice of peritoneal dialysis solutions. Ann Intern Med 78: 144–146, 1973.

49. Shen FH, Sherrard DJ, Scollard D, Merrit A, Curtis FK: Thirst, relative hypernatremia and excessive weight gain in maintenance peritoneal dialysis. Trans Am Soc Artif Intern Organs 24: 142–145, 1978.

50. Oreopoulos DG, Khanna R, McCready W, Katirtzoglou A, Vas S: Continuous ambulatory peritoneal dialysis in Canada. Dial Transpl 9: 224–226, 1980.

51. Twardowski ZJ, Nolph KD, Khanna R, Gluck Z, Prowant BF, Ryan LP: Daily clearances with continuous ambulatory peritoneal dialysis and nightly peritoneal dialysis. Trans Am Soc Artif Intern Organs 32: 575–580, 1986.

52. Twardowski ZJ, Khanna R, Nolph KD: Peritoneal dialysis modifications to avoid CAPD dropouts. In: Khanna R *et al.* (eds). Advances in Continuous Ambulatory Peritoneal Dialysis. Proceedings of the Seventh Annual CAPD Conference, Kansas City, Missouri, February 1987. Peritoneal Dialysis Bulletin, Inc., Toronto. pp 171–178, 1987.

53. Twardowski Z, Ksiazek A, Majdan M, Janicka L, Bochenska-Nowacka E, Sokolowska G, Gutka A, Zbikowska H: Kinetics of continuous ambulatory peritoneal dialysis /CAPD/ with four exchanges per day. Clin Nephrol 15: 119–131, 1981.

54. Vas SI: Microbiologic aspects of chronic ambulatory peritoneal dialysis. Kidney Int 23: 83–92, 1983.

55. Vas SI: Peritonitis. In: Nolph KD (ed), Peritoneal Dialysis. Martinus Nijhoff Publishers. Boston/Dordrecht/Lancaster. Second Edition pp 403–439, 1985.

56. Twardowski ZJ, Khanna R, Nolph KD: Osmotic agents and ultrafiltration in peritoneal dialysis. Nephron 42: 93–101, 1986.

57. Grodstein GP, Blumenkrantz MJ, Kopple JD, Moran JK, Coburn JW: Glucose absorption during continuous ambulatory peritoneal dialysis. Kidney Int 19: 564–567, 1981.

58. Oreopoulos DG, Clayton S, Dombros N, Zellerman G, Katirtzoglou A: Experiences with continuous ambulatory peritoneal dialysis (CAPD). Trans Am Soc Artif Internal Organs 25: 95–97, 1979.

59. Heide B, Pierratos A, Khanna R, Pettit J, Ogilvie R, Harrison J, McNeil K, Siccion Z, Oreopoulos DG: Nutritional status of patients undergoing continuous ambulatory peritoneal dialysis. Perit Dial Bull 3: 138–141, 1983.

60. Chan MK, Baillod RA, Tanner A, Raftery M, Sweny P,

Fernando ON, Moorhead JF: Abdominal hernias in patients receiving continuous ambulatory peritoneal dialsyis. Br Med J 283: 826–826, 1981.

61. Jorkasky D. Goldfarb S: Abdominal wall hernia complicating chronic ambulatory peritoneal dialysis. Am J Nephrol 2: 323–324, 1982.

62. Rubin J, Raju S, Teal N, Hellems E, Bower JD: Abdominal hernias in patients undergoing continuous ambulatory peritoneal dialysis. Arch Intern Med 142: 1453–1455, 1982.

63. Gloor HJ, Nichols WK, Sorkin MI, Prowant B, Kennedy JM, Baker B, Nolph KD: Peritoneal access and related complications in continuous ambulatory peritoneal dialysis. Am J Med 74: 593–598, 1983.

64. Digenis GD, Khanna R, Mathews R, Oreopoulos DG: Abdominal hernias in patients undergoing continuous ambulatory peritoneal dialysis. Peritoneal Dial Bull 2: 115–117, 1982.

65. Spinowitz B, Leggio A, Galler M, Golden R, Rascoff J, Charytan C: Prognostic indicators of hernia development in patients undergoing CAPD. In: Maher JF, and Winchester JF (eds). Frontiers in Peritoneal Dialysis. Proceedings of the III International Symposium on Peritoneal Dialysis. Washington, D.C., 1984, published by Field, Rich & Assoc. Inc., New York, NY, 519–520, 1986.

66. Diaz-Buxo JA: Continuous cyclic peritoneal dialysis. In: Nolph KD (ed), Peritoneal dialysis, Martinus Nijhoff Publishers. Boston/Dordrecht/Lancaster. Second editionn pp 247–266, 1985.

67. Khanna R, Oreopoulos DG, Dombros N, Vas S, Williams P, Meema HE, Husdan H, Ogilvie R, Zellerman G, Roncari DAK, Clayton S, Izatt S: Continuous ambulotory peritoneal dialysis after three years: Still a promising treatment. Peritoneal Dial Bull 1: 24–34, 1981.

68. Twardowski ZJ, Tully RJ, Nichols WK, Sunderrajan S: Computerized tomography in the diagnosis of subcutaneous leak sites during continuous ambulatory peritoneal dialysis ((CAPD). Perit Dial Bull 4: 163–166, 1984.

69. Khanna R, Oreopoulos DG: Peritoneal access using the Toronto Western Hospital permanent catheter. Perspectives in Peritoneal Dialysis 1(No. 2): 4–6, 1983.

70. Fisher J, Calkins WG: Spontaneous umbilical hernia rupture. A report of three cases. Am J Gastroenterol 69: 689–693, 1978.

71. Twardowski ZJ, Prowant BF, Nolph KD, Martinez AJ, Lampton LM: High volume, low frequency continuous ambulatory peritoneal dialysis. Kidney Int 23: 64–70, 1983.

72. Diaz-Buxo JA: CCPD is even better than CAPD. Kidney Int 28:(Suppl. 17): S-26–S-28, 1985.

73. Guazzi M, Polese A, Magrini F, Florentine C, Olivari MT: Negative influences of ascites on the cardiac function of cirrhotic patients. Am J Med 59: 165–170, 1975.

74. Twardowski ZJ, Khanna R, Nolph KD, Scalamogna A, Metzler MH, Schneider TW, Prowant BF, Ryan LP: Intraabdominal pressure during natural activities in patients treated with continuous ambulatory peritoneal dialysis. Nephron 44: 129–135, 1986.

75. Hamodraka-Mailis A: Pathogenesis and treatment of back pain in peritoneal dialysis patients. Perit Dial Bull 3(Suppl 3): S-41–S-43, 1983.

76. Khanna R, Twardowski ZJ, Gluck Z, Ryan LP, Nolph KD: Is nightly peritoneal dialysis (NPD) an effective peritoneal dialysis schedule? Abstracts, American Society of Nephrology – Kidney Int 29: 233, 1986.

77. Nolph KD, Twardowski ZJ, Khanna R: Clinical pathology conference: Peritoneal dialysis. Trans Am Soc Artif Intern Organs 32: 11–16, 1986.

78. Scribner BH: Forward to second ediiton. In: Nolph KD (ed), Peritoneal Dialysis. Martinus Nijhoff Publishers. Boston/Dordrecht/Lancaster. Second edition. pp XI–XII, 1985.

79. Miller JH, Gipstein R, Margules R, Swartz M, Rubini ME: Automated peritoneal dialysis: analysis of several methods of peritoneal dialysis. Trans Am Soc Artif Intern Organs 12: 98–105, 1966.

80. Pirpasopoulos M, Lindsay RM, Rahman M, Kennedy AC: A cost-effectiveness study of dwell times in peritoneal dialysis. Lancet 2: 1135–1136,, 1972.

81. Kablitz C, Stephen RL, Duffy DP, Jacobsen SC, Zelman A, Kolff WJ: Technological augmentation of peritoneal urea clearance: past, present, and future. Dial & Transpl 9(8): 741–778, 1980.

82. Garred LJ, Canaud B, Farrell PC: A simple kinetic model for assessing peritoneal mass transfer in continuous ambulatory peritoneal dialysis. ASAIO J, 6: 131–137, 1983.

83. Popovich RP, Moncrief JW: Transport kinetics. In: Nolph KD (ed), Peritoneal dialysis. Martinus Nijhoff Publishers. Boston/Dordrecht/Lancaster. Second Edition pp 115–158, 1985.

84. Hiatt MP, Pyle WK, Moncrief JW, Popovich RP: A comparison of the relative efficacy of CAPD and hemodialysis in the control of solute concentration. Artif Organs 4: 37–43, 1980.

85. Twardowski ZJ, Nolph KD, Khanna R, Prowant BF, Ryan LP, Moore HL, Nielsen MP: Peritoneal equilibration test. Perit Dial Bull 7: 138–147, 1987.

86. Omong SH, Vellar OD: Analytical error due to concentration gradients in frozen and thawed samples. Clin Chim Acta, 49: 125–126, 1973.

87. Ahmad S, Shen FH, Blagg CR: Intermittent peritoneal dialysis as renal replacement therapy. In: Nolph KD (ed), Peritoneal Dialysis. Martinus Nijhoff Publishers. Boston/Dordrecht/Lancaster. Second edition. pp 179–208, 1985.

88. Diaz-Buxo JA, Chandler JT, Farmer CD, Walker PJ, Holt KL, Burgess WP, Orr SL: Long-term observations of peritoneal clearances in patients undergoing peritoneal dialysis. ASAIO J 6: 21–25, 1983.

89. Twardowski ZJ: Apparently inadequate peritoneal membrane function for solute removal. In: Nissenson AR and Fine RN (eds), Dialysis therapy. Hanley and Belfus, Inc. Philadelphia, The CV Mosby Company, St. Louis, Toronto, London pp 134–137, 1986.

90. Twardowski ZJ: Individualized dialysis for CAPD patient: a review of the experience at the University of Missouri. Uremia Investigation 8(1): 35–43, 1984.

91. Townsend R, Fragola JA: Hydrothorax in a patient receiving continuous ambulatory peritoneal dialysis: successful treatment with intermittent peritoneal dialysis. Arch Intern Med 142: 1571–1572, 1982.

92. Tenckhoff H: Chronic peritoneal dialysis – a manual for patients, dialysis personnel and physicians, Division of Kidney Diseases, Department of Medicine, University of Washington, School of Medicine, Seattle, WA p. 76, 1974.

93. Indraprasit S, Taramas W, Panpakde O: Complete dialysate drainage: an unnecessary step in intermittent peritoneal dialysis. Perit Dial Bull 5: 233–236, 1985.

94. Weiss HA, Mills RL: Treatment of uremia with continuous peritoneal irrigation. US Nav Med Bull 46: 1745–1750, 1946.

95. Lange K, Treser K, Mangalat J: Automatic continuous high flow rate peritoneal dialysis. Archiv f Klin Med 214: 201–206, 1968.

96. Shinaberger JH, Shear L, Barry KG: Increasing efficiency of peritoneal dialysis. Trans Am Soc Artif Internn Organs 11: 76–82, 1965.

97. Shinaberger JH, Shear L, Barry KG: Peritoneal-extracorporeal recirculation dialysis: a technique for improving efficiency of peritoneal dialysis. Invest Urol 2: 555–560, 1965.

98. Stephen RL, Atkin-Thor E, Kolff WJ: Recirculating peritoneal dialysis with subcutaneous catheter. Trans Am Soc Artif Intern Organs 22: 575–584, 1976.

99. Di Paolo N: Semicontinuous peritoneal dialysis. Dial & Transpl 7: 839–842, 1978.

100. Finkelstein FO, Kliger AS: Enhanced efficiency of peritoneal dialysis using rapid, small-volume exchanges. ASAIO J 2: 103–106, 1979.

101. Maher JF, Hirszel P: Pharmacologic manipulation of peritoneal transport. In: Nolph KD (ed), Peritoneal Dialysis. Martinus Nijhoff Publishers. Boston/Dordrecht/Lancaster. Second edition. pp 267–296, 1985.

102. Spencer PC, Farrell PC: Applications of kinetic monitoring in CAPD. In: Continuous ambulatory peritoneal dialysis. In: Weimar W, Fieren MWJA, Diderich PPNN (eds), Proceedings of the Fourth Benelux Symposium, Rotterdam, November 24, op de Hoek CT. pp 9–23, 1984.

103. Twardowski ZJ, Nolph KD, Prowant BF, Moore HL: Efficiency of high volume low frequency continuous ambulatory peritoneal dialysis (CAPD). Trans Am Soc Artif Intern Organs, 29: 53–57, 1983.

104. Krediet RT, Boeschoten EW, Zuyderhoudt FMJ, Arisz L: Differences in the peritoneal transport of water, solutes and proteins between dialysis with two-and with three-litre exchanges. In: Krediet RT: Permeability in Continuous Ambulatory Peritoneal Dialysis Patients. (Thesis) University of Amsterdam, pp 129–146, 1986.

105. Twardowski ZJ, Nolph KD, Khanna R, Prowant BF, Frock J, Dobbie J, Serkes K, Kenley R, Witsoe D, Garber J: Tidal peritoneal dialsyis. Proceedings of the IVth Congress of the International Society for Peritoneal Dialysis. Venice, Italy, June 29 – July 2, 1987 (in press).

CONTINUOUS AMBULATORY PERITONEAL DIALYSIS (CAPD)

JACK W. MONCRIEF and ROBERT P. POPOVICH

1. INTRODUCTION

Continuous Ambulatory Peritoneal Dialysis is the most common form of home dialysis and has become an increasingly utilized alternative method of treatment for patients with end-stage renal disease both in the United States and throughout the world (Figure 1). The increased patient population and renewed scientific interest in peritoneal dialysis is reflected in a major upsurge in scientific publications related to this procedure. A simultaneous decline in the use of home hemodialysis has occurred, and is probably attributable to the tremendous growth in CAPD.

Many of the advantages originally reported with the use of CAPD have been confirmed with large population studies. This includes ease of blood pressure control, improved erythropoesis, stable salt and water balance, decrease dietary restriction, and ease of training and management [1]. This rather spectacular growth has occurred in spite of the continued presence of problems with recurrent infections associated with peritoneal access in the form of catheter exit site and tunnel infections. Recurrent peritonitis is presently felt to be primarily related with these access problems.

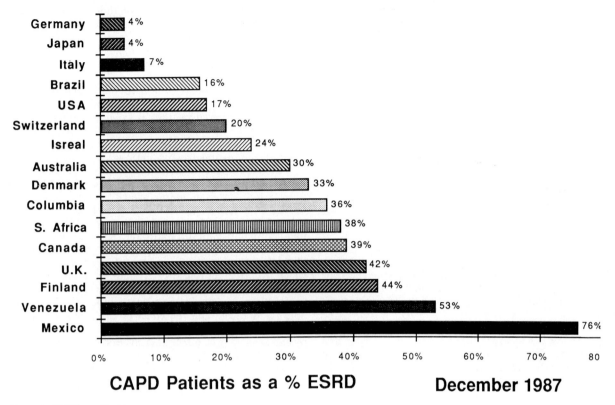

CAPD Patients as a % ESRD   December 1987

Figure 1. CAPD worldwide.

2. CONCEPTS OF CAPD

2.1. Total drain volume and molecular size

2.1.1. Urea removal
The concept of continuous ambulatory peritoneal dialysis modeled by Popovich and Moncrief [2–5] utilizes the smallest volume of dialysate, i.e. lowest dialysate flow ratem, to achievbe the goal of preventing uremia. The remarkable decrease in dialysate volume allows portability during the procedure (Table 1) [6, 7].

If two liters of dialysis solution are placed in the peritoneal cavity and the dwell times extended to allow equilibration (Figure 2), the drained volume of dialysate will then equal trhe urea clearance. If one assumes that adequate urea dialysis is achieved when the blood urea nitrogen is maintained at 70 mg%, the dialysis drained volumes which have equilibrated with the blood urea nitrogen will have 700 mg urea notrogen/l. Urea nitrogen generation in the average 70 kg/man, on a one gram of protein per kilogram body weight diet, will be 7000 mg/day. It is possible, therefore, to remove this quantity of urea nitrogen with a total of 10 l of drained volume if each liter is equilibrated with the blood urea nitrogen of 70 mg%. This can technically be accomplished by the following steps:

1. Infuse two liters of dialysis solution into the peritoneal cavity.
2. Extend the dwell time to allow equilibration of urea nitrogen.
3. Drain this volume and infuse two liters of fresh solution.
4. Exchange the volume four times a day at convenient intervals.
5. Adjust the solution tonicity to produce two liters of ultrafiltrate (two–1.5% glucose, two 4.25% glucose), to achieve a total drained volume of ten liters/day.

The procedure which will adequately remove small molecules (i.e. 60 mw urea) is, therefore, defined. Larger infusion volumes (2.5–3.0 liters) may allow less frequent exchanges and achieve similar results [8]. Increased intra-

Table 1. Calculation of minimal dialysate volume for adequate urea dialysis

Minimal dialysate volume	= Dialysate volume equilibrated with blood urea nitrogen
(Assume – acceptable blood urea nitrogen	= 70 mg%)
Dialysate urea nitrogen concentration	= 700 mg/l
(Measured – urea nitrogen generation rate	= 7.0 g/day)
Minimal dialysate volume	= 10 l/day

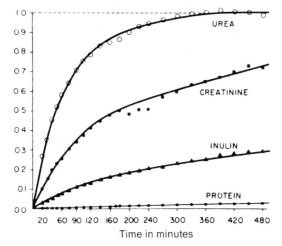

Figure 2. Dialysate concentration, plasma concentration.

abdominal pressure may produce higher incidences of hernias, respiratory embarrassment and pain on infusion, but many patients tolerate these volumes without complications [8].

2.1.2. *Creatinine removal*

When the procedure is evaluated for its efficacy in removing creatinine, it is seen that the larger molecular size (113 daltons) increases resistance of creatinine transfer from the blood to the dialysate compartment (Figure 2). The prolonged dwell time does not reduce the efficiency of creatinine removal as greatly as it does that of urea. Therefore, the procedure is more efficient for the removal of creatinine when compared to urea. Dialysis of creatinine will accrue throughout the prolonged dwell time, and though the rate of creatinine movement from the blood into the dialysate decreases progressively as the concentration gradient between blood and dialysate is lost, dialysis of creatinine continues for 7–8 hr as opposed to urea. In the latter case, dialysis virtually stop at the end of 2–3 hr. CAPD is, therefore, not continuous ambulatory urea dialysis but is continuous ambulatory creatinine dialysis.

2.1.3. *'Middle molecule' removal*

As the molecules of interest increase in weight, higher efficiency is seen with the prolonged dwell time. A molecule of 5200 daltons (inulin) will diffuse from the blood compartment into the dialysate very slowly, and the concentration gradient between the blood and the dialysate will be maintained for an extended period (Figure 2). A single exchange made every twelve hours will produce excellent removal of this size molecule. CAPD is approximately six times better at removing inulin size molecules than is intermittent hemodialysis for 15 hr a week [9, 10].

2.2. Ultrafiltration rate

Although many factors effect ultrafiltration rates during peritoneal dialysis [11–14] – osmotic gradient between blood and dialysate; peritoneal membrane thickness; status of vasoconstriction; hydration of the peritoneal membrane; and total infused volume [15, 16] – the present clinically

controllable factor is the dialysis solution tonicity [17]. As tonicity increases, ultrafiltration rate proportionately increases. Glucose is the osmotic agent in commercially available solutions, and upon instillation of a hypertonic solution of 4.25% glucose, an immediate ultrafiltration rate of approximately 15 to 25 ml/min will occur. As glucose is simultaneously transferred from the dialysate to the blood siude, tonicity will diminish and the ultrafiltration rate will fall proportionately. This transfer will occur at a gradually decreasing rate (related to the concentration gradient between blood and dialysate) and total ultrafiltration will occur over approximately the first 2–4 hr.

A similar but less dramatic ultrafiltration will occur with instillation of a 2.5% or 1.5% glucose solution, and isotonicity will occur at approximately 2–4 hr. The total ultrafiltered volume with instillation of 2000 ml of 1.5% glucose solution will be approximately 300 ml. Five to seven hundred milliliters of ultrafiltration will occur with use of 2000 ml of 2.5% glucose solution. As isotonicity between blood and dialysate is achieved, the reverse flow of isotonic water from the peritoneal cavity into the blood vascular space will occur at a rate of 1 ± 0.5 ml/min [17]. This reverse flow is important in evaluating total volume available for drainage and the effect of the prolonged dwell time. As dwell time increases, drained volume will decrease by approximately 60 ml/hr after the first two to four hours of osmotically controlled ultrafiltration.

There are reports of progressive reversible and irreversible decline in ultrafiltration rate and volume. Some of these appear to be related to peritonitis [18, 19]. A series of reports from Europe indicate that this problem is unrelated to peritonitis [20–23]. There is survey evidence that this problem is limited to patients using fluid manufactured in Europe [24]. Non-glucose osmotic agents are being evaluated but non are clinically available in the United States [25]. Maher has reported a selective incidence in peritoneal ultrafiltration with the addition of Amphotericin B [26]. Diaz-Buxo has reported a decrease in peritoneal clearance in patients with hyperparathyroidism [21]. Increase in solute transport in laboratory animals has been described with the addition of protamine to dialysis solution [27–29] and with dipyridimol by mouth in humans [30]. Verapamil has also been reported to increase ultrafiltration [31, 32]. Mactier and co-workers have reported subdiaphragmatic lymphatic transport of water which substantially affects the recoverable ultrafiltration in CAPD [33].

Dialysis solution with glucose concentrations of 1.5%, 2.5%, 3.5%, and 4.25% are now available for improved control of desired volume of ultrafiltrate. The advantage of these solution concentrations is that they avoid the intermittent symptom of distention frequently created by 4.25% glucose solutions.

2.3. Clinical application of water flux data

2.3.1. *Number of exchanges*

How many exchanges are required to adequately perform CAPD [6, 7]? The primary factor which controls the efficiency of the procedure relative to small molecule removal is not the number of exchanges but the drained volume. The number of exchanges per day is only tangentially related to the total drained volume. If tthree 2 l exchanges of 4.25% glucose solution are performed each day, the total drained volume will be approximately 9 l. If four 2 l exchanges of 1.5% glucose solution are performed per 24 hr, approximately 8 l of drained volume will be achieved.

As the drained volume is decreased from 10–8 l/day, there is some temporary sacrifice in total urea removal (approximately 1.4 g the first day) and urea nitrogen will stabilize at a slightly higher level before removal will again equal production. There is less sacrifice in the removal of creatinine with a decrease in drained volume from 10–8 l/day. The serum creatinine will stabilize approximately 1.5 mg % higher (12.5 ± 1.5 mg % versus 14 ± 1.5 mg %). A 'middle molecule' of 5500 daltons will be removed at approximately the same rate with a drained volume of 10 l/day as compared to 8 l/day. As drained volume (flow rate) requirements are clinically defined, the 'middle molecule' hypothesis should be confirmed or disproved [10, 34].

2.3.2. Dialysis solution tonicity
Vigorous removal of excess salt and water may be used to control edema and hypertension. This can be accomplished rapidly by increasing the frequency of exchanges or through the use of hypertonic solutions.

If intravascular volume depletion or orthostatic hypotension occurs, the patient may be instructed to skip a single exchange. This will prolong the dwell tieme to approximately 10–12 hr and produce an infusion of 60 ml/hr from the abdominal reservoir into the blood vascular space and re-expand the blood volume. This can prevent the need for intravenous fluids. Only a minimal and temporary sacrifice in the dialysis of small molecules will occur.

2.3.3. Glucose absorption
The total glucose absorbed during CAPD depends on the number, and glucose concentration, of the exchanges [35, 36]. If 2 l of 4.25% glucose solution are used twice per day and 2 l of 1.5% glucose solution used twice per day, approximately 900 calories of glucose will be absorbed per 24 hr [35, 37]. Other types of osmotically active agents are being evaluated [38–40]. There is suspicion that this large glucose load is etiologically related to the frequency of obesity and hypertriglyceridemia in patients undergoing CAPD [41].

2.4. Sodium and water balance

Rapid ultrafiltration associated with hypertonic glucose solutions will cause movement of sodium-free water from the blood vascular space into the peritoneal cavity [42]. Hypernatremia will occur if this ultrafiltration continues at a rapid rate. The prolonged dwell time of continuous ambulatory peritoneal dialysis allows near total equilibration between the concentration of sodium in the blood and the dialysate. Thus, 2 l of ultrafiltrate per day will produce a negative sodium balance of 240–280 mEq. This may allow the patient an unrestricted sodium chloride diet.

Since this ultrafiltration volume is a function of the tonicity of the solution used, and the procedure itself is not 'smart', the prescription for the tonicity of the solution must be adjusted to accommodate for the salt and water

ingested by the patient. If rapid ultrafiltration with hypertonic glucose solutions is carried out continuously (each 30 to 60 min), the increased serum sodium will stimulate thirst. A water drinking – ultrafiltration cycle may occur. This may be seen in the early training days during which rapid removal of salt and water is initiated to control blood pressure.

As gradual ultrafiltration procedures salt and water depletion, the intravascular volume will contract and blood pressure will be controlled [43, 44]. The need for antihypertensive medication can often be eliminated simply by continued removal of more salt and water than is ingested until the blood pressure is normal. CAPD allows the body weight to be maintained at a specific level throughout the day. The effects of angiotensin, norepinephrine, and renin do not prevent blood pressure decline produced by intravascular volume depletion, but only narrow the range of weight fluctuation which may occur before hypertension or orthostatic hypotension will occur.

Some patients will require small doses of antihypertensive medication to prevent hypertension. These medications, however, should not be allowed to substitute for adequate management of salt and water balance. There are also a few patients in whom troublesome hypotension will occur in spite of clinical salt and water expansion, including clinical edema. The ideology of this hypotension, usually orthostatic in nature, is not well understood and occurs most commonly in older females.

2.5. Potassium balance

CAPD will prevent most of the signs and symptoms of uremia and move a patient from a state of ESRD to approximately 8–10 ml/min of urea clearance. It is obvious, however, that the limits of the procedure will pose some constraints on the patient's dietary discretion. These limitations are most significant for sodium, water, potassium, and phosphate.

Though it is unusual for any potassium intake to exceed the ability of the procedure to remova potassium, hyperkalemia may occur. On a clinical basis, however, hyperkalemia is uncommon, and a superficial dietary survey will demonstrate the etiology of the potassium load (i.e. two quarts of orange juice per day). Access to potassium within certain limits is prescribed for the patient undergoing the procedure, but frequent serum potassium evaluation during the early training phase should be performed to detect indiscretion.

The amount of potassium removed by the dialysis procedure itself is not adequate to explain the absence of hyperkalemia. In fact, the concentration of potassium in the dialysate is almost invariably lower than the serum potassium [45]. There is, however, an increased quantity of potassium found in the stool [45, 46], an increased total body potassium, and an increased muscle mass associated with anabolism [47, 48]. This combination may serve to explain the absence of the hyperkalemia. A rapid increase in serum potassium does occur in some patients who are temporarily taken off CAPD, and close attention to dietary restriction and potassium evaluation should be paid if CAPD is even temporarily discontinued (12 to 24 hr).

2.6. Phosphare balance

The concentration of phosphate in the drained volume following an eight hour, overnight dwell time is near the serum level of phosphate and can be used as a measure of serum phosphate without resorting to blood sampling [49]. Phosphate dialysis is better with CAPD than with intermittent hemodialysis and many patients require only modest doses (relative to hemodialysis patients) of aluminum hydroxide to maintain acceptabele serum phosphate levels [49–51]. Since calcium carbonate is itself a phosphate binding agent and some patients require calcium supplement to maintain a calcium balance, calcium carbonate may be considered for phosphate control when necessary and may be preferred [50, 52].

Calcium carbonate and calcium citrate are being increasingly recommended as phosphate binding agents as the complications of aluminum and its association with dialysis dementia, progressive osteomalacia, and hypercalcaemia are better understood [53–60].

2.7. Protein loss

High protein diets (1.2 to 1.5 g protein/kg body weight/day) have been recommended because of the protein losses in the dialysate [34, 61–64]. This ranges between 3 and 20 g of protein loss/24 hr. The increased losses occur in patients with recurrent peritonitis [65]. In patients without peritonitis, 3–6 g of protein loss/24 hr has been documented [63]. Positive nitrogen balance has been demonstrated in patients on minimally restricted protein diets [67–69]. As little as 700 mg/kg body weight may allow protein anabolism in some patients [67, 68, 70]. Therefore, protein intakes in excess of 1.0 to 1.5 g/kg do not appear necessary and may increase the requirement for aluminum hydroxide or other phosphate binding agents. Dietary education encouraging the ingestion of high quality protein is essential but supplementation of the protein diet with milk, and milk products will tend to produce hyperphosphatemia which may aggravate itching, suppress serum calcium levels, and stimulate parathyroid hormone secretion.

2.8. Calcium balance

Transport of calcium between blood and dialysate is a function of the concentration of diffusible calcium in the plasma and the calcium concentration in the dialysis solution [71]. With 3.5 milliequivalents of calcium per liter, a diffusion of calcium down the gradient from the solution into the plasma occurs, and a slightly positive calcium balance will accrue [72]. However, ultrafiltration will cause a transport of calcium from the patient into the dialysate and produce a negative calcium balance [73].

The total balance between calcium diffusion and the ultrafiltered calcium will determine the total net calcium flux. Some reports have suggested a positive calcium balance [72]. Others report a negative calcium balance [73]. These differences may reflect a difference in the diffusible calcium in the individual patient population and a variation in the dialysate calcium concentration. (Canada, 2.5 mEq/l vs United States, 3.5 mEq/l). A recent interest in the use of calcium containing phosphate binding agents would suggest

that a zero calcium dialysate solution would be beneficial to allow an increase use of calcium carbonate and calcium citrate as phosphate binding agents while reducing the complication of associated hypercalcaemia.

Dialysate loss of 1.25 dehydroxy vitamin D3 has been reported and small supplemental doses of this vitamin have been suggested [49, 51, 74]. Some patients tend to develop hypercalcaemia and may have poor osteoblastic activity when exposed to oral calcium and vitamin D supplement [75]. Intravenous and intraperitoneal $1.25(OH_2)D_3$ appears to improve bone metabolism and reduce the instance of hypercalcaemia which is associated with oral $1.25(OH_2)D_3$ [54, 60].

3. DIETARY MANAGEMENT

As previously stated, major dietary indiscretion can exceed the removal rate of metabolic toxins, salt and water. However, because CAPD can ultrafilter large volumes of water and remove large quantities of sodium, no major restriction is required. Potassium restriction has been made unnecessary by the presence of large amounts of potassium in the stool [69]. However, adequate dietary instruction is essential to avoid dietary indiscretion.

In patients who are malnourished or protein depleted, a high protein intake of 1.5 g/kg body weight is recommended [47, 73]. When protein repletion has been achieved, free access to protein without supplementation or restriction can be prescribed. The ingestion of very large quantities of salt and water may require the utilization of increasing amounts of hypertonic glucose solutions for removal. This cycle contributes to progressive obesity and hypertriglyceridemia [42, 72]. Salt restriction followed by decreased thirst and, thereby, less water intake may decrease the requirement for hypertonic glucose solutions and alleviate this problem.

It must be remembered, however, that decreasing the ultrafiltration will decrease the total drained volume and, thereby, reduce small molecule dialysis [72]. The prescription for the dialysis solution, therefore, must reach a balance between the need for maximum total drained volumes for adequate dialysis and excessive hypertonic glucose which may produce hypertriglyceridemia and obesity. The practice of using four exchanges per day with one or two consisting dialysis as evaluated by most parameters for up to 5 yr [76]. Dietary calcium and phosphate have been discussed previously.

4. CLINICAL ASPECTS OF CAPD

4.1. Establishing a program

4.1.1. Personnel
Commitment of the nephrologist and nursing personnel to sterile technique, chronic catheter management, and patient training methods is necessary for a successful CAPD program [77, 78]. A well-trained, dedicated staff thoroughly familiar with the concepts of peritoneal dialysis and available for emergency and routine outpatient foolow up should facilitate successful delivery of this system. The

technique is extremely simple. Problems may arise quickly, however, and be demanding on the medical and nursing staff. Thus, adequate personnel, proportionate to the patient population is essential. One nurse to each 8–10 outpatients and a schedule for 24 hr/day coverage is also required [79].

The first week of training should be carried out on a one-to-one basis, with a nurse dedicated to education of each patient. By the end of the first week, the patient is usually performing the technique independently. At that point, troubleshooting and observation can be done in small groups, but no more than one nurse to three patients is practical.

4.1.2. Site of training
Inhospital CAPD training is practiced in some institutions. Out-patient training is preferable, however, because it decreases the cost and prevents the 'ill patient' syndrome that may occur with inhospital procedures [80, 81]. Little equipment is required, and 100–120 square feet of training space per patient is adequate.

4.1.3. Hospital back-up
Although hospitalization has become less frequent [82], good hospital back-up and expert management of the patient is required. Most centers have found that specialized nursing personnel should manage both the outpatient training and follow up, as well as inhospital back-up and management [76, 79, 80].

4.1.4. Team work
Since CAPD replaces only a small amount of the function of the kidneys, a physician who is trained and confident in the care of patients with renal failure must necessarily participate in training and management of the patients. Retraining and support services must be easily accessible to every patient undergoing continuous ambulatory peritoneal dialysis.

4.2. Patient selection

4.2.1. High risk patient population

CAPD is a simple, easily taught technique which lends itself to management of patients willing and able to undergo self-dialysis. The simplicity, however, tends to make it an attractive technique to medical staff with patients who have major difficulties undergoing other types of dialysis. The 'last ditch' effort, 'maybe you ought to try CAPD' approach may produce statistical evidence of a high mortality and an excessive drop out rate of patients who initiate training. Patients in whom there is little left to offer certainly may be 'given a try' on CAPD, but a high failure rate can be expected as well as a high mortality rate [83–85].

4.2.2. Selection
In those patients in whom there is a choice concerning which form of long-term ESRD care is best, selection criteria will be required. Development of these criteria will aid in finding the place that CAPD will best serve the end-stage renal disease population.

CAPD is self-dialysis. It is best offered, therefore, to those patients who are motivated to care for themselves and who

can be expected to accept this responsibility on a long-term basis because of the benefits. A good concept of the relationship between end-stage renal disease and symptoms, a scientific approach to the requirement of dialysis and a belief in the need for this therapy by the patient is essential or failure is inevitable. Internal, rather than external, motivation factors are most beneficial, and the physical and mental capabilities of performing the procedure are required [86]. Personality traits which lead to a desire for personal independence and freedom in a reasonably intelligent individual would make the very best CAPD patient. Studies have demonstrated no difference in the mortality of patients managed with CAPD and in-center hemodialysis when other complicating factors are matched and considered [87–95].

4.2.3. Infants and children
Reports of success with continuous ambulatory peritoneal dialysis in the pediatric population suggest this this modality has become the treatment of choice in the dialysis of infants and small children [14, 96–102]. Adequate clearance to prevent uremia has been reported [103], and preliminary information suggests accelerated linear growth [98, 104, 105]. Aggressive use of intravenous $1.25(OH_2)D_3$ [61] and, more recently, human growth hormone derived by genetic engineering has demonstrated increased and accelerated growth in infants and small children undergoing CAPD [106].

4.3. Contraindications

4.3.1. Transfer surface area
There must be an adequate transfer surface area available for peritoneal dialysis, and clinical evaluation of the adequacy of the surface and blood flow to the peritoneum can be achieved, though it is rarely needed, prior to implantation of a chronic peritoneal catheter.

This information can be obtained by passing a spinal needle through the abdominal wall and infusing two liters of 1.5% glucose solution into the peritoneum. The needle is withdrawn and after a dwell time of 4 hr, a small sample of the dialysate is removed and compared with the serum creatinine. Sixty to 70% equilibration of creatinine in the dialysate as compared to plasma demonstrates normal transfer. Less than 40% may cause concern and less then 30% makes failure of CAPD likely. This technique may be used in those individuals with multiple abdominal surgical procedures including aortic aneurysm repair or previous serious abdominal inflammation, such as pancreatitis or peritonitis secondary to ruptured viscus.

4.3.2. Triglycerides
Severe hypertriglyceridemia not associated with diabetes mellitus is also considered a relative contraindication to CAPD.

4.3.3. Immunosuppression
The requirement of chronic immunosuppressive drugs in patients with conditions such as active systemic lupus erythematosus, have caused concern about the risk of catastrophic results from an episode of peritonitis. Many patients undergoing steriod therapy have now been treated

with CAPD, and no increased mortality has been reported. An improvement in both cellular and hemoral immunity has recently been reported in patients transferred from hemodialysis to CAPD. AIDS patients with ESRD are now being managed with CAPD [83, 107–109].

4.3.4. Ostomies
Chronic abdominal wall infections including open colostomies, ileostomies, and nephrostomies may increase the risk of recurrent peritonitis.

4.3.5. Hernia
Umbilical, inguinal and diaphragmatic hernias as well as hemorrhoids, may be aggravated by increasing intra-abdominal pressure with CAPD and complicate the long-term performance results [73]. The repair of 'large' hernias prior to CAPD appears prudent. The complication appears more commonly in patients using larger volumes of dialysis as suggested by Twardowski and Rubin [8, 10].

4.3.6. Neurological defects
Physical incoordination resulting from progressive neurological disease, cerebrovascular accidents, movement disorders and severe arthritis, may take CAPD impossible to perform.

4.3.7. Back pain
Low back pain may be aggravated by the presence of the fluid in the abdomen with a shift in the center of gravity [73, 111].

4.3.8. Psychological and social problems
A cooperative and compliant patient is essential if CAPD is to be successful. Patients who are psychotic, belligerent or uncooperative cannot be expected to succeed with this form of self-dialysis.

4.4. Peritoneal catheters

4.4.1. Types of catheters
The chronic, indwelling catheter is the lifeline and access for the CAPD patient. Permanent access to the peritoneal cavity as made possible by the development of the dacron felt cuff on the silastic catheter [112]. Various types of catheters, including the single and double cuffed Tenckhoff type, the Toronto Western [113], the Ash (Life) catheter and the Valli catheter [114], lend evidence to the fact that no perfect catheter is available. Past experience with the Tenckhoff catheter has made it the most widely used and successfully employed catheter. The double cuffed catheter may have the advantage of a better seal and make dislodging unlikely and a tunnel infection less likely because the distal cuff is very close to the skin (1 to 2 cm). This, however, increases the risk of distal cuff erosion through the skin which will then produce a chronic tunnel infection. Many investigators feel that the frequency of this complication has made the double cuffed catheter less useful than one with a single cuff [115].

New catheter designs include the curl interperitoneal segment which has reduced in-flow pain and catheter migration, and the Swan-neck (Missouri) design which allows the skin exit to point downward, thereby reducing

debris accumulation at the site and allowing for better cleaning [116].

4.4.2. Methods of implantation
The Tenckhoff catheter can be inserted by a surgical technique or at the patient's bedside. Many nephrologists have practiced the bedside technique in both hospital and office [117]. The majority of physicians prefer these catheters to be implanted in the operating room, however, with the surgical approach allowing direct vision. General anesthesia is preferred by many. Numerous variations have been reported in the position of the catheter cuffs [113, 117, 118]. Kirksey has developed and reported [119] a modification of the technique of cuff placement, in which a single cuffed catheter is used. The cuff is placed superficial to the facia and a non-absorbable suture sewn around the cuff and in the facia. This decreases the tendency toward leakage or displacement in the early phase, prior to tissue ingrowth. It allows early utilization and decreases early failure rate. All catheters except the Tenckhoff require surgical implantation but the latter is much easier to remove.

An evaluation of the integrity of the catheter seal may be performed by the infusion of a large volume of dialysis solution 3 l in the average size adult) while the patient is still on the operating table. If leakage does occur, repair is then easily accomplished while the peritoneum is still accessible [120]. Multiple techniques to eliminate contamination, and thus recurrent infection associated with the bag exchange, have allowed the recognition that many of the recurrent episodes of peritonitis that are continuing to be reported in the CAPD population are related to chronic catheter infection, cuff infection, and a generally inadequate microbiological barrier with present access technology. A new emphasis on the development of new technology for access gives promise to a reduction in the instance of peritonitis if a true bacteriological barrier can be obtained. An excellent discussion of peritoneal catheters and management and exit site treatment was recently published in the Peritoneal Dialysis Bulletin [116].

4.5. Catheters failure

4.5.1. Early catheter failure
Causes of catheter failure include: obstruction secondary to improper placement, folding and bending, occlusion by wrapping of the omentum, and migration of the catheter from the pelvis upward in the peritoneal cavity. Postoperative bleeding into the peritoneal cavity, with fibrin and clot formation and early infection, may also cause obstruction. Early and persistent catheter leakage may require replacement.

4.5.2. Late catheter failure
Late failures (after two weeks' use) are almost invariably associated with peritonitis or catheter displacement, but may be associated with intraabdominal catastrophes unrelated to peritoneal dialysis such as ruptured diverticula, pancreatitis, peptic ulcer, bowel perforation, etc. Fibrin formation can be prevented by the addition of heparin to the solution when peritonitis occurs. Heparin may also be required intermittently in some patients who develop fibrin material in the dialysate unrelated to infection. This latter

problem can usually be documented by a decreasing rate of outflow or partial obstruction. Partial outflow obstruction may be reversed by the early addition of 10 000 units of heparin to the infusion solution and then allowing a prolonged drain time (4–12 hr) during which an increasing rate of flow may occur and the catheter obstruction reversed. Several days of heparin use (2000 units per exchange) may then return the flow to normal. Manipulation of the catheter with Forgarty catheters and trocars yields little more than the potential risk of contamination and subsequent infection with little hope of opening an obstructed catheter.

4.6. Training and follow up

4.6.1. Day 1 to 4
Outpatient and inpatient training has been discussed previously (Section 4.1.2.). Ten to fifteen training sessions are usually required to prepare a patient to manage CAPD [79]. The training sessions are carried out on a daily basis. The sessions are begun after catheter break-in and each sessions consists of 6–8 hr as the patient's physical, emotional, and mental status allows. During the first few days, exchanges are made approximately each 1½ to 2 hr. These rapid exchanges allow better urea and small molecule control and avoid the need for back-up dialysis. It also increases patient learning by repetition and may be used to more rapidly control the expanded intravascular volumes so commonly present. This will bring blood pressure under control as antihypertensive medications are tapered. During these early training days, the patient is taught to make the exchanges using simulation models while the nurse makes the actual exchange. At the end of the training day (4:30 – 5:00 p.m.) 2 l of solution are left in the abdomen overnight. If discomfort occurs during the night, the patient is instructed to drain solution until relief is achieved. One hundred to 300 ml drainage is usually adequate, but some patients may drain as much as 1 l.

4.6.2. Day 4 to 6
After the first few days as technical skills improve, the nurse allows the patient to make the exchanges with supervision. As this practice improves technique, the patient then makes exchanges in the unit without supervision and eventually makes his own exchange at night. When this is accomplished, the patient begins the CAPD regime at a rate of four exchanges per day. This degree of expertise can usually be reached within the first week of training, and the patient is ready to make all four exchanges by Sunday in the absence of the staff.

4.6.3. Day 8 to 12
During the following week, exchange and theory training continue. Repeated documentation of successful adherence to the rigid technique is recorded by the staff. Question and answer sessions also continue with a 'troubleshooting' format and near the end of the second week, the patient is given a battery of examinations to evaluate both the theoretical and practical aspects of accumulated knowledge. These successfully completed, the patient is graduated from the CAPD training program and signs a release stating that CAPD training has included theoretical and practical aspects of the necessary information. The patient is then

given supplies and sent home to perform the technique for two weeks. The nurse accompanies the patient, when feasible, evaluates the home environment, and observes the first exchange performed after graduation.

4.6.4. Follow up
Within 2 to 3 days, contact is made by telephone. At the two week visit, reevaluation of the technique occurs, and suggestion for change are made as clinically indicated. The patient is seen each two weeks for the first three months. With each visit, a complete exchange is observed, and each month a transfer set change is performed by nursing personnel. After three months, the visits are reduced to one per month. During these visits, clinical evaluation by the physician is made and the catheter side is inspected. Compliance and potential theoretical problems are discussed and documented by the staff.

4.6.5. Telephone contact
Close contact with and encouragement of the patient is accomplished with a weekly telephone call which includes specific questions about blood pressure, dry weight, last scale weight, appetite, sense of well-being, catheter site evaluation, and dialysate flow characteristics. The calls serve to detect incipient and slowly developing problems keep the patient aware of the concern of the staff and reduce a reluctance to call if problems arise. The educational process also continues with these calls.

4.6.6. Laboratory tests
During the training phase, laboratory evaluation is obtained on the first day and every other day unless unusual parameters are reported. Hyperkalemia or hypokalemia may require daily testing for serum potassium. If the BUN does not begin to fall or if the blood sugar starts to rise, more frequent evaluation may be necessary. A list of the routine laboratory tests is in Table 2. If the BUN and creatinine are not stable at acceptable levels or slowly declining during the first week, a clinical transport evaluation using the dialysate and serum creatinine comparison as describedd earlier, (Section 4.3.1.) is performed.

Table 2. Routine laboratory tests

Every month:	
BUN	Total protein
Creatinine	Albumin
Sodium	Alk. phosphatase
Potassium	LDH
CO_2	SGOT
Calcium	Hct
Magnesium	HgB
Phosphate	Dialysate protein
Every 3 months	
WBC RBC	Platelet count
Every 6 months:	
Residual renal function	Motor nerve conduction velocity
24 hour urine volume	EKG
Chest X-ray	Bone mineral density

4.6.7. Medications

Medications taken by the patient before beginning dialysis are adjusted with the initiation of CAPD. These include diuretics, phosphate binding agents, and occasionally digitalis preparations. Patients are maintained on water soluble vitamins. Antihypertensive medications are generally tapered during the early phase of training. During this time, intravascular volume is contracted by ultrafiltration. Insulin dosages are adjusted to accommodate the increased glucose load. If the blood sugar is difficult to control or serum triglyceride levels climb over 500, initiation of insulin in the dialysis solution may be required [42, 121]. This latter route of administration has been shown to improve glucose control but a safe technique to add insulin to the dialysis solution is essential [122].

Rarely, a patient who is very compliant and lives a great distance from the center, will be instructed in the technique of adding antibiotics to the dialysis solution and the patient given a starter dose of cephalosporin [123]. The patient is instructed to contact the unit by telephone before using this medication.

5. COMPLICATIONS

5.1. Complications during training

5.1.1. Distension and abdominal pain

Most patients experience some sense of distention and fullness as the CAPD technique is initiated. This is most problematic in young, muscular individuals and less in older multiperous females. These symptoms may be painful and require smaller infusion volumes several days after initiation of training. This may also occur during the overnight dwell time and occasionally cause the patient to question the choice of CAPD as a dialysis technique. These symptoms invariably disappear. The distention symptoms may be most severe in areas where previous surgery has been performed and related to traction on adhesions.

Some patients complain of pain on infusion which may be aggravated by either excessively cold or warm temperatures of solution. This pain is, however, most frequently bicarbonate responsive. The pH of the dialysis solution has been found to be 4.9 to 5.2. The addition of a small amount of 50% bicarbonate solution (5 to 10 ml) will raise the pH to 6.0 to 6.02 and relieve most of the infusion pain. Some patients continue to have bicarbonate responsive pain for several weeks to months, and some require the instillation of small doses of bicarbonate for prevention. With time, however, most patients have discontinued this procedure as the pain is extremely short-lived and usually not worth the trouble required to add the bicarbonate in a sterile manner. Decreasing the rate of infusion by lowering the height of the bag during infusion may also be helpful. This latter maneuver is most helpful in those patients who complain of rectal or peritoneal pain.

5.1.2. Catheter leaks – early

Catheter site leakage is also common during the training period and increases in frequency with early use. These may also develop in patients who experience increased intra-abdominal pressure following catheter implantation. Exam-

ples include straining due to constipation, respiratory distress secondary to asthma or laryngeal edema post anesthesia, or a barium enema performed without draining the abdomen. Most leakage will spontaneously disappear if the abdomen is drained and left empty 1–2 days. Back-up dialysis may be required. Some early leaks may last as long as three weeks before spontaneous closure. Evaluation of continued leakage may be made each three to four days with a small volume of dialysate. When the leakage has ceased, 48 hours should be allowed to pass before CAPD is initiated, with only 1.5% glucose solutions utilized for several days. The incidence of early leakage can be decreased by the 3 l test as described earlier (Section 4.4.2.).

During this delay, training may continue. Exchange technique may be simulated and the theory reinforced in order that the catheter site leakage need not inordinately delay discharge to home. Most early catheter site leakage is not associated with infection but early and empiric treatment of suspected infection may decrease catheter loss and prevent peritonitis. The potential is present for the transmission of organisms from the skin through the exit leakage into the peritoneal cavity.

5.1.3. Catheter leaks – late

Late catheter leakage is usually secondary to a tunnel infection and subsequent to a cuff infection. Diagnosis is established by purulent drainage from the catheter site which is unresponsive to treatment. When cuff infection is present, early catheter removal before dialysate leakage occurs will avoid the peritonitis which invariably follows communication from the peritoneum through an infected catheter cuff.

Rarely, late catheter leakage will occur spontaneously or follow abdominal trauma. Drainage of the dialysate and a dry abdomen for several days will usually allow spontaneous closure and prevent catheter loss.

5.2. Blood pressure control

5.2.1. Hypertension – hypotension

Aggressive attempts to control the blood pressure through blood volume reduction by ultrafiltration will usually produce excellent results [124]. Rapid tapering and discontinuation of antihypertensive medications may allow recrudescence of severe hypertension, and reinstitution of medications for temporary control may be required. Intravascular volume contraction increases the efficacy of any blood pressure medication and even small doses may produce severe orthostatic hypotension. As volume reduction is pursued, spontaneous orthostatic hypotension unrelated to antihypertensive medications may occur in those patients where aggressive ultrafiltration is undertaken for blood pressure control [124, 125]. When this level has been reached, evaluation of body weight and a slight increase in dry weight will produce normotension. If severe hypotension occurs, a reclining posture, increased salt and water intake, and decreased ultrafiltration by the use of only 1.5% glucose solutions will usually suffice (see Section 2.3.). The patient is then placed on a normal diet and the CAPD regimen is prescribed to conform with the usual salt and water intake. Reports of early contraction of extracellular water as a cause of increased hematocrit and orthostatic hypotension have been disputed [126-129].

5.3. Motivation

Patients placed on CAPD who are internally motivated and compliant, do extremely well, learn quickjly and achieve rehabilitation status. There are, however, personality traits and family situations which create a likelihood of failure [130, 131].

Many patients adjust their lives to in-center hemodialysis so completely that their friends, parties and enjoyment are found in this setting. Such patients, who are transferred from hemodialysis because of vascular access or other problems, do poorly on CAPD.

5.3.1. Depression – fatigue

Once training is complete and the patient goes home to an empty house without social contact, the rapid onset of depression and loneliness may be manifested by multiple somatic complaints. Recurring episodes of peritonitis due to lack of compliance should be quickly taken as a signal to make further attempts to establish another vascular access for institution of hemodialysis.

Some patients develop an enthusiasm for CAPD with a misunderstanding of the daily requirements. The enthusiasm soon wanes with the constant demand of a careful, compliant exchange technique, the patient becomes disappointed and disillusioned. This occurs most frequently in patients who have come directly onto CAPD without having undergone other forms of dialytic therapy and can frequently be reversed by a tour through the hemodialysis unit.

In explaining CAPD to patients, a balance must be maintained between enthusiasm and blunt honesty to fully inform the patient of the benefits and side effects of the procedure. This must include the understanding of the possibility of gradual progressive obesity, the need for restriction of carbohydrate intake, strict compliance, tenacious adherence to the protocol and the requirements of long-term self management.

5.3.2. Noncompliance

The failure of patients to comply with the protocols of CAPD is easily detected. This usually manifests itself as recurrent episodes of peritonitis. At this time, a discussion with the patient to explain the risks of noncompliance and the symptoms produced by the infection either produces a turnabout in attitude or a willingness to be removed from CAPD.

Some patients will, however, fail to comply by skipping exchanges or failing to observe even minimal dietary restrictions. For example, an occasional patients may ingest up to 5000 to 6000 ml water/day. These patients usually express amazement that they are drinking excessive water and deny that they are skipping exchanges. BUN and creatinine blood values, however, give evidence of the failure of the patient to comply with the number of required exchanges. If the patient does not perform the number of exchanges prescribed, one or two days of compliance do not significantly change the blood urea nitrogen and creatinine levels. The patient's metabolic product evaluation will reveal this on the routine laboratory tests. The absence

of change in the transfer characteristics of the peritoneal membrane must be ascertained prior to confronting the patient with the evidence of decreased number of exchanges (Section 4.3.1). If the patient is unwilling to comply with the number of exchanges required, another form of dialysis will be necessary. Patients whose motivation and compliance on hemodialysis were marguinal as evaluated by sodium and water balance, phosphate control and potassium control will not necessarily manifest these problems on CAPD. Sodium and water load are rarely a problem, and phosphate balance is often more easily controlled.

5.4. Anorexia and vomiting

Symptoms related to abdonimal distention frequently present with the initiation of CAPD may be manifested by epigastric distress, anorexia and, on occasion, dyspepsia, regurgitation and eructation. The symptomms frequently disappear within 4-5 days and may be related to lingering uremic toxicity prior to dialysis control. The epigastric distress is most likely to persist and is frequently cimetidine responsive. If, after 3-5 days, the symptoms have not abated with cimetidine, psychological support, and decreasing the intra-abdominal volume, then radiographic evaluation should be undertaken. Studies are usually negative but may reveal gastrointestinal pathology such as esophagael reflux, duodenal ulcers or may suggest erosive gastritis.

5.5. Serum potassium abnormality (see previous discussion, Section 2.5.).

5.6. Hyperglycemia

Hyperglycemia may occur in both insulin requiring and non-insulin requiring patients with diabetes mellitus, who were previously controlled by diet or stabilized on insulin [42]. The increased load of glucose from the dialysis solution may produce an increased insulin requirement [121]. In patients known to have diabetes mellitus, daily blood sugar levels should be drawn during the early phase until control is achieved. When insulin is added to the dialysis solution, the amount added to the overnight exchange should be decreased because the rapid glucose absoprtion during the first 2 to 3 hr dwell time, will be followed by a continued absorption of insulin after the glucose is metabolized. Nocturnal hypoglycemia may occur. Many authors now feel that CAPD is the preferred form of dialysis for the diabetic patient [132-137], and report better blood sugar control, improved control of hypertension, steady state control of uremia, and improved hematocrit and cardiac function [138, 139].

5.7. Anemia

A rapid rise in the hemoglobin level with the institution of CAPD has been reported by most investigators [126-129, 140, 141]. The mean hematocrit of 32 volumes percent is significantly higher than the levels reported in hemodialysis patients. There is usually not, however, a complete correction of anemia in patients undergoing CAPD. Blood transfusions are rarely required. Even patients requiring 2-4 units of blood per month on hemodialysis have not required blood while on CAPD. Frequent monitoring of the serum ferritin is indicated to prevent secondary iron deficiency anemia since rapid hemopoiesis may produce a fall in the ferritin level [142]. Increased protein intake and intravenous iron has caused a secondary rise in hematocrit.

5.8. Hernias and hemorrhoids

Increased intra-abdominal volume and pressure may aggravate already present hemorrhoide as well as abdominal and inguinal hernias [73]. Repair of these prior to a commitment of CAPD should be discussed with the patient but neither are a specific contraindication to the initiation of CAPD.

5.9. Back pain

Lumbosacral spine pain in patients who have previously had low back pain may, on occasion, require discontinuation of CAPD. A search for significant symptoms in this area prior to the initiation of CAPD is indicated and should be considered a relative contraindication when present [73, 111].

5.10. Bloody dialysate

Female patients frequently report blood tinged dialysate with each menstrual period. This causes concern because of the turbidity which is created during this time. Symptoms of peritonitis are not present; heparinization has not been required; and spontaneous disappearance occurs.

Rarely a patient will present with spontaneous bleeding into the peritoneal cavity. This appears to be associated with abdominal cramps and diarrhea, and spontaneously disappears. One patient reported grossly bloody dialysate after adding heparin to the dialysate because of fibrin formation. The bleeding into the dialysate did not occur, however, until the patient ingested aspirin, and also disappeared without further treatment.

5.11. Peritonitis

The primary complication which limits the applicability of CAPD to patients with end-stage renal disease is recurrent peritonitis. There has been a rapid decline in the incidence of this complication with the availability of collapsible plastic containers (October, 1978) and materials specifically designed for CAPD (September, 1979).

Peritonitis is the most frequent cause of discontinuation of CAPD; however, many patients have utilized CAPD for 3–4 yr without infection. This suggests that except for the small statistical risk of organisms floating onto the spike at the time of spike exposure during exchanges, the incidence of peritonitis in the patient is related to compliance or an inadequate catheter seal. Material defects may be more common than is currently reported, and recurrent episodes of peritonitis indicate the need for careful examination of both materials and the rigid sterile technique.

The description of continuous ambulatory peritoneal dialysis in 1976 by Popovich and Moncrief also included a recognition of the potential for recurrent peritonitis [143]. This early prediction was confirmed and further studied

in a cooperative effort between these authors and the University of Missouri Medical Center under the direction of Dr. Karl Nolph [65]. Selection of patients who are compliant and motivated and removal of patients from the technique who have recurrent episodes of peritonitis in several programs has decreased the incidence to less than one epidose per patient year. A statistical decrease in the incidence of peritonitis in patients using the Ultraviolet Exchange Device has been found in the 1987 National CAPD Registry Study sponsored by the National Institute of Health [90]; oresently more than 40% of the CAPD population in the United States uses this device.

5.11.1. Diagnosis
Perionitis is diagnosed by an increased number of white blood cells in the dialysate. Rubin *et al.* [123] studied clear dialysate samples and demonstrated 3–25 white blood cells per mm^3 in noninfected dialysate. Cells are predominantly mononuclear. A rapid increase in the dialysate white blood cell count occurs with the onset of peritonitis. Frequently, within 4–8 hr, the white blood cell count may rise to 5000 or more per mm^3. Other symptoms associated with the development of peritonitis include epigastric distress, nausea, vomiting, vague abdominal discomfort, rebound tenderness and fever. These may progress to ileus, lethargy, severe abdominal pain, hypotension and changes in sensorium. None of these symptoms are essential for the diagnosis of peritonitis but should lead to the examination of the dialysate for an increasaed number of white blood cells. A comparison of the white blood cell count using the hemocytometer as opposed to the Coulter.counter demonstrates that the Coulter-counter fails to count all of the cells. Therefore, the hemocytometer white blood cell count is preferred. Random positive cultures without peritonitis suggest that not every incidence of contamination leads to clinical peritonitis [144].

5.11.2. Treatment of peritonitis
Prevention – The single best way to treat peritonitis is prevention. This is best achieved by meticulous development of a technique which, if followed correctly, should produce a patient population with near zero incidence of peritonitis. Once this has been accomplished, peritonitis can then be considered either a materials or patient compliance failure. Each episode of peritonitis should stimulate a search for the etiological factors. Fifty percent of patients (ten) at this institution have performed the technique for greater than one year without peritonitis. The other 50% of patients have had one or more episodes of peritonitis within the first year and 10% of our patients (two) have had 75% of our episodes of peritonitis.

Early treatment. Aerobic culture are obtained the first day prior to initiation of therapy. Table 3 is a suggested clinical approach to decide when to start and adjust therapy.

When the onset of peritonitis is limited to turbid dialysate with mild clinical symptoms, initiation of therapy addition of antibiotics to the dialysis solution on an outpatient basis is usually succesful. The CAPD exchange schedule is continued at the prescribed rate. Seventy-five percent of the peritonitis episodes contracted in the outpatient program are gram positive. Doses of cephalosporin 250 mg

Table 3. Treatment of peritonitis

White blood cell count per cubic meter (unspun dialysate)	Course of action
Day 1 0–50 White blood cells per mm³ Abdominal signs or symptoms present.	Re-examine dialysate visually each hour during next exchange. Repeat white blood cell on dialysate if symptoms persist. No antibiotics.
50–100 White blood cells per mm³	Aerobic culture. repeat white blood cell on next exchange.
No symptoms. 100 or greater white blood cells mm³. With or without symptoms.	Aerobic culture. Cephalosporin 500 mg per exchange for two exchanges. 250 mg per exchange for 4 days 500 mg cephalosporin by mouth for 5 to 7 days thereafter. If symptoms severe, consider hospitalization.
Day 2 Symptoms improved and/or decrease in white blood cells in dialysate.	Continue above – follow by phone.
Symptoms unchanged and mild. White blood cells not decreased or if it is increased.	Culture aerobic, anaerobic, fungal, TBC. Add gentamicin or tobrammycin 100 mg in 2 l for one exchange. 15 mg per exchange for three exchanges cephalosporin by mouth. Consider hospitalization.
Day 3 Symptoms improved. White blood cells decrease to less than 150 mm³ (Check cultures and sensitivity).	Consider only change to oral cephalosporin.
Symptoms improved. White blood cells decreased but greater than 150 (mm³). (Check cultures and sensitivity.)	Continue intraperitoneal. cephalosporin, 250 mg with each exchange.
Symptoms improved after aminoglycocides started 2nd day. Whote blood cells decreased (evaluate sensitivity of positive culture).	Continue gentamicin or tobramycin at 15 mg per two liters for four exchanges. Continue cephalosporin if sensitive.
Symptoms unimproved or worsened. White blood cells unchanged or increased.	Hospitalize. Rapid 15 to 30 min dwell lavage with gentamicin or tobramycin 10 mg per two lityers.

per exchange for four days followed by 5–7 days of oral cephalosporin (i.e. cephalexin 500 mg fopur times per day) has produced complete clearing in 85% of the cases. A starting dose of tobramycin 1.0 mg/kg in the first medicated container, followed by 15 mg/2 l bag until culture results are available, will allow coverage for the less frequent gram negative organisms.

5.11.3. Unresponsive peritonitis

Occasionally, a patient will present one day after the initiation of therapy with progressive symptoms. These include increasing dialysate turbidity and systemic toxicity. This patient should be immediately hospitalized as should any patient presenting initially with severe symptoms. In these patients, repeat aerobic, anaerobic, tuberculose and fungal cultures should be obtained. A gram stain for fungal hyphae and acid fast bacillus to rule out tuberculosis may

occasionally be diagnostic. If evidence of these latter organism is found, immediate steps to drain the abdomen and remove the peritoneal catheter should be undertaken.

Patients who do not rapidly respond to cephalosporin or those with major systemic toxicity should receive aminoglycocide antibiotics. This protocol is frequently documented by a decrease in the number of white blood cells within a 24 hr period and may be interpreted as responsiveness to the antibiotics. Continued intraperitoneal aminoglycosides at 10 mg per exchange in a patient who is clinically responding will usually produce clearing within 3– days. If the patient is unresponsive within 24 to 48 hr or if systemic toxicity persists, drainage of the abdomen and removal of the catheter is indicated. The presence or absence of systemic toxicity, the rapidity of response to empiric cephalosporins, the inclusion of intraperitoneal aminoglycocide antibiotica, and/or a seriously ill patient all influence the therapeutic approach. Drainage of the peritoneal cavity and removal of the catheter in those patients with progressive systemic toxicity or failure to respond may be life saving. The former would be the case in fungal peritonitis, tuberculosis peritonitis and anaerobic peritonitis associated with a perforated bowel. Early surgical correction of the bowel perforation is essential. Though not always fulminent, anaerobic, intestinal tract organisms are virtuallt diagnostic of bowel perforation or leak [145].

5.11.4. Antibiotic therapy
Addition of antibiotics to the dialysis solution is performed via sterile technique. The medication port of the solution container is not quaranteed to be sterile [146] and must be soaked for at least 5 min with povidoneiodine solution prior to the injection of antibiotics. If symptoms and white blood cell counts are diminishing, solutions containing cephalosporin antibiotic are continued for 10 days, or therapy may be changed to oral cephalosporin at day 4. If no improvement is noted, aminoglycocide therapy may be added (after anaerobic, fungal and tuberculosis cultures are obtained). If clearing has not begun after 24 hr, the patient is hospitalized. If clewaring is present, cephalosporin is continued as above, and the patient is contacted by telephone during this interim for evaluation. Most centers continue the treatment for 10 days total.

Any patient who develops peritonitis should be evaluated for materials or compliance failure. After the peritonitis is cleared, the patient should be returned to the training program and several exchanges closely observed. The patient should be closely questioned for possible materials defects. It has been the policy of this facility that a transfer tubing change is always performed during peritonitis treatment. An invisible crack in the spike or a puncture hole in the tubing may produce several episodes of peritonitis before discovery. Clinical and subclinical catheter tunnel infections must also be sought.

5.11.5. Removal of patients from CAPD
In those patients who have more than three episodes of peritonitis within the first six months of CAPD, counseling should determine if compliance is the problem. After the third episode, discontinuation of CAPD and a return to hemodialysis is suggested. Patients are frequently quite willing to discontinue CAPD because of the symptoms and the risk.

5.11.6. Staff induced peritonitis
In the last 18 months, 4 episodes of peritonitis in this

program have been related to contamination by unit personnel. Perforation of the catheter by a clamp during a tubing change was responsible for 2 episodes. Failure of the titanium adapter to seal in the catheter, after replacement of the previous plastic adapter, produced two episodes. Clamping of the catheter should always be achieved with a soft clamo as close to the catheter adapter as is practical since any perforation of the catheter near the skin can cause catheter loss. The change from a plastic to a titanium adapter should include soaking the original adapter for at least ten minutes in povidone-iodine solution, cutting the catheter at the connection site proximal to the portion of the adapter in the catheter, and re-soaking the cut end for 10 min prior to insertion of the titanium adapter. Since adopting this technique, no episodes of peritonitis have been associated with catheter adapter change at this institution [122].

5.11.7. Peritonitis summary
Initiation of theraopy with any elevated dialysate white blood cell count accompanies by close clinical follow-up to demonstrate clearing is critical. Admission tot he hospital when response is slow followed by early removal of the catheter when systemiuc toxicity is present may be life saving. Anaerobic cultures to rule out bowel perforation in patients not responding rapidly to therapy and removal of the catheter in any patient who develops fungal or tuberculosis peritonitis will usually produce clearing and disappearance of symptoms. These complications can be reduced by patient selection and a meticulous teaching program.

6. CONCLUSION

An expanding world-wide experience with continuous ambulatory peritoneal dialysis has demonstrated that this technique has been used to successfully manage patients with end-stage renal disease. The evolutionary use of this technique in the ESRD patient and population, success by dialysis facilities throughout the world, documentation of patient selection criteria have demonstrated that CAPD should be offered as an alternative form of dialysis to those patients capable of and interested in self-dialysis. The declining incidence in the peritonitis rate associated with introduction of techniques and materials is encouraging [145]. Caution must be exercised and adequate personnel availabvle to manage those patients trained on CAPD.

REFERENCES

1. Delano BG: The failure of home hemodialysis. Trans Am Soc Artif Intern Organs (editorial) 33(1): 1, 1987.
2. Popovich RP, moncrief JW: Kinetic modeling of peritoneal transport. In: Trevino-Beccera A, Boen FST, Karger S, Today's Art of Peritoneal Dialysis (eds), Basel, Switzerland 17: 59–72, 1975.
3. Popovich RP, Moncrief JW, Decherd JF: Physiological transport parameters in peritoneal and hemodialysis in 2nd Annual Report No. AM–2–3–2205. Artifical Kidney-Chronic Uremia Program, National Institute of Arthritis, Metabolism and Digestive Diseases. HEW, 1977.
4. Popovich RP, Pyle WK, Moncrief JW, Decgherd JF, Brooks S: Preliminary verification of the low dialysis clearance hypothesis via a novel equilibrium peritoneal dialysis techniquue, Trans Austral Conf Heat and Mass Transfer, Univ of Sidney Press, Sidney, Australia 2: 217, 1977.
5. Popovich RP: Kinetics of peritoneal transport, Peritoneal Dialysis, Wichtig Editore, Milano, 49–62, 1982.
6. Nolph KD: Concluding remarks. In: Trevino-Becerra A, Boen FST, Karger S (eds), Today's Art of Peritoneal Dialysis, Basel... Switzerland 17: 146–148, 1979.
7. Cantarovich F, Perez Loredo J, Chena C, Wolberg R, Vernetti

J, Correa C, Tizado J: CAPD – 3 Daily exchanges. In: Moncrief J, Popovich R (Ed) Proc CAPD Int Symp II, Masson, Pub. Austin, TX, p 125, 1980.

8. Twardowski ZJ, Prowant BF, Nolph KD, Martinez AJ, Lampton LM: High volume, low frequency continuous ambulatory peritoneal dialysis. Kid Intern, 23: 64–70, 1983.

9. Moncrief JW, Popovich RP, Nolph KD: Additional experience with continuous ambulatory peritoneal dialysis (CAPD). Trans Am Soc Artif Intern Organs, 24: 476–483, 1978.

10. Babb AL, Popovich RP, Christopher TG, Scribner BH: The genesis of the square meter-hour hypothesis. Trans Am Soc Artif Intern Organs 17: 81–91, 1971.

11. Rubin J, Nolph KD, Popovich RP, Moncrief JW, Prowant B: Drainage volumes during CAPD. asaio Journal 2: 2, 1979.

12. Miller FN, Nolph KD, Joshua IG: The osmolality component of peritoneal dialysis solutions in Continuous Ambulatory Peritoneal Dialysis, Ed Legrain M, Excerpta Medica. Amsterdam, Holland, pp 12–17, 1980.

13. Henderson LW, Nolph KD: Altered permeability of the peritoneal membrane after using hypertonic peritoneal dialysis fluid. J Clin Invest 48: 992–1001, 1969.

14. Baum M, Powell O, McHenry K, Potter D: Comparison of continuous ambulatory peritoneal dialysis (CAPD) and hemodialysis in children, Abstract, The Am Soc of Neph, p 50A, 1982.

15. Kohaut EC, Alexander SR: Ultrafiltration in the young patient on CAPD, In: Moncrief J, Popovich R (ed), Proc CAPD Int Symp II, Masson, Pub, Austin, Tx, p 125, 1980.

16. Simmons EE, Lockard DT, Moncrief JW, Hiatt MP, McCollough WS, Popovich RP: Experience with continuous ambulatory peritoneal dialysis in the maintenance of a surgically anephric dog. Southwest Vet, 33(2): 129–135, 1980.

17. Pyle WK, Moncrief JW, Popovich RP: Peritoneal transport evaluation in CAPD. In: Moncrief J, Popovich R (ed), Proc CAPD Int Symposium II, Masson, Pub, Austin, Tx, p 35, 1980.

18. Boen ST, Haagsma-Schouten WAG, Birnie RJ: Change in ultrafiltration capacity during peritonitis in CAPD patients, Abstract, 4th ISAO Offic Satel Symp on CAPD, Kyoto, p 30, 1983.

19. Hattori F, Nakamoto M, Milishima C, Fujimi S: Structural change of peritoneum in CAPD, Abstract, 4th ISAO Offic Satel Symp on CAPD, Kyoto, p 38, 1983.

20. Slingeneyer A, Mion C, Mourad G, Canaud B, Faller B, Beraud JJ: Progressive sclerosing peritonitis: a late and severe complication of maintenance peritoneal dialysis, Trans Amer Soc Artif Intern organs, 29: 633–638, 1983.

21. Diaz-Buxco JA, Farmer CD, Walker PJ, Chandler JT, Holt KL: Effects of hyperparathyroidism on peritoneal clearances. Trans Am Soc Artif Intern Organs, 28: 276–278, 1982.

22. Manuel MA: Failure of ultrafiltration in patients on CAPD, Periton DSial Bull – Sup, 3: S38–S40, 1983.

23. Wu G, Khanna R, Oreopoulos DG, Vas SI: Incidence and pathogenesis of ultrafiltration failure among CAPD patients. The Am Soc of Nehp, p 125A, 1983.

24. Nolph KD (*et al*): A survey of ultrafiltration in continuous ambulatory peritoneal dialysis. An International Cooperative Study, Second Righetto F, Scanferla F: Xylitol and low doseages of insulin: new perspectives for diabetic uremic patients on CAPD. Perit Dial Bull, 4: 137–142, 1984.

25. Bazzato G, Coli U, Landini S, Fracasso A, Morachiello P, Righetto F, Scanferla F: Xylitol and low doseages of insulin: new perspectives for diabetic uremic patients on CAPD. Perit Dial Bull, 2: 161–164, 1982.

26. Maher JF, Hirszel P, Bennett RR, Chakrabarti E: Amphorericin B selectively increases peritoneal ultrafiltration. The Am Soc of Nelph, p 121A, 1983.

27. Sacchi VA, Bentzel C J, Mookerjee BK, Beam TB: Protamine Sulfate (PS) augments peritoneal clearances in a rabbit model of CAPD and enhances antimicrobial activity in vitro, Abstracts, Kid Intern, 23: 159,, 1983.

28. Alavi N, Lianos E, Bentzel C: Enhanced peritoneal permeability of the rat, by intraperitoneal use of protamine sulfate. Abstracts, Kid Intern, 16: 880, 1979.

29. Alvai N, Lianos E, Andres G, Bentzel CJ: Effect of protamine on the permeability and structure of rat peritoneum. Kid Int, 21: 44–53, 1982.

30. Rubin J, Adair C, Barnes T, Bower JD: Augmentation of peritoneal clearance bu dipyridamole, Kid Int, 22: 658–661, 1982.

31. Lal SM, Nolph KD, Moore H, Khanna R: Verapamil increases urea transport without increase in protein losses. Abstracts Am Soc Artif Intern Organs, 15: 50, 1986.

32. Lamperi S, Carozzi S, Nasini MG: Calcium antagonists improve ultrafiltration in patients on continuous ambulator peritoneal dialysis (CAPD). Trans Am Soc Artif Intern Organs, 33(33): 657–663, 1987.

33. Mactier RA, Khanna R, Twardowski ZJ, Nolph KD: Role of peritoneal cavity lymphatic absorption in peritoneal dialysis (editorial review), Kid Int, 32(2): 165–172, 1987.

34. Bandiani G, Camaiora E, Nicolini MA, Perotta U: Uremic Polyneuropathy (UPN) progression and myoinositol (MI) in patients undergoing CAPD. Periton Dial Bull – Sup, 7: S3, 1987.

35. Blumenkrantz MJ, Kopple JD, Moran JK, Grodstein GP, Coburn JW: Metabolic balance studies inpatients undergoing continuous ambulatory peritoneal dialysis. Am Soc Neph (Abstract) 112A, 1979.

36. Nolph KD, Rosenfield PS, Powel JT, Danforth E: Peritoneal glucose transport and hyperglycemia during peritoneal dialysis. Am Med Sci 259: 272–281, 1970.

37. Grodstein GP, Blumenkrantz MJ, Kopple JD, Moran JK, Coburn JW: Glucose absorption during continuous ambulatory peritoneal dialysis (CAPD), Abstracts, Kid Intern, 22: 220, 1979.

38. Oreopoulos DG: Further experience with the use of amino acid containg dialysate (Amino-Dianeal), In: Moncrief J, Popovich R (ed), Proc CAPD Int Symp II, Masson Pub, Austin, Tx., p 109, 1980.

39. Cantarovich F, Perez Loredo J, Chena C, Reichart M, Tizado J, castro L, Biana D, Juliamolli V: Additives in CAPD, In: Moncrief J, Popovich R (ed), proc CAPD Int Symp II, Masson, pub, Austin, Tx, p 117, 1980.

40. Bazzato G, Coli U, Landini D, Fracasso A, Morachiello P, Righetto F, Scanferla F, Onesti G: Xylitol as osmotic agent in CAPD: an alternative to glucose for uremic diabetic patiewnts?, Trans Am Soc Artif Intern Organs, 23: 280–285, 1982.

41. Heaton A, Ramos M, Johnston D, Gokal R, Ward MK, Kerr DNS: Glucose and lipid metabolism in continuous ambulatory peritoneal dialysis (CAPD), Abstracts, Kid Intern, 22: 220, 1982.

42. Nolph KD, Hopkins CA, New D, Antwiler GD, Popovich RP: Differences in solute sieving with osmotic vs hydrostatic ultrafiltration. Trans Am Soc Artif Intern Organs 22: 618–626, 1976.

43. Moncrief JW, Popovich RP: Conbtinuous ambulatory peritoneal dialysis. In: Trevino-Becerra A, Boen FST, Karger S (eds), Basel, Today's Art of Peritoneal Dialysis. Switzerland 17: 139–145, 1979.

44. Moncrief JW: Round Table Discussion in Continuous Ambulatory Peritoneal Dialysis, Legrain M (ed), Excerpta Medica, Amsterdam, Holland, p 174–178, 1980.

45. Nolph KD, Moncrief JW, Popovich RP: Multi-center evaluation of CAPD in Annual Report, Artificial Kidney-Chronic Uremia Program, National Institute of Arthritis, Metabolism and Digestive Disease, HEW, 1980.

46. Blumenkrantz MJ: Nutrional aspects of peritoneal aspects

of peritoneal dialysis. Proc of Renal Physicians Assoc Symp Peritoneal Dial, 1979.

47. Nolph KD, Twardowski ZJ, Popovich RP: Equilibration of peritoneal dialysis solutions during long-dwell exchanges. J Lab Cl in Med 93(2): 246–256, 1979.

48. Kobayaski K, Manji T, Hiramatsu S, Maeda K, Uemura J: Nitrogen metabolism in patients on peritoneal dialysis. In: Trevino-Becerra A, Boen FST, Karger S (eds), Today's Art of Peritoneal Dialysis. Basel, Switzerland 17: pp 93–100, 1979.

49. Gokal R, Fryer R, McHugh M, WardMK, Kerr DNS: Calcium and phosphate control in patients on continuous ambulatory peritoneal dialysis. In: Legrain M (ed), Continuous Ambulatory Peritoneal Dialysis. Excerpta Medica, Amsterdam Holland, pp 283–291, 1980.

50. Gokal R, Ellis HA, Ward MK, Kerr DNS: Histological renal bone disease in patients on continuouys ambulatory peritoneal dialysis, In: Moncrief J, Popovich R (eds), Proc CAPD Int Symp II, Masson, pub, Austin, Tx, p 249, 1980.

51. Gokal R: Metabolic Effects (calcium, phosphate, vitamin D, PTH, bone disease and trace metal metabolism) in CAPD, Absrtact, 4th ISAO Offic Satel Symp on CAPD Kyoto, p 84, 1983.

52. Calderaro V, Oreopoulos DG, Meema HE, KHanna R, Quinton S, Carmichael D: Renal Osteodystrophy in patients on continuous ambulatory peritoneal dialysis (CAPD), a biochemical and radiological study. In: Moncrief J, Popovich R (eds), Proc CAPD Int Symp II, Masson, pub, Austin Tx, p 243, 1980.

53. Molitoris BA, Alfrey PS, Miller NL, Hasbargen JA, Kaehney WD, Alfrey AC, Smith BJ (1987), Efficacy of intramuscular and intraperitoneal deferoxamine for aluminum chelation. Kid Int, 31(4): 986–991, 1987.

54. Delmez JA, Dougan CS, Gearing BK, Rothstein M, Windus DW, Rapp N, Slatopolsky E: The effects of intraperitoneal cacitriol on calcium and parathyroid hormone. Kid Int, 31(3): 795–799, 1987.

55. Canavese C, Pacitti A, Salomone M, Pramotton C, Segoloni G, bedino S, Testore G, Lamon S, Vercellone A: Chromatographic studies of aluminum-desferrioxamine complex in uremic patients. Trans Am Soc Artif Intern Organs, 32(1): 367–369, 1986.

56. Dibble JB, Coltman SJ, Gibson J, Brownjohn AM: Acute aluminum toxicity in a CAPD patient: the role of oral aluminium hydroxide. Periton Dial Bul, 7(3): 207–208, 1987.

57. Rahman R, Heaton A, Goodship T, Rodger R, Tapson JS, Sellars L, Ellis HA, Wilkinson R, Ward MK: Renal osteodystrophy in patients on continuous ambulatory peritoneal dialysis: a five year study. Periton Dial Bul, 7(1): 20–26, 1987.

58. Passlick J, Wilhelm M, Grabensee B, Ohnesorge FK: Aluminumfree phosphate binder in patients on CAPD. Perit Dial Bul – Sup, 7(2): S58, 1987.

59. Hamdy NAT, Harris SC, Beneton MNC, Brown CB, Kanis JA: A high incidence of spontaneous hypercalcaemia in continuous ambulatory peritoneal dialysis. Periton Dial Bull – Sup, 7(2): S38, 10987.

60. Salusky IB, Fine RN, Kangarloo H, Gold R, Paunier L, Goodman WG, Brill JE, Gilli G, Slatopolsky E, Coburn JW: 'High-dose' calcitriol for control of renal osteodystrophy in children on CAPD. Kid Intern, 32(1): 89–95, 1987.

61. Blumenkrantz MJ: CAPD: Nutritional concerns – have we learned from the experience in the 1960's and 1970's? UIn: Moncreief J, Popovich R (eds), Proc CAPD Int Symp II, Masson, pub, Austin, Tx, p 83, 1980.

62. Blumenkrantz MJ, Kopple JD, Moran JK, Grodstein GP, Coburn JW: Metabolic balance studies in uremic patients undergoing continuous ambulatory peritoneal dialysis (CAPD), Abstracts, Kid Intern, 16: 882, 1979.

63. Bennett SE, Smith BA, Russell GI, Walls J: The nutritional status of long-term CAPD patients. Periton Dial Bull – Sup,

7(2): S5, 1987.

64. Metcoff J, Pederson J, Gable III J, Llach F: Protein synthesis, cellular amino acids, and energy levels in CAPD patients. Kid Intern – Sup, 32(22): S136–S144, 1987.

65. Popovich RP, Moncrief JW, Nolph KD, Ghods AJ, Twardowski ZJ, Pyle WK: Continuous ambulatory peritoneal dialysis. Ann Intern Med 88(4): 449–456, 1978.

66. Moncrief JW, Popovich RP, Nolph KD, Rubin J, Robson M, Dombros N, DeVeber GA, Oreopoulos DG: Clinical experience with continuous ambulatory peritoneal dialysis. Trans Am Soc Artif Intern Organs, 2(3): 114–119, 1979.

67. Lindholm B, Ahlberg M, Alvestrand A, Furst P, Larlander SG, Gergstrom J: Nutritional aspects of continuous ambulatory peritoneal dialysis. In: Continuous AMbulatory Peritoneal Dialysis, Legrain M (ed), Excerpta Medica, Amsterdam, Holland, pp 199–206, 1980.

68. Gahl GM, Baeyer HV, Riedinger R, Borowzak B, Schurig R, Becker H, Kessell M: Caloric intake, and nitrogen balance in patients undergoing CAPD. In: Moncrief J, Popovich R (ed), Proc CAPD Int Symp II, Masson, Pub., Austin, Tx., p 87, 1980.

69. Lindholm B, Furst P, Alvestrand A, Bergstrom J (intr. by K Nolph): Metabolic effects of continuous ambulatory peritoneal dialysis (CAPD), Abstracts, Kid Inter, 16:892, 1979.

70. von Baeyer H, Gahl GM, Riedinger H, Borowzak R, Averdunk R, Schurig R, Kessel M: Adaptation of CAPD patients to the continuous peritoneal energy uptake. Kid Intern, 23: 29–34, 1983.

71. Medical Letter: Home Peritoneal dialysis for end-stage renal disease, 21–17, Issue 538, 1970.

72. Moncrief JW, Popovich RP, Nolph KD: Additional experience with contunuous ambulatory peritoneal dialysis (CAPD). Trans Am Soc Artif Intern Organs, 24: 476–483, 1978.

73. Oreopoulos DG, Vas S, Zellerman G: Continuous ambulatory peritoneal dialysis. In: Proc 12th Ann Contractors Conf, Artificial Kidney-Chronic Uremia Program, National Institute of Arthritis, Metabolism and Digestive Diseases, January, pp 58–65, 1979.

74. Gokal R, Round table discussion. Legrain M (ed), Excerptia Medica, Amsterdam, Holland, pp 209–313, 1980.

75. Miguel Alonso JL, Martinez ME, Selgas R, Carares M, Gomez P, Sanchez Sicilia L: Peritoneal clearance of parathormone, Abstracts, Kid Intern, 22: 216, 1982.

76. Nolph KD, Sorkin M, Rubin J, Dariush A, Prowant B, Fruto L, Kennedy D: Continuous ambulatory peritoneal dialysis: Three-year experience at one center. Ann of Intern Med, 92(5): 609–613, 1980.

77. Moncrief JW, Sorrels PAJ, Druger VJ, Mullins-Blackson C, Pyle WK, Popovich RP: Development of training programs for CAPD – historical review. In: Legrain M (ed), Continuous Ambulatory Peritoneal Dialysis, Excerpta Medica, Amsterdam, Holland, pp 149–151, 1980.

78. Teehan BP, Schleifer CR, Cupit M, Knapp J, Miles HS: Organized aspects of a continuous ambulatory peritoneal dialysis program. In: Legrain M (ed), Continuous Ambulatory Peritoneal Dialysis, Excerpta Medica, Amsterdam, Holland, pp 152–157, 1980.

79. Sorrels PAJ, Kruger VJ, Moncrief JW, Popovich RP: Austin Diagnostic Clinic, continuous ambulatory peritoneal dialysis training program. In: Legrain M (ed), Continuous Ambulatory Peritoneal Dialysis, Excerpta Medica, Amsterdam, Holland, pp 167–170, 1980.

80. Clayton S, Finer C, Quinton C, Jabaz O, Clark S, Lekman B, Oreopoulos DG: Training patients for continuous ambulatory peritoneal dialysis at the Toronto Western Hospital. In: Legrain M (ed), Continuous Ambulatory Peritoneal Dialysis, Excerptia Medica, Amsterdam, Holland, pp 162–166, 1980.

81. Prowant B, Fruto LV: Inpatient home training for continuous

ambulatory peritoneal dialysis. In: Legrain M (ed), Continuous Ambulatory Peritoneal Dialysis, Excerpta Medica, Amsterdam, Holland, pp 158–161, 1980.

82. Khanna R, Wu G, Vas S, Oreopoulos DG: Mortality and morbidity on continuous ambulatory peritoneal dialysis, Trans Am Soc Artif Intern Organs, 6: 197–204, 1983.

83. Oreopoulos DG: Selection criteria and clinical results of continuous ambulatory peritoneal dialysis. In: Legrain M (ed), Continuous Ambulatory Peritoneal Dialysis, Excerpta Medica, Amsterdam, Holland, pp 101–106, 1980.

84. Price JDE, Moriarty MV: Continuous ambulatory peritoneal dialysis: selection criteria – failures and causes – deaths – diabetes mellitus. In: Legrain M (ed), Continuous Ambulatory Peritoneal Dialysis, Excerpta Medica, Amsterdam, Holland, pp 113–119, 1980.

85. Shaldon S: A cynical critque of continuous ambulatory peritoneal dialysis. In: Legrain M (ed), Continuous Ambulatory Peritoneal Dialysis, Excerpta Medica, Amsterdam, Holland, pp 137–140, 1980.

86. Zapacosta A: Patient selection for CAPD. Seminar on CAPD, Philadelphia, 1980.

87. Di PAolo N, Pula G, Capotondo L, Sansoni E: An index of well being for patients on CAPD. Perite Dial Bul – Sup, 7(2): S24, 1987.

88. Hutchinson TA, Harvey CE: Survival with different forms of dialysis treatment – a prognostically controlled comparison. asaio Journal 8: 13–17, 1985.

89. von Lilien T, Salusky IB, Hall TL, Fine RN: Five years experience of CAPD/CCPD in children with end-stage renal disease (ESRD). Perit Dial Bul – Sup, 7(2): S83, 1987.

90. Nolph K, Lindblad A, Novak J, Cutler S: USA CAPD Registry – 1987 report. Perit Dial Bul – Sup, 7(2): S57, 1987.

91. Ramello A, Malcangi U, Bruno M, Reina E, Ghezzi PM: CAPD or hemodialysis? A comparison after 5 years of first choice treatment. Periton Dial Bull – Sup, 7(2): S62, 1987.

92. Buoncristiani U, Altieri P, Cairo G, Quintaliani G, Ferrara R, Scanziana L: Suitability of CAPD for long term treatment of uremic diabetics. Perit Dual Bul – Sup, 7(2): S11, 1987-

93. Stout JP, Auer J, Kincey J, Hillier VF, Gokal R, Simon LG, Oliver D: Sexual and marital relationships and dialysis – the patients's viewpoint. Perit Dial Bull, 7(2): 97–100, 1987.

94. Nissenson AR, Gentile DE, Soderblom RE, Brax C: Long-term outcome of continuous amculatory peritoneal dialysis, Trans Am Soc Artif Intern Organs, 32(1): 560–563, 1986.

95. Zimmerman SW, Johnson CA, O'Brien M: Survival of diabetic patients on continuous ambulatory peritoneal dialysis for over five years, Perit Dual Bul, 7(1): 26–29, 1987.

96. Nissenson AR, Gentile DE, Soderblum R, Brax C: Long-term outcome of CAPD – regional experience, Dial Transpl, 13: 34–39, 1984.

97. Alexander SR, Tseng CH, Maksym KA, Campbell RA, Talwalkar YB: Clinical parameters in continuous ambulatory peritoneal dialysis for infants and children. In: Moncrief J, popovich R (eds), Proc CAPD Int Symp II, Masso, Pub., Austin, Tx, p 195, 1980.

98. Balfe JW, Irwin MA: Continuous ambulatory peritoneal dialysis in pediatrics. In: Legrain M (ed), Continuous Ambulatory Peritoneal Dialysis, Excerpta Medica, Amsterdam, Holland, pp 131–136, 1980.

99. Baum M, Powell D, McHenry K, Potter D: Comparison of continuous ambnulatory peritoneal dialysis (CAPD) and hemodialysis in children, Abstracts, Kid Intern, 23: 143, 1983.

100. Salusky IB, Kopple JD, Fine RN: Continuous ambulatory peritoneal dialysis in pediatric patients: a 20-month experience, Kid Intern – Sup, 24: S101–S105, 1983.

101. Broyer M, Niaudet P, Champion G, Jean G, Chopin N, Czernichow P: Nutritional and metabolic studies in children on continuous ambulatory peritoneal dialysis, Kid Intern – Sup, 24: S106–110.

102. Salusky IB, Fine RN, Nelson P, Kopple J: Growth and nutritional status (NS) in children receiving CAPD, Abstracts, Kid Intern, 23: 159, 1983.

103. Harmon WE: Continuous ambulatory peritoneal dialysis in children, (Letters) The New Eng Jour of Med, 308: 968, 1983.

104. Gruskin AB, Rosenblum H, Baluarte HJ, Morgenstern BZ, Polinsky MS, Perlman SA: Transperitoneal solute movement in children, Kid Intern – Sup, 24: S95–S100, 1983.

105. Morgenstern B, Pyle WK, Gruskin A, Baluarte HJ, Perlman S, Polinsky M, Kaiser B: Transport characteristics of the pediatric peritoneal membrane, The Am Soc of Neph, p. 122A, 1983.

106. Dr. Richard Fine: personal communication. CAPD Consulents Meeting, 19088.

107. Lee HB, Whang SK, Ihm CG, Chun S: Cell-mediated immunity (CMI) in CAPD patients, The Am Soc of Neph, p 121A, 1983.

108. Giacchino F, Alloatti S, Quarello F, Coppo R, Pellerey M, Piccoli G: The influence of peritoneal dialysis on cellular immunity, Perit Dial Bull, 2: 165, 1982.

109. Williams P, Key R, Harrison J et al: Nutritional and anthropometric assessment oif patients on CAPD over one year: contrasting changes in total body nitrogen and potassium. Perit Dial Bull, 6: 82–87.

110. Rubin J, Raju S, Teal N et al: Abdominal hernia in patients undergoing continuous ambuylatory peritoneal dialysis, Arch Intern Med, 142: 1453–1455, 1982.

111. Hamodraka-Mailis A: Pathogensis and treatment of back pain in peritoneal dialysis patients, Perit Dial Bull – Sup, 3: S41–S43, 1983.

112. Tenchkoff H, Schechter H: A bacteriologically safe peritoneal access device. Trans Am Soc Artif Intern Organs, 14: 181–186, 1968.

113. Oreopoulos DG, Zellerman G, Izatt S: The Toronto Western Hospital permanent peritoneal catheter and continuous ambulatory peritoneal dialysis connector. In: Legrain M (ed), Continuous Ambulatory Peritoneal Dialysis, Excerpta Medica, Amsterdam, Holland, pp 73–78, 1980.

114. Valli A, Comotti C, Torelli, Crescimanno U, Valentini A, Riegler P, Huber W, Borghi M, Gruttadauria C, Scarovanati P, Pecchini F: A new catheter for peritoneal dialysis (two years of experience with Valli Catheter), Transactions, Amer Soc for Artif Internal organs, XXIX: 629–631, 1983.

115. Nolph KD: Personal communication, 1980.

116. Oreopoulos DG, Baird-Heldrich G, Khanna R, Lum GM, Mattheus R, Paulsen K, Twardowski ZJ, Vas SI: Peritoneal catheters and exit-site practices: current recommendations. Perit Dial Bull, 7(3): 130–135, 1987.

117. Tenckhoff H: Chronic Peritoneal Dialysis. In: A Manual for patient, dialysis personnel and physicians, Univ. of Washington School of Medicine, Seattle, Washington.

118. Colombi A, Gianella C: Straight implantation of the Tenckhoff catheter for continuous ambulatory peritoneal dialysis. In: Legrain M (ed), Continuous Ambulatory Peritoneal Dialysis, Excerpta Medica, Amsterdam, Holland, pp 69–72, 1980.

119. Kirksey T: Surgical Implantation of the single-cuff (acute) Tenckhoff catheter. In: Proc CAPD Int Symp II, Masson, 1980.

120. Blumenkrantz MJ: Personal communication, 1984.

121. Flynn CT, Nanson JA: Intraperitoneal insulin with CAPD – an artificial pancreas. Trans Am Soc Artif Intern Organs 25: 114–116, 1979.

122. Going Home with Confidence, Procedure for Continuous Ambulatory Peritoneal Dialysis Staff Program, Baxter Travenol Laboratories Inc., 1979.

123. Rubin J, Rogers WA, Taylor HM, Everett ED, Prowant DB, Fruto LV, Nolph KD: Pertitonitis during continuous ambulatory peritoneal dialysis. Ann Intern Med 92(1): 7–13, 1980.

·124. Moncrief JW: Contunious ambulatory peritoneal dialysis concepts and clinical application. In: Marti M, Locatelli A (eds), Int Symp Chronic Peritoneal Dial, Buenos Aires, Argentina, p 153, 1980.

125. Osmond H, Loh Y, Dombros D, Oreopoulos DG, Paraport A: Effects of CAPD on renin-angiotensin system. Am Soc Neph (Abstract) 67A, 1978.

126. DePaepe M, Sche;straete K, Ringoir S, Lameire NH: influence of continuous ambulatory peritoneal dialysis on the anemia of endstage renal disease, Kid Int, 23: 744–748, 1983.

127. Mehta BR, Mogridge C, Bell JD: Changes in red cell mass, plasma volume and hematocrit in patients in CAPD, Trans Amer Soc Artif Intern Organs, 298: 50–52, 1983.

128. De Paepe M, Lameire N, schelstraete K, Ringoir S: Changes in red cell mass, plasma volume and hemotocrit in patients on continuous ambulatory peritoneal dialysis, Proc Eur Dial Transplant Assoc 18: 286, 1981.

129. Zappacosta AR, Caro J, Erslev A: Normalization of hemotocrit in patients with end-stage renal disease on continuous ambulatory peritoneal dialysis, Am J Med 72: 53, 1982.

130. Lindsay RM, Oreopoulos DG, Burton H, Conley J, Wells G: A comparison of CAPD and hemodialysis in adaptation to home dialysis. In: Moncrief J, Popovich R (eds, Proc CAPD Int Symp II, Masson, Pub., Austin, Tx., p 171, 1980.

131. Moncrief JW, Popovich RP: Peritoneal dialysis for a greater number of patients? In: Schreiner CE (ed), Controversies in Nephrology, Georgetown Universiy, Washington, D.C., pp 31–44, 1979.

132. Flynn CT, Strosahl: Self-care by the blind diabetic on continuous ambulatory peritoneal dialysis, Diab neph, 1: 22–24, 1982.

133. Berger PS, Alpert BE, Longnecker RE: Dialysis therapy for Diabetics, Diab Neph, 2: 22–25, 1983.

134. Sorkin MI, Luger AM, Prowant B, Kennedy J, Moore H, Nolph KD: Histological and functional characteristics of the peritoneal membrane of a diabetic patient after 34 months of CAPD, Perit Dial Bul, 2: 24–27, 1982.

135. Williams C, Belvedere D, Cattran D, Clayton S, Cole E, Fenton S, Gutman K, Khanna R, Knight S, Manuel A, Oreopoulos D, Pierratoss A, Roscoe J, Saiphoo C, Vas S: Experience with CAPD in diabetic patients in Toronto, perit Dial Bul – Sup, 2: S12–S16, 1982.

136. Roscoe JM: Practices of insulin administration in CAPD, Perit Dial Bul – Sup, 2: S27–S29, 1982.

137. Posen G, Lam E, Rappoport A: The management of end-stage renal disease (ESRD) in diabetes mellitus (DM) in Canada in 1981, Trans Amer Soc Artif Intern Organs, 29: 116–118, 1983.

138. Amair P, Khanna R, Leibel B, Pierratos A, Vas S, Meema E, Blair G, Chisholm L, Vas M, Zingg W, Digenis G, Oreopoulos DG: Continuous ambulatory peritoneal dialysis in diabetics with end-stage renal disease. Perit Dial Bul – Sup, 2: S6–S11, 1982.

139. Leenen F, Smith DL, Khanna R, Oreopoulos DG: Changes in left ventricular anatomy and function on CAPD, Perit Dial Bull – Sup, 3: SD26–S28, 1983.

140. Lamperi S, Carozzi S, Icardi A: In vitro and in vivo studies of erthropoesis during continuous ambulatory peritoneal dialysis, Perit Dial Bull, 3: 94–96, 1983.

141. Wideroe TE, Sanengen T, Halvorsen S: Erythropoietin and uremic toxicity during continuous ambulatory peritoneal dialysis. Kidney Intern – Sup, 24(16): S208–S217, 1983.

142. Goldsmith HJ, Forbes A, Gyde OHD, Summerfield G: Hematological aspects of continuous ambulatory peritoneal dialysis. In: Legrain M (ed), Continuous Ambulatory Peritoneal Dialysis, Excerpta Medica, Amsterdam, Holland, pp 302–308, 1980.

143. Popovich RP, Moncrief JW, Decherd JP, Bomar JB, Pyle WK: The definition of a novel portable/wearable equilibrium peritoneal dialysis technique. Trans Am Soc Artif Int Organs (abstr) 5: 64, 1976.

144. Williams PS, Hendy MS, Ackrill P: Routine daily surveillance cultures in the management of CAOPD patients. Perit Dial Bull, 7(3): 183–186.

145. Nolph KD, Sorkin MI: Diagnosis and treatment of peritonitis. In: Moncrief J, Popovich R (eds), Proc CAPD Int Symp II, Masson, Pub, Austin, Tx., p 273, 1980.

146. Baxter Travenol Laboratories, personal communication.

10

CONTINUOUS CYCLIC PERITONEAL DIALYSIS

JOSE A. DIAZ-BUXO

1. INTRODUCTION

Continuous cyclic peritoneal dialysis (CCPD) is based on the concept of continuous equilibration dialysis proposed by Popovich *et al.*, but incorporates the automation provided by a cycler [1, 2]. CCPD uses multiple short nocturnal exchanges, while the patient is connected to the cycler and a long diurnal exchange with the patient ambulatory. Thus, it is a virtual reversal of the CAPD schedule. The primary objective of CCPD is to provide automated, continuous peritoneal dialysis in a convenient manner, freeing the daytime hours from all procedures. The secondary goal is to reduce the rate of peritonitis.

After several years of experience with CCPD we feel that the original goals have been fulfilled. CCPD has been of particular benefit to those patients in need of assistance with procedures due to their poor muscular coordination, blindness and generalized weakness and patients unwilling or unable to perform manual dialysis exchanges. Thus, the interest in CCPD for the very young, the elderly and the diabetic patients.

The growth of CCPD has been modest when compared to that of CAPD. Nonetheless, it is calculated that approximately 2000 patients currently undergo CCPD as their main form of renal replacement therapy. It is likely that the primary deterrent of CCPD growth is the higher cost of treatment. Recent changes in the basic technique of CPPD promise to both simplify the procedure and reduce the cost of provision of therapy.

2. TECHNIQUE

Peritoneal access is provided by a permanent catheter of the straight, curled or column-disk type. CCPD requires an automated cycler capable of delivering variable volumes of dialysate for a prescribed dwell time. The peritoneal catheter is connected to the cycler line before the patient retires at night. Three or four cycles are generally administrated during the night, each lasting two to three hours, using 2 l of commercial dialysate. An additional exchange is effected in the morning, prior to disconnection. The 2 l of dialysate infused in the morning are allowed to dwell intraperitoneally for the next 14–15 hr with the catheter capped. Hypertonic dialysate containing 2.5–4.25% dextrose is recommended for the diurnal cycle in order to prevent significant absorption of the solution. All connections and disconnections take place in the early morning and at night, in the convenience of the patient's home. The average length of time required to set up the equipment and connect the catheter to the cycler is 20 minutes.

A new disconnection technique for CCPD was introduced in 1985 using the principle of external occlusion [3, 4]. A simple, disposable, plastic clamp is used in the morning to occlude the patient's cycler line distal to its connection with the peritoneal catheter (Figure 1). The line is then cut with unsterile scissors. This methodology reduces the disconnection time to a few seconds in the morning, can be easily mastered by most blind patients, the elderly and children, and eliminates the cost of sterile supplies (masks,

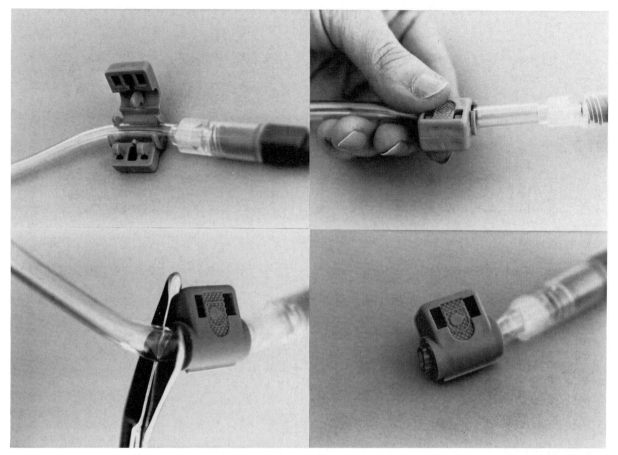

Figure 1. Disposable clamp for disconnection after nocturnal cycle of CCPD using external occlusion.

gloves and desinfectants). The physical and microbiologic tests have shown this technique to be safe. Clinical evaluation with more than 200 patients over two years has shown excellent patient acceptance and no increase in the rate of peritonitis. Only three accidental disconnections have been reported after 36 500 consecutive uses.

Another modification to the CCPD technique designed to reduce the procedural time and the cost of CCPD is the multiple tubing set (MTS™) [5]. The MTS has 12 prongs to accommodate an equal number of dialysate bags and a patient line fitted with three connectors in-series. The equipment is set up with all the dialysate bags required for three consecutive days of CCPD. Only the dialysate lines necessary for one session (24 hr) are open. A new patient line connector is used during each session. Disconnections are performed with two external occluders placed between the last connector used and the connector to be used for the next session. Therefore, the system is never open at the time of disconnection and sterility is preserved for the next CCPD session. The MTS maintains the sterility of the CCPD system, reduces the amount of labor and time associated with cycler setup and decreases the cost of CCPD. No significant difference in the risk of peritonitis has been reported for patients simultaneously treated with conventional CCPD sets and MTS.

2.1. Peritoneal cyclers

The peritoneal cycler was designed to provide automated dialysate exchanges in a safe and simple manner. The principal functions of the cycler are to automatically deliver a prescribed volume of dialysate into the peritoneal cavity and to allow the dialysate to dwell, followed by a period of drainage. All these functions must be precisely timed. In addition, many cyclers incorporate safety and comfort features such as solution heaters and ultrafiltration monitors. Solution heaters are important in preventing administration of cold dialysate which may result in discomfort and lowering of the patient's core temperature. Severe hypothermia can cause cardiac arrhythmias and cardiac arrest [6]. However, these complications are more prone to occur when high flow automated delivery systems are used than with the typical CCPD prescription since equilibration dialysis is a low flow system and the temperature of the inflowing dialysate readily equalizes with that of the patient.

Ultrafiltration monitors are important to prevent overhydration and to keep the patient informed of his volume status at any time during the procedure. Precise ultrafiltration monitors are particularly valuable for cyclers used in the hospital setting during acute dialysis and for patients in need of high ultrafiltration. Some ultrafiltration devices incorporate a continuous digital readout that records the actual net ultrafiltration, while others use an alarm that is activated if the prescribed ultrafiltration goal is not accomplished.

Most cyclers are designed after Lasker's model using gravity for infusion and drainage of dialysate (Figure 2A) [7]. Commercial dialysate in bottles or plastic containers can be utilized. The first step in initiating dialysis is to set the cycler controls to determine the volume of exchanges, length of intraperitoneal dwell, and outflow or drainage time. The dialysate flows from the container to a heating cabinet that will also determine the volume of inflow. Once a temperature of approximately 38°C is accomplished, the fluid is delivered to the peritoneal cavity. After the prescribed dwell time is completed, the cycler automatically shifts into a drain cycle and the fluid is collected in a weight bag to monitor adequate drainage. The spent dialysate finally flows into a disposable drain bag. This basic system can be modified with the use of microcomputerized programs to closely monitor net ultrafiltration.

An offspring of the original cycler concept uses a roller pump to deliver dialysate to a bag placed on a heating cradle which is placed at least 20 cm over the patient's abdomen, thereby preserving the ability to deliver dialysate by gravity while using large dialysate containers (Figure 2B). The roller pump has the dual function of delivering a prescribed volume of dialysate to the heating bag and acting as an occluder to prevent the retrograde transit of bacteria from the final drain container. An advantage of this system is its capability of using less expensive, larger dialysate containers. Large containers of dialysate are difficult to handle by most patients. This system provides active pumping of the dialysate from the floot to the heater plate, eliminating the need to lift the container.

A third type of cycler has been proposed which utilizes roller pumps for both the active infusion and drainage of dialysate into and out of the peritoneal cavity (Figure 2C) [8]. These systems have not found commercial application mainly due to the fear of over distending the abdominal cavity through positive pressure in the event of malfunction and the potential risk associated with application of negative pressure (suction) for drainage. The advantages of this system are the significant reduction in size and weight that a simple set of pumps makes possible and the potential to provide faster inflows and drainage of dialysate.

3. SOLUTIONS FOR CCPD

The recommended dialysate formulation for CCPD is essentially the same as for continuous ambulatory peritoneal dialysis (CAPD). However, for the occasional patient who needs shorter and frequent exchanges in order to accomplish a high rate of ultrafiltration and small solute removal, lower sodium concentrations may be recommended. Where dwell times of short duration and hypertonic glucose solutions are used, proportionately greater removal of extracellular water than sodium often occurs with consequent hypernatremia [9, 10]. This phenomenon is most notable when the dwell times are extremely short, usually less than 30 min, and applies mainly to intermittent peritoneal dialysis (IPD). The standard solutions utilized in most centers for CCPD are given in Table 1. Glucose concentrations of 2.5 or 4.25% are recommended for the long diurnal cycle. The use of lower osmolalities invariably causes absorption of the dialysate which results in overhydration and reduction in solute clearance.

Table 1. Composition of standard solutions for CCPD.

Dextrose	(%)	1.5–4.25
Sodium	(mEq/l)	132
Potassium	(mEq/l)	0
Calcium	(mEq/l)	3.5–4.0
Magnesium	(mEq/l)	0.5–1.5
Lactate	(mEq/l)	35–40

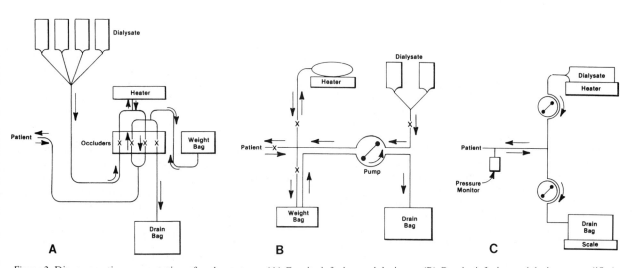

Figure 2. Diagrammatic representation of cycler systems. (A) Gravity infusion and drainage; (B) Gravity infusion and drainage, modified by active transfer of solution; (C)) Active infusion and drainage by roller pumps.

4. PHYSIOLOGIC CONSIDERATIONS

Although the schedule of CCPD is a virtual reversal of CAPD, the use of shorter and more frequent nocturnal exchanges and the introduction of a prolonged diurnal dwell result in physical and kinetic differences that deserve mention.

4.1. Ultrafiltration

The typical patient undergoing CCPD using 8 l of dialysate/day can accomplish a net ultrafiltration of 0.5–3 l with the use of dialysate containing 1.5–4.25% dextrose. In the peritoneal dialysis system, ultrafiltration is mainly a function of transperitoneal osmotic gradient; therefore, increments in the dextrose concentration of the solution can most conveniently increase net ultrafiltration. However, the peritoneal ultrafiltration rate curve exhibits an exponential decay type of configuration. It follows that maximum net ultrafiltration can be achieved by increasing the number of exchanges and reducing the dwell time. Patients with extraordinary ultrafiltration requirements may benefit from additional, shorter nocturnal exchanges.

For practical purposes all net ultrafiltration occurs during the nocturnal exchanges. Even with the use of 4.25% dextrose, most patients will absorb 12–20% of the volume infused for the diurnal cycle after 14 hr of dwell.

4.2. Solute removal

The clearances for small molecules, such as urea and creatinine, for the average patient on four daily exchanges of CCPD (three, 2 l nocturnal exchanges and one 2 l diurnal exchange) are 7.8 l/day for urea and 5.8l for creatinine. These clearances are slightly lower than those of CAPD and superior to IPD. Full equilibration between dialysate and plasma for small molecules is attained within 4 hr of dialysate dwell. Consequently, the long diurnal cycle of CCPD becomes relatively inefficient in clearing small molecules. For patients requiring high small molecular solute removal, the addition of multiple short dwell nocturnal exchanges to enhance small molecular clearances is recommended.

The equilibration of middle molecules is significantly slower. Even at the end of the long diurnal cycle, equilibration is incomplete for larger molecules such as inulin and vitamin B_{12}. For these larger molecules, the time of exposure of dialysate to the peritoneal membrane and the surface area of the peritoneum become the determining factors in solute removal, while manipulation of dialysate flow is of little consequence.

Twardowski et al have suggested the use of high volume dialysate exchanges to increase the rate of solute removal for small molecules [11]. The concept is based on the observation that the rate of transperitoneal equilibration for urea and creatinine is similar for 2 and 3 l dialysate exchanges. Despite the practical advantages offered by this protocol, many patients cannot tolerate high volume dialysate exchanges during the day due to the high intraperitoneal pressure generated by 3 l of dialysate while the patient is in a sitting or standing position. Convenient application of the high volume dialysate exchange concept can be made utilizing the automated nocturnal exchanges of CCPD, since the intraperitoneal pressure generated by the same volume of dialysate is lower when the patient is in the supine position [12, 13, 14]. Forced vital capacity diminishes when dialysate is infused intraperitoneally and has been reported to deteriorate further with increasing intraperitoneal volume in the supine than in the vertical position [13]. Although pulmonary compromise with the use of 3 l of dialysate is rare and only observed in patients with severe obstructive pulmonary disease [15], caution must be exerted in prescribing volumes exceeding 2 l in patients with already restricted vital capacities.

4.3. Contributions of the diurnal cycle

The recognition of a causal relationship between intra-abdominal pressure, body position and certain complications of peritoneal dialysis, has stimulated certain modifications in the CCPD protocol. The most common modifications are the reduction in the volume or total elimination of the diurnal cycle and an increase in the number of nocturnal cycles to partially compensate for the reduction in diurnal clearance of solutes. The elimination of the diurnal cycle of CCPD results in intermittent (IPD) or nightly peritoneal dialysis (NPD) and has a significant impact on solute removal in patients with normal peritoneal permeability.

We have studied the effects of several CCPD protocols on peritoneal urea and creatinine clearances and protein losses in 12 patients with normal peritoneal permeability [16]. Peritoneal permeability was assessed by the standardized equilibration tests proposed by Twardowski et al [17, 18]. The ratio of dialysate glucose concentration at four hours to the initial glucose concentration ranged (D_4/D_0) between 0.33 and 0.42 for the 12 patients studied (Figure 3). Three study protocols were used. The nocturnal exchanges lasted a total of 10 hr and used 1.5% dextrose dialysate. The diurnal exchange lasted for 14 hr and used 4.25% dextrose dialysate. Protocol I consisted of three, 2 l nocturnal exchanges and the diurnal exchange. Protocol II used four, 2 l exchanges and totally eliminated the diurnal exchange and Protocol III used three, 2 l nocturnal exchanges and also eliminated the diurnal cycle. The sequence of the studies was randomized. Figure 4 summarizes the urea and creatinine clearances for the three protocols. Significantly greater clearances for both urea and creatinine were obtained with Protocol I (CCPD) than with Protocols II and III which eliminated the diurnal cycle (NPD). No significant differences in protein losses were observed between the three protocols. These data suggest that an increase in nocturnal dialysate flow only partially compensates for the loss in clearance otherwise provided by the diurnal cycle. The experience is consistent with that of Twardowski et al who demonstrated that NPD required three times the dialysate flow to provide the same urea clearance as CAPD and that creatinine clearance with CAPD was superior to that of NPD patients using 26 l of dialysate over 8 hr for patients with normal peritoneal permeability [19].

Although reductions in diurnal volume may be necessary in some patients due to intolerance or the development of complications associated with increased intra-abdominal

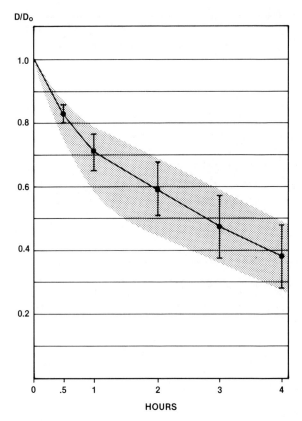

Figure 3. Equilibration curve for glucose for the study population using 2 l of 2.5% dextrose dialysate. D/D_0 refers to glucose concentration in dialysate at time t/glucose concentration in dialysate immediately after instillation. The shaded area represents mean ± 1SD for our total population [16].

pressure (vide infra), most patients on CCPD can tolerate a diurnal volume 50–75% of the nocturnal exchange. Patients with peritoneal hyperpermeability benefit from complete elimination of the diurnal cycle and transfer to NPD. The long-term effects of a 10–20% reduction in the efficiency of solute removal have not been assessed. However, we suspect that these changes may have significant clinical consequences, particularly when consideration is given to the fact that clearances of larger molecules are preferentially affected.

4.4. Relationship between intra-abdominal volume and intra-abdominal pressure

A positive relationship between intra-abdominal pressure and intra-abdominal dialysate volume has been established [12–14]. This relationship is maintained regardless of the patient's position, but the slope of the curve shifts with changes in position (Figure 5). Increments in pressure with a given volume are higher in the upright than in the supine position and further increase in the sitting position [13, 14]. Consequently, the patient is able to tolerate the same or even larger volumes of dialysate at night while in the supine position than during the active hours of the day.

The effects of volume and position on intra-abdominal

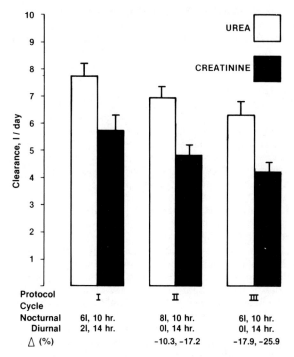

Figure 4. Daily urea and creatinine clearance with different dialysis protocols [16].

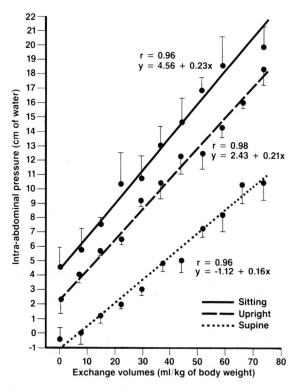

Figure 5. Comparative effect of dialysate volume and patient position on intra-abdominal pressure. Means ± SEM [14].

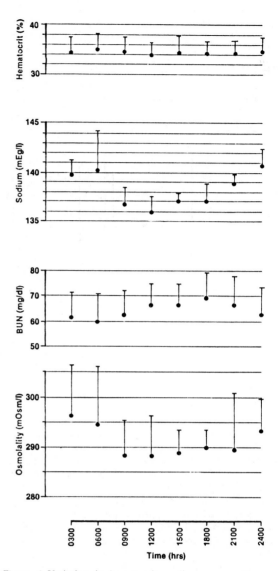

pressure should be kept in mind when prescribing CCPD. Since net ultrafiltration peaks approximately three hours after infusion of hypertonic dialysate for the diurnal cycle, and since this time often coincides with the ingestion of food, which further increases intra-abdominal pressure, it is wise to reduce the volume of diurnal exchange if abdominal discomfort due to increased intra-abdominal pressure is present. In our experience, one third of the patients have complained of abdominal discomfort with intra-abdominal volumes of 28–30 ml/kg body weight, while most patients tolerate 22–25 ml/kg body weight. The appropriate reduction in diurnal intra-abdominal volume has also resulted in a decrease in the incidence of those complications due to increased intra-abdominal pressure.

4.5. Steady physiologic state

One of the desirable features of continuous peritoneal dialysis is the maintenance of a steady physiologic state as reflected by minimal fluctuations in body chemistries. Since most of the ultrafiltration and solute removal during CCPD occurs at night and the bulk of solute and fluid intake occurs during the day, we could expect some fluctuation in the hydration status and body chemistries during a 24-hr period. In practice, this fluctuation should not be a significant limitation since most patients on three times weekly hemodialysis tolerate treatment for many years without obvious disequilibrium symptoms. Furthermore, disequilibrium is rare in patients undergoing intermittent peritoneal dialysis on alternate nights. We have addressed the problem by studying selected biochemical parameters in a series of patients undergoing CCPD (Figure 6). Minimal variations in the blood composition were noted, the most apparent of which were an increase in serum osmolality and sodium at night, and higher BUN levels in the afternoon. These changes are not clinically significant.

4.6. Selection of the optimal schedule for CCPD

In formulating a logical CCPD prescription for a particular patient, the clinician must take into consideration the patient's needs for ultrafiltration and solute clearance together with the aforementioned kinetic principles. The resulting prescription is the 'best compromise' for the specific set of circumstances.

Dwell time is a major determinant of solute removal. Given a fixed volume, the most cost effective prescription uses equal dwell times for all cycles. In clinical practice, nocturnal cycles exceeding ten hours are poorly accepted and those shorter than eight hours significantly reduce solute removal. Thus, a series of nocturnal cycles with equally distributed exchanges over ten hours is recommended. A diurnal cycle is imperative in order to maintain adequate middle molecule clearance.

Variations in the volume of dialysate (flow) significantly affect small solute clearance. Increasing the number of nocturnal exchanges during the 10 hr of automated cycling enhances small solute removal, but does not provide a proportional increase in small solute clearance. Therefore, it is not practical to increase the number of nocturnal cycles beyond four or five in the average patient.

The selection of the optimal exchange volume of dialysate

Figure 6. Variation in hematocrit, sodium, urea, nitrogen and osmolality during a 24-hr period in 5 patients undergoing CCPD.

necessary for adequate therapy should also take into account the age and size of the patient. Most infants will tolerate dialysate volumes of 50 ml/kg of body weight. Older children (weighing 25 kg or more) and adults do best with nocturnal dialysate volumes of 28–35 ml/kg body weight. A 15–25% reduction in the dialysate volume is recommended for the diurnal cycle.

Peritoneal permeability is by far the most important determinant of the optimal CCPD schedule. Patients with average peritoneal permeability and those that fall within one standard deviation of the mean can benefit from CAPD and CCPD using conventional schedules. However, patients with extremely high peritoneal transport rates ($D_4/D_0 < 0.15$) will absorb most of their dialysate with dwell times exceeding three hours and should be transferred to nocturnal peritoneal dialysis. Some patients with high peritoneal transport rates (high permeability) can maintain adequate or superior solute removal and satisfactory ultrafiltration with NPD. Conversely, patients with extremely low peritoneal transport ($D_4/D_0>0.6$) usually require transfer to hemodialysis due to poor solute clearance.

5. CLINICAL EXPERIENCE WITH CCPD

5.1. Hematologic and biochemical parameters

The experience with the hematologic and biochemical profiles of pediatric and adult patients undergoing CCPD has been previously reported [2, 4, 14, 20–27]. Although the results are essentially the same as those observed in patients undergoing CAPD, reference should be made to a few selected parameters which have been studied in greater detail or which have shown characteristic behavior in the CCPD patient population

5.1.1. Hematologic parameters
The hemoglobin concentrations have uniformly improved among patients undergoing CCPD. The extent of the increments in hemoglobin concentration are similar to those reported by other groups with CAPD [28–30]. The factors responsible for the improvement have not been fully delineated. The most likely explantations for this phenomenon are a decrease in plasma volume, an increase in red cell life, or a combination of these factors. A characteristic pattern of rapid improvement in hematocrit and hemoglobin concentrations is usually noted during the first three months of therapy followed by a very slow increase during the subsequent 6 months. This is often accompanied by a drop in weight at the initiation of dialysis, probably reflecting contraction of plasma volume and removal of edema fluid, and progressive weight gain thereafter, possibly due to an accumulation of adipose tissue and/or an increase in muscle mass. This pattern is consistent with the observations of DePaepe et al, who reported an increase in hematocrit during the first 6 months of CAPD treatment concomitant with a decrease in plasma volume followed by an increase in red cell mass during the subsequent months of observation [30]. Lamperi *et al.* have shown an improvement in hematocrit, hemoglobin, and reticulocyte values and a strong correlation with the recovery of the erythroid cell proliferative activity in patients undergoing CAPD [31]. No change in the level of serum erythropoietin was reported by these authors, suggesting that the improvement in bone marrow function is due to better clearance of substances which inhibit the response of bone marrow to erythropoietin. During the first six months of peritoneal dialysis, it is likely that a concomitant decrease in plasma volume and a gradual increase in red cell mass takes place, which accounts for the dramatic improvement in hemoglobin and hematocrit values. In our experience the hemoglobin concentration has remained relatively stable after nine months of CCPD, but can be drastically affected by severe and prolonged episodes of peritonitis and concomitant malnutrition.

5.1.2. Nitrogenous waste products
Marked interpatient variation has been noted in nitrogenous waste product concentration. We have seen a small increase in BUN and creatinine concentrations among CCPD patients when compared to CAPD patients using the same dialysate flows. A similar increase in serum creatinine concentrations in CCPD has been reported among pediatric patients [26].

5.1.3. Calcium, phosphorus and renal osteodystrophy
No significant differences have been noted between calcium and phosphorus concentrations or the dosage of phosphate binders required between CAPD and CCPD patients in our program. Most patients were dialyzed with a dialysate calcium concentration of 4 mEq/l. Vitamin D supplementation (1,25-dihydroxycholecalciferol) was used in 30% of the patients who presented with hypocalcemia at the beginning of CCPD therapy. During the first six months of treatment 65% of the patients required calcium carbonate supplement in order to maintain their serum calcium levels in the range of 8.5–9.5 mg%. After one year however, only 15% of the patients required oral calcium supplementation, while most were able to maintain a normal serum calcium level. Since calcium carbonate has been used as our primary phosphate binder during the past 2 yr, more than 90% of the patients remain on oral calcium supplements at the end of one year. Eighty-five percent of the patients have required phosphate binders and only 15% were capable of maintaining a normal phosphate level without binders. The serum alkaline phosphatase levels have been slightly elevated without apparent trends.

Renal osteodystrophy manifested by osteitis fibrosa, osteomalacia and aluminum deposition in the ossification front has been observed among patients undergoing CCPD. Nonetheless, we have been impressed by the lower incidence of fractures and clinically significant renal osteodystrophy requiring parathyroidectomy among the CAPD and CCPD patients compared to our hemodialysis population. Circulating parathyroid hormone levels have also proven significantly lower among CCPD patients than in hemodialysis patients, even when the data are adjusted for duration of uremia, age and sex (unpublished observations). Rahman et al have reported significant reductions in serum parathyroid hormone concentrations among CAPD patients [32]. Among their patients with secondary hyperparathyroidism, 82% showed histologic improvement in their bone biopsies. Delmez et al also concluded that CAPD generally enhances the mineralizing capacity of osteoblasts and support that CAPD is beneficial to the uremic skeleton [33]. Since a lower incidence of hyperparathyroidism has been reported among diabetic uremic patients and the proportion of diabetics was higher among our CCPD than hemodialysis patients, it is possible that the etiologic factors leading to end-stage renal disease may have played a role in this difference [34, 35].

It is premature to reach conclusions regarding the development of renal osteodystrophy in patients undergoing CCPD due to the limited number of patients studied. However, the improved and constant maintenance of an adequate acid-base balance when compared to patients undergoing hemodialysis could also play a role in the prevention of renal osteodystrophy.

5.1.4. Nutritional status
In our experience very few patients ingest the recommended

1.2 gm of protein/kg of body weight/day as estimated from nutritional histories and protein counts on a selective menu diet. The mean consumption for our population is 0.75 gm protein/kg of body weight/day with more than 75% of patients ingesting less than the recommended daily allowance. No specific caloric restrictions have been recommended unless the patient develops obesity or is diabetic. On this dietary program, 40 patients observed for a period of at least one year have shown a mean calculated dry weight increase in body mass of 3.95 ± 1.21 kg. Twenty-two to 35% of the energy intake was estimated to be provided by dialysate glucose.

Fine and Salusky have also reported a deficient energy and protein intake among children undergoing chronic peritoneal dialysis for more than one year [27]. In their experience, it was energy intake that was mostly affected. Among the children studied the total energy intake (oral plus dialysate) of the prepubertal patients was 75 ± 22% of the prescribed intake, with 50% of the patients consuming less than 75% of the amount prescribed. In the pubertal patients, the estimated intake was 54 ± 9% of that prescribed. Protein intake was 96 ± 30% of that prescribed in the prepubertal children, with 36% of the children consuming less than 75% of the prescribed intake. The pubertal children consumed 72 ± 19% of the amount prescribed, with 56% consuming less than 75%.

We should consider three circumstances, inherent to continuous peritoneal dialysis, which contribute to malnutrition: 1) protein losses through the peritoneal effluent; 2) the constant intraperitoneal glucose infusion and, 3) the effects of increased intraperitoneal pressure on appetite. Marked interpatient variations in peritoneal protein losses are observed. However, the typical protein losses for noninfected patients vary between 6 and 12 gm/day [36]. Most CCPD patients maintain low normal or mildly depressed serum albumin levels similar to those reported for CAPD. In our experience and that of others the total daily peritoneal protein losses bear no correlation to the peritoneal dialysis schedule, number or length of dialysate exchanges or dialysate flow [16]. However, slightly higher peritoneal protein losses are often observed in patients using hypertonic dextrose solutions. Leichter *et al.* have reported their experience with multiple CCPD protocols in children and were unable to find a clear-cut relationship between protein losses and the number of exchanges [37]. Although the daytime dwell contributed significantly to the protein loss, the total loss did not increase when a daytime dwell was used. Peritonitis can cause drastic increases in protein losses [36]. Combined with the anorexia typically seen with peritonitis and the hypercatabolic state generated by sepsis, the protein loss acquires new significance. Katirtzoglou *et al.* have noted that the influence of peritonitis on protein losses can be persistent [38]. Patients who had never experienced peritonitis had a protein loss averaging 5.69 gm/day, compared with 9.7 gm/day in patients who had had at least one episode of peritonitis in the previous three months.

The use of glucose as an osmotic agent in peritoneal dialysis can be considered a blessing or a curse in disguise. On the one hand, glucose provides a significant caloric load, occasionally contributing as much as one third of the energy requirements for the patient [39]. On the other hand, the constant glucose load may result in hyperglycemia among diabetics, hypertriglyceridemia, obesity and poor protein intake. An adult type of kwashiorkor can develop in some patients due to protein malnutrition in the presence of excessive energy intake. CCPD has the advantage of providing increased net ultrafiltration per gram of glucose absorbed during the shorter nocturnal cycles. However, the diurnal cycle results in a considerable glucose load due to its length and the use of hypertonic solutions

The increased intra-abdominal pressure generated by intraperitoneal dialysate also interferes with food intake by causing early satiety or aggravating symptoms of gastrointestinal reflux. If these symptoms are present, intra-abdominal pressure can be reduced by a proportional decrease in the volume of the diurnal dialysate exchange. Hypercholesterolemia has not been a significant problem in most patients. As is the case with CAPD, a small percentage of CCPD patients have developed hypertriglyceridemia. In most cases, the serum concentration of triglycerides were already high at the initiation of CCPD. Among diabetic patients with hypertriglyceridemia, significant improvent in serum triglycerides can be achieved with the addition of intraperitoneal insulin in doses of 5–15 units/l of dialysate (Figure 7). The correction of hyperlipidemia in diabetic patients is consistent with the experience of Moncrief *et al.* [40]. Nondiabetic patients usually fail to respond to intraperitoneal insulin. Beardsworth *et al.* have also concluded that there is no significant change in any lipid parameter in nondiabetic hyperlipidemic patients on CAPD treated with insulin despite a significant fall in fasting and postprandial glucose values [41].

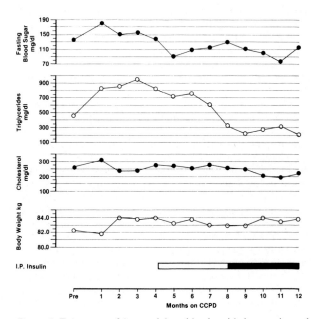

Figure 7. Treatment of hypertriglyceridemia with intraperitoneal insulin in a Type II diabetic patient undergoing CCPD. Open bar represent the addition of regular insulin, 5 units/2 l of 1.5% D and 10 units/2 l of 4.25% D dialysate; solid bar denotes addition of 10 units/2 l of 1.50% D and 15 units/2 l of 4.25% D dialysate.

5.2. Blood pressure control

Excellent blood pressure control can be attained with manipulation of the hydration state in most patients. Approximately 80% of patients suffered from hypertension requiring multiple drug therapy prior to treatment with CCPD, but only 10% of the patients have required antihypertensive agents after six months of therapy. Postural hypotension has been very infrequent among nondiabetic patients. However, 30% of diabetics suffered from severe postural hypotension, despite adequate or excessive hydration and normal or elevated blood pressure in the supine position. Postural hypotension under these circumstances is characteristic of autonomic neuropathy secondary to diabetes.

5.3. Selected complications of CCPD

The complications of CCPD are, generally speaking, the same as those observed with CAPD. However, due to the inherent differences in technique between these two modalities of therapy, the incidence of certain complications have been reported to be different.

5.3.1. Peritonitis

Peritonitis remains the most frequent complication of chronic peritoneal dialysis and the single most common cause of hospitalization for this population of patients. Technical advances in connecting devices and improvements in the teaching of aseptic technique to patients have significantly reduced the incidence of peritonitis among patients undergoing CAPD. However, most centers still experience one episode of peritonitis per patient per year. The incidence of peritonitis in our CCPD experience has been significantly lower than that observed among CAPD patients [42]. Our average incidence of peritonitis has been 0.4 episodes/yr or one episode every 2.5 yr. The introduction of new connectology, disconnection techniques, the use of various disinfectants and modifications in the cycler sets do not seem to have had an influence on the incidence of peritonitis during our six year experience (Figure 8) [43].

The probability of developing the first episode of peritonitis for CCPD patients during the first year varies between 35 and 52% (Figure 9) [43, 44]. The most recent report from the NIH U.S.A. CAPD Registry showed a peritonitis rate of 1.0 episode/yr which is lower than that reported for CAPD [44]. Likewise, other programs caring for adult patients have reported significantly lower rates of peritonitis for CCPD [21, 23, 45]. The experience in children undergoing CAPD and CCPD so far has not shown significant differences in the rate of peritonitis between the two modalities [25–27].

There are multiple potential factors that could be responsible for the low incidence of peritonitis in CCPD. The number of connections required between the peritoneal catheter and the system is reduced to two per day with the standard technique and one per day when external occlusion is used. Although there are multiple connections between the system lines and the bottles or bags, the likelihood of contaminating two disposable sterile parts seems minimal compared with a connection with the permanent catheter. All connections in CCPD take place at

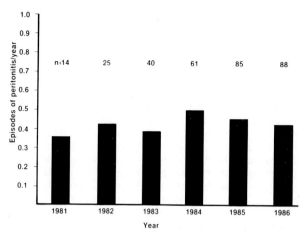

Figure 8. Incidence of peritonitis for CCPD patients according to calendar year of experience.

a convenient time or location, which probably improves the patient's concentration and minimizes fatigue. Better aseptic control of the environment can also be accomplished in the patient's home than in unfamiliar surroundings.

The direction of dialysate flow following a connection in CCPD is another potential factor influencing the incidence of peritonitis. In the cases of IPD and CAPD, dialysate is immediately infused into the peritoneal cavity following a connection. In contrast, with CCPD, the peritoneal fluid is drained into the connecting bag following a connection. If bacterial contamination were to occur during the connecting procedure, it is likely that the transit of bacteria into the peritoneum will be facilitated by inflowing dialysate in the case of CAPD, but bacteria will

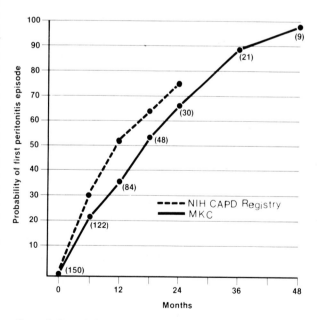

Figure 9. Cumulative probability of experiencing the first episode of peritonitis. The interrupted line represents the total experience of the NIH CAPD Registry [44] and the solid line refers to the Metrolina Kidney Center population [43].

be washed out by drainage of spent dialysate in the case of CCPD. It is of interest that CCPD shares the same flow sequence as bagless CAPD which also has been reported to have a very low rate of peritonitis [46–49]. The low incidence of peritonitis with bagless CAPD has been common to most programs whether a desinfectant is used or not [50]. Verger and Luzar have studied the effects of dialysate flush on peritoneal lines and catheters contaminated with organisms of different adhesiveness [50]. They reported a high success rate in clearing lines pre-contaminated with low-adhesiveness microorganisms (S. epidermidis), provided the contact time between bacteria and plastic line is short. Since most instances of contamination are due to these organisms and the contact time is relatively short, it is likely that a simple dialysate flush is effective in preventing peritonitis in CCPD and bagless CAPD.

Finally, the prolonged diurnal dwell of CCPD should potentially allow repopulation of the peritoneal resident macrophages and provide a better host immune defense. We have observed an increased number of round cells in the effluent from diurnal exchanges in CCPD patients that often exceeds 100 cells/m^3 in noninfected patients [4].

5.3.2. Exit site infections and catheter replacements

The incidence of exit site infections for our population and for the total population of the NIH CAPD Registry has been 0.4 and 0.5 episodes/patient year of observation [44]. These results are identical to those reported for CAPD. Since the frequency of exit site infection is similar for CAPD and CCPD patients, it is an unlikely factor to account for the lower rate of peritonitis among CCPD patients. The frequency of catheter replacement among CCPD patients has also been similar to that reported for CAPD (0.2–0.3 replacements/patient year of observation).

5.3.3. Hernias and other complications due to increased intra-abdominal pressure

The increased intra-abdominal pressure generated by the continuous presence of dialysate in the peritoneal cavity probably plays a significant role in the development or aggravation of certain complications of CAPD and CCPD. Our early experience with CCPD revealed no difference in the incidence of these complications between the two modalities of therapy. However, since the volume of dialysate for the diurnal cycle has been reduced, the incidence of these complications, particularly hernias, has been lower [52]. The maximum diurnal volume used in our program is 2 l or 28 ml/kg body weight. For patients who are at high risk of developing these complications or who are symptomatic at the initiation of therapy, a 25–35% reduction in the diurnal volume is recommended.

Hernias have been described with higher frequency among patients undergoing CAPD than those on IPD, NPD or CCPD with reduced diurnal volumes. Umbilical, inguinal, abdominal and diaphragmatic hernias have been described with several centers reporting de novo development of hernias in 9–24% of patients undergoing CAPD [53–56]. The incidence is 2–3% among patients on IPD and those on CCPD with reduced diurnal volumes [52]. During our initial 30 months of experience with CCPD, 9% of patients developed hernias. Most patients were multiparous, elderly females with weak anterior abdominal walls. Fol-

lowing surgical repair all patients returned to CCPD using reduced dialysate volumes for the diurnal exchange (1000–1500 ml) without recurrence of hernias.

Dialysate leaks are often the result of increased intra-abdominal pressure. Depending on the location of the leak it can manifest as genital edema, anterior wall edema or in the case of a pericatheter leak, a pseudohernia. Pseudohernias are hernia-like distentions around or in proximity to the catheter exit site which are easily reducible and collapse when the abdominal cavity is empty. Exploration of the hernial sac reveals a dilated structure of fibrous tissue and muscle not lined by peritoneum. There is simple accumulation of fluid that has dissected the peritoneal space at the pont where the catheter pierces the peritoneum. The transit of peritoneal fluid around the catheter and into the hernial sac can be demonstrated with the use of intra-abdominal contrast material injected while the patient is in the hands-knees position [57]. This complication has been seen more often with single cuff peritoneal catheters than with double cuff catheters [52]. All patients have been treated by simple removal of the catheter, replacement with a double cuff device and a resting period of 10–14 days without peritoneal dialysis to allow healing. CCPD has been reinstituted using volumes of up to 2 l at night and 1.5 l during the day without recurrence of the complication.

Low back pain, gastroesophageal reflux, and other complications resulting from increased intra-abdominal pressure have been managed in a similar manner by reducing the diurnal intra-abdominal volume. Very few patients have required transfer to NPD due to any of these complications. In fact, some patients can tolerate higher intra-abdominal volumes during the night which compensate for the reduction in daytime dialysate flow.

5.3.4. Catheter-related complications

The incidence of catheter-related complications in CCPD has been essentially the same as that reported for CAPD. Catheter outflow obstruction has been less frequent in CAPD and CCPD than with IPD and is usually corrected by conservative means. One-way obstruction is most often due to omental wrapping around the intraperitoneal portion of the catheter, or to catheter migration. Conservative treatment consisting of simple exercise and stimulation of the bowel by enemas corrects the problem in the majority of patients.

Loss of ultrafiltration from increased peritoneal solute transport rates has been documented with both CAPD and CCPD. Although at present we are conducting initial and serial peritoneal equilibration tests in all patients, the data are limited and do not allow a definitive statement regarding the incidence of loss of ultrafiltration. It is imperative to document the presence of hyperpermeability or increased solute transport rate in any patient presenting with inability to maintain an adequate hydration status, despite the use of hypertonic solution, with peritoneal permeability studies. Aside from peritoneal hyperpermeability with rapid absorption of dialysate glucose there are several circumstances that may interfere with the effective removal of fluid in the presence of a normal peritoneal membrane including: 1) an increase in sodium intake, 2) an increase in the sodium concentration of the dialysate, 3) a significant decrease in residual renal function resulting in increased weight gain and edema without an actual drop in peritoneal ultrafiltration, 4) mechanical problems with the catheter resulting in reduced surface area available for transperitoneal exchange, 5) uncontrolled hyperglycemia in diabetics which may decrease the transperitoneal osmotic gradient, and 6) severe hypoalbuminemia that may result in edema and difficulty with mobilization of fluid from the interstitial tissue. It is imperative to evaluate the patient who experiences difficulty with fluid removal in order to determine a real versus apparent ultrafiltration loss.

5.4. Morbidity and mortality

The mean total number of days of hospitalization per year for patients undergoing CCPD has been reported to be 20.8 by the NIH CAPD Registry [44]. Eight days were due to specific CCPD complications (peritonitis, exit site and tunnel infections, catheter replacement). These figures are not significantly different from those reported for patients undergoing CAPD.

Technique survival for patients undergoing CCPD has also been comparable to those patients on CAPD. Figure 10 provides the cumulative probability of transfer to another modality of therapy (hemodialysis, IPD, CAPD, NPD, or off dialysis without return of renal function) for patients at our institution and for the total population reported by the NIH CAPD Register. The probability of transfer at the end of one year is 18–19% and after two years of therapy 24–34%. Suki *et al.* have recently reviewed the outcome of their CCPD population during the past seven years and the causes of dropout in these patients [58]. Faced with the fact that only a small percentage of the patients trained on CCPD remained on therapy at the end of two years, the authors concluded that the losses from CCPD for reasons of dissatisfaction with peritoneal dialysis were

actually small. They identified three high risk factors for termination of therapy: 1) age (50% of their patients were over 50 yr of age); 2) comorbid factors which rendered 56% of the patients partially or totally dependent upon a partner and; 3) diabetes (one third of the patients were diabetic). Only 12.5% of the patients transferred to hemodialysis. The major causes of dropout from CCPD were death and transplantation, rather than transfer to an alternate modality of therapy.

Patient survival is also similar for CAPD and CCPD. Our survival rate after three years for nondiabetic patients is 83% [23]. Figure 11 provides the cumulative probability of death for our diabetic and nondiabetic population. The CAPD Registry has reported survival rates of 77% at one year and 62% at two years for all patients undergoing CCPD [44].

6. TREATMENT OF DIABETICS WITH CCPD

Continuous peritoneal dialysis has provided a new and physiologic route for insulin administration, sparing the patient multiple daily injections. It is quite feasible to obtain tight blood sugar control in the patient undergoing CAPD, due to the multiple exchanges during the day which allow divided and variable doses of insulin at the required times. It has been more difficult to design a uniform method for intraperitoneal insulin administration in the patient undergoing CCPD, due to the fact that most of the caloric load takes place during the day while only one peritoneal dialysis exchange is administered. Nevertheless, excellent glycemic control can be obtained in the majority of patients if the time is spent to calculate the precise dose of insulin required, and if a regular and predictable caloric intake is maintained with little day to day variation.

All insulin-dependent diabetic patients should be instructed in intraperitoneal insulin administration and regular

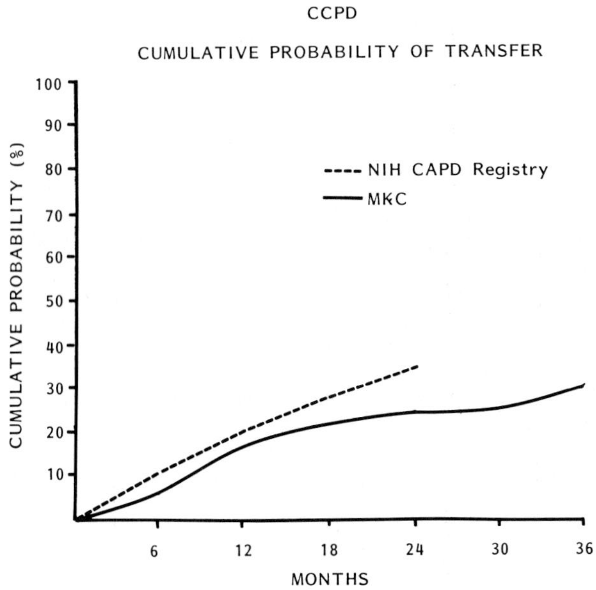

CCPD

CUMULATIVE PROBABILITY OF TRANSFER

Figure 10. Cumulative probability of transfer to hemiodialysis, IPD, CAPD or off dialysis without return of renal function for patients on CCPD.

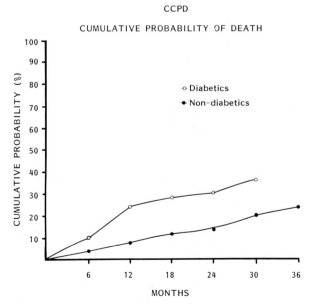

CCPD

CUMULATIVE PROBABILITY OF DEATH

Figure 11. Cumulative probability of death for patients on CCPD.

blood sugar determinations using fingerprick technique and a glucometer. Since the dialysate containers often do not drain simultaneously during the nocturnal exchanges, it is recommended that the insulin dose be divided among all containers in order to avoid a sudden and massive infusion of insulin and consequent hypoglycemia. The average intraperitoneal insulin dose required for good control of glycemia has been three times the previous total subcutaneous dose. In most cases, 50% of the intraperitoneal dose has been used for the long-dwell diurnal cycle with the remaining 50% equally divided among nocturnal exchanges. While the patient is in the hospital, blood sugars are determined four times daily, or more often if required. All subcutaneous insulin injections are discontinued and an initial dose of regular insulin, equivalent to two times the previous total 24-hr subcutaneous insulin dose, is prescribed for intraperitoneal use. Fifty percent of the regular insulin is added to the diurnal dialysate container (4.25% dextrose) and the other 50% is equally divided among the three bottles used for the nocturnal exchanges. This dose often requires adjustment with the final daily dose closer to three times the previous total insulin doses required for good glycemic control. If additional intraperitoneal insulin is needed, the guidelines suggested by the Toronto Western Hospital protocol are followed [59].

The one-year patient survival for diabetic patients in our population is 76% (Figure 11). This survival rate is definitely lower than for the nondiabetic population. However, it is significantly better than that reported for diabetic patients undergoing IPD [60, 61]. Amair *et al.* have reported survival rates for diabetic patients undergoing CAPD which are comparable or superior to the survival rates obtained by other programs for nondiabetic patients undergoing CAPD or hemodialysis [62]. Several investigators have reported two year survival rates of 60–80% among diabetics undergoing CAPD [63–68]. A factor that may influence the lower survival rate for our diabetic population is a high rate of transplantation, both living related and cadaveric, for most young diabetic patients entering our program; thereby eliminating this relatively healthy population from our statistics. We have also depended heavily on CCPD for older, blind, and dependent diabetics who require a partner for their treatment at home.

7. TREATMENT OF CHILDREN WITH CCPD

It has been estimated that approximately 75% of children requiring renal replacement therapy are treated with various forms of peritoneal dialysis [68]. The fact that chronic peritoneal dialysis does not require venipuncture nor heparinization makes it an attractive choice for the treatment of the pediatric patient. Children comprise a significant proportion of the patients being treated with CCPD. Several features of CCPD make it particularly useful for the therapy of children: 1) it offers adequate dialysis with minimal medical contact since the frequency and length of the procedure is relatively short; 2) increases the amount of free time for recreation and study during the day; and 3) allows the use of a partner, usually the parents, without significant restriction of their productive time. Although most series describing the experience with CCPD in children

are small, the proliferation of reports during the past five years attest to the interest in CCPD for pediatric use and the efficacy of this therapy in treating uremic children while awaiting renal transplantation [25–27, 37, 68–71]. From the review of the data accumulated from these experiences we can reach the following conclusions: 1) CCPD has facilitated and simplified the therapy of children by allowing the participation of parents or guardians; 2) the adequacy of dialysis compares with CAPD and hemodialysis; 3) the rate of dropout has been low with very few patients transferring to hemodialysis or CAPD; 4) the hematologic and biochemical parameters are comparable to CAPD and those observed in adults undergoing CCPD; 5) the rate of peritonitis has been similar to that observed with CAPD and; 6) the rate of growth has remained below the normal mean, but has been maintained in most cases.

Together with all the complications inherent to uremia, the pediatric patient faces growth retardation as a common problem. The growth rates observed in children on different modalities of therapy have varied greatly. In comparison with hemodialysis it has been suggested that children on peritoneal dialysis may have a slightly higher, although not significantly different growth rate [72, 73]. The experience with CCPD uniformly has shown that most uremic children are growth retarded (less than fifth percentile for height [27]) at the initiation of dialysis and maintain the same growth velocity during the period of CCPD (Figure 12). No correlation between energy and protein intake and growth velocity has been documented. We await with interest the outcome of pediatric patients undergoing peritoneal dialysis treated with erythropoietin and growth hormone.

8. CCPD IN THE TREATMENT OF ACUTE RENAL FAILURE

Continuous equilibration peritoneal dialysis (CEPD) has been successfully used for the treatment of confined patients with acute renal failure [74, 75]. A peritoneal cycler with peritoneal dwell times of 2–6 hr can be utilized providing a steady physiologic state and continuous ultrafiltration according to the patient's needs. Hypercatabolic patients can be treated with shorter cycles and higher dialysate flows, which will enhance ultrafiltration and small solute removal. Patients with postoperative acute renal failure, sepsis, rhabdomyolysis and acute intoxications are often hypercatabolic, requiring total parenteral nutrition. The need for continuous ultrafiltration in the presence of oliguria mandates continuous dialytic therapy if a steady physiologic state is to be maintained. Peritoneal dialysis has the additional advantage of providing a significant and constant glucose infusion. In the presence of a high catabolic rate, early dialysis is recommended in order to maintain adequate biochemical profiles.

9. RENAL TRANSPLANTATION IN CCPD PATIENTS

A successful renal transplant is undoubtedly the ideal treatment for end-stage renal disease. Some concern has been expressed about the influence of peritoneal dialysis

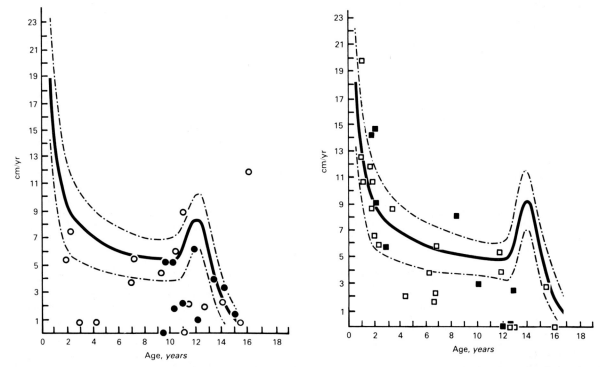

Figure 12. Growth velocity for female (left) and male (right) children tested with CAPD and CCPD [26]. Symbols: circles, females; squares, males; open symbols, CAPD; solid symbols, CCPD. Points represent the cumulative averages for each patient while on dialysis therapy related to the age at time of analysis. Dark line and thinner broken lines represent the mean ± 2 SD for the normal population.

on the outcome of transplantation. The basis for these concerns rest on laboratory and clinical investigations suggesting enhanced immunologic responses among peritoneal dialysis patients compared to those observed in patients undergoing hemodialysis [76, 77]. E-rosette formation and skin reactions to DNCB have been reported to improve in some patients on CAPD, but not on hemodialysis patients, suggesting improved cellular immunity among CAPD patients [78, 79]. It has also been suggested that the protective effect of pretransplant blood transfusions is less marked in peritoneal dialysis patients [76, 77, 80]. An increased ratio of helper to suppressor T-cells among CAPD patients has also been reported to be associated with lower one year survival rates [76, 77]. In spite of these clinical and theoretical considerations, most centers' experience with hemodialysis and peritoneal dialysis have failed to see a difference in the success of transplants performed in peritoneal versus hemodialysis patients [81-86]. Our experience with both IPD and CCPD have shown similar results in the outcome of renal transplantation among these patients and those on hemodialysis [86].

The presence of a peritoneal catheter is a source of potential infection in the immunosuppressed host. Peritonitis has been reported to result in septicemia and subsequent death of peritoneal dialysis patients following transplantation [86]. Thus, it is imperative to observe strict catheter care in all peritoneal dialysis patients following transplantation. The following recommendations ase useful in maintaining a peritoneal access until adequate renal allograft function has been established and in preventing

septic complications: 1) the abdomen should be drained prior to transplantation surgery, 2) a peritoneal fluid cell count, differential and culture should be obtained, 3) the catheter exit site should be cleaned daily, 4) the catheter should be irrigated every 48 hours to assure a patent lumen and, 5) the catheter should be removed within two weeks after surgery, or as soon as adequate graft function is established. In our experience, these simple steps have allowed the adequate use of the peritoneal access whenever required in the immediate post-transplantation period and has prevented peritonitis in all instances.

10. CONCLUSIONS

CCPD has provided an alternative form of continuous peritoneal dialysis for patients who need automated treatment during the night without interruptions in the daily routine for dialysis exchanges, and those patients requiring the assistance of a partner. The clinical experience has shown comparable results to CAPD. Although the rate of peritonitis has been impressively low in many programs caring for adults, the experience has not been duplicated in children. No differences in the outcome of transplantation between CCPD, CAPD, and hemodialysis have been documented. In the final choice of peritoneal therapy, the patient's lifestyle, psychologic needs, and preferences should be considered over all other factors in order to attain the highest level of rehabilitation.

REFERENCES

1. Popovich RP, Moncrief JW, Decherd JF *et al.*: The definition of a novel portable/wearable equilibrium peritoneal dialysis technique. (Abstract) Am Soc Artif Intern Organs 5: 64, 1976.
2. Diaz-Buxo, Walker PJ, Farmer CD *et al.*: Continuous cyclic peritoneal dialysis – a preliminary report. Artif Organs 5: 157–161, 1981.
3. Diaz-Buxo JA, Kay DA, Holt KL: Safe, simple, inexpensive disconnecting device for CCPD. Kidney Int 27: 179, 1985.
4. Diaz-Buxo JA: Continuous ambulatory and continuous cycling peritoneal dialysis. In: La Greca G, Chiaramonte S, Fabris A, Ferriani M, Ronco C (eds), Peritoneal Dialysis. Milano: Wichtig Editore 257–264, 1985.
5. Diaz-Buxo JA, Burgess WP, Farmer CD, Chandler JT, Walker PJ, Adcock A: Multiple tubing set (MTS™) – making CCPD safe, simple and cost effective. Perit Dial Bull 7: S22, 1987.
6. Tenckhoff H: Chronic peritoneal dialysis manual. University of Washington, School of Medicine, Seattle, Washington, 1974.
7. Lasker N, McCawley EP, Passarotti CT: Chronic peritoneal dialysis. Trans Am Soc Artif Intern Organs 12: 94, 1966.
8. Blumenkrantz MJ, Gordon A, Roberts M *et al.*: Applications of the Redy Sorbent System to hemodialysis and peritoneal dialysis. Artif Organs 3: 230–236, 1979.
9. Shen FH, Sherrard DJ, Scollard D *et al.*: Thirst, hyponatremia and excessive weight gain in maintenance peritoneal dialysis. Trans Am Soc Artif Intern Organs 24: 142–145, 1978.
10. Nolph KD, Sorkin ML, Moore H: Autoregulation of sodium and potassium removal during continuous ambulatory peritoneal dialysis. Trans Am Soc Artif Intern Organs 26: 334–338, 1980.
11. Twardowski ZJ, Nolph KD, Prowant B, Moore HL: Efficiency of high volume, low frequency continuous ambulatory peritoneal dialysis. Trans Am Soc Artif Intern Organs 29: 53–57, 1983.
12. Gotloib L, Mines M, Garmizo L *et al.*: Hemodynamic effects of increasing intra-abdominal pressure in peritoneal dialysis. Perit Dial Bull 1: 41–43, 1981.
13. Twardowski ZJ, Prowant BF, Nolph KD *et al.*: High volume, low frequency continuous ambulatory peritoneal dialysis. Kidney Int 23: 64–70, 1983.
14. Diaz-Buxo JA: CCPD is even better than CAPD. Kidney Int 28 : S26–28, 1985.
15. O'Brien AAJ, Power J, O'Brien L, Clancy L, Keogh JAB: The effect of 2 L dialysate on respiratory function. Perit Dial Bull 7: S57, 1987.
16. Diaz-Buxo JA, Farmer CD, Chandler JT, Walker PJ, Burgess WP: CCPD – wet is better than dry. Perit Dial Bull S22, 1987.
17. Twardowski ZJ, Nolph KD, Khanna R *et al.*: Peritoneal equilibration test. Perit Dial Bull 7: 138–147, 1987.
18. Diaz-Buxo JA: The importance of the peritoneal equilibration test – a plea for uniformity. Perit Dial Bull 7: 118, 1987.
19. Twardowski ZJ, Nolph KD, Khanna R *et al.*: Daily clearances with continuous ambulatory and nightly peritoneal dialysis. Trans Am Soc Artif Intern Organs 32: 575–580, 1986.
20. Diaz-Buxo JA, Walker PJ, Chandler JT *et al.*: Continuous cyclic peritoneal dialysis. In: Gahl GM, Kessel M, Nolph KD (eds), Advances in Peritoneal Dialysis. Amsterdam: Excerpta Medica pp 126–130, 1981.
21. Price CG, Suki WN: Newer modification of peritoneal dialysis: options in the treatment of patients with renal failure. Am J Nephrol 1: 97–104, 1981.
22. Diaz-Buxo JA: Continuous cyclic peritoneal dialysis (CCPD). In: Franz HE (ed), Blood Purification, 3rd edition (German). Stuttgart: Georg Thieme Verlag, pp 458–463, 1985.
23. Diaz-Buxo JA, Walker PJ, Chandler JT *et al.*: Experience with intermittent peritoneal dialysis and continuous cyclic peritoneal dialysis. Am J Kidney Dis 4: 242–248, 1984.
24. Walls J, Smith BA, Feehally J *et al.*: CCPD – An improvement

on CAPD. In: Gahl GM, Kessel M, Nolph KD (eds), Advances in peritoneal dialysis. Amsterdam: Excerpta Medica 141–143, 1981.
25. Brem AS, Toscano AM: Continuous cycling peritoneal dialysis for children: An alternative to hemodialysis treatment. Pediatrics 74: 254–258, 1984.
26. Southwest Pediatric Nephrology Study Group: continuous ambulatory and continuous cyclic peritoneal dialysis in children. Kidney Int 27: 558–564, 1985.
27. Fine RN, Salusky IB: CAPD/CCPD in children: Four year's experience. Kidney Int 30: S7–10, 1986.
28. Moncrief JW, Popovich RP, Nolph KD *et al.*: Clinical experience with continuous ambulatory peritoneal dialysis. ASAIO J 2: 114–118, 1979.
29. Lamperi S, Icardi A, Carozzi S *et al.*: Effect of CAPD on renal anemia. Int J Nephrol Urol Androl 1: 43–52, 1981.
30. De Paepe MBJ, Schelstraete KHG, Ringoir SMG *et al.*: Influence of continuous ambulatory peritoneal dialysis on the anemia of end-stage renal disease. Kidney Int 23: 744–748, 1983.
31. Lamperi S, Carozzi S, Icardi A: In vitro and in vivo studies of erythropoiesis during continuous ambulatory peritoneal dialysis. Perit Dial Bull 3: 94–96, 1983.
32. Rahman R, Heaton A, Goodship THJ *et al.*: Renal osteodystrophy in patients on continuous ambulatory peritoneal dialysis: a five-year study. Perit Dial Bull 7: 20–25, 1987.
33. Delmez JA, Fallon MD, Bergfeld MA *et al.*: Continuous ambulatory peritoneal dialysis and bone. Kidney Int 30: 379–384, 1986.
34. Vincenti F, Hattner R, Amend WJ Jr *et al.*: Decreased secondary hyperparathyroidism in diabetic patients receiving hemodialysis. JAMA 245: 930–933, 1981.
35. Vincenti F, Arnaud SB, Recker R *et al.*: Parathyroid and bone response of the diabetic patient to uremia. Kidney Int 25: 677–682, 1984.
36. Blumenkrantz MJ, Gahl GM, Kopple JD: Protein losses during peritoneal dialysis. Kidney Int 19: 593–602, 1981.
37. Leichter HE: The optimal CCPD regimen for children. Perspect Perit Dial 5: 5–8, 1987.
38. Katirtzoglou A, Oreopoulos DG, Husdan H *et al.*: Reappraisal of protein losses in patients undergoing continuous ambulatory peritoneal dialysis. Nephron 26: 230–233, 1980.
39. Grodstein GP, Blumenkrantz MJ, Kopple JD *et al.*: Glucose absorption during continuous ambulatory peritoneal dialysis. Kidney Int 19: 564–567, 1981.
40. Moncrief JW, Pyle WK, Simon P *et al.*: Hypertriglyceridemia, diabetes mellitus and insulin administration in patients undergoing CAPD. In: Moncrief JW, Popovich RP (eds), CAPD update. Proc 2nd Int Symp, Mason, New York, pp 143–165, 1981.
41. Beardsworth SF, Goldsmith HJ, Stanbridge BR: Intraperitoneal insulin cannot correct hyperlipidemia of CAPD. Perit Dial Bull 3: 126–127, 1983.
42. Diaz-Buxo JA: Does CCPD lower the peritonitis rate? Contributions to Nephrol 57: 191–196, 1987.
43. Diaz-Buxo JA, Walker PJ, Burgess WP *et al.*: Current status of CCPD in the prevention of peritonitis. In: Khanna R, Nolph KD, Prowant B, Twardowski ZJ, Oreopoulos DG (eds), Advances in continuous ambulatory peritoneal dialysis. Toronto: Perit Dial Bull 145–148, 1986.
44. National CAPD Registry of the National Institute of Health, Bethesda, Maryland, 1987.
45. Cavoretto L, Jackson F: A decrease in peritonitis with CCPD: one unit's experience. Nephrol Nurse 5: 33–37, 1983.
46. Bazzato G, Landini S, Coli U, Lucatello S, Fracasso A, Moracchiello M: A new technique of continuous ambulatory peritoneal dialysis (CAPD): double-bag system for freedom to the patient and significant reduction of peritonitis. Clin Nephrol 13: 251–254, 1980.
47. Maiorca R, Cancarini GC, Broccoli R *et al.*: Prospective controlled

controlled trial of a Y-connector and disinfectant to prevent peritonitis in continuous ambulatory peritoneal dialysis. Lancet ii: 642–644, 1983.

48. Suki WN, Walshe JJ, Ashebrook DW, Gentile DE, Tucker CT, Ash SR, Ahmad S: Multicenter evaluation of a bagless CAPD system. Trans Am Soc Artif Intern Organs 32: 572–574, 1986.

49. Diaz-Buxo JA, Walshe JJ, Flanigan M: Multicenter experience with Y-set CAPD system (Freedom Set). Perit Dial Bull S23, 1987.

50. Verger C, Faller B, Ryckelynck JPH, Cam G, Pierre D: Comparison between the efficacy of CAPD Y-lines without 'in line' disinfectant and standard systems: A multicenter prospective controlled trial. Perit Dial Bull 7: S82, 1987.

51. Verger C, Luzar MA: In vitro study of CAPD Y-line system. In: Khanna R et al. (eds), Advances in peritoneal dialysis. Toronto: Perit Dial Bull 160–164, 1986.

52. Diaz-Buxo JA, Geissinger WT: Single cuff versus double cuff Tenckhoff catheter. Perit Dial Bull 4: S100–102, 1984.

53. Chan MK, Baillod RA, Tanner A et al.: Abdominal hernias in patients receiving continuous ambulatory peritoneal dialysis. Br Med J 283: 826, 1981.

54. Digenis GE, Khanna R, Oreopoulos DG: Abdominal hernias in patients undergoing continuous ambulatory peritoneal dialysis. Perit Dial Bull 2: 115–117, 1982.

55. Jorkasky D, Goldfarb S: Abdominal wall hernia complicating chronic ambulatory peritoneal dialysis. Am J Nephrol 2: 323–324, 1982.

56. Rubin J, Raju S, Teal N et al.: Abdominal hernia in patients undergoing continuous ambulatory peritoneal dialysis. Arch Intern Med 142: 1453–1455, 1982.

57. Tucker CT, Cunningham JT, Nichols AM et al.: Cannulography with peritoneal air contrast study. Contemp Dial 3: 9–13, 1982.

58. Suki WN, Muniz E, Nishioka J: Drop-out in patients undergoing continuous cyclic peritoneal dialysis. In: Khanna R, Nolph KD, Prowant B, Twardowski ZJ, Oreopoulos DG (eds), Advances in Continuous Ambulatory Peritoneal Dialysis. Toronto: Perit Dial Bull, Inc, pp 183–185, 1987.

59. Khanna R, Liebel B: The Toronto-Western protocol. Perit Dial Bull 6: 101–102, 1981.

60. Katirtzaglou A, Elzatt S, Oreopoulos D et al.: Chronic peritoneal dialysis in diabetics with end-stage renal failure. In: Friedman EA, L'Esperance FA (eds), The Diabetic Renal-retinal Syndrome. New York: Grune and Stratton, pp 317–331, 1980.

61. Mitchell JC, Frohnert PP, Kurtz SB et al.: Chronic peritoneal dialysis in juvenile-onset diabetes mellitus: a comparison with hemodialysis. Mayo Clin Proc 53: 775–781, 1978.

62. Amair P, Khanna R, Liebel B et al.: Continuous ambulatory peritoneal dialysis in diabetics with end-stage renal disease. N Eng J Med 306: 625–630, 1982.

63. Williams C, Belvedere D, Cattran D et al.: Experience with CAPD in diabetic patients in Toronto. Perit Dial Bull 2: S12–15, 1982.

64. Khanna R, Wu G, Chisholm L et al.: Further experience with CAPD in diabetics with end-stage renal disease. Diabetic Nephropathy 2: 8–12, 1983.

65. Legrain M, Rottembourg J, Bentchikou H et al.: Dialysis treatment of insulin dependent diabetic patients: ten year's experience. Clin Nephrol 21: 72–81, 1984.

66. Mejia G, Zimmerman SW: Comparison of continuous ambulatory peritoneal dialysis and hemodialysis for diabetics. Perit Dial Bull 5: 7–11, 1985.

67. Coronel F, Hortal L, Naranjo P: Analysis of factors in prognosis of diabetics on CAPD – Long term experience. Perit Dial Bull 7: S18, 1987.

68. Fine RN: Choosing a dialysis therapy for children with endstage renal disease. Am J Kidney Dis 4: 249–252, 1984.

69. Alliapoulos JC, Salusky IB, Hall T et al.: Comparison of continuous cycling peritoneal dialysis with continuous ambulatory peritoneal dialysis in children. J Pediatrics 105: 721–725, 1984.

70. Warady BA, Campoy SF, Gross SP et al.: Peritonitis with continuous ambulatory peritoneal dialysis and continuous cycling peritoneal dialysis. J Pediatrics 105: 726–730, 1984.

71. Chormann ML, Staccone M, Edd P, Andrus CH, Ornt DB: Experience with automated peritoneal dialysis (APD) in a pediatric population. In: Khanna R, Nolph KD, Prowant B, Twardowski ZJ, Oreopoulos DG (eds), Advances in Continuous Ambulatory Peritoneal Dialysis. Toronto: Perit Dial Bull, Inc, pp 66–72, 1987.

72. Baum M, Powell D, Calvin D et al.: Continuous ambulatory peritoneal dialysis in children, comparison with hemodialysis. N Eng J Med 307: 1537–1540, 1982.

73. Potter DE: Comparison of peritoneal dialysis and hemodialysis in children. Dial and Transplant 7: 800–802, 1978.

74. Posen GA, Luiscello J: Continuous equilibration peritoneal dialysis in the treatment of acute renal failure. Perit Dial Bull 1: 6, 1980.

75. Katirtzoglou A, Kontesis P, Myopoulou-Synvoulidis D, Digenis GE, Synvoulidis A, Komminos Z: Continuous equilibration peritoneal dialysis (CEPD) in hypercatabolic renal failure. Perit Dial Bull 3: 178–180, 1983.

76. Guillou PJ, Will EJ, Davison AM, Giles GR: CAPD – a risk factor in renal transplantation? Br J Surg 71: 878–880, 1984.

77. Gelfand M, Kois J, Quillan B et al.: CAPD yields inferior transplant results compared to hemodialysis (HD). Perit Dial Bull 4: S26, 1984.

78. Giacchino F, Alloatti S, Quarello F et al.: The influence of peritoneal dialysis on cellular immunity. Perit Dial Bull 2: 165–168, 1982.

79. Giangrande A, Cantu P, Limido A, de Francesco D, Malacrida V: Continuous ambulatory peritoneal dialysis and cellular immunity. Proc EDTA 19: 372–377, 1982.

80. Walker JF, Oreopoulos DG, Uldall PR et al.: The effect of pre-transplant blood transfusion on graft outcome in patients on peritoneal dialysis prior to renal transplantation. Trans Proc 17: 687–689, 1982.

81. Cardella CJ: Renal transplantation in patients on peritoneal dialysis. Perit Dial Bull 2: 165–168, 1982.

82. Gokal R, Ramos JM, Veitch P et al.: Renal transplantation in patients on continuous ambulatory peritoneal dialysis. Proc EDTA 18: 222–227, 1981.

83. Stefanidis C, Balfe JW, Arbus GS et al.: Renal transplantation in children treated with continuous ambulatory peritoneal dialysis. Perit Dial Bull 1: 5–8, 1983.

84. Leichter HE, Salusky IB, Fine RN: Renal transplantation in patients on CAPD and CCPD – special focus in pediatrics. Perspect in Perit Dial 4: 12–15, 1986.

85. Wood C, Thomson NM, Scott DF et al.: Results of renal transplantation in patients on CAPD. Perit Dial Bull 4: S72, 1984.

86. Diaz-Buxo JA, Walker PJ, Burgess WP et al.: The influence of peritoneal dialysis on the outcome of transplantation. Int J Artif Organs 9: 359–362, 1986.

11

PHARMACOLOGIC ALTERATION OF PERITONEAL TRANSPORT RATES

PRZEMYSLAW HIRSZEL and JOHN F. MAHER

Peritoneal dialysis has become an increasingly popular alternative to hemodialysis for therapy of chronic renal failure [1–3]. Concurrently, the effect of pharmacological and physiological manipulations on peritoneal transport have been explored seeking enhanced understanding of transport mechanisms and clinically useful methods to augment transport.

1. RATIONALE FOR AUGMENTING TRANSPORT RATES

Mass transport rates of small solutes by peritoneal dialysis are slower than those by hemodialysis. Hence, peritoneal dialysis consumes more time to achieve a given control of the plasma concentration of a solute such as urea. Inefficient transport can contribute to the risk of peritonitis because more exchanges of dialysis solution are required. Once peritonitis occurs, solute transport may increase, but the ultrafiltration rate decreases because of more rapid dissipation of the osmotic gradient. Thereafter, transport should return to baseline rates unless inadequate treatment allows loss of peritoneal surface area or decreased permeability. Marginal transport rates after peritonitis may lower the ultrafiltration capacity to an unacceptable level [4]. Moreover, for hypercatabolic or hyperkalemic patients the transport inefficiency for small solutes may be quite significant, even when the peritoneal surface area and permeability have not been reduced.

The efficiency of peritoneal mass transport may be particularly impaired by systemic vascular disease [5]. Often, diseases such as diabetes mellitus and scleroderma become so widespread as to affect all the vasculature, including the splanchnic bed, before causing terminal renal failure.

Continuous ambulatory peritoneal dialysis (CAPD) does not have the disadvantage of time consumption because treatment time does not inhibit rehabilitation [6]. But CAPD also requires adequate efficiency to be clinically satisfactory. With coexistent vascular disease or after many episodes of peritonitis, peritoneal mass transport may be so borderline as to render the procedure inadequate unless more frequent exchanges are used, with the attendant hazards of multiple tubing disconnections. Moreover, some patients undergoing CAPD have low rates of ultrafiltration across the peritoneum or acquire this abnormality. Under other circumstances increased catabolism may increase the nitrogen load. Despite continuous peritoneal dialysis, augmented transport may be required whenever there is decreased transport efficiency or increased catabolism.

When peritoneal dialysis is used to remove exogenous toxins, it is usually mandatory that removal rates be maximal. Conversely, when protein loss is excessive it can be judicious to decrease the transport rates, at least of larger solutes. Hence, further understanding of the mechanisms of mass transport and the influence of pharmacologic and physiologic manipulations on them is important fundamental information for accelerating or decreasing transport rates as clinically indicated. Recent evidence suggests that the major sites of ultrafiltration and of diffusion across the peritoneum differ [7] and these transport sites can be modulated selectively [8, 9]. Frequently, patients undergoing peritoneal dialysis also require a variety of drugs that have specific vasoactive or membrane effects. Knowledge of the effects of such agents on transport parameters can influence the appropriate choice of a drug for a particular indication.

2. MECHANISMS OF TRANSPORT

A dialysis solution in the peritoneal cavity approaches concentration equilibrium with plasma by diffusion. Additionally, net osmotic and hydrostatic forces promote the movement of water, usually from plasma to dialysate. Such ultrafiltration also convectively removes solutes. Solutes also can enter dialysate from adjacent tissue rather than from plasma [10]. Finally, solutes absorbed from peritoneal dialysate into the portal vasculature may undergo hepatic metabolism before reaching the systemic circulation decreasing the absorbed concentration [11]. The bulk of absorption presumably occurs through lymphatics.

3. DIFFUSION

Diffusion occurs by random kinetic movement of molecules and tends to spread any substance evenly throughout the space available to it. This process is not affected by drugs directly, but the barriers to diffusion can be influenced pharmacologically. Diffusion rates correlate directly with temperature, however.

The rate of linear diffusion of a solute in any direction throughout a cross-sectional area, expressed as mass transport or quantity per unit time, is proportional to the concentration gradient. Interposing a membrane with pores that are large in relation to the diffusing molecules merely restricts the total area available for free diffusion. Dividing the mass transport rate by the gradient, or more simply by the plasma concentration, yields a clearance value. Prolonged intraperitoneal dwell dissipates the concentration gradient decreasing the mass transport rate. Hence, unless clearances are calculated on short-term exchanges, e.g., hourly, they are misleadingly low and the dialysance [12] or mass transfer coefficient must be determined [13].

Free diffusion across capillary walls becomes progressively restricted as the square root of the molecular mass of the solute increases [14]. Accordingly, peritoneal permeability area coefficients decrease as the square root of the molecular mass increases, while clearances bear a slightly different relationship as concentration equilibrium is approached [15]. Many other factors affect the multiple diffusion coefficients that characterize multicomponent mass transfer across macroscopic biologic membranes.

Water soluble solutes traverse intercellular channels, whereas lipid soluble solutes dissolve in plasma membranes readily permeating cells. The diffusion of small water soluble solutes is so rapid that the observed peritoneal transport rates can be accounted for by intercellular pores that total only 0.2% of the estimated surface area [16]. At the usual exchange rate of dialysis solution of 2 1 hourly and with a peritoneal blood flow rate of 60–100 ml/min [17] the clearances of small solutes such as urea and creatinine are much lower than by hemodialysis, but large solutes like inulin are removed relatively faster, which suggests that the total pore area of the peritoneum is less than that of cellulosic membranes but that the pores are larger [18]. Studies of the transport of neutral dextrans are consistent with heteroporosity of the peritoneum with some pores larger than 40 Å [19]. Larger solutes such as polypeptides and small proteins appear to traverse the capillary wall in vesicles adjoining or contiguous with intercellular clefts [20–22]. The effective size of the pores in capillaries can be influenced by the protein concentration of the perfusate, by the capillary blood pressure and volume, and by drugs.

The thickest layer of transport resistance is the dense interstitial connective tissue between the capillary endothelium and the mesothelium. This unstirred layer of gelatinous fluid impedes transport of solutes that permeate the capillary wall. Dehydration increases this resistance because of the resultant distortion of the porous channels of this layer [23].

Studies of transport across isolated mesentery suggest that the mesothelial cells also contribute to transport resistance [24]. The validity of such measurements requires that the membrane remains both intact (scanning electron microscopy) and viable (dye studies). Mesothelial cells are flattened and overlapping with tight junctions [22]. They lie on a continuous basement membrane and contain numerous intracytoplasmic vesicles. Permeation of solutes into the isolated hemidiaphragm is lower in areas covered by the mesothelium compared to bare areas. This impedance is offset by the addition of a redox dye to the system and is restored by adding malate or succinate, but lost again when malonate is added [25]. These results suggest that oxidative metabolism and ATP formation are intimately linked in regulating diffusion through this cell layer; it should respond to pharmacologic manipulation.

4. DIALYSATE FLOW RATE

The diffusive transport rate of any given solute depends mostly on the electrochemical concentration gradient. This gradient dissipates as solute leaves the plasma and accumulates in dialysate. Obviously impractical, infinitely high blood and dialysate flow rates would maintain maximal concentration gradients. Large poorly diffusible solutes accumulate in dialysate so slowly that increasing the rate of dialysis solution exchange above 2 1 per hour adds little to the gradient and the clearance. With intermittent peritoneal dialysis the usual drainage rate of dialysate is about 2100 ml/hr or 35 ml/min. Under this circumstance the clearance of a small, highly diffusible solute such as urea is about 20 ml/min indicating incomplete equilibration, i.e., a dialysate/plasma concentration ratio of 20/35 or about 0.6. Increasing the dialysate exchange rate can only increase the clearance by about 30% [26]. When dialysate volume is insufficient to contact the entire peritoneal surface, however, clearances are suboptimal until the exchange volume is increased [27]. Accordingly, clearance decreases as fluid is being exchanged and can be augmented by leaving a residual volume in the peritoneum as the excess volume is exchanged [28]. But, greatly improved mass transport must depend on augmentation of blood flow or peritoneal permeability or area, just as hemodialyzer efficiency has increased with larger surface area dialyzers, more permeable membranes and higher blood flow rates. Recognition of the limited value of high dialysate flow rates prompted Popovich and colleagues [6] to develop CAPD which prolongs diffusion time rather than increasing the volume or exchange rate of dialysis solution. The procedural variant, continuous cyclic peritoneal dialysis (CCPD), com-

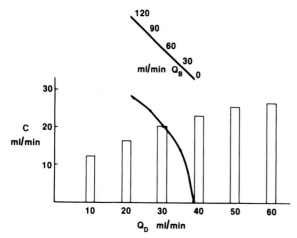

Figure 1. As dialysate flow rate (Q_D), or volume exchanged, increases, peritoneal clearance (C) of a highly diffusible solute (bars) increases rapidly until flow rate is high and thereafter gradually. At any given dialysate flow rate, increases in blood flow (Q_B) induce a curvilinear increase in clearance (dots).

bines this concept with intermittent, more rapid exchanges [29, 30]. The effect of dialysis solution flow rate and of blood flow rate on peritoneal clearances are shown in Figure 1.

5. MESENTERIC BLOOD FLOW

Blood flow to the visceral peritoneum derives predominantly from the mesenteric circulation. The parietal peritoneum has a small surface area and is perfused by vasculature of the abdominal wall. Mesenteric blood flow rates average about 10% of the cardiac output or 40 ml/min/100 g [31, 32], while the effective blood flow rate to the human peritoneum averages 60 to 100 ml/min [17]. When mesenteric blood flow is doubled, the clearances of small solutes such as urea increase by 30 to 50% [33], consistent with a resting blood flow that exceeds the maximal rate at which the capillary diffusion capacity can completely clear the perfusing blood [34].

The splanchnic vascular bed can sequester blood, excluding it from or releasing it into the circulation as systemic volume changes. Thus, hemodynamic effects of drugs can influence splanchnic blood volume and flow rate considerably. Because drugs usually affect the splanchnic blood flow and volume *pari passu*, changes in peritoneal transport that result from the altered volume can be misinterpreted as flow rate mediated. The mesenteric vasculature is accompanied by autonomic neuroelements from the celiac plexus with primary neurocontrol by sympathetic innervation. Both alpha- and beta-adrenergic receptors are located in mesenteric vessels [35]. These vessels also contain dopaminergic receptors. Vasoactive responses of the mesenteric vascular bed to pharmacologic manipulations are well established. The vasoconstrictor response that normally occurs with appropriate stimuli can be prevented by blocking alpha receptors of the mesenteric vascular bed with phenoxybenzamine. Moreover, prostaglandins are intimately involved in the fine control of vascular dynamics

by modifying vasoconstrictor responses [36]. Indeed, during peritonitis peritoneal generation of prostaglandins (especially vasodilators) increases contributing importantly to the protein loss and other flux abnormalities [37]. The opportunities for increasing peritoneal mass transport by pharmacologic modulation of blood flow to the peritoneum are numerous [38].

6. CONVECTIVE TRANSPORT

Solute is also convected into the peritoneum by ultrafiltration. The pores through capillary walls restrict the passage of protein but little compositional change occurs with smaller solutes such as urea. Solutes as large as inulin are sieved appreciably during peritoneal ultrafiltration. The hydrostatic pressure of the blood, which decreases from 32 to 15 mm Hg from the arterial to the venous end of the capillary, is opposed by the plasma oncotic pressure, normally 25 mm Hg, and by the interstitial hydrostatic pressure minus the interstitial osmotic pressure. Hence, the ultrafiltration rate through mesenteric capillaries at normal pressures is only about 3.0 ml/min/M^2 of surface area. This ultrafiltrate normally returns promptly to venules and lymphatics. Normally, peritoneal fluid resembles lymph from the leg rather than from the hepatic or thoracic duct [39] and is derived from mesenteric capillaries. With increased hepatic venous pressure the surface of the liver contributes predominately to ascites formation.

When 2 l of isotonic fluid is infused intraperitoneally, it raises extravascular hydrostatic pressure promoting the absorption of fluid at a rate of about 10% of residual volume per hour [40]. Added dextrose raises the dialysate osmotic pressure sufficiently to induce net ultrafiltration in proportion to the dextrose concentration of the instilled fluid. Because of the restricted diffusion coefficient of dextrose relative to the solvent, 1.5% dextrose dialysis fluid yields about 3.0 ml/min/M^2 of ultrafiltrate. Inward diffusion of dextrose dissipates the osmotic pressure gradient rapidly despite metabolism of the absorbed glucose. Hence, the ultrafiltration rate decreases with time. The ultrafiltration rate can be increased by using a higher concentration of dextrose, a less permeant solute of comparable osmotic activity, or by drugs that increase the capillary filtration coefficient [41] or raise the capillary hydrostatic pressure by venular constriction, which may be the case with dopamine [42].

In uremic patients hypertonic dextrose dialysis solution increases rates of solute loss, which has been attributed to enhanced permeability [41]. Most of the increased solute removal with hypertonic dextrose dialysis fluid can be accounted for by increased convective transport, however. Moreover, plasma volume expansion due to retention of absorbed dextrose contributes importantly to the higher mass transport rates [44]. Indeed, in the intact rabbit convective transport increases but diffusion does not as the volume expansion by hypertonic dialysis fluid is promptly excreted. Unlike diffusion which separates solutes according to molecular size, convection does not discriminate by size until sieving occurs as the dimensions of the effective pores are approached. Since convection adds more to the transport rate of slowly diffusible solutes, it mimics an increase in permeability of the diffusion barrier.

Biologic membranes have interstices and discontinuities between their lipid and protein complexes so that pores of a sort exist for diffusion and ultrafiltration. The Pappenheimer theory of restricted diffusion across capillaries takes into account 1) the stearic hindrance at the entrance of a pore, 2) friction between molecules moving within a pore and 3) molecular friction with the stationary walls of a pore as factors impeding the passage of molecules through pores of molecular dimensions. Such pores are lined by the fixed ionic groups of protein (amino-, imino-, and carboxyl) and of lipid (phosphate and choline) [45].

Anionic sites predominantly composed of heparan sulfate and chondroitin sulfate are a constant feature of basement membranes of the microvasculature [46]. They are particularly abundant in fenestrated capillaries, some of which have been identified in human parietal and diaphragmatic peritoneum [47]. Anionic sites are also found on the luminal surface of fenestrated endothelia, in the amorphous interstitial connective substance and at the peritoneal surface of the mesothelial plasmalemma, all of which contribute to the structure of peritoneal membrane [47]. Lastly, the lymphatic endothelium and intercellular clefts of lymphatic endothelial cells contain abundant anionic sites [48].

These ionic charges restrict the diffusive and convective passage of charged solutes through the membrane. For example, the rate of absorption of acids and bases from peritoneal fluid decreases to the extent of the ionization at physiological pH [40]. Diffusive rates of potassium, lithium and phosphate into the peritoneum are slower than the rates of uncharged solutes of similar size, unlike the transport across synthetic hemodialysis membranes [15]. Moreover, in the absence of a diffusion gradient the sodium concentration of osmotically induced peritoneal ultrafiltrate is much lower than that of plasma, i.e., about 75 mEq/l [49]. The addition of furosemide to the dialysis solution raises the peritoneal ultrafiltrate sodium concentration [50], consistent with a drug effect on the membrane.

There is a paucity of data concerning the influence of the peritoneal membrane anionic sites on transport of charged macromolecules across the peritoneum. Peritoneal transfer of heparin is negligible, which may relate to its negative charge [51]. With higher amounts of intraperitoneal heparin absorption may reach 15% to 20% of the administered dose [52].

The charge issue is further complicated by the presence of a surface active material lining the peritoneal membrane which is mostly composed of phosphatidylcholine (lecithin) [53]. A decrease in dialysate phospholipids was reported in patients with a low ultrafiltration capacity and in those with peritonitis [54]. Intraperitoneal phosphatidylcholine promptly raised the ultrafiltration rate while the oral route required about 30 days to achieve this effect. The authors suggest that lecithin administration restored the normal peritoneal surfactant lining [54]. To explain augmentation of ultrafiltration after phosphatidylcholine, another group proposed that these phospholipid molecules bind to the anionic sites on the luminal side of the mesothelium creating a water repellent surface which diminishes the thickness of the unstirred dialysate. This would augment diffusion of solutes from blood to the peritoneum while the hydrophobic lecithin molecules would impede water absorption,

favoring ultrafiltration [55].

7. TRANSPORT OF LIPIDS

Transport of fatty acids into peritoneal fluid does not proceed by simple diffusion and convection from plasma. These lipids rapidly diffuse through cell membranes reaching concentration equilibrium across biological membranes within a few minutes. The concentration ratio dialysate/plasma water, however, is far above unity for several fatty acids. Diffusion equilibrium does not occur from plasma to dialysate or from gastrointestinal luminal contents to dialysate and is uninfluenced by circulating concentrations of lipases [10]. Rather, non-esterified fatty acids flux from adjacent adipose tissue to peritoneal fluid and thereafter into portal venous blood [56]. Moreover, peritoneal absorption of barbiturates of comparable size depends on their lipid partition coefficient [40]. Whether lipid soluble drugs can be removed from fat stores in the mesentery by this process remains to be established and methods to exploit this transport mechanism should be studied.

8. LYMPHATIC ABSORPTION

Lymphatics are the primary route for absorption from the peritoneum of isotonic dialysate including macromolecules, particles and formed blood elements [57]. Most absorption occurs via the subdiaphragmatic lymphatics with lesser amounts via the mesenteric lymphatic vessels [58]. Absorption from the peritoneum of macromolecules such as albumin and fibrinogen has been reported [59–61] and used as a measure of peritoneal lymphathic flow rates [61, 62].

The peritoneal absorption of polydispersed neutral dextrans does not show size discrimination, adding evidence that the major route is by lymphatic transport [63]. The rate of lymphatic flow from the peritoneum correlates positively with ventilation (diaphragmatic movement) and negatively with end expiratory pressure; it decreases with erect posture and with dehydration [64]. Lymphatic absorption subtracts from the gross peritoneal ultrafiltration volume and may be an especially important negative quantity in patients with clinically significant loss of net ultrafiltration. In preliminary studies, neostigmine increased net ultrafiltration and solute transport in peritoneal dialysis in rats and diminished dialysate absorption measured by loss of instilled albumin [65]. In another study, phophatidylcholine augmented net ultrafiltration without increasing flux of water into the peritoneal cavity, presumably by reducing lymphatic reabsorption [66]. These preliminary studies suggest that limiting lymphatic absorption is a potential mechanism for augmenting peritoneal clearances that should be explored further.

9. MECHANISMS OF ACCELERATING PERITONEAL TRANSPORT

An adequate rate of transport by peritoneal dialysis requires enough blood flow to the dialyzing surface, sufficient area

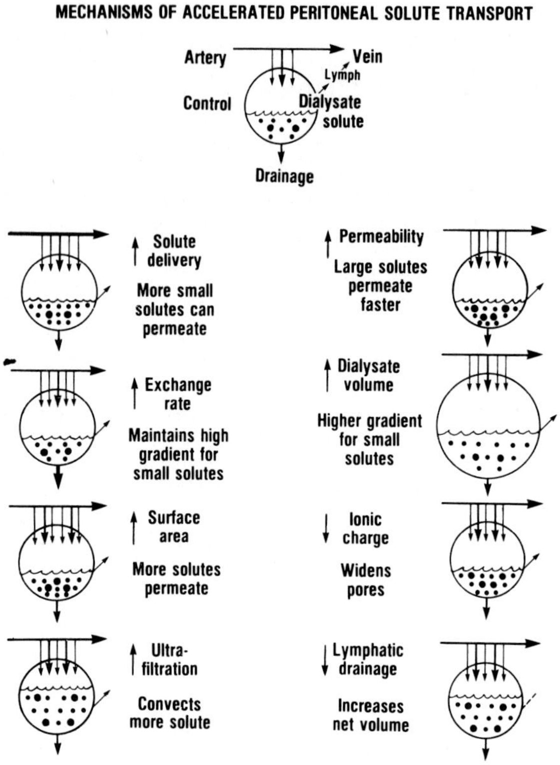

MECHANISMS OF ACCELERATED PERITONEAL SOLUTE TRANSPORT

Figure 2. A schematic representation of solute removal by peritoneal dialysis. The circles represent the peritoneum containing small solutes (dots) and larger compounds. The long horizontal arrow above the circle represents peritoneal blood flow. Vertical arrows above the circle display transfer of small (thin lines) and large (thick lines) solutes. The lower arrow indicates drainage, and the side arrow indicates lymphatic absorption.

and permeability of the membrane for rapid permeation of solutes and ultrafiltration of fluid, as well as rapid diffusion throughout the dialysate which is periodically replaced thereby maintaining electrochemical gradients.

Mechanisms whereby peritoneal transport might be augmented are outlined below and conceptually presented in Figure 2. Increasing blood flow to the peritoneum accelerates the rate of solute delivery to the membrane augmenting transport of small highly diffusible solutes, but only modestly.

Increased splanchnic perfusion, however, augments peritoneal clearances of larger solutes at least as much as the transport of smaller solutes. This suggests an increase in peritoneal surface area or permeability resulting from vasodilation, attributed to dilation of the functional peritoneal capillaries combined with perfusion of more capillaries. Spreading the same wall mass over a larger circumference decreases the wall thickness and stretches pores. Intercellular junctions widen accelerating mass transport [23]. Raising blood flow by local application of vasodilators also opens previously closed capillaries, increasing the surface area available for transport [67, 68]. In the resting state blood may circulate predominantly through metarterioles. Enhanced perfusion opens more capillaries exposing blood to a more permeable surface. Furthermore,

vasodilators with a predominant venular site of action may cause greater increases in diffusion rates but arteriolar dilators may increase the ultrafiltration rate. By increasing blood flow, diffusion and ultrafiltration may occur throughout a greater length of the capillaries than occurs under resting conditions.

Depending on the nature of the vasodilating agent there may be an increase (arteriolar relaxation), decrease (lowered venular tone), or no change (balanced effects) in capillary hydrostatic pressure. This hydrostatic pressure may affect capillary diameter, volume and permeability and is a major determinant of the filtration rate through the capillary. Certain drugs can affect specifically the capillary filtration coefficient, i.e., the volume filtered per unit of pressure per unit of time (ml/mm Hg/min). The rate of ultrafiltration under the artificial circumstances of intraperitoneal fluid administration is largely determined, however, by the osmotic gradient across the peritoneum customarily induced by dextrose. As dextrose diffuses, the gradient dissipates rapidly. Increased solute permeability of the peritoneum increases the rate of glucose absorption so a constant fluid flux may represent increased fluid flux/gradient.

The gross ultrafiltration rate is offset by dialysate absorption; hence lowering lymphatic flow rates raises net ultrafiltration.

Specific drugs may affect directly the permeability of the capillary or the mesothelium [69]. Drugs that influence membrane charge, cell volume, cell metabolism or intercellular junction may directly influence peritoneal permeability without affecting flow rates.

The flow rate of dialysate determines the transport rate, at least of very diffusible solutes by maintaining the chemical gradient. Transport requires dialysate contact with the membrane, which is adequate when fluid volume reaches 1.5 l/M² [27]. Rapid exchange of small volumes enhances mixing and increases transport by decreasing the impedance due to unstirred layers. Tidal exchange techniques that leave a residual volume of dialysate in the peritoneum maintain peritoneal surface contact throughout the fluid exchange, also increasing efficiency.

Finally, the transport rate of specific solutes may be accelerated, e.g., by chelating agents or adsorbents, by changing pH thereby influencing nonionic diffusion, by adding protein to dialysate to bind toxins, or by intraperitoneal charged macromolecules [70]. It is likely that maximal transport rates will only be achieved by combinations of maneuvers affecting different resistances to transport as exemplified by the additive transport acceleration effects of intraperitoneal nitroprusside, increased dialysis fluid flow rate, temperature and dextrose concentration [71].

10. RESTORATION OF DECREASED TRANSPORT RATES TOWARD NORMAL

When peritoneal blood flow and clearances have been reduced by disease, transport rates may be restored toward normal by treating the specific abnormality. For example, the mesenteric blood flow rate varies directly with cardiac output. Treatment of heart failure should improve peritoneal clearances, although digoxin is a mesenteric vasoconstrictor. Treatment of heart failure in our patients increased mean clearances of creatinine and urea by 37% and 47% respectively. Chronic congestive heart failure with hepatic congestion may raise portal venous pressure, however, increasing splanchnic volume, capillary diameter and peritoneal permeability.

Loss of blood volume by hemorrhage reduces peritoneal transport of urea and potassium in the dog [72]. When blood pressure and volume are restored toward normal by infusing blood or saline, clearances return to normal. After hemorrhagic hypotension, clearances are not increased by raising blood pressure with norepinephrine nor is transport affected adversely by lowering the blood pressure further with phenoxybenzamine [73]. These studies suggest that blood pressure per se does not influence importantly the efficiency of peritoneal dialysis which does depend, however, on adequate splanchnic volume and perfusion.

Several vascular diseases can impair the mesenteric arterial circulation, so reducing peritoneal transport rates [5]. Vascular damage secondary to diabetes mellitus is not considered reversible and the vasculitis of systemic lupus erythematosus does not readily respond to therapy. Some diseases that cause renal failure such as malignant hypertension and hemolytic uremic syndrome cause widespread vascular endothelial injury inducing platelet thrombi [74]. Reduced peritoneal transport rates complicating these diseases are improved by dipyridamole [75]. The augmentation of peritoneal transport rates persists after dipyridamole vasodilation abates and is attributed to its antiplatelet aggregating effect. Peritoneal clearances of patients with normal vasculature improve only minimally and transiently with dipyridamole administered orally or intraperitoneally and only a modest increment in peritoneal solute transport occurs in animals given dipyridamole intraperitoneally or intravenously [76].

The impaired peritoneal transport that complicates irreversible systemic vascular lesions can also improve toward normal with the local application of vasodilators such as isoproterenol [77, 78]. There is no evidence that increased clearances result from improvement in the vascular disease but rather may be attributed to vasodilation of diseased vessels.

11. INCREASING PERITONEAL TRANSPORT ABOVE NORMAL VALUES

Drugs may increase peritoneal transport rates to values exceeding normal, both in patients without vascular disease [79] and in animal models [80–82]. Evidence against a nonspecific effect due to an intraperitoneal inflammatory reaction includes the following. Effects on mass transport can be separated from those on fluid flux and solvent drag [8, 9, 50, 83]. Transport rates increase without the vasodilator inducing an intraperitoneal inflammatory exudate [79]. Certain drugs accelerate transport when given either intravenously or intraperitoneally [76, 84]. Peritoneal transport rates respond in accord with the known vasoactive properties, increasing with vasodilators and decreasing with vasoconstrictor agents [84, 85]. Solute response may be selective, based for example on ionic charge. Finally, inactive metabolites and drug vehicles do not affect peritoneal transport rates [8, 85].

Many studies suggest that peritoneal clearances will increase only if a vasodilator selectively affects the splanchnic vasculature or is applied locally, e.g., by intraperitoneal instillation. Intravenously such drugs may cause widespread vasodilation decreasing blood pressure, splanchnic perfusion and splanchnic volume, thereby lowering peritoneal transport rates. To date membrane-active agents have only augmented transport when applied locally, i.e., instilled intraperitoneally.

12. ISOPROTERENOL ENHANCEMENT OF PERITONEAL MASS TRANSPORT

In patients with reduced peritoneal clearance, Nolph *et al* improved transport rates by adding isoproterenol (0.06 mg/l) to the dialysis solution [77, 78]. Mean clearances increased to the lower range of normal but only transiently and not all patients improved significantly [86]. No systemic effects of intraperitoneal isoproterenol were detected even with cardiac monitoring. Such use of isoproterenol has been explored in greater detail in animals. In acute studies in anesthetized dogs intraperitoneal isoproterenol increased urea and creatinine clearances by 45% and 30%, respectively, but subpressor intravenous doses of isoproterenol did not augment transport [81]. In normal unanesthetized rabbits 0.04 μmol/kg of intraperitoneall isoproterenol raised urea and creatinine clearance by 50%, but osmotically induced water flux was unaffected [87]. No systemic effects were observed. On exposure to light and air isoproterenol rapidly became ineffective.

Despite raising mesenteric blood flow to 188% of control by intravenous isoproterenol, Felt *et al.* [33] showed that clearances did not increase. With intraperitoneal isoproterenol a comparable flow increase raised peritoneal inulin and creatinine clearances by 27% and 18%, respectively. The disparity in blood flow and clearance changes suggests that capillary blood volume may be as important as blood flow in mediating changes in permeability.

Isoproterenol, a beta adrenergic agonist, relaxes the mesenteric vascular bed. When used clinically to accelerate peritoneal transport, no systemic toxicity was shown despite continuous use of isoproterenol for 20 exchanges [88]. Yet, a better transport accelerator continues to be sought because of the potential cardiotoxicity and the need to apply the drug topically.

13. EFFECTS OF THEOPHYLLINE ON PERITONEAL FLUXES

In rabbits, changes in solute transport and in osmotic water flux were inconsistent, both after intraperitoneal and intravenous aminophylline, despite doses (30 to 150 μmol/kg) sufficient to achieve blood theophylline concentrations exceeding the therapeutic range [89]. Theophylline acts as a nonselective antagonist of two types of adenosine receptors which mediate opposite effects on vascular tone [90]. Hence, with normal hemodynamics a selective vasodilation may not be as apparent. Moreover, the high flux rate of this xanthine could have induced widespread vasodilation because of rapid absorption with no net gain in splanchnic blood flow or volume.

14. NITROPRUSSIDE AUGMENTATION OF PERITONEAL MASS TRANSFER

The observations by Nolph et al. [86] that intraperitoneal nitroprusside increases peritoneal mass transport have been confirmed in multiple laboratories in several species [91–94]. Urea and creatinine clearances increase as much as 50% above control with greater increments in inulin clearances and protein loss, consistent with enhanced peritoneal permeability or area or both rather than simply increased solute delivery. Osmotic ultrafiltration increases slightly [72] or not at all as rapid glucose absorption dissipates the osmotic gradient. Nitroprusside-induced increases in mass transport are dose dependent and can be seen with as little as 1.0 mg/kg [95]. It has also been suggested that increments in peritoneal mass transfer coefficients with topical nitroprusside can indicate peritoneal vascular reserve [96]. Systemic effects of nitroprusside have not been detected in most studies and intravenously the drug does not accelerate peritoneal mass transport. The transport increment is sustained for serveral exchanges and on discontinuation may persist somewhat for up to 2 hr [97]. Augmented transport represents an increase in permeance of the peritoneum (mass transfer coefficient × area) due to capillary, especially venular, dilation and from opening of previously nonperfused capillaries [95, 98]. Although it is metabolized to thiocynate, this toxic metabolite is rapidly dialyzed and no evidence of accumulation has been observed with repeated nitroprusside instillation.

15. DIPYRIDAMOLE EFFECTS ON PERITONEAL EFFICIENCY

Dipyridamole is an orally effective general smooth muscle relaxant with pharmacologic properties similar to those of papaverine. It rapidly but transiently vasodilates [99] and has a sustained antiplatelet aggregating effect, which may explain the restoration of clearances toward normal in patients with intravascular platelet aggregations [76]. Peritoneal transport of urea and creatinine increase by 43% and 70%, respectively, in patients with normal vasculature given 300 mg/day of dipyridamole orally [100, 101]. The clearance of radiolabeled EDTA and DPTA increase by 75% and 41%, respectively [101]. Modest increments in the clearances of uric acid and inulin also occur but are delayed for a few days [102]. In normal rabbits dipyridamole given intravenously (0.5 mg/kg) or intraperitoneally (2.5 mg/kg) increased urea and creatinine clearances by 39% and 16%, respectively [76, 103]. The limited effectiveness and the transient vasodilator response of dipyridamole are reflected by two randomized control studies which did not demonstrate significant increases in peritoneal transport [104, 105]. Nevertheless, dipyridamole may be useful for selected patients when systemic disease with platelet thrombi affects mesenteric vessels and an oral agent is preferred.

16. INFLUENCE OF CATECHOLAMINES ON PERITONEAL TRANSPORT KINETICS

To explore further vasoactive effects on peritoneal transport catecholamines have been studied in animals undergoing peritoneal dialysis. Gutman et al. [81] noted lower increments in dialysate urea with large intraperitoneal doses of dopamine in dogs but did not measure dialysate volume. Because blood pressure increased, the lower urea accumulation in the dialysate was attributed to splanchnic vasoconstriction. To offset vasoconstriction Parker et al. [106] added an alpha adrenergic blocker to the dialysis fluid. With intraperitoneal phentolamine and intravenous dopamine peritoneal clearances increased in dogs. In patients, however, Chan et al. [107] observed no effect of low (4 mg/l) or high doses (20–160 mg/l) of intraperitoneal dopamine on dialysate urea, creatinine or phosphate. They did not measure dialysate volume, so the effect on ultrafiltration rate could not be discerned. In rabbits, intraperitoneal dopamine caused dose related (0.6 to 1.8 mg/kg) increases in peritoneal urea clearance [84]. The increments occurred with lower doses than those used by Gutman et al. [81] and drug concentrations (10 to 30 mg/l) within the range studied by Chan et al [107]. Species differences may account for the discrepant results.

Intravenous l-norepinephrine significantly decreased peritoneal clearances of urea and creatinine in unanesthetized rabbits [84, 107]. Dose dependent decrements correlated with the pressor response [108]. Comparable pressor doses of intravenous dopamine increased clearances of urea and creatinine to 145% of control values, whereas low doses had minimal and inconsistent effects [108]. Osmotic water flux increased only slightly (from 0.18 to 0.24 ml/kg/min) but significantly (p<0.02). Because dopamine vasoconstricts venules relatively more than arterioles as compared to norepinephrine [42], augmented water flux could be mediated by increased hydrostatic pressure rather than a change in hydraulic permeability. Dopamine augmented solute transport was unaffected by concurrent beta blockade with propranolol, was decreased by simultaneous alpha adrenergic receptor blockade by phentolamine, and was abolished by haloperidol blockade of dopaminergic receptors [108]. Accordingly the augmented transport is attributed to dopamine receptor mediated mesenteric vasodilation and in part, alpha adrenergic somatic vasoconstriction increasing blood pressure while mesenteric blood flow is maintained. Although dopamine may not be suitable for augmenting efficiency of routine peritoneal dialysis, these data argue strongly that it should be preferable to l-norepinephrine when vasopressor therapy is required during peritoneal dialysis. Seeking an effective oral agent we studied the influence of ibopamine, an analogue. Only minimal increments in fluid and solute flux occurred with ibopamine whether given by mouth, intravenously or intraperitoneally to normal rabbits [109].

17. OTHER VASODILATORS THAT AFFECT PERITONEAL TRANSPORT

No consistent change in peritoneal clearance of urea or creatinine was observed in patients given 20 to 40 mg of hydralazine intraperitoneally which decreased blood pressure slightly [86]. Hydralazine (168 daltons) should be rapidly absorbed from the peritoneal fluid, but its pharmacologic action may depend on biotransformation to an active compound. Hence, widespread vasodilation may occur despite local application with no preferential effect on splanchnic blood flow or volume.

Diazoxide caused a modest increase in peritoneal clearances of urea and creatinine and a significant decrement in blood pressure when administered intraperitoneally to patients at a dose of 100 to 300 mg [86]. An increase in ultrafiltration rate approaching 50% of control values was found inconsistently. In another study, 150 mg of diazoxide increased peritoneal clearances of urea, creatinine and phosphate by 58%, 48% and 39%, respectively [101].

The intraperitoneal administration of 5 mg of phentolamine did not influence peritoneal solute transport rates in five patients so investigated, nor did it affect osmotic water flux [86].

In anesthetized rats, histamine (4 or 8 μg) raised only modestly (9% to 16%) the clearances of urea and inulin, whereas 3 μg of bradykinin augmented these clearances by 13% and 25%, respectively [91]. Histamine cause overt capillary dilation and increased permeability with protein exudation which can be blocked in rabbits by both H_1 and H_2 receptor antagonists [110]. Minimal effects of histamine on small solute transport may reflect decreased plasma volume due to protein loss. In isolated rat mesentery, viewed by television microscopy after fluorescein labelling, protein exudation is also demonstrable [23]. Dilation is most prominent in the venous end of the capillary and similar changes are noted with nitroprusside.

In preliminary studies of a few unanesthetized animals tolazoline increased peritoneal urea clearances to more than 150% of control values [111]. Tolazoline, a substituted imidazole which can be given by mouth, is a potent adrenergic blocker somewhat similar to phentolamine.

The calcium channel blockers, verapamil and diltiazem, given intraperitoneally modestly but significantly increased peritoneal urea clearances despite causing a marked fall in systemic blood pressure [112]. Protein exudation did not increase leading to the interpretation that the arteriolar end of the capillary dilated and blood flow increased but surface area and venular permeability were unaffected.

Modest increases in urea clearance and glucose absorption and a marked exaggeration of protein loss followed intraperitoneal instillation of captopril, an angiotension converting enzyme inhibitor in rats [113]. These increments despite drug induced systemic hypotension may reflect increased blood flow, surface area or permeability due to blockade of a baseline level of angiotension II activity.

It is thus apparent that many vasoactive drugs can affect peritoneal transport rates. Some have been studied in a limited number of species, only in a few animals or at only one dose. Isoproterenol and nitroprusside consistently augmented clearances in several studies from multiple laboratories. Dipyridamole advantageously can be given by mouth and is particularly effective when platelet aggregation limits capillary filling.

Norepinephrine as anticipated consistently decreased clearances, whereas dopamine not only did not but at certain doses appreciably increased transport rates. Interestingly,

dihydroergotamine, an agent that accelerates blood flow by causing somatic venoconstriction, reduces peritoneal ultrafiltration rates and urea clearance presumably due to the decreased plasma volume [109, 114].

Because numerous other drugs are administered for various indications to patients undergoing peritoneal dialysis, the influences of a variety of other agents on peritoneal mass transport have been explored.

18. PROSTAGLANDIN MODULATION OF PERITONEAL TRANSPORT

Prostaglandins control regional blood flow by virtue of their capability of modulating vasoconstrictor responses [36]. The prostaglandins are unsaturated 20 carbon lipids biosynthesized from arachidonic acid and other precursors by prostaglandin synthetase, an enzyme present in tissues [88]. Depending on the local concentration of the specific terminal enzyme, e.g. endoperoxide reductase leading to $PGF_{2\alpha}$ or endoperoxide isomerase leading to PGE_2, a given product predominates in a given tissue. Regional blood flow is one determinant of enzyme activity. In circulation the prostaglandins are degraded during a single passage through the lung thereby acting only locally with the exception of prostacyclin and thromboxanes which have half-lives of a few minutes. Biosynthesis of these compounds can be inhibited by various drugs at varied sites in the synthetic pathway. Prostaglandins of the PGA, PGE or PGI series vasodilate whereas $PGF_{2\alpha}$ and thromboxanes are potent vasoconstrictors [116, 117]. These prostaglandins act locally in arterial walls to influence vascular tone and modulate the response of vascular smooth muscle to other vasoactive agents [118].

Intraperitoneal instillation of PGA_1 or PGE_1 increased peritoneal clearances of urea and creatinine modestly in alert normal rabbits, whereas 125 μg/kg of PGE_2 significantly raised creatinine clearance to 132% and urea clearance to 180% of control values [80, 85, 119]. In contrast, intraperitoneally the vasoconstrictor $PGF_{2\alpha}$ (125 μg/kg) decreased peritoneal clearances to 80% (urea) and 82% (creatine) of control [85]. These prostaglandins did not affect fluid flux and were totally ineffective when given intravenously. Neither intravenous nor intraperitoneal administration of prostacyclin affected peritoneal solute or water transport significantly over a dose range from 25 to 125 μg/kg [65]. It is interpreted that prostacyclin caused widespread vasodilation so that mesenteric blood flow and volume were not selectively increased. Hence, transport remained unaffected.

Prostaglandin synthetase stimulators and inhibitors have not had pronounced effects on peritoneal transport under baseline conditions. Oral pretreatment with 10 to 21 mg/kg of sulfinpyrazone, a potent stimulator of prostaglandin synthetase, did not alter peritoneal clearances significantly [119]. When mefenamic acid, a potent prostaglandin synthetase inhibitor, is administered intravenously or intraperitoneally to alert, intact rabbits in doses sufficient to inhibit platelet function, neither the peritoneal clearances of creatinine or urea nor water flux changed [119]. Oral pretreatment of rabbits with indomethacin blocked platelet aggregation but did not change clearances or ultrafiltration rates significantly [119]. Intraperitoneal indomethacin increases the size of pinocytotic vesicles and narrows intercellular spaces in the rabbit, however [120]. Alteration of prostaglandin synthetase affects both vasoconstrictor and vasodilator prostaglandins. Hence, regional blood flow may not change. Imidazole specifically blocks the synthesis of vasoconstrictor thromboxanes but an intraperitoneal dose of 5 mg/kg did not augment clearances in rabbits. Yet, when vasodilator prostaglandin activity predominates to compensate for increased renin-angiotensin activity or ischemic vascular disease, aspirin or indomethacin decreases regional blood flow [121]. However, the reduction of clearances induced by intravenous l-norepinephrine, which should be accompanied by vasodilator prostaglandin stimulation, is exaggerated by pretreatment with indomethacin in only half of the animals so studied. These results suggest that endogenous prostaglandins do not play a major role in regulating peritoneal blood flow under ordinary circumstances. But in patienst that depend on vasodilator prostaglandins to maintain organ perfusion, blockade of prostaglandin synthetase could impair transport and a history of exposure to such drugs should be sought if clearances are low. Intraperitoneally, the prostaglandin precursor arachidonic acid (1.5 to 5.6 mg/kg) increased creatinine clearance by 36% and urea clearance by 24%, however, suggesting an effect of endogenous prostaglandins, but systemic use of indomethacin did not block this increase [119, 122]. With peritonitis the increased solute transport rates are accompanied by augmented prostaglandin release, abnormalities that can be blocked by indomethacin [37].

19. VASODILATOR GASTROINTESTINAL HORMONES

Glucagon and secretin are structurally similar polypeptide gastrointestinal hormones that increase mesenteric blood flow by as much as 100% above baseline when pharmacologic doses are given but augment different gastrointestinal functions [98]. Secretin, like cholecystokinin, increases predominantly hepatic blood flow but glucagon has the more potent effect on the mesenteric circulation. Gastrin, structurally similar to cholecystokinin, also increases mesenteric blood flow [98]. The augmented mesenteric circulation can be induced by intraduodenal instillation of corn oil, l-phenylalanine or acid, after a short latency consistent with the physiologic release of secretin or cholecystokinin [124]. Similar changes can be induced by low intravenous doses of these hormones. The effects of secretin and cholecystokinin on mesenteric blood flow are additive and potentiated by theophylline [125]. This hormonal mesenteric vasodilation is attributed to direct relaxation of vascular tone presumably mediated by cyclic AMP.

When administered intravenously immediately predialysis, 30 µg/kg of glucagon significantly increased peritoneal clearances of urea and creatinine in alert rabbits [83, 126]. The same dose of glucagon intraperitoneally did not augment clearances significantly. Since this large peptide should traverse the peritoneum slowly, hormonal activity presumably occurs at the endothelial rather than the mesothelial surface. Nevertheless, much higher doses given intraperitoneally do increase clearance somewhat.

Bolus administration of these hormones is more effective than continuous infusion despite their short half-lives [127]. Nevertheless, intravenous infusion of about 30 µg/kg/hr increased mesenteric arterial blood flow and peritoneal inulin clearance (but not creatinine) in dogs, unlike intraperitoneal instillation [33]. Slight increments in urea and creatinine clearances occurred with intravenous secretin or cholecystokinin [83]. Intravenously, but not intraperitoneally, secretin (10 U/kg) increased osmotic water flux in rabbits from 0.19 to 0.29 ml/kg/min [83]. The endogenous release of cholecystokinin or secretin or their intra-arterial infusion relaxes precapillary sphincters and increases the capillary filtration coefficient from 0.05 to 0.10 ml/min/mm Hg/100 g [128]. Secretin also increases the capillary filtration coefficient in the mesenteric vasculature of the cat [41]. Neither glucagon nor cholecystokinin affected peritoneal water flux during dialysis in rabbits, however [83]. The separation of the effects of gastrointestinal hormones on diffusive and on convective transport suggests the possible use of separate pharmacologic agents acting additively.

20. OTHER HORMONES AND DRUGS AFFECTING PERITONEAL BLOOD FLOW AND DIFFUSION

Parenteral administration of vasopressin to anesthetized dogs decreased peritoneal clearances of small solutes, consistent with a hormonally mediated reduction in mesenteric blood flow [129, 130]. Since inulin clearance increased slightly under such circumstances, a concurrent increase in membrane permeability has been postulated [105], in accord with the accelerated transport that occurs in isolated membrane preparations [131].

In preliminary studies in rabbits and patients, large doses of methyl prednisolone increased peritoneal clearances by as much as 69%, but such augmented transport was observed inconsistently [132].

The peritoneal transport rates of potassium and [131] iodide increased when streptokinase or serotonin were administered systemically to anesthetized dogs [129]. Whether these agents affect peritoneal permeability directly or augment blood flow remains to be determined.

In sedated rabbits dialyzed with a hypertonic dialysis solution containing 0.25% procaine hydrochloride, peritoneal urea and inulin clearances increased by more than 60% [133]. The effect persisted for at least an hour after procaine was discontinued. Procaine vasodilates, which may augment transport. However, the addition of procaine to either side of the isolated mesothelium increased transport after a transient decrease. This effect may be due to disruption of the microfilaments of tight junctions between cells.

Variations in electrolyte concentrations also influence peritoneal blood flow and permeability. For example, topically applied low potassium solutions vasoconstrict several vascular beds including the mesenteric, interfering with normal Na-K-ATPase activity and should thereby decrease peritoneal transport efficiency. Modest increments in potassium concentration vasodilate, an effect that is inhibited by oubain [134].

The dialysis solution itself affects the peritoneal vasculature. Miller and colleagues [67, 135] have shown that the mesenteric vasculature transiently vasoconstricts and then vasodilates when exposed to peritoneal dialysis solution. The prolonged vasodilation depends on the presence of hyperosmolar dialysis fluid containing either acetate or lactate. Bicarbonate buffered isotonic Krebs solution did not induce vasodilation.

21. MEMBRANE SURFACE-ACTIVE AGENTS

Penzotti and Mattocks [82, 136, 137] accelerated peritoneal transport of labelled urea and creatinine in sedated rabbits by adding a variety of surface-acting agents including dioctyl sodium sulfosuccinate, cetyl trimethyl ammonium chloride and N-myristyl-ß-amino-proprionate. These compounds have not been employed clinically but may help identify agents for clinical use. More recently, Dunham *et al.* [138] verified a dose-dependent rise in creatinine and urea clearances when docusate sodium was given intraperitoneally to tranquilized rabbits. The effect persisted for 5 hr.

The solvent dimethyl sulfoxide did not augment clearance of potassium or urea in rabbits, however, except to the extent that large doses intraperitoneally created an osmotic gradient and increased convective transport [139].

Cytochalasins disrupt microfilaments of cellular junctions. Cytochalasin D given intraperitoneally raises the clearances of creatinine and urea in the rabbit, consistent with augmented diffusion through intercellular gaps [8]. Concurrently the ultrafiltration rate decreases, attributed to accelerated glucose transport diminishing the osmotic gradient more rapidly, as occurs in acute peritonitis [140]. Similarly, cytochalasins B, D and E increased permeability of the peritoneum to urea, inulin and albumin in rats [141]. Only cytochalasin B actions were significantly reversible which may relate to its unique ability to affect carrier proteins of the cell membrane.

The addition of 1 mg/kg of furosemide to hypertonic peritoneal dialysis solution augmented sodium movement accompanying osmotically induced water flux in rabbits [50]. Normally, electrolytes do not accompany water in the same concentration as exists in plasma water suggesting that membrane charge impedes transport, a phenomenon that is interrupted by furosemide. Intraperitoneal furosemide also caused a 27% increase in peritoneal urea clearance but no demonstrable changes in transport rates occur in patients undergoing intermittent peritoneal dialysis when treated systemically with this diuretic. Moreover, oral use of furosemide did not affect sodium, potassium or water transport in patients undergoing continuous ambulatory peritoneal dialysis [142]. But, furosemide does increase the peritoneal transport of uric acid and of barbiturates [143]. Intraperitoneally, 1.25 mg/kg of ethacrynic acid did not affect sodium flux with the bulk flow of water across the peritoneum but augmented urea clearance to about 165% of baseline [50]. Patients treated by CAPD may experience a restoration of lost ultrafiltration capacity after treatment by furosemide or by hemofiltration [144]. A specific effect of furosemide has been postulated, but correction of an overexpanded splanchnic volume by decreasing glucose absorption could restore ultrafiltration capacity.

Charged macromolecules may also interact with peri-

toneal anionic sites, altering membrane ultrastructure and permeability. In rats local administration of protamine, a polycation, markedly increases peritoneal permeability to inulin and to a lesser extent to urea, associated with a partial disruption of the mesothelial junctions [145]. Similarly, in rats cationic poly-l-lysine augments peritoneal permeability for urea, inulin and albumin, while with the anionic poly-l-glutamic acid there was an opposite trend [146]. Another group of authors [147] showed that cationic ferritin applied *in vitro* at the mesothelial side of the membrane decreases permeability of water, glucose and inulin without affecting the transport of urea. In contrast, anionic ferritin had no effect on water and solute movement.

22. INCREASED ULTRAFILTRATION RATES

Because the peritoneal ultrafiltration rate is normally low compared to the clearance of low molecular weight solutes (10% to 20%) even doubling this rate has only a modest effect on removal of such substances as urea and drugs [148]. Ultrafiltration contributes importantly, however, to the removal of large, poorly diffusible solutes as occurs with hemodialysis [149].

The ultrafiltration rate can be increased by raising the capillary hydrostatic pressure, by venular constriction, or by arteriolar relaxation. Few drugs appear to increase capillary hydrostatic pressure but this mechanism can account for increased ultrafiltration by dopamine [108]. Surface-active agents can increase ultrafiltration by narrowing the stagnant dialysate layer and creating a water-repellant lining on the surface of the peritoneum [55]. Factors that diminish peritoneal lymph flow raise net ultrafiltration rates by minimizing the loss of fluid by absorption [65].

Secretin increases the hydraulic permeability of the peritoneal membrane [83]. This selective action on the splanchic bed occurs from the vascular side only. The amino-nucleoside of puromycin, which causes glomerular lesions with increased macromolecular permeability, also induces this effect on peritoneal capillaries [150]. After a few days, puromycin causes a proteinaceous ascites in rats with faster permeation of labelled test solutes than in control rats. The prolonged effect of such a permeability augmenting drug could be commendable, but other nonglomerular capillary beds are probably also affected, which would make it hazardous even in anephric patients.

Amphotericin B increases the rate of ultrafiltration per osmotic gradient, i.e., the ultrafiltration coefficient [9]. Above 0.5 mg/kg there is no dose effect and it is effective only from the serosal side [9, 151]. Amphotericin B creates channels in biological membranes for solute and water penetration. Increments in peritoneal solute clearances with amphotericin B are only modest and can be accounted for by enhanced convection [9]. However, peritoneal mass transport of sodium also increases. Because osmotic ultrafiltrate during peritoneal dialysis is hyponatric, the sodium gradient so established is an impediment to water transport that amphotericin B cancels [151]. Amphotericin B or safer analogues could help treat the reduced ultrafiltration capacity that occasionally complicates long-term peritoneal dialysis.

Phosphatidylcholine increases ultrafiltration rates in patients with peritonitis and those who acquire low filtration capacity, presumably by restoring mesothelial surfactant [54]. In rabbits phosphatidylcholine increases net ultrafiltrate volume [55], an effect that only becomes significant after hours of peritoneal dialysis in accord with our studies showing ineffectiveness during hourly exchanges. Rather than the surfactant effect, phosphatidylcholine may impede lymphatic absorption [66].

Chlorpromazine (2 mg/l) intraperitoneally also increases the ultrafiltration rate and solute clearances, largely by increased convection and presumably by its surfactant effect [152]. This drug decreased surface tension of the dialysate.

Neostigmine decreases the rate of lymphatic flow and thereby increases net ultrafiltration in rate [65]. Anticholinesterase agents also have complex hemodynamic effects which could influence peritoneal transport and increase gastrointestinal motility which would enhance dialysate mixing.

The osmotic gradient across the peritoneum is the major determinant of the rate of ultrafiltration per surface area. This gradient depends mainly on the dialysate dextrose concentration but is also influenced by sodium and urea gradients, plasma oncotic pressure and the rate of dextrose absorption. Recently, Ronco *et al.* [153] suggested that maximal rates of ultrafiltration are inhibited by the steep curvilinear rise in plasma protein oncotic pressure in the peritoneal capillaries, reflecting the limited blood flow rate. Nitroprusside vasodilation did not raise the ultrafiltration ceiling, however, [154]. We recently showed that the ultrafiltration coefficient decreases in rabbits as intraperitoneal dwell is prolonged, suggesting some concentration polarization, which could be corrected by increasing turbulence at the membrane interface [155]. Increased absorption of dextrose will accompany most manipulations that enhance solute permeability and hence dissipate the glucose osmotic gradient faster reducing ultrafiltration. Insulin is required to maintain low plasma glucose levels and achieve the maximal gradient. Exogenous insulin added intraperitoneally does not increase the glucose mass transfer coefficient [156]. Because excessive glucose absorption can be hazardous, alternative osmotic agents have been evaluated. Amino acids added to the dialysate offer a nutritional advantage but may be costly. Dextrans, glucose polymers and cross-linked gelatins are large enough to permeate the peritoneum poorly thereby maintaining the osmotic gradient throughout long dwell exchanges [157], but are eliminated slowly after absorption. An ideal agent for achieving maximal ultrafiltration has not been identified.

23. TRANSPORT ACCELERATION OF SPECIFIC SOLUTES

Removal of barbiturates may be accelerated by increasing dialysate pH with tris buffer thereby influencing the rate of non-ionic diffusion [158]. Alkalinization of peritoneal dialysate by THAM also raises uric acid transport [159]. Drugs that counteract the membrane anionic charge should enhance removal of charged solutes. For example, hexadimethrine bromide increases peritoneal phosphate clearances but does not affect urea or glucose transport [109] and a polycation especially augments phosphate transfer [70]. Adding albumin to peritoneal dialysis solution enhances removal of barbiturates [160], ethchlorvynol [161] and salicylate [162], and predictably should augment the clearance of numerous other drugs that circulate bound to plasma proteins, such as some aminoglycoside antibiotics, quinine and phenytoin. Increases in peritoneal clearance of barbiturates, phenytoin and salicylates have been achieved by agents that displace protein binding [163]. Albumin enriched peritoneal dialysis fluid also augments removal of trace metals such as copper [164]. Enhanced removal of trace elements can also be accomplished by chelation [165–167]. For lipophilic drugs such as glutethimide and short-acting barbiturates, transport can be enhanced by adding lipid to the dialysate [168]. In general, the removal of drugs is too slow by peritoneal dialysis for treating severe overdosage. These specific effects such as chelation, however, may influence therapeutic drug concentrations and certain uremic metabolites.

24. CONCLUSIONS

It is easy for clinicians as well as bioengineers to forget that the peritoneum unlike synthetic hemodialysis membranes is alive. The mesenteric circulation is remarkable for its size and complexity and until recently for the paucity of knowledge about its physiology. The numerous drugs and hormones that affect mesenteric blood flow and membrane physiology should have predictable effects on peritoneal transport parameters [38, 169]. Patients undergoing chronic dialysis characteristically receive several drugs regularly, many of which have hemodynamic and membrane transport effects. The influence of these agents on the peritoneum must be ascertained. Those treated for acute problems, for example in an intensive care unit, are exposed to even a greater abundance of drugs potentially altering transport. Rational use of drugs and other physiological manipulations in patients maintained by peritoneal dialysis requires an understanding of their effects on peritoneal blood flow and permeability. It is naive to consider the peritoneum as an inert membrane with constant blood flow and transport characteristics. Further investigation of the interactions of drugs and the peritoneum may identify optimal methods of augmenting transport efficiency safely.

ACKNOWLEGEMENT

This work was supported by the Uniformed Services University of the Health Sciences Protocol No. R08318. The opinions or assertions contained herein are the private views of the authors and should not be construed as official or as necessarily reflecting the views of the Department of Defense or the Uniformed Services University of the Health Sciences. The experiments reported herein were conducted according to the principles set forth in the 'Guide for the Care and Use of Laboratory Animals,' Institute of Animal Resources, National Research Council, DHEW Pub. No (NIH) 78–23.

REFERENCES

1. Broyer M, Brunner FP, Brynger H, Donckerwolcke RA, Jacobs C, Kramer P, Selwood NH, Wing AJ: Combined report on regular dialysis and transplantation in Europe, XII, 1981. Proc Eur Dial Transplant Assoc 19: 3, 1982.
2. Oreopoulos DG: Chronic peritoneal dialysis. Clin Nephrol 9: 165, 1978.
3. Nolph KD: Continuous ambulatory peritoneal dialysis. Am J Nephrol 1: 1, 1981.
4. Verger C, Brunschvicg O, Le Charpentier Y, Lavergne A, Vantelon J: Structural and ultrastructural peritoneal membrane changes and permeability alterations during continuous ambulatory peritoneal dialysis. Proc Eur Dial Transpl Assoc 18: 199, 1981.
5. Nolph KD, Stoltz ML, Maher JF: Altered peritoneal permeability in patients with systemic vasculitis. Ann Intern Med 75: 753, 1973.
6. Popovich RP, Moncrief JW, Nolph KD, Ghods AJ, Twardowski ZJ, Pyle WK: Continuous ambulatory peritoneal dialysis. Ann Intern Med 88: 449, 1978.
7. Nolph KD, Miller FN, Pyle WK, Popovich RP, Sorkin MI: An hypothesis to explain the ultrafiltration characteristics of peritoneal dialysis. Kidney Int 20: 543, 1981.
8. Hirszel P, Dodge K, Maher JF: Acceleration of peritoneal solute transport by cytochalasin D. Uremia Invest 8: 85, 1985.
9. Maher JF, Hirszel P, Bennett RR, Chakrabarti E: Amphotericin B selectively increases peritoneal ultrafiltration. Am J Kidney Dis 4: 285, 1984.
10. Maher JF, Hirszel P, Hohnadel DC, Abraham J, Lasrich M: Fatty acid removal during peritoneal dialysis. Mechanisms, rates and significance. asaio J 1: 8, 1978.
11. Dedrick RL, Myers CE, Bungay PM, DeVita VT Jr: Pharmacokinetic rationale for peritoneal drug administration in the treatment of ovarian cancer. Cancer Treat Rep 62: 1, 1978.
12. Henderson LW, Cheung AK, Chenoweth DE: Choosing a membrane. Am J Kidney Dis 3: 5, 1983.
13. Garred LJ, Canaud B, Farrell PC: A simple kinetic model for assessing peritoneal mass transfer in chronic ambulatory peritoneal dialysis. asaio J 6: 131, 1983.
14. Pappenheimer JR, Renkin EM, Borrero LM: Filtration, diffusion and molecular sieving through peripheral capillaries; a contribution to the pore theory of capillary permeability. Am J Physiol 167: 13, 1951.
15. Lasrich M, Maher JM, Hirszel P, Maher JF: Correlation of peritoneal transport rates with molecular weight: a method for predicting clearances. asaio J 2: 107, 1979.
16. Gosselin RE, Berndt WO: Diffusional transport of solutes through mesentery and peritoneum. J Theor Biol 3: 487, 1962.
17. Aune S: Transperitoneal exchange II: Peritoneal blood flow estimated by hydrogen gas clearances. Scand J Gastroenterol 5: 99, 1970.
18. Nolph KD: The first hemodialyzer. asaio J 1: 2, 1978.
19. Hirszel P, Chakrabarti EK, Bennett RR, Maher JF: Permselectivity of peritoneum to neutral dextrans. Trans Am Soc Artif Intern Organs 30: 625, 1984.
20. Casley-Smith JR: An electron microscopical study of the passage of ions through the endothelium of lymphatic and blood capillaries and through the mesothelium. Q J Exp Physiol 52: 105, 1967.
21. Cotran RS, Karnovsky MJ: Ultrastructural studies of the permeability of the mesothelium to horseradish peroxidase. J Cell Biol 57: 123, 1968.
22. Gotloib L, Digenes GE, Rabinovich S, Medline A, Oreopoulos DG: Ultrastructure of normal rabbit mesentery. Nephron 34: 248, 1983.
23. Wayland H: Transmural and interstitial molecular transport. In: Legrain M (ed), Proc Int Symposium Continuous Ambulatory Peritoneal Dialysis, Excerpta Medica, Amsterdam, p 18, 1980.
24. Breborowicz A, Knapowski J: Studies on the resistance of the peritoneal mesothelium to solute transport. Peritoneal Dial Bull 4: 37, 1984.
25. Cascarano J, Rubin AD, Chick WL, Zweifach BW: Metabolically induced permeability changes across mesothelium and endothelium. Am J Physiol 206: 373, 1964.
26. Robson, M, Oreopoulos DG, Izatt S, Ogilvie R, Rapaport A, deVeber GA: Influence of exchange volume and dialysate flow rate on solute clearance in peritoneal dialysis. Kidney Int 14: 486, 1978.
27. Twardowski Z, Nolph KD, Prowant BF, Moore HL: Efficiency of high volume low frequency continuous ambulatory peritoneal dialysis (CAPD). Trans Am Soc Artif Intern Organs 29: 53, 1983.
28. Ratnu KS, Haldia KR, Panicker S, Mathur AS: A new technique – semicontinuous rapid flow, high volume exchange for effective peritoneal dialysis in shorter periods. Nephron 31: 159, 1982.
29. Diaz-Buxo JA, Walker PJ, Farmer CD, Chandler JT, Holt KL, Cox P: Continuous cyclic peritoneal dialysis. Trans Am Soc Artif Intern Organs 27: 51, 1981.
30. Nakagawa D, Price C, Steinbaugh B, Suki W: Continuous cycling peritoneal dialysis: a viable option in the treatment of chronic renal failure. Trans Am Soc Artif Intern Organs 23: 55, 1981.
31. Grayson J, Mendel D: Physiology of the Splanchnic Circulation. Williams and Wilkins Co, Baltimore, 1965.
32. Lanciault G, Jacobson ED: The gastrointestinal circulation. Gastroenterology 71: 851, 1976.
33. Felt, J, Richard C, McCaffrey C, Levy M: Peritoneal clearance of creatinine and inulin during dialysis in dogs: effect of splanchnic vasodilators. Kidney Int 17: 459, 1979.
34. Renkin EM: Exchange of substances through capillary walls. In: Wolstenholme GEW (ed), Ciba Foundation Symposium, Little, Brown and Co, Boston, p 50, 1969.
35. Swan KG, Reynolds DG: Adrenergic mechanisms in the canine mesenteric circulation. Am J Physiol 220: 1779, 1971.
36. Messina EJ, Weiner R, Kaley G: Prostaglandins and local circulatory control. Fed Proc 35: 2367, 1976.
37. Steinhauer HB, Gunter B, Schollmeyer P: Enhanced peritoneal generation of vasoactive prostaglandins during peritonitis in patients undergoing CAPD. In: Maher JF, Winchester JF (eds), Frontiers in Peritoneal Dialysis, Field, Rich and Assoc, New York, p 604, 1986.
38. Maher JF: Blood flow to the peritoneum: physiological and pharmacological influences. In: Moncrief JW, Popovich RP (eds), CAPD Update Continuous Ambulatory Peritoneal Dialysis, Masson Publ USA, New York, p 53, 1981.
39. Courtice FC, Roberts DCK: Peritoneal fluid in the rabbit: permeability of the mesothelium to proteins, lipoproteins and acid hydrolases. Lymphology 8:1, 1975.
40. Torres IJ, Litterst CL, Guarino AM: Transport of model compounds across the peritoneal membrane in the rat. Pharmacology 17: 330, 1978.
41. Richardson PDI: The actions of natural secretin on the small intestinal vasculature of the anesthetized cat. Br J Pharmacol 58: 127, 1976.
42. Goldberg LI: Cardiovascular and renal actions of dopamine: potential clinical applications. Pharmacol Rev 24: 1, 1972.
43. Henderson LW, Nolph KD: Altered permeability of the peritoneal membrane after using hypertonic peritoneal dialysis. J Clin Inves 48: 992, 1969.
44. Maher JF, Bennett RR, Hirszel P, Chakrabarti E: The mechanism of dextrose-enhanced peritoneal mass transport rates. Kidney Int 28: 16, 1985.
45. Harris EJ: Transport and Accumulation in Biological Systems, Third Edition. Butterworths, London, 1972.

46. Charonis AS, Wissig SL: Anionic sites in basement membranes. Differences in their electrostatic properties in continuous and fenestrated capillaries. Microvasc Res 25: 265, 1983.
47. Gotloib L, Shustack A, Jaichenko J: Ruthenium-red-stained anionic charges of rat and mice mesothelial cells and basal lamina: The peritoneum is a negatively charged dialyzing membrane. Nephron 48: 65, 1988.
48. Leak LV: Distribution of cell surface charges on mesothelium and lymphatic endothelium. Microvasc Res 31: 18, 1986.
49. Ahearn DJ, Nolph KD: Controlled sodium removal with peritoneal dialysis. Trans Am Soc Artif Intern Organs 18: 423, 1972.
50. Maher JF, Hohnadel DC, Shea C, DiSanzo F, Cassetta M: Effects of intraperitoneal diuretics on solute transport during hypertonic dialysis. Clin Nephrol 7: 96, 1977.
51. Furman KI, Gomperts ED, Hockley J: Activity of intraperitoneal heparin during peritoneal dialysis. Clin Nephrol 9: 15, 1978.
52. Canavese C, Salomone M, Mangiorotti G, Pacitti A, Trucco S, Scaglia C, Assone F, Lunghi F, Vercellone A: Heparin transfer across the rabbit peritoneal membrane. Clin Nephrol 26: 116, 1986.
53. Grahame GR, Torchia MG, Dankewich KA, Ferguson IA: Surface-active material in peritoneal effluent of CAPD patients. Peritoneal Dial Bull 5: 109, 1985.
54. DiPaolo N, Buoncristiani U, Capotundo L, Saggiotti E, DeMia M, Rossi P, Sansoni E, Bernini M: Phosphatidylcholine and peritoneal transport during peritoneal dialysis. Nephron 44: 365, 1986.
55. Breborowicz A, Sombolos K, Rodela H, Ogilvie R, Bargman J, Oreopoulos D: Mechanism of phosphatidylcholine action during peritoneal dialysis. Peritoneal Dial Bull 7: 6, 1987.
56. Mermier P, Baker H: Flux of free fatty acids among host tissues, ascitic fluid and Ehrlich ascites carcinoma cells. J Lipid Res 15: 339, 1971.
57. Dumont AE, Robbins E, Martelli A, Iliescu H: Platelet blockade of particle absorption from the peritoneal surface of the diaphragm. Proc Soc Exp Biol Med 167: 137, 1981.
58. Flessner MF, Dedrick RL, Fenstermacher JD, Blasberg RG, Sieber SM: Peritoneal absorption of macromolecules. In: Maher JF, Winchester JF (eds), Frontiers in Peritoneal Dialysis, Field Rich and Assoc, New York, p 41, 1986.
59. Daugirdas JT, Ing TS, Gandhi VC, Hano JE, Chen WT, Yan L: Kinetics of peritoneal fluid absorption in patients with chronic renal failure. J Lab Clin Med 95: 351, 1980.
60. Flessner MF, Parker RJ, Sieber SM: Peritoneal lymphatic uptake of fibrinogen and erythrocytes in the rat. Am J Physiol 244: H89, 1983.
61. Rippe B, Stelin G, Ahlmén J: Lymph flow from the peritoneal cavity in CAPD patients. In: Maher JF, Winchester JF (eds), Frontiers in Peritoneal Dialysis, Field, Rich and Assoc, New York, p 24, 1986.
62. Mactier RA, Nolph KD, Khanna R, Twardowski ZJ, Moore H, McGary T: Lymphatic absorption in peritoneal dialysis in the rat. Lymphology 20: 47, 1987.
63. Hirszel P, Shea-Donohue T, Chakrabarti E, Montcalm E, Maher JF: The role of the capillary wall in restricting diffusion of macromolecules. A study of peritoneal clearance of dextrans. Nephron 1988 49: 58, 1988.
64. Khanna R, Mactier R, Twardowski ZJ, Nolph KD: Peritoneal cavity lymphatics. Peritoneal Dial Bull 6: 113, 1986.
65. Mactier RA, Khanna R, Nolph KD, Twardowski ZJ, Moore H: Neostigmine increases ultrafiltration and solute clearances in peritoneal dialysis by reducing lymphatic drainage. Peritoneal Dial Bull 7: S50, 1987.
66. Mactier R, Khanna R, Moore H, Twardowski Z, Nolph K: Phosphatidylcholine enhances the efficiency of peritoneal dialysis by reducing lymphatic reabsorption. Abstracts Am Soc Nephrol 20: 100A, 1987.
67. Miller FN, Joshua IG, Harris PD, Wiegman DL, Jauchem JR: Peritoneal dialysis solutions and the microcirculation. Contrib Nephrol 17: 51, 1979.
68. Nolph KD: Peritoneal anatomy and transport physiology. In: Drukker W, Parsons FM, Maher JF (eds), Replacement of Renal Function by Dialysis, Second edition, Martinus Nijhoff, The Hague, p 440, 1983.
69. Breborowicz A, Knapowski J: Local anesthetic-bupivicaine increases the transperitoneal transport of solutes. Part II: In vitro study. Peritoneal Dial Bull 4: 224, 1984.
70. McGary TJ, Nolph KD, Moore HL, Kartinos NJ: Polycation as an alternative osmotic agent and phosphate binder in peritoneal dialysis. Uremia Invest 8: 79, 1984.
71. DeSanto NG, Capodicasa G, Capasso G, Giordano C: Development of means to augment peritoneal urea clearances: The synergistic effects of combining high dialysate temperature and high dialysate flow rates with dextrose and nitroprusside. Artif Organs 5: 409, 1981.
72. Erbe RW, Green JA Jr, Weller JM: Peritoneal dialysis during hemorrhagic shock. J Appl Physiol 22: 131, 1967.
73. Greene JA Jr, Lapco L, Weller JM: Effect of drug therapy of hemorrhagic hypotension on kinetics of peritoneal dialysis in the dog. Nephron 7: 178, 1970.
74. Kincaid-Smith P: Participation of intravascular coagulation in the pathogenesis of glomerular and vascular lesions. Kidney Int 7: 242, 1975.
75. Maher JF, Hirszel P: Augmentation of peritoneal clearances by drugs. In: Legrain M (ed), Proc Int Symposium Continuous Ambulatory Peritoneal Dialysis, Excerpta Med, Amsterdam, p 42, 1980.
76. Maher JF, Hirszel P, Abraham JE, Galen MA, Chamberlin M, Hohnadel DC: The effect of dipyridamole on peritoneal mass transport. Trans Am Soc Artif Intern Organs 23: 219, 1977.
77. Brown ST, Ahearn DJ, Nolph KD: Reduced peritoneal clearance in scleroderma increased by intraperitoneal isoproterenol. Ann Intern Med 78: 891, 1973.
78. Nolph KD, Miller L, Husted FC, Hirszel P: Peritoneal clearance in scleroderma and diabetes mellitus: effects of intraperitoneal isoproterenol. Int Urol Nephrol 8: 161, 1976.
79. Nolph KD, Ghods AJ, Brown PA, Twardowski ZJ: Effects of intraperitoneal nitroprusside on peritoneal clearance in man with variations of dose, frequency of administration and dwell times. Nephron 24: 114, 1979.
80. Maher JF, Hirszel P, Lasrich M: An experimental model for study of pharmacologic and hormonal influences on peritoneal dialysis. Contrib Nephrol 17: 131, 1979.
81. Gutman RA, Nixon WP, McRae RL, Spencer HW: Effect of intraperitoneal and intravenous vasoactive amines on peritoneal dialysis: study in anephric dogs. Trans Am Soc Artif Intern Organs 22: 570, 1976.
82. Penzotti SC, Mattocks AM: Effects of dwell time, volume of dialysis fluid and added accelerators on peritoneal dialysis of urea. J Pharm Sci 60: 1520, 1971.
83. Maher JF, Hirszel P, Laasrich M: The effects of gastrointestinal hormones on transport by peritoneal dialysis. Kidney Int 16: 130, 1979.
84. Hirszel P, Lasrich M, Maher JF: Divergent effects of catecholamines on peritoneal mass transport. Trans Am Soc Artif Intern Organs 25: 110, 1979.
85. Maher JF, Hirszel P, Lasrich M: Modulation of peritoneal transport rates by prostaglandins. Adv Prostaglandin Thromboxane Res 7: 695, 1980.
86. Nolph KD, Ghods AJ, Van Stone J, Brown PA: The effects of intraperitoneal vasodilators on peritoneal clearances. Trans Am Soc Artif Intern Organs 22: 586, 1976.
87. Maher JF, Shea C, Cassetta M, Hohnadel DC: Isoproterenol enhancement off peritoneal permability. J Dial 1: 319, 1977.

88. Vanichayakornkul S, Nimmanit S, Chirawong P, Nilwarangkur S: Accelerated peritoneal dialysis with intraperitoneal isoproterenol. J Med Assoc Thailand 61 (Suppl 1): 127, 1978.

89. Maher JF, Cassetta M, Shea C, Hohnadel DC: Peritoneal dialysis in rabbits. A study of transperitoneal theophylline flux and peritoneal permeability. Nephron 20: 18, 1978.

90. Londos C, Cooper DMF, Wolff J: Subclasses of external adenosine receptors. Proc Natl Acad Sci USA 77: 2551, 1980.

91. Brown EA, Kliger AS, Goffinet J, Finkelstein FO: Effect of hypertonic dialysate and vasodilators on peritoneal dialysis clearances in the rat. Kidney Int 13: 271, 1978.

92. Nolph K, Ghods A, Brown P, Miller F, Harris P, Pyle K, Popovich R: Effects of nitroprusside on peritoneal mass transfer coefficients and microvascular physiology. Trans Am Soc Artif Intern Organs 23: 210, 1977.

93. Hirszel P, Maher JF, Chamberlin M: Augmented peritoneal mass transport with intraperitoneal nitroprusside. J Dial 2: 131, 1978.

94. Raja RM, Kramer MS, Rosenbaum JL: Enhanced clearance with intraperitoneal nitroprusside in high flow recirculation peritoneal dialysis. Trans Am Soc Artif Intern Organs 24: 133, 1978.

95. Nolph KD, Ghods AJ, Brown PA, Twardowski PA: Effects of intraperitoneal nitroprusside on peritoneal clearances in man with variations of dose frequency of administration and dwell times. Nephron 24: 114, 1979.

96. Selgas R, Carmona AR, Martinez ME, Perez-Fontan M, Salinas M, Conesa J, Martinez Ara J, Sicilia LS: Peritoneal vascular reserve characterization through nitroprusside-induced modification of peritoneal mass transfer coefficients. Int J Artif Organs 8: 181, 1985.

97. Riembau E, Lloveras J, Aubia J, Masramon J, Garcia C, Orfila MA, Llorach M: Sequential intraperitoneal administration of nitroprusside in patients maintained on peritoneal dialysis. J Dial 4: 203, 1980.

98. Miller FN, Nolph KD, Harris PD, Rubin J, Wiegman DL, Joshua IG, Twardowski ZJ, Ghods AJ: Microvascular and clinical effects of altered peritoneal dialysis solutions. Kidney Int 15: 630, 1979.

99. Sano N, Satoh S, Hashimoto K: Differences among dipyridamole, carbochromen and lidoflazine in responses of the coronary and the renal arteries. Jpn J Pharmacol 22: 857, 1972.

100. Ryckelynck JP, Pierre D, DeMartin A, Rottembourg J: Amelioration des clairances péritonéales par le dipyridamole. Nouv Presse Med 7: 472, 1978.

101. Limido A, Cantu P, Allaria P, Colombo L, Giangrande G: Velocita di flusso ed effetto dei farmaci nella valutazione dell efficienza della dialisi peritoneale. Minerva Nephrol 26: 161, 1979.

102. Rubin J, Adair C, Barnes T, Bower JD: Augmentation of peritoneal clearance by dipyridamole. Kidney Int 22: 658, 1982.

103. Maher JF, Hirszel P: Augmenting peritoneal mass transport. Int J Artif Organs 2: 59, 1979.

104. Reams GP, Young M, Sorkin M, Twardowski Z, Gloor H, Moore H, Nolph KD: Effects of dipyridamole on peritoneal clearances. Uremia Invest 9: 27, 1986.

105. Rubin J, Adair C, Bower J: A double-blind trial of dipyridamole in CAPD. Am J Kidney Dis 5: 262, 1985.

106. Parker HR, Schroeder JP, Henderson LW: Influence of dopamine and Regitine on peritoneal dialysis in unanesthetized dogs. Abstracts Am Soc Artif Intern Organs 7:43, 1978.

107. Chan MK, Varghese Z, Baillod RA, Moorhead JF: Peritoneal dialysis: effect of intraperitoneal dopamine. Dial Transplant 9: 380, 1980.

108. Hirszel P, Lasrich M, Maher JF: Augmentation of peritoneal mass transport by dopamine. Comparison with norepinephrine and evaluation of pharmacologic mechanisms. J Lab Clin Med 94: 747, 1979.

109. Maher JF, DiPaolo B, Shostak A, Hirszel P: Pharmacology of peritoneal transport. In: Khanna R, Nolph DK, Prowant B, Twardowski ZJ, Oreopoulos DG (eds), Advances in Continuous Ambulatory Peritoneal Dialysis, Toronto, Univ Toronto Press, p 3, 1987.

110. Shostak A, Hirszel P, Maher JF: Histamine and antagonists influence peritoneal permeability. Abstracts Am Soc Nephrol 20: 103A, 1987.

111. Maher JF: Principles of dialysis and dialysis of drugs. Am J Med 62: 475, 1977.

112. Lal SM, Nolph KD, Moore HL, Khanna R: Effects of calcium channel blockers (Verapamil, Diltiazem) on peritoneal transport. Trans Am Soc Artif Intern Organs 32: 564, 1986.

113. Lal SM, Moore HL, Nolph KD: Effects of intraperitoneal captopril on peritoneal transport in rats. Peritoneal Dial Bull 7: 80, 1987.

114. Shostak A, Hirszel P, Chakrabarti E, Maher JF: Dihydroergotamine lowers peritoneal transfer rates: A hypovolemic transport decrease. Peritoneal Dial Bull 7: S69, 1987.

115. Pace Asciak CR: Oxidative biotransformation of arachidonic acid. Prostaglandins 13: 811, 1977.

116. Nakano J, McCurdy JR: Hemodynamic effects of prostaglandins E_1, A_1 and F_2 in dogs. Proc Soc Exp Biol Med 128: 39, 1968.

117. Messina EJ, Kaley G: Microcirculatory responses to prostacyclin and PGE_2 in the rat cremaster muscle. Adv Prostaglandin Thromboxane Res 7: 719, 1980.

118. Vane JR, McGiff JC: Possible contributions of endogenous prostaglandins to the control of blood pressure. Circ Res 36, 37(suppl 1): 68, 1975.

119. Maher JF, Hirszel P, Lasrich M: Prostaglandin effects on peritoneal transport. Proc 2nd Int Symposium on Peritoneal Dial 2: 65, 1981.

120. Mileti M, Bufano G, Scaravonati P, Pecchini F, Carnevale G, Lanzarini P: Effect of indomethacin on the peritoneum of rabbits on peritoneal dialysis. Peritoneal Dial Bull 3: 194, 1983.

121. Strong CG, Romero JC: Effects of indomethacin in rabbit renovascular hypertension. Clin Sci Mol Med 51: 249s, 1976.

122. Hirszel P, Lasrich M, Maher JF: Arachidonic acid increases peritoneal clearances. Trans Am Soc Artif Intern Organs 27: 61, 1981.

123. Thulin L, Samnegård H: Circulatory effects of gastrointestinal hormones and related peptides. Acta Chir Scand (Suppl) 482: 73, 1978.

124. Fara JW, Rubenstein EH, Sonneschein RR: Intestinal hormones in mesenteric vasodilation after intraduodenal agents. Am J Physiol 223: 1058, 1972.

125. Farah JW: Effects of gastrointestinal hormones on vascular smooth muscle. Am J Dig Dis 20: 346, 1975.

126. Hirszel P, Maher JF, LeGrow W: Increased peritoneal mass transport with glucagon acting at the vascular surface. Trans Am Soc Artif Intern Organs 24: 136, 1978.

127. Farini R, Del Favero G, Adorati M, Pedrazzoli S, Fabris G, Giordano P, D'Angelo A, Zotti E, Lise M, Chiaramonte M, Salvagnini M, Naccarato R: Comparison between bolus injection and infusion of Secretin and Pancreozymin in the diagnosis of chronic pancreatic disease (one-hour test). Acta Hepatogastroenterol (Stuttg) 24: 462, 1977.

128. Biber B, Farah J, Lundgren O: Vascular reactions in the small intestine during vasodilation. Acta Physiol Scand 89: 499, 1973.

129. Hare HG, Valtin H, Gosselin RE: Effect of drugs on peritoneal dialysis in the dog. J Pharmacol Exp Ther 145: 122, 1964.

130. Henderson LW, Kintzel JE: Influence of antidiuretic hormone on peritoneal area and permeability. J Clin Invest 50: 2437, 1971.

131. Shear L, Harvey JD, Barry KG: Peritoneal sodium transport:

enhancement by pharmacologic and physical agents. J Lab Clin Med 67: 181, 1966.

132. Maher JF, Hirszel P LeGrow W: Enhanced peritoneal permeability with methyl prednisolone. Clin Res 26: 64A, 1978.

133. Breborowicz A, Knapowski J: Augmentation of peritoneal dialysis clearance with procaine. Kidney Int 26: 392, 1984.

134. Haddy F: The mechanism of potassium vasodilation. In: Vanhoutte PM, Leusen I (eds), Mechanisms of Vasodilation, S Karger, Basel, p 200, 1978.

135. Miller FN, Nolph KD, Joshua IG, Wiegman DL, Harris PD, Anderson DB: Hyperosmolality, acetate and lactate: Dilatory factors during peritoneal dialysis. Kidney Int 20: 397, 1981.

136. Penzotti SC, Mattocks AM: Acceleration of peritoneal dialysis by surface-active agents. J Pharm Sci 57: 1192, 1968.

137. El-Bassiouni EA, Mattocks AM: Acceleration of peritoneal dialysis with minimal N-myristyl-ß-amino-proprionate. J Pharm Sci 62L: 1314, 1973.

138. Dunham CB, Hak LJ, Hull JH, Mattocks AM: Enhancement of peritoneal permeability of the rat by intraperitoneal use of docusate sodium. Kidney Int 20: 563, 1981.

139. Maher JF, Chakarabarti E: Ultrafiltration by hyperosmotic peritoneal dialysis fluid excludes intracellular solutes. Am J Nephrol 4: 169, 1984.

140. Raja RM, Kramer MS, Rosenbaum JL, Bolisay C, Krug M: Contrasting changes in solute transport and ultrafiltration with peritonitis in CAPD patients. Trans Am Soc Artif Intern Organs 27: 68, 1981.

141. Alavi N, Lianos E, Van Liew JB, Mookerjee BK, Bentzel CJ: Peritoneal permeability in the rat: Modulation by microfilament-active agents. Kidney Int 27: 411, 1985.

142. Scarpioni L, Ballacchi S, Bergonzi G, Fontana F, Poisetti P, Zanazzi MA: High-dose diuretics in CAPD. Peritoneal Dial Bull 2: 177, 1982.

143. Grzegorzewska A, Baczyk K: Furosemide-induced increase in urinary and peritoneal excretion of uric acid during peritoneal dialysis in patients with chronic uremia. Artif Organs 6: 220, 1982.

144. Bazzato G, Coli U, Landini S, Lucatello S, Fracasso A, Righetto F, Scanferla F, Morachiello P: Restoration of ultrafiltration capacity of peritoneal membrane in patients on CAPD. Int J Artif Organs 7: 93, 1984.

145. Alavi H, Lianos E, Andres G, Bentzel CJ: Effect of protamine on the permeability and structure of rat peritoneum. Kidney Int 21: 44, 1982.

146. Capodicasa G, Capasso G, Anastasio P, Lanzetti N, Giordano C: Changes on peritoneal permeability by charged poly-amino acids. Peritoneal Dial Bull 7: S13, 1987.

147. Breborowicz A, Rodela H, Bargman J, Oreopoulos DG: Effect of cationic molecules on the permeability of the mesothelium in vitro. Peritoneal Dial Bull 7: S9, 1987.

148. Lau AH, Chow Tung E, Assadi FK, Fornell L, John E: Effect of ultrafiltration on peritoneal dialysis drug clearances. Pharmacology 31: 284, 1985.

149. Nolph KD, Nothum RJ, Maher JF: Ultrafiltration: a mechanism for removal of intermediate molecular weight substances in coil dialyzers. Kidney Int 6: 55, 1974.

150. Avasthi PS: Effects of aminonucleoside on rat blood-peritoneal barrier permeability. J Lab Clin Med 94: 295, 1979.

151. Maher JF, Hirszel P, Bennett RR, Chakrabarti E: Augmentation of peritoneal hydraulic permeability by amphotericin B: locus of action. Peritoneal Dial Bull 4: 229, 1984.

152. Indrapasit S, Sooksriwongse C: Effect of chlorpromazine on peritoneal clearances. Nephron 40: 341, 1985.

153. Ronco C, Brendolan A, Bragantini L, Chiaramonte S, Feriani M, Fabris A, LaGreca G: Studies on ultrafiltration in peritoneal dialysis: influence of plasma proteins and capillary blood flow. Peritoneal Dial Bull 6: 93, 1986.

154. Levin TN, Rigden LR, Nielsen LH, Moore HL, Twardowski ZJ, Khanna R, Nolph KD: Maximal ultrafiltration rates during peritoneal dialysis in rats. Kidney Int 31: 731, 1987.

155. Maher JF, Hirszel P, Shostak A, DiPaolo B, Chakrabarti E: Prolonged intraperitoneal dwell decreases ultrafiltration coefficient in rabbits. Am J Kidney Dis 12: 62, 1988.

156. Rubin J, Reed V, Adair C, Bower J, Klein E: Effect of intraperitoneal insulin on solute kinetics in CAPD: insulin kinetics in CAPD. Am J Med Sci 291: 81, 1986.

157. Twardowski ZJ, Khanna R, Nolph KD: Osmotic agents and ultrafiltration in peritoneal dialysis. Nephron 42: 93, 1986.

158. Knochel JP, Clayton LE, Smith WL, Barry KG: Intraperitoneal THAM: an effective method to enhance phenobarbital removal during peritoneal dialysis. J Lab Clin Med 64: 257, 1964.

159. Knochel JP, Mason AD: Effect of alkalinization on peritoneal diffusion of uric acid. Am J Physiol 210: 1160, 1966.

160. Campion DAS, North JDK: Effect of protein binding of barbiturates on their rate of removal during peritoneal dialysis. J Lab Clin Med 66: 549, 1965.

161. Schultz JC, Crouder DG, Medart WS: Excretion studies in ethchlorvynol (Placidyl) intoxication. Arch Intern Med 117: 409, 1966.

162. Etteldorf JN, Dobbins WT, Summit RL, Rainwater WT, Fischer RL: Intermittent peritoneal dialysis using 5% albumin in the treatment of salicylate intoxication in children. J Pediatr 58: 226, 1961.

163. Kudla RM, El-Bassiouni EA, Mattocks AM: Accelerated peritoneal dialysis of barbiturates, diphenylhydantoin and salicylate. J Pharm Sci 60: 1065, 1971.

164. Cole DEC, Lirenman DS: Role of albumin enriched peritoneal dialysate in acute copper poisoning. J Pediatr 92: 955, 1978.

165. Mehbod H: Treatment of lead intoxication. Combined use of peritoneal dialysis and edetate calcium disodium. JAMA 201: 972, 1967.

166. Lowenthal DT, Chardo F, Reidenberg MM: Removal of mercury by peritoneal dialysis. Arch Intern Med 134: 139, 1974.

167. Falk RJ, Mattern WD, Lamanna RW, Gitelman HJ, Parker NC, Cross RE, Rastall JR: Iron removal during continuous ambulatory peritoneal dialysis using desferrioxamine. Kidney Int 24: 110, 1983.

168. Shinaberger JH, Shear L, Clayton LE, Barry KG, Knowlton M, Goldbaum LR: Dialysis for intoxication with lipid soluble drugs: enhancement of glutethimide extraction with lipid dialysate. Trans Am Soc Artif Intern Organs 11: 173, 1965.

169. Maher JF: Characteristics of peritoneal transport: physiological and clinical implications. Mineral Electrolyte Metab 5: 201, 1981.

12

COMMENTS ON DIALYSIS SOLUTION, ANTIBIOTIC TRANSPORT, POISONINGS, AND NOVEL USES OF PERITONEAL DIALYSIS

JACK RUBIN

1. INTRODUCTION

In this chapter we will review the nature of the dialysis solutions added to the peritoneal cavity, discuss concepts of intraperitoneal nutrition, and review the transport of antibiotics and other drugs into and out of the peritoneal cavity. We will not discuss chemotherapy. Excellent drug reviews for dosage modification in uremia are available [1–13].

2. DIALYSIS SOLUTIONS

Dr.'s Ward, Klein, and Watham, submitted their report on The Investigation of the Risks and Hazards with Devices Associated with Peritoneal Dialysis. Table 1, taken from their report, summarizes the risks asscoiated with peritoneal dialysis solutions [14].

2.1. Electrolytes

Peritoneal dialysis solutions are formulated with electrolytes including: sodium, chloride, calcium and magnesium, either acetate or lactate as potential bicarbonate, and an osmotically active agent, usually glucose. Solutions are supplied premixed or in concentrate of 30% and 50% glucose for use with reverse-osmosis dialysis machines. The ideal dialysis solution is not known but it is unrealistic to expect a separate solution for each patient. Nevertheless, attempts have been made to modify the peritoneal dialysis solutions administered to patients.

2.2. Magnesium

The recent surge of interest in metabolic bone disease has prompted a reconsideration of dialysate magnesium concentration. Many believe that serum magnesium concentrations are too high among patients undergoing CAPD and this has lead to the marketing of a 'low magnesium' solution. This may be because removal is inhibited by an excessively high dialysate concentration [15–19]. This high magnesium concentration may lead to an excessive body burden and potentially inhibit bone remodelling. A dialysate concentration of 0.5 mEq/l may normalize the serum concentration and decrease the body burden of magnesium [17]. Magnesium is an important cation involved in several enzymatic reactions. In the laboratory, it is almost impossible to show abnormalities related to modestly elevated magnesium concentrations, but one can readily demonstrate abnormalities in the presence of lowered serum magnesium.

Table 1. Summary of risks and hazards associated with peritoneal dialysis solutions (with permission from ref. 14)

Event	Risk (R) or hazard (H)*	Underlying cause	Clinical consequences
1. Bacterial contamination of dialysate	H	Contaminated water bath for heating bottles; Pin hole leaks in dialysate bags; contamination during spiking of dialysate container	Peritonitis
2. Impurities in dialysate (particulate matter, endotoxin formaldehyde)	R, H	Inadequate quality assurance, incomplete rinsing of on-line proportioning machines after desinfection	Pain, peritonitis, sclerosis of peritoneum, loss of clearance
3. Trace chemicals in water used for dialysate preparation	R	Inadequate water purification	Clinical significance unknown
4. Hypertriglyceridemia	R	Use of glucose as an osmotic agent	Long-term effects on patient morbidity are unknown
5. Hyperosmolarity and hyperglycemia	R, H	Use of glucose as an osmotic agent	Hyperosmolar coma (with 70 g/l glucose) high glucose loads in diabetes requiring additonial insulin therapy, hypovolemia and hypotension
6. Hypermatremia	R	Formation of hypotonic ultrafiltrate, high sodium concentration in dialysate	Hypertension, cerebral edema
7. Acidic dialysate	R, H	Need to keep pH in range 5.0–5.5 to avoid glucose caramelization during heat sterilization	Pain, sclerosis of peritoneum, loss of clearance
8. Hyperosmolarity	H	Use of sorbitol as an osmotic agent	Hyperosmolar coma, death
9. Use of glass bottles for dialysate	R, H	Weight, bulk and brittleness of bottle	Increased peritonitis in continuous ambulatory peritoneal dialysis from increased connect-disconnect, over balancing of carousels, bottle breakage
10. Use of incorrect dialysate composition	R	Inadequate quality assurance, operator error	Poor control of fluid balance, hypovolemia, hypernatremia
11. Abdominal pain	R, H	Instillation of dialysate under pressure, prolonged use of hypertonic dialysates, acidic dialysates (see 7 above)	Pain, discomfort, buffer loss by patient
12. Hepatitis positive dialysate	H	Treatment of hepatitis B positive patients	Hepatitis outbreak amongst staff

* A hazard is defined as an actual occurrence detrimental to patient safety, while a risk is an event which has not occurred but which is considered likely to occur and to have detrimental clinical consequences.

Recently magnesium depletion has been found among hemodialysis patients submitted to three years of dialysis with no magnesium in the dialysate [19].

2.3. Calcium

Calcium absorption is dependent on the unbound serum concentration, dialysate protein concentration and the degree to which water entry into the peritoneal cavity diminishes the concentration gradient for absorption. Ultrafiltration will dilute dialysate and diminish the concentration gradient for absorption, or even cause a reversal of the diffusion gradient. Although protein concentrations are low in dialysate effluent, it is possible that intraperitoneal protein binds a small amount of calcium.

The level of ionized calcium in dialysate and plasma are likely the major determinants of absorption. The rate of ionized calcium absorption in general parallels the rate of total calcium absorption. Patients undergoing CAPD may be in slightly positive calcium balance [16, 22–30]. Calcium free dialysate may be used as an adjunct to treat patients with hypercalcemia [27–28]. Hourly dialysate exchange times yield removal rates of 10–17 ml/min for 1.5% glucose solutions and 12–24 ml/min for 7% solutions. Clearances of calcium vary inversely with serum protein concentration. Calcium free dialysate is not commercially available but dextrose and saline may be used [29–30]. We have found it occasionally useful to add an ampule of calcium chloride to the dialysate of the hypocalcemic recently parathyroidectomized CAPD patient.

2.4. Sodium

Sodium has been added to dialysate in varying concentrations ranging from 120–140 mEq/l. Hypernatremia may occasionally occur because the sodium concentration in the ultrafiltrate approximates 70 mEq/l [31–34]. Nolph has suggested that sodium losses from patients undergoing continuous ambulatory peritoneal dialysis are to some extent regulated by intravascular volume with smaller losses when patients are intravascularly depleted [35]. Raja suggested that the increase in serum sodium concentrations could be avoided, and an isonatric ultrafiltrate achieved with a dialysate sodium concentration of 115–120 mEq/l in 7% dextrose dialysate, and 125–130 mEq/l for a 4.25% dextrose dialysate [32]. The hyponatric ultrafiltrate permits treatment of hyponatremia. Dialysis both protects the patient from further volume expansion if hypertonic saline is used and removes more water than sodium [31–37].

Delivered sodium concentration can vary, depending upon the manufacturing process. If a 5% variation is possible, then the sodium content of 140 mEq/l can vary between 135–148 mEq/l. It is possible to induce net absorption of sodium in hyponatric patients [38–39].

Sodium transport across rabbit omentum can be modified by pharmacologic and physical agents [40]. Sodium is likely transported between rather than through cells. Transport has not been shown to require metabolic activity but transport across mesentery was enhanced when calcium was removed from dialysate [40].

Dialysis has also been used to treat salt poisoning in infancy [41]. Here the dialysate was 5% glucose in distilled water. This dialysate was hypo-osmolar compared to serum concentrations of the infants being treated and fluid was absorbed.

2.5. Potassium

Potassium chloride is commonly added to dialysate to prevent potassium depletion. Spital showed that if 20 mEq/l were added to dialysate, one could expect a net absorption of 15 mEq [47]. One should note that their data shows 12 mEq may have been absorbed during the first 15 min. If one added 40 mEq/l KCL abdominal pain occurred.

Potassium is cleared via peritoneal dialysis. Rapid cycle 7% glucose exchanges obtained removal rates of 26 ml/min [43]. Studies of potassium diffusion show that serum and dialysate do not reach equilibration during long intraperitoneal dwells [44]. It has been suggested that, since potassium may leach from red cells during serum separation in vitro, serum potassium concentrations may be spuriously elevated, thus accounting for this observation.

3. DIALYSIS SOLUTION BASE

3.1. Acetate, lactate and bicarbonate

Acetate formulated dialysate solutions demonstrate an antibacterial activity not found with lactate solutions. However these differences are not found after dialysate is added to the peritoneal cavity [45–47]. One group compared their rates of peritonitis from their own dialysis population

treated with either acetate or lactate solutions manufactured by the same company [48]. They observed lower peritonitis rates with acetate solutions. Low pH and high osmolability inhibit peripheral blood leukocytes [49–51]. These changes are present within the peritoneal cavity for approximately 10–30 min after intraperitoneal instillation of dialysate. Neutrophils incubated in dialysate effluent which had been present within the peritoneal cavity for one hour showed no loss of activity [52–55]. The major determinant of neutrophil activity appears to be whether sufficient immunoglobins and organisms enter the peritoneal cavity following the bacterial infection [56].

3.2. Alkalinizing agents

Racemic lactate is used in commercially available solutions. Solutions containing 45 mEq/l of lactate have raised serum bicarbonate above physiologic concentrations. Lower concentrations have not maintained serum bicarbonate and have been associated with a negative base balance [57–58]. D-lactate is as quantitatively as important as L-lactate in bicarbonate generation and does not accumulate in the patient [59–61]. Hourly dialysate exchanges yield clearance rates of 6.2 ml/min for D-lactate and 8.7 ml/min for L-lactate respectively. Lactate removal rates may be increased by nitroprusside and bicarbonate.

Dialysis solutions formulated with acetate yield peritoneal clearances similar to those formulated with lactate [65]. The microvascular effects are similar to lactate solutions. Loss of ultrafiltration during CAPD has been associated with acetate solutions but likely other factors, rather than acetate are important [67–68]. Observations in man, but not confirmed in rats, suggested that dialysate takes longer to reach physiologic pH with acetate solutions as compared to lactate [69–71]. This delay was postulated to be a cause of abdominal pain and was due to greater titratable acidity in the acetate solutions.

Both acetate and bicarbonate solutions may be helpful in the treatment of lactic acidosis as they do not add to the systemic concentration of lactate [72–78]. There is only one pathway for lactate removal – to pyruvate – but there are many pathways available for acetate. The main thrust in the treatment of lactic acidosis should be directed to the primary cause. Systemic pH correction should be administered with dialysis reserved for correction of an overexpanded intravascular space. Bicarbonate in the dialysate prevents diffusion into dialysate, and although less effective, may also be used to administer bicarbonate to the patient when the serum concentration is low. Dialysate cycling machines that allow multiprong tubing may be used to formulate a bicarbonate solution at the bedside. For example, 4 l of 0.9% saline and 3 l of 5% dextrose and 0.45% saline to which is added 5 vials of sodium bicarbonate, 45 mEq in 50 ml, will yield a solution containing 131 mEq/l sodium and 28 mEq/l bicarbonate. Calcium and magnesium supplementation may be necessary. The converse has also been observed. Severe systemic alkalosis may occur when peritoneal dialysis and nasogastric suction are combined for a prolonged period. Chloride rich dialysate has been used to treat metabolic alkalosis [79]. A recent review of parenteral solutions makes a plea for a physiologic composition [80].

A method for preparing bicarbonate buffered dialysate has been described for chronic dialysis. Dialysate solutions containing bicarbonate did not yield improvement in peritoneal clearances even though these solutions lacked vasoactive properties [81–84]. The solution was associated with enhanced protein leakage into dialysate [84]. Alkalinization of dialysate will serve to trap solutes within the peritoneal cavity and may be used to enhance barbiturate, salicylate and uric acid excretion [85, 86].

4. GLUCOSE AS AN OSMOTIC AGENT

Glucose is the agent commonly used for inducing water movement into the peritoneal cavity. Glucose must be formulated at an acid pH or it caramelizes. This acid pH occasionally causes pain on inflow of dialysate, may damage the activity of leukocytes mobilized into the peritoneal cavity due to infection, and impedes aluminum removal from the patient [87, 88]. Since 5–10 gr of glucose may be expected to be absorbed from 2 1 of dialysate when 1.5% glucose is exchanged hourly and between 35–40 g when 4.25% glucose is used, glucose may be a contributing factor in the elevation in serum lipids observed in patients undergoing peritoneal dialysis [87, 88]. In our CAPD population we found that serum lipids were elevated but did not find further elevation in serum cholesterol or triglycerides over a two year period [9]. Some investigators have suggested that glucose intolerance may eventually develop because the pancreas fails. Providing only occasional 4.25% solutions are used there should be little risk of pancreatic exhaustion [92]. Dialysate accounts for 15–30% of the total caloric intake of CAPD patients [93–96]. Although many patients increase their weight with CAPD, it is unclear whether they are all becoming obese or returning to their usual body weight [97]. Hyperglycemia may occur with frequent hypertonic exchanges and a reactive hypoglycemia may occur post dialysis [98–100]. Glucose induced water movement into the peritoneal cavity is through extracellular pathways [101, 102]. Clearances have been found to increase in the dialysis exchange following a 7% exchange in man and 4.25% exchange in rats. This is thought to occur through 'alteration' of the extracellular pathway [103, 104], which to some extent may be altered by an expanded extracellular volume from the absorbed glucose. Investigators, using man as subject, have had difficulty demonstrating this with 4.25% glucose dialysate exchanges [105]. Although the rate of glucose absorption from the peritoneal cavity is not influenced by the presence of intraperitoneal insulin [106] or removal of the omentum [107], peritoneal inflammation enhances glucose absorption [108]. Following instillation of glucose, water rapidly enters the dialysate and dilutes the remaining glucose thus lowering the concentration gradient [109, 110]. The ultrafiltration rate parallels these intraperitoneal changes in osmolality and glucose [111].

There are occasional patients in whom usual concentrations of dialysate glucose fail to yield sufficient ultrafiltration. We have seen this among patients with frequent episodes of peritonitis. We have had the patients increase their concentration of glucose in dialysate by adding hypertonic dialysate, decreasing the duration of exchanges,

and in one patient who refused to discontinue CAPD dialyzing the patient once weekly by hemodialysis to remove retained extravascular fluid. This patient did not have an episode of peritonitis during this time and was able to return to CAPD without requiring hemodialysis after eight months. Hypertonic solutions lead to peritoneal membrane thickening but these changes resolve when glucose is withdrawn [112, 113].

5. NON-GLUCOSE OSMOTIC AGENTS

Dialysate has been formulated with sorbitol or mannitol in an attempt to improve blood glucose control in diabetic patients. These substances accumulate in the blood. Although periodic use is possible if the concentration is less than 2%, there is no advantage to the patient since glucose control can be accomplished by an additional dose of insulin. Their use is not recommended [114–121]. Xylitol has been used to dialyze patients. Toxic effects occur at absorption rates over 150 g/day. Large doses may cause calcium oxalate deposition if infused rapidly and prolonged use may cause hyperuricemia. There are no proven benefits for using xylitol and only potential toxicities [122, 123]. Fructose may be useful as dialysis properties of fructose are similar to glucose. However, there are no proven benefits for the use of fructose as an osmotic agent and it may cause a hyperosmolal state [124–126].

Glycerol may be used as an osmotically active agent to induce ultrafiltration. It is less active than glucose and there is a greater amount of caloric uptake per unit of ultrafiltration. There are no significant advantages and substitution for glucose is not recommended [127–134].

Polymers as osmotically active agents in dialysate would permit a longer maintenance of the transmembrane concentration gradient. The caloric load per unit of ultrafiltration should be better then glucose. The agents must be capable of being metabolized and also be non-immunogenic. Neutral dextran has been tried unsuccessfully [125–136]. A glucose polymer of 900 average molecular weight was found to accumulate in serum. Recently, a polymer of glucose of mean m.w. =20 000 has been tried as well as peptides [135–142].

Gelatin was one of the first agents used to induce ultrafiltration into the peritoneal cavity but it was more difficult to use than glucose [143–146]. Polyelectrolytes have also been used to induce ultrafiltration but only acute studies are available for these relatively toxic agents [147–149].

6. AMINO-ACIDS AS OSMOTIC AGENTS

The peritoneal dialysis patient is exposed to nutritional risk [150]. Many patients complain of anorexia. They are commonly prescribed a diet containing 1–1.2 g/kg body weight of protein yet self selected diets in elderly patients, often the best suited to CAPD for medical reasons, are often deficient in protein of high biologic value. It has been suggested that to maintain nitrogen balance the older patient may have an increased requirement for essential amino acids when total nitrogen intake is increased [151]. Patients tend to gain weight but without increases in muscle mass, especially if frequent peritonitis occurs [152, 153]. The dialysate losses contain protein and amino acids which increase the dietary protein requirement [154, 155]. Amino acid concentrations in the blood of uremic patients were often similar to patterns found in malnourished patients [156]. Because of these nutritional risks and the potential benefit to the patient, investigators have sought to either supplement or provide the total food intake using intra-peritoneal feeding [157]. Animals maintained on portal infusions have been shown to do as well as those maintained systemically. Thus nutrients absorbed from the peritoneal cavity will be utilized appropriately [158–161]. It seemed sensible to many to administer amino-acids via the perit-oneal cavity. They could then act as an osmotically active agent, serve to diminsh amino-acid losses, and perhaps, as less glucose would be required to induce ultrafiltration into the peritoneal cavity, have a salutary effect on serum lipids [162–173].

Amino-acids can be substituted for glucose. But use of amino-acids for one month failed to improve serum lipids. Also their use may impair appetite [174]. They do not block diffusion of solute into the peritoneal cavity. Except for the newborn and the cirrhotic, there is little risk of toxicity [75–181]. Amino-acid solutions appear to be compatible with aminoglycoside antibiotics but penicillins may be significantly inactivated if not used within a 24 hr period after addition to an amino-acid containing solution [182, 183]. Combining penicillins with amino-acids may increase the immunogenic potential of penicillin. While the steri-lization cycles of amino acids and glucose are not com-patable, amino acids can be autoclaved with glycerol [184].

Are amino acids worth using in peritoneal dialysate? The major stimulus for evaluating amino-acids was their po-tential for adding nitrogen to the malnourished patient. Unfortunately, definitive studies have not yet been under-taken in a sufficient number of patients to prove that these agents work. Alterations in serum amino-acid patterns or serum to muscle tissue concentration gradients do not evaluate long term improvement in nutritional status [185–191]. Most studies have utilized commercially available amino-acid preparations. These preparations are suitable since patients are receiving other protein and caloric sources and the risk, if any, of amino-acid imbalance should be minimal.

Fat solutions have been instilled intraperitoneally but are insufficiently absorbed to be clinically useful. In studies to be reported, repeated instillation, of 10% Liposyn (Tra-venol Lab, Deerfield IL.) into the peritoneal cavity of rats was associated with both peritoneal inflammation and inspissation within intestinal folds and death [192–195] of the experimental rat.

7. DEFICIENCIES IN PREPARATION OF DIALYSATE

Peritoneal dialysate is now purchased in soft or firm plastic containers. These containers have torn resulting in con-taminated dialysate [196]. Aseptic peritonitis secondary to endotoxins, eosinophilic peritonitis secondary to plastici-zers, and an allergic reaction to ethylene oxide from dialysis tubing have been reported [197–200]. Recently, elevated serum chromium and aluminum concentrations in serum

have been attributed to absorption from dialysate [200–1204]. Zinc may leach from dialysate bags and may account for 25% of the recommended dietary intake [205, 206]. Bisulfite is often added to dialysate but at concentrations employed is of no risk to the patient since most of the added bisulfite is destroyed in the sterilization process [207–210]. Dialysate contains particulates which may cause granulomata within the peritoneal cavity and it is unclear if they play a role in sclerosing peritonitis or peritoneal ultrafiltration loss [211, 212]. Warming dialysate in water and careless drying of the packaged dialysate may lead to peritonitis if the contaminated water spills on the connecting apparatus [213].

8. AGENTS TO AUGMENT PERITONEAL TRANSPORT

The sites offering resistance to peritoneal transport are not fully defined. Peritoneal membranes have differing perme-abilities and the contributions of the various membranes to peritoneal transport are unknown [214–218]. Blood flow is not limiting for small solutes [221–223]. Peritoneal transport rates of urea and potassium are only modestly decreased during hypotension and hypothermia. Vasodi-lator and vasopressor therapy in this situation do not alter peritoneal clearances [224, 225]. When blood flow was increased in the superior mesenteric artery after intrape-ritoneal administration of isoproterenol, but not systemic intravenous administration, creatinine and inulin peritoneal clearances improved. When mesenteric artery blood flow was kept at control levels by a clamp, clearances did not increase. Glucagon, only effective systemetically, improved inulin clearances but not creatinine, suggesting its site of activity is at the endothelial rather than the mesenteric surface [226–228]. Again, control of blood flow returned clearances to control levels [228].

Although dialysate osmolality, pH, or the presence of acetate or lactate may alter selected areas of the peritoneal microcirculation, modifications of dialysate have had little success in improving peritoneal transport [229–232]. Fur-thermore, inhibitors of prostaglandin synthesis may alter anatomy of the microcirculation [233, 234] but prostag-landins have only modest effects on transport [235, 236]. The effective peritoneal area is unknown and may be limiting for larger solutes. The interstitium may selectively inhibit transport since charged solutes may be repelled by carboxyl and amino groups of proteins. This would explain the low concentration of sodium in peritoneal ultrafiltrate [237, 238]. Furosemide has been reported to increase the sodium and barbiturate concentration in ultrafiltrate, sug-gesting that it may alter these postulated charges [239–242]. Heparin, negatively charged, is poorly absorbed from the peritoneal cavity [243]s. The mesentery is equally permeable to iodide and cationic rubidium suggesting that inhibition to transport may be endothelial for selected solutes [244]. Transport may be racemically selective [245]. Recently, chlorpromazine has been suggested as an agent that im-proves ultrafiltration and peritoneal urea and inulin cle-arances by decreasing the thickness of the stagnant fluid film [246]. Lowering surface tension by surface active agents, either anionic, cationic or neutral, improves transport [247–250].

Effects may be additive in improving transport. Intraperitoneal THAM, which through unknown mechanisms improve urea transport [251], added to dialysate with polysorbate further improved transport. Modest effects may be lost. Furosemide augmentation of peritoneal clearance is only evident during isotonic dialysis [252]. Although some have suggested that altering stagnant layers by surface active agents improves transport, more than one mechanism may be altered [253, 254]. Disrupting the tight junctions of cells alters transport, suggesting that this may be an important cause of peritoneal resistance [255, 256]. Preserving the concentration gradient for diffusion by binding the solute of interest with either albumin, for indirect bilirubin [257–260], or with b-cyclodextrin [261] may improve transfer into the peritoneal cavity. Alkalinizing agents act to trap barbiturates, salicylates, or uric acid within the peritoneal cavity [262]. Vasoactive agents have been most widely used. Here again, results have been contradictory and gains only modest [263, 264]. Dopamine has been reported to have some effect or no effect, depending on the concentration infused [265–267]. Dipyridamole has been reported effective when administered intraperitoneally but not orally [268–271]. Nitroprusside generally, but not always, augments peritoneal transport [272–276].

In summary, numerous agents can augment peritoneal transport. To date none are clinically in common use.

9. ANTIBIOTIC COMPATABILITY IN PERITONEAL DIALYSATE

Antibiotics are often added to dialysate to treat peritonitis. In the absence of peritonitis, they may be added to dialysate to treat systemic infection in a peritoneal dialysis patient.

Dialysate concentrate is available for use with proportioning machines. These machines dilute 1 part concentrate and 19 parts water. Antibiotics are added to the concentrate which, of necessity contains 30 to 50% dextrose. Aminoglycosides retain 80% activity over a 24 hr period in dialysate concentrate. Tombramycin was found to be the most labile and should be used withn 12 hr [277–279]. Vancomycin and amikacin activities were not impaired in dialysate concentrate. Concentrate was found to impair the activity of gentamicin and tobramycin, cephalothin, cefamandole, moxalactam, pencicillin, carbenicillin, and ampicillin [289–281].

Antibiotics are added to commercially formulated dialysate at concentrations similar to their bacterial inhibitory concentrations [282–293]. It may be convenient to formulate these solutions 24–48 hr in advance of use, especially if they are given to the patient to use at home, and hence compatability and inactivation become considerations. Dialysate is similar in composition to intravenous solutions, 5% dextrose and Ringer's lactate, and much information should be available in the hospital pharmacy. Many years of experience in the treatment of peritoneal dialaysis related peritonitis have shown that antibiotics, added alone or in combination to dialysate, are effective in eradicating the infecting organisms. Most studies added antibiotics just prior to use and little data are available regarding the treatment of patients with dialysate to which antibiotics had been added 24 hr previously.

Treatment of Gram negative peritonitis with a combination of an aminoglycoside and penicillin may lead to inactivation of the aminoglycoside if the concentration of penicillin is more than 20/l that of the aminoglycoside. The reaction is slow and requires these concentrations for 24 hr. Antibiotic activity and chemical stability are not a major clinical problem if solutions are used within 24 hr. Measured antibiotic activity in Mueller-Hinton broth is greater than fresh dialysate or dialysate effluent. This may explain the common clinical observation that Gram negatives organisms causing peritonitis among CAPD patients are not always eradicated by one antibiotic. Heparin and insulin do not interfere with antibiotic activity. Both insulin and cefuroxime may bind to the plastic dialysate bag and thus change the amount of drug deliverd [294–298].

10. ANTIBIOTICS

Peritoneal dialysis offers the advantage of a ready route of drug administration which may be used both in the treatment of peritonitis as well as drug delivery to ill dialysis patients. Intraperitoneal administration permits high local concentration of antibiotic. This is especially useful when highly protein bound drugs that slowly penetrate the peritoneal cavity are used [299].

Prophylactic therapy has been employed in an attempts to reduce peritonitis rates during intermittent peritoneal dialysis but has been found to be ineffective [300–305].

Peritoneal dialysis patients receiving antibiotic therapy rarely need the dose of antibiotic supplemented. The anephric dose is often satisfactory for the peritoneal dialysis patient.

Reviews of antibiotic kinetics and doses exist [306–320]. Tables 11 and 12 in Chapter 14 list guidelines for antibiotic dosage during peritonitis complicating peritoneal dialysis [320].

10.1. Cephalosporins (first generation)

Cephalothin was administered intraperitoneally every 6 hr at a dose of 100 mg/l, 75% was absorbed and serum levels reached 3.5–5.6 mg/l over 4–48 hr. In one report peritonitis did not enhance peritoneal uptake of cephalotin [321, 322].

Cefazolin has been used in both intermittent and long dwell peritoneal dialysis. Kinetics are similar to cephalothin [323–326].

Since cephalosporin penetrance into the peritoneal cavity yields satisfactory drug levels, oral treatment regimens have been proposed. Cephradine failed to provide satisfactory antibiotic coverage [327–328]. Cephalexin has also been used. Although penetrance was poor in non-infected patients, penetrance improved with peritonitis [325, 330–332].

10.2. Cephalosporins (second generation)

The peritoneal clearances of these agents range from 1–4 ml/min. Their half life in serum ranges from 8–12 hr and their volume of distribution is approximately extracellular fluid space.

Cefoxitin is 75% absorbed during a 6 hr residence within

the peritoneal cavity. Peritoneal clearance is less than 10% of plasma clearance [333–334].

Cefuroxime has been used in intermittent peritoneal dialysis and CAPD. However, one observer suggested that it may bind to the plastic dialysate container resulting in erratic drug delivery. Transport from serum into the peritoneal cavity increases with peritonitis [329, 335–339].

Cefamandole penetrates the peritoneal cavity in the active form when given intravenously and is also readily absorbed from the peritoneal cavity. About 75% of the administered dose is absorbed during a 6 hr intraperitoneal residence [340–346]. Peritonitis did not significantly enhance transport into the peritoneal cavity.

Cefonicid has a prolonged half-life of 48 hr in CAPD patients and only poorly penetrates the peritoneal cavity of non-infected patients [347].

10.3. Cephalosporins (third generation)

Ceftizoxime administered intravenously yields antibacterial levels in the peritoneal cavity within an hour of a 1 g dose. During a 6 hr intraperitoneal residence of dialysate, 75% of the drug is absorbed [348–351].

Ceftazidime has been used alone and in combination with vancomycin to provide Gram positive coverage. Its properties are similar to other cephalosporins. About 20% are absorbed from a 2 l hourly exchange of dialysate, 40% from a 4 hr cycle and 75% from a 6 hr cycle (352–354].

Moxalactam, lamoxactam and latamoxef are the same drug. The antibiotic exists as a stereoisomer. The kinetics of these isomers are similar. Peritoneal clearance provided about 10% of the plasma clearance. Intravenous therapy alone does not provide adequate dialysate levels, except for the most sensitive organisms, and intraperitoneal supplementation is necessary [355–359].

Cefotiam and Cefoperazone have been used to treat peritonitis during CAPD with moderate success. They are primarily eliminated by the liver and may be given once daily as a 1 g dose [360–362].

Cefotaxime also undergoes hepatic metabolism to a desacetyl derivative that prevents accumulation of the parent drug during therapy. Transport into the peritoneal cavity is enhanced during peritonitis [363–369]. In non infected CAPD patients 75% of an ip administered dose was absorbed after 6 hr. Intraperitoneal and intravenous administration yield equivalent serum concentrations.

Ceftriaxone is readily absorbed from the peritoneal cavity. Effective serum and dialysate levels were obtained with an intraperitoneal dose of 200 mg/2 l of dialysate exchanged four times daily. Seventy-five percent of the drug is absorbed during a 6 hr dwell [370].

Cefotetan poorly penetrates the peritoneal cavity. Less then 10% of an intravenous dose was removed from the dialysate of patients undergoing CAPD. To prevent accumulation among patients udnergoing CAPD, one group recommended maintenance therapy be half the normal dose every 24 hr [371]. Both Cefmenoxime, intravenously administered, and Cefixime, orally administered, have similar kinetics and only poorly penetrate into dialysate [372, 373].

10.4. Monobactam

Aztreonam is similar in spectrum and activity to the third generation cephalosporins. Experience with the drug is limited in peritoneal dialysis. However therapy using 500 mg/l in the first bag and 250 mg/l in subsequent bags, in combination with vancomycin has been reported to be highly successful [374–376].

10.5. Quinolones

These antibiotics have a spectrum of activity similar to the cephalosporins. They diffuse into the peritoneal cavity so that therapeutic concentrations are obtained using oral therapy. Experience with these agents in the treatment of dialysis related peritonitis is limited [377–380].

10.6. Penicillins

The new broad spectrum penicillins have been an important advance in the treatment of peritonitis related to peritoneal dialysis. A broad spectrum penicillin in conjunction with vancomycin as first line therapy prior to the culture result avoid the toxicity of the aminoglycosides. High glucose concentrations may degrade penicillins and they should be mixed just prior to addition to the dialysate [381]. Prolonged exposure of an aminoglycoside and a penicillin lead to inactivation of the aminoglycoside. This may occur in the serum of uremic patients. The penicillins have the greatest antagonistic effect on tobramycin followed by gentamicin and sisomicin. Amikacin was least effected. Azlocillin, as compared to mezlocillin and piperacillin which were equal, caused the greatest loss of aminoglycoside activity. The reaction is time dependent and at least 6 hr are required before significant loss of activity occurs. A concentration ratio of penicillin to aminoglycoside of 200/l seems to be associated with the greatest loss of activity.

Methicillin is well absorbed from the peritoneal cavity [382]. Peritoneal dialysis does not alter the dosage requirements of patients receiving systemic oxacillin therapy [383]. Peritonitis does not alter the kinetics of dicloxacillin [384, 385].

Ampicillin's half life is not changed by peritoneal dialysis performed hourly with 2 l volumes. It is absorbed from dialysate and absorption is enhanced with peritonitis. Amoxicillin administered orally during peritoneal dialysis yields 'therapeutic' dialysate concentrations but it is unclear whether the patients improve on this therapy [386–391]. Carbenicillin, ticarcillin and piperacillin half lives are prolonged during uremia. Carbenicillin, in a dose of 8 g daily, ticarcillin, in a dose of 4 g daily and piperacillin, in a dose of 3 g daily, provide effective serum levels. These antibiotics are effective when added into the peritoneal cavity to treat peritonitis. Peritoneal clearance of carbenicillin is 6 ml/min and insufficient drug is transported into the dialysate to be therapeutic, thus intraperitoneal supplementation is necessary [392–399]. Recently clavulinic acid, and inhibitor of B-lactamases, has been combined with ticarcillin and ampicillin [400].

Azlocillin is poorly transported into peritoneal dialysate. Treatment of peritonitis with this agent probably requires intraperitoneal supplementation [401, 402].

We could not find a report of peritonitis treated by mecillinam nor mezlocillin. Both of these agents are readily cleared during hemodialysis with significant (50 ml/min) non-renal clearance of the drug and both are transported poorly into dialysate. Therefore, therapy of peritonitis with either of these agents would require intraperitoneal supplementation [403, 404].

10.7. Aminoglycosides

The aminoglycosides are effective broad spectrum agents suitable for initial intraperitoneal therapy of peritonitis. Intraperitoneal administration yields high local concentration and after 12 to 24 hr serum concentrations will reach therapeutic levels. Absorption is enhanced during peritonitis. Our main concern with intraperitoneal therapy is that this regimen results in prolonged steady state levels which in combination with repeated exposure to aminoglycosides, may cause oto or vestibular toxicity. Furthermore it may compromise residual renal function. This has lead to dosing schedules that permit peak and through serum levels [405]. If feasible, drug concentrations should be monitored. Aminoglycosides are distributed in the extracellular fluid space. They are not protein bound. Their half lives are 2–3 days in patients without renal function. Peritoneal dialysis with hourly exchange cycles decreases the half life to 24 hr. Peritoneal clearance rates during hourly dialysis are 2–17 ml/min. Even though synergy between aminoglycosides and penicillins exists prolonged exposure of aminoglycosides to penicillins leads to inactivation [406, 407]. This reaction is thought to occur between the b-lactam ring of the penicillin and the methylamino group. Penicillins must be present for several hours in concentrations at least fivefold greater than the aminoglycoside. This occurs when uremic patients receive high dose carbenicillin therapy. If drugs are to be added to dialysate, they should be mixed just prior to instillation [408–415].

Intraperitoneal administration of neomycin was reported to cause apnea in children with peritonitis [416]. This was due to a neuromuscular block of the nondepolarizing type similar to that caused by d-tubocurarine. Ether may potentiate the block. Neomycin may be absorbed from the peritoneal cavity. Currently, it has no place in routine therapy of peritoneal dialysis peritonitis.

Kanamycin has also been reported to cause apnea, which was reversed by calcium gluconate [417]. Kanamycin and amikacin have been used to treat peritonitis. Since these are potentially the most toxic agents their use should be reserved for absolute indications [418–425].

Gentamicin transport from serum to dialysate and absorption from dialysate increases with peritonitis although sisomicin kinetics were not altered by peritonitis [426–438].

Tombramycin and Netilmicin kinetics are similar to those of gentamicin [439–449].

10.8. Vancomycin, erythromycin, clindamycin, metronidazole

CAPD has generated a need for effective antibiotic therapy of methicillin resistant staphylococci. Vancomycin therapy provides effective antibiotic coverage [450–469]. Thirty to 50 mg/l of Vancomycin added to dialysate eventually provide effective serum levels without a loading dose. About 50% of the amount instilled is absorbed during a six hour dwell. We have found that vancomycin administred during peritonitis at a dose of 50 mg/l (4 exchanges daily) yields serum levels of 10–15 mg/l after 3 days. The concentration increases to 40 mg/l after 7 days of therapy. Some administer an intravenous or intraperitoneal loading dose of 250 to 500 mg followed by maintainence doses of 15 mg/l. A 500 to 1000 mg intravenous dose may be expected to provide adequate drug levels for 4–7 days. It is unclear if intraperitoneal administration is more effective than intravenous administration. Peritoneal clearance during hourly dialysis ranges between 2–9 ml/min. Drug levels are readily available and can be measured if needed. Because of the accumulation of degredation products the fluorescence polarization immunoassay may overestimate drug concentration [450–469].

Recently a new glycopeptide antibiotic, Teicoplanin, has been introduced. Only 7% of an administered intravenous dose was recovered in the dialysate but therapeutic concentrations were maintained in serum and dialysate for two days following a 3 mg/kg dose [470].

Erythromycin in a dose of 125 mg/l of dialysate, in combination with sodium fusidate, was associated with transient deafness. Serum levels were between 60–80 mg/l [471].

Clindamycin phosphate must be enzymatically activated. During peritonitis sufficient protein is present in dialysate to activate the drug. As peritonitis improves and protein concentrations diminish, so may drug activation. Intravenous dosage does not provide adequate intraperitoneal levels. A dose of 167 mg/l of dialysate has been proposed for intraperitoneal treatment [472–476].

Metronidazole does not require dosage adjustment during CAPD. It reaches effective concentration in dialysate [477–480].

10.9. Polymyxins

Colistin has been used to treat Gram negative peritoneal infections. Peritoneal clearance is in the range of 1 ml/min with hourly peritoneal exchanges. Apnea has been reported with colistin [481–484].

10.10. Tetracycline and chloramphenicol and others

Tetracycline is readily absorbed from the peritoneal cavity [485–488]. The peritoneal clearance (serum to dialysate) was 6 ml/min. Peritoneal dialysis has been used to treat an overdose in a child [489].

Chloramphenicol sodium succinate, like clindamycin phosphate, requires hydrolysis to the active form. Little is removed by peritoneal dialysis [490–491]. Systemic therapy is not influenced by peritoneal dialysate losses. Thiamphenicol, an analogue of chloramphenicol, has similar kinetics. It is poorly absorbed from dialysate [492–494].

Sulfa derivitives have been administered intraperitoneally to treat post operative peritonitis and bacterial peritonitis as well as peritonitis caused by Nocardia asteroides [495–503]. Concentrations in serum over 200–250 mg/l may be associated with nausea. In patients undergoing CAPD, the half life of trimethoprim was 33 hr and the half life of sulfamethoxazole was 14 hr. A dose of 320 mg of trimethoprim and 1600 mg of sulfamethoxazole was recommended for systemic infections, 4 tablets daily. This may yield excessive serum levels of trimethoprim and subtherapeutic concentration of sulfamethoxazole in dialysate. Intraperitoneal therapy has been recommended at doses of 80 mg of trimethoprim and 400 mg of sulfamethoxazole to each of four 2 l daily dialysate bags. Susceptability testing may not predict a therapeutic response [504–511].

Quinine is slowly removed by peritoneal dialysis [24–31]. Peritoneal clearance is 1–3 ml/min with 2 l hourly exchanges of dialysate. Poor clearance is due to the 70% protein binding. Since quinine is a weak base, peritoneal clearance would be increased by maintaining a lower pH in dialysate although dialysate pH rapidly equilibrates with serum pH.

Chloroquine is poorly removed by peritoneal dialysis [512].

Isoniazid may be administered in full dosage to patients with renal failure. Isoniazid intoxication has been treated with peritoneal dialysis [513]. Some authors report substantial drug removal but this has not been found by all investigators [513–515].

Cycloserine poisoning has been treated by peritoneal dialysis [516]. Although the authors reported rapid reduction in serum concentrations, they were unable to measure dialysate concentrations.

Amantadine and Acyclovir are only slightly removed with peritoneal dialysis, less than 10–15% of an administered dose [517–520]. An intravenous dose of 2.5 mg/kg a day of acyclovir has recently been recommended [521].

10.11. Antifungal agents

Fungal peritonitis is difficult to treat and is frequently associated with excessive mortality. Although some have treated patients with intraperitoneal instillation of antifungal agents, we favor dialysis catheter removal and systemic therapy. It is unclear why intraperitoneal therapy has been relatively unsuccessful, especially as compared to treatment of bacterial peritonitis. However it is possible that the dialysis catheter protects the organisms from the antifungal agent [522–525].

Amphotericin B has been used to treat fungal peritonitis during peritoneal dialysis. Intraperitoneal administration of amphotericin may cause severe pain when instilled in doses from 0.5–3 mg/l of dialysate [526]. The drug tends to flocculate at a pH of 5, although calcium and sodium chloride may also contribute to flocculation. This flocculation may impair its intraperitoneal distribution [527]. One could consider raising the pH of the dialysate by adding 10–20 meq of sodium bicarbonate. Intraperitoneal administration may selectively increase peritoneal ultrafiltration [528, 529] but this has been associated with the development of peritoneal adhesions. The drug is highly protein bound and slowly penetrates into ascitic fluid. Therefore, less than 50% of serum levels are achieved after 3–5 days of daily intravenous therapy in the range of 50 mg [527, 530–533]. Miconazole, a parenterally given imidazole antifungal agent, and its analoge ketoconazole, which may be administered orally, have been used to treat fungal peritonitis [534–542]. Miconazole also induces pain when administered intraperitoneally at dosages of 7–15 mg/l. Although ketoconazole concentrations are low in peritoneal dialysate after oral administration, some suggest that protein binding is altered in uremia and thus free serum concentrations are similar to non-uremic patients.

5-fluorocytosine may be used alone or in combination with amphotericin B or miconazole [543–547]. This drug readily penetrates the peritoneal cavity. Peritoneal clearance is 14 ml/min. A dosage of 40 mg/kg/day for two days tapering to 30 mg/kg for two more days and 15 mg/kg for maintenance has been proposed [543]. An intraperitoneal preparation has been used successfully at a dose of 50 mg/l [548–552]. Drug levels should be monitored and maintained between 20–75 mg/l.

11. ANTISEPTICS AND SCLEROSING PERITONITIS

Intraperitoneal instillation of antiseptics, including a preparation that acts through conversion to formaldehyde, have been used in the treatment of grossly contaminated abdominal surgeries [553]. A saline-iodine flush was advocated for treatment and prevention of peritonitis during peritoneal dialysis. The consequences of repeated exposure and enhanced iodine absorption are unknown and this treatment has been associated with intraperitoneal adhesions [554–561]. Some investigations have suggested that povidone-iodine is rapidly inactivated within the peritoneal cavity causing an inflammatory response which accounts for the antibacterial effect.

Chlorhexidine has been used to treat peritonitis during CAPD but causes pain. It has also been associated with sclerosing peritonitis [562–565].

Sodium hypochlorite is used with selected Y connection devices. To date no complications except pain related to intraperitoneal infusions have been reported [566].

Clinicians are concerned that the peritoneal membrane will eventually be destroyed by prolonged exposure to hypertonic solutions, particulate matter found in dialysate containers, antiseptics and recurrent episodes of peritonitis. Some investigators have found that peritoneal clearance falls during prolonged therapy others have not [567–574]. Recently, some patients have experienced a loss of ultrafiltration capacity while undergoing CAPD which has been attributed to rapid absorption of glucose. There is no way of knowing which patient is at risk, although acetate dialysate and frequent peritonitis episodes have been implicated [575–577].

Phosphatidylcholine has been found in dialysate effluent. Preliminary reports suggest that replenishing phosphatidylcholine may correct ultrafiltration failure, although in our experience this has not been effective [578–580]. Sclerosing peritonitis has also been associated with prolonged dialysis using acetate solutions [581–585]. The bowel wall becomes encapsulated by a diffuse sclerosis of the serosal membranes. The pathology resembles that found with the early B-blocker practolol. We have seen this experimentally in dogs maintained on dialysis with chronic peritonitis as well as in humans with methicillin resistant Staphyloccus epidermidis peritonitis ineffectively treated for a 2–3 week period and following fungal peritonitis.

12. POISONING

12.1. Heavy metals

Before dialysis became available on a routine basis, there were many case reports of intoxications treated with the use of peritoneal dialysis. These included such diverse substances as mushrooms and arsine [586–590]. Peritoneal dialysis functions primarily to support the patient through acute renal failure. Several reviews of the dialysis of poisons are available [591–594]. The following sections will focus on poisoning and the use of peritoneal dialysis as treatment for this.

The emerging importance of aluminum has generated interest in desferoxamine. Athough peritoneal dialysate contains little aluminum, contamination of dialysate has been reported. The acidic pH of dialysate favors absorption [595–601]. Aluminum bone disease and encephalopathy have been treated by desferoxamine [602–603]. Desferoxamine may be administered intravenously, intramuscularly, or intraperitoneally and for similar doses one can expect similar amounts of aluminum to be removed [604–606]. There are no reported side effects with intraperitoneal instillation although we have had patient complaints of occasional muscle aches following intraperitoneal instillation. Hypotension has been reported after rapid intravenous infusion.

Iron intoxication has also been treated with chelating agents. In the past calcium disodium EDTA administered systemically has increased iron removal rates [607–609]. More recently, desferoxamine has been used [610–612].

Copper poisonings as well as acute hemolytic crises of Wilson's disease have been treated with peritoneal dialysis [613–618]. The chelating agents D-penicillamine, either orally, intramusculary, or intraperitoneally, and dimercaprol (BAL) have been used. Not all studies confirm the efficacy of D-penicillamine. Albumin may be added to trap copper in the dialysate.

Mercury poisoning has been treated with the chelating agent added systemically or intraperitoneally and albumin added to dialysate to trap the metal [618–623].

Chromium has been reported as a contaminant of dialysate. The peritoneal clearance of chromium is approximately 1 ml/min. Removal by hemodialysis is approximately three times more efficient then peritoneal dialysis but similar amounts may be removed since therapy is readily extended with peritoneal dialysis [595, 624, 625].

Both lead and gold are removed with peritoneal dialysis although the reported peritoneal clearances for gold are inconsistent, ranging from 1–14 ml/min at flow rates of 2 l/hr [623, 626–630].

12.2. Alcohols, lithium, bromide

Methanol intoxication is often fatal. Peritoneal dialysis has been used in therapy but does not appear to be as useful as hemodialysis. Several case reports have suggested full recovery with hemodialysis whereas recovery with peritoneal dialysis was associated with residual blindness. The unfavorable clinical outcomes may have been the result of using peritoneal dialysis to treat the more unstable patient. However it appears that a rapid drop in serum concentration may be important and hemodialysis is recommended [631–636].

Ethylene glycol poisoning has been treated with peritoneal dialysis. Peritoneal oxalate removal rate, at 2 l intraperitoneal volumes and hourly exchanges, was about half the urea rate [637–640]. The removal rate using CAPD dialysis cycles is similar to creatinine [641].

Peritoneal dialysis has also been used in the removal of iso-propyl alcohol and ethanol. Although less efficient than hemodialysis, therapy may be prolonged and thus substantial drug may be removed [642, 643].

Lithium is used as an anti-psychotic. Although peritoneal dialysis is less efficient than hemodialysis, 90 ml/min vs 10–15 ml/min, the amounts removed over a 12 hr period have been reported to be similar [644–647]. As lithium is distributed in both intracellular and extracellular space, the limiting factor is the rate of transfer from the intracellular to the extracellular space. A patient has been treated by intraperitoneal lithium therapy [648].

Bromide renal excretion is similar to chloride. Peritoneal clearance rates are similar to the rates for creatinine, 15 ml/min. Hemodialysis is more efficient. Saline infusion coupled with diuretic therapy is the therapy of choice [649–651].

Cesium-137, a radioactive agent, is removed with peritoneal dialysis. Studies in rabbits yielded removal rates of 5–10 ml/min [652].

12.3. Analgesics and sedatives

Salicylate intoxication is common. Peritoneal dialysis is useful in the critically ill infant. This therapy not only removes salicylate but it also corrects acid base abnormalities. Efficiency is increased by alkalinizing the dialysate and by adding albumin. Alkalinizing the dialysate after addition of albumin may be necessary to alleviate 'inflow' pain [653–660].

Paracetamol is not readily removed by dialysis. Dialytic therapy is often needed for control of renal failure while awaiting hepatic recovery [661].

Peritoneal dialysis has been used to remove propoxyphene but is much less efficient than hemodialysis, 9 vs 170 ml/min, respectively. Dialysis is of little benefit because of the minimal concentration in blood. Renal excretion is urine flow dependent and may reach 28 ml/min with forced diuresis [662–664].

The half-life of the non-tricyclic antidepressant fluoxetine and of the tricyclic antidepressants are not extended among patients undergoing both intermittent peritoneal dialysis or CAPD and poisonings are not effectively treated by peritoneal dialysis [665–669].

Barbiturate intoxication is best treated with intensive nursing and forced diuresis although peritoneal dialysis may be used as an adjunct. Removal rates are increased by alkalinization of dialysate, the addition of albumin, and perhaps by the addition of furosemide (20 mg/l) to the dialysate. Peritoneal dialysis will also warm the hypothermic patient [670–684].

Meprobamate intoxication is generally characterized by a short duration of coma. The host metabolizes approximately 8% of the ingested dose per hour. It is approximately 50% protein bound. Peritoneal removal rates are approximately 15–20 ml/min. Clearance is not enhanced by albumin or alkalinization of dialysate [685–688].

Glutethimide is most efficiently removed with a lipid dialysate. The host metabolizes approximately 2% of the ingested dose per hour. Peritoneal dialysis with 5% albumin improves clearance from the peritoneal cavity [689–693].

Methyprylon (Noludar) is not effectively removed by peritoneal dialysis [694–696]. Methyprylon and glutethimide are most efficiently removed by microcapsule hemoperfusion [694].

Ethchlorvynol (Placidyl) half life ranges from 50–100 hr. Peritoneal removal rates are reported to be 18 ml/min. The addition of albumin to dialysate does not enhance removal [691, 697–699].

Peritoneal dialysis has been used in the treatment of pargyline hydrochloride (Eutonyl) poisoning. Although clinical improvement occurred during peritoneal dialysis in one study, no clearance data were reported [700].

Methaqualone is only transported into the peritoneal cavity at 5 ml/min and therefore peritoneal dialysis is not useful. Microcapsule hemoperfusion effeciently removes methaqualone [694, 701, 702].

Amphetamine removal may be enhanced with the aid of peritoneal dialysis [703–705].

12.4. Miscellaneous

After ingestion, fluoride is rapidly bound to bone and then slowly excreted [706]. Dialysis does not remove significant amounts of fluoride. Net transfer from dialysate was observed suggesting that the dialysate may have been formulated with fluoridated water.

Thallium is ineffectively removed with peritoneal dialysis [707]. In potassium ferrocyanide poisoning, cyanide is the toxic agent. Peritoneal dialysis has been used to maintain the patient during acute renal failure [708].

Oral hypoglycemics are occasionally ingested accidently or as a suicide attempt. They are not dialyzable, although peritoneal dialysis may help by providing glucose to the host [709, 710].

Antihistamine preparations are ineffectively removed with peritoneal dialysis. The delayed release capsule and the frequent formulation of these agents with other medications may complicate management [711, 712]. Gallamine neuromuscular blockade has been reversed by peritoneal dialysis although removal rates were not reported [713].

Weed poisons are frequently used as agents for suicide attempts. Peritoneal dialysis is useful in treating the renal failure that ensues with paraquat poisoning. Peritoneal dialysis has been used as adjunctive therapy in the treatment of organophosphorus poisoning and, although metabolites were found in dialysate, the amount removed was unclear [714–717].

Poisoning from volatile oils can occur. Eucalyptus oil poisoning has been reported and inference of dialyzability was made from the odor of the dialysate and clinical improvement [718]. Peritoneal dialysis has been used to manage the acute renal failure seen in a case of toluene intoxication. In this instance, a bleeding diathesis associated with hepatic failure made this the therapy of choice [719].

Although phenols have been reportedly removed with peritoneal dialysis, the rate was insufficient to be of benefit during a case of 'Lysol' poisoning (cresol 10% in soap) [720–721].

Poisoning with boric acid, a weak antiseptic, occurs primarily in infants. Peritoneal dialysis is effective although clearance rates have been reported to be only 1–2 ml/min [722–725].

Chlorate may be mistaken for chloride and accidental ingestion may occur. This oxidizing agent induces an acute renal failure secondary to intravascular hemolysis and nephrotoxicity. Peritoneal dialysis has been used effectively to treat the acute renal failure associated with this type of poisoning [726, 727].

Hexachlorophene is poorly eliminated by peritoneal dialysis [728].

As dialysate contains thyroid binding globulin, attempts have been made to enhance removal rates of thyroid hormone during thyroid storm with peritoneal dialysis. Clinical experience is limited [728–733].

Amino-acid toxicity may account for much of the harm to infants suffering from maple-syrup-urine disease. In this disease, branched chain amino-acids accumulate. Peritoneal dialysis has also been used as an adjunct in the therapy of leucinosis [734]. Peritoneal clearances of valine, leucine, isoleucine and several keto acids are reported to range between 1–3 ml/min [735–737]. CAPD has been used to treat a patient with methyl-malonyl-CoA mutase apoenzyme deficiency [738, 739]. Peritoneal dialysis has been used to treat the hyperammonemia found in Ornithine transcarbamylase deficiency [740–744].

13. CARDIO-ACTIVE AGENTS

Digoxin and digitoxin are not removed from the body in significant amounts by peritoneal dialysis [745–753].

Quinidine dosage adjustment is not needed for patients undergoing either intermittent peritoneal dialysis or CAPD [754, 755].

Amiodarone and its desethyl metabolite are not removed with peritoneal dialysis [756].

Nifedipine removal is negligible with peritoneal dialysis [757].

Propranolol, and its glucuronide conjugate are negligibly removed with peritoneal dialysis [758, 759]. No dosage modification is required for Atenolol [760].

Procaine has been used to enhance peritoneal transport [761]. Lidocaine has been used to alleviate dialysate inflow discomfort (5 cc in 2 l). Peritoneal clearance during CAPD, 8 to 10 l of dialysate effluent daily, has been reported at 5 ml/min. During hourly exchanges the peritoneal clearance may approach that of creatinine. Due to variable rates of acetylation in uremic patients, this drug appears to accumulate and it is best avoided when other agents are available [762–765]. Tocainide dosage should be adjusted as if the peritoneal dialysis patient had severe renal failure, the T1/2 being 25 hr [766].

The anti-hypertensive agents alpha-methyldopa, diazoxide and clonidine do not require dosage modification [767–769]. The anti-anginal medication isosorbide-5-nitrate does not require dosage modification during peritoneal dialysis [770].

14. MISCELLANEOUS DRUGS

14.1. Agents to relieve dyspepsia

Cimetidine and metoclopramide peritoneal clearances are too low to require alteration of the renal failure dosage [771–778].

14.2. Corticosteroids

Prednisolone kinetics are not altered by dialysis but consideration should be given to supplementing the dose of methylprednisolone after hemodialysis. There are no data available for methylprednisolone use during peritoneal dialysis [779, 780].

14.3. Anti-epileptic agents

Peritoneal dialysis removes little of the administered dose of phenytoin or valproic acid [781–786].

14.4. Anti-fibrinolytic agents

Epsilon-aminocaproic acid requires dosage adjustment in the patient undergoing intermittent peritoneal dialysis. Total body removal of the drug is only 25% that of a non-uremic patient. Peritoneal dialysis accounted for about half the amount removed. Recommendations for the CAPD patient are not available [787].

14.5. Anti-thrombotic agents

Heparin is poorly absorbed from the peritoneal cavity. It is used to prevent adhesions during peritonitis and also facilitates peritoneal drainage when there is a large amount of ascitic protein. Some investigators claimed that it increases dialysate effluent volume and possibly peritoneal clearance rates. It is recommended that high concentrations of heparin are not mixed in the same bag as aminoglycosides. For example, in dialysis delivery systems that use multi-pronged tubing connected to multiple dialysate bags one should add the medications to separate bags. Selective manufacture of specific subfractions may soon be a reality [788–798].

14.6. Anti-lipid agents

Clofibrate may induce rhabdomylysis and hyperkalemia. Protein binding of the drug is altered in uremia. Peritoneal clearance is minimal during CAPD. The drug should be avoided [799].

14.7. Bronchodilators

Theophylline is commonly used as a bronchodilator. Peritoneal removal rates have been reported to be approximately 1 to 9 ml/min. In the event of theophylline toxicity, charcoal hemoperfusion is most efficient [800–805].

14.8. Radiographic contrast agents

Sodium diatrizoate peritoneal clearance is half that of urea and has been reported to range from 5–12 ml/min with a mean of 9 ml/min [806, 807].

Sodium iodide peritoneal clearance has been measured at 12 ml/min [808]. Diethylenetriaminepentacetate (DTPA) is a chelating agent that may be used in heavy metal intoxications. It is commonly labelled with technetium-99m. and is removed from the peritoneal cavity at 65% of the rate of creatinine [809].

Radiogallium is highly protein bound and a negligible amount is cleared by peritoneal dialysis [810].

Methylene blue causes pain when instilled into the peritoneal cavity [811].

15. DIALYSATE LOSSES OF VITAMINS

Serum folate and B-12 are removed during peritoneal dialysis [812, 813]. Vitamin C is removed at a rate ranging from 11–22 ml/min for 2 l intraperitoneal volumes infused for 10 min, allowed to dwell for 30 min, and drained for 20 min [814] and losses may be sufficient to require supplementation [815]. Thiamine (B1), riboflavin (B2) and pyridoxine (B6) also require supplementation [813, 816]. Although vitamin A may be found in dialysate, serum and tissue concentrations remain normal [817, 818]. Vitamin E was not found in dialysate [819]. Vitamin D is lost in dialysate and consideration should be given to supplementing children on peritoneal dialysis [820].

REFERENCES

1. Johnson CA, Zimmerman SW, Rogge M: The pharmacokinetics of antibiotics used to treat peritoneal dialysis-associated peritonitis. Am J Kidney Dis 4: 3-17, 1984.
2. Lasrich M, Maher JM, Hirszel P, Maher JF: Correlation of peritoneal transport rates with molecular weight: A method for predicting clearances. ASAIO J 2: 107–113, 1979.
3. Bunke CM, Aronoff GR, Luft FC: Pharmacokinetics of common antibiotics used in continuous ambulatory peritoneal dialysis. Am J Kidney Dis 3: 114–117, 1983.
4. Paton TW, Cornish WR, Manuel MA, Hardy BG: Drug therapy in patients undergoing peritoneal dialysis: Clinical pharmacokinetic considerations. Clin Pharmacokin 10: 404–426, 1985.
5. Bennett WM, Muther RS, Parker RA, Feig P, Morrison G, Golper TA, Singer I: Drug therapy in renal failure: Dosing guidelines for adults. Part I: Antimicrobial agents, analgesics. Ann Intern Med 93: 62–89, 1980.
6. Bennett WM, Muther RS, Parkr RA, Feig P, Morrison G, Golper TA, Singer I: Drug therapy in renal failure: Dosing guidelines for adults. Part II: Sedatives, hypnotics, and tranquilizers; cardiovascular, antihypertensive, and diuretic agents; miscellaneous agents. Ann Intern Med 93: 286–325, 1980.
7. Maher JF: Pharmacokinetics in patients with renal failure. Clin Nephrol 21: 39–46, 1984.
8. Watanabe AS: Pharmocokinetic aspects of the dialysis of drugs. Drug Intell Clin Pharm 2: 407–416, 1977.
9. Reidenberg MM: Drug metabolism in uremia. Clin Nephrol 4: 83–85, 1975.
10. Jackson EA, McLeod DC: Pharmacokinetics and dosing of

antimicrobial agents in renal impairment, Part 1. Am J Hosp Pharm 31: 36–52, 1974.

11. Jackson EA, McLeod DC: Pharmacokinetics and dosing of antimicrobial agents in renal impairment, Part 2. Am J Hosp Pharm 31:137–148, 1974.

12. Janknegt R, Nube MJ: A simple method for predicting drug clearances during CAPD. Periton Dial Bull 5: 254–255, 1985.

13. Gibson TP: Renal Disease and drug metabolism: An overview. Am J Kidney Dis 8: 7–17, 1986.

14. Ward RA, Klein E, Wathen RL: Investigation of the risks and hazards with devices associated with peritoneal dialysis and sorbent regenerated dialysate delivery systems. Periton Dial Bull, Apr-June Supplement 3(2): S1–S52, 1983.

15. Brautbar N, Gruber HE: Magnesium and bone disease. Nephron 44: 1–7, 1986.

16. Parker A, Nolph KD: Magnesium and calcium mass transfer during continuous ambulatory peritoneal dialysis. Trans Am Soc Artif Intern Organs 26: 194–196, 1980.

17. Nolph KD, Prowant B, Serkes KD, Morgan L, Baker B, Charytan C, Gham K, Hamburger R, Husserl F, Kleit S, McGuinness J, Moore H, Warren T: Multicenter evaluation of a new peritoneal dialysis solution with a high lactate and a low magnesium concentration. Periton Dial Bull, April-June 3(2): 63–65, 1983.

18. Kohaut EC, Balfe JW, Potter D, Alexander S, Lum G: Hypermagnesemia and mild hypocarbia in pediatric patients on CAPD. Periton Dial Bull 3(1): 40, 1983.

19. Kenny MA, Casillas E, Ahmad S: Magnesium, calcium and pth relationships in dialysis patients after magnesium repletion. Nephron 46: 199–205, 1987.

20. Gonella M, Moriconi L, Buzzigoli G, Urbano, Bartolini V, Bonaguidi F, Rossi G, Mariani G: Patterns of bone mineralization in chronic uremia patients on long-term hemodialysis with low magnesium in the dialysis fluid, Parts 1 & 2. Contr Dial 4: 38–42, 1983.

21. Burnell JM, Teubner E: Effects of decreasing dialysate magnesium in patients with chronic renal failure. Rev Interam Radio 6: 191–197, 1976.

22. Kwong MBL, Lee JSK, Chan MK: Transperitoneal calcium and magnesium transfer during an 8-hour dialysis. Periton Dial Bull 7: 85–89, 1987.

23. Blumenkrantz MJ, Kopple JD, Moran JK, Coburn JW: Metabolic balance studies and dietary protein requirements in patients undergoing continuous ambulatory peritoneal dialysis. Kidney Int 21: 849–861, 1982.

24. Garrett JJ, Cuddihee RE: Calcium absorption during peritoneal dialysis. Trans Am Soc Artif Intern Organs 14: 372–375, 1968.

25. Rubin J, Rust P, Brown P, Popovich RP, Nolph KD: A Comparison of peritoneal transport in patients with psoriasis and uremia. Nephron 29(3&4): 185–1189, 1981.

26. Anderson KEH: Calcium transfer during intermittent peritoneal dialysis. Nephron 29: 63–67, 1981.

27. Stoltz ML, Nolph KD, Maher JF: Factors affecting calcium removal with calcium-free peritoneal dialysis. J Lab Clin Med 78: 389–398, 1971.

28. Nolph KD, Stoltz M, Maher JF: Calcium free peritoneal dialysis: Treatment of vitamin D intoxication. Arch Intern Med 128: 809–814, 1971.

29. Lemann J, Donatelli AA: Calcium intoxication due to primary hyperparathyroidism. Ann Intern Med 60: 447–461, 1964.

30. Miach PJ, Dawborn JK, Martin TS, Moon WJ: Management of the hypercalcemia of malignancy by peritoneal dialysis. Am J Med 21: 782–784, 1975.

31. Raja RM, Cantor RE, Boreyko C, Bushchri H, Kramer MS, Rosenbaum JL: Sodium transport during ultrafiltration peritoneal dialysis. Trans Am Soc Artif Intern Organs 18: 429–435, 1972.

32. Raja RM, Kramer MS, Rosenbaum JL, Manchanda R, Lazaro

N: Evaluation of hypertonic peritoneal dialysis solutions with low sodium. Nephron 11: 342–353, 1973.

33. Daniel J, Ahearn, Nolph KD: Controlled sodium removal with peritoneal dialysis. Trans Am Soc Artif Intern Organs 18: 423–428, 1972.

34. Nolph KD, Hano JE, Teschan PE: Peritoneal sodium transport during hypertonic peritoneal dialysis. Ann Intern Med 70: 931–941, 1969.

35. Nolph KD, Sorkin MI, Moore H: Autoregulation of sodium and potassium removal during continuous ambulatory peritoneal dialysis. Trans Am Soc Artif Intern Organs 26: 334–338, 1980.

36. Quellhorst E, Lowitz HD, Scheler F: The influence of dialysate osmolarity on the effectiveness of peritoneal dialysis. Klin Wschr (Berlin) 49: 583–587, 1971.

37. Cundy T, Trafford JAP: Efficacy of peritoneal dialysis in severe thiazide-induced hyponatraemia. Postgrad Med J 57: 734–735, 1981.

38. Swales JD: Sodium uptake in peritoneal dialysis. Brit Med J 3: 345–347, 1967.

39. Bisson PG, Bailey KM: Sodium in peritoneal dialysis solutions. Brit Med J 6174: 1322–1323, 1979.

40. Shear L, Harvey JD, Barry KG: Peritoneal sodium transport: Enhancement by pharmacologic and physical agents. J Lab Clin Med 67: 181–188, 1966.

41. Finberg L, Kiley J, Luttrell CN: Mass accidental salt poisoning in infancy. JAMA 184: 121–124, 1963.

42. Spital A, Sterns RH: Potassium supplementation via the dialysate in continuoius ambulatory peritoneal dialysis. Am J Kidney Dis 6: 173–176, 1985.

43. Brown ST, Ahearn DJ, Nolph KD: Potassium removal with peritoneal dialysis. Kidney Int 4: 67–69, 1973.

44. Nolph KD, Twardowski ZJ, Popovich RP, Rubin J: Equilibration of peritoneal dialysis solutions during long-dwell exchanges. J Lab Clin Med 93: 246–256, 1979.

45. Richardson, JA, Borchardt EA: Adverse effect on bacteria of peritoneal dialysis solutions that contain acetate. Brit Med J 3: 749–750, 1969.

46. Gjessing J: Bacterial growth in the dialysate fluid and the reaction of peritoneum to peritoneal dialysis. Acta Med Scand 182: 509–512, 1967.

47. Richardson JA, Borchardt KA: Antibacterial effect to different dialysis. Brit Med J 2: 468–469, 1972.

48. Binswanger U, Keusch G, Bammatter F, Heule H, Kiss D: Peritonitis during continuous ambulatory peritoneal dialysis: Improving patient defense by type of buffer of dialysate? Nephron 28: 300–302, 1981.

49. Diskin CJ, Coplon N, Feldman C, Vosti K: Antimicrobial activity in continuous ambulatory peritoneal dialysis. Periton Dial Bull 3: 150–154, 1983.

50. Flournoy DJ, Perryman FA, Quadri SMH: Growth of bacterial clinical isolates in continuous ambulatory peritoneal dialysis fluid. Periton Dial Bull 3: 144–145, 1983.

51. Panzetta G, Loschiavo C, Bertazzoni EM: Effects of various peritoneal dialysis solutions on bacterial growth in vitro. Periton Dial Bull 4: 27–29, 1984.

52. Marichal JF, Faller B, Brignon P, Degoulet P, Aime F: Peritonitis in Continuous Ambulatory Peritoneal Dialysis: A role for dialysate? Nephron 42: 167–170, 1986.

53. Duwe AK, Vas SI, Weatherhead JW: Effects of the composition of peritoneal dialysis fluid on chemiluminescence, phagocytosis, and bacterial activity in vitro. Infect Immunol 33: 120–125, 1981.

54. Gallimore B, Gagnon RF, Stevenson MM: Cytotoxicity of commercial peritoneal dialysis solutions towards peritoneal cells of chronically uremic mice. Nephron 43: 283–289, 1986.

55. Rubin J, Lin LM, Lewis R, Cruse J, Bower JD: Host defense mechanisms in continuous ambulatory peritoneal dialysis. Clin Nephrol 20: 140–144, 1983.

56. Harvey DM, Sheppard KJ, Morgan AG, Fletcher J: Effect of dialysate fluids on phagocytosis and killing by normal neutrophils. J Clin Microbiol 25(8): 1424–1427, 1987.

57. Nolph KD, Prowant B, Serkes KD, Morgan L, Baker B, Charytan C, Gham K, Hamburger R, Husserl F, Kleit S, McGuinness, Moore H, Warren T: Multicenter evaluation of a new peritoneal dialysis solution with a high lactate and a low magnesium concentration. Periton Dial Bull 3: 63–65, 1983.

58. Teehan BP, Reichard GA, Sigler MH, Schleifer CR, Cupit MC, Haff AC: Acid-base balance in continuous ambulatory peritoneal dialysis. Proc Clin Dial Transplant Forum 10: 100–104, 1980.

59. Richardson RMA, Roscoe JM: Bicarbonate, l-lactate and d-lactate balance in intermittent peritoneal dialysis. Periton Dial Bull 6: 178–185, 1986.

60. Vaziri ND, Warner AS: Peritoneal dialysis clearance of endogenous lactate. J Dial 3: 107–113, 1979.

61. Lee HA, Hill LF, Hewitt V, Ralston AJ, Berlyne GM: Lactic acidaemia in peritoneal dialysis. Proc EDTA 4: 150–155, 1967.

62. Breborowicz A, Szulc R: Removal of endogenous lactates via the peritoneum in experimental lactic acidosis. Intern Care Med 7: 297–300, 1981.

63 Robson M, Pinto T, Kao E, Oren A: The metabolism of lactate and bicarbonate in CAPD, In: Atkins RC, Thomson NM, Farrell PC (eds), Peritoneal Dialysis, New York, Churchill Livingstone, pp 211–216, 1981.

64. La Greca G, Biasioli S, Chiaramonte S, Fabris A, Feriani M, Pisani E, Ronco C: Acetate, lactate and bicarbonate kinetics in peritoneal dialysis, In: Atkins RC, Thomson NM, Farrell PC (eds), Peritoneal Dialysis, New York, Churchill Livingstone, pp 217–221, 1981.

65. Dixon SR, McKean WI, Pryor JE, Irvine ROH: Changes in acid-base balance during peritoneal dialysis with fluid containing lactate ions. Clin Sci 39: 51–60, 1970.

66. Rubin J, Nolph KD, Arfaania D, Wiefma DL, Miller FN, Harris PD: Comparison of the effects of lactate and acetate on clinical peritoneal clearances. Clin Nephrol 12: 145–147, 1979.

67. Faller B, Marichal JF: Le dialysat a l'acetate: responsable de la perte de l'ultrafiltration en dialyse peritoneale continue ambulatoire.

68. Pedersen FB, Ryttov N, Deleuran P, Dragsholt C, Kildeberg P: Acetate versus lactate in peritoneal dialysis solution. Nephron 39: 55–58, 1985.

69. Ing TS, Gandhi VC, Daugirdas JT, Reid RW, Hunt J, Popli S: Peritoneal dialysis using bicarbonate-buffered dialysate. Int J Artif Organs 7: 166, 1984.

70. Kwong MBL, Wu GG, Rodella H, Brandes L, Oreopoulos DG: Effect of the peritoneal dialysate buffer on ultrafiltration: Studies in normal rabbits. Periton Dial Bull 5: 182–185, 1985.

71. Cullon ET, Moore HL, Nolph KD, Keller RS: pH Equilibration with acetate and lactate solutions during peritoneal dialysis. Periton Dial Bull 5: 123–126, 1985.

72. Hayat JC: The treatment of lactic acidosis in the diabetic patient by peritoneal dialysis using sodium acetate: A report of two cases. Diabetologia 10: 485–487, 1974.

73. Vaziri ND, Ness R, Wellikson L, Barton C, Greep N: Bicarbonate-buffered peritoneal dialysis: An effective adjunct in the treatment of lactic acidosis. Am J Med 67: 392–396, 1979.

74. Naparstek Y, Rubinger D, Friedlaender MM, Popovtzer MM: Lactic acidosis and peritoneal dialysis. Isr J Med Sci 18: 513–514, 1982.

75. Foulks Maj CJ, Wright Maj LF: Successful repletion of bicarbonate stores in ongoing lactic acidosis: A role for bicarbonate-buffered peritoneal dialysis. Southern Med J 74: 1162–1163, 1981.

76. Rossen B, Ladefoged J: A comparison between the effects of acetate and lactate in peritoneal dialysis solutions. Scand J Urol Nephrol 16: 279–281, 1982.

77. Nash MA, Russo JC: Neonatal lactic acidosis and renal failure: The role of peritoneal dialysis. J Ped 91: 101–105, 1977.

78. Sheppard JM, Lawrence JR, Oon RCS, Thomas DW, Row RG, Wise PH: Lactic acidosis: Recovery associated with use of peritoneal dialysis. Aug N Z J Med 4: 389–392, 1972.

79. Vilbar RM, Ing TS, Shin KD, Gandhi VC, Viol GW, Chen WT, Geisd WP, Hano JE: Treatment of metabolic alkalosis with peritoneal dialysis in a patient with renal failure. Artif Organs 2: 421–422, 1978.

80. Veech RL: The toxic impact of parenteral solutions on the metabolism of cells: A hypothesis for physiological parenteral therapy. Am J Clin Nutr 44: 519–551, 1986.

81. Feriani M, Biasioli S, Brion D, Brendolan A, Gargantini L, Chiaramonte S, Fabris A, Ronco C, LaGreca G: Bicarbonate solutions for peritoneal dialysis: A reality. Int J Artif Organs 8: 57–58, 1985.

82. Ing TS, Humayun HM, Daugirdas JT, Reid RW, Hano JE, Gandhi VC, Popli S: Preparation of bicarbonate-containing dialysate for peritoneal dialysis. Int J Artif Organs 6: 217–218, 1983.

83. Biasioli S, Feriani M, Chiarmonte S, La Greca G: Buffers in peritoneal dialysis. Int J Artif Organs 10: 3–8, 1987.

84. Rubin J, Nolph KD, Arfania D, Joshua IG, Miller FN, Wiegman DL, Harris PD: Clinical studies with a nonvasoactive peritoneal dialysis solution. J Lab Clin Med 93: 910–915, 1979.

85. Knochel JP, Mason AD: Effect of alkalinization on peritoneal diffusion of uric acid. Am J Physiol 210: 1160–1164, 1966.

86. Nahas GG, Giroux JJ, Gjessing J, Verosky M, Mark LC: The use of THAM in peritoneal dialysis. Trans Am Soc Artif Intern Organs 10: 345–349, 1964.

87. Duwe AK, Vas SI, Weatherhead JW: Effects of the composition of peritoneal dialysis fluid on chemiluminescence, phagocytosis, and bacterial activity in vitro. Infect Immunol 33: 120–125, 1981.

88. Gilli P, Bastiani P De, Fagioli F, Buoncristiani U, Carobi C, Stabellini N, Squerzanti R, Rosati G, Farinelli A: Positive aluminium balance in patients on regular peritoneal treatment: An effect of low dialysate ph? Proc EDTA 17: 219–225, 1980.

89. Nolph KD, Rosenfield PS, Powell JT, Danforth E: Peritoneal glucose transsport hyperglycemia during peritoneal dialysis. Am J Med Sci 259: 272–281, 1970.

90. Anderson G, Bergquist-Poppen M, Collste LG, Hultman E: Glucose absorption from the dialysis fluid during peritoneal dialysis. Scand J Urol Nephrol 5: 77–79, 1971.

91. Rubin J, Walsh D, Bower J: Diabetes, dialysate losses and serum lipids during continuous ambulatory peritoneal dialysis. Am J Kidney Dis 10(2): 104–108, 1987.

92. Armstrong VW, Creutzfeldt W, Ebert R, Fuchs C, Hilgers R, Scheler F: Effect of dialysate glucose load on plasma glucose and glucoregulatory hormones in CAPD patients. Nephron 39: 141–145, 1987.

93. Grodstein GP, Blumenkrantz MJ, Kopple JD, Moran JK, Coburn JW: Glucose absorption during continuous ambulatory peritoneal dialysis. Kidney Int 19: 564–567, 1981.

94. DeSanto NG, Capodicasa G, Senatore R, Cicchetti T, Cirillo D, Damiano M, Torella R, Giugliano D, Improta L, Giordano C: Glucose utilization from dialysate in patients on continuous ambulatory peritoneal dialysis (CAPD). Int J Artif Organs 2: 119–124, 1979.

95. Gahl GM, Baeyer V, Averdunk R, Riedinger H, Borowzak B, Schurig R, Becker H, Kessel M: Outpatient evaluation of dietary intake and nitrogen removal in continuous ambulatory peritoneal dialysis. Ann Intern Med 94: 643–646, 1981.

96. Thames KA, Rubin J, Teal N, Bower J: Do CAPD dialysate

losses reflect a patients dietary history? CRN Quart 10(4): 13–16, 1986.

97. Rubin J, Kirchner K, Barnes T, Teal N, Ray R, Bower J: Evaluation of continuous ambulatory peritoneal dialysis. Am J Kidney Dis 3: 199–204, 1983.

98. Handa SP, Cushner GB: Hyperosmolar hyperglycemic non-ketotic coma during peritoneal dialysis. Southern Med J 61: 700–702, 1968.

99. Greenblatt DJ: Fatal hypoglycaemia occuring after peritoneal dialysis. Brit Med J 2: 270–271, 1972.

100. Peitzman SJ, Agarwal BN: Spontaneous hypoglycemia in end-stage renal failure. Nephron 19: 131–139, 1977.

101. Maher JR, Chakrabarti E: Ultrafiltration by hyperosmotic peritoneal dialysis fluid excludes intracellular solutes. Am J Nephrol 4: 169–172, 1984.

102. Maher JF, Bennett RR, Hirszel P, Chakrabarti E: The mechanism of dextrose-enhanced transport rates. Kidney Int 28: 16–20, 1985.

103. Henderson LW: Peritoneal ultrafiltration dialysis: Enhanced urea transfer using hypertonic peritoneal dialysis fluids. J Clin Invest 45: 950–955, 1966.

104. Brown EA, Kliger AS, Goffinet J, Finkelstein FO: Effect of hypertonic dialysate clearances in the rat. Kidney Int 13: 271–277, 1978.

105. Rubin J, Klein E, Bower J: Investigation of the net sieving coefficient of the peritoneal membrane during peritoneal dialysis. ASAIO J 5: 9–15, 1982.

106. Rubin J, Reed V, Adair C, Bower J, Klein E: Effect of intraperitoneal insulin on solute kinetics in CAPD: Insulin kinetics in CAPD. Am J Med Sci 291: 81–87, 1986.

107. Albert A, Takamatsu H, Fonkalsrud EW: Absorption of glucose solutions from the peritoneal cavity in rabbits. Arch Surg 19: 1247–1251, 1984.

108. Rubin J, McFarland S, Hellems EW, Bower JD: Peritoneal dialysis during peritonitis. Kidney Int 19: 460–464, 1981.

109. Nolph K, Twardowski Z, Popovich R, Rubin J: Equilibration of peritoneal dialysis solutions during long dwell exchanges. J Lab Clin Med 93: 246–256, 1979.

110. Rubin J, Nolph K, Popovich R, Moncrief J, Prowant B: Drainage volumes during continuous ambulatory peritoneal dialysis. ASAIO J 2: 54–60, 1979.

111 Kreidet RT, Boeschoten EW, Zuyderhoudt FMJ, Arisz L: The relationship between peritoneal glucose absorption and body fluid loss by ultrafilatration during continuous ambulatory peritoneal dialysis. Clin Nephrol 27: 51–55, 1987.

112. Cunningham RS: Studies on absorption from serous cavities: The effect of dextrose upon the peritoneal mesothelium. Am J Physiol 53: 488–494, 1920.

113. Selby R, Gilsdorf R, Potter D, Schon D: Systemic appearance of nutrients used in peritoneal nutritional support. J Parent Nutr 8: 93, 1984.

114. Phanichphant S, Govithrapong: Short term effect of 4% hypertonic glucose as compared to 4% mixed hypertonic mannitol solution in conventional peritoneal dialysis. Nephron 40: 322–328, 1985.

115. Aviram A, Pfau A, Czaczkes JW, Ullmann TD: Hyperosmolality with hyponatremia, caused by inappropriate administration of mannitol. Am J Med 42: 648–650, 1967.

116. Quellhorst E, Mietzsch G, Doht B, Fernandez-Redo E, Kubosch J, Leititis U, Volles E, Thorwirt V, Scheler F: Sorbithaltige Spullosung als Ursache schwerer unvertraglichkeitsercheinungen bei der peritonealdialyse. Dtsch Med Wschr 100: 1431–1435, 1975.

117. Quellhorst E, Lowitz HD, Scheler F: Einflub der osmolaritat in der spulflussigkeit auf die effektivitat der peritonealdialyse. Klin Wschr 49: 583–587, 1971.

118. Bischel MC, Barbour BH: Peritoneal dialysis with sorbitol versus dextrose dialysate: Clinical findings and alterations of blood and cerebrospinal fluid. Nephron 12: 449–463, 1974.

119. Raja RM, Moros JG, Kramer MS, Rosenbaum JL: Hyperosmotic coma complicating peritoneal dialysis with sorbitol dialysate. Ann Intern Med 73: 993–994, 1970.

120. Yutuc W, Ward G, Shilipetar G, Tenckhoff H: Substitution of sorbiton for dextrose in peritoneal irrigation fluid: A preliminary report. Trans Am Soc Artif Intern Organs 13: 168–171, 1967.

121. Olmsted WH: The metabolism of mannitol and sorbitol: Diabetes 2: 132–137, 1953.

122. Yen TS: Experimental study on peritoneal dialysis using xylitol-containing solution. J Formosa Med Assoc 69: 292–303, 1970.

123. Bazzato G, Coli U, Landini S, Fracasso A, Morachiello P, Righetto F, Scanferla R, Onesti G: Xylitol as osmotic agent in CAPD: An alternative to glucose for uremic diabetic patients? Trans Am Soc Artif Intern Organs 28: 280–286, 1982.

124. Kiyasu JY, Chaikoff IL: On the manner of transport of absorbed fructose. J Biol Chem 2: 935–939, 1957.

125. Raja RM, Kramer MS, Manchanda R, Lazaro N, Rosenbaum JL: Peritoneal dialysis with fructose dialysate – prevention of hyperglycemia and hyperosmolality. Ann Intern Merd 79: 511–517, 1973.

126. Robson MD, Levy J, Rosenfeld JB: Hyperglycemia and hyperosmolality in peritoneal dialysis: Its prevention by the use of fructose. Proc EDTA 6: 300–306, 1969.

127. Heaton A, Ward MK, Johnston DG, Nigholson DV, Alberti KGMM, Kerr DNS: Short term studies on the use of glycerol as an osmotic agent in continuous ambulatory peritoneal dialysis (CAPD). Clin Sci 67: 121–130, 1884.

128. Heaton A, Ward MK, Johnston DG, Alberti KGMM, Kerr DNS: Evaluation of glycerol as an osmotic agent for continuous ambulatory peritoneal dialysis in end stage renal failure. Clin Sci 70: 23–29, 1986.

129. Daniels FH, Leonard EF, Cortell S: Glucose and glycerol compared as osmotic agents for peritoneal dialysis. Kidney Int 25: 20–25, 1984.

130. De Paepe M, Matthijs E, Dolkart R, Lameire N: Experience with glycerol as the osmotic agent in peritoneal dialysis in diabetic and non-diabetic patients, In: Keen H, Legrain M (eds), Prevention and treatment of diabetic nephropaty, MTP Press Limited, Boston 1983.

131. Lin ECC: Glycerol utilization and its regulation in mammals. Ann Rev Biochem 46: 765–795, 1977.

132. Lindholm B, Werynski A, Bergstrom J: Kinetics of peritoneal dialysis with glycerol and glucose as osmotic agents. Trans Am Soc Artif Intern Organs 33: 19–27, 1987.

133. Matthys E, Dolkart R, Lameire N: Extended use of a glycerol-containing dialysate in diabetic CAPD patients. Periton Dial Bull 7: 10–15, 1987.

134. Matthys E, Dolkart R, Lameire N: Potential hazards of glycerol dialysate in diabetic CAPD patients. Periton Dial Bull 7: 16–19, 1987.

135. Gjessing J: The use of dextran as a dialyzing fluid in peritoneal dialysis. Acta Med Scand 185: 237–239, 1969.

136. Jirka J, Kotkova E: Peritoneal dialysis by iso-oncotic dextran solution in anaesthetized dogs: Intraperitoneal fluid volume and protein concentration in the irrigation fluid. Proc Eur Dail Transplant Assoc 4: 141–145, 1967.

137. Young EA, Fletcher JT, Cioletti LA, Hollrah LA, Weser E: Metabolism of parenteral glucose oligo saccharides in man. J Parent Nutr 5: 369–377, 1981.

138. Higgins JT, Gross ML, Somani P: Patient tolerance and dialysis effectiveness of a glucose polymer-containing peritoneal dialysis solution. Periton Dial Bull (Supp) 4: 131–133, 1984.

139. Rubin J, Jones Q, Planch A, Bower J, Klein E: Evaluation of a peritoneal dialysis solution containing polymer. Am J Med Sci 289: 12–16, 1985.

140. Rubin J, Jones Q, Planch A, Bower J, Klein E: Substitution of a starch polymer for glucose in peritoneal dialysis. Nephron 39: 40–46, 1985.

141. Mistry CD, Mallick NP, Gokal R: Ultrafiltration with an isosmotic solution during long peritoneal dialysis exchanges. Lancet 25: 178–182, 1987.

142. Klein E, Ward RA, Williams TE, Feldhoff PW: Peptides as substitute osmotic agents for glucose in peritoneal dialysate. Trans Am Soc Artif Intern Organs 32: 550–553, 1986.

143. Fine J, Frank HA, Seligman AM: The treatment of acute renal failure by peritoneal irrigation. Ann Surg 124: 857–878, 1946.

144. Frank H, Seligman AM, Fine J: Further experiences with peritoneal irrigation for acute renal failure. Ann Surg 128: 561–608, 1948.

145. Twardowski ZJ, Moore HL, McGary TJ, Poskuta M, Stathakis C, Hirzel P: Polymers as osmotic agents for peritoneal dialysis. Periton Dial Bull (Supp) 4: 125–131, 1984.

146. Martis L, Deleo M, Tolburst T, Bock F, Chapman J: Oxypolygelatin as an osmotic agent for peritoneal dialysis. Abstracts ASAIO, p. 31, 1986.

147. Daniels F, Nedev N, Cataldo T, Leonard E, Cortell S: A macromolecular polyelectrolyte (gelifundol) as an osmotic agent. Abstracts Am Soc Nephrol, p. 81A, 1985.

148. Nolph K, Hopkins C, Rubin J, Twardowski Z, Popovich R, Van Stone J: Polymer induced ultrafiltration in dialysis: High osmotic pressure due to impermeant polymer sodium. Trans Am Soc Artif Intern Organs 24: 162–168, 1978.

149. Mcgary TJ, Nolph KD, Kartinos NJ: Polyanions as osmotic agents in a simulated in vitro model of peritoneal dialysis. ASAIO J 4: 108–116, 1981.

150. Schilling H, Wu G, Pettit J, Harrison J, McNeill K, Siccion Z, Oreopoulos DG: Nutritional status of patients on long-term CAPD. Periton Dial Bull5: 12–18, 1985.

151. Tuttle SG, Swendseid ME, Mulcare D, Griffith WH, Bassett SH: Essential amino acid requirements of older men in relation to total nitrogen intake. Metab Clin Exp 8: 61–72, 1959.

152. Rubin J, Kirchner K, Barnes T, Teal N, Ray R, Bower J: Evaluation of continuous ambulatory peritoneal dialysis. Am J Kidney Dis 3: 199–-204, 1983.

153. Rubin J, Flynn M, Nolph K: Total body potassium: A guide to nutritional health in patients undergoing continuous ambulatory peritoneal dialysis. Am J Clin Nutr 34: 94–98, 1981.

154. Giordano C, DeSanto NG, Capodicasa G, DiLeo VA, DiSerafino A, Cirillo D, Esposito R, Fiore R, Damiano M, Buonadonna L, Cocco F, DiIoria B: Amino acid losses during CAPD. Clin Nephrol 14: 230–232, 1980.

155. Khanna R, Wu G, Rodella H, Oreopoulous DG: Use of amino acid containing solution in CAPD. Periton Dial Bull (Supp) 4: 121–125, 1984.

156. Young GA, Parsons FM: The effect of peritoneal dialysis upon the amino acids and other nitrogenous compounds in the blood and dialysates from patients with renal failure. Clin Sci 37: 1–10, 1969.

157. Terry R, Sandrock WE, Nye RE, Whipple GH: Parenteral plasma protein maintains nitrogen equilibrium over long periods. J Exp Med 87: 547–559, 1948.

158. Gusberg RJ, Gump FE, Kinney JM: The demands of hyperalimentation on splanchinc blood flow and oxygen consumption. Surgt Forum 25: 56–58, 1974.

159. Fairman RM, Crosby LO, Stein TP, Buzby GP, Mullen JL: Prehepatic total parenteral nutrition in the chair-adapted primate. J Parent Enteral Nutr 7: 237–243, 1982.

160. Oren A, Wu G, Andersen GH, Marliss E, Khanna R, Pettit J, Mupas L, Rodella H, Brandes L, Roncari DA, Kakis G, Harrison J, McNeil K, Oreopoulos DG: Effective use of amino acids dialysate over four weeks in CAPD patients. Periton Dial Bull 3: 66–73, 1983.

161. Joyeux H, Astruc B, Solassol C: Total parenteral nutrition by portal vein in canine pregnancy. Acta Clin Scand (Supp) 466: 105, 1976.

162. Oreopoulos DG, Crassweller P, Katirtzoglou A, Ogilvie R, Zellerman G, Rodella H, Vas SI: Amino acids as an osmotic agent (instead of glucose) in continuous ambulatory peritoneal dialysis, In: Legrain (ed), Continuous Ambulatory Peritoneal Dialysis, Proceedings of an International Symposium, Amsterdam, Excerpta Medica, pp 335–340, 1979.

163. Furst P, Bergstrom J, Lindholm: Studies of amino acid metabolism in continuous ambulatory peritoneal dialysis patient's preliminary results, in Continuous Ambulatory Peritoneal Dialysis, Legrain (ed), Proceedings of an International Symposium, Amsterdam, Excerpta Medica, 1979, pp. 292–297.

164. Wells IC, Durr MP, Grabner BJ, Holladay FP, Campbell AS, Zielinski CM: Experimental study of chronic ambulatory peritoneal dialysis: Inhibition of protein and amino acid losses by single amino acids. Clin Physiol Biochem 3: 8–15, 1985.

165. Randerson DH, Chapman GV, Farrell PC: Amino acid and dietary status in CAPD patients, in Peritoneal Dialysis, Atkins RC, Thomson NM, Farrell PC (eds), New York, Churchill Livingstone, 1981, pp. 179–191.

166. Oreopoulos DG, Marliss E, Anderson GH, Sombros N, Williams P, Khanna R, Rodella H, Brandes L: Nutritional aspects of CAPD and the potential use of amino acid containing dialysis solution. Periton Dial Bull (Supp) 3: 10–12, 1983.

167. Williams PD, Marliss EB, Anderson GH, Oren A, Stein AN, Khanna R, Petitt J, Brandes L, Rodella H, Mupa L, Dombros N, Oreopoulos DG: Amino acid absorption following intraperitoneal administration in CAPD patients. Periton Dial Bull 2: 124–130, 1982.

168. Dombros N, Oren A, Marliss EB, Anderson GH, Stein AN, Khanna R, Petit J, Brandes L, Rodella H, Leibel BS, Oreopoulos D: Plasma amino acid profiles and amino acid losses in patients undergoing CAPD. Periton Dial Bull 2: 27–32, 1982.

169. Jackson MA, Thomas DW, Talbot S, Lee HA: Prevention of amino acid losses during peritoneal dialysis. Postgrad Med J 55: 533–536, 1979.

170. Pedersen FB, Dragsholt C, Frifelt JJ, Trostmann AF, Ekelund SS, Paaby P: Alternative use of amino acid and glucose solutions in CAPD. Periton Dial Bull 5: 215–218, 1985.

171. McGale EHF, Pickford JC, Aber GM: Quantitative changes in plasma amino acids in patients with renal disease. Clin Chim Acta 38: 395–403, 1972.

172. Kowalewski J, Tomaszewski J, Hanzlik J, Zawislak H: The elimination of free, peptide-bound and protein-bound hydroxyproline into dialysate during peritoneal dialysis in patients with renal failure. Clin Chim Acta 34: 123–126, 1971.

173. Gjessing J: Addition of amino acids to peritoneal dialysis fluid. Lancet 2: 812, 1968.

174. Yound GA, Keogh JB, Parsons FM: Plasma amino acids and protein levels in chronic renal failure and changes caused by oral supplements of essential amino acids. Clin Chim Acta 61: 205–213, 1975.

175. Kopple JD, Jones MP: Amino acid metabolism in patients with advanced uremia and in patients undergoing chronic dialysis. Adv Nephrol 8: 233–268, 1979.

176. Cernacek P, Becvarova H, Gerova Z, Valek A, Spustova V: Plasma tryptophan level in chronic renal failure. Clin Nephrol 14: 246–249, 1980.

177. Daniel RG, Waisman HA: Adaptation of the weanling rat to diets containing excess methionine. J Nutr 99: 299–306, 1969.

178. Zimmerman RA, Scott HM: Interrelationship of plasma amino acid levels and weight gain in the chick as influenced by suboptimal and superoptimal dietary concentrations of single amino acids. Nutrition 87: 13–18, 1965.

179. Stegink LD, Baker GL: Infusion of protein hydrolysates in the newborn infant: Plasma amino acid concentrations. J Ped 78:: 595–602, 1971.

180. Olney JW, Ho OL: Brain damage in infant mice following oral intake of glutamate, aspartate or cysteine. Nature 227: 609–611, 1970.

181. Heird WC, Nicholson JR, Driscoll JM, Schullinger JN, Winters RW: Hyperammonemia resulting from intravenous alimentation using a mixture of synthetic L-amino acids: A preliminary report. J Ped 81: 162–165, 1972.

182. Laegeler WL, Tio JM, Blake MI: Quality control and drug analysis: Stability of certain amino acids in a parental nutrition solution. Am J Hosp Pharm 31: 776–779, 1974.

183. Colding H, Andersen GE: Stability of antibiotics and amino acids in two synthetic 1-amino acid solutions commonly used for total parental nutrition in children. Antimicrob Agents Chemother 13: 555–558, 1978.

184. Lameire N: An evaluation of the dialysate solutions for continuous ambulatory peritoneal dialysis. Netherlands J Med 30: 301–307, 1987.

185. Bergstrom J, Furst P, Noree LO, Vinnars E: The effect of peritoneal dialysis on intracellular free amino acids in muscle from uraemic patients. Proc Eur Dial Transplant Assoc 9: 393–401, 1972.

186. Kopple JD, Blumenkrantz MJ, Jones MR, Moran JK, Coburn JW: Plasma amino acid levels and amino acid losses during continuous ambulatory peritoneal dialysis. Am J Clin Nutr 36: 395–402, 1982.

187. Giordano C, De Santo NG, Capodicasa G, Di Serafino A, Di Leo VA, Fiore R, Damiano M, Buonadonna L, Iorio B: Studies on amino acids in diabetic patients undergoing CAPD. Int J Artif Organs 4: 62–67, 1981.

188. Furst P, Bergstrom J, Josephson B, Noree LO: The effect of dialysis and administration of essential amino acids on plasma and muscle protein synthesis, studied with N in uraemic patients. Proc Eur Dial Transplant Assoc 7: 175–180, 1970.

189. Bergstrom J, Furst P, Noree LO, Vinnaars E: Intracellular free amino acids in muscle tissue of patients with chronic uraemia: Effect of peritoneal dialysis and infusion of essential amino acids. Clin Sci Mol Med 54: 51–60, 1978.

190. Hanning RM, Balfe JW, Zlotkin SH: Effectiveness and nutritonal consequences of amino acid based vs glucose based dialysis solutions in infants and children receiving CAPD. Am J Clin Nutr 46: 22–30, 1987.

191. De Alvaro, Jimeno A, Perez-Diaz V, Largo E, Ibanes E, Martin del Rio R, Latorre A, Anllo F, Ortiz O: Parenteral nutrition via the peritoneum with dextrose and amino acids. Nephron 46: 49–56, 1987.

192. Mitwalli A, Rodella H, Brandes L. Wanless I, Wu G, Ogilvie R, Schilling H, Dobbie JW, Wilson LS, Oreopoulos DG: Is fat absorbed through the peritoneum? Periton Dial Bull 5: 165–168, 1985.

193. Coran AG, Herman CM: The use of parental alimentation in renal failure: The effect of an intravenous fat emulsion and essential amino acids on dogs undergoing bilateral nephrectomy. J Ped Surg 7:21–26, 1972.

194. Gjessing J: Absorption of amino acids and fat from the peritoneum. Opuse Med Bd 13: 251–252, 1968.

195. Rubin J, Jones Q, Planch A, Bower J: Intraperitoneal feeding. Trans Am Soc Artif Intern Organs, June 1988, (in press).

196. Stewart WK, Anderson DC, Wilson MI: Hazard of peritoneal dialysis: Contaminated Fluid. Brit Med J 1: 606–607, 1967.

197. Karanicolas S, Oreopoulos DG, Inzatt SH, Shimizu A, Manning RF, Sepp H, DeVeber GA, Darby T: Epidemic of aseptic peritonitis caused by endotoxin during chronic peritoneal dialysis. New Engl J Med 296: 1336–1337, 1976.

198. Solary E, Cabanne JF, Tanter Y, Rifle G: Evidence for a role of plasticizers in 'eosinophilic' peritonitis in continuous ambulatory peritoneal dialysis. Nephron 4 341–342, 1986.

199. Patterson R, Lerner C, Roberts M, Moel D, Grammer LC: Ethylene oxide (ETO) as a possible cause of an allergic reaction during peritoneal dialysis and immunologic detection of eto from dialysis tubing. Am J Kidney Dis 8: 64–66, 1986.

200. Nassberger L, Arbin A, Ostelius J: Exposure of patients to phthalates from polyvinyl chloride tubes and bags during dialysis. Nephron 45: 286–290, 1987.

201. Cumming AD, Simpson G, Bell D, Cowie J, Winney RJ: Acute aluminium intoxication in patients on continuous ambulatory peritoneal dialysis. Lancet 1: 103–104, 1982.

202. Thomson NM, Stevens BJ, Humphre TJ, Atkins RC: Comparison of trace elements in peritoneal dialysis, hemodialysis, and uremia. Kidney Int 23: 9–14, 1983.

203. Leung A, Henderson I, Halls D, Fell G, Kennedy AC: Trace element abnormalities in continuous ambulatory peritoneal dialysis. Proc EDTA 22: 410–414, 1985.

204. Wallaeys B, Cornelis R, Mees L, Lameire N: Trace elements in serum, packed cells and dialysate of CAPD patients. Kidney Int 30: 599–604, 1986.

205. Tamura T, Cornwell PE, Vaughn WH, Waldo FB, Kohaut EC. Zinc levels in peritoneal dialysate. Am J Clin Nutr 41: 865, 1985.

206. Zlotkin SH, Rundle MA, Hanning RM, Buchanan BE, Balfe JW: Zinc absorption from glucose and amino acid dialysis solutions in children on continuous ambulatory peritoneal dialysis (CAPD). J Am Coll Nutr 6: 345–350, 1987.

207. Halaby SF, Mattocks AM: Absorption of sodium bisulfate from peritoneal dialysis solutions. J Pharm Sci 54: 52–55, 1965.

208. Bhaghat B, Lockett MF: The absorption and elimination of metabisulphite and thiosulphate by rats. J Surg Res 25: 232–235, 1978.

209. Wilkins JW, Rivecca JN: Measurement of bisulfite in biologic solutions. Clin Chem 15: 997–1001, 1969.

210. Wilkins JM, Greene JA, Weller JM: Toxicity of intraperitoneal bisulfite. Clin Pharm Ther 9: 328–332, 1968.

211. Lasker N, Burker JF, Patchefsky A, Haughey E: Peritoneal reactions to particulate matter in peritoneal dialysis solutions. Trans Am Soc Artif Intern Organs 21: 342–345, 1975.

212. Verger C, Berry JP, Galle P, Lavergne A, Hoang C, LeCharpentier Y: Foreign material inclusions in the peritoneum of CAPD patients: A study with x-ray microanalysis. Periton Dial Bull 2: 138–139, 1982.

213. Abrutyn E, Goodhart GL, Ross K, Anderson R, Buxton A: Acinetobacter calcoaceticus outbreak associated with peritoneal dialysis solutions. Am J Epidemiol 107: 328–335, 1978.

214. Breborowicz A, Knapowski J, Breborowicz G: Intracellular calcium ions modulate permeability of the peritoneal mesothelium in vitro. Periton Dial Bull 5: 105–108, 1985.

215. Knapowski JB, Simon MP, Feder EM: Preparation of parietal peritoneum for measurements of in vitro permeability. Artif Organs 3: 219–223, 1979.

216. Knapowski J, Baczyk K, Goral R, Adam W: Effect of ethacrynic acid on water transfer and sodium transfer across human peritoneal membrane. Curr Prob Clin Biochem 4: 126–130, 1975.

217. Berndt WO, Gosselin RE: Rubidium and creatinine transport across isolated mesentery. Biochem Pharmacol 8: 359–366, 1961.

218. Berndt WO, Gosselin RE: Action of vasopressin on the permeability of mesentery. Science 134: 1987–1988, 1961.

219. Berndt WO, Gosselin RE: Differential changes in permeability of mesentery to rubidium and phosphate. Am J Physiol 202: 761–767, 1962.

220. Shear L, Castollot JJ, Barry KG: Peritoneal fluid absorption: Effects of dehydration on kinetics. J Lab Clin Med 66: 232, 1965.

221. Nolph KD, Popovich RP, Ghods AJ: Determinants of low

clearances of small solutes during peritoneal dialysis. Kidney Int 13: 117–123, 1978.

222. Aune S: Transperitoneal exchange: Peritoneal blood flow estimated by hydrogen gas clearance. Scand J Gastroenterol 5: 99, 1970.

223. Henderson LW, Kintzel JE: Influence of antidiuretic hormone on peritoneal membrane area and permeability. J Clin Invest 50: 237–244, 1971.

224. Patton JF, Doolittle WH, Hamlet MP: Peritoneal clearance of urea and potassium following experimental hypothermia. J Appl Physiol 36: 403–406, 1974.

225. Greene JA, Lapco L, Weller JM: Effect of drug therapy of hemmorrhagic hypotension on kinetics of peritoneal dialysis in the dog. Nephron 7: 178–183, 1970.

226. Hirszel P, Naher JF, LeGrow W: Increased peritoneal mass transport with glucagon acting at the vascular surface. Trans Am Soc Artif Intern Organs 24: 136–138, 1978.

227. Maher JF, Hirszel P, Lasrich M: Effects of gastrointestinal hormones on transport by peritoneal dialysis. Kidney Int 16: 130–136, 1979.

228. Felt J, Richard C, McCaffrey C, Levy M: Peritoneal clearance of creatinine and inulin during dialysis in dogs: Effect of splanchnic vasodilators. Kidney Int 16: 459–469, 1979.

229. Miller FN, Nolph KD, Joshua IG, Wiegman DL, Harris PD, Andersen DB: Hyperosmolality, acetate, and lactate: Dilatory factors during peritoneal dialysis. Kidney Int 20: 397–402, 1981.

230. Rubin J, Nolph K, Arfania D, Wiegman D, Miller F, Harris F: Comparison of the effects of lactate and acetate on clinical peritoneal clearances. Clin Nephrol 12: 145–147, 1979.

231. Nolph K, Rubin J, Wiegman D, Harris P, Miller F: Peritoneal clearances with three types of commercially available peritoneal dialysis solutions: Effects of pH adjustment and intraperitoneal nitroprusside. Nephron 24: 35–40, 1979.

232. Rubin J, Nolph K, Arfania D, Miller F, Wiegman D, Joshua L Harris P: Studies on non-vasoactive peritoneal dialysis solutions. J Lab Clin Med 93: 901–915, 1979.

233. Mileti M, Bufano G, Scaravonati P, Pecchini F, Carnevale G, Lanzarini P: Effect of indomethacin on the peritoneum of rabbits on peritoneal dialysis. Periton Dial Bull 3:4–194, 1983.

234. Steinhauer HB, Schollmeyer P: Prostaglandin mediated loss of proteins during peritonitis in continuous ambulatory peritoneal dialysis. Kidney Int 29: 584–590, 1986.

235. Hirszel P, Lisrich M, Maher JF: Arachidonic acid increases peritoneal clearances. Trans AM Soc Artif Intern Organs 27: 61–63, 1981.

236. Maher JF, Hirszel P, Lasrich M: Prostaglandin effects on peritoneal transport, In: Gahl GM, Kessel M, Nolph KD, (eds), Advances in Peritoneal Dialysis, Proceedings of the Second International Symposium on Peritoneal Dialysis, Amsterdam, Excerpta Medica, pp 65–72, 1981.

237. Rubin J, Klein E, Bower J: Investigation of the net sieving coefficient of the peritoneal membrane during peritoenal dialysis. ASAIO J 5: 9–15, 1982.

238. Ahearn DJ, Nolph KD: Controlled sodium removal with peritoneal dialysis Trans Am Soc Artif Intern Organs 18: 423–428, 1972.

239. Exaire E, Becerra AT, Monteon F: An overview of treatment with peritoneal dialysis in drug poisoning: Contr Nephrol 17: 39–43, 1979.

240. Maher JF, Hohnadel DC, Shea C, Disanzo F, Cassetta M: Effect of intraperitoneal diuretics on solute transport during hypertonic dialysis. Clin Nephrol 7: 96–100, 1977.

241. Grzegorzewska A, Baczyk K: Furosemide-induced increase in urinary and peritoneal excretion of uric acid during peritoneal dialysis in patients with chronic uremia. Artif Organs 6: 220–224, 1983.

242. Boutron HF, Brocard JF, Singlas E: Pharmacokinetic of

furosemide in CAPD, In: Gahl GM, Kessel M, Nolph KD (eds), Advances in Peritoneal Dialysis, Proceedings of the Second International Symposium on Peritoneal Dialysis, Amsterdam, Excerpta Medica, pp 90–92, 1981.

243. Furman KL, Gomperts ED, Hockley J: Activity of intraperitoneal heparin during peritoneal dialysis. Clin Nephrol 9: 15–18, 1978.

244. Hare HG, Valtin H, Gosselin RE: Effect of drugs on peritoneal dialysis in the dog. J Pharmacol Exp Ther 145: 122–129, 1964.

245. Rubin J, Adair C, Johnson B, Bower J: Stereospecific lactate absorption during peritoneal dialysis. Nephron 31: 224–228, 1982.

246. Indraprasit S, Sooksriwongse C: Effect of chlorpromazine on peritoneal clearances. Nephron 40: 341–343, 1985.

247. El-Bassiouni EA, Mattocks AM: Acceleration of peritoneal dialysis with minimal N-Myristyl-B-Aminopropionate. J Pharm Sci 62: 1314–1317, 1973.

248. Kudla RM, El-Bassiouni EA, Mattocks AM: Accelerated peritoneal dialysis of barbiturates, diphenylhydantoin, and salicylate. J Pharm Sci 60: 1065–1067, 1971.

249. Mattocks AM, Penzotti SC: Acceleration of peritoneal dialysis with minimum amounts of dioctyl sodium sulfosuccinate. J Pharm Sci 61: 475–476, 1972.

250. Mattocks AM: Accelerated removal of salicylate by additives in peritoneal dialysis fluid. J Pharm Sci 58: 595–598, 1969.

251. McLean WM, Poland DM, Cohon MS, Penzotti SC, Mattocks AM: Effect of Tris (hydroxymethyl) aminomethane on removal of urea by peritoneal dialysis. J Pharm Sci 56: 1614–1621, 1967.

252. Grzegorzewska A, Beczy K: Furosemide induced discrepancy between peritoneal clearnace of uric acid and potassium in terminal uraemic, In: Gahl GM, Kessel M, Nolph KD, (eds), Advances in Peritoneal Dialysis, Proceedings of the Second International Symposium, Amsterdam, Excerpta Medica, pp 93–95, 1981.

253. Penzotti SC, Mattocks AM: Acceleration of peritoneal dialysis by surface-active agents. J Pharm Sci 57: 1192–1195, 1968.

254. Hirszel P, Chakrabarti E, Maher J: Exaggerated protein loss complicating sterile peritonitis results from increased diffusion. Periton Dial Bull 6: 141–143, 1986.

255. Alavi N, Lsaianos E, van Liew JB, Mookerjee BK, Bentzel CJ: Peritoneal permeability in the rat: Modulation by microfilament-active agents. Kidney Int 27: 411–419, 1985.

256. Hirszel P, Dodge K, Maher JF: Acceleration of peritoneal solute transport by cytochalasin D. Uremia Invest 8: 85–88, 1984.

257. Etteldorf JN, Dobbins WT, Summitt RL, Rainwater WT, Fischer RL: Intermittent peritoneal dialysis using 5 per cent albumin in the treatment of salicylate intoxication in children. J Ped 58: 226–236, 1961.

258. Christoforov B, Ingrand J, Petite JP, Foliot A: Captation de la bilirubine non conjuguee par des dialyses peritoneales avec une solution de serum albumine humaine. Path Biol 17: 985–990m 1969.

259. Grollman AP, Odell GB: Removal of bilirubin by albumin binding during intermittent peritoneal dialysis. New Engl J Med 267: 279–282, 1962.

260. Hobolth N, Devantier M: Removal of indirect reacting bilirubin by albumin binding during intermittent peritoneal dialysis in the newborn. Acta Poediat Scand 58: 171–172, 1969.

261. Perrin JH, Field FP, Hansen DA, Mufson RA, Totosian G: B-cyclodextrin as an aid to peritoneal dialysis: Renal toxicity of B-cyclodextrin in the rat. Res Comm Chem Pathol Pharmacol 19: 373–376, 1978.

262. Nahas GG, Gjessing J, Giroux JJ, Verosky M, Mark LC: The passage of THAM across the peritoneum during dialysis. Clin Pharm Ther 6: 560–567, 1965.

263. Nolph KD, Miller L, Husted FC, Hirszel P: Peritoneal

clearances in scleroderma and diabetes mellitus: Effects of intrapertitoneal isoproterenol. Int Urol Nephrol 8: 161–169, 1976.

264. Brown ST, Ahearn DJ, Nolph KD: Reduced peritoneal clearances in scleroderma increased by intraperitoneal isoproterenol. Ann Intern Med 78: 891–894, 1973.

265. Gutman RA, Nixon WP, McRae RL, Spencer HW: Effect of intraperitoneal and intravenous vasoactive amines on peritoneal dialysis: Study in anephric dogs. Trans Am Soc Artif Intern Organs 22: 570–573, 1976.

266. Chan MK, Varghese A, Baillod RA, Moorhead JF: Peritoneal Dialysis: Effect of intraperitoneal dopamine. Dial Transplant 9: 382–384, 1980.

267. Hirszel P, Lasrich M, Naher JF: Augmentation of peritoneal mass transport by dopamine: Comparison with norepinephrine and evaluation of pharmacologic mechanisms. J Lab Clin Med 94: 747–754, 1979.

268. Maher JF, Hirszel P, Galen MA: Enhanced transport with dipyridamole. Trans Am Soc Artif Intern Organs 23: 219–223, 1977.

269. Ryckelynck J, Pierre D, Demartin A: Enhancement of peritoneal clearance with dipyridamole. Nouv Presse Med 7: 472, 1978.

270. Rubin J, Adair C, Barnes T, et al: Augmentation of peritoneal clearance by dipyridamole. Kidney Int 22: 658–661, 1982.

271. Rubin J, Adair C, Bower J: A double blind trial of dipyridamole in CAPD. Am J Kidney Dis 5: 262–266, 1985.

272. Selgas R, Carmona AR, Martinez ME, Perez-Fontan M, Salinas M, Conesa J, Ara JM, Sicilia LS: Peritoneal vascular reserve characterization through nitroprusside-induced modification of peritoneal mass transfer coefficients. Int J Artif Organs 8: 181–186, 1985.

273. Nolph KD, Ghods AJ, Brown PA, Twardowski ZJ: Effects of intraperitoneal nitroprusside on peritoneal clearances in man with variations of dose, frequency of administration and dwell times. Nephron 24: 111–120, 1979.

274. DeSanto NG, Capodicasa G, Capasso G, Giordano C: Development of means to augment peritoneal urea clearances: The synergistic effects of combining high dialysate temperature and high dialysate flow rates with dextrose nitroprusside. Artif Organs 5: 409–414, 1981.

275. Finkelstein FO, Yap P, Kliger AS: Effect of nitroprusside on peritoneal dialysis clearances. Yale J Biol 53: 127–132, 1980.

276. Riambau E, Lloveras J, Orfila MA, Masramon J, Llorach N: Significance of the sequential intraperitoneal administration of nitroprusside in intermittent peritoneal dialysis, In: Gahl GM, Kessel M, Nolph KD (eds), Advancs in Peritoneal Dialysis, Proceedings of the Second International Symposium on Peritoneal Dialysis, Amsterdam, Excerpta Medica, pp 82–84, 1981.

277. Guttman RA: Automated peritoneal dialysis for home use. Quart J Med 47: 261–280, 1978.

278. Nance KS, Matzke GR: Stability of gentamicin and tobramycin in concentrate solutions for automated peritoneal dialysis. Am J Nephrol 4: 240–243, 1984.

279. Glew RH, Pavuk RA: Stability of vancomycin and aminoglycoside antibiotics in peritoneal dialysis concentrate. Nephron 28: 241–243, 1981.

280. Rubin J, Humphries H, Smith G, Bower G: Antibiotic activity in peritoneal dialysate. Am J Kidney Dis 3:205–208, 1983.

281. Appleby DH, John JF: Effect of peritoneal dialysis solution on the antimicrobial activity of cephalosporins. Nephron 30: 341–344, 1982.

282. Grise G, Lemeland JF, Fillastre JP: Etude De la stabilite de huit cephalosporines de deuxieme et troisieme generations dans le liquide de dialyse peritoneale. Path Biol 33: 335–339, 1985.

283. McCormick EM, Echols RM: Effect of peritoneal dialysis

fluid pH on bactericidal activity of ciprofloxacin. Anitmicrobial agents and chemotherapy 31: 657–659, 1987.

284. Schwartz MA, Bara E, Rubycz I, Granatek AP: Stability of methicillin. J Pharm Sci 54: 149–150, 1965.

285. Zost ED, Uanghick VA: Compatibility and stability of disodium carbenicillin in combination with other drugs and large volume parenteral solutions. Am J Hosp Pharm 29: 135–140, 1972.

286. Janknegt R, Koks CHW, Nube MJ: Stability of antibiotics in CAPD fluid. Periton Dial Bull 5: 78–79, 1985.

287. Sewell DJ, Golper TA, Brown SD, Nelson E, Knower M, Kimbrough RC: Stability of single and combination antimicrobial agents in various peritoneal dialysates in the presence of inulin and heparin. Am J Kidney Dis 3: 209–212, 1983.

288. Pickering LK, Rutherford I: Effect of concentration and time upon inactivation of tobramycn, gentamicin, netilmicin and amikacin by azlocillin, carbenicillin, mecillinam, mezlocillin and piperacillin. J Pharm Exp Ther 217: 345–349, 1980.

289. Sewell DL, Golper TA: Stability of antimicrobial agnets in peritoneal dialysate. Antimicrob Agents Chemother 21: 528–529, 1982.

290. Loeppky C, Tarka E, Everett ED: Compatibility of cephalosporins and aminoglycosides in peritoneal dialysis fluid. Periton Dial Bull 3: 127–129, 1983.

291. Walker PC, Kaufmann RE, Massoud N: Compatability of cefazolin and gentamicin in peritoneal dialysis solutions. Drug intelligence and Clinical Pharmacy 20: 697–700, 1986.

292. Shalit I, Welch DF, Joaquin VHS, Marks M: In vitro antibacterial activities of antibiotics against Pseudomonas aeruginosa in peritoneal dialysis fluid. Antimicrob Agents Chemother 27: 908–911, 1985.

293. Chan MK, Browning AK, Poole CJM, Matheson LA, Li CS, Baillod RA, Moorhead JF: Cefuroxime pharmacokinetics in continuous and intermittent peritoneal dialysis. Nephron 41: 161–165, 1985.

294. Kane M, Jay M, DeLuca PP: Binding of insulin to a continuous ambulatory peritoneal dialysis system. Am J Hosp Pharm 43: 81–88, 1986.

295. Johnson CA, Amidon GA, Reichert JE, Porter WR: Adsorption of insulin to the surface of peritoneal dialysis solution containers. Am J Kidney Dis 3: 224–228, 1983.

296. Twardowski ZJ, Nolph KD, McGary TJ, Moor HL: Nature of insulin binding to plastic bags. Am J Hosp Pharm 40: 579–582, 1983.

297. Twardowski ZJ, Nolph KD, McGary TJ, Moore HL: Influence of temperature and time on insulin adsorption to plastic bags. Am J Hosp Pharm 40:583–586, 1983

298. Twardowski ZJ, Nolph KD, McGary TJ, Moore HL, Collin P, Ausman RK, Slimack WS: Insulin binding to plastic bags: A methodologic study. Am J Hosp Pharm 40: 575–579, 1983.

299. Ryan DM: Influence of surface area/volume ratio on the kinetics of antibiotics in different tissues and tissue fluids. Scand J Infect Dis (Supp) 44: 24–33, 1985.

300. Low DE, Vas SI, Oreopoulos DG, Manuel MA, Saiphoo MM, Finer C, Dombros N: Prophylactic cephalexin ineffective in chronic ambulatory peritoneal dialysis. Lancet 2:753–754, 1970.

301. Axelrod J, Meyers BR, Hirschman SZ, Stein R: Prophylaxis with cephalothin in peritoneal dialysis. Arch Intern Med 132: 368–371, 1973.

302. Schwartz FD, Kallmeyer J, Dunea G, Kark RM: Prevention of infection during peritoneal dialysis. JAMA 199: 115–117, 1967.

303. Eremin J, Marshall VC: The place of prophylactic antibiotic in peritoneal dialysis. Austral Ann Med 18: 264–266, 1969.

304. D'Ocon, Fereres J, Maqueda S, Prats D, Touchard A: Uso Profilactico De Antibioticos en dialisis peritoneal. Pevista Clinica Espanola 126: 333–336, 1972.

305. Manuel MA, Paton TW, Cornish WR: Drugs and peritoneal

dialysis. Periton Dial Bull 3: 117–125, 1983.

306. Gibson TP: Dialyzability of common therapeutic agents. Dial Transplant 8: 24–40, 1979.

307. Bunke CM, Aronoff GR, Luft FC: Prediction of antibiotic concentrations in patients receiving continuous ambulatory peritoneal dialysis, In: Proceedings of the 13th International Congress of Chemotherapy, Spitzy KH, Karrer K (eds), Vienna, Austria, pp 81–82, 1983.

308. Jackson EA, McLeod DC: Pharmacokinetics and dosing of antimicrobial agents in renal impairment. Am J Hosp Pharm 31: 36–52, 1974.

309. Jackson EA, McLeod DC: Pharmacokinetics and dosing of antimicrobial agents in renal impairment. Am J Hosp Pharm 31: 137–148, 1974.

310. Johnson CA, Zimmerman SW, Rogge M: The pharmacokinetics of antibiotics used to treat peritoneal dialysis-associated peritonitis. Am J Kidney Dis 4: 3–17, 1984.

311. Bennett WM: Drug prescribing in renal failure. Drugs 17: 111–123, 1979.

312. Bunke CM, Aronoff GR, Luft FC: Pharmacokinetics of common antibiotics used in continuous ambulatory peritoneal dialysis. Am J Kidney Dis 3: 114–117, 1983.

313. Paton TW, Cornish WR, Manuel MA, Hardy BG: Drug therapy in patients undergoing peritoneal dialysis: Clinical pharmacokinetic considerations. Clin Pharm 10: 404–426, 1985.

314. Bennett WM, Muther RS, Parker RA, Feig P, Morrison G, Golper TA, Singer I: Drug therapy in renal failure: Dosing guidlines for adults. Ann Intern Med 93: 62–89, 1980.

315. Bennett WM, Muther RS, Parker RA, Feig P, Morrison G, Golper TA, Singer I: Drug therapy in renal failure: Dosing guidelines for adults. Ann Intern Med 93: 286–325, 1980.

316. Maher JF: Pharmacokinetics in patients with renal failure. Clin Nephrol 21: 39–46, 1984.

317. Watanabe AS: Pharmacokinetic aspects of the dialysis of drugs. Drug Intell Clin Pharm 2: 407–416, 1977.

318. Reidenberg MM: Drug metabolism in uremia. Clin Nephrol 4: 83–85, 1975.

319. Janknegt R, Nube MJ: A simple method for predicting drug clearances during CAPD. Periton Dial Bull 5: 254–255, 1985.

320. Keane WF, Everett ED, Fine R, Golper TA, Vas SI, Peterson PK: CAPD related peritonitis management and antibiotic therapy recommendations travenol peritonitis management advisory group. Periton Dial Bull 7: 55–62, 1987.

321. Munch R, Seurer J, Siegenthaler W, Kuhlmann U: Serum and dialysate concentrations of intraperitoneal cephalothin in patients undergoing continuous ambulatory peritoneal dialysis. Clin Nephrol 20: 40–43, 1983.

322. Rubin J, Adair C: Nitrogen losses and cephalotin absorption in peritonitis treated by hourly peritoneal dialysis. Am J Kidney Dis (in press).

323. Kayer D, Wenger N, Agarwal B: Pharmacology of intraperitoneal cefalozin in patients undergoing peritoneal dialysis. Antimicrob Agents Chemother 14: 318–312, 1978.

324. Bunke CM, Aronoff GR, Brier ME, Sloan RTS, Luft FC: Cefalozin and cephalexin kinetics in continuous ambulatory peritoneal dialysis. Clin Pharmacol Ther 33: 66–72, 1983.

325. Levison ME, Levison SP, Kies K, Kaye D: Pharmacology of cefalozin in patients with normal and abnormal renal function. J Ineft Dis (Supp) 128: 354–357, 1973.

326. Chow Tung E, Lau AH, Vidyasagar D, John EG: Effect of peritoneal dialysis on serum concentrations of three drugs commonly used in pediatric patients. Dev Pharmacol 8: 85–95, 1985.

327. Johnson CA, Welling PG, Zimmerman SW: Pharmacokinetics of oral cephradine in continuous ambulatory peritoneal dialysis patients. Nephron 38: 57–61, 1984.

328. Boeschoten EW, Rietstra PJGM, Krediet RT, BVVisser MJ, Arisz L: CAPD peritonitis: A prospective randomized trial of oral versus intraperitoneal treatment with cephradine. J Antimicrob Chemother 16: 789–797, 1985.

329. Searle M, Raman GV: Oral treatment of peritonitis complicating continuous ambulatory peritoneal dialysis. Clin Nephrol 23: 241–244, 1985.

330. Drew PJT, Casewell MW, Desai N, Houang ET, Simpson CN, Marsh FP: Cephalexin for the oral treatment of CAPD peritonitis. J Antimicrob Chemother 13: 153–159, 1984.

331. Ritzerfeld VW, Westerboer S, Trappe H: Cephalexin in serum, dialysat und urin nierengeschadigter patienten. Arzneim Forsch Jahrgang 20: 1881–1884, 1970.

332. Davis GM, Forland SC, Cutler RE: Serum and dialysate concentrations of cephalexin following repeated dosing in CAPD patients. Am J Kidney Dis 6: 177–180, 1985.

333. Greaves WL, Kreeft JH, Ogilvie RI, Richards GK: Cefoxitin disposition during peritoneal dialysis. Antimicrob Agents Chemther 19: 253–255, 1981.

334. Arvidsson, Alvan G, Tranaeus A, Malmborg AS: Pharmacokinetic studies of cefoxitin in continuous ambulatory peritoneal dialysis. Eur J Clin Pharmacol 28: 333–337, 1985.

335. McIntosh ME, Smith WGJ, Junor BJR, Forrest G, Brodie MJ: The effect of peritonitis on the distribution of cefuroxime in patients undergoing continuous ambulatory peritoneal dialysis. Scot Med J 29: 117–118, 1984.

336. Chan MK, Browning AK, Poole CJM, Matheson LA, Li CS, Baillod RA, Moorhead JF: Cefuroxime pharmacokinetics in continuous and intermittent peritoneal dialysis. Nephron 41: 161–165, 1985.

337. Local FK, Munro AJ, Kerr DNS, Sussman M: Pharmacokinetics of intravenous and intraperitoneal cefuroxime in patients undergoing peritoneal dialysis. Clin Nephrol 16: 40–43, 1981.

338. LaGreca G, Biasioli S, Chiaramonte S, Fabris A, Feriani M, Pisanti E, Ronco C, Xerri L: Pharmacokinetics of intravenous and intraperitoneal cefuroxime during peritoneal dialysis. Int J Clin Pharmacol Ther Toxicol 20: 92–94, 1982.

339. McIntosh ME, Smith WGJ, Junor BJR, Forrest G, Brodie MJ: The effect of peritonitis on the distribution of cefuroxime in patients undergoing continuous ambulatory peritoneal dialysis. Scott Med J 29: 117–118, 1984.

340. Pancorbo S, Comty C: Pharmacokinetics of cefamandole in patients undergoing continuous ambulatory peritoneal dialysis. Periton Dial Bull 3: 135–137, 1983.

341. Yamasaku F, Rsuchida R, Usuda Y: A study of the kinetics of cephalosporins in renal impairment. Postgrad Med J 46: 57–59, 1970.

342. Bliss M, Mayerson M, Arnold T, Logan J, Michael UF, Jones W: Disposition kinetics of cefamandole during continuous ambulatory peritoneal dialysis. Antimicrob Agents Chemother 29: 649–653, 1986.

343. Meyers BR, Hirschman SZ: Pharmacokinetics of cefamandole in patients with renal failure, Antimicrob Agents Chemother 11: 248–250, 1977.

344. Ahern MJ, Finkelstein FO, Andriole VT: Pharmacokinetics of cefamandole in patients undergoing hemodialysis and peritoneal dialysis. Antimicrob Agents Chemother 10: 457–461, 1976.

345. Janicke DM, Morse GD, Apicella MA, Jusko WJ, Walshe JJ: Pharmacokinetic modeling of bidirectional transfer during peritoneal dialysis. Clin Pharmacol Ther 40: 209–218, 1986.

346. Morse GD, Rowinski C, Lieveld PE, Walshe JJ: Drug-protein binding during continuous ambulatory peritoneal dialysis. Periton Dial Bull 6: 144–147, 1986.

347. Morse GD, Lane T, Nairn DK, Deterding J, Curry J, Gal P: Peritoneal transport of cefonicid. Antimicrob Agents Chemother 31: 292–294, 1987.

348. Burgess ED, Blair AD: Pharmacokinetics of ceftizoxime in patients undergoing continuous ambulatory peritoneal dialysis. Antimicrob Agents Chemother 24: 237–239, 1983.

349. Johnson CA, Zimmerman SW, Bayer W, Craig WA: Pharmacokinetics of intravenous ceftizoxime in patients on continuous ambulatory peritoneal dialysis. Clin Nephrol 23: 120–124, 1985.

350. Gruer LD, Bartlett R, Ayliffe GAJ: Species identification and antibiotic sensitivity of coagulase negative staphylococci from CAPD peritonitis. J Antimicrob Agents Chemother 13: 577–583, 1984.

351. Gross MJ, Somani P, Ribner BS, Raeader R, Freimer EH, Higgins JT: Ceftizoxime elimination kinetics in continuous ambulatory peritoneal dialysis. Clin Pharmacol Ther 34: 673–680, 1983.

352. Tourkantonis A, Nicolaidis P: Pharmacokinetics of ceftazidime in patients undergoing peritoneal dialysis. J Antimicrob Chemother 12: 263–267, 1983.

353. Comstock TJ, Straughn AB, Krauss AP, Meyer MC, Finn AL, Chubb JM: Ceftazidime (CAZ) (GR20263) pharmacokinetics during continuous ambulatory peritoneal dialysis (CAPD) and intermittent peritoneal dialysis (IPD). Drug Intell Clin Pharm 17: 453, 1983.

354. Gray HH, Goulding S, Eykyn SJ: Intraperitoneal vancomycin and ceftazidime in the treatment of CAPD peritonitis. Clin Nephrol 23: 81–84, 1985.

355. Konigshausen T, Nachtigall W, Putzhofen G, Rosin H: Pharmacokinetics of lamoxactam in patients using continuous ambulatory peritoneal dialysis (CAPD), In: Spitzy KH, Karrer K (eds), Proceedings of the 13th International Congress of Chemotherapy, Vienna, Austria, pp 6–10, 1983.

356. Ragnaud JM, Albin H, Wone C: Pharmacokinetics of latamofex (moxalactam) in patients on CPAD. Periton Dial Bull 5: 208, 1985.

357. Singlas E, Boutron HF, Merdjan H, Brocard JF, Pocheville M, Fries D: Moxalactam klinetics during chronic ambulatory peritoneal dialysis. Clin Pharmacol Ther 34: 403–407, 1983.

358. Morse G, Janicke D, Cafarell R, Piontek K, Apicella M, Jusko WJ, Walshe J: Moxalactam epimer disposition in patients undergoing continuous ambulatory peritoneal dialysis. Clin Pharmacol Ther 38: 150–156, 1985.

359. Jones TE, Milne RW, Mudaliar Y, Sansom LN: Moxalactam kinetics during continuous ambulatory peritoneal dialysis after intraperitoneal administration. Antimicrob Agents Chemother 28: 293–298, 1985.

360. Ragnaud JM, Roche-Bezian MC, Marceau C, Demothes-Mainard F, Albin H, Prevost D, Wone C: Traitement des peritonites en dialyse peritoneale continue ambulatoire par une dose quotidienne de 1g de cefotiam par voie intraperitoneale. Path Biol 34: 512–516, 1986.

361. Hodler JE, Galeazzi RL, Rudhardt M, Seiler AJ: Pharmacokinetics of cefoperazone in patients undergoing chronic ambulatory peritoneal dialysis: Clinical and pathophysiological implications. Eur J Clin Pharmacol 26: 609–612, 1984.

362. Keller E, Jansen A, Pelz K, Hoppe-Seyler G, Schollmeyer P: Intraperitoneal and intravenous cefopereazone kinetics during continuous ambulatory peritoneal dialysis. Clin Pharmacol Ther 35: 208–213, 1984.

363. Petersen J, Stewart RDM, Catto GRD, Edward N: Pharmacokinetics of intraperitoneal cefotaxime treatment of peritonitis in patients on continuous ambulatory peritoneal dialysis. Nephron 40: 79–82, 1985.

364. Matousovic K, Moravek J, Vitko S, Prat V, Horcickova M: Pharmacokinetics of intravenous and intraperitoneal cefotaxime in patients undergoing CAPD. Periton Dial Bull 5: 33–35, 1985.

365. Lewis DA, Chapman ST, Kingswood JC, White LO, Banks RA, Reeves DS: Pharmacokinetics of cefotaxime in continuous ambulatory peritoneal dialysis (CAPD), In: Spitzy KH, Karrer K (eds), Proceedings of the 13th International Congress of Chemotherapy, Vienna, Austria, pp 15–18, 1983.

366. Schurig R, Kampf D, Spieber W, Wiehermuller K, Becker H: Cefotaxime pharmacokinetics in peritoneal dialysis, In: Gahl GM, Kesel M, Nolph KD (eds), Advances in Peritoneal Dialysis, Proceedings of the Second International Symposium on Peritoneal Dialysis, Amsterdam. Excerpta Medica, pp 96–98, 1981.

367. Albin HC, Demotes-Mainard FM, Bouchet JL, Vincon GA, Martin-Dupont C: Pharmocokinetics of intravenous and intraperitoneal cefotaxime in chronic ambulatory peritoneal dialysis. Clin Pharmacol Ther 38: 285–288, 1985.

368. Heim KL, Halstenson CE, Comty CM, Affrime MB, Matzke GR: Disposition of cefotaxime and desacetyl cefotaxime during continuous ambulatory peritoneal dialysis. Antimicrob Agents Chemother 30: 15–19, 1986.

369. Overgaard S, Lkkegaard N, Scrder S, Fugleberg S, Nielsen-Kudsk F: Cefotaxime disposition pharmacokinetics during peritoneal dialysis. Pharmacol Toxicol 60: 321–324, 1987.

370. Koup JR, Keller E, Neumann H, Stoeckel K: Ceftriaxone pharmacokinetics during peritoneal dialysis. European J Clin Pharmacol 30: 303–307, 1986.

371. Browning MJ, Holt A, White LO, Chapman ST, Banks RA, Reeves DS, Yates RA: Pharmacokinetics of cefotetan in patients with end-stage renal failure on maintenance dialysis. J Antimicrob Chemother 18: 103–106, 1986.

372. Sica DA, Polk RE, Kerkering TM, Patterson P, Baggett J: Cefmenoxime kinetics during continuous ambulatory peritoneal dialysis. Eur J Clin Pharmacol 30: 713–717, 1986.

373. Guay DRP, Meatherall RC, Hardin GK, Brown: Pharmacokinetics of cefixime (CL 284, 635; Fk 027) in healthy subjects and patients with renal insufficiency. Anitmicrob Agents Chemother 30: 485–490, 1986.

374. Hortling L, Sipila R: Multiresistant Serratia marcescens peritonitis in a patient on continuous ambulatory peritoneal dialysis (CAPD) successfully treated with aztreonam (S26, 776) a new monobactam antibiotic. Clin Nephrol 21: 355, 1984.

375. Gerig JS, Bolton ND, Swabb EA, Scheld WM, Bolton WK: Effect of hemodialysis and peritoneal dialysis on aztreonam pharmacokinetics. Kidney Int 26: 308–318, 1984.

376. Drawta M, Glupczynski Y, Lameire N, Matthys D, Verschraegen G, Van Eeckhoute M, Boelaert J, Schurger M, Van Landuyt, Verbeelen D, Lauwers: Aztreonam in CAPD peritonitis. Lancet 25: 213–214, 1987.

377. Fleming LW, Moreland TA, Scott AC, Stewart WK, White LO: Ciprofloxacin in plasma and peritoneal dialysate after oral therapy in patients on continuous ambulatory peritoneal dialysis. J Antimicrob Chemother 19: 493–503, 1987.

378. Shalit I, Greenwood RB, Marks MI, Pederson JA, Frederick DL: Pharmacokinetics of single-dose oral ciprofloxacin in patients undergoing chronic ambulatory peritoneal dialysis. Antimicrob Agents Chemother 30: 152–156, 1986.

379. McCormick EM, Echols RM: Effect of peritoneal dialysis fluid and pH on bactericidal activity of ciprofloxacin. Antimicrobial Agents Chemother 31: 657–659, 1987.

380. Fillastre JP, Leroy A, Humbert G: Ofloxacin pharmacokinetics in renal failure. Antimicrobial Agents Chemother 31: 156–160, 1987.

381. Adam D, Haneder J: Studies of the inactivation of aminoglycoside antibiotics by acylureidopenicillins and piperacillin. Infection 9: 182–185, 1981.

382. Shear L, Shinaberger JH, Barry KG: Peritoneal transport of antibiotics in man. New Engl J Med 272: 666–669, 1965.

383. Ruedy J: The effects of peritoneal dialysis on the physiological disposition of oxacillin, ampicillin and tetracycline in patients with renal disease. Can Med Assoc J 94: 258–261, 1966.

384. Thomae U, Boos W, Adam D: Transperitoneale resorption von oxacillin, azlocillin und sisomicin unter kontinuierlicher ambulanter peritonealdialyse (CAPD) bei patienten mit und ohne peritonitis. Med Welt Bd 32: 1365–1367, 1981.

385. Derensinski SC, Stevens DA: Clinical evaluation of parenteral

dicloxacillin. Curr Ther Res 18: 151–162, 1975.

386. Bulger RJ, Bennett JV: Intraperitoneal administration of broad spectrum antibiotics in patients with renal failure. JAMA 194: 140–144, 1965.

387. Buck AC, Cohen SL: Absorption of antibiotics during peritoneal dialysis in patients with renal failure. J Clin Pathol 21: 88–92, 1968.

388. Ruedy J: The effects of peritoneal dialysis on the physiological disposition of oxacillin, ampicillin and tetracycline in patients with renal disease. Can Med Assoc J 94: 257–261, 1966.

389. Thomae U, Boos W, Adam D: Transperitoneale resoprtion von ampicillin, cefuroxim und gentamicin unter kontinuierlicher ambulanter peritonealdialyse. Med Welt Bd 33: 182–184, 1982.

390. Briedigkeit VH, Schroter R: Antibiotikaspiegelbestimmungen bei patienten mit niereninsuffizienz wahrend der peritonealdialyse. Das deutsche gesundheitswesen 8: 337–341, 1986.

391. Jones RH, Cundy R, Bullock R, Brown CW, Dufton J, Majer R, Bridgman KM: Concentrations of amoxycillin in serum and dialysate of uraemic patients undergoing peritoneal dialysis. J Infect 1: 235–242, 1979.

392. Eastwood JB, Curits JR: Carbenicillin administration in patients with severe renal failure. Brit Med J 1: 486–487, 1968.

393. Hoffman TA, Bullock WE: Pharmacokinetics of carbenicillin in patients with hepatic and renal failure. J Infect Dis (Sup) 122: 75–77, 1970.

394. Bodey GP, Rodriquez V, Stewart D: Clinical pharmacological studies of carbenicillin. Am J Med Sci 257: 185–190, 1969.

395. Shattil SJ, Bennett JS, McDonough M, Turnbull J: Carbenicillin and penicillin G inhibit platelet function in vitro by impairing the interaction of agonists with the platelet surface. J Clin Invest 65: 329–337, 1980.

396. Brumfitt W, Percival A, Leigh DA: Clinical and laboratory studies with carbenicillin: A new penicillin active against pseudomonas pyocyanea. Lancet 1: 1289–1293, 1967.

397. Wise R, Reeves DS, Parker AS: Administration of ticarcillin, a new antipseudomonal antibiotic, in patients undergoing dialysis. Antimicrob Agents Chemother 5: 119–120, 1974.

398. Whelton A, Carter GG, Bryant HH, Porteous LA, Walker WG: Carbenicillin concentrations in normal and diseased kidneys: A therapeutic consideration. Ann Intern Med 78: 659–662, 1973.

399. Dalet F, Amado E, Cabrera E, Donate T, del Rio G: Pharmacokinetics of the combination of ticarcillin with clavulanic acid in renal insufficiency. J Antimicrob Agents Chemother 17: 57–64, 1986.

400. Watson ID, Boulton-Jones M, Stewart MJ, Henderson I, Payton CD: Pharmacokinetics of clavulanic acid-potentiated ticarcillin in renal failure. Ther Drug Monitor 9: 139–147, 1987.

401. Leung ACT, Orange G, Henderson IS, Sleigh JD: Successful use of combined intraperitoneal azlocillin and aminoglycoside in the treatment of dialysis associated pseudomonas peritonitis. Periton Dial Bull 4: 98–101, 1984.

402. Whelton A, Stout R, Delgado FA: Azlocillin kinetics during extracorporeal haemodialysis and peritoneal dialysis. J Antimicrob Chemother 11(8): 89–95, 1983.

403. Kampf D, Schurig R, Weihermuller K, Forster D: Effects of impaired renal function, hemodialysis, and peritoneal dialysis on the pharmacokinetics of mezlocillin. Antimicrob Agents Chemother 18: 81–87, 1980.

404. Schapira A: Single dose kinetics and dosage of mecillinam in renal failure and haemodialysis. Clin Pharmacol 9: 364–370, 1984.

405. Walshe JJ, Morse GD, Janicke DM, Apicella MA: Crossover pharmacokinetic analysis comparing intravenous and intraperitoneal administration of tobramaycin. J Infect Dis 153: 645–815, 1986.

406. Smith CB, Dans PE, Wilfert JN, Finland M: Use of gentamicin in combination with other antibiotics. J Infect Dis 119: 370–377, 1969.

407. Smith IM: Supplemental antibiotics to enhance the action of gentamicin in pseudomonas and mixed infections. J Infect Dis 198: 201, 1971.

408. Ervin RF, Bullock WE, Nuttall CE: Inactivation of gentamicin by penicillins in patients with renal failure. Antimicrob Agents Chemother 9: 1004–1011, 1976.

409. Riff LJ, Jackson GG: Laboratory and clinical conditions for gentamicin inactivation by carbenicillin. Arch Inern Med 130: 887–891, 1972.

410. McLaughlin JE, Reeves DS: Clinical and laboratory evidence for activation of gentamicin by carbenicillin. Lancet 1: 261–264, 1971.

411. Noone P, Pattison JR: Therapeutic implications of interaction of gentamicin and penicillins. Lancet 2: 575–578, 1971.

412. Eykyn S, Phillips I, Ridley M: Gentamicin plus carbenicillin. Lancet 1: 545–546, 1971.

413. Riff L, Jackson GG: Gentamicin plus carbenicilin. Lancet 1: 592, 1971.

414. Flournoy DJ: The inactivation of gentamicin and netilmicin by carbenicillin: Its effect on Serratia marcescens. J Antibiot 31: 868–871, 1978.

415. Welbert R, Keane W, Shapiro F: Carbenicillin inactivation of aminoglycosides in patients with severe failure. Trans Am Soc Artif Intern Organs 22: 440–441, 1976.

416. Masur H, Whelton PK, Whelton A: Noemycin toxicity revisited. Arch Surg 111: 822–825, 1976.

417. Mullett RD, Keats AS: Apnea and respiratory insufficiency after intraperitoneal administration of kanamycin. Surgery 49: 530–533, 1960.

418. Atkins RC, Mion C, Despaux E, Van-Hai N, Julien C, Mion H: Peritoneal transfer of kanamycin and its use in peritoneal dialysis. Kidney Int 3: 391–396, 1973.

419. Cohn I, Cotlar AM: Intraperitoneal kanamycin. Ann Surg 155: 532–537, 1962.

420. Divincenti FC, Cohn I: Prolonged administration of intraperitoneal kanamycin in the treatment of peritonitis. Am J Surg 37: 177–180, 1971.

421. Matzke GR, Salem N, Bockbrader H, Blevins R: The effect of peritoneal dialysis on the pharmacokinetics of amikacin. Proc Clin Dial Transplant Forum 10: 302–304, 1980.

422. Madhavan T, Yar emchuk K, Pohlod LD, Burch K, Fisher E, Cox F, Quinn EL: Effect of renal failure and dialysis on the serum concentration of the aminoglycoside amikacin. Antimicrob Agents Chemother 10: 464–466, 1976.

423. Regeur L, Colding H, Jensen H, Kampmann JP: Pharmacokinetics of amikacin during hemodialysis and peritoneal dialysis. Antimicrobial Agents Chemother 11: 214–218, 1977.

424. Coles GA, Roberts D: The recommended dosage of amikacin for CAPD is too high. Periton Dial Bull 2: 191, 1982.

425. Slingeneyer A, Liendo-Liendo C, Despaux E, Balmeyer B, Perez C, Mion C: Transfert peritoneal de lamikacine son utilisation en dialyse peritoneale de supplance. La Nouvelle Press Medicale 31: 3432–3435, 1979.

426. Smithivas Thana, Hyams PJ, Matalon R, Simberkoff MS, Rahal JJ: The use of gentamicin in peritoneal dialysis: Pharmacologic results. J Infect Dis 124: 77–83, 1971.

427. Blouin RA, Bauer LA, Piecoro JJ, Holland NH: Decreased gentamicin half-life during peritoneal dialysis. Drug Intell Clin Pharm 14: 218–219, 1980.

428. DePaepe M, Lameire N, Ringoir S, Belpaire F, Bogaert M: Peritoneal pharmacokinetics of gentamicin in man and rabbit, In: Gahl GM, Kessel M, Nolph KD (eds), Advances in Peritoneal Dialysis, Proceedings of the Second International Symposium on Peritoneal Dialysis, Amsterdam, Excerpta Medica, pp 99–101, 1981.

429. Hamann SR, Oeltgen PR, Shank WA, Blouin RA, Natarajan L: Evaluation of gentamicin pharmacokinetics during perit-

oneal dialysis. Ther Drug Monitor 4: 297–300, 1982.

430. Pancorbo S, COmty C: Pharmacokinetics of gentamicin in patients undergoing continuous ambulatory peritoneal dialysis. Antimicrob Agents Chemother 19: 605–607, 1981.

431. DePaepe M, Belpaire F, Bogaert M, Lamiere N, Ringoir S: Gentamicin for treatment of peritonitis in continuous ambulatory peritoneal dialysis. Lancet 2: 424–425, 1981.

432. Gary NE: Peritoneal clearance and removal of gentamicin. J Infect Dis 124: 96–97, 1971.

433. Fuquay D, Koup J, Smith AL: Brief clinical and laboratory observations J Ped 99: 473–476, 1981.

434. DePaepe La, Lameire N, Belpaire F, Bogaert M: Peritoneal pharmacokinetics of gentamicin in man. Clin Nephrol 19: 107–109, 1983.

435. Jusko WJ, Baliah T, Kim KH, Gerbracht LM, Yaffe SJ: Pharmacokinetics of gentamicin during peritoneal dialysis in children. Kidney Int 9: 430–438, 1976.

436. Somani P, Shapiro RS, Stockard H, Higgings JT: Undirectional absorption of gentamicin from the peritoneum during continuous ambulatory peritoneal dialysis. Clin Pharmacol Ther 32: 113–121, 1982.

437. Indraprasit S, Ukaravichien V, Pummangura C, Kaojarern: Gentamicin removal during intermittent peritoneal dialysis. Nephron 44: 18–21, 1986.

438. Thomae U, Boos W, Adam D: Transperitoneal resorption von oxacillin, azlocvillin, sisomicin unter kontinuierlicher ambulanter peritonealdialyse (CAPD) bei patienten mit und ohne peritonitis. Med Welt Bd 37: 1365–1367, 1981.

439. Regamy C, Gordon RC, Kirby WMM: Comparative pharmacokinetics of tobramycin and gentamicin. Clin Pharm 14: 396–403, 1972.

440. Paton T, Manuel A, Cohen LB, Walker SE: The disposition of cefazolin and tobramycin following intraperitoneal administration in patients on continuous ambulatory peritoneal dialysis. Periton Dial Bull 3: 73–76, 1982.

441. Bunke CM, Aronoff GR, Brier ME, SLoan RS, Luft FC: Tobramycin kinetics during continuous ambulatory peritoneal dialysis. Clin Pharmacol Ther 34: 110–116, 1983.

442. Gokal R: Risks of tobramycin use in CAPD patients with peritonitis. Periton Dial Bull 2: 139–142, 1982.

443. Cujec B, Wu G, Vas S, Lawson V, Khanna R: Accidental tobramycin overdose in a CAPD patient treated by intermittent peritoneal dialysis. Periton Dial Bull 4: 266–267, 1984.

444. Malcoff RF, Finkelstein RO, Andriole VT: Effect of peritoneal dialysis on serum levels of tombramycin and clindamycin. Antimicrob Agents Chemother 8: 574–580, 1975.

445. Weinstein AJ, Karchmer AW, Moellering RC: Tobramycin concentrations during peritoneal dialysis. Antimicrob Agents Chemother 4: 432–433, 1973.

446. Rubin J, Deraps GD, Walsh D, Adair C, Bower J: Protein losses and tobramycin absorption in peritonitis treated by hourly peritoneal dialysis. American Journal of Kidney Diseases 8: 124–127, 1986.

447. Dahlager JI, Ekelund B: Netilmicin in treatment of peritonitis in patients on continuous ambulatory peritoneal dialysis – CAPD, In: Spitzy KH, Karrer K (eds), Proceedings of the 13th International Congress of Chemotherapy, pp 24–27, 1983.

448. Grefberg N, Danielson BG, Nilsson P: Netilmicin in CAPD peritonitis. Periton Dial Bull 4: 186–187, 1984.

449. Keogh JA, Carr ME, Falkiner FR, Martin P, Grant G, Keane DT: Pharmacokinetics of netilmicin in CAPD patients. Pertion Dial Bull 3: 172–175, 1983.

450. Blevins RD, Halstenson CE, Salem NG, Matzke GR: Pharmacokinetics of vancomycin in patients undergoing continuous ambulatory peritoneal dialysis. Antimicrob Agents Chemother 25: 603–606, 1984.

451. Ayus JC, Eneas JFF, Tong TG, Benowitz NL, Schoenfeld PY, Hadley KL, Becker CE, Humphreys MH: Peritoneal clearance and total body elimination of vancomycin during chronic intermittent peritoneal dialysis. Clin Nephrol 11: 129–132, 1979.

452. Pancorbo S, Comty C: Peritoneal transport of vancomycin in 4 patients undergoing continuous ambulatory peritoneal dialysis. Nephron 31: 37–39, 1982.

453. Gray HH, Goulding S, Eykyn SJ: Intraperitoneal vancomycin and ceftazidime in the treatment of CAPD peritonitis. Clin Nephrol 23: 81–84, 1985.

454. Magera BE, Arroyo JC, Rosansky SJ, Postic B: Vancomycin pharmacokinetics in patients with peritonitis on peritonbeal dialysis. Antimicrob Agents Chemother 23: 710–714, 1983.

455. Krothapalli RK, Senekjuan HO, Ayus JC: Efficacy of intravenous vancomycin in the treatment of gram-positive peritonitis in long term peritoneal dialysis. Am J Med 75: 345–348, 1983.

456. Glew RH, Pavuk RRA, Shuster A, Alfred HJ: Vancomycin pharmacokinetics in patients undergoing chronic intermittent peritoneal dialysis. Int J Clin Pharmacol Ther Toxicol 20: 559–563, 1982.

457. Nielsen HE, Sorensen I, Hansen HE: Peritoneal transport of vancomycin during peritoneal dialysis. Nephron 24: 274–277, 1979.

458. Mounier M, Benevent D, Denis F: Pharmacocinetique de la vancomycione chez les patients insuffisans renaux chroniques en dalyse peritoneale continue ambulatoire (DPCA) apres administration intra-abdominale. Path Biol 33: 542–544, 1985.

459. Rogge MC, Johnson CA, Ximmerman SW, Welling PG: Vancomycin disposition during continuous ambulatory peritoneal dialysis: A pharmacokinetic analysis of peritoneal drug transport. Antimicrob Agents Chemother 27: 578–582, 1985.

460. Gruer LD, Turney JH, Curley J, Michael J, Adu D: Vancomycin and tobramycin in the treatment of CAPD peritonitis. Nephron 41: 279–282, 1985.

461. Brauner L, Kahlmeter G, Lindholm T, Simonsen O: Vancomycin and netilmycin as first line treatment of peritonitis in CAPD patients. J Antimicrob Chemother 15: 751–758, 1985.

462. Bunke CM, Aronoff GR, Brier ME, Sloan RS, Luft FC: Vancomycin kinetics during continuous ambulatory peritoneal dialysis. Clin Pharmacol Ther 34: 631–637, 1983.

463. Morse GD, Farolino DF, Apicella MA, Walshe JJ: Comparative study of intraperitoneal and intravenous vancomycin pharmacokinetic during continuous ambulatory peritoneal dialysis. Antimicro Agents Chemother 31: 173–177, 1987.

464. Whitby M, Edwards R, Aston E, Finch RG: Pharmacokinetics of single dose intravenous vancomycin in CAPD peritonitis. J Antimicrob Chemother 19: 351–357, 1987.

465. Harford AM, Sica DA, Tartaglione T, Polk RE, Dalton HP, Poynor W: Vancomycin pharmacokinetics in continuous ambulatory peritoneal dialysis patients with peritonities. Nephron 43: 217–222, 1986.

466. Bennett-Jones D, Wass V, Mawson P, Taube D, Neild D, Ogg C, Cameron JS, Williams DG: A comparison of intraperitoneal and intravenous/oral antibiotics in CAPD patients. Periton Dial Bull 7: 31–33, 1987.

467. Hekster YA, Vree TB, Weemaes CMR, Rotteveel: Toxicologic and pharmacokinetic evaluation of a case of vancomycin intoxication during continuous ambulatory peritoneal dialysis. Pharm Weekbl [Sci] 8: 293–297, 1986.

468. Morse GD, Nairn DK, Bertino JS, Walshe JJ: Overestimation of vancomycin concentrations utilizing fluorescence polarization immunoassay in patients on peritoneal dialysis. Ther Drug Monit 9: 212–215, 1987.

469. Bailie GR, Morton R, Ganguli L, Keaney M, Waldek S: Intravenous or intraperitoneal vancomycin for the treatment of continuous ambulatory peritoneal dialysis associated gram positive peritonitis? Nephron 46: 316–318, 1987.

470. Traina GL, Fellin G, Rosina R, Cavenagji L, Buniva G, Bonati M: Pharmacokinetics of teicoplanin in patients on continuous ambulatory peritoneal dialysis. Eur J Clin Pharmacol 31: 501–504, 1986.

471. Taylor R, Schofield IS, Ramos JM, Bint AJ, Ward MK: Otoxicity of erytrhomycin in peritoneal dialysis patients. Lancet 2: 935–936, 1981.

472. Cohen L, Bailey D: Efficacy of intraperitoneal clindamycin in refractory peritonitis: Report of two cases. Periton Dial Dull 4: 92–94, 1984.

473. Reinarz JA, McIntosh DA: Lincomycin excretion in patients with normal renal function, severe azotemia and with hemodialysis and peritoneal dialysis. Antimicrob Agents Chemother 165: 232–238, 1965.

474. Malacoff RF, Finkelstein FO, Andriole VT: Effect of peritoneal dialysis on serum levels of tobramycin and clindamycin. Antimicrob Agents Chemotherapy 8: 574–580, 1975.

475. Golper TA, Sewell DL, Fisher PB, Wolfson M: Incomplete activation of intraperitoneal clindamycin phosphate during peritoneal dialysis. Am J Nephrol 4: 38–42, 1984.

476. Schwartz MT, Kowalsky SF, McCormick EM, Parker WA, Echols RM: Clindamycin phosphate kinetics in subjects undergoing CAPD. Clin Nephrol 26: 303–306, 1986.

477. Holten E, Erichsen NS: Concentration of metronidazole in serum during peritoneal dialysis. Chemother 27: 414–415, 1981.

478. Bush A, Holt JE, Sankey MG, Kaye CM, Gabriel R: Penetration of metronidazole into continuous ambulatory peritoneal dialysate. Periton Dial Bull 3: 176–177, 1983.

479. Cassey JG, Clark DA, Merrick P, Jones B: Pharmacokinetics of metronidazole in patients undergoing peritoneal dialysis. Antimicrob Agents Chemother 24: 950–951, 1983.

480. Guay DR, Meatherall RC, Baxter H, Jack WR, Penner B: Pharmacokinetics of metronidazole in patients undergoing continuous ambulatory peritoneal dialysis. Antimicrob Agents Chemother 25: 306–309, 1984.

481. Parisi AF, Kaplan MH: Apnea during treatment with sodium colistimethate. JAMA 194: 298–299, 1965.

482. Goodwin NJ, Friedman EA: The effects of renal impairment, peritoneal dialysis, and hemodialysis on serum sodium colistimethate levels. Ann Intern Med 68: 984–994, 1968.

483. Swick HM, Maxwell E, Charache P, Sevin S: Peritoneal dialysis in colistin intoxication: Report of a case. Ped Pharmacol Ther 74: 976–980, 1969.

484. MacKay DN, Kaye D: Serum concentrations of colistin in patients with normal and impaired renal function. New Engl J Med 270: 394–397, 1964.

485. Greenberg PA, Sanford JP: Removal and absorption of antibiotics in patients with renal failure undergoing peritoneal dialysis. Ann Intern Med 66: 465–479, 1967.

486. Shear L, Shinaberger JH, Barry KG: Peritoneal transport of antibiotics in man. New Engl J Med 272: 667–669, 1965.

487. Rose H, Roth DA, Koch ML: Serum tetracycline levels during peritoneal dialysis. Am J Med Sci 250: 66–68, 1965.

488. Bulger RJ, Bennett JV: Intraperitoneal administration of broad-spectrum antibiotics in patients with renal failure. JAMA 194: 140–144, 1965.

489. Morton KC: Peritoneal dialysis in acute poisoning: Successful treatment of 15 month old child ingesting 30 times the adult dose of achrocidin. Clin Ped 5: 565–567, 1966.

490. Weber J, Dockum R, Taylor J: Intraperitoneal administered chloraphenicol. Periton Dial Bull 4: 266, 1984.

491. Menz VHP, Hartmann I, Oldershausen HF: Zur pharmakokinetik von thiamphenical. Arzneim-Forsch 24: 102–104, 1974.

492. Furman KI, Koornhof HJ, Kilroe-Smith TA, Landless R, Robinson RG: Peritoneal transfer of thiamphenicol during peritoneal dialysis. Antimicrob Agents Chemother 9: 557–560, 1976.

493. Milek JF, Kalfopoulos P, Merier G: La cinetique des tetracyclines chez l'homme. Scheiz Med Wschr 101: 625–633, 1971.

494. Bulger RJ, Bennett JV: Intraperitoneal administration of braod-spectrum antibiotics in patients with renal failure. JAMA 194: 140–144, 1965.

495. Fremont JF, Dkhissi H, Thomas D, Tolani M, Laurence G, Coevoet B, Fournier A, Orfila J: Traitement des peritonitis en dialyse peritoneale. Path Biol 31: 544–547, 1983.

496. Halstenson CE, Blevins RB, Salem NG, Matzke GR: Trimethoprim sulfamethoxazole pharmacokinetics during continuous ambulatory peritoneal dialysis. Clin Nephrol 22: 239–243, 1984.

497. Rothenberg S, SIlvani H, Chester S, Warmer H, McCorkle HJ: Comparison of the efficacy of therapeutic agents in the treatment of experimentally induced diffuse peritonitis of intestinal origin. Ann Surg 123: 1148–1163, 1948.

498. Glasson P. Favre F: Treatment of peritonitis in continuous ambulatory peritoneal dialysis patient with co-trimoxazole. Nephron 36: 65–67, 1984.

499. Rottembourg AM, Untersinger ESB: Administration intraperitoneale de sulfamethoxazole-trimethoprime dans le traitement des infections compliquant les dialyses peritoneales chroniques. La Nouvelle Presse Medicale 7: 3932, 1978.

500. Craig WA, Kunin CM: Trimethoprin-sulfamethoxazole: Pharmacodynamic effects of urinary pH and impaired renal function. Ann Intern Med 78: 491–497, 1973.

501. Adam WR, Brown DJ, Dawborn JK: The use of sulphadimidine (Sulphamezathine) in patients with renal failure. Med J Aust 1: 936–938, 1973.

502. Martea M, Hekster YA, Vree TB, Voets AJ, Berden JHM: Pharmacokinetics of cefradine, sulfamethoxazole and trimethoprim and their metabolites in a patient with peritonitis undergoing continuous ambulatory peritoneal dialysis. Pharm Weekbl [Sci] 9: 110–116, 1987.

503. Ojo O, Jones C, Stevens DL: The antimicrobial implications of the pharmacokinetics of cotrimoxazole in CAPD patients. Periton Dial Bull 7: 74–77, 1987.

504. Held H: Uber die wirksamkeit der peritonealdialyse bei der behandlung der chininvergiftung. Disch Med Wschr 97: 1793–1795, 1972.

505. Donadio JV, Whelton A, Gilliland PF, Cirksena WJ: Peritoneal dialysis in quinine intoxication. JAMA 204: 182, 1968.

506. Markham TN, Dodson VN, eckberg DL: Peritoneal dialysis in quinine sulfate intoxication, JAMA 202: 128–129, 1967.

507. McKenzie IFC, Mathew TH, Bailie MJ: Peritoneal dialysis in the treatment of quinine overdose. Med J Aust 1: 58–59, 1968.

508. Donadio JV, Whelton A: Quinine therapy and peritoneal dialysis in acute renal failure complicating malarial haemoiglobinuria. Lancet 1: 375–379, 1968.

509. Brooks MH, Hano JE, Clayron LE, Kazyak L, Barry KG: Quinine extraction during peritoneal dialysis: The role of nonionic diffusion. Invest Urol 7: 510–516, 1970.

510. Sabto J, Pierce RM, West RH, Gurr FW: Hemodialysis, peritoneal dialysis, plasmapheresis and forced diuresis for the treatment of quinine overdose. Clin Nephrol 15: 264–268, 1981.

511. Gold CH, Buchanan N, Tringham V, Viljoen M, Strickland B, Moodley GP: Isoniazid pharmacokinetics in patients in chronic renal failure. Clin Nephrol 6: 365–368, 1976.

512. McCann WP, Permisohn R, Palmisano PA: Fatal chloroquine poisoning in a child: Experience with peritoneal dialysis. Pediatr 55: 536–538, 1975.

513. Wattel F, Gosselin B, CHopin C, Durocher A: Intoxication massive par l'isoniazide: Traitement par dialyse peritoneale. La Nouvelle Presse Medicale 12: 1134–1135, 1975.

514. Bowersox DW, Winterbauer RH, Stewart GL, Orme B, Barron E: Isoniazid dosage in patients with renal failure. New Engl J Med 289: 84–87, 1973.

515. Gloger P. Vogt O, Lange H: Dialyse bei vergiftung mit isoniazid. Dtsch Med Wschr 96: 1307–1309, 1971.
516. Atkins R, Cutting CJ, Mackintosh TF: Acute poisoning by cycloserine. Brit Med J 1: 907–908, 1965.
517. Ing TS, Mahurkar SD, Dunea G, Hayashi JA, Klawans HL: Removal of amandatine dydrochloride by dialysis in patients with renal insufficiency. CMA Journal 115: 515, 1976.
518. Shah GM, Robert L, Winer RL, Krasny HC: Acyclovir pharmacokinetics in a patient on continuous ambulatory peritoneal dialysis. Am J Kidney Dis 7: 507–510, 1986.
519. Seth SK, Visconti JA, Hebert LA, Krasny HC: Acyclovir pharmacokinetics in a patient on continuous ambulatory peritoneal dialysis. Clin Pharm 4: 320–322, 1985.
520. Rubin J: Overdose with acyclovir in a CAPD patient. Periton Dial Bull 7: 42, 1987.
521. Boelaert J, Schurgers M, Daneels R, Van Landuyt HW, Weatherly BC: Multiple dose pharmacokinetics of intravenous acyclovir in patients on continuous ambulatory peritoneal dialysis. J Antimicrob Chemother 20: 69–76, 1987.
522. DeVault GA, Brown ST, King JW, Fowler M, Oberle A: Tenckhoff catheter obstruction resulting from invasion curvularia lunata in the absence of peritonitis. Am J Kidney Dis 6: 124–127, 1985.
523. Horisberger JD, Wauters JP: Fungal eosinophilic peritonitis due to Alternatia in a patient on continuous ambulatory peritoneal dialysis. Periton Dial Dull 4: 255–256, 1984.
524. Pearson JG, McKinney TD, Stone WJ: Penicillium peritonitis in a CAPD patient. Periton Dial Bull 3: 20–21, 1983.
525. McNeely DJ, Vas SI, Dombros N, Oreiopoulos DG: Fusarium peritonitis: Periton Dial Bull 1: 94–96, 1981.
526. Bayer AS, Blumenkrantz MJ, Montgomerie JZ, Galpin JE, Coburn JW, Guze LB: Candida peritonitis. Am J Med 61: 832–840, 1976.
527. Loeppky CB, Sprouse RF, Carlson JV, Everett ED: Trichoderma viride peritonitis. Southern Med J 76: 798–799, 1983.
528. Smith WGJ, Tsakiris D, Briggs JD, Junor BJR: The high morbidity of fungal peritonitis in continuous ambulatory peritoneal dialysis. Proc EDTA-ERA 22: 397–400, 1985.
529. Maher JF, Hirszel P, Chakrabarti E, Bennett RR: Contrasting effects of amphotericin and the solvent sodium desoxycholate on peritoneal transport. Nephron 43: 38–42, 1986.
530. Muther RS, Bennett WM: Peritoneal clearance of amphotericin B and 5-flurocytosine. Western Med J 133: 157–160, 1980.
531. Polak A: Pharmacokinetics of amphotericin B and flucytosine. Postgrad Med J 55: 67–670, 1979.
532. Peterson LR, Hall WH, Kelty RH, Votava HJ: Therapy of candida peritonitis: penetration of amphotericin B into peritoneal fluid. Postgrad Med J 54: 340–342, 1978.
533. Kerr CM, Perfect JR, Craven PC, Jorgensen JH, Drutz DJ, Shelburne JD, Gallis HA, Gutman RA: Fungal peritonitis in patients on continuous ambulatory peritoneal dialysis. Ann Int Med 99: 334–337, 1983.
534. Nunan TO, Roe Y, Hilton PJ: Candida albicans peritonitis in a CAPD patient with dystrophic nails. Periton Dial Bull 4: 268, 1984.
535. Johnson R, Blair A, Ahmad S: Ketoconazole in the fungal peritonitis. Periton Dial Bull 5: 136, 1985.
536. McGuire NM, Port FK, Kauffman CA: Ketoconazole pharmacokinetics in continuous ambulatory peritoneal dialysis. Periton Dial Bull 4: 199–201, 1984.
537. Chapman JR, Warnock DW: Ketoconazole and fungal CAPD peritonitis. Lancet 1: 510–511, 1983.
538. Borelli D, Fuentes J, Leiderman E, Restrepo A, Bran JL, Legendre R, Levine HB, Stevens DA: Ketoconazole, an oral antifungal laboratory and clinical assessment of imidazole drugs. Postgrad Med J 55: 657–661, 1979.
539. Fabris A, Biasioli S, Borin D, Brendolan A, Chiaramonte S, Feriani M, Pisani E, Ronco C, La Greca G: Fungal peritonitis in peritoneal dialysis: Our experience and review of treatments. Periton Dial Dull 4: 75–77, 1984.
540. Lempert KD, Jones JM: Flucytosine-miconazole treatment of Candida peritonitis. Arch Intern Med 142: 577–578, 1982.
541. Plempel M: Pharmacokinetics of imidazole antimycotics. Postgrad Med J 55: 662–666, 1979.
542. Johnson RJ, Blair AD, Ahmad S: Ketoconazole kinetics in chronic peritoneal dialysis: Clin Pharmacol Ther 37: 325–329, 1985.
543. Cecchin E, DeMarchi S, Panarello G, Franceschin A, Chiaradia V, Santini G, Tesio F: Torulopsis glabrata peritonitis complicating continuous ambulatory peritoneal dialysis: Successful management with oral 5-fluoracytosine. Am J Kidney Dis 4: 280–284, 1984.
544. Davies SJ, Wessels DJ, Gibson J, Pattison J, Turney JH: Successful oral treatment of Candida peritonitis. Periton Dial Bull 5: 257, 1985.
545. Wang F: Cryptococcus peritonitis. Periton Dial Bull 5: 78, 1985.
546. Vandevelde AG, Mauceri AA, Johnson JE: 5-fluorocytosine in the treatment of myocotic infections. Ann Intern Med 77: 43–51, 1972.
547. Steer PL, Marks MI, Klite PD, Eickhoff TC: 5-fluorocytosine: An oral antifungal compound: A report on clinical and laboratory experience. Ann Intern Med 76: 15–22, 1972.
548. Drouhet D, Babinet P, Chapusot JP, Kleinknecht: 5-fluorocytosine in the treatment of candidiasis with acute renal insufficiency: Its kinetics during haemodiolysis and peritoneal dialysis. Biomedicine 19: 408–414, 1973.
549. Pocheville M, Charpentier B, Brocard JF, Benarbia S, Hammouche M, Fries D: Successful in situ treatment of a fungal peritonitis during CAPD. Nephron 37: 66–67, 1984.
550. Giangrande A, Tortorano AM, Limido A, Viviani MA: Management of Candida peritonitis in a CAPD patient by fluorocytosine therapy: Importance of drug level monitoring in body fluids. Boll Lst Sieroter Milan 62: 478–481, 1983.
551. Andersen K, OlsenH: Candida peritonitis in a patient receiving chronic intermittent peritoneal dialysis. Scand J Infect Dis 10: 91–92, 1978.
552. Holdsworth SR, Atkins C, Scott DF, JAckson R: Management of candida peritonitis by prolonged peritoneal lavage containing 5-fluorocytosine. Clin Nephrol 4: 157–159, 1975.
554. Lavelle KJ, Doedens DJ, Sleit SA, Forney RB: Iodine absorption in burn patients treated tropically with povidone-iodine. Clin Pharmacol Ther 17: 355–362, 1974.
555. Stephen RL, Kablitz C, Kitahara M, Nelson JA, Duffy DP, Kolff WJ: Peritoneal dialysis: Peritonitis: Saline-Iodine flush. Dial Transplant 8: 584–655, 1979.
556. Lavigne JE, Brown CS, Machiedo GW, Blackwood JM, Rush BF: The treatment of experimental peritonitis with intraperitoneal betadine solution. J Surg Res 16: 307–311, 1974.
557. Ahrenholz DH, Simmons RL: Povidone-iodine in peritonitis. J Surg Res 26: 458–463, 1979.
558. Yee E, Foss K, Schimdt RW: Use of povidone iodine in continuous ambulatory peritoneal dialysis (CAPD) – A technique to reduce the incidence of infectious peritonitis. Trans Am Soc Artif Intern Organs 26: 223–224, 1980.
559. Gilmore OJA, Reid C, Houang E, Shaw EJ: Intraperitoneal povidone-iodine in peritonitis. J Surgh Res 25: 471–476, 1978.
560. Furman KI, Ninin DT, Block JD: Reason for failure of saline-iodine flushes, In: Gahl GM, Kessel M, Nolph KD (eds), Advances in Peritoneal Dialysis, Proceedings of the Second International Symposium, Amsterdam, Excerpta Media, pp 281–286, 1981.
561. Browne MK, MacKenzie M: A controlled trial of taurolin in establshed bacterial peritonitis. Surg Gyn Ob 146: 721–724, 1978.
562. Junor BJR, Briggs JD, Forwell MA, Dobbie JW, Henderson I: Sclerosing peritonitis – The contribution of chlorhexidine

in alcohol. Periton Dial Bull 5: 101–104, 1985.

563. Somerville PJ, Kaye M: Chlorhexidine is unsuitable for long term use in patients on CAPD. Periton Dial Bull 2: 195, 1982.

564. Putnam TJ: The living peritoneum as a dialyzing membrane. Am J Physiol 18: 548–565, 1923.

565. Cunningham RS: The physiology of the serous membranes. Physiol Rev 6: 242–280, 1926.

566. Cantaluppi A, Scalamogna A, Castelnovo C, Graziani G: Peritonitis prevention in continuous ambulatory peritoneal dialysis: Long-term efficacy of a Y-connector and disinfectant. Periton Dial Bull 6: 58–61, 1986.

567. Lasker N, Burke JF, Patchefsky A, Haughey E: Peritoneal reactions to particular matter in peritoneal dialysis solutions. Trans Am Soc Artif Intern Organs 21: 342–345, 1975.

568. Huertas VE, Weller JM, Rosenwieg J, Weller JM: Starch peritonitis following peritoneal dialysis. Nephron 30: 82–84, 1982.

569. Verger C, Berry JP, Galle P, Laverggne A, Hoang C, Le Charpentier YL: Foreign material inclusions in the peritoneum of CAPD patients: A study with x-ray microanalysis. Periton Dial Bull 2: 138–139, 1982.

570. Kaw JL, Beck EG, Bruch J: Studies of quartz cytotoxicity on peritoneal macrophages of guinea pigs pretreated with polyvinylpyridine N-Oxide. Environ Res 9: 313–320, 1975.

571. Verger C, Brunschvigg O, Le Charpentier Y, Lavergne A, Vantelon J: Peritoneal structure alterations on CAPD, In: Gahl GM, Kessel M, Nolph KD (eds), Advances in Peritoneal Dialysis, Proceedings of the Second International Symposium on Peritoneal Dialysis, Amsterdam, Excerpta Media, pp 10–15, 1981.

572. Finkelstein FO, Kliger AS, Bastl C, Yap P: Sequential clearance and dialysance measurements in chronic peritoneal dialysis patients. Nephron 18: 342–347, 1977.

573. Randerson DH, Farrell PC: Long term peritoneal clearances in CAPD, In: Atkins RC, Thomson NM, Farrell PC (eds), Peritoneal Dialysis, New York, Churchill Livingstone, pp 30–40, 1981.

574. Rubin J, Nolph K, Arfania D, Brown P: Follow-up of hourly peritoneal clearances with and without nitroprusside augmentation in patients undergoing CAPD. Kidney Int 16: 619–623, 1979.

575. Nolph KD, Ryan L, Moore H: Factors affecting ultrafiltration in continuous ambulatory peritoneal dialysis. Periton Dial Bull 4: 14–19, 1984.

576. Faller B, Marichal JF: Loss of ultrafiltration in continuous ambulatory peritoneal dialysis: A role for acetate. Periton Dial Bull 4: 10–13, 1984.

577. Slingeneyer A, Canaud B, Mion C: Permanent loss of ultrafiltration capacity of the peritoneum in long term peritoneal dialysis: An epidemiological study. Nephron 33: 133–138, 1983.

578. Grahame GR, Torchia MG, Dankewich KA, Ferguson IA: Surface-active material in peritoneal effluent of CAPD patients. Periton Dial Bull 5: 109–111, 1985.

579. Breborowicz A, Sombolos K, Rodela H, Ogilvie R, Bargman J, Oreopoulos D: Mechanism of phosphatidylcholine action during dialysis. Periton Dial Bull 7: 6–9, 1987.

580. Di Paolo, Buoncristini U, Capotondo L, Gaggiotti E, De Mia M, Sansoni E, Rossi P, Bernini: Phosphatidylcholine and peritoneal transport during peritoneal dialysis. Nephron 44: 365–370, 1986.

581. Hauglustaine D, Meerbeek J, Monballyu J, Goddeeris P, Lauwerijns J, Michielsen P: Sclerosing peritonitis with mural bowel fibrosis in a patient on long term CAPD. Clin Nephrol 22: 158–162, 1984.

582. Slingeneyer A, Mion C, Mourad G, Canaud B, Faller B, Beraud JJ: Progressive sclerosing peritonitis: A late and severe complication of maintenance peritoneal dialysis. Trans Am

Soc Artif Intern Organs 22: 633–640, 1983.

583. Grefberg N, Nilsson P, Andreen T: Sclerosing obstructive peritonitis beta-blockers and continuous ambulatory peritoneal dialysis. Lancet 733–734, 1983.

584. Shaldon S, Koch KM, Quelhorst E, Dinarello CA: Pathogenesis of sclerosing peritonitis in CAPD. Trans Am Soc Artif Intern Organs 30: 193–194, 1984.

585. Pusateri R, Ross R, Marshall R, Meredith JH, Hamilton R: Sclerosing encapsulating peritonitis: report of a case with small obstruction managed by long-term home hyperalimentation and a review of the literature. Am J Kidney Dis 8: 56–60, 1986.

586. Steyn DG: The treatment of cases of amanita phalloides and amanita capensis poisoning. S A Med J 40: 405–406, 1966.

587. Costantino D, Damia G: L'Intoxication phalloidienne; Resultats de diverses therapeutiques chez 47 malades. La Nouvelle Presse Medicale 25: 23125–2317, 1977.

588. Myler RK, Lee JC, Hopper J: Renal tubular necrosis caused by mushroom poisoning. Arch Intern Med 114: 196–204, 1964.

589. Halilbasic A, Pasic I, Martinovic K, Perkovic, Salatic M, Muminhodzic TK: Mjesto peritonealne dijalize u terapiji akutnih egzogenih trovanja. Arch Hig Rada Toksikol 31: 247–249, 1980.

590. Levinsky WJ, Smalley RV, Hillyer PJ, Shindler RI: Arsine hemolysis. Environ Health 20: 436–440, 1970.

591. Arena JM: Poisoning – general treatment and prevention. JAMA 233: 358–363, 1975.

592. Winchester JF, Gelfand MC, Knepshield JH, Schreiner GE: Dialysis and hemoperfusion of poisons and drugs – Update. Trans Am Soc Artif Intern Organs 23: 762–842, 1977.

593. Dutz VH, Eckard D: Die dialysebehandlung bei akuten intoxikationen. Ber Ges Inn Med 7: 183–185, 1970.

594. Arieff AI, Freidman EA: Coma following nonnarcotic drug overdosage: Management of 208 adult patients. Am J Med Sci 266: 405–426, 1973.

595. Thomson NM, Stevens BJ, Humphrey TJ, Atkins RC: Trace elements in patients on continuous ambulatory peritoneal dialysis, In: Gahl GM, Kessel M, Nolph KD (eds), Advances in Peritoneal Dialysis, Proceedings of the Second International Symposium, Amsterdam, Excerpta Mediaca, pp 473–477, 1981.

596. Sorkin MI, Nolph KD, Anderson HO, Morris JS, Kennedy J, Prowant B, Moore H: Aluminum mass transfer during continuous ambulatory peritoneal dialysis. Periton Dial Bull 1: 91–93, 1981.

597. Rottembourg J, Gallego JL, Jaudon MC, Clavel JP, Legrain M: Serum concentration and peritoneal transfer of aluminum during treatment by continuous ambulatory peritoneal dialysis. Kidney Int 25: 919–924, 1984.

598. Gilli P, Bastiani PD, Fagiolo F, Buoncristiani U, Carobi C, Stabellini N, Squerzanti R, Rosati G, Farinelli A: Positive aluminum balance in patients on regular peritoneal treatment: An effect of low dialysate ph? Proc EDTA 17: 219–225, 1980.

599. Williams P, Khanna R, McLachlan DRC: Enhancement of aluminum removal by desferrioxamine in a patient on continuous ambulatory peritoneal dialysis with dementia. Periton Dial Bull 1: 73, 1981.

600. Andreoli SP, Dunn D, DeMyer W, Sherrard DJ, Bergstein JM: Intraperitoneal deferoxamine therapy for aluminum intoxication in a child undergoing continuous ambulatory peritoneal dialysis. J Ped 107: 76–763, 1985.

601. Mion C: Aluminum in continuous ambulatory peritoneal dialysis and post dilutional hemofiltration. Clin Nephrol 24(1): 88–93, 1985.

602. Warady BA, Ford DM, Gaston CE, Sedman AB, Huffer WE, Lum GM: Aluminum intoxication in a child: treatment with intraperitoneal desferrioxamine. Pediatr 78: 651–655, 1986.

603. Payton CD, Junor BJR, Fell: Succesful treatment of aluminum encephalopathy by intraperitoneal desferrioxamine.

Lancet 19: 1132–1133, 1984.

604. Hercz G, Salusky IB, Norris KC, Fine RN, Coburn J: Aluminum removal by peritoneal dialysis: intravenous vs. intraperitoneal deferoxamine. Kidney Int 30: 944–948, 1986.

605. Molitoris BA, Alfrey P, Miller NL, Hasbargen JA, Kaehney WD, Alfrey A, Smith BJ: Efficacy of intramuscular and intraperitoneal deferoxamine for aluminum chelation. Kidney Int 31: 986–991, 1987.

606. O'Brien AA, Mc Pharland C, Keogh JA: The use of intravenous and intraperitoneal desferrioxamine in aluminum osteomalacia. Nephrol Dial Transplant 2: 117–119, 1987.

607. Lavender S, Bell JA: Iron intoxication in an adult. Brit Med J 2:: 406, 1970.

608. Covey TJ: Ferrous sulfate poisoning. J Ped 64: 218–226, 1964.

609. Greengard J: Iron poisoning in children. Clin Toxicol 8: 575–597, 1975.

610. Falk RJ, Mattern WD, Lamanna RW, Gitelman HJ, Parker NC, Cross RE, Rastall JR: Iron removal during continuous ambulatory peritoneal dialysis using deferoxamine. Kidney Int 24: 110–112, 1983.

611. Stanbaugh GH, Holmes AW, Gillit D, Reichel GW, Stranz M: Iron chelation therapy in CAPD: A new and effective treatment of iron overload disease in ESRD patients. Periton Dial Bull 3: 99–101, 1983.

612. McCarthy JT, Kurtz SB, Mussman GV: Deferoxamine enhanced fecal losses of aluminum and iron in a patient undergoing continuous ambulatory peritoneal dialysis. Am J Med 82: 367–370, 1987.

613. Cole EC, Lirenman DS: Role of albumin-enriched peritoneal dialysate in acute copper poisoning. J Ped 92: 955–957, 1978.

614. Chugh KS, Singhal PC, Sharm BK, Das KC, Datta BN: Acute renal failure following copper sulphate intoxication. Postgrad Med J 53: 18–23, 1977.

615. Hamlyn AN, Gollan JL, Douglas AP, Sherlock S: Fulminant Wilson's disease with haemolysis and renal failure: Copper studies and assessment of dialysis regimens. Brit Med J 2: 660–663, 1977.

616. Cole DE: Peritoneal dialysis for removal of copper. Brit Med J 7: 50–51, 1978.

617. De Bont B, Moulin D, Stein F, Van Hoof F, Lauwerys R: Peritoneal dialysis with d-penicillamine in Wilson disease. J Ped 107: 545–547, 1985.

618. Aronow R, Fleischmann LE: Mercury poisoning in children. Clin Ped 15: 936–945, 1976.

619. Batson R, Peterson CJJ: Acute mercury poisoning: Treatment with bal and in anuric states with continuous peritoneal lavage. Ann Intern Med 29: 278–293, 1948.

620. Robillard JE, Rames LK, Jensen RL, Roberts RJ: Peritoneal dialysis in mercurial diuretic intoxication. J Ped 88: 79–81, 1976.

621. Kahn A, Denis R, Blum D: Accidental ingestion of mercuric sulphate in a 4 year old child. Clin Ped 16: 956–958, 1977.

622. Lowenthal DDT, Chardo F, Reidenberg MM: Removal of mercury by peritoneal dialysis. Arch Intern Med 134: 139–141, 1974.

623. Felton JS, Kahn E, Salick B, Van Natta FC, Whitehouse MW: Heavy metal poisoning: Mercury and lead. Ann Intern Med 76: 779–792, 1972.

624. Kaufman DB, DiNicola WD, McIntosh R: Acute potassium dichromate poisoning. Am J Dis Child 119: 374–376, 1970.

625. Schiffl H, Weidmann P, Weiss M, Massry SG: Dialysis treatment of acute chromium intoxication and comparative efficacy of peritoneal versus hemodialysis in chromium removal. Mineral Electrolyte Metab 7: 28–35, 1982.

626. Mehbod H: Treatment of lead intoxication. JAMA 201: 152–154, 1967.

627. Mirouze J, Mion C, Mathieu-Daude P, Monnier L, Selam JL: Nephropathie chronique au cours d'un saturnisme. La Nouvelle Presse Medicale 31: 1642–1644, 1975.

628. Bezerra JBG, Scheinberg MA, Abuchan R: Agranulocitose severa induzida por sais de ouro: Reversao atraves da dialise peritonial. Rev Ass Med Brasil 24: 377–378, 1978.

629. Combs RJ, Dentino MM, Lehrman L, Szred JJ: Gold toxicity and peritoneal dialysis. Arth Rheumatol 19: 936–938, 1976.

630. Garland JS, Sheth KJ, Wortmann DW: Poor clearance of gold using peritoneal dialysis for the treatment of gold toxicity. Arth Rheumatol 29: 450–451, 1986.

631. Keyvan-Larijarni H, Tannerberg AM: Methanol intoxication: Comparison of peritoneal dialysis and hemodialysis treatment. Arch Intern Med 134: 293–296, 1974.

632. Wenzl JE, Mills SD, McCall JT: Methanol poisoning in an infant. Am J Dis CHild 116: 445–447, 1968.

633. Stinebaugh BJ: The use of peritoneal dialysis in acute methyl alcohol poisoning. Arch Intern Med 105: 613–617, 1960.

634. Humphrey TJ: Methanol poisoning: Management of acidosis with combined haemodialysis and peritoneal dialysis. Med J Aust 1: 833–835, 1974.

635. Setter JG, Singh R, Brackett NC, Randall RE: Studies on the dialysis of methanol. Trans Am Soc Artif Intern Organs 13: 178–182, 1967.

636. Litovitz T: The alcohols: Ethanol, methanol, isopropanol, ethylene glycol. Ped Clin North Am 33: 311–323, 1986.

637. Parry MF, Wallach R: Ethylene glycol poisoning. Am J Med 57: 143–150, 1974.

638. Vale JA, Widdop B, Bluett NH: Ethylene glycol poisoning. Postgrad Med J 2: 598–602, 1976.

639. Joly JB, Huault G, Frossarrd C, Fabiani P, Thieffry S: Communications. Societe Medicale Des Hopitaux de Paris 119: 27–45, 1968.

640. Zarembski PM, Rosen SM, Hodgkinson A: Dialysis in the treatment of primary hyperoxaluria. Brit J Urol 41: 530–533, 1969.

641. Yamauchi A, Fujii M, Shirai D, Mikami H, Okada A, Imai E, Ando A, Orita Y, Kamada T: Plasma concentration and peritoneal clearance of oxalate in patients on continuous ambulatory peritoneal dialysis (CAPD). Clin Nephrol 4: 181–185, 1986.

642. Dua SL: Peritoneal dialysis for isopropyl alcohol poisoning. JAMA 230: 235, 1974.

643. Grubbauer HM, Schwarz R: Peritoneal dialysis in alcohol intoxication in a child. Arch Toxicol 43: 317–320, 1980.

644. Wilson JHP, Doner AJM, Van Der Hem GK, Wientjes J: Peritoneal dialysis for lithium poisoning. Brit Med J 2: 749–750, 1971.

645. Humbert G, Fillastre JP, Leroy J, Maitrot B, Toberlem G, Leroux G, Lavoine A: Intoxication par le lithium. Sem Hop Paris 50: 509–514, 1974.

646. Brown EA, Pawlikoski TRB: Lithium intoxication treated by peritoneal dialysis. Brit J Clin Pract 35: 90–91, 1981.

647. Sauder AJ, Kopferschmitt J, Jaegle ML: Toxicokinetics of lithium intoxication treated by hemodialysis. Clin Toxicol 23: 501–517, 1985–1986.

648. Flynn CT, Chandran PKG, Taylor MJ, Shadur CA: Intraperitoneal lithium administration for bipolar affective disorder in a patient on continuous ambulatory peritoneal dialysis. Int J Artif Organs 10: 105–107, 1987.

649. Rumpf KW, Fuchs Ch, Poser W, Scheler F: Bromcarbamidintoxikation mit akutem nierenversagen und beidseitigen oberschenkelvenenthrombosen. Med Klin 72: 993–997, 1977.

650. Schmitt GW, Maher JF, Schreinder GE: Ethacrynic acid enhanced bromuremis: A comparison with peritoneal and hemodialysis. J Lab Clin Med 68: 913–922, 1966.

651. Grosse G, Hofer W, Gruska H, Beyer KH, Kubicki St, Schirop TH: Zur klinik der schweren carbromal intoxication. Klin Wschr 52: 39–49, 1974.

652. Dziuk E: Experimental studies on removal of cesium-137 by peritoneal dialysis. Polish Med J 11: 1596–1601, 1972.

653. Schlegel RJ, Altstatt LB, Canales L, Goiser JL, Alexander

JL, Gardner LI: Peritoneal dialysis for severe salicylism: An evaluation of indications and results. J Ped 69: 553–562, 1966.

654. Etteldorf JN, Dobbins WT, Summitt RL, Rainwater WT, Fischer RL: Intermittent peritoneal dialysis using 5 per cent albumin in the treatment of salicylate intoxication in children. J Ped 58: 226–236, 1961.

655. Halle MA, Collipp PJ: Treatment of methyl salicylate poisoning by peritoneal dialysis. N Y State J Med 69: 1788–1789, 1969.

656. Kloss JL, Boeckman CR: Methyl salicylate poisoning: Case report and discussion of treatment by peritoneal dialysis. Ohio State Med J 63: 1064–1065, 1966.

657. Etchart LW, Billings MD: Peritoneal dialysis in salicylate intoxication. Rocky Mountain Med J, Nov, pp 55–56, 1965.

658. Hayat JC: L'Intoxication salicylee. La Nouvelle prese Medicale 17: 715–719, 1973.

659. Hill JB: Current concepts: Salicylate Intoxication. New Engl J Med 288: 1110–1113, 1973.

660. Buselmeier TJ, Mauer SM, Merino GE, Rodrigo F, Simmons RL, Najarian JS, Kjellstrand CM: Therapy of severe salicylate intoxication. Crit Care Med 1: 64–70, 1976.

661. Maclean D, Peters TJ, Brown RAG, McGathie M, Baines GF, Robertson PGC: Treatment of acute paracetamol poisoning. Lancet 1: 849–852, 1968.

662. McCarthy WH, Keenan RL: Propoxyphene hydrochloride poisoning: Report of the first fatality. JAMA 187: 460–461, 1964.

663. Gary NE, Maher JF, DeMyttenaerre MH, Liggero SH, Scott KG, Matusiak W, Schreiner GE: Acute propoxyphene hydrochloride intoxication. Arch Intern Med 121: 453–457, 1968.

664. Karliner JS: Propoxyphene hydrochloride poisoning: Report of a casae treated with peritoneal dialysis. JAMA 199: 1006–1009, 1967.

665. Tasset JJ, Singh S, Pesce A: Evaluation of amitriptyline pharmacokinetics during peritoneal dialysis: Therapeutic Drug Monitoring 7: 255–257, 1985.

666. Aronoff GR, Bergstrom RF, Pottratz ST, Sloan RS, Wolen RL, Lemberger L: Fluoxetine kinetics and protein binding in normal and impaired renal function. Clin Pharmacol Ther 36: 138–144, 1984.

667. Royds RB, Knight AH: Tricyclic antidepressant poisoning. Practitioner 204: 282–286, 1970.

668. Oreopoulos DG: Recovery from massive amitriptyline overdose. Lancet 2: 221, 1968.

669. Sunshine P, Yaffe SJ: Amitriptyline poisoning: Clinical and pathological findings in a fatal case. Am J Dis Child 106: 501–506, 1963.

670. Exaire E, Becerra AT, Monteon F: An overview of treatment with peritoneal dialysis in drug poisoning: Contr Nephrol 17: 39–43, 1979.

671. Hadden J, Johnson K, Smith S, Price L, Giardina E: Acute barbiturate intoxication. JAMA 209: 893–900, 1969.

672. Robinson RR, Gunnels JC, Clapp JR: Treatment of acute barbiturate intoxications. Modern Treat 8: 461–479, 1971.

673. Setter JG, Maher JF, Schreiner GE: Barbiturate intoxication: Arch Intern Med 117: 224–236, 1966.

674. Whiting EG, Barrett OM, Inmon TW: Treatment of barbiturate poisoning: The use of peritoneal dialysis. California Med 102: 367–369, 1965.

675. Henderson LW, Merrill JP: Treatment of barbiturate intoxication: With a report of recent experience at Peter Bent Brigham Hospital. Ann Intern Med 64: 876–891, 1966.

676. Knochel JP, Clayton LE, Smith WL, Barry KG: Intraperitoneal THAM: An effective method to enhance phenobarbital removal during peritoneal dialysis. J Lab CLin Med 64: 257–268, 1964.

677. Setter JG, Freeman RB, Maher JF, Schreiner GE: Factors influencing the dialysis of barbiturates. Trans Am Soc Artif Int Organs 10: 340–344, 1964.

678. Berman LB, Vogelsang P: Removal rates for barbiturates using two types of peritoneal dialysis. New Engl J Med 270: 77–80, 1964.

679. Campion DS, North JDK: Effect of protein binding of barbiturates on their rate of removal during peritoneal dialysis. J Lab Clin Med 66: 549–563, 1965.

680. Rosenbaum JL, Mandanas R: Treatment of phenobarbital intoxication in dogs with an anion-recirculation peritoneal dialysis technique. Trans Am Soc Artif Intern Organs 13: 183–189, 1967.

681. Lash RF, Burdette JA: Accidental profound hypothermia and barbiturate intoxication: A report of rapid 'Core' rewarming by peritoneal dialysis. JAMA 201: 123–124, 1967.

682. Fell RH, Gunning AJ, Bardhan KD, Triger DR: Severe hypothermia as a result of barbiturate overdose complicated by cardia arrest. Lancet 1: 392–394, 1968.

683. Nahas GG, Girouz JJ, Gjessing J, Verosky M, Mark LC: The use of THAM in peritoneal dialysis. Trans Am Soc Artif Intern Organs 10: 345–349, 1964.

684. Monsallier JF, Pocidalo JJ, Vachon F: Le Traitement De L'Intoxication Barbiturique Aigue 7: 2031– 2036, 1967.

685. Maddock RK, Bloomer HA: Meprobamate Overdosage: Evaluation of its severity and methods of treatment. JAMA 201: 999–1003, 1967.

686. Castell DO, Sode JS: Meprobamate intoxication treated with peritoneal dialysis. Illinois Med J 131: 298–299, 1967.

687. Hardy W, Pas AT, Nixon RK: Meprobamate intoxication treated by peritoneal dialysis. Henry Ford Hosp Med Bull 11: 347–349, 1963.

688. Mouton DE, Cohen RJ, Barrett O: Meprobamate poisoning: Successful treatment with peritoneal dialysis. Am J Med Sci 253: 706–709, 1967.

689. Rice AJ, Gruhn SW, Gibson TP, Delle M, Dibona GF: Effect of saline infusion on the renal excretion of secobarbital, glutethimide, meprobamate, and chlordiazepoxide. J Lab Clin Med 80: 56–62, 1972.

690. McDonald DF, Greene WM, Kretchmar L, OBrien G: Experiences in acute glutethimide (doriden) intoxication: Superiority of extracorporeal dialysis over peritoneal dialysis. Invest Urol 1: 127–133, 1963.

691. Arieff AI, Friedman EA: Coma following nonnarcotic drug overdosage: Management of 208 adult patients. Am J Med Sci 266: 405–426, 1973.

692. Ozdemir AI, Tannenberg AM: Peritoneal and hemodialysis for acute glutethimide overdosage. N Y State J Med 72: 2076–2079, 1972.

693. Demytenaere M, Schoenfeld L, Maher JF: Treatment of glutethimide poisoning: A comparison of forced diuresis and dialysis. JAMA 203: 885–887, 1968.

694. Chang TMS, Coffey JF, Taroy E, Lister C, Stark A: Methaqualone, methyprylon, and glutethimide clearance by the ACAC microcapsule artificial kidney: In vitro and in patients with acute intoxication. Trans Am Soc Artif Intern Organs 19: 87–91, 1973.

695. Polin RA, Henry D, Pippinger CE: Peritoneal dialysis for severe methyprylon intoxication. J Ped 90: 831–833, 1977.

696. Collins JM: Peritoneal dialysis for methyprylon intoxication. J Ped 92: 519–520, 1978.

697. Ogilvie RI, Douglas DE, Lochead JR, Moscovich MD, Kaye M: Ethchlorvynol (placidyl) intoxication and its treatment by hemodialysis. Can Med Assoc J 95: 954–956, 1966.

698. Teehan BP, Maher JF, Carey JJH, Flynn PD, Schreinre GE: Acute ethchlorvynol (placidyl) intoxication. Ann Intern Med 72: 875–882, 1970.

699. Schultz JC, Crowder DG, Medart WS: Excretion studies in ethchlorvynol (placidyl) intoxication. Arch Intern Med 117: 409–411, 1966.

700. Lipkin D, Kushnick T: Pargyline hydrochloride poisoning in a child. JAMA 201: 135–136, 1967.

701. Demarco V, Bear R, Kapur BM: Peritoneal dialysis in methaqualone overdose. CMA J 113: 823, 1975.

702. Proudfoot AT, Noble J, Nimmo S, Brown SS, Cameron JC: Peritoneal dialysis and haemodialysis in methaqualone (mandrax) poisoning. Scot Med J 13: 232–236, 1968.

703. Wallace HE, Neumayer F, Gutch CF: Amphetamine poisoning and peritoneal dialysis. Am J Dis Child 108: 657–661, 1964.

704. Zalis EG, Cohen RJ, Lundberg GD: Use of peritoneal dialysis in experimental amphetamine poisoning. Proc Soc Exp Biol Med 12: 278–281, 1965.

705. Espelin DE, Done AK: Amphetamine poisoning: Effectiveness of chlorpromazine. New Engl J Med 278: 1361–1365, 1968.

706. Yolken R, Koneony P, McCarthy P: Acute fluoride poisoning. Pediatr 58: 90–93, 1976.

707. Koshy KM, Lovejoy FH: Thallium ingestion with survival: Ineffectiveness of peritoneal dialysis and potassium chloride diuresis. Clin Toxicol 18: 521–525, 1981.

708. Nagarantnam N, Alagarathnam K, Thambapillai AJ, Wijemanne HSR: Acute renal failure following potassium ferrocyanide poisoning treated with peritoneal dialysis. Forensic Sci 4: 87–89, 1974.

709. Skoutakis VA, Black WD, Acchiardo SR, Wood GC: Peritoneal dialysis in the treatment of acetohexamide-induced hypoglycemia. Am J Hosp Pharm 34: 68–70, 1977.

710. Graw RG: Chlorpropamide intoxication – treatment with peritoneal dialysis. Pediatr 45: 106–109, 1970.

711. Meadow SR, Leeson GA: Poisoning with delayed-release tablets: Treatment of debendox poisoning with purgation and dialysis. Arch Dis Child 49: 310–312, 1974.

712. Diekmann L, Hosemann RR, Dibbern HW: Pheniramin (avil) intoxication bei einem kleinkind. Arch Toxikol 29: 317–324, 1972.

713. Lowenstein E, Goldfine C, Flacke WE: Administration of gallamine in the presence of renal failure – reversal of neuromuscular blockade by peritoneal dialysis. Anesthiology 33: 556–558, 1970.

714. Kann VV, Burgermeister W, Wawschinek O: Standardisierte forcierte diurese und peritoneal dialyse in der behandlung einer alkylphosphatvergiftung. Wien Med Wochenschr 23: 667–669, 1979.

715. Guyon F, Bismuth C, Leclerc JP, Dauchy F: Intoxication massive par le paraquat mortelle en moins de 24 h donnees toxicologiques et anatomocliniques. J Europeen De Toxicologie 7: 182–187, 1974.

716. Hargreave T, Gresham GA, Karayannopoulos S: Paraquat poisoning. Postgrad Med J 45: 633–635, 1969.

717. Fisher HK, Humphries M, Bails R: Paraquat poisoning: Recovery from renal and pulmonary damage. Ann Intern Med 75: 731–736, 1971.

718. Gurr FW, Scroggie JG: Eucalyptus oil poisoning treated by dialysis and mannitol infusion: With an appendix on the analysis of biological fluids for alcohol and eucalyptol. Austral Ann Med 14: 238–249, 1965.

719. O'Brien ET, Yeomas WB, Hobby JAE: Hepatorenal damage from toluene in a glue sniffer. Irish Med J 2: 29–30, 1971.

720. Thomas BB: Peritoneal dialysis and lysol poisoning. British Med J 3: 720, 1969.

721. Wengle B, Hellstrom K: Volatile phenols in serum of uraemic patients. Clin Sci 43: 493–498, 1972.

722. Martin GI: Asymptomatic boric acid intoxication: Value of peritoneal dialysis. N Y State J Med 21: 1842–1844, 1971.

723. Segar WE: Peritoneal dialysis in the treatment of boric acid poisoning. New Engl J Med 262: 798–800, 1960.

724. Baliah T, Macleish H, Drummond KN: Acute boric acid poisoning: Report of an infant successfully treated by peritoneal dialysis. Can Med Assn J 101: 166–168, 1969.

725. Wong LC, Heimbach MD, Truscott DR, Duncan BD: Boric

726. Knight RK, Trounce JR, Cameron JS: Suicidal chlorate poisoning treated with peritoneal dialysis. Brit Med J 3: 601–602, 1967.

727. Klendshoj NC, Burke WJ, Authone R, Anthone S: Chlorate poisoning. JAMA 180: 107–108, 1962.

728. Boehm RM, Czajka PA: Hexachlorophene poisoning and the ineffectiveness of peritoneal dialysis. Clin Toxicol 14: 257–262, 1979.

729. Hermann J, Schmidt HJ, Kruskemper HL: Thyroxine elimination by peritoneal dialysis in experimental thyrotoxicosis. Horm Metab Res 5: 180–183, 1973.

730. Hermann J, Beisenherz W, Gillieh KH, Jester HG, Kluge R, Nissen P, Kruskemper HL: Peritoneal dialysis in the treatment of thyrotoxic crisis. Germ Med Mth 14: 616–617, 1969.

731. Schaible UM, Durr F, Kallee E: Accelerated elimination of thyroxine by peritoneal dialysis. Klin Wsch 50: 1112–1113, 1972.

732. Herrmann J, Kruskemper HL, Grosser KD, Bohn W: Peritonealdialyse in der behandlung der thyeotoxischen krise. Dtsche Med Wochenschr 17: 742–745, 1971.

733. Inaba M, Nishizawa Y, Nishitani H, Miki T, Onishi Y, Mizutani Y, Yamakawa M, Morii H: Concentrations of thyroxine-binding globulin in sera and peritoneal dialysates in patients on chronic peritoneal ambulatory dialysis. Nephron 42: 58–61, 1986.

734. Rey F, Rey J, Cloup M, Feron JF, Dore F, Labrune B, Frezel J: Traitement d'urgence d'une forme aigue de leucinose par dialyse peritoneale. Arch Franc Ped 26: 133–137, 1969.

735. Gaull GE: Pathogenesis of maple-syrup-urine disease: Observations during dietary management and treatment of coma by peritoneal dialysis. Biochem Med 3: 130–149, 1969.

736. Wendel U, Becker K, Przyrembel H, Bulla M, Manegold C, Hoinowski A, Langenbeck U: Peritoneal dialysis in maple-syrup urine disease: Studies on branched-chain amino and keto acids. Eur J Ped 134: 557–63, 1980.

737. Russell G, Thom H, Tarlow MJ, Gompertz D: Reduction of plasma propionate by peritoneal dialysis. Pediatr 53: 281–283, 1974.

738. Sanjurjo P, Jaquotot C, Vallo A, Uriarte R, Prats JM, Ugarte M, Rodriguez J: Tratamiento combinado de exanguinotransfusion dialisis peritoneal en un caso neonatal de acidemia metil-malonica con hiperamoniemmia severa. En Esp Pedi 17: 317–320, 1982.

739. Martin JF, Hamdy N, Nicholl J, Lewtas N, Bergvall U, Owen P, Syder D, Middlebrook A: Prostacyclin in cerebral infaction. New Engl J Med 312: 1641–1642, 1985.

740. Snyderman SE, Sansaricq C, Phansalkar SV, Schacht RG, Norton PM: The therapy of hyperammonemia due to ornithine transcarbamylase defiency in a male neonate. Pediatr 56: 56–73, 1975.

741. Wiegand C, Thompson T, Bock GH, Mathis RK, Kjellstrand CM, Mauer SM: The management of life-threatening hyperammonemia: A comparison of several therapeutic modalities. J Ped 96: 142–144, 1980.

742. Dunn SE, Swartz RD, Thoene JG: Comparison of exchange transfusionm peritoneal dialysis, and hemodialysis for the treatment of hyperammonemia in an anuric newborn infant. J Ped 95: 67–70, 1979.

743. Siegal NJ, Brown RS: Peritoneal clearance of ammonia and creatinine in a neonate. J Ped 82: 1044–1046, 1973.

744. Nyhan WL, Wolff J, Kulovich S, Shumacher AE: Intestinal obstruction due to peritoneal adhesions as a complication of peritoneal dialysis for neonatal hyperammonemia. Eur J Ped 143: 211–213, 1985. ·

745. Gloor HJ, Moore H, Nolph KD: The peritoneal handling of digoxin during CAPD. Periton Dial Bull 2: 13–16, 1982.

746. Doherty JE, Ackerman GL, Kane JJ: Treatment of digoxin intoxication. Lancet 1: 494–495, 1973.

747. Doherty JE, Bissett JK, Kane JJ, Soyza N, Murphy ML, Flanigan WJ, Dalrymple GV: Tritiated digoxin: Studies in renal disease in human subjects. Int J Clin Pharmacol 12: 89–95, 1975.

748. Kramer P, Quellhorst E, Horenkamp J, Scheler F: Dialysance und prozentuale elimination verschiedener herzglykoside wahrend der hamo und peritonealdialyse. Klin Wschr 50: 609–613, 1972.

749. Depaepe M, Belpaire F, Bogaert Y: Pharmacokinetics of digoxin in CAPD. Clin Exp Dial Apheresis 6: 65–73, 1982.

750. Pancarbo S, Comty C: Digoxin pharmacokinetics in continuous peritoneal dialysis. Ann Intern Med 93: 639, 1980.

751. Ackerman GL, Doherty JE, Flanigan WJ: Peritoneal dialysis and hemodialysis of tritiated digoxin. Ann Intern Med 67: 718–723, 1967.

752. Risler T, Peters U, Pablick J, Grabensee B, Krokou: Pharmacokinetics of digoxin and digitoxin in patients on continuous ambulatory peritoneal dialysis (CAPD), In: Gahl GM, Kessel M, Nolph KD (eds), Advances in Peritoneal Dialysis, Proceedings of the Second International Symposium on Peritoneal Dialysis, Amsterdam, Excerpta Medica, pp 88–89, 1981.

753. Lameire N, Belpaire F, Bogaert M, Bogaerts Y, DePaepe M, Ringoir S: Peritoneal pharmacokinetics: A review and studies on digoxin and gentamicin, In Atkins RC, Thomson NM, Farrell PC (eds), Peritoneal Dialysis, New York, Churchill Livingstone, pp 30–40, 1981.

754. Chin TWF, Pancorbo S, Comty C: Quinidine pharmacokinetics in continuous ambulatory peritoneal dialysis. Clin Exp Dial Apheresis 5: 391–397, 1981.

755. Hall K, Meatherall B, Krahn J, Penner B, Rabson JL: Clearance of quinidine during peritoneal dialysis. Am Heart J 104: 646–647, 1982.

756. Harris L, Hind CRK, McKenna WJ, Savage C, Krinkler SJ, Storey GCA, Holt DW: Renal elimination of amoidaroine and is desethyl metabolite. Postgrad Med J 59: 440–442, 1983.

757. Spital A, Scandling JD: Nifedipine in continuous ambulatory peritoneal dialysis. Arch Intern Med 143: 2025, 1983.

758. Parrott KA, Alexander SR, Stennett DJ: Loss of propranolol via CAPD in two patients. Periton Dial Bull 4: 110, 1984.

759. Parrott KA: Determination of propranolol in peritoneal dialysis fluid by high performance liquid chromatography without extraction. J Chrom 274: 171–178, 1983.

760. Campese VM, Feinstein EI, Guara V, Mason WD, Massry SG: Pharmocokinetics of atenolol in patients treated with chronic hemodialysis or peritoneal dialysis. J Clin Pharmacol 25: 393–395, 1985.

761. Breborowicz A, Knapowski J: Augmentation of peritoneal dialysis clearance with procaine. Kidney Int 26: 392–396, 1984.

762. Pimentel LV, Epstein LM, Sellers EM, Foster JR, Bennion LJ, Nadler LM, Bough EW, Weser JK: Survival after massive procainamide ingestine. Am J Cardiol 32: 727–730, 1973.

763. Kroboth PD, Mitchum K, Puschett JB: Use of procainamide in chronic ambulatory peritoneal dialysis: Report of a case. Am J Kidney Dis 4: 78–79, 1984.

764. Raehl Cl, Moorthy AV, Beirne GJ, Pitterle ME: Procainamide administration during continuous ambulatory peritoneal dialysis. Am Heart J 110: 1306–1308, 1985.

765. Thomson PD, Melmon KL, Richardson JA, Cohn K, Steinbrunn W, Cudihee R, Rowland M: Lidocaine pharmacokinetics in advanced heart failure, liver disease, and renal failure in humans. Ann Intern Med 78: 499–508, 1973.

766. Braun J, Sorgel F, Engelmaier F, Gessler U: Peritoneal dialysis clearance of tocainide in a patient on continuous ambulatory peritoneal dialysis. Periton Dial Bull 5: 139, 1985.

767. Roots, I, Hilderbrandt AG, Baethke R, Glass U, Molzahn M: Influence of haemo and peritoneal dialysis on pharma-

cokinetics of diazoxide. Nauyn Schiedeberg Arch Pharmacol 287: 289, 1975.

768. Hulter HN, Licht JH, Ilnicki LP: Clinical efficacy and pharmacokinetics of clonidine in hemodialysis and renal insufficiency. J Lab Clin Med 94: 223–231, 1979.

769. Yeh BK, Dayton PG, Waters WC: Removal of alpha-methyldopa (aldomet) in man by dialysis (35155). Proc Soc Exp Biol Med 135: 840–843, 1970.

770. Evers J, Bonn R, Boertz A, Cawello W, Lucklow V, Fey M, Aboudan F, Dickmans HA: Pharmacokinetics of isosorbide-5-nitrate during haemodialysis and peritoneal dialysis. Eur J Clin Pharmacol 32: 503–505, 1987.

771. Vaziri ND, Ness RL, Barton CH: Peritoneal dialysis clearance of cimetidine. Am J Gastroenterol 71: 572–576, 1979.

772. Kogan FJ, Sampliner RE, Mayersohn M, Kazama RM, Perrier D, Jones W, Michael UF: Cimetidine disposition in patients undergoing continuous ambulatory peritoneal dialysis. J Clin Pharmacol 23: 252–256, 1983.

773. Pizzella KM, Moore MC, Schultz RW, Walshe J, Schentag JJ: Removal of cimetidine by peritoneal dialysis, hemodialysis, and charcoal hemoperfusion. Ther Drug Monitor 2: 273–281, 1980.

774. Hyneck ML, Murphy JF, Lipschultz DE: Cimetidine clearance during intermittent and chronic peritoneal dialysis. Am J Hosp Pharm 38: 1760–1762, 1981.

775. Bodemar G, Norlander B, walan A: Pharmacokinetics of cimetidine after single doses during continuous treatment. CLin Pharmacokin 6: 306–315, 1981.

776. Paton TW, Manuel MA, Walker SE: Cimetidine disposition in patients on continuous ambulatory peritoneal dialysis. Peritoneal Dialysis Bulletin 2: 73–76, 1982.

777. Berardi RR, Cornish LA, Hyneck ML: Metoclopramide removal during continuous ambulatory peritoneal dialysis. Drug Intell Clin Pharm 20: 154–155, 1986.

778. Myre SA, Singh S, Kawamoto D, Marshall L, Wright GJ: Metoclopramide kinetics during continuous ambulatory peritoneal dialysis. Drug Intell Clin Pharm 20: 508, 1986.

779. Bjorck S, Ahlmen J, Mellstrand T, Stelin G: Influence of dialysis on prednisolone kinetics. Acta Med Scand 215: 379–382, 1984.

780. Sherlock JE, Letteri JM: Effect of hemodialysis on methylprednisolone plasma levels. Nephron 18: 208–211, 1977.

781. Blair AAD, Hallipike JF, Laselles PT, Wingate DL: Acute diphenylhydantoin and primidone poisoning treated by peritoneal dialysis. J Neurol Neusorug Psychiat 31: 520–523, 1968.

782. Tenckhoff H, Sherrard DJ, Hickman RO, Ladda RL: Acute diphenylhydantoin Intoxication. Am J Dis Child 116: 422–425, 1968.

783. Lindahl S, Westerling D: Detoxification with peritoneal dialysis and exchange transfusion after diphenylhydantoin intoxication. Acta Poediatr Scand 71: 665–666, 1982.

784. Hess B, Keusch G, Fluckiger J, Binswanger U: Zur Pharmakokinetik von phenytoin bei kontinuierlicher ambulanter peritonealdialyse. Schweiz Med Wschr 114: 16–19, 1984.

785. Hays DP, Primack WA, Abroms IF: Phenytoin clearance by continuous ambulatory peritoneal dialysis. Drugg Intell Clin Pharm 19: 429–431, 1985.

786. Orr JM, Farrell K, Abbott FS, Ferguson S, Godolphin: The effects of peritoneal dialysis on the single dose and steady state pharmacokinetics of valproic acid in a uremic epileptic child. Eur J Clin Pharmacol 24: 387–390, 1983.

787. Fish SS, Pancorbo S, Berkseth R: Pharmacokinetics of epsilon-aminocaproic acid during peritoneal dialysis. J Neurosurg 54: 736–739, 1981.

788. Regamy C, Schaberg D, Kirby WMM: Inhibitory effect of heparin on gentamicin concentrations in blood. Antimicrob Agents Chemother 1: 329–332, 1972.

789. Thayssen P, Pindborg T: Peritoneal dialysis and heparin.

Scand J Urol Nephrol 12: 73–74, 1978.

790. O'Leary JP, Malik FS, Donahoe RR, Johnston AD: The effects of a minidose of heparin on peritonitis in rats. Surg Gyn OB 148: 571–575, 1979.

791. Mion CM, Beon ST, Scriber P: Analysis of factors responsible for the formation of adhesions during chronic peritoneal dialysis. Am J Med Sci 250: 675–679, 1965.

792. Ponce SP, Barata JDF, Santos JR: Interference of heparin with peritoneal solute transport. Nephron 39: 47–49, 1985.

793. Furman KI, Gomperts ED, Hockley J: Activity of intraperitoneal heparin during peritoneal dialysis. Clin Nephrol 9: 15–18, 1978.

794. Vas S; Questions, answers. Periton Dial Dull 1: 67, 1981.

795. Schrader J, Tonnis H-J, Schler F: Long term intraperitoneal application of low molecular weigth heparin in a continuous ambulatory peritoneal dialysis patient with deep vein thrombosis. Nephron 42: 83–84, 1986.

796. Greis E, Paar D, Graben N, Bock KD: Intraperitoneal fibrin-formation and its inhibition in CAPD. Clinical Nephrology 26: 209–212, 1986.

797. Canavese C, Salomone M, Mangiarotti G, Pacitti A, Trucco S, Scaglia C, Assone F, Lunghi F, Vercellone A: Heparin transfer across the rabbit peritoneal membrane. Clinical Nephrology 26: 116–120, 1986.

798. Stiekema JCJ: Heparin and its biocompatibility. Clinical Nephrology Suppl 1: 53–58, 1986.

799. Demedts W, Desager JP, Belpaire F, Lameire N: Life-threatening hyperkalemia associated with clofibrate induced myopathy in a CAPD patient. Periton Dial Bull 3: 15–16, 1983.

800. Lee CSC, Peterson JC, Marbury TC: Comparative pharmacokinetics of theophylline in peritoneal dialysis and hemodialysis. J Clin Pharmacol 23: 274–280, 1983.

801. Levy G, Gibson TP, Whitman W, Procknal J: Hemodialysis clearance of theophylline. JAMA 237: 1466–1467, 1977.

802. Emonds AJG, Driessen MJ: Treatment of theophylline intoxication: A model study utilizing peritoneal dialysis. Clin Toxicol 13: 505–511, 1978.

803. Weinberger M, Hendeles L: Role of dialysis in the management and prevention of theophylline toxicity. Dev Pharmacol Ther 1: 26–30, 1980.

804. Miceli JN, Clay B, Fleischmann LE, Sarnaiek AP, Aronow R, Done AK: Pharmacokinetics of severe theophylline intoxication managed by peritoneal dialysis. Dev Pharmacol Ther 1: 16–25, 1980.

805. Miclei JN, Bidani A, Aronow R: Peritoneal dialysis of theophylline. Clin Toxicol 14: 539–544, 1979.

806. Ackrill P, McIntosh CS, Nimmon C, Baker LRI, Cattell WR: A comparison of the clearance of urographic contrast medium (sodium diatrizoate) by peritoneal and haemodialysis. Clin Sci Mol Med 50: 69–74, 1976.

807. Milman N, Christensen E: Elimination of diatrizoate by peritoneal dialysis in renal failure. Acta Radiol 15: 265–272, 1973.

808. Brooks MH, Barry KG: Removal of iodinated contrast material by peritoneal dialysis. Nephron 12: 10–14, 1973.

809. Wainer E, Boner G, Lubin E, Rosenfield JB: Clearance of tc-99m DTPA in hemodialysis and peritoneal dialysis: Concise communication. J Nucl Med 22: 768–771, 1981.

810. Karimeddini MK: Ga-67 Scanning during peritoneal dialysis. J Nucl Med 22: 479–480, 1981.

811. Steiner RW: Adverse effects of intraperitoneal methylene blue: Periton Dial Bull 3: 43, 1983.

812. Sevitt LH, Hoffbrand AV: Serum folate and vitamin B_{12} levels in acute and chronic renal disease: Effect of peritoneal dialysis. Brit Med J 2: 18–21, 1969.

813. Blumberg A, Hanck A, Sander G: Vitamin nutrition in patients on continuous ambulatory peritoneal dialysis (CAPD). Clin Nephrol 20: 244–250, 1983.

814. Tsapas G, Magoula I, Paletas K, Concouris L: Effect of peritoneal dialysis on plasma levels of ascorbic acid. Nephron 33: 34–37, 1983.

815. Mydlik M, Derziova K, Havris S, Mizla P: Vitamin C: A nepretrizita ambulantna peritonealna dialyza. Vnitrni lekarstvi 29: 249–253, 1983.

816. Henderson IS, Leung ACT, Shenkin A: Vitamin status in continuous ambulatory peritoneal dialysis. Periton Dial Bull 3: 143–145, 1984.

817. Vahlquist A, Berne B, Danielson BG, Grefberg N, Berne C: Vitamin A losses during continuous ambulatory peritoneal dialysis. Nephron 41: 179–183, 1985.

818. Parrott KA, Stockberger RA, Alexander SR, Miller LT, Leklem JE, Jenkins RD: Plasma vitamin-a levels in children on CAPD. Periton Dial Bull 7: 90–92, 1987.

819. Mydlik M, Derzsiova K, Valek A, Szabo T, Dandar V, Takac M: Vitamins and continuous ambulatory peritoneal dialysis (CAPD). Int Urol Nephrol 17: 281–286, 1985.

820. Guillot M, Lavocat C, Garabedian M, Sachs C, Balsan S, Gagnadoux MF, Broyer M: Evaluation of 25 (OH) D loss in dialysate of children on continuous ambulatory peritoneal dialysis. Proc EDTA 18: 290–292, 1981.

13

NUTRITIONAL MANAGEMENT OF PATIENTS UNDERGOING PERITONEAL DIALYSIS

BENGT LINDHOLM AND JONAS BERGSTRÖM

1. INTRODUCTION

Patients with chronic renal failure display a variety of metabolic and nutritional abnormalities and a large proportion of the patients demonstrate signs of protein-energy malnutrition [1–20]. This may be a consequence of multiple factors including disturbances in protein and energy metabolism, hormonal derangements, infections and other superimposed illnesses, and poor food intake because of anorexia, nausea and vomiting, caused by uremic toxicity. With maintenance dialysis therapy, some of these factors, but far from all, can be partly or fully corrected. On the other hand, metabolic and nutritional problems are caused by the method of dialysis. For example, the hemodialysis procedure per se may induce protein catabolism [8, 15, 16], peritoneal dialysis is associated with large protein losses into the dialysate [18, 19], and both dialysis methods are associated with dialytic losses of amino acids, vitamins, and other essential small solutes [20]. Futhermore, peritoneal dialysis is associated with absorption of large quantities of glucose from the dialysate. These factors, superimposed on the metabolic abnormalities and inadequate nutritional state of patients with chronic renal failure, may have serious consequences in the form of aggravated malnutrition, susceptibility to infection, anemia, cardiovascular dysfunction, progressive neuropathy, hyperlipidemia, failure of rehabilitation, and increased morbidity and mortality [12, 20, 21, 22].

1.1. Intermittent peritoneal dialysis

Although peritoneal dialysis in a patient was first described by Ganter in 1923 [23], it was not until the early 1960s that peritoneal dialysis was accepted as a longterm therapy in uremic patients [24, 25]. For long, its use remained rather limited, however, and it never became as universally accepted as hemodialysis, mainly because of the need for repeated abdominal puncture and the high incidence of peritonitis [25]. During the 1970s the introduction of devices that secure a safe permanent access to the peritoneal cavity, and the development of automatic peritoneal dialysis systems aroused a new interest in peritoneal dialysis [25–27]. However, in comparison to hemodialysis, peritoneal dialysis is a relatively inefficient method for removal of uremic waste products. Various schedules have been proposed for chronic intermittent peritoneal dialysis, e.g., 9-15 hr or more per dialysis, mostly adding up to 20-45 hr/week, with an exchange of dialysate ranging from 70 to 240 l/week, all schedules resulting in a much lower weekly urea clearance than in patients on intermittent hemodialysis. Unless the patients have significant residual renal function this frequency of dialysis is usually inadequate and patients often remain symptomatically uremic. Due to weakness, anorexia and vomiting, nutrient intake is often insufficient during the interdialytic period. During intermittent peritoneal dialysis most patients are confined to the bed for long periods of time and thus inactive, which may further contribute to loss of muscle mass and hamper rehabilitation. Intermittent peritoneal dialysis has to a large extent been reserved for older patients, patients with cardiovascular disease, and temporarily for patients waiting for a place in a chronic hemodialysis program or as a permanent substitute for hemodialysis when hemodialysis facilities are lacking.

The long-term experiences with maintenance intermittent peritoneal dialysis for the definitive management of patients with end-stage renal failure generally are not favourable in terms of nutritional aspects (Table 1). Although capable of transiently improving uremic symptoms, intermittent peritoneal dialysis is frequently associated with progressive tissue wasting and malnutrition. Dialysate protein, amino acid and trace mineral losses are substantial and the combination of insufficient dialysis and inadequate nutrient intake are major factors contributing to the frequently observed development of malnutrition and wasting.

1.2. Continuous ambulatory peritoneal dialysis (CAPD)

In 1976, a team from Austin, Texas, USA, led by Popovich and Moncrief described 'a novel portable/wearable equilibrium peritoneal dialysis technique' which was based on a kinetic model predicting that 'acceptable blood metabolite levels will result if 10 l of dialysate per day are allowed to continuously equilibrate with body fluids' [28]. The idea suggested that the continuous presence of two liters of peritoneal dialysis fluid in the peritoneal cavity, interrupted only intermittently by brief periods for drainage and instillation of fresh dialysis solution five times per day, could represent a continuous ambulatory, primarily internal dialysis system [28–30]. Clinical tests showed that this concept was valid and the name of the technique was changed to continuous ambulatory peritoneal dialysis (CAPD) [29, 30]. Initially, dialysis fluid in glass bottles were used and the technique was therefore cumbersome and time consuming and associated with a high incidence of peritonitis due to the need of connections and disconnections of bottles and tubing to the Tenckhoff catheter at each exchange [29, 30]. A major improvement of the technique was introduced in 1977 when a team in Toronto, Canada, led by Oreopoulos started to use dialysis fluid in polyvinylchloride bags [31]. Following instillation of the fluid by gravity, the collapsible plastic bag was folded, and carried with the patient under clothing for 4-8 h while the patient conducted his or her normal activities. The bag was then unfolded and the dialysate was drained by gravity into the same bag without disconnecting the tube from the catheter [31]. During CAPD, the patient is thus being dialyzed 7 days a week, 24 h a day, and, as the name indicated, CAPD is designed primarily for home treatment of patients with chronic renal failure.

CAPD implies that the patients are continuously dialyzed against fluid instilled into the peritoneal cavity and exchanged 3-5 times per day. This method has now gained widespread acceptance as an alternative to hemodialysis for chronic renal replacement therapy [107]. It is simple, can be handled by the patient himself, and is, therefore, cost effective. In CAPD, the relative insufficiency of peritoneal dialysis for removal of waste products is partly compensated for by the fact that the process is continuous over 24 h, 7 days a week. Following the preliminary experiences with CAPD in the late 1970s, several favourable effects were reported (Table 2). The patients starting on CAPD appeared to thrive, their body weight and hematocrit increased and the control of serum biochemistries, acid-base equilibrium, and fluid balance was reported to be comparable to, or better than, in patients undergoing other forms of dialysis therapy [29–31]. These effects, which suggested an anabolic state, were attributed to the continuous dialytic process and to an effective removal of uremic middle molecules [29–30]. However, CAPD also involves several catabolic factors such as loss of appetite, loss of proteins and amino acids into the peritoneal dialysate, and recurrent peritonitis [29-32]. The continuous supply of glucose and lactate or acetate from the dialysate represents a sizable and perhaps undesirable energy load that may induce or accentuate hyperglycemia, hyperinsulinemia, hypertriglyceridemia, and other metabolic abnormalities

Table 1. Nutritional problems with intermittent peritoneal dialysis

1. Anorexia due to insufficient dialysis of small solutes.
2. High dialysate protein and amino acid losses.
3. Physical inactivation (bedridden during long dialysis sessions).
4. High incidence of peritonitis.
5. Hyperglycemia.

Table 2. Nutritional advantages with CAPD

1. Stable metabolite levels due to continuous dialysis.
2. Prevention of hyperkalemia and other electrolyte disorders.
3. Improved control of metabolic acidosis.
4. Effective removal of middle molecules.
5. Continuous energy supply.
6. Intradialytic catabolism (such as in HD) is avoided.

Table 3. Nutritional problems with CAPD

1. High incidence of peritonitis.
2. Loss of protein (5–15 g/d) and amino acids (2–4 g/d).
3. Anorexia (due to glucose absorption, abdominal filling, insufficient dialysis).
4. Hyperglycemia and hyperinsulinemia.
5. Hyperlipidemia and dyslipoproteinemia.
6. Obesity.

Table 4. Evidence of malnutrition in uremic patients

1. Subjective global assessment of nutritional status indicates a high prevalence of malnutrition.
2. Body weight (% relative body weight, % pre-uremic body weight) is low.
3. Skinfold thickness (triceps, biceps, subscapular, suprailliac) is low.
4. Midarm muscle circumference is low.
5. Visceral proteins (serum total protein, albumin, transferrin, immunoglobins, C_3, C_4) are low.
6. Essential amino acids (plasma, leucocytes, muscle) are low.
7. Non-essential amino acids (plasma, leucocytes, muscle) are high.
8. Muscle intracellular alkali-soluble protein (ASP): DNA is low.

(Table 3). These observations raised questions about the long-term metabolic and nutritional consequences of CAPD [27]. Later, with an increasing number of patients being maintained on long-term CAPD, several potentially adverse metabolic effects have emerged, which might limit its more widespread use [18, 33–36].

This chapter will focus on metabolic and nutritional problems of the adult non-diabetic patient undergoing continuous ambulatory peritoneal dialysis (CAPD). After describing the syndrome of malnutrition in patients with chronic renal failure including when appropriate a brief description of the situation in hemodialyzed patients as a general background, we describe specific metabolic and nutritional problems in CAPD patients. Finally, recommendations are given for the nutritional assessment and nutritional management of these patients.

2. MALNUTRITION IN CHRONIC RENAL FAILURE

Several reports have documented that protein-energy malnutrition and wasting are frequently present in nondialyzed as well as in patients undergoing maintenance dialysis therapy even in those patients who appear to be normal and who have had a succesful clinical course [1–22]. The evidence for malnutrition in uremic patients (Table 4) includes: 1) Reduced 'dry weight' or postdialysis weight compared to the weight of normal subjects of the same age, sex, and height or in comparison with the preuremic weight of the patient. 2) Low values for triceps and subscapular skinfold thickness indicating reduced body fat stores. 3) Midarm muscle circumference (calculated from triceps skinfold thickness and midarm circumference) is reduced indicating reduced muscle mass. 4) Visceral proteins such as serum albumin, transferrin, immunoglobulins, and complement components are reduced indicating reduced body protein stores. 5) Muscle intracellular noncollagen (alkali-soluble) protein content relative to the DNA content in muscle is reduced indicating protein depletion on the cellular level. 6) The plasma amino acid pattern and the intracellular muscle amino acid pattern are abnormal and include various alterations such as reduced concentrations of essential amino acids that are commonly observed in chronic malnutrition.

When evaluating the nutritional effects of dialysis therapies it should be kept in mind that the patient starting on maintenance dialysis therapy is often suffering from severe malnutrition and wasting. During the period prior to the institution of dialysis therapy the patients are often treated with low protein diets and a variety of drugs that may worsen anorexia and interfere with the absorption of

specific nutrients. In addition, complications such as infections, pericarditis, congestive heart failure, complications of therapy, in particular corticosteroid therapy, may result in the patient initiating dialysis being in an already severely debilitated state.

Once dialysis therapy is begun, accompanied by reduction of uremic symptoms and liberalization of the diet, some patients may show improved nutritional status. However, many of the indicators of malnutrition that are present at the onset of therapy remain abnormal and some aspects of malnutrition may become even more severe.

Several studies suggest that malnutrition is an important factor for morbidity and mortality in dialysis patients [12, 21, 37, 38]. In a study of 120 hemodialysis patients, Acchiardo *et al.* [21] found that a subgroup with a mean protein intake of 0.63 g/kg/day (calculated from urea appearance rate) had a mortality of 14% per year, while groups of patients with higher intakes, 0.93, 1.02, and 1.29 g/kg/day, had mortalities of only 4, 3, and 0%, respectively. The number of hospitalizations per year was also much higher in the group of patients with the lowest intake of protein with higher frequencies of heart disease, pericarditis, infection, and gastrointestinal manifestations than in the other patient groups. The authors concluded that protein malnutrition is the main factor in morbidity and mortality of hemodialysis patients. However, it cannot be ruled out that in some patients increased morbidity was the primary event, and low protein intake was a secondary phenomenon.

Thus it is generally accepted that suboptimal nutritional status is associated with increased morbidity and may contribute to poor rehabilitation and quality of life. Cutaneous anergy and other immune alterations strikingly similar to those observed in malnutrition have also been documented in hemodialysis patients [39, 40, 41], suggesting that protein-energy malnutrition may be a risk factor for infection and septicemia. The incidence of peritonitis and length of stay in hospital have been found to be greater in CAPD patients who were hypoalbuminemic [42, 43]. Infection is a common complication in uremic patients which may in itself lead to malnourishment. If improved nutritional status could improve host defenses in uremia, this might have important clinical consequences. Whether or not immunologic dysfunction is related to nutritional status in uremic patients or is secondary to uremia per se is not established.

2.1. Causes of protein-energy malnutrition in uremia

A variety of causes (Table 5) contribute to impaired nutritional status in uremic patients [1–22]. The most important are: 1) Abnormal protein and amino acid metabolism secondary to the influence of uremia per se, loss of renal tissue, and proteinuria. 2) Poor food intake because of anorexia, nausea, and vomiting, caused by uremic toxicity. 3) Intercurrent illnesses such as infections, hyperparathyroidism, pericarditis, and congestive heart failure resulting in increased metabolic stress and sometimes profound hypercatabolism. 4) Decreased biological activity of anabolic hormones such as insulin and somatomedins and increased circulating levels of catabolic hormones such as glucagon and parathyroid hormone. 5) Dialytic losses of amino acids, water-soluble vitamins and other essential small molecular solutes. 6) Protein losses into the dialysate (in peritoneal dialysis). 7) Catabolic effects of the dialytic procedure (in hemodialysis). 8) Frequent blood sampling. 9) Low physical activity. 10) Abnormal cell energy metabolism, carbohydrate intolerance, and impaired lipid metabolism, contributing to negative energy balance.

3. PROTEIN AND AMINO ACID METABOLISM

It is well recognized that patients with advanced chronic renal failure have a tendency towards negative nitrogen balance and muscle wasting. This may be a consequence of several catabolic factors affecting protein and amino acid metabolism. These factors are to a large extent fundamental components of the uremic condition and are only slightly modified by the mode of dialysis therapy whereas other factors, e.g. dialytic losses of protein and amino acids, are introduced by the method of dialysis.

3.1. Increased protein catabolism

There is evidence that uremia per se is a catabolic state and that the uremic condition promotes net degradation of protein and amino acids [20, 44–49]. Thus impaired protein synthesis as well as enhanced protein catabolism may contribute to diminution of lean body mass in uremia. Protein synthesis in vitro is impaired in the presence of

Table 5. Causes of protein-energy malnutrition and wasting in uremic patients

---

1. Increased net protein catabolism (uremic toxicity).
2. Anorexia, nausea, vomiting (uremic toxicity).
3. Intercurrent illnesses such as infections resulting in hypercatabolism.
4. Decreased biological activity of anabolic hormones (insulin, somatomedins).
5. Increased circulating levels of catabolic hormones (glucagon, PTH).
6. Impaired cell energy metabolism and negative energy balance.
7. Urinary protein loss.
8. Frequent blood drawing.
9. Dialytic losses of amino acids and vitamins (HD, PD).
10. Intradialytic hypercatabolism (HD).
11. Dialysate protein loss (PD).

---

uremic plasma dialysate [44]. Increased protein synthesis is observed in the presence of postdialysis as compared to predialysis plasma dialysate, indicating that factors in uremia inhibit protein synthesis and that dialysis removes a great part of the inhibitory effect which appears to be related to dialyzable molecules. The amino acid transport is also inhibited by uremic plasma in vitro [47].

Increased muscle release of amino acids in experimental chronic uremia in rats [48, 49] suggests that muscle protein catabolism is enhanced. In contrast, the observation of a general tendency towards decreased net amino acid release from leg tissues in uremic patients [50] is consistent with a reduced protein turnover and in line with the observation of lower protein flux, i.e., a lower rate of breakdown and synthesis of protein in relation to protein intake in nondialyzed uremic children than in normal children [51]. Protein turnover was lower in a group of uremic patients before and after treatment with CAPD than in normal subjects although this difference did not reach statistical significance, but the balance between synthesis and breakdown was significantly increased and was maintained high after 3 months on CAPD [52]. However, it cannot be excluded that the decreased net release of amino acids and the low protein turnover observed in these studies reflect adaptive responses to depletion of muscle protein and intracellular amino acid pools, respectively.

It has been suggested that release of interleukin 1 (IL-1) or endogenous pyrogen plays a role by stimulating lysosomal protein breakdown in muscle tissue, an effect mediated through liberation of prostaglandin E [53]. Other catabolic factors in hypercatabolic renal failure may be increased release of protein-catabolic enzymes into the circulation [54].

As will be discussed later protein requirements of CAPD patients, although variable, seem to be at least 1 g/kg body weight/day and in some patients probably higher. This is about twice as much as the minimum requirements in normal subjects of 0.5 g/kg body weight/day. The protein and amino acid losses of 8-18 g/day in CAPD correspond to about 0.2-0.3 g/kg body weight which has to be compensated for by increased intake of high-quality protein. However, it is questionable whether the protein losses during CAPD (without peritonitis) might totally account for the increased protein requirements compared to normal subjects and nondialyzed uremic patients. In addition to the unfavourable effects of low energy intake and recurrent peritonitis, there is a possibility that the dialytic procedure per se stimulates protein catabolism by substances other than live bacteria. These substances could be microbial products (endotoxins), acetate, plasticizers, silicon, glucose, or other products from the system which elute into the peritoneal cavity.

Shaldon *et al.* [55] have reported that CAPD is associated with a production of IL-1 and have proposed this mechanism as an explanation for why some patients develop so-called sclerosing peritonitis. There is a possibility that chronic stimulation of peritoneal macrophages, induced by endotoxin, acetate, plasticizers, silicon, etc., may have effects beyond the peritoneal cavity, i.e., induce protein catabolism in skeletal muscle by the action of IL-1. This might be an additional explanation of why patients on CAPD need much more protein than normal subjects and nondialyzed uremic patients.

3.2. Abnormal amino acid pattern

There are numerous reports of abnormal plasma amino acid concentrations in patients with chronic renal failure [3, 56, 57]. Among the consistent findings are high concentrations of several nonessential amino acids and low concentrations of essential amino acids, including the branched chain amino acids valine, isoleucine, and leucine. The plasma concentration of tyrosine is low and the phenylalanine/tyrosine ratio is high. Many of the plasma amino acid abnormalities found in uremia are similar to those observed in protein malnutrition, and it has been suggested that they are in part attributable to dietary inadequacy.

The largest pool of free amino acids, however, is not in the extracellular fluid, but in skeletal muscle. In untreated uremic patients a typical muscle intracellular amino acid pattern is observed with low concentration of valine, but normal concentrations of leucine and isoleucine and low concentrations of threonine, lysine, and histidine [2].

Some of the observed changes are thought to be due to metabolic alterations in uremia or due to impaired degradation or decreased urinary excretion by the diseased kidneys, whereas other abnormalities may reflect inadequate nutritional intake [2, 3, 11]. Since shortage of one of the essential amino acids is enough to critically limit protein synthesis these amino acid abnormalities may have a crucial role in the syndrome of malnutrition of uremia.

3.3. Hormonal derangements

Insulin is an anabolic hormone that enhances amino acid transport and stimulates protein synthesis. Insulin-mediated glucose metabolism is severely impaired in uremic subjects, and the primary site of this insulin resistance resides in peripheral tissues, mainly muscle [58]. Fasting plasma insulin concentrations are increased. In vitro studies of the effect of insulin on muscle metabolism of amino acids have given somewhat controversial results in as much as the ability of insulin to stimulate transport of amino acids into muscle has been observed to be impaired [48, 59], whereas inhibition by insulin of muscle release of tyrosine and phenylalanine has been reported to be normal [49] and that of alanine even to be enhanced [48] when compared to controls. However, in chronically uremic subjects with markedly impaired insulin-mediated glucose metabolism, physiologic hyperinsulinemia was observed to decrease net release of amino acids from leg tissues to the same extent as in control subjects [50].

Decreased biological activity of other anabolic hormones such as somatomedins [60, 61] as well as increased circulating levels of catabolic hormones such as glucagon [62] and parathyroid hormone [63] may contribute to protein wasting, although their exact roles in this respect are not well understood.

3.4. Anorexia and gastrointestinal disorders

Uremic patients often have poor dietary intake because of anorexia, nausea, and vomiting [20]. Although these symptoms are usually less severe with the commencement of dialysis therapy, they are often not completely reversed. Treatment with CAPD may even worsen anorexia due to a chronic sense of abdominal fullness and continuous peritoneal absorption of glucose. The hemodialysis procedure itself is also often associated with nausea and vomiting, possibly related to rapid shifts of fluid and electrolytes. Patients undergoing hemodialysis usually consume less food on days they dialyze, and their eating pattern is often different on these days with reduced protein intake.

In addition, hemodialysis patients have delayed gastric emptying which may exacerbate anorexia [64]. Futhermore, impaired intestinal absorption of fat and other nutrients may contribute to malnutrition in uremic patients [65].

3.4.1. Decreasing protein and energy intake with time in CAPD patients

Nutritional problems may occur in CAPD patients due to a decreased intake of both protein and total energy with time on CAPD [66–70]. After 1 year on CAPD the average dietary protein intake is reported to fall to about 1.0 g/kg/day and the average total energy intake to about 30 kcal/kg/day [66, 67, 69, 70]. Although some patients may exhibit positive nitrogen balance even with this relatively low nutritional intake, it is probably inadequate for many patients undergoing long-term CAPD. Our group has observed that the nitrogen balance decreases with time on CAPD in parallel with decreasing protein and energy intakes [71].

The reduced nutritional intake during CAPD seems to be caused by a decrease in appetite, probably due to absorption of dialysate glucose and abdominal distension by the dialysis fluid [68, 72, 73]. Another explanation is that CAPD patients may become underdialyzed. As the total solute clearance falls (due to a decrease in residual renal function), the patients may develop uremic symptoms including anorexia with reduced nutritional intake as a consequence.

3.5. Intercurrent illness

Patients with end-stage renal disease also develop frequent intercurrent illnesses. Infection, especially of the vascular access and peritonitis, cardiac disease, and pulmonary edema, as well as gastrointestinal diseases such as peptic ulcer, are frequent complications of uremia. Whenever a patient develops an intercurrent illness there is a high likelihood that his eating habits will change and his appetite will decrease. Serious illness in uremic patients results in metabolic stress that may lead to negative nitrogen balance [74].

3.5.1. Recurrent peritonitis

One of the most serious complications of CAPD is recurrent peritonitis. Adverse effects of recurrent peritonitis on nutritional status were demonstrated by Rubin *et al.* [75, 76] who observed that changes in total body potassium correlated negatively with episodes of peritonitis per month and that patients with a high incidence of peritonitis had lower arm muscle circumference and lower plasma protein than patients with a lower incidence of peritonitis.

Peritonitis is associated with increased losses of protein in the dialysate which in intermittent peritoneal dialysis may amount to 100 g of protein in 24 hr or more. In CAPD patients with mild peritonitis the dialysate protein losses increased to an average of 15.1 ± 3.6 g/day [77]. In addition bacterial infection in the peritoneal cavity with inflammation may be a strong catabolic stimulus superimposed on the enhanced protein losses, thus contributing to negative nitrogen balance. A few nitrogen balance studies have been performed in CAPD patients with peritonitis and the results show that the nitrogen balance became strongly negative [74, 78]. Contributing factors are abdominal pain, anorexia, nausea, and vomiting which may hamper nutrition by the oral route.

3.6. Protein losses

Substantial loss of protein into the dialysate is a major drawback with peritoneal dialysis. Loss of protein in intermittent peritoneal dialysis amounts to about 13 g/10 hr [77], but may increase to 38-40 g/10 hr or more during peritonitis [18, 77] with elevated protein losses persisting for weeks following a period of peritonitis.

In CAPD, the reported average loss of protein into the dialysate varies between 5 and 15 g in different studies with large interindividual differences [66, 67, 76, 78–89]. The daily losses are relatively constant in the individual patient [83, 85]. However, interpatient variability in protein loss is considerable; some patients have as little as 3 g/day of protein losses, while others have losses of 20 g/day or more [84–86]. Thus, dialysate protein loss may vary between 20 and 140 g/week in different patients. In addition, some patients may have a large urinary loss of protein [86]. Dialysate protein losses are reported to be stable during long-term treatment [67, 76, 80, 81, 88, 90]; however, the combined urine and dialysate protein losses may decrease over time [66].

The effluent dialysate contains a spectrum of proteins that are principally derived from serum proteins [87]. The loss of a given protein is to some extent predictable on the basis of its molecular weight; the lower the molecular weight of the protein, the higher its concentration in the dialysate compared to the plasma [87]. In addition, the amount lost of a given protein will depend on its serum concentration and the permeability of the peritoneum. Other factors such as the rate of biosynthesis of proteins and the reabsorption rate by the lymphatics may also influence the losses of proteins [87].

Proteins diffuse into the peritoneal cavity at a relatively constant rate; the transperitoneal transport of serum proteins is principally membrane and permeability dependent [84, 85, 87]. Conditions which might be expected to release histamine in the tissues to the peritoneal cavity (allergic reactions, inflammation, septicemia, certain drugs) may increase the peritoneal permeability and result in increased protein losses [91]. The presence of factors such as intraperitoneal exposure to endotoxin during dialysis [55, 92] or systemic endotoxins [91] might explain the large interindividual variation in protein loss.

The type of dialysis protocol cannot explain the large interindividual differences in protein loss. Variations of the total outflow volume of dialysate per day have only a marginal effect [85], or no effect at all [84], on protein losses.

The major protein fraction found in the effluent dialysate is albumin which accounts for, on the average, 48-65% of total protein losses [83, 84, 89, 92]. Randerson *et al.* [79] note that mean serum albumin was 49 ± 2% of serum total protein, while the loss of albumin accounted for 56 ± 7% of total dialysate protein loss; this demonstrates the preferential loss of this lower molecular weight protein.

IgG accounts for about 15% of total protein losses [79, 84]. Blumenkrantz *et al.* [84] observed that losses of IgG and IgM correlated with their concentrations in serum. Large losses of IgG may predispose patients to peritonitis [93,94].

Protein losses may increase considerably, usually by 50-100% [84, 95], during peritonitis and may remain elevated for several weeks [66, 136]. This is mainly due to increased peritoneal permeability. In addition, intraperitoneal sources of dialysate protein may be of importance [87]. Albumin is the predominant protein loss during peritonitis [96].

The nutritional significance of protein losses during CAPD are mainly related to their impact on body protein stores and the need to replace losses by increased synthesis of serum proteins. In addition, proteins of lower molecular weight may become depleted possibly too quickly for the patients biosynthetic system to compensate resulting in depletion of specific proteins [87]. On the other hand, the lowering effect on certain serum proteins, such as PTH, may be beneficial. Moreover, middle molecular weight uremic toxins are efficiently removed by CAPD due to the high permeability of the peritoneum and the continuous dialytic process. Finally, plasma constituents found in CAPD effluent are similar to those found in urine from nephrotic patients and it is possible that the peritoneal loss of plasma constituents such as proteins and lipoproteins might be linked to the hypertriglyceridemia in CAPD patients [97].

3.7. Amino acid losses

Whereas protein losses during peritoneal dialysis are unparalleled in hemodialysis, the losses of free amino acids into the dialysate during peritoneal dialysis are of the same magnitude (per week) as with HD, or less. Variable amounts of free amino acids have been reported to be lost in patients on intermittent peritoneal dialysis: about 4-6 g/dialysis [98–100]; in another study [101] much higher: 17.3 g/36 hr of dialysis. Conjugated amino acid losses are about 2.4 g/dialysis [100].

During CAPD, the reported average dialysate losses of free amino acids vary between 1.2 to 3.4 g per 24 hr in different studies [79, 102–107]. The highest values for amino acids, 3.4 ± 1.2 g per day, are reported by Kopple *et al.* [104]. Their patients were all men and had a rather high dietary protein intake; however, amino acid losses did not increase when their dietary protein intake increased from 1.0 to 1.4 g of protein/kg body weight/24 hr.

About 29% of the amino acids lost into the dialysate are essential amino acids [104]. The amino acids losses are reported to average only 5.3% of the total dialysate nitrogen losses [108]. This loss of amino acid nitrogen is not great and should easily be replaced by ingestion of food. On the other hand, dialysate losses for certain amino acids might aggravate deficiencies of specific amino acids in patients on CAPD.

The major factors that determine the loss of a given amino

acid are its concentration in plasma and the volume of dialysate outflow per 24 hr [104, 107, 109]. The amino acid concentrations in plasma and in dialysate tend towards equilibrium with a passive diffusion gradient [79, 104, 107, 109]. The molar ratio of dialysate to plasma amino acid concentrations approaches one for most amino acids, provided that the dwell time is sufficiently long; after 4 to 8 hr the reported average molar ratios vary between 0.7 and 0.9 for most amino acids [79, 104, 107, 109].

Since the size of most of the amino acids (on the average, roughly, 140 daltons) is only slightly higher than that of creatinine (113 daltons) one would expect the peritoneal clearances for individual amino acids to be about 20% lower than the clearance of creatinine. This appears to be true for most of the amino acids. Randerson *et al.* [79] report that after a dwell time of 4.5 hr the molar dialysate/plasma ratios varied between 0.51 (taurine) and 0.90 (asparagine); the corresponding ratio for creatinine was 0.83. In the study by Kopple *et al.* [104], the average dialysate (collected over 24 hr, 3-5 exchanges) to plasma (postabsorptive) ratio for amino acids was 0.72; range, 0.47 (taurine) to 0.90 (threonine).

These observations show that there are large variations between different amino acids. Moreover, for some amino acids the dialysate/plasma ratios may exceed unity. Fürst *et al.* [106] found ratios exceeding one for several amino acids; for example, alanine (1.1), aspartic acid (2.7), glutamic acid (1.6), hydroxyproline (5.3) and proline (1.1). The high dialysate concentrations of alanine, aspartic acid, and glutamic acid have been attributed to the high portal-vein concentrations of these amino acids, which are selectively handled (transaminated) in the splanchnic area [106]. Dombros *et al.* [107] found a mean dialysate/plasma ratio of 0.86; however, there were large variations between different amino acids, from 0,62 (taurine) to 3.31 (aspartate), and high values were found also for proline (1.13) and methionine (1.10).

4. ENERGY METABOLISM

Several studies indicate that energy malnutrition is a major component of the commonly observed wasting syndrome of chronically uremic patients [2, 3, 5-7]. Abnormalities in energy metabolism in uremia include carbohydrate intolerance in combination with hyperinsulinemia and hyperglucagonemia, hyperlipidemia and other lipid abnormalities, and various signs of abnormal cell energy metabolism [1-5]. In addition, dietary energy intake is commonly reduced contributing to negative energy balance and to negative nitrogen balance [20, 33, 36, 110, 111].

Alterations in carbohydrate metabolism in uremia are of particular importance in peritoneal dialysis due to the impact of glucose absorption by the peritoneal route. Thus, peritoneal dialysis is often associated with hyperglycemia, accentuated hyperinsulinemia and hyperlipidemia. Despite the absorption of glucose, however, energy malnutrition appears to be a common problem also in patients undergoing peritoneal dialysis although some patients undergoing CAPD may become obese.

4.1. Abnormal cell energy metabolism

Several observations in uremic patients indicate that their cell energy metabolism is abnormal [110-120]. Defects in post-receptor events in uremia may result in decreased muscle insulin-mediated glucose uptake, glycogen synthesis, and, possibly, glucose oxidation [112-114]. Reduced activities of key glycolytic enzymes have also been observed in the skeletal muscle of uremic patients [115] and both ATP and energy charge levels have been found to be reduced in leucocytes of uremic patients [116, 120]. In addition, muscle carnitine deficiency in patients undergoing hemodialysis [117] may result in impaired beta-oxidation of fatty acids which is the main energy source in skeletal muscle. Lipid accumulation has been observed in the quadriceps muscle in uremic patients and has been attributed to deficient utilization of lipids by muscle perhaps due to deficient muscle carnitine pools, or decreased activity of carnitine-palmytil transferase [121].

Uremic patients frequently complain of muscle weakness and may show degenerative changes in skeletal muscle [112]. These symptoms and signs, which have been reported to be typical for the so-called uremic myopathy also have been thought to relate to abnormal energy metabolism in uremia [12].

We have studied muscle high-energy phosphates and glycogen stores in 30 patients who had been on CAPD for 17 ± 15 months [118, 119]. Percutaneous muscle biopsies were carried out in the morning with the patients fasting after an overnight dwell with 1.36% glucose dialysis fluid. The biopsy material was immediately frozen and analyzed for its content of ATP, phosphocreatine, free creatine, and total creatine, as well as of glycogen. The high-energy phosphate stores in skeletal muscle, i.e. ATP and phosphocreatine, were found to be reduced in CAPD patients compared to normal subjects whereas glycogen was not significantly changed. The results suggest that skeletal muscle in CAPD patients are in a low-energy state relative to normal. There was a similar decrease in both ATP and phosphocreatine content indicating defective energy production or defective energy expenditure in the cells. ATP is the immediate source of energy for muscle contraction and active ion transport; ATP is resynthesized by oxidative phosphorylation, by anaerobic glycolysis and by transphosphorylation of phosphocreatine. Although the clinical significance is unclear, the observed abnormalities in cell energy metabolism might contribute to symptoms such as muscle fatigue in CAPD patients. Del Canale *et al.* [122] report similar findings in non-dialyzed uremic patients.

4.2. Carbohydrate metabolism in uremia

Chronic renal failure is associated with glucose intolerance and other abnormalities reflecting impaired glucose metabolism [1, 4, 123-125]. Although fasting blood glucose levels are often normal, most uremic patients show an abnormal oral or intravenous glucose tolerance test [124]. Impaired beta-cell response to glucose is observed in some patients, but the predominant abnormality is peripheral resistance to the action of insulin [123-125], which is attributed to a postreceptor defect in insulin action [58]. Glucose intolerance in uremia is mainly due to a reduction in tissue utilization of glucose due to the inability of insulin to stimulate glucose uptake by peripheral tissues [4, 125]. In addition, increased hepatic production of glucose from gluconeogenesis may also contribute to hyperglycemia [48, 126]. The circulating levels of several hormones such as insulin, glucagon, growth hormone and parathyroid hormone are often elevated [4, 62, 127, 128], mainly due to their impaired degradation by the diseased kidneys [1].

4.3. Glucose absorption

During intermittent peritoneal dialysis substantial quantities of glucose are absorbed from the dialysis fluid, often resulting in marked hyperglycemia [158–161]. About 38 g of glucose are absorbed each hour when dialysis fluid containing glucose 42.5 g/l is used [160].

The reported mean daily absorption of glucose in CAPD in different studies varies between 100 to 200 g of glucose [79, 129–134]. The rate of glucose absorption varies considerably between patients, indicating large interindividual differences in peritoneal permeability; however, within the individual patient the amount of glucose absorbed per day on any given dialysis regimen is quite constant [130, 131]. Grodstein *et al.* [130] report that the correlation between the amount of glucose absorbed each day and the average concentration of glucose in the dialysis fluid is so close that the net uptake of glucose may be predicted from the average concentration in the instilled dialysis fluids. The uptake in individual patients may vary between 52 g [131] and 316 g [130] and, if hypertonic solutions are exchanged every 75 min, the absorption of glucose may even exceed 700 g per 24 hr [129]. About 60-80% to the amount of glucose instilled into the peritoneal cavity is absorbed during an exchange of about 6 hr [130, 132]. Thus, during a 6 hr cycle, 45-60 g of glucose are absorbed from the 3.86% solution, 24-40 g are absorbed from the 2.27% solution, and 15-22 g are absorbed from 1.36% solution.

4.3.1. Glucose absorption during peritonitis
The rate of glucose absorption is markedly increased during episodes of peritonitis due to increased peritoneal permeability and enhanced diffusive transperitoneal transport of glucose [135–139]. The accelerated rate of glucose absorption results in a rapid decrease of the concentration of glucose in the dialysate, and hence in a rapid loss of the osmotic driving force for water removal [140]. Since these alterations may necessitate the use of more hypertonic solutions, or more frequent exchanges of dialysis fluid to maintain daily ultrafiltration at a constant level, glucose absorption may increase markedly during peritonitis.

4.3.2. Long-term changes in glucose absorption
The amount of glucose that is absorbed each day appears to be stable in most patients undergoing long-term CAPD treatment in the United States [76]. However, glucose absorption have been reported to increase with time on CAPD among certain groups of patients undergoing CAPD in Europe [141, 142]. This discrepancy is thought to be related to unknown components in dialysis fluids manufactured by some of the European companies [142]. It is possible that these impurities are identical with potentially irritant glucose metabolites including 5-hydroxymethylfur-

fural which have been identified in unused dialysis fluids [143, 144].

4.4. Metabolic effects of a single dialysis cycle

During CAPD, a single dialysis cycle with hypertonic dialysate (anhydrous dextrose 3.86 g/dl) results in peak blood glucose and plasma insulin levels within 45-90 min, whereas the elevated glucagon levels decrease only slightly [68, 129, 133, 145–148]. These changes are similar to those observed after an oral glucose load in CAPD patients [147, 149, 150]. However, an intraperitoneal supply of glucose is reported to result in a more marked hyperglycemia and in a more long-lasting hyperinsulinemia than when the same amount of glucose is given orally [147]. Blood glucose and serum insulin levels remain significantly raised 6 hr after the onset of hypertonic dialysis [145]. Exchanges with isotonic dialysis fluid have only a marginal effect on blood glucose and serum insulin levels [145, 148].

Basal lactate and alanine levels are raised in CAPD patients, but – despite the absorption of lactate – the concentrations of these gluconeogenic precursors do not change significantly after instillation of the dialysis fluid [145]. This may indicate that the endogenous production of lactate is increased in CAPD patients, perhaps due to increased glycolysis, coupled with reduced lactate utilization by gluconeogenesis. The blood concentrations of ketone bodies and non-esterified fatty acids are lowered throughout dialysis, indicating suppression of both lipolysis and ketogenesis. Thus, CAPD results in the following changes: (1) hyperglycemia, (2) hyperinsulinemia, (3) reduced gluconeogenesis, (4) inhibition of lipolysis, and (5) suppression of ketogenesis.

By contrast, hemodialysis with glucose-free dialysate results in marked decreases in blood glucose, insulin, lactate and pyruvate levels along with profound increases in acetoacetate and betahydroxy butyrate levels [16, 151]. These intradialytic alterations, which resemble the physiological response to fasting for 48 to 72 hr, are thought to be due to losses of about 20-30 g of glucose into the dialysate [16, 151]. The observed metabolic responses during glucose-free hemodialysis indicate that oxidation of fatty acids is increased to meet the increased energy demand and to counteract the development of hypoglycemia.

4.5. Glucose intolerance

In the 1960s, several investigators reported that institution of HD resulted in markedly improved glucose intolerance [152, 153]. However, nonspecific glucose measurements were used and the reported favourable effects of HD may probably in part be attributed to removal of non-glucose reducing substances that can interfere with measurements of glucose [154]. Most recent studies, in which glucose specific methods have been used, indicate that following HD glucose intolerance improves only marginally, or not at all [154–157].

The alterations in carbohydrate metabolism in uremia are of particular importance in peritoneal dialysis in view of the impact of glucose absorption from the dialysate. The normal pancreatic response to overcome the peripheral insulin resistance in uremia is to further increase the secretion of insulin; however, if the insulin response is inadequate glucose intolerance may become overtly impaired [4]. A potential hazard with peritoneal dialysis is therefore that the intraperitoneal glucose load might exhaust the secretory capacity of the pancreatic beta-cells. Indeed, deterioration in the insulin response to oral glucose has been reported to occur in patients on CAPD [102]. The serum insulin response to an oral glucose load is reported to decrease in the first few days after a session of intermittent peritoneal dialysis, indicating that the peritoneal glucose load may induce a temporary exhaustion of the pancreatic beta-cells [162].

The effects of CAPD on glucose tolerance and serum immunoreactive insulin and glucagon responses to oral glucose were studied in 13 patients undergoing their first year of therapy [150]. The patients were studied at the start of CAPD, and again after 3 and 12 months on CAPD. Before the start of CAPD, about 50% of the patients displayed decreased glucose tolerance characterized by: an increased peak glucose concentration and a delayed return of blood glucose towards the fasting level; normal fasting blood glucose (< 6.7 mmol/l); and, either normal or high serum immunoreactive insulin and glucagon levels. These alterations represent typical findings in uremic patients [1, 4].

The follow-up studies after 3 and 12 months treatment with CAPD showed no significant changes of any of these variables [150]. The blood glucose concentration over time curves during the tests were, in fact, almost inseparable. Thus, the treatment with CAPD for one year appeared to have no effect on glucose tolerance and insulin secretory response. Also, there was no statistically significant relationship between the peritoneal glucose supply and any of the variables expressing glucose tolerance (fasting blood glucose, blood glucose during tests, and total and incremental areas under the glucose curve).

These data therefore seem to refute the hypothesis that the contionuous glucose load during CAPD results in further impairment of glucose tolerance by exhausting insulin secretion capacity as observed in patients undergoing intermittent peritoneal dialysis [162].

It should be noted that the oral glucose tolerance tests in our studies [150] were performed after a 10-14 h interruption of dialysis. In patients performing regular CAPD the presence of glucose intolerance together with the hyperglycemic stress of the continuous absorption of glucose may result in manifest diabetes mellitus (see below).

Several observations including the observed inhibitory effect of middle molecules on glucose utilization in several tissues and cells suggest that accumulation of uremic toxins may be responsible for the impaired glucose metabolism in uremia [4, 163, 164, 165]. If these toxins are dialysable one might expect that dialysis should lead to improved glucose metabolism. The finding that the impaired glucose tolerance does not improve during CAPD may suggest that such toxins – if they exist – are inadequately removed by CAPD and show that CAPD is not an optimal treatment as regards glucose intolerance. Thus, neither CAPD [150], nor HD [4] restores glucose metabolism to normal. However, Heaton et al. [166] found that 24 hr mean blood glucose levels fell after 3 months' dialysis whereas insulin levels were unchanged; this may imply that insulin sensitivity

had improved.

4.5.1. Hyperglycemia and hyperinsulinemia in CAPD

Although exchanges with isotonic dialysate have only a marginal effect on blood glucose and insulin levels, there is a constant tendency in CAPD patients towards hyperglycemia along with hyperinsulinemia [102, 145]. This tendency is reflected by increased plasma C-peptide levels as well as by an increased ratio between C-peptide and insulin in CAPD patients compared with HD patients, indicating that CAPD patients have continuously increased production of proinsulin [147].

Some patients on CAPD may develop manifest diabetes mellitus due to the continuous hyperglycemic stress of the absorption of glucose. Kurtz et al. [167] report that 3 out of 40 CAPD patients, without a history of diabetes mellitus, required intraperitoneally administered insulin to control plasma insulin levels. We have observed development of manifest diabetes mellitus de novo in 5 out of 95 non-diabetic CAPD patients [36]. Similarly, other workers have observed that patients with non-insulin dependent diabetes mellitus may develop an insulin-dependent state during CAPD [168].

We have observed that patients who developed manifest diabetes mellitus during CAPD had markedly increasing body weight – possibly due to increased peritoneal absorption of glucose – and hyperinsulinemia [36]. These findings suggest that the occurrence of manifest diabetes mellitus during CAPD may be due to increased peritoneal permeability to glucose (for example, after repeated episodes of peritonitis as observed in two of our patients); however, a further impairment of tissue sensitivity to insulin might also play a role in individual patients.

Since sustained hyperinsulinemia may possibly increase atherogenenis [169], the elevated circulating insulin levels – rather than the relatively small de novo incidence of insulin-dependent diabetes mellitus – constitute a potential risk factor for the majority of the patients during long-term treatment with CAPD. In addition, hyperglycemia in CAPD may lead to formation of both abnormal circulating proteins [169] and abnormal – and potentially atherogenic – structural proteins in the capillary basement membrane [4]. Possible effects of glucose absorption in CAPD are summarized in Table 6.

4.6. Lipid metabolism

Chronic renal failure is associated with deranged lipid metabolism [1, 170–173] resulting in typical serum lipoprotein abnormalities and an increased prevalence of hypertriglyceridemia [174–179]. The 'uremic dyslipoproteinemia' which shares several similarities with both the type III and type IV hyperlipoproteinemia [180–182], is characterized by: an increased concentration of lipids concurrently with a relative cholesterol-enrichment of very low density lipoproteins (VLDL); an increased concentration and a relative enrichment of triglycerides in low density lipoproteins (LDL); a decreased concentration of cholesterol in high density lipoproteins (HDL); and, accumulation of an electrophoretic subclass of VLDL, late pre-beta lipoproteins, which are thought to represent triglyceride depleted remnants of VLDL and/or chylomicrons [180, 181, 183, 184]. These changes usually result in elevated

Table 6. Glucose absorption in CAPD

Benefits

Continuous energy supply resulting in improved energy balance.
Hyperinsulinemia may promote anabolism.
Continuous glucose supply may prevent hypoglycemia.
Continuous dialysis with potassium free solutions with glucose contributes to improved control of hyperkalemia.

Disadvantages

Hyperglycemia results in formation of abnormal glucosylated proteins.
Hyperinsulinemia may promote atherogenesis.
Hyperglycemic stress may result in exhaustion of pancreatic be-tacells.
Hyperlipidemia due to continuous glucose supply and hyperinsulinemia.
Obesity.
Anorexia.
Amino acid alterations.
Toxic effects on peritoneum.

---

serum triglycerides, where the serum cholesterol level often is normal.

Other abnormalities include an altered composition of lipoproteins as regard their relative content of apoproteins [178, 179, 185, 186]. Hyperapobetalipoproteinemia appears to be the major dyslipoproteinemia in patients undergoing CAPD [187]. Altered composition of body fat is also reported [188]. In uremia, the fatty esters in the body are composed of an increased proportion of saturated fatty acids, whereas the relative content of linoleic acid is markedly reduced [188].

Serum lipoprotein abnormalities are reported to occur early in the course of progressive chronic renal failure; and, except for transitory alterations during each hemodialysis session [189], they are only marginally affected by hemodialysis or conservative treatment with low protein diets [180, 183, 190–192].

Although the mechanism(s) behind the uremic hypertriglyceridemia are unknown, evidence has been provided for both an increased hepatic production and an impaired removal of circulating triglyceride-rich VLDL-particles [170, 183, 193–196]. Low enzymatic activity of both serum lipoprotein lipase and hepatic lipase are thought to contribute to the impaired removal of triglycerides from the circulation [170].

An excessive supply of carbohydrates and derangements of glucose metabolism (including hyperinsulinemia and peripheral insulin resistance) may lead to increased hepatic production of triglycerides [197, 198]. In addition, the mechanism of carbohydrate-induced hypertriglyceridemia may involve not only increased hepatic production of VLDL, but also impaired removal of circulating VLDL [199, 200].

4.7. Hyperlipidemic effect of CAPD

Several of the reported lipid abnormalities in uremia including the low concentration of HDL cholesterol [201], high serum cholesterol levels [201], the abnormal accumulation of VLDL remnants [180, 181, 202], hyperapobeta-

lipoproteinemia [187], and the low relative content of linoleic acid in fatty esters [188], are all thought to be factors that may promote arteriosclerosis. These risk factors are affected by nutritional factors such as protein and energy intake, which can change considerably in patients undergoing CAPD.

In uremic patients, an increased dietary intake of carbohydrates results in markedly increased serum triglyceride levels [203–205]. Conversely, a reduction of the proportion of carbohydrates in the diet results in decreasing serum triglyceride levels [205, 206]. These observations show that serum VLDL and total triglyceride levels in uremic patients are strongly correlated to the quantity of carbohydrates consumed.

A hyperlipidemic effect of CAPD was demonstrated in several studies after introduction of CAPD, and it became apparent that hypertriglyceridemia and serum lipoprotein abnormalities were accentuated within the first months of the treatment [131, 132, 207–210].

In a study from our group, the effects of CAPD on serum lipids and lipoproteins over the initial year of therapy were studied in 23 patients who were investigated before the start of CAPD, and again after 3 months (17 patients) and 13 months on CAPD [211]. The baseline investigation showed lipoprotein abnormalities, including increased VLDL-CHOL and VLDL-TG, increased LDL-TG, and decreased HDL-CHOL resulting in an increased serum TG level but normal serum CHOL. This abnormal serum lipoprotein pattern, which is typical for the 'uremic dyslipoproteinemia', was further accentuated during CAPD. The patients showed a significant and persistent increase of the VLDL-fraction and a smaller, and transitory, increase in LDL-CHOL. These changes resulted in a significant increase of both serum CHOL and serum TG during the first months of the treatment, and the rise in serum CHOL remained statistically significant also after one year on CAPD. VLDL-TG, VLDL-CHOL, and serum TG, and the changes of these variables over the study period, correlated with the amount of glucose supplied intraperitoneally in the dialysis fluid. The results of this study indicate that the continuous peritoneal absorption of glucose (100-200 g/24 hr) during CAPD contributes to potentially atherogenic changes in serum lipids and lipoproteins. However, these changes were, in part, transitory, indicating an adaptation to the peritoneal glucose load in CAPD.

Other studies have demonstrated a hyperlipidemic effect on CAPD; however, the results differ considerably between different reports due to large interindividual variations, varying energy intakes and fluctuations of serum lipids over time in the individual patient [167, 212–218]. Nevertheless, the results may be summarised as follows. At the start of CAPD, many patients show hypertriglyceridemia, while most have normal serum cholesterol levels. During the first year of CAPD both serum triglycerides and serum cholesterol levels usually increase, at least during the initial months of the treatment. These changes are due to currently increased lipid concentrations in the VLDL and LDL fractions, whereas the changes in HDL usually are less marked. These changes are more marked in patients already hyperlipidemic at the start of CAPD [215]. A positive correlation between serum triglycerides and insulin levels in CAPD have been demonstrated implying a role of insulin in hypertriglyceridemia [166].

4.7.1. Hypertriglyceridemia

The prevalence of hypertriglyceridemia in patients undergoing long-term treatment with CAPD is reported to be 60-80% [216, 217]. Although many patients on CAPD may develop very high triglyceride concentrations [209, 216], the changes of this variable often fail to reach statistical significance due to large interindividual differences.

The fractional removal rate of (exogenous) triglycerides from the blood (k_2) at intravenous fat tolerance tests, as well as the changes of k_2 during the treatment, vary considerably between the patients [209]. We found that patients with stable or decreasing triglyceride levels after 1 yr on CAPD often show increasing k_2 values, whereas patients with continuously increasing triglycerides often 'fail' to improve the fractional removal rate of exogenous triglycerides [209]. The average fractional removal rate of triglycerides, however, does not change significantly during the first year of CAPD [212].

Differences in circulating lipid levels between patients, and within individual patients over time, may be due also to varying energy intake of the patients. Many centres recommend to their patients a restricted use of hypertonic PD fluid, as well as a decreased dietary energy intake. These interventions seem to effectively reduce the development of hypertriglyceridemia [212].

4.7.2. Hypercholesterolemia in CAPD

The initial hyperlipidemic effect of CAPD involves all three lipoprotein fractions. About 15-30% of the patients develop hypercholesterolemia de novo during their first year on CAPD [211, 216]. The rise in serum cholesterol levels are due to increased levels of both VLDL cholesterol and LDL cholesterol [210].

In addition, an increased HDL cholesterol level has also been observed [213, 214]. This is in keeping with observations of a positive correlation between HDL cholesterol levels and energy intake in uremic patients [219].

Many patients are treated with low protein diets containing 20-40 g of protein/day before the start on CAPD. During CAPD, their dietary protein intake increase to, on the average, about 80 g/day. Since both the quantity and the quality of protein intake [220, 221] are reported to affect serum cholesterol levels it is possible that changes in dietary protein intake may contribute to the observed hypercholesterolemia in the CAPD patients.

This is supported by the finding of a positive correlation between serum albumin and VLDL cholesterol levels, suggesting and interrelationship between protein and lipid status [211]. On the other hand, it has been suggested that protein losses into the dialysate during the CAPD may induce a hypercholesterolemia similar to that observed in the nephrotic syndrome [210]. This suggestion is supported by observations of a significant correlation between serum cholesterol levels and dialysate protein losses in children undergoing CAPD [221]. However, Breckenridge *et al.* [214] found little indication that loss of apolipoproteins, or lipoproteins, into the dialysate could account for any changes in plasma lipoproteins during CAPD.

4.7.3. Transitory changes of serum lipoprotein levels during CAPD

Changes in serum lipid concentrations during CAPD are transitory, except in a small group of patients who show steadily increasing concentrations especially of the VLDL fraction [132]. Peak levels of serum cholesterol and triglycerides are usually reached within 3-12 months, with a subsequent fall during the following months to pretreatment levels as noted previously [211, 215, 216].

Thus, the uremic dyslipoproteinemia remains essentially unchanged after 1 yr of CAPD compared to the pretreatment status, with the exception of a small group of patients in whom serum triglyceride levels increase significantly [215]. In fact, serum lipid levels after one year on CAPD are approximately the same in HD and CAPD patients; CAPD patients may even show better (less reduced) HDL cholesterol levels than HD patients [222].

The finding that the hyperlipidemic effect of CAPD is transitory in many patients may indicate a metabolic adaptation to the glucose load during CAPD but it may also be due to changes in energy intake over time. Baeyer *et al.* [103] have suggested that the total carbohydrate intake in CAPD patients is regulated by a spontaneous decrease of the oral carbohydrate intake. This suggestion is supported by results in CAPD patients showing a low relative content of dietary energy derived from carbohydrates [103, 223].

Atherogenic changes during CAPD

Treatment with CAPD seems to induce potentially atherogenic alterations, especially during the initial months of the treatment. Thus, the ratios between LDL and HDL cholesterol, as well as the ratio between VLDL plus LDL cholesterol and HDL cholesterol – which are considered to be atherogenic indices – increase significantly during the first year of the treatment [211]. On the other hand, patients undergoing CAPD appear to have lower rates of accumulation of free cholesterol in peripheral tissues and this might result in a lower incidence of atherosclerotic vascular disease in CAPD [224].

The incidence of cardiovascular diseases during CAPD appears to be similar to that reported in patients of HD and serum lipid levels do not seem to discriminate between CAPD patients with and without these complications [225, 226]. Furthermore, the long-term effects of the deterioration of uremic dyslipoproteinemia during CAPD are still uncertain as the drop-out rate from CAPD is high. Therefore, it still remains necessary to evaluate the effects of various therapeutic approaches to lower serum lipid levels in CAPD patients such as the restricted use of hypertonic dialysis fluid [212], attempts to replace glucose with other osmotic agents [68], lipid-lowering drugs including L-carnitine [227], dietary modification [212] and exercise [228].

5. NUTRITIONAL STATUS

5.1. Nutrional status in patients undergoing intermittent peritoneal dialysis

It is a common experience, although rarely communicated in scientific papers, that patients on intermittent peritoneal dialysis frequently show evidence of protein-energy malnutrition and protein wasting [17–19, 229, 230]. Signs of malnutrition, often unrecognized, have been described as the depletion syndrome and are characterized by progressive loss of lean body mass often masked by over hydration giving a false impression of stable body weight [230]. Underlying factors may be poor nutrional intake (anorexia due to insufficient small-molecule removal, old age, and systemic disease), loss of protein and amino acids in the dialysate, recurrent peritonitis, and inactivity.

In a comparative study of hemodialysis versus intermittent peritoneal dialysis the hemodialysis patients maintained better nutritional status as reflected in body weight and arm muscle circumference than the intermittent peritoneal dialysis patients who also tended to have a lower protein intake as reflected in their urea appearance [229].

The plasma amino acid pattern in intermittent peritoneal dialysis patients often resembles that seen in patients with malnutrition [230, 231]. Patients on intermittent peritoneal dialysis also showed gross abnormalities in muscle intracellular free amino acids, indicating that the amino acid abnormalities of chronic uremia were, if anything, aggravated [232].

5.2. Nutritional status in CAPD patients

Despite losses of protein, amino acids, and other vital substances, there are several signs indicating net anabolism in CAPD patients during their 1st year of the treatment. Thus, the average weight gain may exceed 5 kg without any clinical signs indicating fluid overload [66, 79, 80, 167]. The total body potassium content is reported to increase [66, 67, 75] although this is not a consistent finding [75, 233].

Anthropometric assessments have shown stable values or slight improvements [76, 234]. Visceral protein levels in serum often rise [78], and hematocrit and hemoglobin levels usually increase [80, 235] during the initial months of the treatment.

Until recently there have been relatively few reports on clinically overt malnutrition in CAPD patients, despite the losses of protein and the relatively low – and decreasing – dietary intake of protein and energy. In earlier reports, only a few patients were reported to develop severe hypoproteinemia or other clear-cut signs of severe protein-energy malnutrition [81, 167, 236] although serum protein levels, body weight and several other nutrional parameters were frequently reduced compared with normal subjects. However, in several recent reports signs of malnutrition have been demonstrated in a large proportion of CAPD patients. Based on the subjective global assessment [237, 238] malnutrition was present in 41.6% of patients on CAPD for less than three months and was present in 18.1% of patients on CAPD for longer than 3 months [239]. In a cross-sectional study, protein-energy malnutrition, assessed from a score system based on triceps skinfold, midarm muscle circumference, serum transferrin and relative body weight, was recorded in 56% of CAPD patients (9/16 patients) and in 53% of HD patients (17/32 patients) [240]. Furthermore, as discussed in the following sections, a large portion of CAPD patients have signs of subclinical malnutrition, including low alkali-soluble protein content relative to DNA in muscle, and gradual reduction of total

body nitrogen, reflecting a loss of lean body mass and body protein [7, 66, 67, 75, 76, 241]. Poor nutrional status has been reported also in children undergoing CAPD [242] who fail to grow at a normal rate [243]. Abnormal plasma and muscle free amino acid concentrations are also observed in CAPD patients [78, 79, 104–107]. The plasma amino acid abnormalities suggest that malnutrition persists in CAPD patients. However, sustained hyperinsulinemia stimulated by the glucose uptake from the dialysate [244–246] may also have contributed to the reduced plasma amino acid concentrations.

5.3. Plasma amino acid levels in CAPD patients

Plasma amino acid concentrations are not restored to normal in CAPD patients. The reported abnormalities include decreased plasma levels of valine, leucine, lysine, threonine, tyrosine, serine, and glutamine, and increased concentrations of several of the non-essential amino acids [52, 78, 79, 104–107, 245, 246]. However, in some of the studies the plasma amino acid pattern was relatively well maintained. For example, Kopple *et al.* [104] found a normal sum of plasma essential, non-essential, and total amino acid concentrations although plasma valine, leucine, and serine concentrations were significantly decreased. Kopple *et al.* noted that this may reflect a rather high protein and energy intake in their patients [104].

The observed plasma amino acid abnormalities – which are similar to those observed in untreated uremic patients – probably reflect metabolic and nutritional derangements of uremia rather than depletion due do dialysate amino acid losses. Decreased concentrations of valine [11] and taurine [11], and a decreased ratio of valine to glycine [3] are thought to be useful as indicators of malnutrition; the presence of these abnormalities in the CAPD patients may therefore indicate protein deficiency. However, the sustained hyperinsulinemia during CAPD may also have contributed to the reduced plasma amino acid concentrations, all the more so as insulin resistance in uremia does not appear to extend to the stimulating effect of the hormone on cellular amino acid uptake [2, 245, 246].

Administration of glucose to non-uremic subjects tends to lower plasma concentrations of large neutral (methionine, phenylalanine, tyrosine, and tryptophan) and branched-chained amino acids (valine, leucine, and isoleucine); however, the effect on tryptophan is relatively small [244]. These changes have been reported to be associated with suppression of the elective consumption of carbohydrates, possibly a consequence of a relative increase of tryptophan levels in the brain and enhanced synthesis and release of serotonin [244]. It is of interest to note that augmented activity of serotonergic and dopaminergic systems with increased concentrations of 5-hydroxyindoleacetic acid (5-HIAA) and homovanillic acid (HVA) in the cerebrospinal fluid (CSF) have been observed in patients undergoing peritoneal dialysis whereas low CSF concentrations of 5-HIAA and HVA were found in HD patients [247]. It is possible that these alterations may relate to the reported loss of apetite, and tiredness in many CAPD patients. Recent studies in our laboratory have shown that CAPD patients have markedly reduced plasma total tryptophan levels whereas the free tryptophan level appears to be only slightly reduced. By contrast, muscle tryptophan was found to be high [248].

5.4. Muscle free amino acids in CAPD

We have investigated the effect of CAPD on the muscle free amino acid status [245, 246]. In muscle, taurine was significantly reduced, whereas none of the essential amino acids were significantly decreased. By contrast, most of the essential amino acids and several of the non-essential amino acids showed significantly reduced plasma concentrations. Thus, plasma valine, leucine, lysine, threonine, tyrosine, and histidine levels were all low as were plasma taurine, serine, glutamine, and ornithine. The ic/ec gradient was increased for most essential and several non essential amino acids. These results suggest that, except for taurine, the intracellular free amino acid pattern in muscle is less abnormal in CAPD patients than in patients undergoing other forms of therapy in whom muscle valine, threonine, tyrosine, lysine, histidine as well as taurine levels are frequently reduced [2, 245, 246, 255]. Graziani *et al.* [250] found low muscle valine, tyrosine, leucine, phenylalanine, and serine concentrations in their CAPD patients.

The finding of low intracellular pools of taurine indicates depletion of this amino acid in the CAPD patients [245, 246]. The muscle intracellular concentration of taurine in normal man is high (20-23 mmol/l) and the intra- to extracellular gradient (about 200:1) is higher than that of any other free amino acid [249]. Taurine has many important biological functions. It seems to stabilise the transmembrane potential, enhance calcium transport into the cells and increase calcium binding to intracellular membranes; it has anti-arrhytmic properties and exerts a positive inotropic effect in the heart [251]. Taurine seems to be an essential amino acid in the cat, in which taurine deficiency induces retinal degeneration with blindness [252]. Taurine may also be indispensable for growth and development in infant primates [253]. Taurine metabolism and nutritional requirements for taurine in man are largely unknown. However, Geggel *et al.* [254] have recently reported that children, and possibly adults, receiving long-term parenteral nutrition may develop abnormally low plasma taurine levels along with an abnormal electroretinogram which improved after taurine supplementation. Previous results in uremic patients [255] undergoing other forms of therapy suggest that taurine may be an essential amino acid in uremia. Low plasma concentrations of taurine in CAPD patients have been reported by others [105, 256]; however, an increased concentration was found in one study [104].

The low intracellular taurine concentration found by us in CAPD patients and in other uremic patients occurs despite normal or increased intra- and extracellular methionine pools and a normal or high cysteine concentration in plasma, i.e. precursor sulphuric amino acids are available for synthesis. A critical enzyme for taurine synthesis is cysteinesulfinic acid decarboxylase (CSAD), pyridoxal-5-phosphate being required as a coenzyme [251]. Low exogenous supply of taurine as well as low CSAD-activity, possibly due to pyridoxine deficiency, might be factors which contribute to taurine depletion in uremic patients.

The consequences of taurine depletion in uremia are unknown, but it may conceivably contribute to such symptoms as muscular fatigue, arrhythmia, cardiomyopathy, and, in children, growth retardation.

Serum protein levels in CAPD patients.

Despite the large losses of protein most CAPD patients maintain serum total protein and albumin levels that are usually only slightly reduced [67, 76, 79, 80, 86]. Serum transferrin and C_3 levels may even increase to normal values during the initial months of CAPD treatment [67]. However, serum albumin, IgG, IgM and total protein levels are usually slightly lower than in patients on HD [222, 256]. Farrell and Randerson [257] noted that serum albumin levels decreased significantly in patients who were transferred from HD to CAPD. Nolph *et al.* [80] reported significant decreases in serum IgG, albumin and total protein levels during the initial 6 months of CAPD and Goodship *et al.* [52] observed a significant fall of serum albumin after 3 months on CAPD. Thomson *et al.* [258] observed that serum albumin concentrations fell by, on the average, 6 g/l within one month of commencing CAPD, whereas Rubin *et al.* [256] found that serum protein concentrations fell only in patients with a high frequency of peritonitis.

Kaysen and Schoenfeld have reported that plasma albumin mass, total albumin mass and the distribution of albumin are normal in CAPD patients and that albumin homeostatis is maintained through decreased catabolism and increased synthesis of albumin [86]. This may explain why only few patients develop severe hypoproteinemia during long-term treatment with CAPD. However, during episodes of peritonitis serum albumin levels may fall below 25 g/l [258].

Serum protein levels are commonly used as indicators of protein nutritional status. However, it should be noted that the serum concentration of any protein is determined by a number of factors including the rates of its synthesis and catabolism, the distribution within extra- and intravascular compartments, and losses into peritoneal cavity [6, 18, 259]. Low molecular weight proteins such as prealbumin and retinol-binding protein are usually increased in uremia due to decreased renal degradation.

There is no constant relationship between any transport protein and the total amount of protein in the body relative to an appropriate standard [259]. Moreover, decreased serum protein concentrations probably do not assess specific protein malnutrition [260]. Also, imbalances in the composition of nutritional intakes may probably affect serum protein levels. Lunn and Austin [261] have reported that excess energy intake in rats fed on low-protein diets may promote the development of hypoalbuminemia. Thus, it is possible that the peritoneal glucose load during CAPD may have a lowering effect on serum protein levels.

Many factors other than the dialysate protein loss affect serum protein levels. A poor nutritional intake and intercurrent illnesses, especially peritonitis, probably contribute more to low serum protein levels than does the continuous protein loss. Albumin, transferrin, prealbumin and retinol-binding protein have been reported to decrease in CAPD patients eating less than 1.3 g/protein/kg/day [43].

Protein losses may indirectly contribute to various nutritional and metabolic disturbances in patients on CAPD; for example, hypercholesterolemia, altered amino acid metabolism, metabolic bone disease due the losses of vitamin D binding protein [36, 87, 262, 263].

5.6. Total body nitrogen

Indirect evidence of a gradual deterioration of the nutritional status of CAPD patients has emerged from prospective studies on total body nitrogen [66, 67]. Oreopoulos and co-workers have reported that total body nitrogen – which is an indicator of total body protein mass – decreases during the initial two years of CAPD treatment, concomitantly with a stable nitrogen output and a decreasing protein intake. By contrast, body weight and total body potassium are reported to increase significantly in the same patients. The Toronto group [66, 67] concluded that the increase of body weight and total body potassium may reflect an increase of intracellular water, and that the combination of a stable nitrogen output and a declining protein intake may result in long-term negative nitrogen balance – reflected by decreasing total body nitrogen.

Total body nitrogen first decreases significantly (within one year), but then remains stable at a lower level for up to 3 yr [233]. Decreased total body nitrogen was only seen in male patients, whereas total body nitrogen in female patients did not change significantly. After one year or more, total body nitrogen remained on the lower level; about 75% of the normal mean value in the men and about 85% of normal in the women. These changes were positively correlated with the initial values of total body nitrogen; the higher the initial value, the more marked was the decrease. These findings indicate that adaptive changes occur during CAPD, resulting in lower body protein mass [233]. Especially big men with large protein stores risked a large loss of body nitrogen, probably because they did not succeed in consuming an adequate diet. Losses in total body nitrogen occurred mainly in patients who ingested less than 0.9 to 1.0 g protein and less than 23 to 24 kcal/kg body weight per day. In another study from the Toronto group, seven (35%) of 20 randomly selected CAPD patients had subnormal values of total body nitrogen indicating reduced body protein stores [264].

5.7. Muscle intracellular protein content

Although most authors agree that patients undergoing CAPD, as well as uremic patients undergoing other forms of therapy, often are malnourished, conventional methods for the assessment of nutritional status in CAPD patients have shown diverging results as regards the long-term nutritional effects of the treatment. Protein malnutrition is a concept that often is difficult to define in uremic patients due to the possible influence of several factors other than the nutritional status per se, such as day-to-day fluctuations of metabolites and uremic toxins as well as of fluid overload. This is especially evident when analyzing various plasma constituents such as serum proteins and plasma amino acids; however, similar problems may also arise when analyzing and interpreting anthropometric data in uremic patients.

Skeletal muscle protein is the largest store of nitrogen and non-fat energy in the body. Breakdown of muscle protein occurs in catabolic conditions thereby providing free amino acids to the liver for gluconeogenesis and for synthesis of visceral proteins. Changes in muscle cell metabolism may not always be revealed by analysis of plasma constituents, but can be studied by percutaneous needle biopsy of the quadriceps femoris muscle [265]. This is a rapid and simple procedure that can be used for routine assessment of the muscle protein status.

The need of muscle biopsy studies in CAPD patients are stressed by the findings that muscle cell mass evaluated anthropometrically is reported to be stable in most studies despite signs of muscle protein depletion as evaluated by measurements of total body nitrogen in patients undergoing long-term therapy with CAPD [66, 67]. On the other hand, total body potassium has been reported to increase in the same patients which could suggest that potassium might accumulate in spite of decreased protein stores [66].

In protein malnutrition, the number of nuclei in muscle is only slightly affected and the muscle DNA content may therefore serve as a reference standard for various muscle constituents [7, 246]. The ratio of muscle alkalisoluble protein (non-collagen intracellular protein) (ASP) to DNA provides a measure of the amount of protein per cell unit, and the use of this nutritional index may therefore be used to evaluate the muscle protein status at the cellular level [7, 246].

We have evaluated the muscle content of ASP and DNA in 18 CAPD patients who had been maintained on CAPD for 4-62 months, and, in addition, analyzed the muscle content of potassium and creatine to determine whether the relative amounts of ASP, potassium, and creatine might be altered in patients undergoing CAPD [246]. This study showed reduced values of ASP/DNA, potassium/DNA and creatine/DNA compared to normals indicating muscle cellular protein deficiency. This was mainly due to an increased muscle content of DNA suggesting shrinkage of the mean cell mass due to cytoplasmatic reduction. There were strong intercorrelations between creatine/DNA, potassium/DNA, and ASP/DNA indicating that changes in creatine, potassium and ASP occur in parallel within the muscle cells [265]. These findings suggest that total body potassium should reflect the size of lean body mass (protein mass) in CAPD patients, provided that the patients are not suffering from potassium depletion which was not the case in our patients. Guarnieri *et al.* [7], also found reduced ASP/DNA as well as a low RNA/DNA ratio in muscle of their CAPD patients indicating reduced ribosomal capacity for protein synthesis. Similar results were obtained in uremic patients undergoing other forms of therapy [7].

6. WATER AND ELECTOLYTE METABOLISM

Chronic renal failure is associated with disturbances in water and eletrolyte metabolism, the predominant alterations being an increase in total body water, and increased plasma sodium, chloride, potassium, and magnesium concentrations [266–268]. By studying the composition of muscle tissue obtained by percutaneous needle biopsy it is possible to assess changes in water and electrolyte metabolism on the cellular level [265, 269]. Muscle biopsy studies in uremic patients undergoing intermittent dialysis therapy or conservative treatment have shown increased muscle water, chloride, and sodium contents, and diverging results concerning muscle potassium and magnesium contents [265, 269–277]. The increase in muscle water content in uremic patients is due to an increase of both intra- and extracellular water contents [277].

Most authors agree that muscle potassium content is either normal or increased in intermittently dialyzed patients [271–274, 277], whereas non-dialyzed patients may show a low or a normal muscle potassium content [271, 272, 275, 277]. Paired observations in patients before and after 6 weeks of HD demonstrating a significant rise of muscle potassium content from low to normal values suggest that dialysis per se may lead to restoration of muscle potassium stores [271]. However, the observed improvement in muscle potassium status following commencement of dialysis may be due also to increased protein intake, resulting in increased potassium intake, and possibly a more positive potassium balance [271].

6.1. Plasma electrolytes in CAPD

Patients on CAPD appear to be well-controlled with regard to acid-base equilibrium and fluid balance, and plasma electrolyte levels are maintained almost at steady state levels [29, 30, 278]. However, the use of dialysis fluid containing magnesium 0.75 mmol/l and no potassium is associated with hypermagnesemia [279], and in some patients, hypokalemia [280]. Normokalemia and hypokalemia are significantly more common in CAPD than in HD patients whereas hyperkalemia is more frequent in HD patients [281].

Many centers are now using dialysis fluids containing magnesium 0.25 mmol/l, resulting in lower serum magnesium concentrations [279]. It should be noted, however, that hypermagnesemia does not appear to result in any clinical complications. Patients with a poor nutritional intake may develop lowered serum magnesium levels on dialysis with low magnesium dialysis fluid and this might result in long-term magnesium depletion. On the other hand, lower serum magnesium levels may increase the acceptable upper limits of dietary magnesium intake and magnesium-containing phosphate binders can therefore be used more freely.

6.2. Muscle water and electrolytes in CAPD

We have studied the effect of CAPD on muscle water and electrolytes in 33 patients undergoing CAPD for 1–38 months [282]. The patients showed an increase in total muscle water, extracellular water, intracellular water, sodium, and chloride relative to fat free solids (FFS). The muscle potassium content was increased, both relative to FFS and to magnesium, whereas the intracellular potassium concentration was normal. The muscle magnesium content was normal despite hypermagnesemia.

The muscle content of sodium, chloride, and extracellular water were significantly lower in the CAPD patients undergoing intermittent peritoneal dialysis or being conservatively treated [277, 282]. The values in the CAPD patients also tended to be lower than those observed in hemodialysis patients [277, 282]. Thisdc finding is in keeping with observa-

tions that the state of hydration and blood pressure may be better controlled by CAPD than by other forms of dialysis.

The muscle potassium content was slightly increased in the CAPD patients, both relative to fat-free solids and to magnesium, whereas the intracellular potassium concentrations was normal [282]. This finding indicates that the potassium stores were well maintained on the cellular level in the CAPD patients despite continuous dialysis against potassium-free dialysis fluid. It is possible that high circulating insulin levels may have contributed to the well-maintained muscle potassium stores in our patients. Since insulin mediated potassium uptake is reported to be normal in uremia [283] the hyperinsulinemia in the CAPD patients should promote a shift of potassium from the extracellular to the intracellular space. This suggestion is supported by observations of an insulin dependent increase in cellular uptake of potassium during intraperitoneal supply of glucose in the uremic rat [284].

Progressive accumulation of intracellular water and potassium during CAPD has been suggested [66, 67] to explain apparently contradictory results showing increasing total body potassium but decreasing total body nitrogen with time in the same patients [66]. However, we found a negative correlation between muscle total water content and the duration of CAPD, and no correlation between muscle potassium content and duration of treatment [282].

Thus, our results from muscle biopsy studies in the CAPD patients [282] are not keeping with intracellular water and potassium accumulating with time on CAPD; however, it should be pointed out that these measurements of muscle composition concern changes on the cellular level and do not take into account changes in lean body mass, associated with muscle wasting or hypertrophy.

Panzetta *et al.* [285] have reported that cell overhydration was a distinctive feature in their CAPD patients, whereas extracellular water was significantly lower than the predicted value. They speculated that there was a shift of body water from the extracellular to the intracellular compartment [285]. The results of our study show that the muscle intracellular water content tended to be lower in the CAPD patients than in 161 non-dialyzed and dialyzed uremic patients [277, 282] although the patients still showed an increase in the intracellular muscle water content; this is a typical feature of muscle in chronically uremic patients, regardless of the mode of therapy [277].

Despite hypermagnesemia in our CAPD patients during treatment with dialysis fluids containing magnesium 0.75 mmol/l, the muscle content of magnesium was not altered [282]. Magnesium appears not to accumulate in excess together with intracellular water as is the case with potassium, presumably because muscle magnesium is mainly present as a complex, bound to ATP and other energy-rich phosphagens in the cell, and not as a free ion [286]. The present observation that the muscle magnesium content in CAPD patients is essentially normal may therefore suggest that the intracellular energy metabolism was not grossly deranged. On the other hand, we have observed (vide supra) that muscle adenosine triphosphate and phosphocreatine were slightly decreased in CAPD patients, without any significant change in free creatine and total creatine in muscle [246]. These results suggest that the skeletal muscle in CAPD patients are in a low-energy state [246].

7. NUTRITION AND ADEQUACY OF DIALYSIS

Routine biochemical measures such as urea, creatinine, albumin, and hemoglobin levels, which are widely used as indicators of the adequacy of dialysis, are all influenced by nutritional factors, in particular by protein intake [12, 18, 287]. Furthermore, signs and symptoms of uremia in inadequately dialyzed patients are often difficult to distinguish from signs and symptoms of malnutrition. Therefore, an evaluation of the nutritional status and dietary protein intake in dialysis patients necessitates an assessment of the adequacy of dialysis (and vice versa). The importance of nutritional factors for the outcome of dialysis therapy is vindicated by the reported association between poor nutritional status and increased morbidity in hemodialysis patients [12, 14, 21, 22].

Adequacy of dialysis, however, is a concept which is not easy to define. No one measure, clinical or biochemical, has proven acceptable to measure the adequacy of dialysis treatment [12, 163, 164, 287–289]. Most authors agree that good appetite with a sufficient intake of nutrients, and a well maintained nutritional status, should be present to classify a patient on dialysis as adequately treated [12, 18, 287–289]. Thus, the nutritional status and the clinical and biochemical control of uremia in dialysis patients are closely interrelated. Protein intake – and its rate of catabolism and generation of urea and other nitrogenous compounds – forms a major determinant of the dialysis therapy needed. Conversely, the adequacy of dialysis therapy may directly influence nutrient intake; for example, underdialysis may lead to anorexia and inadequate intake of nutrients. This may result in malnutrition and wasting which, in turn, may contribute to many aspects of the uremic syndrome, including progressive neuropathy, muscle weakness, anemia, impaired wound healing and susceptibility to infection [12, 18, 163, 164, 287, 290].

7.1. Control of uremia in CAPD

The well-being of uremic patients is reported to often improve after the start of CAPD, and this appears to be the case also for patients who are transferred from HD to CAPD [29–31, 34, 291]. Most authors report that CAPD results in an adequate control of uremic signs and symptoms [29–31, 34[. For example, Wu *et al.* [34] contend that CAPD provides adequate dialysis according to several criteria including adequate biochemical control and amelioration of uremic complications.

There is evidence that CAPD in some respects may lead to improved control of uremic toxicity in comparison to HD. For example, platelet function [292], immunological competence [293, 294], and control of anemia [295–297] are reported to be better with CAPD than with HD. These beneficial effects of CAPD have been attributed to the efficient rewmoval of middle molecules with CAPD (see below).

On the other hand, there are several uremic symptoms and complications that appear not to be adequately controlled by CAPD. For example, many patients on CAPD complain of tiredness, insomnia [298], muscle weakness [299] and anorexia [134]. The occurence of such symptoms may lead to inadequate nutrient intake and impaired nutritional status. Furthermore, as discussed in the previous sections, much of the metabolic and nutritional abnormalities in uremia persist during CAPD. These observations show that the control of uremia is far from optimal by CAPD.

7.2. Adaptive decrease of protein intake in underdialyzed patients

A high protein intake seems to be a requirement for patients on regular dialysis treatment to maintain nitrogen equilibrium and avoid loss of body protein. It may, however, be difficult to fulfill these requirements since some dialysis patients seem to lose appetite and reduce their protein intake spontaneously. This is especially common in patients who are underdialyzed with regard to small molecules. Experiences from the National Cooperative Study on Dialysis Prescription [12], conducted in the USA, show that those hemodialysis patients who were dialyzed according to a schedule which implied a low total weekly clearance of urea had a significantly lower urea appearance rate and consequently a lower blood urea nitrogen level than might have been expected if the protein intake had been as high as prescribed. This strongly suggests that patients underdialyzed with regard to small molecules tend to reduce their protein intake spontaneously, thereby compensating for insufficient removal of urea and other small molecules. One explanation may be that urea and other uremic toxins adversely influence the appetite. A high morbidity in the subgroup of patients with low weekly small-molecule clearance in the National Cooperative Study [12] may, thus, rather be a consequencve of protein malnutriton than a direct effect of small-molecule toxicity. Supporting evidence are the data of Shapiro *et al.* [38] and Acchiardo *et al.* [21] demonstrating that patients with the lowest protein intake and lowest blood urea nitrogen level had the highest morbidity and mortality.

In patients switched from hemodialysis to low-efficiency hemofiltration and vice versa, it has been observed that blood urea tended to increase less during the hemofiltration periods than expected, if the protein intake was constant [300, 301], and that the urea appearance rate was lower during hemofiltration than during hemodialysis [301], suggesting that the patients had lowered their protein intake during hemofiltration as an adaption to the lower removal of small molecules.

The dietary protein intake has been reported to decrease in patients after transfer from hemodialysis to CAPD while it increases in patients transferred from CAPD to hemodialysis [257]. This might be due to less efficient removal of small molecules in CAPD.

Most CAPD patients have a total urea clearance of about 8 to 12 ml/min [18]. If some residual renal function exists, it will make a major contribution to total urea clearance. If the residual renal function decreases, for example from 2 ml/min to 1 ml/min, the effluent dialysate volume must be increased by 1.44 l/day to yield the same total urea clearance [18]. However, if the patient in the foregoing example became underdialyzed, developed anorexia, and therefore maintained a stable stable serum urea level, the deterioration in residual renal function might pass undetected, and the patient may develop an insidious, downhill path with progressive protein malnutrition and 'failure to thrive' [18].

7.3. Uremic middle molecules in CAPD

The middle molecule hypothesis states that middle molecular toxins in the molecular weight range of 350–5000 daltons/molecule accumulate in uremia and are a major cause of various uremic complications [163, 164]. In comparison to HD, CAPD is a very inefficient method with regard to removal of small molecules although this low efficiency is in part compensated for by the long duration and the continuous dialysis process in CAPD [29, 30]. On the other hand, the peritoneal membrane has a higher permeability for molecules within the middle molecular weight range than the membranes commonly used in hemodialyzers. Moreover, the long dwell times in CAPD, which lead to fairly rapid equilibration between body fluids and the peritoneal dialysate of small molecules like urea and creatinine, and thus less efficient removal of these substances, are favourable from the point of view of removal of middle molecules [29, 302–304].

As a result of higher clearances of middle molecules in CAPD, one would expect that patients on CAPD should have lower plasma concentrations of middle molecules than patients on intermittent dialysis. Indeed, this has been confirmed by direct determination of middle molecules using combined gel filtration and ion-exchange chromatography [304]. Thus, we observed that, in CAPD, the peritoneal clearance of four different middle molecule fractions, 7a, 7b, 7c and 7d was, on the average, 89% of the creatinine clearance in the same patients [304]. The corresponding figures for intermittent peritoneal dialysis and HD were 65% and 40%, respectively, of the creatinine clearance. These observations confirm the superiority of CAPD over intermittent forms of dialysis as regards the removal of middle molecules. This finding agrees with results showing that the vitamin B_{12} peritoneal clearance (which is similar to the clearances of middle molecules) was higher in patients on CAPD (6.6 ml/min) than in patients on intermittent peritoneal dialysis (2.4 ml/min), and that the peritoneal clearance of vitamin B_{12} in CAPD was approximately 60% of the creatinine clearance [303].

Furthermore, we observed that the generation rate of the middle molecule fraction 7c was approximately the same in the CAPD patients as in normal subjects, whereas in non-dialyzed uremic patients the urinary excretion (generation) of this fraction was considerably higher than normal [304]. In view of our observation that high plasma levels of 7c, which presumably reflect increased generation of this middle molecule fraction, frequently are associated with uremic complications both in non-dialyzed and dialyzed chronic uremic patients [163, 164], the finding of a normal 7c generation rate might imply that the metabolic control of uremia is better in patients on CAPD than in uremic patients undergoing other forms of therapy [304].

Various beneficial effects of CAPD, for example, improved platelet function [292], improved immunological competence [293, 294], and improved control of anemia [295–297], have been attributed to the efficient removal of middle molecules in CAPD. On the other hand, the reported deterioration of peripheral nerve function during CAPD [305, 306] seems to contradict the middle molecule hypothesis. However, recent findings that middle molecules may have lower molecular weights than earlier thought would imply that their elimination by standard intermittent HD is adequate and that CAPD offers no appreciable advantage with regard to middle molecule removal [304].

8. NUTRITIONAL MANAGEMENT

Patients undergoing CAPD require relatively few restrictions concerning their dietary intakes of water, salt, and other nutrients. In fact, this is one of the main advantages with CAPD as compared to intermittent dialysis. However, a major problem is that many CAPD patients have insufficient nutritional intakes. Individualized dietary prescriptions are therefore necessary. *Ad libitum* diets should be discouraged. Recommended nutritional intakes in patients undergoing CAPD are given in Table 7.

8.1. Dietary protein requirements

It has long been recognized that dietary requirements of protein are higher in dialysis patients than in normal subjects and nondialyzed uremics [307]. However, there is no consensus about the amount of dietary protein that is necessary to maintain nitrogen balance in patients in intermittent hemodialysis. Results of nitrogen balance studies in patients on maintenance hemodialysis twice a week suggested that approximately 0.75 g/kg/day of high biological value protein is necessary to maintain nitrogen equilibrium or a slightly positive nitrogen balance [308, 309]. According to more recent long-term studies this amount of protein may not, however, be adequate. Signs of malnutrition have been observed in substantial fractions of apparently well-rehabilitated patients on maintenance hemodialysis, who had a daily intake of about 1 g protein/kg body weight/day [310, 311].

In contrast, subjects with normal renal function have a minimum daily protein requirement of about 0.5 g protein/kg/day [312] and nondialyzed uremic patients may be in nitrogen balance on 0.5–0.6 g/kg/day of high-quality

Table 7. Recommended nutritional intakes in patients undergoing CAPD

Dietary energy intake	≥ 30 kcal/kg/d
Total energy intake	≥ 35 kcal/kg/d
Dietary protein intake	≥ 1.2 g/kg/d
Water and sodium chloride	As tolerated by fluid balance
Potassium	60–80 mmol/d
Magnesium	200–300 mg/d
Calcium	1.0–1.4 g/d
Phosphate	0.7–1.2 g/d
Supplemental vitamins	
Ascorbic acid	100–200 mg/d
Vitamin B_1	10–40 mg/d
Vitamin B_6	5–15 mg/d
Folic acid	0.5–1.0 mg/d
Vitamins B_{12}, A, E, and K	None
Vitamin D	See text
Trace elements	See text

protein [313] or less, if the diet is supplemented with essential amino acids [314] or their keto analogues [315]. Hence, the increased protein requirements of hemodialysis patients cannot be attributed to uremia, but must be a consequence of the hemodialysis treatment.

Another important factor may be the energy intake (vide infra). It has been recommended that maintenance hemodialysis patients should ingest about 35 kcal/kg body weight/day, but it is conceivable that many patients have a lower energy intake which can contribute to decreased utilization of protein. Children on maintenance hemodialysis frequently ingest less energy than the recommended daily allowances and increasing the energy intake may be associated with a positive growth response [316] .

Several studies show that nitrogen equilibrium can be maintained, or positive nitrogen balance be achieved during the initial year on CAPD [78, 103, 108, 317, 318, 319]. The daily intake of protein of the patients in these studies varied between 0.7 and 2.1 g/kg body weight. The nitrogen balance has been found to be positively correlated to protein intake [78, 108] and to total energy intake [78]. Some patients with an intake of less than 1.0 g protein/kg body weight/day exhibited a clearly positive nitrogen balance [78], whereas other patients with a protein intake of about 1.0 g/kg/day were in negative nitrogen balance [108].

In patients undergoing CAPD, a dietary protein intake of 1.0–1.2 g/kg/day has been reported to be associated with several signs indicating protein malnutrition; for example, decreasing total body nitrogen, intracellular protein depletion, and abnormal concentrations of plasma and muscle free amino balance studies therefore indicate that CAPD patients should have a dietary protein intake exceeding 1.2. g/kg/day, The increased requirement of protein in CAPD patients, compared with non-dialyzed uremic patients, is to a large extent due to protein loss into the dialysate, which may vary between 0.05–0.3 g/kg/day. In CAPD patients with frequent episodes of peritonitis or other intercurrent illnesses the requirement of protein is further increased.

Several CAPD patients have a dietary protein intake of 1.5 g/kg/day or more, and some patient ingest more than 1.8 g/kg/day during the initial months of CAPD. A high protein intake may lead to increased serum phosphate levels, and may accentuate acidosis due to increased generation of acidic products from protein metabolism. Thus, patients with a high protein intake may require additional administration of phosphate binders and sodium bicarbonate. However, we have not observed any adverse clinical effects of protein intakes above 1.8 g/kg/day and there appears to be no reason to institute protein restriction in patients with high nutritional intakes.

It is essential that patients on CAPD understand the importance of maintaining a high protein intake. Protein derived from animal sources (meats, fish, egg, milk) are of the highest biological value whereas vegetables and grain provide protein of lower quality. At least 50% of the protein intake should be of high biological protein value to provide a surplus of essential amino acids. Patients with a protein intake of 1.0 g/kg/day, or lower, should be considered at risk, and should receive additional training and advice concerning nutrition. If this does not result in increased protein intake one may consider oral or peritoneal sup-

plementation with essential amino acids.

8.1.1. Amino acid supplementation

Attempts have been made to compensate for the amino acid losses and increased protein requirements in regular hemodialysis patients by supplementation orally with essential amino acids [320–323] or mixtures of essential amino acids and keto acid analogues [324] or intravenously with essential amino acids or mixtures of nonessential amino acids [325–327]. On the basis of measurement of visceral proteins as well as plasma amino acids, some authors conclude that the effect of essential amino acid supplementation is questionable, at least in hemodialysis patients with a relatively high protein intake [322, 324, 327]. However, positive results have also been reported, especially in one study where there was evidence that the patients were inadequately nourished prior to the start of essential amino acid therapy [78].

It has been suggested that amino acids should be substituted for glucose as osmotic agents in peritoneal dialysis [68, 328]. By now, there are several reports on the use of amino acid solutions in CAPD [329–332]. The potential benefits of using amino acids as osmotic agents include: 1) Compensation for protein and amino acid losses into the dialysate, 2) Compensation for inadequate dietary protein intake, 3) Improvement of amino acid abnormalities, 4) Elimination, or amelioration, of harmful metabolic and nutritional effects of glucose absorption, 5) Elimination of harmful effects of glucose and glucose metabolites on the peritoneal membrane, 6) The ultimate goal is to improve the nutritional status.

In the study by Oren *et al.* [330] the use of a 1% amino acid solution given twice per day in 6 CAPD patients over four weeks resulted in significantly increased serum transferrin levels as well as in increased total body nitrogen. The study by Oren *et al.* [330] showed for the first time that daily use of amino acid solutions for peritoneal dialysis can be performed without adverse clinical effects. The authors concluded that the daily use of amino acid solutions may result in improved nutritional status in patients undergoing CAPD. However, the observed average change in total body nitrogen (corrected for changes in BUN levels) was only + 3.5% [19]. Moreover, changes in serum transferrin levels may be due to other factors than improved nutritional status.

Nevertheless, the results from the Toronto group are promising. It now remains to investigate how the amino acid composition should be optimized for a solution intended for peritoneal use in order to obtain both an efficient osmotic effect and the best possible nutritive effect with improvement or normalization of plasma and muscle aminograms. Furthermore, the effect of amino acid solutions on nutritional status has to be evaluated in long-term studies in CAPD patients.

8.2. Energy requirements

Several observations indicate that energy malnutrition is a major component of the commonly observed wasting in chronically uremic patients [2, 3, 5, 6, 7]. The energy malnutrition could be due to inadequate nutrient intake, increased energy expenditure, or a combination of these two factors. Clinically stable chronically uremic patients who ingest diets providing about 0.55 to 0.60 g protein/ kg/day have been reported to need approximately 35 kcal/ kg/day to ensure that they will be in neutral or positive nitrogen balance and maintain body weight and fat mass [110]. Measurements by indirect calorimetry in nondialyzed uremic patients and patients undergoing maintenance hemodialysis suggest that for a given physical activity, energy expenditure is not different from normal [111]. Dietary histories reveal that, as a group, dialysis patients have low energy intake and consume only about 23 to 27 kcal/kg/ day [10, 11], far less than the 35 kcal/kg/day usually prescribed. The reduction in energy intake in uremic patients does not appear to be an adaptive response to a lower energy need but, more likely, constitutes a maladaptive state which may contribute to malnutrition [111]. Kopple and co-workers [110] have reported that the resting energy expenditure did not decrease in uremic patients when they were fed lower energy intakes. They suggested that chronic renal failure patients may not be able to conserve energy expenditure normally when energy intake is restricted and that this might be another cause of the wasting and malnutrition in renal failure [110].

Energy malnutrition appears to be an overlooked problem in CAPD patients. Deficient muscle energy stores [118, 119], inadequate energy intake in CAPD patients, and anthropometric data, indicate that more attention should be given to the assessment of energy balance in CAPD.

In CAPD, glucose absorption from dialysate averages about 8 kcal/kg/day; however, it may vary between 5 kcal/ kg/day to 20 kcal/kg/day (see previous text). Glucose absorption should therefore be measured, or estimated [130], so that an appropriate dietary energy intake can be established. Despite the peritoneal glucose load, many CAPD patients have a total energy intake below 35 kcal/ kg/day. As discussed above this level of the energy intake has been reported to be associated with various signs indicating malnutrition in the CAPD patients. This strongly underlines the importance of high energy intakes to maintain neutral or positive nitrogen balance during CAPD. Dietary manipulations designed to increase energy intake are recommended except for obese patients and patients with marked hypertriglyceridemia. It is recommended that dietary energy intake should exceed 30 kcal/kg/day.

8.3. Vitamins

Inadequate dietary intake, altered metabolism in uremia, and vitamin loss into dialysate may lead to vitamin deficiences, in particular deficiencies of water-soluble vitamins [333–338].

Blumberg *et al.* [335] studied vitamin status in 10 CAPD patients who were on an unrestricted diet and not receiving vitamin supplements. The fat-soluble vitamin A and E showed increased plasma levels, while vitamin B_1, vitamin B_6, folic acid, and vitamin C levels were low or borderline low due to losses into the dialysate and inadequate dietary intake of these vitamins. Vitamins B_2 and B_{12} were normal. Blumberg *et al.* [335] suggested that CAPD patients should receive 30–40 mg of vitamin B_1, 10–15 mg of vitamin B_6, 0.5–1 mg of folic acid and 100–200 mg of vitamin C.

Henderson *et al.* [336] studied 9 patients who were investigated before starting CAPD, after 6 months of CAPD with oral water-soluble vitamin supplementation and after a further 6 month without vitamin supplementation. They observed normal plasma levels of vitamins A and E. Vitamin C levels were increased before the commencement of CAPD and did not change after 6 months of dialysis with supplementation of 100 mg of vitamin C. After a further 6 month period without supplementation, levels fell significantly. Vitamin B_1 and B_2 levels were normal during the study period, but vitamin B_6 levels decreased significantly after 6 months of CAPD without any supplementation. Vitamin B_{12} status and serum and red-cell folate levels were either normal or increased. Henderson *et al.* [336] suggested that CAPD patients should receive vitamins C and B_6, but probably not folic acid.

Boeschoten *et al.* [337] investigated vitamin status and dialysate losses of vitamins in 31 patients whio had been maintained on CAPD for 0.5 to 36 months. The patients did not receive vitamin supplements for at least 4 weeks before sampling. In 24 h dialysates only losses of vitamin C (8.7 ± 2.4 mg) and folic acid (9.4 ± 0.4 ug) exceeded their excretions in the urine of healthy subjects. Deficiencies of vitamin B_6 – which could not be explained by increased loss via dialysates – were found in 58% of the patients, vitamin C was deficient in 50%, and folic acid in 17% of the patients. The authors concluded that CAPD patients should be given vitamin B_6, vitamin C and folic acid [337].

These results show that depletion of vitamin C, vitamin B_1, vitamin B_6 and folic acid may occur during CAPD and that the patients should receive supplementation with these vitamins. However, the need of supplemental folic acid appears to be low (0.5–1 mg/day).

Polyvitamin preparations containing vitamin A should be avoided because of the possibility of vitamin A toxicity. No supplemental vitamin K or E is recommended. Digenis *et al.* [338] suggest that vitamin B_{12} should be supplemented; however, most authors have found normal vitamin B_{12} status in CAPD (see above). Vitamin D requirements are discussed elsewhere in this book.

8.4. Carnitine

Recent studies have shown low concentrations of carnitine in plasma and muscle in patients undergoing hemodialysis [339]. Carnitine deficiency has been reported to occur also in patients undergoing CAPD [340, 341] although this is not a consistent finding [339, 342].

Deficient carnitine stores in patients on maintenance dialysis have been attributed to: (1) losses of carnitine into the dialysate, (2) deficient stores of the carnitine precursors lysine and methionine, (3) inadequate dietary protein intake, and (4) impaired carnitine biosynthesis [339–349].

It is possible that the elevation in serum lipids in uremic patients, particularly triglycerides, in dialysis patients might be related to a carnitine deficit [343–347]. Supplementation of carnitine by mouth or by addition to the dialysis fluid has been reported to be useful in treatment of hypertriglyceridemia in hemodialysis patients [334, 343–345]. In addition, carnitine replacement therapy may result in decreased serum cholesterol levels and increased HDL cholesterol levels [345, 346, 348, 349].

The role, if any, of L-carnitine supplementation in CAPD

remains to be elucidated. Patients eating well will probably have well-maintained carnitine stores due to an adequate intake of both carnitine and the carnitine precursors, lysine and methionine, in the food. However, CAPD patients with a poor nutritional intake may be at risk of developing a carnitine deficiency.

8.5. Trace elements

Uremic patients show altered blood and tissue concentrations of many trace elements [350]. High levels have been attributed to impaired renal elimination or contamination of dialysis fluid, and low levels of trace elements may occur due to inadequate dietary intake or loss of protein bound trace elements into the peritoneal dialysate [350, 351]. The single most important abnormality is the consistent finding of accumulation of aluminium in uremic patients; this problem is discussed elsewhere in this book.

Thomson *et al.* [351] investigated trace element status in 31 patients who were on CAPD for at least 3 months. The predominant abnormalities were a marked reduction in red cell concentrations of zinc and copper; however, the clinical significance, if any, of these alterations could not be established. Whole blood chromium concentrations were increased to twice normal in the CAPD patients.

Wallaeys *et al.* [352] observed major deviations from normality for bromine (low), chromium (high) and cobalt (high serum concentrations). Danielsson *et al.* [353] have also reported on the abnormal trace element status in CAPD patients with significantly increased blood levels of selenium and cadmium whereas the concentrations of manganese, tin, zinc and nickel were reduced.

The clinical significance of these alterations have not been established as yet. However, supplementation with zinc has been suggested in patients with hypogeusia, anorexia and muscle weakness [351].

8.6. Sodium and water

Sodium and water can be removed easily with CAPD and most patients can therefore be allowed a liberal intake of salt and water. Some patients may require a high dietary intake of salt to prevent hypotension. A large dietary intake of sodium, (4–8 g/day) and water (1500–3000 ml/day) may enable the patient to use more hypertonic exchanges. This results in increased dialysate outflow volumes, increased dialysate clearances of small molecules, and increased energy intake in the form of glucose absorption. However, this treatment may be undesirable in obese patients or in patients with marked hypertriglyceridemia.

8.7. Sodium bicarbonate and acid-base balance

Acidosis in uremic patients is mainly caused by accumulation of phosphate, sulphate, and organic acids, by impaired ammonia excretion, and by bicarbonate loss in urine and dialysate. The major source of acid is dietary protein, in particular its sulphur contents.

Acidosis is reported to be better controlled by CAPD than by other forms of dialysis [278]. Acidosis in CAPD patients should be controlled by additional supplementation with sodium bicarbonate and not by attempts to reduce

dietary protein intake.

8.8. Potassium and magnesium

The minimum requirements for potassium and magnesium are probably met by any diet that meets energy and protein requirements. Hypokalemia may indicate a poor nutritional intake. Hyperkalemia is often due to excessive intake of fruits or vegetables. However, elimination of fruit and vegetables from the diet introduces problems of diet palatability and potential vitamin deficiencies. It is therefore preferable to administer potassium-binding ion exchange resins to patients with hyperkalemia.

Potassium balance was neutral with a protein diet of 1.0 g/kg/day and significantly positive with a diet containing 1.5 g/kg/day [108]. Potassium balance was positive when potassium intake was 67 mmol/day or greater [108]. Dialysate losses accounted for approximately 70% of potassium output and about 30% was from feces [108].

In the same study [108], dietary magnesium intake and balance were greater with the higher protein diet and magnesium balance was significantly positive with both diets (see above). Patients using dialysis fluids containing 0.75 mmol/l have only small losses of magnesium into the dialysate [108].

8.9. Calcium and phosphorous

Uremia is associated with accumulation of phosphorous, mainly in the form of phosphate, and reduced intestinal absorption of calcium caused by vitamin D deficiency and resistance to the actions of vitamin D. The goal of management is the achievement of normal serum calcium and phosphate levels, reduction of secondary hyperparathyroidism, and restoration of normal vitamin D activity. This is discussed elsewhere in this book.

Both calcium and phosphorous balances were greater with the higher protein diet (1.5 g/kg/day) in the study by Blumenkrantz *et al.* [108]; calcium balance was always neutral or positive when dietary intake was equal to 720 mg/day ir greater. Calcium uptake, or loss, from dialysate was rather small compared with the calcium intake from the diet [108].

These observations concerning mineral metabolism in CAPD show that adult patients undergoing CAPD may go into positive mineral balance, especially with high protein diets [108].

The observation that neutral or positive balance was attained in CAPD patients with a dietary calcium intake equal to 720 mg/day, or greater, may suggest that net calcium absorption is higher in CAPD patients than in other categories or uremic patients [223]. Thus, the need of oral calcium supplements may be lower in CAPD patients than in other uremic patients. However, oral calcium supplementation, e.g. in the form of calcium carbonate (40% calcium), may reduce intestinal phosphate absorption and correct mild acidosis. Therefore oral calcium supplementation is recommended for CAPD patients as tolerated by serum calcium.

The minimum requierement of phosphorous is probably met by any diet that meets energy and protein requirements. Hypophosphatemia may suggest insufficient intakes of protein and energy.

Hyperphosphatemia may be due to excessive intakes of milk or cheese, and some dietary restrictions may be necessary. In general, however, restrictions of dietary phosphorous intake may be difficult to combine with a sufficient dietary protein intake. The use of oral phosphate binders to combat hyperphosphatemia and the related problem of aluminium toxicity is discussed elsewhere in this book.

9. ASSESSMENT OF NUTRITIONAL STATUS

Nutritional status should be assessed in all patients undergoing CAPD to identify those patients who may need nutritional support and so that the effects of the treatement can be monitored. Most of the commonly used methods for nutritional assessment in non-uremic individuals can, with some modifications, be applied to uremic patients [2, 3, 5, 6, 11, 12, 18]. The assessment of nutritional status should include anthropometric measurements and biochemical and other laboratory studies as well as an evaluation of nutrient intake (Table 8).

9.1. Assessment of nutrient intake

Dietary assessments are necessary to determine whether a patient is adhering to the prescribed diet. This is often not the case. Current eating habits and patients' intakes of specific nutrients should be assessed, preferably by a skilled dietitian. Dietary histories along with diet records compiled by the patients can provide valuable information regarding patient compliance with the prescribed diet [2, 6, 18]. In addition, dietary protein intake can be estimated also by calculating the urinary plus dialysate urea nitrogen appearance. Protein loss into dialysate, and glucose absorption from dialysate, must be considered when evaluating nutrient intake.

9.2. Anthropometric measurements

Patients with chronic renal failure have increased body water and reduced fat stores and reduced muscle mass [5, 6, 10–12, 14]. Since body water, in particular extracellular fluid, may fluctuate considerably in dialysis patients, body weight gives only an approximative estimate of tissue weight. A careful evaluation to determine the 'dry', edema-free, post-drain body weight is therefore necessary. The results of several studies show that increased body weight during the first year on CAPD is probably due to a combination of increased body fat, body protein, and, body water. However, it should be noted that few patients reach a body weight than exceeds their premorbid non-uremic weight.

9.3. Biochemical monitoring of nutritional status

Several biochemical parameters can be used for routine assessment of nutritional status. Urea nitrogen appearance, which can be used to estimate total nitrogen output, should be determined at frequent intervals. Total nitrogen output correlates closely with nitrogen intake provided that dialysate protein loss is relatively constant and that patients

Table 8. Assessment of nutritional status

Medical history
Changes in body weight?
Pre-uremic weight?
Current appetite status and changes in appetite?
Gastrointestinal symptoms? (vomiting? diarrhea?)
Complicating diseases resulting in metabolic stress?
Functional capacity? (bedridden?)
Medication? (steroids? insulin?)

Physical examination
Muscle wasting?
Loss of subcutaneous fat?
Edema?
Subjective global assessment of nutritional status

Evaluation of nutrient intake
Diet records and dietetic interviews
Urea nitrogen appearance (urine plus dialysate) and calculation of dietary protein intake

Anthropometric measurements
Body weight (post-drain)
Height: weight ratio, e.g. Broca's index
% Relative body weight
% Desirable body weight
% Usual pre-uremic weight
Skinfold thickness (triceps, biceps, subscapular, suprailiac) and calculation of % body fat
Midarm muscle circumference and calculation of midarm muscle circumference

Biochemical monitoring
Serum urea and creatinine
Serum sodium, potassium, magnesium, standard bicarbonate, calcium and phosphorous
Serum total protein, albumin, transferrin (IgG, IgA, IgM, C_3, C_4, prealbumin, pseudocholinesterase)
Blood glucose
Serum triglycerides, cholesterol (apolipoprotein B, VLDL, LDL, HDL)
Hb, hematocrit, and ferritin
Urine and dialysate outflow volumes per 24 hr
Urine and dialysate protein loss
Total (renal plus dialysate) creatinine and urea clearances and calculation of urea nitrogen appearance
Plasma amino acids
(Muscle and leucocyte amino acids)
(Muscle alkali-soluble protein: DNA)

are not markedly anabolic or catabolic [354, 355]. Thus, urea nitrogen appearance can be used to estimate dietary protein intake in clinically stable CAPD patients.

A major problem in CAPD, as well as in other forms of dialysis, is that the appearance of signs and symptoms related to inadequate dialysis or malnutrition often is insidious, and that the results of biochemical measurements that are used to assess changes in the state of uremia during dialysis are difficult to interpret correctly over a short time-period. Thus, it is not easy to delineate cause and effect relationships as regard inadequate control of uremia and malnutrition in dialysis patients. In the underdialyzed patient, the occurence of anorexia with subsequently reduced protein intake may result in reduced formation of urea and thus a lower serum urea level. If one fails to recognize this relationship such changes may be misinterpreted as an expression of adequate dialysis.

Similarly, it is necessary to consider the significance of alterations in the serum creatinine level. It is necessary to appreciate that the generation of creatinine is proportional to the total muscle mass, and that muscle wasting therefore may result in a reduced serum creatinine level.

Obviously, single measurements of serum urea and creatinine provide far from ideal guides for determining the need of dialysis or the need of changes in protein intake. However, frequent assessments and analyses of trends for these variables over a longer time period may allow correct prescriptions of dialysate flow rate to achieve adequate dialysis. Also, repeated measurements of serum urea and creatinine levels may increase the value of these variables as indicators of the nutritional status, especially if combined with analyses of the 24 hr flows of urea and creatinine.

ACKNOWLEDGEMENTS

We thank Ms M. Berndtsson for excellent secretarial work.

10. SUMMARY

Protein-energy malnutrition and wasting are common in patients undergoing maintenance dialysis. The main causes are poor food intake and the impaired metabolism of protein and energy in uremia. Energy malnutrition appears to be a major component of the uremic wasting syndrome. Insufficient dialysis is a major cause of anorexia. The nutritional and metabolic abnormalities in CAPD appear to be similar to those found in patients undergoing hemodialysis. It is important that CAPD patients are prescribed an adequate amount of protein (> 1.2 g protein/kg/day) and energy (total energy intake > 35 kcal/kg/day) and sufficient dialysis to enable ingestion of the diet. Despite glucose absorption many CAPD patients have signs of energy malnutrition. The nutritional management of CAPD patients should include frequent assessment of their nutritional status.

REFERENCES

1. Emmanouel DS, Lindheimer MD, Katz Al: Metabolic and endocrine abnormalities in chronic renal failure, In: Brenner BM, Stein JH (eds), Chronic Renal Failure, New York, Churchill Livingstone, p 46–83, 1981.
2. Alvestrand A, Bergström J: Nutritional management, In Suki WN, Massry SG (eds), Therapy of Renal Diseases and Related Disorders, Boston, Martinus Nijhoff Publishers, p 459–480, 1984.
3. Kopple JD: Abnormal amino acid and protein metabolism in uremia. Kidney Int 14: 340–348, 1978.
4. Smith D, DeFronzo RA: Endocrine dysfunction in chronic renal failure, In Nissenson AR, Fine RN, Gentile DF (eds), Clinical Dialysis, Norwalk, Connecticut, Appleton-Century-Crofts, p 451–497, 1984.
5. Guarnieri G, Faccini L, Lipartiti T, Ranieri F, Spangaro F, Giuntini D. Toigo G, Dardi F, Vivaldi FB, Raimondi A: Simple methods for nutritional assessment in hemodialyzed patients. Am J Clin Nutr 33: 1598–1607, 1980.
6. Blumenkrantz MJ, Kopple JD, Gutman RA, Chan YK, Barbour GL, Roberts C, Shen FH, Gandhi VC, Tucker CT, Curtis FK, Coburn JW: Methods for assessing nutritional status of patients with renal failure. Am J Clin Nutr 33: 1567–1585, 1980.
7. Guarnieri G, Toigo G, Situlin R, Faccini L, Coli U, Landini S, Bazzato G, Dardi F, Campanacci L: Muscle biopsy in chronically uremic patients: Evidence for malnutrition. Kidney Int 24, Suppl 16: S187–193, 1983.
8. Borah M, Schoeneld PY, Gotch FA, Sargent JA, Wolfson M, Humphreys MH: Nitrogen balance in intermittent hemodialysis therapy. Kidney Int 14: 491–500, 1978.
9. Kluthe R, Luttgen FM, Capetianu T, Heine V, Katz N, Sudhoff A: Protein requirements in maintenance hemodialysis. Am J Clin Nutr 31: 1812–1820, 1978.
10. Thunberg BJ, Swamy AP, Cestero RV: Cross-sectional and longitudinal nutritional measurements in maintenance hemodialysis patients. Am J Clin Nutr 34: 2005–2012, 1981.
11. Young GA, Swanepoel CR, Croft MR, Hobson SM: Anthropometry and plasma valine, amino acids and proteins in the nutritional assessment of hemodialysis patients. Kidney Int

21: 492–499, 1982.
12. Schoenfeld PY, Henry RR, Laird NM, Roxe DM: Assessment of nutritional status of the national cooperative dialysis study population. Kidney Int 23, Suppl 13: S-80–S-88, 1983.
13. Bergström J, Alvestrand A, Fürst P, Hultman E, Widstam-Attorps U: Muscle intracellular electrolytes in patients with chronic uremia. Kidney Int 24, Suppl 16: S-153–S-160, 1983.
14. Wolfson M, Strong CJ, Minturn D, Gray DK, Kopple JD: Nutritional status and lymphocyte function in maintenance hemodialysis patients. Am J Clin Nutr 37: 547–555, 1984.
15. Farrell PC, Hone PW: Dialysis-induced catabolism. Am J Clin Nutr 33: 1417–1422, 1980.
16. Ward RA, Shirlow MJ, Hayes JM, Chapman GV, Farrell PC: Protein catabolism during hemodialysis. Am J Clin Nutr 32: 2443–2449, 1979.
17. Ahmad S, Gallagher N, Shen F: Intermittent peritoneal dialysis: Status reassessed. Trans Am Soc Artif Intern Organs 25: 86–88, 1979.
18. Blumenkrantz MJ, Salusky IB, Schmidt RW: Managing the nutritional concerns of the patient undergoing peritoneal dialysis, In: Nolph KD (ed), Peritoneal dialysis. Boston, Martinus Nijhoff Publishers, pp 345–401, 1985.
19. Khanna R, Oreopoulos DG: Complications of peritoneal dialysis other than peritonitis, In: Nolph KD (ed), Peritoneal Dialysis. Boston, Martinus Nijhoff Publishers, pp 441–524, 1985.
20. Bergström J: Protein catabolic factors in patients on renal replacement therapy. In-depth Review. Blood Purif 3: 215–236, 1985.
21. Acchiardo SR, Moore LW, Latour PA: Malnutrition as the main factor in morbidity and mortality of hemodialysis patients. Kidney Int 24, Suppl 16: S-199–S-203, 1983.
22. Harter HR: Review of significant findings from the national cooperative dialysis study and recommendations. Kidney Int 23, Suppl 13: S-107–S-112, 1983.
23. Ganter G: Über die Beseitigung giftiger Stoffe aus dem Blut durch Dialysis. Munch Med Wochenschr 70: 1478–1480, 1923.
24. Boen ST: Peritoneal dialysis. Thesis. University of Amsterdam, The Netherlands, 1959.
25. Gokal R: Historical development and clinical use of continuous ambulatory peritoneal dialysis, In: Gokal R (ed), Continuous Ambulatory Peritoneal Dialysis. London, Churchill Livingstone, pp 1–13, 1986.
26. Tenckhoff H, Schechter H: A bacteriologically safe peritoneal access device. Trans Am Soc Artif Intern Organs 14: 181–186, 1968.

27. Oreopoulos DG: Chronic peritoneal dialysis. Clin Nephrol 9:165–173, 1978.

28. Popovich RP, Moncrief JW, Decherd JF, Bomar JB, Pyle WK: The definition of a novel portable/wearable equilibrium peritoneal dialysis technique. Abstr. Trans Am Soc Artif Intern Organs 5: 64, 1976.

29. Popovich RP, Moncrief JW, Nolph KD, Ghods AJ, Twardowski ZJ, Pyle WK: Continuous ambulatory peritoneal dialysis. Ann Intern Med 88: 449–456, 1978.

30. Nolph KD, Popovich RP, Moncrief JW: Theoretical and practical implications of continuous ambulatory peritoneal dialysis. Nephron 21: 117–122, 1978.

31. Oreopoulos DG, Robson M, Izatt S, Clayton S, De Veber GA: A simple and safe technique for continuous ambulatory peritoneal dialysis (CAPD). Trans Am Soc Artif Intern Organs 24: 484–489, 1979.

32. Bergström J: Potential metabolic problems associated with continuous ambulatory peritoneal dialysis, In: Legrain M (ed), Continuous Ambulatory Peritoneal Dialysis. Amsterdam, Excerpta Medica, pp 277–282, 1980.

33. Kopple JD, Blumenkrantz MJ: Nutritional requirements for patients undergoing continuous ambulatory peritoneal dialysis. Kidney Int 24, Suppl 16: S-295–S-302, 1983.

34. Wu G, Kim D, Oreopoulos DG: Efficacy and adequacy of continuous ambulatory peritoneal dialysis. In: Robinson RR (ed), Nephrology. Vol. II, New York, Springer-Verlag, pp 1581–1610, 1984.

35. Lindholm B, Alvestrand A, Norbeck HE, Tranaeus A, Bergström J: Long-term metabolic consequences of continuous ambulatory peritoneal dialysis, In: Robinson RR (ed), Nephrology. Vol. II, New York, Springer Verlag, pp 1611–1626, 1984.

36. Lindholm B, Bergström J: Nutritional aspects of CAPD, In: Gokal R (ed), Continuous Ambulatory Peritoneal Dialysis. London, Churchill Livingstone, pp 228–264, 1986.

37. Degoulet P, Legrain M, Reach I, Aime F, Devries C, Rojas P, Jacobs C: Mortality risk factors in patients treated by chronic hemodialysis. Nephron 31: 103–110, 1982.

38. Shapiro JI, Argy WP, Rakowski TA, Chester A, Siemsen AS, Schreiner GE: The unsuitability of BUN as a criterion for prescription dialysis. Trans Am Soc Artif Intern Organs 29: 129–134, 1983.

39. Bansal VK, Popli S, Pickering J, Ing TS, Vertuno LL, Kano JF: Protein-calorie malnutrition and cutaneous anergy in hemodialysis maintained patients. Am J Clin Nutr 33: 1608–1611, 1980.

40. Mattern WD, Hak LJ, Lamanna RW, Teasley KM, Laffell MS: Malnutrition, altered immune function, and the risk of infection in maintenance hemodialysis patients. Am J Kidney Dis 1: 206–218, 1982.

41. Sengar DPS, Rashid A, Harris JF: In vitro cellular immunity and in vivo delayed hypersensitivity in uremic patients maintained on hemodialysis. Int Archs Allergy appl. Immun 47: 839, 1974.

42. Corey PN, Steele C: Risk factors associated with time to first infection and time to failure on CAPD. Perit Dial Bull 3 (Suppl 3): S14–S18.

43. Young GA, Young JB, Young SM, Hobson SM, Hildreth B, Brownjohn AM, Parsons FM: Nutrition and Delayed Hypersensitivity during Continuous Ambulatory Peritoneal Dialysis in Relation to Peritonitis. Nephron 43: 177–186, 1986.

44. Delaporte C, Gros F, Anagnostopoulos T: Inhibitory effects of plasma dialysate on protein synthesis in vitro influence of dialysis and transplantation. Am J Clin Nutr 33: 1407–1410, 1980.

45. Flugel-Link RM, Salusky IB, Jones MR, Kopple JD: Protein and amino acid metabolism in posterior hemicorpus of acutely uremic rats. Am J Physiol 244: E615–623, 1983.

46. Kopple JD: Nutrition in renal failure. Causes of catabolism and wasting in acute or chronic renal failure. In: Robinson R (ed), Nephrology. Vol. II, Proc IXth Int Cong Nephrol, New York, Springer-Verlag, pp 1499–1515, 1985.

47. Cernaeck P. Spustova V, Dzurik R: Inhibitor(s) of protein synthesis in uremic serum and urine: partial purification and relationship to amino acid transport. Biochem Med 27: 305–316, 1982.

48. Garber AJ: Skeletal muscle protein and amino acid metabolism in experimental chronic uremia in the rat. J Clin Invest 62: 623–632, 1978.

49. Harter HR, Karl IE, Klahr S, Kipnis DM: Effects of reduced renal mass and dietary protein intake amino acid release and glucose uptake by rat muscle in vitro. J Clin Invest 64: 513–523, 1979.

50. DeFronzo RA, Smith D, Alvestrand A: Insulin resistance in uremia is specific for glucose metabolism. Kidney Int 23: 222, 1983.

51. Conley SB, Rose GM, Robson Am, Bier DM: Effects of dietary intake and hemodialysis on protein turnover in uremic children. Kidney Int 17: 827–846, 1980.

52. Goodship THJ, Lloyd S, Clague MB, Bartlett K, Ward MK, Wilkinson R: Whole body leucine turnover and nutritional status in continuous ambulatory peritoneal dialysis. Clin Sci 73: 463–469, 1987.

53. Baracos V, Rodemann HP, Dinarello CA, Goldberg AL: Stimulation of muscle protein degradation and prostaglandin E_2 release by leukocytic pyrogen (interleukin 1). New Engl J Med 308: 553–558, 1983.

54. Hörl WH, Stepinski J, Schäfer RM, Wanner C, Heidland A: Role of proteases in hypercatabolic patients with renal failure. Kidney Int 24: suppl 16, pp 37–42, 1983.

55. Shaldon S, Koch KM, Quellhorst E, Dinarello CA: Pathogenesis of sclerosing peritonitis in CAPD. Trans Am Soc Artif Internal Organs 30: 193–194, 1984.

56. Gulyassy PF, Aviram A, Peters JH: Evaluation of amino acid and protein requirements in chronic uremia. Archs Intern Med 126: 855–859, 1970.

57. Young GA, Parsons FM: Plasma amino acid imbalance in patients with chronic renal failure on intermittent dialysis. Clinica chim. Acta 27: 491–496, 1970.

58. DeFronzo RA, Alvestrand A, Smith D, Hendler R, Hendler F, Wahren J: Insulin resistance in uremia. J Clin Invest 67: 563–568, 1981.

59. Arnold W, Holliday MA: In vitro suppression of insulin-mediated amino acid uptake in uremic skeletal muscle. Am J Clin Nutr 33: 1428–1432, 1980.

60. Phillips LS, Pennisi AJ, Belosky DC: Somatomedin activity and in-organic sulfate in children undergoing dialysis. J Clin Endocr Metab 46: 165–168, 1978.

61. Phillips LS, Kopple JD: Circulating somatomedin activity and sulfate levels in adults with normal and impaired kidney function. Metabolism 30: 1091–1095, 1981.

62. Sherwin RS, Basil C, Finkelstein FO, Fisher M, Black H, Hendler R, Felig P: Influence of uremia and hemodialysis on the turnover and metabolic effects of glucagon. J Clin Invest 57: 722–731, 1976.

63. Moxley MA, Bell NH, Wagle SR, Allen DO, Ashmore J: Parathyroid hormone stimulation of glucose and urea production in isolated liver cells. Am J Physiol 227: 1058–1061, 1974.

64. Grodstein GP, Harrison A, Roberts C, Ippitili A, Kopple JD: Impaired gastric emptying in hemodialysis patients (Abstract). Kidney Int 16: 952A, 1979.

65. Drukker A, Levy E, Bronza N, Stankiewich H, Goldstein R: Impaired intestinal fat absorption in chronic renal failure. Nephron 30: 154–160, 1982.

66. Williams P, Kay R, Harrison J, McNeil K, Petit J, Kelman B, Mendez M, Klein M, Ogilvie R, Khanna R, Carmichael D, Oreopoulos DG: Nutritional and anthropometric assess-

ment of patients on CAPD over one year: contrasting changes in total body nitrogen and potassium. Peritoneal Dial Bull 1: 82–87, 1981.

67. Heide B, Pierratos A, Khanna R, Petit J, Ogilvie R, Harrison J, McNeil K, Siccion Z, Oreopoulos DG: Nutritional status of patients undergoing continuous ambulatory peritoneal dialysis (CAPD). Peritoneal Dial Bull 3: 138–141, 1983.

68. Oreopoulos DG, Marliss E, Anderson GH, Oren A, Dombros N, Williams P, Khanna R, Rodella H, Brandes L: Nutritional aspects of CAPD and the potential use of amino acid containing dialysis solutions. Peritoneal Dial Bull 3: 10–15, 1983.

69. Lindholm B, Karlander SG, Norbeck HE, Bergström J: Hormonal and metabolic adaptation to the glucose load of CAPD in non-diabetic patients; in Keen, Legrain, Prevention and treatment of diabetic nephropathy, pp 353–359, MTP Press, Boston, 1983.

70. Randerson DH, Farrell PC: Metabolic generation and clearance variation in long-term CAPD; In: Moncrief, Popovich, CAPD Update, pp 75–81 (Masson, New York 1981).

71. Lindholm B, Ahlberg M, Alvestrand A, Fürst P, Tranaeus A, Bergström J: Nitrogen balance and protein and energy intake during CAPD, (Abstract). 4th Int Congr on Nutrition and Metabolism in Renal Disease, Williamsburg, 1985.

72. Von Baeyer H, Gahl GM, Riedinger H, Borowzak R, Averdonk R, Schurig R, Kessel M: Adaptation of CAPD patients to the continuous peritoneal energy uptake. Kidney Int 23: 29–34, 1983.

73. Gahl GM, Von Baeyer H, Riedinger R, Borowzak B, Schurig R, Becker H, Kessel M: Caloric intake and nitrogen balance in patients undergoing CAPD; In: Moncrief, Popovich, CAPD Update, pp 87–93 (Masson, New York 1981).

74. Grodstein GP, Blumenkrantz MJ, Kopple JD: Nutritional and metabolic response to catabolic stress in uremia. Am J Clin Nutr 33: 1411–1416, 1980.

75. Rubin J, Flynn MA, Nolph KD: Total body potassium – a guide to nutritional health in patients undergoing continuous ambulatory peritoneal dialysis. Am J Clin Nutr 34: 94–98, 1981.

76. Rubin J, Kirchner K, Barnes T, Teal N, Ray R, Bower JD: Evaluation of continuous ambulatory peritoneal dialysis. Am J Kidney Dis 3: 199–204, 1983.

77. Blumenkrantz MJ, Gahl GM, Kopple JD, Kamdar AV, Jones MR, Kessel M, Coburn JW: Protein losses during peritoneal dialysis. Kidney Int 19: 593–602, 1981.

78. Lindholm B, Alvestrand A, Fürst P, Tranaeus A, Bergström J: Efficacy and clinical experience of CAPD – Stockholm, Sweden; In: Atkins, Thomson, Farrell, Peritoneal Dialysis, pp 147–161 (Churchill Livingstone, Edinburgh 1981).

79. Randerson DH, Chapman GV, Farrell PC: Amino acid and dietary status in CAPD patients. In: Atkins, Thomson, Farrell, Peritoneal Dialysis, pp 179–191 (Churchill Livingstone, Edinburgh 1981).

80. Nolph KD, Sorkin M, Rubin J, Arfania D, Porwant B, Fruto L, Kennedy D: Continuous ambulatory peritoneal dialysis. Three-year experience at one center. Ann. Intern Med 92: 609–613, 1980.

81. Randerson DH, Farrell PC: Clinical assessment of CAPD. Dial Transplant 10: 389–398, 1981.

82. Gahl GM, Schurig R, Becker H, Sorge F, Pustelnik A, Borowzak B, Riedinger R, Von Baeyer H, Kessel M: Clinical and metabolic aspects of continuous ambulatory peritoneal dialysis (CAPD). Int J Artif Organs 3: 245–249, 1980.

83. Katirtzoglou A, Oreopoulos DG, Husdan H, Leung M, Ogilvie R, Dombros N: Reappraisal of protein losses in patients undergoing continuous ambulatory peritoneal dialysis. Nephron 26: 230–233, 1980.

84. Blumenkrantz MJ, Gahl GM, Kopple JD, Kamdar AV, Jones MR, Kessel M, Coburn JW: Protein losses during peritoneal dialysis. Kidney Int 19: 593–602, 1981.

85. Rubin J, Nolph KD, Arfania D, Prowant B, Fruto L, Brown P, Moore H: Protein losses in continuous ambulatory peritoneal dialysis. Nephron 28: 218–221, 1981.

86. Kaysen GA, Schoenfeldt PY: Albumin homeostasis in patients undergoing continuous ambulatory peritoneal dialysis. Kidney Int 25: 107–114, 1984.

87. Dulaney JT, Hatch FE: Peritoneal dialysis and loss of proteins: a review. Kidney Inty 26: 253–262, 1984.

88. Diaz-Buxo JA: Intermittent, continuous ambulatory and continuous cycling peritoneal dialysis. In: Nissenson, Fine, Gentile, Clinical dialysis, pp 263–306 (Appleton-Century-Crofts, Norwalk 1984).

89. Young GA, Brownjohn AM, Parsons FM: Protein Losses in Patients Receiving Continuous Ambulatory Peritoneal Dialysis. Nephron 45: 196–201, 1987.

90. Rubin J, Walsh D, Bower JD: Diabetes, Dialysate Losses, and Serum Lipids During Continuous Ambulatory Peritoneal Dialysis. Am J Kidney Dis 10: 104–108, 1987.

91. Miller FN, Hammerschmidt DE, Anderson GL, Moore JN: Protein loss induced by complement activation during peritoneal dialysis. Kidney Int 25: 480–485, 1984.

92. Shaldon S: Peritoneal macrophage – the first line of defense, In: La Greca G (ed), Proc Second Int Course on Peritoneal Dialysis. Milano, Wichtig Editore, 1985 (in press).

93. Leichter HE, Salusky IB, Wilson M, Hall T, Jordan SC, Ettenger RB, Fine RN: 3 1/3 years experience with peritonitis in children undergoing CAPD and CCPD (Abstract) Perit Dial Bull 4 (suppl): S36, 1984.

94. Boesken WH, Schuppe HC, Seidler A, Schollmeyer P: Peritoneal membrane permeability for high and low molecular weight protein (H/LMWP) under CAPD, In: Maher JF, Winchester JF (eds), Frontiers in Peritoneal Dialysis. New York, Field, Rich and Assoc., Inc., pp 47–52, 1986.

95. Bannister DK, Acchiardio SR, Moore LW, Kraus AP: Nutritional effects of peritonitis in continuous ambulatory peritoneal dialysis (CAPD) patients. J Am Diet Ass 87: 53–56, 1987.

96. Rubin J, Deraps GD, Walsh D, Adair C, Bower J: Protein Losses and Tobramycin Absorption in Peritonitis Treated by Hourly Peritoneal Dialysis. Am J Kidney Dis 8: 124–127, 1986.

97. Staprans I, Piel CF, Felts JM: Analysis of Selected Plasma Constituents in Continuous Ambulatory Peritoneal Dialysis Effluent. Am J Kidney Dis 7: 490–494, 1986.

98. Berlyne GM, Lee HA, Giordano C, Pascale C de, Esposito R: Amino acid loss in peritoneal dialysis. Lancet i: 1339, 1967.

99. Noree LO, Bergström J, Fürst P, Hallgren B: The effect of essential amino acid administration on nitrogen metabolism during dialysis. Proc Eur Dial Transplant Ass 8: 182, 1971.

100. Young GA, Parsons FM: The effect of peritoneal dialysis upon the amino acids and other nitrogenous compounds in the blood and dialysate of patients with renal failure. Clin Sci 37: 1, 1968.

101. Finkelstein AS, Kliger AS: Chronic peritoneal dialysis in diabetic patients with end-stage renal failure. Proc Clin Dial Transplant Forum 5: 142, 1975.

102. Armstrong VW, Buschmann U, Ebert R, Fuchs C, Rieger J, Scheler F: Biochemical investigations of CAPD: plasma levels of trace elements and amino acids and impaired glucose tolerance during the course of treatment. Int J Artif Org 3: 237–241, 1980.

103. Von Baeyer H, Gahl GM, Riedinger H, Borowzak B, Kessel M: Nutritional behaviour of patients on continuous ambulatory peritoneal dialysis. Proc EDTA 18: 193–198, 1981.

104. Kopple JD, Blumenkrantz MJ, Jones MR, Moran JK, Coburn JW: Plasma amino acid levels and amino acid losses during continuous ambulatory peritoneal dialysis. Am J Clin Nutr 36: 395–402, 1982.

105. Giordano C, De Santo NG, Capodicasa G, Die Leo VA, Di Serafino A, Cirillo D, Esposito R, Fiore R, Damiano M, Buonadonna L, Cocco F, Di Iorio B: Amino acid losses during CAPD. Clin Nephrol 14: 230–232, 1980.

106. Fürst P, Bergström J, Lindholm B: Studies of amino-acid metabolism in continuous ambulatory peritoneal dialysis patients – preliminary results, In: Legrain M (ed), Continuous Ambul;atory Peritoneal Dialysis. Amsterdam, Excerpta Medica, pp 292–2907, 1980.

107. Dombros N, Oren A, Marliss EB, Anderson GH, Stein AN, Khanna R, Petit J, Brandes L, Rodella H, Leibel BS, Oreopoulos D: Plasma amino acid profiles and amino acid losses in patients undergoing CAPD. Perit Dial Bull 2: 27–32, 1982.

108. Blumenkrantz MJ, Kopple JD, Moran JK, Coburn JW: Metabolic balance studies and dietary protein requirements in patients undergoing continuous ambulatory peritoneal dialysis. Kidney Int 21: 849–864, 1982.

109. De Santo NG, Capodicasa G, Di Leo VA, Di Serafino A, Cirillo D, Esposito R, Fiore R, Cucciniello E, Damiano M, Buonadonna L, Di Iorio R, Capasso G, Giordano C: Kinetics of amino acids equilibration in the dialysate during CAPD. Int J Artif Organs 4: 23–30, 1981.

110. Kopple JD, Monteon FJ, Shaib JK: Effect of energy intake on nitrogen metabolism in nondialyzed patients with chronic renal failure. Kidney Int 29: 734–742, 1986.

111. Monteon FJ, Laidlaw SA, Shaib JK, Kopple JD: Energy expenditure in patients with chronic renal failure. Kidney Int 30: 741–747, 1986.

112. Brautbar N: Skeletal myopathy in uremia: Abnormal energy metabolism. Kidney Int 24 (Suppl 16): S81–S86, 1983.

113. Smith D, DeFronzo RA: Insulin resistance in uremia mediated by postbinding defects. Kidney Int 22: 5462, 1982.

114. May RC, Clark AS, Goheer MA, Mitch WE: Specific defects in insulin-mediated muscle metabolism in acute uremia. Kidney 28: 490–497, 1985.

115. Guarnieri G, Toigo G, De Marchi S *et al*: Muscle hexokinas and phosphofructokinase activity in chronically uremic patients. In: Giordano C, Friedman EA (eds). Uremia: Pathobiology of patients treated for 10 years or more, Milano: Wichtig Editore, 278–282, 1981.

116. Metcoff J, Dutta A, Burns G *et al*: Effects of amino acid infusions on cell metabolism in hemodialyzed patient with uremia. Kidney Int 24 (Suppl 16): 87–92, 1983.

117. Bertoli M, Baltistella PA, Vergani *et al*: Carnitine deficiency induced during hemodialysis and hyperlipidemia: effect of replacement therapy. Am J Clin Nutr 34: 1496–1500, 1981.

118. Bergström J, Lindholm B, Alvestrand A, Hultman E: Muscle composition in CAPD patients. In: La Greca G, Chiaramonte S, Fabris A, Feriani M, Ronco C (eds), Peritoneal Dialysis. Milano: Wichtig Editore, pp 107–110, 1986.

119. Lindholm B, Hultman E, Bergström J: Skeletal muscle low-energy state in CAPD. In: Proc. IV Congr Int Soc Perit Dial, 1987 (in press).

120. Metcoff J, Pederson J, Gable J, Llach F: Protein synthesis, cellular amino acids, and energy levels in CAPD patients. Kidney Int 32 (Suppl 22): S136–S144, 1987.

121. Quintanilla AP, Sahgal V. Uremic myopathy. Int J of Artif Organs 7: 239–242, 1984.

122. Del Canale S, Fiaccadori E, Ronda N, Söderlund K, Antonucci C, Guariglia A: Muscle energy metabolism in uremia. Metabolism 35: 981–983, 1986.

123. Westervelt FB: Insulin effect in uremia. J Lab Clin Med 74: 79–84, 1969.

124. DeFronzo RA, Andres R, Edgar P, Walker WG: Carbohydrate metabolism in uremia: A review. Medicine 52: 469–481, 1973.

125. DeFronzo RA, Tobin JD, Rowe JW, Andres R: Glucose intolerance in uremia. Quantification of pancreatic beta cell sensitivity to glucose and tissue sensitivity to insulin. J Clin Invest 62: 425–435, 1978.

126. Rubenfeldt S, Garber AJ: Abnormal carbohydrate metabolism in chronic renal failure. The potential role of accelerated glucose production, increased gluconeogenesis, and impaired glucose disposal. J Clin Invest 62: 20–28, 1978.

127. Massry SG: The toxic effects of parathyroid hormone in uremia. Sem in Nephrol 3: 306–328, 1983.

128. Bilbrey GL, Faloona GR, White MG, Knochel JP: Hyperglucagonemia of renal failure. J Clin Invest 53: 841–847, 1974.

129. De Santo NG, Capodicasa G, Denatore R, Cicchetti T, Cirillo D, Damiano M, Torella R, Giugliano D, Improta L, Giordano C: Glucose utilization from dialysate in patients on continuous ambulatory peritoneal dialysis (CAPD). Int J Artif Org 2: 119–124. 1979.

130. Grodstein GP, Blumenkrantz MJ, Kopple JD, Moran JK, Coburn JW: Glucose absorption during continuous ambulatory peritoneal dialysis. Kidney Int 19: 564–567, 1981.

131. Keusch G, Bammatter F, Mordasini R, Binswanger U: Serum lipoprotein concentrations during continuous ambulatory peritoneal dialysis (CAPD), In: Gahl GM, Kessel M, Nolph KD (eds), Advances in Peritoneal Dialysis. Amsterdam, Excerpta Medica, pp 427–429, 1981.

132. Lindholm B, Karlander SG, Norbeck HE, Fürst P, Bergström J: Carbohydrate and lipid metabolism in CAPD patients, In: Atkins R, Thomson N, Farrell P (eds), Peritoneal Dialysis. Edinburgh, Churchill Livingstone, pp 198–210, 1981.

133. Splendiani G, Acitelli S, Albano V, Gianforte A, Tancredi M: Metabolic aspects of CAPD, In: Gahl GM, Kessel M, Nolph KD (eds), Advances in Peritoneal Dialysis. Amsterdam, Excerpta Medica, pp 449–451, 1981.

134. Von Baeyer H, Gahl GM, Riedinger H, Borowzak R, Averdunk R, Schurig R, Kessel M; Adaptation of CAPD patients to the continuous peritoneal energy uptake. Kidney Int 23: 29–34, 1983.

135. Rubin J, Ray R, Barnes T, Bower J: Peritoneal abnormalities during infectious episodes of continuous ambulatory peritoneal dialysis. Nephron 29: 124–127, 1981.

136. Verger C, Larpent L, Dumontet M: Prognostic value of peritoneal equilibration curves (EC) in CAPD patients, In: Maher JF, Winchester JF (eds), Frontiers in Peritoneal Dialysis. New York, Field, Rich and Assoc., Inc., pp 88–93, 1986.

137. Smeby LC, Wideröe TE, Jörstad S: Individual differences in water transport during continuous peritoneal dialysis. ASAIO J 4: 17–27, 1981.

138. Passlick J, Frank A, Berger M,. Grabensee B: Alteration in glucose absorption during peritonitis and its effects in diabetic and nondiabetic patients undergoing CAPD. (Abstract) Perit Dial Bull 4 (suppl): S48, 1984.

139. Manuel MA: Failure of ultrafiltration in patients on CAPD. Perit Dial Bull 3 (suppl): S38–40, 1983.

140. Henderson L: Ultrafiltration with peritoneal dialysis, In: Nolph KD (ed), Peritoneal Dialysis. Boston, Martinus Nijhoff Publishers, pp 158–177, 1985.

141. Nolph KD, Ryan L, Moore RH, Legrain M, Mion C, Oreopoulos DG: Factors affecting ultrafiltration in continuous ambulatory peritoneal dialysis. Perit Dial Bull 4: 14–19, 1984.

142. An international cooperative study – second report. A survey of ultrafiltration in continuous ambulatory peritoneal dialysis. Perit Dial Bull 4: 137–142m, 1984.

143. Henderson IS, Couper I, Lumsden A: Potentially irritant glucose metabolites in unused CAPD fluid, In: Maher JF, Winchester JF (eds), Frontiers in Peritoneal Dialysis. New York, Field, Rich and Assoc., Inc., pp 261–264, 1986.

144. Arbin A: Release of chemicals from dialysis-bags and tubes of PVC-plastics. (Abstract) Perit Dial Bull 5: 90, 1985.

145. Heaton A, Johnston DG, Burrin JM, Orskov H, Ward MK,

Alberti KGMM, Kerr DNS: Carbohydrate and lipid metabolism during continuous ambulatory peritoneal dialysis (CAPD): the effect of a single dialysis cycle. Clin Sci 65: 5329–545, 1983.

146. Armstrong VW, Fuchs C, Scheler F: Biochemical studies on patients undergoing continuous ambulatory peritoneal dialysis. Klin Wochenschr 58: 1065–1069, 1980.

147. Wideröe TE, Smeby LC, Myking OL: Plasma concentrations and transperitoneal transport of native insulin and C-peptide in patients on continuous ambulatory peritoneal dialysis. Kidney Int 25: 82–87, 1984.

148. Armstrong VW, Creutzfeldt W, Ebert R, Fuchs C, Hilgers R, Scheler F: Effect of dialysis glucose load on plasma and glucoregulatory hormones in CAPD patients. Nephron 39: 141–145, 1985.

149. Lindholm B, Bergström J, Karlander SG: Glucose metabolism in patients on continuous ambulatory peritoneal dialysis (CAPD). Trans Am Soc Artif Intern Organs 17: 58–60, 1981.

150. Lindholm B, Karlander SG: Glucose tolerance in patients undergoing continuous ambulatory peritoneal dialysis. Acta Med Scand 220: 477–483, 1986.

151. Wathen RL, Keshaviah P, Hommeyer P, Cadwell K, Comty CM: The metabolic effects of hemodialysis with and without glucose in the dialysate. Am J Clin Nutr 31: 1870–1875, 1978.

152. Hampers CL, Soeldner JS, Doak PB, Merill JP: Effect of chronic renal failure and hemodialysis on carbohydrate metabolism. J Clin Invest 45: 1719–1731, 1966.

153. Alfrey AC, Sussman KE, Holmes JH: Changes in glucose and insulin metabolism induced by dialysis in patients with chronic uremia. Metabolism 16: 733–740, 1967.

154. Swenson RS, Weisinger J, Reavan GM: Evidence that hemodialysis does not improve the glucose intolerance of patients with chronic renal failure. Metabolism 23: 929–936, 1974.

155. Davidson MB, Dabir-Vaziri N, Schaffer M: Effect of protein intake and dialysis on the abnormal growth hormone. glucose, and insulin homeostasis in uremia. Metabolism 25: 455–464, 1976.

156. Ferranini E, Pilo A, Tuoni M: The response to intravenous glucose of patients on maintenance hemodialysis: effects of dialysis. Metabolism 28: 125–136, 1979.

157. Marumo F, Sakai T, Sato S: Response of insulin, glucagon and growth hormone to arginine infusion in patients with chronic renal failure. Nephron 24: 81–84, 1979.

158. Boyer J, Gill GN, Epstein FH: Hyperglycemia and hyperosmolality complicating peritoneal dialysis. Ann Intern Med 67:568–572, 1967.

159. Nolph KD, Rosenfeld PS, Powell JT, Danforth JR E: Peritoneal glucose transport and hyperglycemia during peritoneal dialysis. Am J Med Sci 259: 272–281, 1970.

160. Anderson G, Bergquist-Poppen M, Bergström J, Collste LG, Hultman E; Glucose absorption from the dialysis fluid during peritoneal dialysis. Scand J Urol Nephrol 5: 77–79, 1971.

161. Brown JD, Adam WR, Dawborn JK: Glucose absorption and hyperglycaemia during peritoneal dialysis. Aust N Z J Med 1: 1–5, 1973.

162. Spitz I, Rubinstein AH, Bersohn I, Lawrence AM, Kirsteins L: The effect of dialysis on the carbohydrate intolerance of chronic renal failure. Horm Metab Res 2: 86–93, 1970.

163. Bergström J, Fürst P: Uremic toxins, In: Drukker W, Parsons FM, Maher JF (eds), Replacement of Renal Function by Dialysis. Boston, Martinus Nijhoff Puiblishers, pp 354–390, 1983.

164. Bergström J: Clinical implications of middle molecules, In: Nissenson AR, Fine RN, Gentile DE (eds), Clinical dialysis. Norwalk, Connecticut, Appleton-Century-Crofts, pp 577–589, 1984.

165. McCaleb ML, Izzo MS, Lockwood DH: Characterization and partial purification of a factor from uremic human serum that induces insulin resistance. J Clin Invest 75: 391–396, 1985.

166. Heaton A, Johnston DG, Haigh JW, Ward MK, Alberti KGMM, Kerr DNS: Twenty-four hour hormonal and metabolic profiles in ureamic patients before and during treatment with continuous ambulatory peritoneal dialysis. Clin Sci 69: 449–457, 1985.

167. Kurtz SB, Wong VH, Anderson CF, Vogel JP, McCarthy JT, Mitchell JC: Continuous ambulatory peritoneal dialysis. Three years' experience at the Mayo Clinic. Mayo Clin Proc 58: 633–639, 1983.

168. De Fremont JF, Bataille P, Moriniere P, Kaczmareck P, Fievet P, Fournier A; Metabolic tolerance of continuous ambulatory peritoneal dialysis (CAPD), In: Gahl GM, Kessel M, Nolph KD (eds), Advances in Peritoneal Dialysis. Amsterdam, Excerpta Medica, pp 446–448, 1981.

169. Stout RW: The relationship of abnormal circulating insulin levels to atherosclerosis. Atherosclerosis 27: 1–13, 1977.

170. Chan NK, Varghese Z, Moorhead JF: Lipid abnormalities in uremia, dialysis and transplantation. Kidney Int 19: 625–637, 1981.

171. Heuck CC, Ritz E: Hyperlipoproteinemia in renal insufficiency. Nephron 25: 1–7, 1980.

172. Bagdade JD: Hyperlipidemia and atherosclerosis in chronic dialysis patients, In: Drukker W, Parsons FM, Maher JF (eds), Replacement of Renal Function by Dialysis. Boston, Martinus Nijhoff Publishers, pp 588–594, 1983.

173. Sakhrani L: Lipoprotein abnormalities in uremia, In: Nissenson AR, Fine RN, Gentile DE (eds), Clinical Dialysis. Norwalk, Connecticut, Appleton-Century-Crofts, pp 439–450, 1984.

174. Bagdade JD, Albers JJ: Plasma high-density lipoprotein concentrations in chronic hemodialysis and renal transplant patients. N Engl J Med 296: 1436–1439, 1977.

175. Brunzell JD, Albers JJ, Haas LB, Goldberg AP, Agadoa L, Sherrard DJ: Prevalence of serum lipid abnormalities in chronic hemodialysis. Metabolism 26: 903–910, 1977.

176. Attman PO, Gustafson A: Lipid and carbohydrate metabolism in uraemia. Eur J Clin Invest 9: 285–291, 1979.

177. Ibels LS, Simons LA, King JO, Williams PF, Neale FC, Stewart JH: Studies on the nature and causes of hyperlipidemia in uremia, maintenance dialysis and renal transplantation. Q J Med 176: 601–614, 1975.

178. Rapaport J, Aviram M, Chaimovitz C, Brook JG: Defective high density lipoprotein composition in patients on chronic hemodialysis. N Engl J Med 299: 1326–1329, 1978.

179. Nestel PJ, Fidge NH, Tan MH: Increased lipoprotein-remnant formation in chronic renal failure. N Engl J Med 307: 329–333, 1982.

180. Norbeck HE, Carlson LA: The uremic dyslipoproteinemia: Its characteristics and relations to clinical factors. Acta Med Scand 209: 489–503, 1981.

181. Norbeck HE, Carlson LA: Increased frequency of late pre-beta lipoproteins (LP-beta) in isolated serum very low density lipoproteins in uraemia. Eur J Clin Invest 10: 423–426, 1980.

182. Norbeck HE: Lipoprotein metabolism in chronic renal failure, In: Noseda G, Fragiacomo C, Fumagalli R, Paoletti R (eds), Lipoproteins and Coronary Atherosclerosis. Amsterdam, Elsevier Biomedical Press B.V., pp 337–342, 1982.

183. Norbeck HE: Serum lipoproteins in chronic renal failure (Thesis). Acta Med Scand Suppl 649: 1–49, 1981.

184. Norbeck HE, Orö L, Carlson LA: Serum lipid and lipoprotein concentrations in chronic uremia. Acta Med Scand 200: 487–492, 1976.

185. Drüeke T, Lacour B, Roullet JB, Funck-Brentano JL: Recent advances in factors that alter lipid metabolism in chronic renal failure. Kidney Int 24 (suppl 16): S134–138, 1983.

186. Staprans I, Felts JM, Zacherie B: Apoprotein composition in plasma lipoproteins in uremic patients on hemodialysis.

Clin Chim Acta 93: 135–143, 1979.

187. Sniderman A, Cianflone K, Kwiterovich PO, Hutchinson T, Barre P, Prichard S: Hyperapobetalipoproteinemia: the major dyslipoproteinemia in patients with chronic renal failure treated with chronic ambulatory peritoneal dialysis. Atherosclerosis (Elsevier Scientific Publishers) 65: 257–264, 1987.

188. Norbeck HE, Walldius G: Fatty acid composition of serum and adipose tissue lipids in males with chronic renal failure. Acta Med Scand 211: 75–85, 1982.

189. Norbeck HE, Olsson AG: Effect of intravenous heparin on serum lipoprotein in uremic man, In: Lundblad RL, Brown WV, Mann KG, Roberts HR (eds), Chemistry and Biology of Heparin. Amsterdam Elsevier North Holland, Inc., pp 217–223, 1982.

190. Attman PO, Gustafson A, Alanpovic P, Wang CS: Effect of protein-reduced diet on plasma lipids, apolipoproteins and lipolytic activities in patients with chronic renal failure. Am J Nephrol 4: 92–98, 1984.

191. Frank WM, Sreepada Rao TK, Manis T, Delano BG, Avram MM, Saxena AK, Carter AC, Friedman EA: Relationship of plasma lipids to renal function and length of time on maintenance hemodialysis. Am J Clin Nutr 31: 1886–1892, 1978.

192. Haas LB, Wahl PW, Sherrard DJ: A longitudinal study of lipid abnormalities in renal failure. Nephron 33: 145–149, 1983.

193. Norbeck HE, Rössner S: Intravenous fat tolerance test with intralipid in chronic renal failure. Acta Med Scand 211: 69–74, 1982.

194. Chan MK, Varghese Z, Persaud JW, Naillod RA, Moorhead JF: Hyperlipidemia in patients on maintenance hemo- and peritoneal dialysis: the relative pathogenic roles of triglyceride production and triglyceride removal. Clin Nephrol 17: 183–190, 1982.

195. Attman PO, Gustafson A: Lipid and carbohydrate metabolism in uraemia. Eur J Clin Invest 9: 285–291, 1979.

196. Russel GI, Davies TG, Walls J: Evaluation of the intravenous fat tolerance test in chronic renal disease. Clin Nephrol 13: 282–286, 1980.

197. Olefsky J, Farquhar JW, Reavan GM: Reappraisal of the role of insulin in hyperglyceridemia. Am J Med 57: 551–560, 1974.

198. Coulston AM, Liu GC, Reaven GM: Plasma glucose, insulin and lipid response to high-carbohydrate low-fat diets in normal humans. Metabolism 32: 52–56, 1983.

199. Mancini M. Mattock M, Rabaya E, Chait A, Lewis B: Studies of the mechanisms of carbohydrate-induced lipaemia in normal man. Atherosclerosis 17: 445–454, 1973.

200. Lewis B: The Hyperlipidaemias. Clinical and Laboratory Practice, Oxford, Blackwell Scientific Publications, p 147, 1976.

201. Kannel WB, Castilli WP, Gordon T: Cholesterol in the prediction of atherosclerotic disease. New perspective based on Framingham study. Ann Intern Med 90: 85–91, 1979.

202. Ron D, Oren H, Aviram M, Better OS, Brook JG: Accumulation of lipoprotein remnants in patients with chronic renal failure. Atherosclerosis 46: 67–75, 1983.

203. Sorge F, Castro LA, Nagel A, Kessel M: Serum glucose, insulin, growth hormone, free fatty acids and lipids responses to high carbohydrate and to high fat isocaloric diets in patients with chronic, non-nephrotic renal failure. Horm Metab Res 7: 118–127, 1975.

204. Sanfelippo ML, Swenson RS, Reavan GM: Response of plasma triglycerides to dietary change in patients on hemodialysis. Kidney Int 14: 180–186, 1978.

205. Cattran DC, Steiner GS, Fenton SSA, Ampil M: Dialysis hyperlipemia: response to dietary manipulations. Clin Nephrol 13: 177–182, 1980.

206. Okubo M, Tsukamoto Y, Yoneda T, Homma Y, Nakamura H, Marumo F: Deranged fat metabolism and the lowering effect of carbohydrate poor diet on serum triglycerides in patients with chronic renal failure. Nephron 25: 8–14, 1980.

207. Lindholm B, Alvestrand A, Fürst P, Karlander SG, Norbeck HE, Ahlberg M, Tranaeus A, Bergström J: Metabolic effects of continuous ambulatory peritoneal dialysis. Proc EDTA 17: 283–289, 1980.

208. Lindholm B, Bergström J, Norbeck HE: Lipoprotein (LP) metabolism in patients on continuous ambulatory peritoneal dialysis (CAPD), In: Gahl GM, Kessel M, Nolph KD (eds), Advances in Peritoneal Dialysis. Amsterdam, Excerpta Medica, pp 434–436, 1981.

209. Lindholm B, Karlander SG, Norbeck HE, Bergström J: Glucose and lipid metabolism in peritoneal dialysis, In: La Greca G, Biasoli S, Ronco C (eds), Peritoneal Dialysis. Wichtig Editore, pp 219–230, 1982.

210. Gokal R, Ramos JM, McGurk JG, Ward MK, Kerr DNS: Hyperlipidaemia in patients on continuous ambulatory peritoneal dialysis. In: Gahl GM, Kessel M, Nolph KD (eds), Advances in Peritoneal Dialysis. Amsterdam, Excerpta Medica, pp 430–433, 1981.

211. Lindholm B, Norbeck HE: Serum lipids and lipoproteins during continuous ambulatory peritoneal dialysis. Acta Med Scand 220: 143–151, 1986.

212. Turgan C, Feehally J, Bennett S, Davies TJ, Walls J: Accelerated hypertriglyceridemia in patients on continuous ambulatory peritoneal dialysis – A preventable abnormality. Int J Artif Organs 4: 158–160, 1981.

213. Roncari DAK, Breckenridge WC, Khanna R, Oreopoulos DG: Rise in high-density lipoprotein-cholesterol in some patients treated with CAPD. Perit Dial Bull 1: 136–137, 1981.

214. Breckenridge WC, Roncari DAK, Khanna R, Oreopoulos DG: The influence of continuous ambulatory peritoneal dialysis on plasma lipoproteins. Atherosclerosis 45: 249–258, 1982.

215. Khanna R, Breckenridge C, Roncari D, Digenis G, Oreopoulos DG: Lipid abnormalities in patients undergoing continuous ambulatory peritoneal dialysis. Perit Dial Bull 3 (suppl): S13–15, 1983.

216. Ramos JM, Heaton A, McGurk JG, Wark MK, Kerr DNS: Sequential changes in serum lipids and their subfractions in patients receiving continuous ambulatory peritoneal dialysis. Nephron 35: 20–23, 1983.

217. Nolph KD, Ryan KL, Prowant B, Twardowski Z: A cross sectional assessment of serum vitamin D and triglyceride concentrations in a CAPD population. Perit Dial Bull 4: 232–237, 1984.

218. Chan MK, Persaud JW, Varghese Z, Baillod RA, Moorhead JF: Postheparin lipolytic enzymes in patients on CAPD, in Frontiers in Peritoneal Dialysis, edited by Maher JF, Winchester JF, New York, Field, Rich and Assoc., Inc., p. 437–442, 1986.

219. Tsukamoto Y, Okubo M, Yoneda T, Marumo F, Nakamura H: Effects of a polyunsaturated fatty acid-rich diet on serum lipids in patients with chronic renal failure. Nephron 31: 236–241, 1982.

220. Tripathy K, Lotero H, Bolanos O: Role of dietary protein upon serum cholesterol levels in malnourished subjects. Am J Clin Nutr 23: 1160–1168, 1970.

221. Broyer M, Niaudet P, Champion G, Jean G, Chopin N, Czernichow P: Nutritional and metabolic studies in children on continuous ambulatory peritoneal dialysis. Kidney Int 24 (suppl 15): S106–110, 1983.

222. Chan MK, Baillod RA, Chuah P, Sweny P, Raftery MJ, Varghese Z, Moorhead JF: Three years' experience of continuous ambulatory peritoneal dialysis. Lancet 1: 1409–1412, 1981.

223. Lindholm B, Karlander SG, Norbeck HE, Bergström J: Hormonal and metabolic adaptation to the glucose load of

CAPD in non-diabetic patients, In: Keen H, Legrain M (eds), Prevention and Treatment of Diabetic Nephropathy. Boston, MTP Press Ltd, pp 353–359, 1983.

224. Dieplinger H, Schoenfeld PY, Fielding CJ: Plasma cholesterol metabolism in end-stage renal disease. Difference between treatment by hemodialysis or peritoneal dialysis. J Clin Invest 77: 1071–1083, 1986.

225. Khanna R, Wu G, Vas S, Oreopoulos DG: Mortality and morbidity on continuous ambulatory peritoneal dialysis. ASAIO J 6: 197–204, 1983.

226. Wu G et al; Cardiovascular deaths among CAPD patients. Perit Dial Bull 3 (suppl): S23–26, 1983.

227. Bertoli M, Battistella PA, Vergani L, Naso A, Gasparotto ML, Romagnoli GF. Angelini C: Carnitine deficiency induced during hemodialysis and hyperlipidemia: effect of replacement therapy. Am J Clin Nutr 34: 1496–1500, 1981.

228. Cattran DC: The significance of lipid abnormalities in patients receiving dialysis therapy. Perit Dial Bull 3 (suppl): S29–32, 1983.

229. Gutman RA, Blumenkrantz MJ, Chan YK, Barbour GL, Gandhi VC, Shen FK, Tucker T, Murawski BJ, Coburn JW, Curtis FK: Controlled comparison of hemodialysis and peritoneal dialysis: Veterans Administration Multicenter Study. Kidney Int 26: 459–470, 1984.

230. Palmer RA, Newell JE, Gray ES, Quinton WE: Treatment of chronic renal failure by prolonged peritoneal dialysis. New Engl J Med 274: 248, 1966.

231. Bergström J, Fürst P, Noree LO: The effects of peritoneal dialysis on intracellular free amino acids in muscle from uremic patients. Proc Eur Dial Transplant Ass 9: 393, 1972.

232. Bergström J, Fürst P, Noree LO, Vinnars E: Intracellular free amino acids in muscle tissue of patients with chronic uremia: effect of peritoneal dialysis and infusion of essential amino acids. Clin Sci mol Med 54: 51–60, 1978.

233. Schilling H, Wu G, Petit J, Harrison J, McNeil M, Siccion Z, Oreopoulos DG: Nutritional status of patients on long-term CAPD. Perit Dial Bull 5: 12–18, 1985.

234. Bouma SF, Dwyer JT: Glucose absorption and weight change in 18 months of continuous ambulatory peritoneal dialysis. J Am Diet Ass 84: 194–197, 1984.

235. Summerfield GP, Gyde OHB, Forbes AMW, Goldsmith HJ, Bellingham AJ: Haemoglobin concentration and serum erythropoietin in renal dialysis and transplant patients. Scand J Haematol 30: 389–400, 1983.

236. Thomson NM, Atkins RC, Humphry TJ, Agar JM, Scott DE: Continuous ambulatory peritoneal dialysis (CAPD): an established treatment for end-stage renal failure. Aust NZ J Med 13: 489–496, 1983.

237. Baker JP, Detsky AS, Wesson DE, Wolman SL, Stewart S, Whitewell J, Langer B, Jeejeebhoy KN: Nutritional assessment. A comparison of clinical judgement and objective measurements. New Eng J Med 306: 969–972, 1982.

238. Detsky AS, McLaughlin JR, Baker JP, Johnston N, Whittaker S, Mendelson RA, Jeejeebhoy KN: What is subjective global assessment of nutritional status? J Parent Ent Nutr 11: 8–13, 1987.

239. Fenton SSA, Johnston N, Delmore T, Detsky AS, Whitewell J, O'Sullivan R, Cattran DC, Richardson RMA, Jeejeebhoy KN: Nutritional assessment of continuous ambulatory peritoneal dialysis. Trans Am Soc Artif Intern Organs 33: 650–653, 1987.

240. Marckmann P: Nutritional status of patients on hemodialysis and peritoneal dialysis. Clin Nephrol 29: 75–78, 1988.

241. Panzetta G, Guerra U, D'Angelo A, Sandrini S, Terzi A, Oldrizzi L, Maiorca R: Body composition and nutritional status in patients on continuous ambulatory peritoneal dialysis (CAPD). Clin Nephrol 23: 18–25, 1985.

242. Salusky IB, Fine RN, Nelson P, Blumenkrantz MJ, Kopple JD: Nutritional status of children undergoing continuous ambulatory peritoneal dialysis. Am J Clin Nutr 38: 599–611, 1983.

243. De Santo NG, Gilli G, Capasso G, Di Leo Va, Giordano C: Growth during continuous ambulatory peritoneal dialysis (CAPD). Int J Artif Organs 5: 331–332, 1982.

244. Martin-Du Pan R, Mauron C, Glaeser B, Wurtman RJ: Effect of various oral glucose doses on plasma neutral amino acid levels. Metabolism 31: 937–943, 1982.

245. Lindholm B, Bergström J, Alvestrand A: Muscle free amino acids in patients treated with CAPD, in: Maher JF, Winchester JF (eds), Frontiers in Peritoneal Dialysis, New York, Field, Rich, and Associates, p. 400–404, 1986.

246. Bergström J, Lindholm B, Alvestrand A, Hultman E: Muscle composition in CAPD patients, in: La Greca G, Chiaramonte S, Fabris A, Feriani M, Ronco C (eds), Peritoneal Dialysis, Milano, Wichtig Editore, p. 107–110, 1986.

247. Biasioli S, D'Andrea G, Chiaramonte S, Farbis A, Feriani M, Ronco C, Borin D, Brendolan A, La Greca G: The role of neurotransmittors in the genesis of uremic encephalopathy. Int J Artif Organs 7: 101–106, 1984.

248. Lindholm B, Garcia E, Qureshi GA, Henriksson S, Bergström J: High muscle and low plasma tryptophan in CAPD. (Abstract) Fifth Int Congr on Nutr and Metab in Renal Dis, Strasbourg, 1988.

249. Bergström J, Fürst P, Notee LO, Vinnars E: Intracellular free amino acid concentration in human muscle tissue. J Appl Physiol 36: 693–697, 1974.

250. Graziani G, Cantaluppi A, Casati S, Citterio A, Ponticelli C, Trifiro A, Borghi L, Sani F, Simoni I, Montanari A, Novarani A: Branched chain and aromatic free amino acids in plasma and skeletal muscle of uremic patients undergoing hemodialysis and CAPD. Int J Artif Organs 7: 85–88, 1984.

251. Hayes KC: Taurine in metabolism. Ann Rev Nutr 1: 401–425, 1981.

252. Knopf K, Sturman JA, Armstrong M, Hayes KC: Taurine: An essential nutrient for the cat. J Nutr 108: 773–778, 1978.

253. Hayes KC, Stephan ZF, Sturman JA: Growth depression in taurine depleted infant monkeys. J Nutr 110: 2058–2064, 1980.

254. Geggel HS, Ament ME, Heckenlively JR, Martin DA, Kopple JD: Nutritional requirements for taurine in patients receiving long-term parenteral nutrition, New Engl J Med 312: 142–146, 1985.

255. Alvestrand A, Fürst P, Bergström J: Intracellular amino acids in uremia. Kidney Int 24 (Suppl 16): S9–S16, 1983.

256. Rubin J, Barnes T, Burns P, Ray R, Teal N, Hellems E, Bower J: Comparison of home hemodialysis to continuous ambulatory peritoneal dialysis. Kidney Int 23: 51–56, 1983.

257. Farrell PC, Randerson DH: Comparison of CAPD with HD and IPD, in: Gahl GM, Kessel M, Nolph KD (eds), Advances in Peritoneal Dialysis. Amsterdam, Excerpta Medica, pp 131–137, 1981.

258. Thomson NM, Atkins RC, Humphry TJ, Agar JM, Scott DE: Continuous ambulatory peritoneal dialysis (CAPD): An established treatment for endstage renal failure. Aust N Z J Med 13: 489–496, 1983.

259. Flynn MA: Nutritional problems in continuous ambulatory peritoneal dialysis. Perit Dial Bull 4 (suppl): S142–146, 1984.

260. Golden MH: Transport proteins as indices of protein status. Am J Clin Nutr 35: 1159–1165, 1982.

261. Lunn PG, Austin S: Excess energy intake promotes the development of hypoalbuminaemia in rats fed on low-protein diets. Br J Nutr 49: 9–16, 1983.

262. Delmez JA, Slatopolsky E, Martin KJ, Gearing BN, Harter HR: Minerals, vitamin D, and parathyroid hormone in continuous ambulatory peritoneal dialysis. Kidney Int 21: 862–867, 1982.

263. Aloni Y, Shany S, Chainovitz C: Losses of 25-hydroxyvitamin D in peritoneal fluid: possible mechanism for bone disease in uremic patients treated with chronic ambulatory peritoneal

dialysis. Min Electr Metab 9: 82–86, 1983.

264. Somnolos K, Berkelhammer C, Baker J, Wu G, McNamee P, Oreopoulos DG: Nutritional assessment and skeletal muscle function in patients on continuous ambulatory peritoneal dialysis. Perit Dial Bull 6: 53–58, 1986.

265. Bergström J: Muscle electrolytes in man. (Thesis) Scand J Clin Lab Invest 14 (Suppl 68), 1962.

266. Bourgoignie JJ, Jacob AI, Salman AL, Pennell JP: Water, electrolyte, and acid-base abnormalities in chronic renal failure. Seminars in Nephrol 1: 91–111, 1981.

267. Mitch WE, Wilcox CS: Disorders of body fluids, sodium and potassium in chronic renal failure. Amer J Med 72: 536–550, 1982.

268. Coles GA: Body composition in chronic renal failure. Q J Med 41: 25–47, 1972.

269. Bergström J: Percutaneous needle biopsy of skeletal muscle in physiological and clinical research. Scand J Clin Lab Invest 35: 609–6165, 1975.

270. Graham JA, Lamb JF, Linton AL: Measurement of body water and intracellular aelectrolytes by means of muscle biopsy. Lancet II: 1172–1176, 1967.

271. Bilbrey GL, Carter NW, White MG, Schilling JF, Knochel JP: Potassium deficiency in chronic renal failure. Kidney Int 4: 423–430, 1973.

272. Montanari A, Graziani G, Borghi L, Cantaluppi A, Simoni I, Lorenzano E, Ponticelli C, Novarini A: Skeletal muscle water and electrolytes in chronic renal failure. Effects of long-term regular dialysis treatment. Nephron 39: 316–320, 1985.

273. Broyer M, Delaporte C, Maziere B: Water, electrolytes and protein content of muscle obtained by needle biopsy in uremic children. Biomedicine 21: 278–285, 1974.

274. Bergström J, Hultman E: Water, electrolyte and glycogen content of muscle tissue in patients undergoing regular dialysis therapy. Clin Nephrol 2: 24–33, 1974.

275. Montanari A, Borghi L, Canali M, Novarinia A, Borghetti A: Studies on cell water and electrolytes in chronic renal failure. Clin Nephrol 9: 200–204, 1978.

276. Cotton JR, Woodward T, Carter NW, Knochel JP: Correction of uremic cellular injury with a protein restricted, amino acid supplemented diet. Kidney Int 14: 673, 1978.

277. Bergström J, Alvestrand A, Fürst P, Hultman E, Widstam-Attorps U: Muscle intracellular electrolytes in patients with chronic uremia. Kidney Int 24 (suppl 16): S153–160, 1983.

278. Nissenson AR: Acid-base homeostasis in peritoneal dialysis patients. Int J Artif Organs 7: 175–176, 1984.

279. Nolph KD, Prowant B, Serkes KD, Morgan L, Baker B, Charytan C, Gham K, Hamburger R, Husserl F, Kleit D, McGuinness J, Moore H, Warren T: Multicenter evaluation of a new peritoneal dialysis solution with a high lactate and a low magnesium concentration. Perit Dial Bull 3: 63–65, 1983.

280. Lameire N, Ringoir S: Introductory remarks: An overview of peritonitis and other complications of continuous ambulatory peritoneal dialysis, In: Legrain M (ed), Continuous Ambulatory Peritoneal Dialysis. Amsterdam, Excerpta Medica, p 229, 1980.

281. Tazamaloukas AH, Avasthi PS: Temporal profile of serum potassium concentration in nondiabetic and diabetic outpatients on chronic dialysis. Am J Nephrol 7: 101–109, 1987.

282. Lindholm B, Alvestrand A, Hultman F, Bergström J: Muscle water and electrolytes in patients undergoing continuous ambulatory peritoneal dialysis. Acta Med Scand 219: 323–330, 1986.

283. Alvestrand A, Wahren J, Smith D, DeFronzo RA: Insulin-mediated potassium uptake is normal in uremic and healthy subjects. Am J Physiol 246: F174–180, 1984.

284. Oren A, Bernhard R, Riley LJ, Mojaverian P, Ferguson RK: Effect of increased insulin secretion during CAPD on potassium metabolism, In: Maher JF, Winchester JF (eds),

Peritoneal Dialysis. New York, Field, Rich and Associates Inc, pp 409–415, 1986.

285. Panzetta GG, Guerra U, D'Angelo A, Sandrini S, Terzi A, Oldrizzi L, Maiorca R: Body composition and nutritional status in patients on continuous ambulatory peritoneal dialysis (CAPD). Clin Nephrol 23: 18–25, 1985.

286. Nanninga LB: Calculation of free magnesium, calcium and potassium in muscle, Biochem Biophys Acta 54: 338–344, 1961.

287. Delano BG: Regular dialysis treatment, In: Drukker W, Parsons FM, Maher JF (eds), Replacement of Renal Function by Dialysis, Boston, Martinus Nijhoff Publishers, pp 391–409, 1983.

288. Blass CR: Adequacy of dialysis. Am J Kidney Dis 4: 218–223, 1984.

289. Twardowsky ZJ: Individualized dialysis for CAPD patients: a review of the experience at the University of Missouri. Uremia Invest 8: 35–43, 1984.

290. Bergström J, Lindblom U, Noree LO: Preservation of peripheral nerve function in severe uremia during treatment with low protein high calorie diet and surplus of essential amino acids. Acta Neurol Scand 51: 99–109, 1975.

291. Simmons RG, Anderson C, Kamstyra L: Comparison of quality of life of patients on continuous ambulatory peritoneal dialysis, hemodialysis, and after transplantation. Am J Kidney Dis 4: 253–255, 1984.

292. Arends JP, Krediet RT, Boeschoten WE, Van der Lelie J, Veenhof CHN, Von dem Borne AEGK: Improvement of bleeding time, platelet aggregation and platelet count during CAPD treatment. Proc EDTA 18: 280–285, 1981.

293. Giacchino F, Alloatti S, Belardi P, Quarello F, Bosticardo GM, Pozaato M, Aprato A, Segoloni G, Piccoli G: Continuous ambulatory peritoneal dialysis and cellular immunity, In: Gahl GM, Kessel M, Nolph KD (eds), Advances in Peritoneal Dialysis. Amsterdam Excerpta Medica, pp 214–219, 1981.

294. Giacchino F, Pozzato M, Piccoli G: Evaluation of the influence of peritoneal dialysis on cellular immunity by the E-rosette inhibition test. Artif Organs 8: 156–160, 1984.

295. Summerfield GP, Gyde OHB, Forbes AMW, Goldsmith HJ, Bellingham AJ: Haemoglobin concentration and serum erythropoietin in renal dialysis and transplant patients. Scand J Haematol 30: 389–400, 1983.

296. De Paepe MBJ, Schelstraete KGH, Ringoir SMG, Lameire NH: Influence of continuous ambulatory peritoneal dialysis on the anemia of endstage renal disease. Kidney Int 23: 744–748m 1983.

297. Zappacosta AR, Caro J, Erslev A: Normalization of hematocrit in patients with end-stage renal disease on continuous ambulatory peritoneal dialysis. The role of erythropoietin. Am J Med 72: 53–57, 1982.

298. Moldofsky H, Krueger JM, Walter J, Dinarello CA, Lue FA, Quance G, Oreopoulos DG: Sleep-promoting material extracted from peritoneal dialysate of patients with end-stage renal disease and insomnia. Perit Dial Bull 5: 189–193, 1985.

299. Gomez-Fernandez P, Sanchez Agudo L, Caltrava JM, Escuin F, Selgas R, Martinez ME, Montero A, Sanchez-Sicilia L: Respiratory muscle weekness in uremic patients under continuous ambulatory peritoneal dialysis. Nephron 36: 219–223, 1984.

300. Quellhorst EA: Ultrafiltration and haemofiltration – practical applications; In: Drukker W, Parsons FM, Maher JF (eds), Replacement of Renal Function by Dialysis, Boston, Martinus Nijhoff Publishers, pp 265–274, 1983.

301. Baldamus CA, Knobloch M, Sachoeppe W, Koch KM: Hemodialysis/hemofiltration: a report of a controlled crossover study. Int J Artif Organs 3: 211–214, 1980.

302. Bergström J: Serum middle molecules and CAPD. Perit Dial Bull 2: 59–61, 1982.

303. Randerson DH, Farrell PC: Mass transfer properties of the human peritoneum. ASAIO J 3: 140–146, 1980.
304. Bergström J, Asaba H, Fürst P, Lindholm B: Middle molecules in chronic uremic patients treated with continuous ambulatory peritoneal dialysis. Perit Dial Bull 3 (suppl): S7–9, 1983.
305. Lindholm B, Tegnér R, Tranaeus A, Bergström J: Progress of peripheral uremic neuropathy during continuous ambulatory peritoneal dialysis (CAPD). Trans Am Soc Artif Organs 28: 263–268, 1982.
306. Tegner R, Lindholm B: Uremic polyneuropathy: Different effects of hemodialysis and continuous ambulatory peritoneal dialysis. Acta Med Scand, 218: 409–416, 1985.
307. Comty CA: Long-term dietary management of dialysis patients. J Am Diet Ass 54: 439–444, 1968.
308. Ginn HE, Frost A, Lary WW: Nitrogen balance in hemodialysis patients. Am J Clin Nutr 21: 385–393, 1968.
309. Kopple JD, Shinaberger JH, Coburn JW, Sorensen MK, Rubini ME: Optimal dietary protein treatment during chronic hemodialysis. Trans Am Soc Artif Intern Organs 15: 302–307, 1969.
310. Schaeffer G, Heinze V, Jontofsohn R, Katz N, Rippich TH, Schäfer B, Sudhoff A, Zimmerman W, Kluthe R: Amino acid and protein intake in RDT patients. A nutritional and biochemical analysis. Clin Nephrol 3: 228–233, 1975.
311. Kluthe R, Luttgen FM, Capetianu T, Heinze V, Katz N, Sudhoff A: Protein requirements in maintenance hemodialysis. Am J Clin Nutr 31: 1812–1820, 1978.
312. Shrimshaw NW: An analysis of past and present recommended daily allowances for protein in health and disease. New Engl J Med 294: 136–142, 1976.
313. Kopple JD, Coburn JW: Metabolic studies of low protein diets in uremia. Medicine 52: 583–595, 1973.
314. Alvestrand A, Ahlberg M, Bergström J, Fürst P: Clinical results of long-term treatment with low protein diet and a new amino acid preparation in chronic uremic patients. Clin Nephrol 19: 67–73, 1983.
315. Bergström J, Ahlberg M, Alvestrand A, Fürst P: Metabolic studies with keto acids in uremia. Am J Clin Nutr 31: 1761–1766, 1978.
316. Simmons JM, Wilson CJ, Potter DE, Holliday MA: Relation of calorie deficiency to growth failure in children on hemodialysis and the growth failure in children on hemodialysis and the growth response to calorie supplementation. New Engl J Med 285: 653–656, 1971.
317. Giordano C, De Santo NG, Pluvio M, Di Leo VA, Capodicasa G, Cirillo D, Esposito R, Damiano M: Protein requirement of patients on CAPD: a study on nitrogen balance. Int J Artif Organs 3: 11–14, 1980.
318. Brzostowicz M, Schoenfeld P, Kaysen G, Mapes D, Newhouse Y, Piercy L, Humphreys M: Continuous ambulatory peritoneal dialysis (CAPD): nitrogen balance is maintained or improved during initiation of therapy. (Abstract 37 A). 13th Ann Meet Am Soc of Nephrology, Washington, DC, 1980.
319. Gahl GM, Von Baeyer H, Averdunk R, Riedinger H, Borowzak B, Schurig R, Becker H, Kessel M: Outpatient evaluation of dietary intake and nitrogen removal in continuous ambulatory peritoneal dialysis. Ann Intern Med 94: 643–646, 1981.
320. Llach F, Franklin SS, Maxwell MH: Dietary management of patients in chronic renal failure. Nephron 14: 401–412, 1975.
321. Philips ME, Havard J, Howard JP: Oral essential amino acid supplementation in patients on maintenance hemodialysis. Clin Nephrol 9: 241–248, 1978.
322. Hecking E, Köhler J, Zobel R, Lemmel EM, Mader H, Opferkuch W, Prellwitz W, Keim HJ, Müller D: Treatment with essential amino acids in patients on chronic hemodialysis: a double blind cross-over study. Am J Clin Nutr 31: 1821–1826, 1976.
323. Acchiardo S, Moore L, Cockrell S: Effect of essential amino acids (EAA) on chronic hemodialysis (CHD) patients (PTS). Trans Am Soc Artif Intern Organs 28: 608–613, 1982.
324. Neuhäuser M, Ulm A, Leber HW, Schütterle G: Influence of essential amino acids and keto acids on protein metabolism and the anaemia of patients on chronic intermittent haemodialysis. Proc Eur Dial Transplant Ass 14: 557–562, 1978.
325. Piraino AJ, Firpo JJ, Powers DV: Prolonged hyperalimentation in catabolic chronic dialysis therapy patients. J Parent Ent Nutr 5: 463–477, 1981.
326. Heidland A, Kult J: Long-term effects of essential amino acid supplementation in patients on regular dialysis treatment. Clin Nephrol 3: 234–239, 1975.
327. Guarnieri G, Faccini L, Lipartit T, Rainieri F, Spangaro F, Giuntini D, Toigo G, Dardi F, Berquier-Vivaldi F, Raimondi A: Simple methods for nutritional assessment in hemodialyzed patients. Am J Clin Nutr 33: 1598–1607, 1980.
328. Gjessing J: Addition of amino acids to peritoneal dialysis fluid. Lancet 2: 812, 1968.
329. Goodship THJ, Lloyd S, McKenzie PW, Earnshaw M, Smeaton I, Bartlett K, Ward MK, Wilkinson R: Short-term studies on the use of amino acids as an osmotic agent in continuous ambulatory peritoneal dialysis. Clin Sci 73: 471–478, 1987.
330. Oren A, Wu G, Anderson GH, Marliss E, Khanna R, Petit J, Mupas L, Rodella H, Brandes L, Roncari DA, Kakis G, Harrison J, McNeil K, Oreopoulos DG: Effective use of amino acid dialysate over four weeks in CAPD patients. Perit Dial Bull 3: 66–73, 1983.
331. Pedersen EB, Dragsholt C, Laier E, Frifelt JJ, Trostman AF, Ekelund S, Paaby P: Alternate use of amino acid and glucose solutions in CAPD. Perit Dial Bull 5: 215–218, 1985.
332. Lindholm B, Werynski A, Bergström J: Peritoneal dialysis with amino acid solutions; Fluid and solute transport kinetics. Artif Organs 12: 2–10, 1988.
333. Kopple JD, Swendseid ME: Vitamin nutrition in patients undergoing maintenance hemodialysis. Kidney Int suppl 2: S79–84, 1975.
334. Kopple JD, Mercurio K, Blumenkrantz MJ, Jones MR, Tallos J, Roberts C, Card B, Saltzman R, Casciato DA, Swendseid ME: Daily requirement for pyridoxine supplements in chronic renal failure. Kidney Int 19: 694–704, 1981.
335. Blumberg A, Hanck A, Sander G: Vitamin nutrition in patients on continuous ambulatory peritoneal dialysis (CAPD). Clin Nephrol 20: 244–250, 1983.
336. Henderson IS, Leung ACT, Shenkin A: Vitamin status in continuous ambulatory peritoneal dialysis. Perit Dial Bull 4: 143–145, 1984.
337. Boeschoten EW, Schrijver J, Krediet RT, Arisz L: Vitamin deficiencies in CAPD patients. Abstract. Perit Dial Bull 4: suppl S7, 1984.
338. Digenis GE, Dombros N, Charytan C, Oreopoulos DG: Supplements for the CAPD patient (Vitamins, folic acid, zinc, iron, and anabolic steroids). Perit Dial Bull 7: 219–223, 1987.
339. Moorthy AV, Rosenblum M, Rajaram R, Shug AL: A comparison of plasma and muscle carnitine levels in patients on peritoneal or hemodialysis for chronic renal failure. Am J Nephrol 3: 205–208, 1983.
340. Buoncristiani U, DiPaolo N, Carobi C, Cozzari M, Quintaliani G, Bracaglia R: Carnitine depletion with CAPD. In: Gahl GM, Kessel M, Nolph KD (eds), Advances in peritoneal dialysis. Excerpta Medica, Amsterdam, pp 441–445, 1981.
341. Buoncristiani U, Carobi C, DiPaolo N, Cozzari M, Burgnamo R: Progression of carnitine depletion in patients on long-term CAPD. Abstract. Perit Dial Bull 4: suppl S10.
342. Amair P, Gregoriadis A, Rodela H, Ogilvie R, Khanna R, Brandes L, Roncari DAK, Oreopoulos DG: Serum carnitine in patients on continuous ambulatory peritoneal dialysis (CAPD). Perit Dial Bull 2: 11–12, 1982.

343. Maebashi M, Imamura A, Yosinaga K, Sato T, Funyu T, Ishidoya Y, Hirayama N: Carnitine depletion as a probable cause of hyperlipidemia in uremic patients on maintenance hemodialysis. Tohoku J Exp Med 139: 33–42, 1983.

344. Bertoli M, Battistella PA, Vergani L, Naso A, Gasparotto ML, Romagnoli GF, Angelini C: Carnitine deficiency induced during hemodialysis and hyperlipidemia: effect of replacement therapy. Am J Clin Nutr 34: 1496–1500, 1981.

345. Guarnieri GF, Ranieri F, Toigo G, Vasile A, Climan M, Rizzoli V, Moracciello M, Campanacci L: Lipid lowering effect of carnitine in chronically uremic patients treated with maintenance hemodialysis. Am J Clin Nutr 33: 1489–1492, 1980.

346. Lacour B, Di Giulio S, Chanard J, Ciancioni C, Haguet M, Lebkiri B, Basile C, Drüeke T, Assan R, Funck-Brentano JL: Carnitine improves lipid anomalies in haemodialysis patients. lancet II: 763–764, 1980.

347. Vacha GM, Ciorcelli G, Siliprandi N, Corsi M: Favourable effects of L-carnitine treatment on hypertriglyceridemia in hemodialysis patients: decisive role of low levels of high-density lipo-protein-cholesterol. Am J Clin Nutr 38: 532–540, 1983.

348. Caruso U, Cravotto E, Tisone G, Elli M, Stortoni F, D'Iddio S, Pola P. Savi L, Tondi P, Casciani CU: Long-term treatment with L-carnitine in uremic patients undergoing chronic hemodialysis: effects on the lipid pattern. Curr Ther Res 33: 1098–1104, 1983.

349. Casciani CU, Caruso U, Cravotto E, D'Iddio S, Corsi M, Pola P, Savi L, Grilli M: L-carnitine in haemodialysed patients. Changes in lipid pattern. Arzneim Forsch Drug Res 32: 293–297, 1982.

350. Alfrey AC, Smythe WR: Trace metals and regular dialysis. In: Drukker W, Parsons FM, Maher JF (eds), Replacement of Renal Function by Dialysis. Martinus Nijhoff, Boston, pp 804–810, 1983.

351. Thomson NM, Stevens BJ, Humphrey TJ, Atkins RC. Comparison of frace elements in peritoneal dialysis, hemodialysis, and uremia. Kidney Int 23: 9–14, 1983.

352. Wallaeys B, Cornelis R, Lameire N: The trace elements Br, Co, Cr, Cs, Cu, Fe, Mn, Rb Se and Zn in serum, packed cells and dialysate of CAPD patients. Abstract. Perit Dial Bull 4: suppl S70, 1984.

353. Danielson BG, Grefberg N, Nilsson P, Weiss L: Trace elements in patients on CAPD. Abstract. Kidney Int 23: 146, 1983.

354. Blumenkrantz MJ, Kopple JD, Moran JK, Grodstein GP, Coburn JW: Nitrogen and urea metabolism during continuous ambulatory peritoneal dialysis. Kidney Int 20: 78–82, 1981.

355. Farrell PC: Kinetic modeling in peritoneal dialysis, In: Nissenson AR, Fine RN, Gentile DE (eds), Clinical Dialysis. Norwalk, Connecticut, Appleton-Century-Crofts, pp 307–318, 1984.

14

PERITONITIS

STEPHEN I. VAS

1. INTRODUCTION

The frequent occurrence of peritonitis, – one of the major complications of peritoneal dialysis, – has hindered the development and acceptance of this technique.

In the mid-1940's, Seligman [1], Frank [2] reported a method of continuous peritoneal lavage, but the high incidence of infection and technical difficulties, as well as the introduction of the artificial kidney, discouraged its supporters. In 1951, Grollman [4] drew attention again to the value of peritoneal dialysis in the treatment of acute renal failure when he introduced intermittent peritoneal lavage. Later, Doolan [5] confirmed its safety and effectiveness in human subjects. Another major advance, the introduction of the stylet catheter which allowed safe access to the peritoneal cavity [6, 7], made possible intermittent peritoneal dialysis with infection rates of 5.2 to 7.5 episodes of peritonitis per patient year of dialysis [8, 9].

In 1964 Palmer and associates [10] began to provide longterm intermittent peritoneal dialysis employing an indwelling silicone rubber irrigating catheter device which Tenckhoff [11] later modified to its present form. This technique reduced infection rates to 0.23 to 1.2 episodes of peritonitis per patient year (12–18).

In 1976 Popovich and colleagues [19] described the technique of continuous ambulatory peritoneal dialysis (CAPD) for the treatment of chronic renal failure. The incidence of peritonitis with this method, employing bottled dialysate, was 4.6 episodes of peritonitis per patient year [20]. This technique was subsequently modified and replaced the bottled dialysate with a plastic dialysate bag [21]. This arrangement was more convenient for the patients and substantially reduced the number of manipulations of the catheter and therefore the infection rate. Subsequently, many workers using this technique have reported rates of peritonitis varying from 1.2 to 6.3 episodes per patient year (20–26). As noted above, these high rates of infection have been the major criticism of the procedure [27–30], but with increasing control of peritonitis, CAPD could become the dialysis of choice for many patients with endstage renal disease.

In fact with appropriate training, selection of patients and precautionary measures, peritonitis rates can be reduced to one episode every 18 to 24 months. Some units report even better results than this.

The U.S. CAPD Registry [31] – which follows data from over 20 000 patients reports a peritonitis rate of 1.07 to 1.47 episodes/patient year. This rate is an average rate including peritoneal dialysis units which perform the procedure on very few patients and very large units. Similarly it includes units which are just starting with the program as well as units which have many years experience.

It appears that peritonitis rates can be reduced by careful training, use of appropriate equipment, etc. to a rate of approximately one episode of peritonitis every 2 yr. If this rate becomes the generally obtained rate, CAPD will have a much better acceptance for the treatment of endstage renal failure.

Intermittent peritoneal dialysis has a lower rate of peritonitis. It is not unusual to observe peritonitis rates of one every 3 to 5 yr. The reason for this difference is not quite clear. It is tempting to speculate that the shorter time patients are on peritoneal dialysis the less number of connections the volume of the fluid has something to do with this decreased rate. This argument is fallacious. If one compares certain parameters of intermittent peritoneal dialysis with continuous ambulatory peritoneal dialysis it becomes obvious that the number of connections made during intermittent peritoneal dialysis is larger, the total volume of fluid used is more and therefore none of these factors may be important in the development of peritonitis. The only factor which is different in the two populations is that intermittent peritoneal dialysis patients do not have dialysis fluid in the abdominal cavity for the major part of their program (usually 2 days off, 12 to 18 hr on). It is speculative but plausible that peritoneal defense mechanisms are operating better when the peritoneum does not contain large volumes of fluid (see discussion on defense mechanisms below).

CCPD or continuous cycling peritoneal dialysis has peritonitis rates reported in-between CAPD and IPD [32], though the recent report of the National CAPD Registry of the US [31] does not substantiate this claim. This modality of treatment is generally less accepted.

2. PATHOGENESIS OF PERITONITIS

Initially those who had to deal with peritonitis episodes in peritoneal dialysis patients conceived peritonitis as similar to the experience with surgical peritonitis [33]. While this was a reasonable approach, it became clear soon that peritonitis developing in dialysis patients has considerable differences from that of surgical peritonitis.

While small amounts of contamination do not usually cause surgical peritonitis as evidenced by the large number of laparotomies which heal without any evidence of clinical peritonitis, minor contaminations in the peritoneal dialysis patients will lead to peritonitis. Similarly, surgical peritonitis develops mainly when the abdominal cavity has a major soil, usually by fecal content and therefore removal of the contaminating material is essential. In peritoneal dialysis, such large amounts of contaminations are rare. Finally, in surgical peritonitis about 30% of the patients will show bacteremia as part of the disease [60], while in peritonitis of peritoneal dialysis patients positive blood cultures are the rare exception rather than a frequent event and when positive blood cultures are observed, they are usually the harbinger of a haematogenous source of peritoneal infection [70]. Finally, the distribution of organisms isolated from CAPD shows predominantly gram positive organisms.

It is for these reasons that peritonitis of CAPD patients has now been accepted as a special disease entity and its management requires a different approach.

More similar to peritonitis in PD patients is the disease called spontaneous bacterial peritonitis [34–39] which is occasionally seen in patients suffering from cirrhosis of the liver with ascites. It is believed that in these patients the lack of reticuloendothelial function of the liver is the primary reason why these patients develop spontaneous peritonitis. These patients also have large volumes of fluid in their abdominal cavity which may also explain some of the similarities.

2.1. Portals of entry

Microbial environment and host are living in a symbiotic relationship. The occasional penetrations of infectious organisms into an intact host are met with defense and usually the small number of invaders is destroyed [40, 184, 185].

Table 1. Distribution of organisms isolated from peritonitis episodes

Coagulase negative Staphylococci	30–40%
Staphylococcus aureus	10–20%
Streptococcus sp	10–15%
Neisseria sp	1–2 %
Diphtheroid sp	1–2 %
E. coli	5–10%
Pseudomonas sp	5–10%
Enterococcus	3–6 %
Klebsiella sp	1–3 %
Proteus sp	3–6 %
Acinetobacter sp	2–5 %
Anaerobic organisms	2–5 %
Fungi	2–10%
Other (Mycobacteria. etc)	2–5 %
Culture negative	0–30%

The outcome therefore is dependent on delicate balance of the number of invaders vs. defense. Bacterial penetration is probably a frequent event (it is known for example that minor exertions like brushing of teeth or bowel movements will lead to transient shortlasting bacteremias in many normal individuals) and will only rarely lead to major infections.

We do not know how frequently infectious events occur in peritoneal dialysis patients. It is well conceivable that these events are more frequent than the episodes of peritonitis [184, 185]. Since the conditions which lead to peritonitis are not known, all portals of entry have to be considered seriously and to reduce peritonitis all of them have to be managed with great care.

Surveyance cultures from abdominal skin site, throat and hands done on peritoneal dialysis patients before they enter a dialysis program have been done in our unit. The results of such surveyance are shown in Table 2. These are the areas from which incidental contaminations of peritoneal dialysis patients can more frequently occur. In fact, if one compares the Staphylococcus aureus phage type or the Staphylococcus epidermidis biotype isolated from the peritoneal fluid of these patients during peritonitis episodes with the skin biotype as shown in Table 3, it is obvious that the patients are at high risk from their own flora rather than acquiring infections from the environment of other people. This observation has been confirmed by others [234].

It is therefore possible to generate a probable listing (see Table 4) estimating from the type of organisms isolated from peritonitis the probable route of entry. This is a speculative listing making an educated guess on the route through which infections may occur. For example it is assumed that 2/3 of S. epidermidis infections occur through the intraluminal route while only 1/2 of S. aureus infections occur through the same route. Such a listing is helpful (and by experience close to accurate) in understanding the role of various portals of entry.

2.1.1. Intraluminal infections

Intraluminal infections occur when bacteria enter the internal pathway of peritoneal dialysis tubing through the internal surface or through cracks developed in the tubing. The commercial dialysis fluids are prepared with great care and they can be considered sterile. There have been no episodes ascribed to peritoneal dialysis from commercial sources in the last few years [41]. Additions through the port to the peritoneal dialysis bag have to be made with sterile precautions and fresh vials of drugs should be used for each addition.

Intraluminal infection may occur more frequently than

Table 3. Correlation of isolates of skin and peritonitis of CAPD patients

Organism	Same type	Different type
Staph epi (biotype)	45(96%)	
Staph epi (plasmid type)	3(50%)	3(50%)
Staph aureus (phage type)	19(86%)	3(14%)

Table 4. Routes of infections in CAPD patients

Route	Organism	%
Transluminal	Staph epi	
	Staph aureus	30–40
	Acinetobacter	
Periluminal	Staph epi	
	Staph aureus	
	Pseudomonas	20–30
	Yeast	
Transmural	Enteric org	
	Anaerobes	25–30
Hematogenous	Streptococcus	
	M tuberculosis	5–10
Ascending	Yeast	
	Lactobacillus	2–5

believed, but do not result in peritonitis. In a study done by us [184], it was shown that if one cultures routinely clear bags from patients not showing signs of peritonitis a certain number will grow organisms. These organisms usually are Propionobacteria though occasionally other organisms can be grown. The common factor in these cultures that the require prolonged growth (usually 8–12 days) indicating that their number is very small. The patients do not require treatment. This observation emphasizes the experience that routine surveillance cultures of bags from patients not showing symptoms are unnecessary and misleading [185].

Most of the intraluminal infections develop after accidental contamination of the spike by touch contamination or disconnects of the dialysis tubing. Touch contaminations can be reduced by devices which provide no touch mechanisms and accidental disconnects have been reduced considerably with the introduction of titanium locking connectors. Various other devices (see section 11.1.) have been devised to reduce intraluminal infections.

2.1.2. Periluminal infections

The Silastic catheter never forms a completely sealed

Table 2. Surveillance cultures of 47 CAPD patients

Organism	Hand	Abdomen	Nose	Total
Coagulase neg Staph	66(76%)	56(69%)	59(63%)	181(69%)
Staph aureus	3(3%)	4(5%)	7(7%)	13(5%)
Gram negative bacilli	3(3%)	4(5%)	8(9%)	15(6%)
Diphtheroids, yeast, etc	15(7%)	18(22%)	20(21%)	53(20%)
Total	87	81	94	262

junction with the skin or subcutaneous tissues [42]. While the purpose of the cuffs (single or double) was to reduce the penetration of bacteria around the catheter, it does not always achieve its goal. Therefore, bacterial penetration around the catheter is a possibility. Casual penetration of bacteria around the catheter is probably not a factor, to develop peritonitis from a periluminal source either an exit site infection or a tunnel infection has to develop. Studies in our unit have shown that while originally the exit site was kept under occlusive dressings, the removal of such occlusive dressing in fact permitting the patient to daily showers without any cover of the exit site does not lead to increased incidence of peritonitis. It is therefore probable that an infectious process has to establish itself in the tissues of the exit site or the subcutaneous tunnel to produce a peritoneal infection. Bacteria may enter from these subcutaneous infections occasionally leading to clinical symptoms.

2.1.3. Transmural (intestinal) infections
The isolation of multiple intestinal organisms from peritoneal dialysis fluid, especially if they belong to more than one group of bacteria or if anaerobic organisms are isolated, is indicative of a fecal leak. There is some evidence that bacteria may migrate through intact intestinal wall [43]; rarely an ischemic bowel disease may lead to more frequent penetration [36]. It is more likely that the source of intestinal leak is pre-existing diverticulosis in these patients. It is known that diverticulosis increases with age and also there is an increased incidence in diverticulosis in polycystic disease. A study done by us showed that diverticulosis was a major source of faecal peritonitis [44].

2.1.4. Hematogenous infections
It has been shown that hematogenous peritonitis develops frequently in the spontaneous bacterial peritonitis of cirrhotics [34, 35]. We have observed in a few patients that Streptococcus viridans peritonitis developed in patients who had acute upper respiratory infections. Some of these patients preceded development of peritonitis with positive blood cultures from which the same organism usually Streptococcus viridans was isolated. It is also probable that tuberculous peritonitis develops through this route [45].

2.1.5. Other endogenous infections
Rarely, other sources can be implicated in the development of peritonitis. We [46] and others [47, 48, 69] have observed women who had a vaginal leak of peritoneal dialysis fluid. Some of these developed Candida peritonitis. Tubal ligation was indicated in some of these patients after which the vaginal leak disappeared and there was no recurrence of peritonitis. Intrauterine contraceptive devices [183] were also recognized as a possible source of infection. Women on CAPD therefore should be advised of different contraceptive practices.

2.1.6. Environmental infections
Peritonitis from which Pseudomonas maltophilia, Acinetobacter [49] or other environmental bacteria are isolated, are observed sometimes. It is possible that these infections develop by contact with water [50] (showering, swimming pool) entering through the exit site. In peritoneal dialysis patients, episodes of infections with Mycobacterium chelonei [51, 52] have been described where the source was ascribed to tap water entering the peritoneal cavity.

2.1.7. Biofilm
The formation of a biofilm may be a property of certain organisms and surfaces [188]. Biofilms on peritoneal catheters have been described [153, 154]. The biofilm appears to be present on catheter surfaces regardless of the peritonitis history of the patient [187]. The role of the biofilm in initiating peritonitis is questioned [189]. It appears that the presence of biofilm on the catheters does not necessarily lead to peritonitis and an added injury (decrease in defense mechanisms, chemical injury etc.) is needed. Further studies on the formation and role of biofilms are needed to answer this question. The presence of the biofilm is also stimulating research for better non-adhesive catheter material.

2.2. Inflammatory response

The normal homeostatis of the peritoneal cavity is disrupted if bacteria or chemical stimuli enter the peritoneal cavity.

2.2.1. Inflammatory mediators
Bacteria combining with normal opsonins present in the peritoneal cavity in the presence of complement will result in the release of chemotactic factors which will stimulate the outflow of polymorphonuclear cells thus increasing the cell number present in the peritoneal cavity and shifting it from a predominantly mononuclear cell population [143] to a polymorphonuclear cell population [33]. Other inflammatory mediators will be released, like histamine, serotonin etc. [53], which will result in vasodilatation leading to increase in protein, outflow and some of the mediators will produce the typical peritoneal pain.

2.2.2. Fibrin, fibronectin
The normal peritoneal cavity fluid contains fibrinogen and fibrinolysin [54] which breaks down the fibrin formed and maintains the shiny slippery surface of the peritoneum. During inflammation, the fibrinolysis is affected and while increased amounts of fibrinogen enters the peritoneal cavity, the resulting fibrin will not be broken down rapidly because of the lack of fibrinolysis. The result of this is the formation of fibrin filaments and fibrin clots.

Myhre-Jensen [55] and Porter [56] have shown that the fibrinolytic activity of the mesothelial surface of the peritoneum resides in the mesothelial cells. The presence of fibrinolytic activities suggests that fibrinolysis may assist in removing fibrin deposits from these surfaces. However, it has been demonstrated that certain stimuli such as cuts, abrasions and ischemia are associated with local depression of peritoneal fibrinolytic activity [57–59]. Also, Hau et al [60] were able to decrease fibrinolytic activity by inducing bacterial peritonitis. Thus it appears that the depression of fibrinolytic activity of the peritoneum is an important mechanism in the development of fibrin formation and probably in intraperitoneal adhesions.

Fibronectin, a normal constituent of biological fluids, has been studied in CAPD patients [180, 181]. While its concentration increases in peritoneal fluid of CAPD patients during peritonitis, it has no predictive value for susceptibility to peritonitis.

2.2.3. Cellular response

The normal peritoneal cell population is primarily mononuclear cells, probably macrophages of blood origin and some mesothelial cells from the peritoneal lining [202, 205]. With inflammation, rapid migration of polymorphonuclear cells occurs [143]. The rapidity of this migration is truly amazing. It may take only a few hours for a completely clear peritoneal fluid to turn cloudy. The evaluation of the peritoneal cell population is a useful adjunct in the diagnosis of peritonitis [143]. The cellular response also follows the improvement of peritonitis on therapy and is a good clinical sign to follow therapeutic success. Occasionally, eosinophilic cells enter the peritoneal cavity (see Section 7.3.2.).

Abscess formation is an infrequent complication of peritonitis of peritoneal dialysis patients. Onderdonk *et al.* [84] demonstrated that intra-abdominal abscess formation appeared to be related to a synergy between anaerobes and gram negative aerobic bacteria. Since isolation of anaerobes is a rare occurrence in peritonitis in peritoneal dialysis patients. Abscess formation in peritonitis due to faecal flora should also be suspected. Also Staphylococcus aureus is a organism which is associated with frequent abscess formation due to its effect on fibrin around the organisms [144].

3. DEFENSE MECHANISMS OF THE PERITONEUM

The peritoneal membrane lines the interior of the abdominal wall (parietal peritoneum) and the abdominal viscera (visceral peritoneum) forming a potential space of the peritoneal cavity. The peritoneal membrane consists of a surface layer of mesothelial cells which lie on a basement membrane with deeper layers of capillaries and lymphatics. Transport through the peritoneal membrane, moves from the capillaries through the basement membrane through intercellular junctions. Small particles may have two methods for transport: moving through cellular junctions or through pinocytosis by mesothelial cells [148, 149]. The principal route for movement of small particles from the peritoneum is via the lymphatics, primarily through the lymphatics below the diaphragmatic surface [150]. The exact mechanism of this movement is not clear although Courtice and Simmonds [151] have postulated that openings exist between the peritoneal cavity and the diaphragmatic lymphatics. These lymphatics may be important components of host defences. This may explain the extremely low rate of bacteremia in peritoneal dialysis patients during peritonitis. In secondary surgical peritonitis the rate of bacteremia is 30% [152]. In cirrhotic patients with spontaneous peritonitis the rate of bacteremia is between 39 to 76% [34, 355, 61]. The rate of bacteremia in patients on intermittent peritoneal dialysis is about 15% [8]. We have not observed a single positive blood culture in several hundred episodes of bacterial peritonitis in CAPD patients except as noted above where the bacteremia preceded peritonitis. The defense mechanism of the peritoneum is probably the single most important factor in the removal of small amounts of microorganisms from the peritoneal cavity.

3.1. Humoral factors

It has been shown that the immunoglobulins and complement are present in the peritoneal fluid though the normal level of these components is not established. The serum immunoglobulin levels of these patients are not severely compromised [62]. Some patients may have a decreased level of opsonins and probably other factors needed for immunological reactions in the peritoneal cavity [63, 207, 208]. The relative lack of opsonins as a cause of repeated episodes of peritonitis in the peritoneal dialysis fluid of socalled high risk patients is proposed [208, 209]. This is not dependent on the origin of the causative organism [198]. The lack of ability to produce adequate amounts of interleukin-1 and the release of large amounts of prostaglandin E2 by the macrophages of certain patients as the cause of recurrent peritonitis has also been postulated [197].

3.2. Cellular factors

While the normal self-clearing mechanism of the peritoneum is primarily dependent on mesothelial cells and mononuclear cells in the peritoneal cavity during inflammation a large number of active phagocytic polymorphonuclear cells enter the peritoneal cavity participating in the removal of bacteria. Whether these cells have a reduced bactericidal capacity is subject to controversy [201, 203, 204]. Under the conditions of peritoneal dialysis, patients have instead of the normal few milliliters of fluid, 2 l of dialysis fluid with a low pH and high osmolality. We have shown that low pH and high osmolality decrease the efficiency of phagocytic cells which may not be fully functional at least during the initial periods of peritoneal dialysis [64, 193–195]. In addition, urea, creatinine and other low molecular weight substances enter the peritoneal cavity during peritoneal dialysis. We have examined the effect of these molecules and did not find them deleterious to phagocytosis in the concentrations present in the peritoneal dialysis fluid. Similarly, heparin, which is added to reduce fibrin formation did not appear to inhibit phagocytosis.

The relative ratio of bacteria to cell is also important in the efficiency of phagocytosis. The large volume present in the peritoneal cavity during peritoneal dialysis dilutes this ratio and the chance of phagocytosis is diminished. It is therefore preferable to use smaller volumes of peritoneal dialysis fluid during the therapy of acute peritonitis.

The role of the eosinophils in peritoneal dialysis fluid is not established. While some phagocytosis is performed by eosinophilic cells, they probably represent reaction to inflammatory agents rather than a primary defense mechanism.

The role of lymphocyte mediators in peritoneal defenses is not clear. While it is known that end stage renal failure inhibits cellular immune functions, the role of such inhibition is not established in peritonitis [65, 66]. Patients with renal failure are considered more susceptible to infections [72]. This may be connected with lack of mediators or production of inhibitors [197], but the role of various immune functions requires reinvestigation.

4. MICROBIOLOGICAL DIAGNOSIS OF PERITONITIS

4.1. Specimen

In order to establish accurate microbiological diagnosis of peritonitis, the following points are important:

a) Cultures should be taken as early as possible from suspected cases of peritonitis.

b) Large volumes should be concentrated for improving recovery rate.

c) Washing of the specimens with sterile saline may be necessary in patients while on antibiotic therapy.

d) Aggressive microbiological methods should be used to identify the organisms as soon as possible to achieve rational antibiotic therapy [67].

Several studies have dealt in the recent past with the conditions necessary for improved diagnosis in CAPD peritonitis [155–159]. In the Toronto Western Hospital, patients are instructed to bring their first cloudy bag with them to establish diagnosis. This first bag is delivered immediatly to the laboratory. Initially it was believed that culturing or organisms should be done immediately after drainage of the fluid. In a small study we established that even several hours or days will not decrease the accuracy of bacteriological diagnosis from these fluids. Therefore, the sample which arrives at night can be safely kept till the morning for bacteriological identification [68].

4.2. Gram stain

Gram stain from the sediment of the peritoneal dialysis bag established the presence of microorganisms only in about 20 to 30% of the cases. This is not a sufficiently high ratio and does not permit rational therapy. While gram stains are customarily done, the therapy of these patients will have to be started on speculative therapy rather than based on the gram stain. The only time where a gram stain may be helpful is the establishment of fungal peritonitis which frequently can be seen in the initial gram stain, thus, preventing the patient from receiving unnecessary antibiotic therapy.

4.3. Culture procedure

The microbiological culturing of peritoneal dialysis samples is of utmost importance to establish the proper etiological agent and the appropriate antibiotic therapy. In addition the type of organism indicates the possible source of infection, therefore helping in the epidemiology of the disease. Culture methods have been review recently [159]. Initially peritoneal dialysis fluid was handled in the laboratories as any other specimen, sampling small amounts of fluid [157, 158]. It became evident that the culturing of large amounts of fluid improves the accuracy of diagnosis [73, 22]. Most methods presently employed incorporate a concentration method [156], filtration or centrifugation. In addition, the removal of possible antibiotics present in the specimen further improved the isolation rate [155].

Dialysis bag sampling protocol
Toronto Western Hospital
Medical Microbiology
The efficiencies of various methods are expressed as percentage of the antibiotic removal resin (ARD) method taken as the gold standard (100%)

Sample collection
Mix contents of bag well before sampling.
Flood port with methyl alcohol and leave for 60 seconds.
Allow approximately 20 ml to run from sampling port to clear it of alcohol.

Conventional method for culturing CAPD bags
15 ml of peritoneal fluid is centrifuged and the sediment plated on:
Blood agar
McConkey agar
Pre-reduced medium (Chopped meat-carbohydrate)
Brain heart infusion broth (BHI)
Sabourod's agar (if necessary).
Plates are followed for 5–7 days. Cultures identified and antibiotic sensitivities done as routine procedures.
The efficiency of this method is about 64%.

Concentration method for culturing CAPD bags

I. Cloudy bag procedure
A.
1) Aseptically fill two 25 × 150 mm screw cap tubes (approximately 50 ml each).
2) Centrifuge the 2–50 ml tubes for 30 min at top speed.
3) Aseptically decant supernatants. Vortex to resuspend sediment.
4) Do Gram stain from sediment.

AA1. Patient not on antibiotics
The sediments of two tubes of 50 ml are injected using a sterile 1 ml syringe into 100 ml thioglycollate broth each (BBL No. 135/C thioglycollate with 0.05% SPS (Liquoid) added). Tubes are incubated and subcultures identified with routine methodology.
   The efficiency of this method is about 72%.

Alternate method
One 50 ml sediment is aspirated into a 1 ml syringe and injected into BACTEC 6B bottle the other 50 ml sediment similarly into a BACTEC 7D bottle. They are read daily according to BACTEC methodology for 14 days. If growth index rises, subcultures are identified with routine methodology.
   The efficiency of this method is about 73%.

AA2. Patient on antibiotics
Sediment in tubes (Step A2) should be resuspended in 50 ml sterile saline and centrifuged for 30 min at top speed. (Washing) Aseptically decant the supernatants. Sediment of two tubes processed as in AA1.
   The efficiency of this method using thioglycollate medium is about 75%, using the BACTEC methodology it is 94%.

Alternate method
The washing of the sediment can be omitted and the sediment injected into BACTEC 16B and 17D, containing antibiotic removal resin directly. This method is the gold standard (100%) resulting in the highest yield of positive cultures.

II. Clear bag procedure
Clear bags cannot be sedimented since no sediment will form. The concentration of these samples are based on filtration. No efficiencies can be established for these cultures since many of these fluids come from suspected (but not proven) infectious episodes.

B1. Use of Addichek filtration system (Millipore Corp. Bedford, Mass)

Spike Addichek into the sampling port and allow chamber to fill with approximately 100 ml of effluent. Clamp bag, remove Addichek and replace spike cover. Remove yellow cap on base of Addichek and connect to vacuum Clamp off vacuum flask when Addichek is empty.

BB1. Patient on antibiotics

Spike a minibag of sterile saline (100 ml) and allow chamber to fill. Connect Addichek to vacuum flask and allow saline to run through filter. Spike 100 ml bottle of TWH thioglycollate and allow chamber to fill.

BB2. Patient not on antibiotics

A bottle of 100 ml TWH thioglycollate is spiked and chamber allowed to fill.

Incubation and examination

Addichek: Incubated at 36°C 2–3 weeks and checked daily. BACTEC: Incubate at 36°C 7 days. If radioactive counts increase, do Gram stained smear and subcultures.

Table 5 is from Vas and Low [155].

Table 5. Numbers of positive cultures from 160 dialysis fluid samples from 51 patients

Culture	No. of cultures	No. of positives	%
BHI	110	50	45.5
Thio	110	60	54.5
Straight	160	80	50.0
Aerobic		(77)	
Anaerobic		(3)	
Washed	160	109	68.1
Aerobic		(105)	
Anaerobic		(4)	
Resin	50	36	72.0
Aerobic		(34)	
Anaerobic		(2)	

Organisms isolated from 107 positive dialysis fluids.*

Organism	No. of isolates
S. epidermidis	17
S. aureus	18
S. bovis	9
Neisseria sp.	1
E. coli	26
M. morgani	5
K. pneumoniae	2
P. vulgaris	6
Enterococcus	7
Hafnia sp.	4
Acinetobacter sp.	2
P. aeruginosa	5
Enterobacter sp.	5
S. marcescens	6
Candida sp.	19
Bacteroides fragilis	3
Total	135

* Cultures done from the same peritoneal fluid recovered by different methods are listed only once. Some fluids had multiple organisms.

Recently several reports have suggested the use of Limulus lysate test for the diagnosis of Gram negative peritonitis [160, 161, 162]. This test appears to identify with good accuracy the Gram negative peritonitis cases making the initial use of aminoglycosides unnecessary thereby reducing potential toxicity. These reports require further evaluation [163].

The speed with which bacteriological diagnosis can be established is important [70]. The concentration method increases not only the possible proper identifications but also reduces the length necessary for bacteriological cultures. The majority of cultures will become positive after the first 24 hr and in over 75% of cases diagnosis can be established in less than 3 days.

4.4. Antibiotic sensitivities

Antibiotic sensitivities of the isolated organisms are established by normal laboratory procedures against the primary and secondary antibiotics used in the treatment of peritonitis. It is important to be informed of local antibiotic sensitivity patterns of organisms since this varies from hospital to hospital. Such knowledge of local sensitivity patterns is useful in establishing the initial antibiotic treatment until sensitivity results become available (Table 6).

4.5. Cell count

Cell counts are routinely established from the first dialysis fluid and preferably daily afterwards to follow the efficiency of therapy [143]. We use centrifugal (Cytospin) smears for differential cell counts in judging the clinical course of peritonitis. Normal white cell count in the peritoneal dialysis fluid is considered 0–100 cells per cubic millimeter. Above 100 white blood cells per cubic millimeter, the peritoneal dialysis fluid is visibly cloudy. Therefore no cell count has to be done on an emergency basis to establish so called 'cloudy fluid'.

5. PRESENTING SIGNS AND SYMPTOMS OF PERITONITIS

The literature contains only general reference to presenting signs and symptoms of patients presenting with peritonitis [16]. These manifestations include mild abdominal pain, low grade temperature, and usually mild abdominal tenderness. Conn [35] described clinical features of patients with spontaneous peritonitis. Fever was present in these patients in 81%, abdominal pain in 78% and physical signs of peritonitis in 65%. We have reviewed presenting symptoms and signs in 103 episodes of peritonitis of CAPD patients. Fever of >37.5° was present in 53%, abdominal pain was present on admission in 79%. 31% experienced nausea and 7% complained of diarrhea. All but 1 patient had cloudy fluid before admission but only 78% had cloudy fluid on admission. 70% showed abdominal tenderness and 50% rebound pain.

We use a practical definition [73] of peritonitis which requires the presence of two of the following criteria in any combination:

a) Presence of organisms on Gram stain or culture of

Table 6. Antibiotic sensitivities (MIC mg/l-90%) of various organisms isolated from CAPD patients. Nov 1984 – Apr 1985. Toronto Western Hospital

Gr + organisms (N)	KEF	CFZ	MET	CTM	VAN	RIF	MAN
Coag. neg. Staph. (34)	1	<1	.5	<6	<2	<.01	<.1
S. aureus (25)	<.5	<1	1	<6	<1	<.01	<.5
Enterococcus (5)	>32	>32	>16	6	<1	>.16	>32
Str. viridans (2)	<.5	<1	<.2	<6	<1	.04	<.5
Str. Group B.	<.5	<1	<.2	<6	<1	>.25	<.5

Gr – organisms (N)	TOB	CFZ	AMP	CTM	PIP	PER	MAN
E coli (12)	<1	<1	2	<6	<4	<8	<1
Pseudomonas sp. (16)	4	>32	>32	>100	<4	<8	>32
K. pneumoniae (4)	<1	2	32	<6	<4	<8	<1
K. oxytoca (8)	<1	<1	32	<6	<4	<8	2
S. marcescens (4)	<1	>32	>32	<6	<4	<8	>32
M. morgani (5)	<1	>32	>32	<6	<4	<8	8
Enterobacter sp. (1)	<1	2	8	<6	<4	<8	4
Acinetobacter sp. (1)	<1	4	<1	<6	<4	<8	<1
Alcaligenes sp. (1)	>16	32	8	>100	<4	<8	4

KEF = Cephalothin, CFZ = Cefazoline, MET = Methicillin, CT = Cotrimoxazole, VAN = Vancomycin, RIF = Rifampin, MAN = Cefamandole, T = Tobramycin, AMP = Ampicillin, PIP = Piperacillin, PER = Cefoperazone.

PD fluid.
b) Cloudy fluid with predominantly polymorphonuclear cells.
c) Symptoms of peritoneal inflammation.

We find this working definition reliable since we have established that > 100 cells in the fluid are visibly cloudy. No emergency cell counts have to be done therefore to establish the diagnosis of peritonitis.

Besides the above mentioned presenting signs and symptoms patients sometimes present with profound hypotension and shock. This presentation is usually a sign of either Staphylococcus aureus peritonitis or faecal peritonitis.

Many of the patients will have only very mild symptoms and do not require hospitalization.

6. CLINICAL COURSE OF PERITONITIS

6.1. Incubation period

The incubation period of peritonitis in peritoneal dialysis is not well known. It is estimated from touch contamination incidents that the incubation period usually is 24 to 48 hr. Occasionally, incubation periods may be as short as 6 to 12 hr.

The appearance of the symptoms may be very rapid [70] and develop during one peritoneal dialysis exchange.

The incubation period of endogenous infections is not known but probably is much shorter, than exogenous infections.

6.2. Length of symptoms

In most cases of peritonitis the symptoms decrease rapidly after initiation of therapy and disappear within 2 to 3 days. During this period the cell counts decrease and bacterial cultures become negative. In the majority of the cases positive peritoneal cultures are present only for 3 to 4 days [70]. Any prolongation of symptoms is indicative of a complicated course or a possible organism which does not respond well to antibiotics used and requires further investigation.

6.3. Exit site and tunnel infections

Exit site and tunnel infections are rarely symptomatic. Usually they are discovered on routine investigation of the exit site or the patient complaining of some purulent discharge. The exit site is inflamed with a serous or purulent discharge and sometimes painful infiltrate can be seen. Tunnel infections are much more difficult to diagnose if they are present without exit site infections and recently radioactive scanning [142] has been recommended as a diagnostic procedure. Exit site and tunnel infections may be present for prolonged periods without leading to peritonitis but they are always a potential danger for the development of the disease [74].

6.4. Relapse, recurrence of reinfection

These concepts are not well defined in the peritoneal dialysis population. Relapse is the reappearance of symptoms, the appearance of positive cultures after cultures have become negative or an increase of polymorphonuclear cells in the peritoneal dialysis fluid after they have declined; relapse occurs while the patient is still on therapy. It indicates either inadequate treatment or possibly the opening of an abscess cavity which was previously inaccessible to treatment.

Recurrence is the term used of reappearance of symptoms of infection after the therapy has been stopped but within a two week period. It indicates probably either inadequate therapy or the presence of an endogenous focus like exit site or tunnel infection from which seeding occurred.

Re-infection is a new peritonitis episode beyond the 2 week period either with the same organism or a different organism. If reinfection happens with the same organism as before an internal focus should be suspected.

7. CAUSATIVE ORGANISMS OF PERITONITIS

The overwhelming majority of peritonitis episodes are caused by bacteria. While a small number (4 to 8%) of peritonitis episodes are caused by fungi, most of them belonging to the species Candida a few of them caused by Torulopsis and some of them caused by filamentous fungi (Dermatophyton, Mucor, Penicillium, Fusarium, etc.) [75, 81].

7.1. Viruses

The role of viruses in peritoneal dialysis patients is not certain. One report [210] has claimed viral peritonitis, a culture negative peritonitis with concomitant rise in Enterovirus serum titer. Certainly if viral peritonitis would be a more common event, evidence would have by now surfaced.

More interesting is the observation that viral infections predispose to peritonitis [211]. While this is a coincidental observation it would deserve further study.

Dialysis of a patient infected with a virus is occasionally necessary when the patient develops renal failure. This does not present a problem generally.

Table 7. Bacteria isolated from peritonitis of CAPD patients

Acinetobacter sp	Micrococcus mucilaginous
Actinomyces israeli	Mycobacterium chelonei
Aeromonas hydrophylia	Mycobacterium fortuitum
Alcaligenes fecalis	Mycobacterium tuberculosis
Bacillus cereus	Neisseria
Bacteroides fragilis	Neisseria gonorrhoeae
Bordetella bronchiseptica	Pasteurella multocida
Campylobacter fetus	Propionobacteria
Campylobacter jejuni	Proteus sp
Citrobacter sp	Pseudomonas aeruginosa
Corynebacteria	Pseudomonas cepacia
Corynebacterium aquaticum	Pseudomonas maltophilia
Clostridium difficile	Pseudomonas stutzeri
Clostridium perfringens	Serratia sp
E. coli	Staphylococcus aureus
Enterobacter agglomerans	Staphylococcus epidermidis
Enterococcus	Stomatococcus mucilaginous
Gardnerella vaginalis	Streptococcus faecalis
CDC Group IV c-2	Streptococcus pneumoniae
CDC Group Ve-1	Streptococcus pyogenes
CDC Group Ve-2	Streptococcus viridans
Klebsiella sp	Vibrio alginolyticus
Listeria monocytogenes	

While attempt has been made to make the listing comprehensive it may not be complete (from [174]).

The dialysis of Hepatitis B surface antigen positive patients presented problems even in dialysis units which had experience in the hemodialysis of HBsAg positive patients. The precautions developed for hemodialysis were not suitable for PD. Special precautions became especially important with the demonstration [212, 213] of surface antigen in the dialysis fluid.

Small outbreaks of infections have been reported from PD units [214]. Adequate precautions have been developed in most units to cover this risk [215]. Both patients and staff are recommended to be vaccinated against hepatitis B with resulting decrease of contact risk to patients or staff.

More important is the recent controversy of nonA nonB hepatitis and AIDS in dialysis centers [163–168]. This controversy relates to several problems:

a) AIDS is presently an incurable, fatal disease.

b) Dialysis patients may have a higher incidence of AIDS or nonA nonB hepatitis due to previous multiple transfusions.

c) Previous outbreaks of hepatitis B in hemodialysis units sensitized staff to risks.

The incidence AIDS antibodies in dialysis patients is not adequately established. While there are limited studies, no national or international figures are available [166, 167]. Relatively high percentages of false positive tests are reported.

The incidence of renal failure appears to be slightly increased in AIDS patients. Some of these patients may require dialysis [168]. The precautions necessary to dialyse AIDS patients are not difficult. Precautions already in place to prevent the spread of hepatitis B are adequate [171, 172].

A special problem is the recent observation that patients who have AIDS antibodies or are Hepatitis B antigen carriers may have a higher incidence of transplant rejection [170, 173]. Since many dialysis patients are transplant candidates, this may result in reduced chances for successful transplantation.

Routine serological screening of dialysis patients or staff is not justified at present.

Table 8. Yeasts, fungi, algae isolated from peritonitis of CAPD patients

Yeasts	*Filamentous fungi*
Candida albicans	Alternaria alternans
Candida guillermondii	Aspergillus fumigatus
Candida krusei	Aspergillus flavus
Candida parapsilopsis	Curvularia lunata
Candida tropicalis	Drechslera spicifera
Coccidioidomyces immitis	Exophiala jenselmei
Pityrosporum ovale	Fusarium moniliforme
Pityrosporum pachydermatis	Fusarium oxysporum
Cryptococcus neoformans	Fusarium verticilloides
Rhodotorula rubra	Lecythophora mutabilis
Torulopsis glabrata	Mucor
	Penicillium sp.
Algae	Trichisporon cutaneum
	Trichoderma koningii
Prothotheca wickerhamii	Trichoderma viride

While attempt has been made to make the listing comprehensive it may not be complete (from [174]).

7.2. Protozoa, parasites

No protozoan or parasitic peritonitis has as yet been described.

7.3. Bacteria

7.3.1. Gram positive organisms

S. Epidermidis. Staphylococcus epidermidis peritonitis is the most frequent event. It is generally a benign form of peritonitis. Its origin is from the skin by the transluminal route or from an exit site infection periluminally. It responds well to appropriate antibiotic treatment and usually it is symptomless within 2 to 3 days. This is a form of peritonitis most suitable for home treatment with oral antibiotics. The organisms belong to the coagulase negative Staphylococcus group (generally called Staphylococcus epidermidis). Table 9 shows a selection of coagulase negative staphylococci isolated in our hospital which were biotyped [76] indicating that Staphylococcus epidermidis proper is the leading cause of peritonitis in these patients. The role of slime formation of this group of organisms in the attachment to the catheter deserves further study [77, 154, 175, 176].

S. Aureus. Staphylococcus aureus peritonitis is a much more alarming infection. Patients who are admitted with this infection usually are hypotensive, some of them in outright shock and they complain of extensive abdominal pain. Patients with Staphylococcus aureus peritonitis showing symptoms of toxic shock syndrome have been reported [70, 78]. While the infection presents with alarming symptoms, it usually responds well to antibiotic treatment. The improvement is much slower than Staphylococcus epidermidis infections. We have found it useful to treat these patients with a combination of a penicillin type antibiotic (penicillin or cloxacillin depending on the sensitivity of the organisms) and rifampin which shows synergy against this organism [70]. The infection subsides slower and sometimes residual abscesses are found [144]. It is important that patients with exit site infections and tunnel infections will frequently recur and catheter removal may be necessary.

S. Viridans. Streptococcus viridans peritonitis is a milder form of peritonitis though patients often complain of severe pain. The name of this infection is probably a misnomer.

Table 9. Biotypes of coagulase negative staphylococci isolated from CAPD peritonitis

Biotype	Vas %	Gruer et al. [175] %
Staph epidermidis	77	79
Staph warneri	7	5
Staph haemolyticus	6	5
Staph hominis	4	5
Staph capitis	2	0
Staph simulans	2	5
Staph saprophyticus	1	0
Staph xylosus	1	0
No. of strains	91	43

We analyzed a few alpha hemolytic streptococci isolated from peritonitis episodes as shown in Table 10 indicating that several alpha hemolytic streptococci may be participating in these infections [79]. We assume that this infection is caused by hematogenous spread as well as direct intraluminal infection from the oral flora. While it is possible that this infection is preceded by upper respiratory infections, antibiotic prophylaxis for this purpose has not been investigated.

Enterococcus. Enterococcus, while Gram-positive clearly is a fecal organism and indicates transmural infection. Peritonitis caused by this organism has no distinguishing features from Gram-negative peritonitis (see below).

Diphtheroids, propionobacteria. Diphtheroids, or the anaerobic variety Propionobacteria, are skin organisms indicating intraluminal infections. They may be insignificant contaminants [184]. While some of them are quite resistant to antibiotics, most of them respond quite readily to antibiotic treatment [80].

7.3.2. Gram negative organisms

Enterobacteria. Gram negative enterobacteria are an indication of fecal contamination of the peritoneal cavity. While a small number of Gram negative organisms may colonize the skin (Table 2) it is more likely that peritonitis with these organisms indicates direct faecal contamination. If more than a single gram negative organism is isolated from the peritoneal fluid, it is a strong indication of a perforation. They usually respond well to appropriate treatment with aminoglycosides or cephalosporins.

Pseudomonas. Pseudomonas infections are usually more resistant to treatment, often cause multiple abscesses in the patient and therefore require careful evaluation [82]. Patients with this infection may become hypotensive. Besides S. aureus, this infection is the most frequent cause of catheter removal. Treatment with aminoglycoside and a penicillin derivative like piperacillin should be started. The piperacillin should be given intravenously to avoid inactivation of the aminoglycoside.

Acinetobacter. Acinetobacter [49], while it has no special distinguishing features, may be an indication of environmental contamination usually from water. Its treatment does not represent any problems.

Miscellaneous organisms. Single episodes of peritonitis cau-

Table 10. Biotypes of alpha-hemolytic streptococci isolated from CAPD peritonitis

Biotype	No.
Strep sanguinis II	12
Strep bovis (var)	2
Strep anginosus (constellatus)	1
Strep mg (intermedius)	1
Strep mitis	1

sed by a large number of various organisms (Hemophilus, Neisseria, Campylobacter etc.) were described (Table 1) showing that most organisms have the capability to cause infections if inoculated into the peritoneal cavity of CAPD patients.

7.3.3. Anaerobic organisms

Clostridia, bacteroides. Clostridium and bacteroides species are isolated from a small percentage of peritoneal fluids and therefore some centers question the importance of doing anaerobic cultures on peritoneal fluids [83]. While they are only present in a small number of infections, our experience with infections containing anaerobic organisms indicated they are very severe infections usually requiring laparotomy and there is a high propensity for abscess formation [84]. Aggressive surgical management is necessary [85-87] and therefore we consider it important to culture peritoneal fluids for these organisms.

7.3.4. Mycobacteria

M. Tuberculosis. Mycobacterium tuberculosis a rare organism causing peritonitis in peritoneal dialysis patients requires special consideration. It is not a primary organism causing peritonitis but usually settles on the peritoneum from a distant site by hematogenous spread. It occurs in patients who have had a previous infection with this organism and their disease was inadequately treated. It is therefore a disease to be considered in high risk groups [88]. It is difficult to diagnose because the organism grows very slowly on artificial media and therefore the microbiology laboratory may not be of much help initially. The index of suspicion should be high if a patient comes to the hospital with pain and cloudy fluid which is predominantly mononuclear in composition and repeated cultures do not yield a bacteriological answer [89, 90]. Since the treatment of the disease requires long term anti-tuberculous chemotherapy and the removal of the catheter, the establishment of this diagnosis is rather important. If a high index of suspicion exists, peritoneal biopsy through direct laparotomy of laparoscopy is indicated [91, 92]. A histological diagnosis with caseous granulomas with or without the presence of acid fast organisms is an indication for catheter removal and chemotherapy.

One should consider anti-tuberculous prophylactic chemotherapy of patients who have a positive tuberculin test [93]. This consideration is even more important in view of the fact that many of the patients who are on peritoneal dialysis will enter later a transplant program and therefore are at high risk for reactivation of tuberculosis.

Other mycobacteria. Peritoneal infections with Mycobacterium chelonei have been observed in intermittent peritoneal dialysis units from contamination of dialyzers from water sources [51, 52]. M. fortuitum infection has also been observed [233].

7.4. Fungi

Yeasts. Yeast are the most common organisms causing fungal peritonitis in peritoneal dialysis patients [75, 81, 94, 95, 218-221]. They probably enter the peritoneal cavity intraluminally or periluminally though in a few cases vaginal infection was noted.

The importance of yeast infections of the peritoneal cavity lies in the fact that they are very difficult to treat with antifungal antibiotics [75, 95, 216-221]. They are also rather resistant to normal immune mechanisms like phagocytic killing [225]. These antibiotics do not show good penetration into the peritoneal cavity and cannot be administered intraperitoneally because they are very irritating and painful. 5-fluorocytosin, an antifungal agent often used in the treatment of Candida cystitis is not suitable for treatment alone since resistance emerges against it fairly rapidly. Treatment with amphotericin, miconazole, ketoconazole – with or without 5-fluorocytosine – while described in a few cases, is erratic, therefore catheter removal has to be considered early in these patients [75, 95-98, 216-221]. After catheter removal, the symptoms subside rapidly with or without chemotherapy. If the patient cannot be considered for catheter removal and antibiotic therapy has to be attempted, the placing of the patient on intermittent peritoneal dialysis may be considered on the basis of increasing peritoneal defenses as discussed above.

Filamentous Fungi. Filamentous fungi rarely invade the catheter and cause peritoneal infections [75, 81, 95, 99, 221]. Since most filamentous fungi are resistant to antifungal antibiotics early catheter removal has to be considered.

The importance of fungal infections also lies in the fact that most of the fungi including Candida can colonize the surface of the silastic material of the catheter and therefore elimination of this infection without catheter removal appears to be rather futile [153].

7.5. Cryptogenic

7.3.1. 'Sterile' or aseptic peritonitis

This condition is usually due to inappropriate culture procedures or specimens taken while the patient is on antibiotics. The incidence of sterile peritonitis varies among units from 2 to 20% [70, 100] depending on the methods used in the laboratory.

Chemical peritonitis which is an aseptic peritonitis has been described early in the peritoneal dialysis experience [145]. It has been recently reported as a consequence of antibiotic therapy with vancomycin [191].

7.5.2. Eosinophylic peritonitis

This is an alarming complication usually observed early after catheter implantation [101, 120]. It may or may not be associated with peripheral eosinophilia. It is not a true infectious peritonitis since there is no causative organism isolated. Usually these patients do not have pain or other signs or symptoms of peritonitis, only cloudy fluid. The condition subsides in a couple of days without further complications and without therapy. It is assumed to be associated with chemical stimuli leached from the catheter or the equipment for peritoneal dialysis [102]. Eosinophilia in the peritoneal fluid may be observed with use of antibiotics or other drugs in patients who are hypersensitive to these drugs. Air in the peritoneal cavity may produce an eosinophil response in dialysate.

7.5.3. Neutrophylic peritonitis

Diarrhea. Neutrophilia in the peritoneal fluid has been observed during diarrhea of patients without having any bacteria isolated from the peritoneal fluid.

Endotoxin. Endotoxin is also associated with neutrophilia in the peritoneum [145].

7.5.4. Bloody fluid

Menstruation, ovulation. During menstruation of ovulation, some patients will observe bloody peritoneal dialysis fluid. While initially this is alarming it has no consequences and will be present in a few exchanges.

Intraperitoneal hemorrhage. True intraperitoneal hemorrhage, especially in patients who are on anticoagulants may be an alarming problem. If patients are on intraperitoneal heparin it should be suspended for a few days. Careful monitoring of PT and PTT in patients who are on anticoagulants and peritoneal dialysis is necessary. If the intraperitoneal hemorrhage is very profuse, intraabdominal hemostasis through surgical intervention may be considered.

8. TREATMENT OF PERITONITIS

Treatment of peritonitis has to be initiated in the absence of appropriate diagnostic information and therefore certain arbitrary decisions have to be taken on the appropriateness of the antibiotic treatment based on the considerations discussed above on causative organisms.

8.1. Antibiotics

The antibiotics selected for initial treatment should be effective against the most frequent organisms observed in peritonitis. It is important to know and develop such approaches jointly with the infectious disease specialist in each hospital (see Table 6) since certain differences in the sensitivities against antibiotics of various organisms can be observed depending on the hospital.

Recommended antibiotic dosages as modified for peritoneal use are listed in Tables 11 and 12.

First choice of antibiotics should cover the majority of the organisms present in these infections. Therefore it should give coverage against most gram positive organisms as well as gram negative organisms. Most centers use as initial choice cephalothin or cephazolin in appropriate concentrations. These antibiotics show a good coverage for Staphylococcus epidermidis and some coverage for Staphylococcus aureus while covering a certain number of gram negatives. If one wants to cover the more threatening intestinal organisms the addition of an aminoglycoside is justified. If the patient is hypersensitive to cephalosporins, the use of vancomycin in conjunction with aminoglycoside is the first choice. Also, in areas where methicillin resistance of staphylococci is increased, vancomycin is a proper choice initially. After the organisms have been identified and an antibiotic sensitivity is available, adjustments should be made to the therapy.

Penetration of antibiotics from the peritoneal cavity to serum is good and rapid [103, 104]. It is therefore not necessary in most cases to give an intravenous loading dose since peritoneal administration of antibiotics will achieve high enough concentrations in the serum in a few hours.

Recently two expert committees [178, 179] made therapeutic recommendations. While very similar, they reflect regional preferences to treatment.

The pharmaceutical literature generally frowns upon a mixture of antibiotics in the same fluid. This question has been investigated and has been found that the commonly used antibiotics do not interact deleteriously in peritoneal dialysis fluid. Moreover, other additions like heparin and insulin do not interfere with the antibiotics [[105–109].

8.2. Length of treatment

There is no general agreement how long peritonitis should be treated. In our hospital we administer antibiotics for 7 days after the last positive culture has been obtained. Since antibiotic elimination will be slow after cessation of treatment and this adds another probable two days of effective therapy, the effective length of treatment in our patients is probably for 10–14 days. If the cultures turn negative later or the patients symptoms subside slowly, more prolonged treatment is necessary. If no clinical improvement and/or decrease in cell count is evident after 4–5 days, repeat cultures are necessary and change in antibiotics should be considered.

8.3. Side effects

Hypersensitivity reactions against antibiotics have been observed in peritoneal dialysis patients. If antibiotics are used intraperitoneally in these patients, eosinophilia in the peritoneal fluid may be observed. Skin rash may appear in patients with antibiotic hypersensitivity from peritoneal application only and the use of such drugs must be discontinued. Recently chemical peritonitis after use of a preparation of vancomycin (Vancoled) has been reported [191].

Aminoglycosides are known to have nephrotoxic and ototoxic effects as well as vestibular toxicity. In the concentrations used in our hospital (8 mg/l peritoneal dialysis fluid) we have not observed nephrotoxicity, though evaluation of nephrotoxicity in the patients with small residual renal functions is difficult. All attempts should be made to preserve residual functions since the loss of such functions may necessitate one extra peritoneal dialysis cycle per day [110].

Ototoxicity has been observed in patients where gentamicin was used. Tobramycin, netilmicin or amikacin is believed to have less ototoxicity or vestibular toxicity. We have rarely observed vestibular or ototoxicity except in patients who accidentally overdose themselves severalfold with intraperitoneal antibiotics. Under normal use such side effects are not frequent.

The use of rifampin occasionally results in elevation of liver enzymes or nausea, necessitating the discontinuation of the drug. In our hospital we use a dose of 600 mg of

Table 11. Antibiotic dosing guidelines – 2L bag dose schedule (with permission of the publisher from [178])

| | Half-life (H) | | | Dose | | | |
| | | | | Initial | | Maintenance | |
	Normal	ESRD	CAPD	mg/kg	mg/2l bag	mg/l	mg/each 2l/bag
Aminoglycosides							
Amikacin	1.6	39	ND	5.0–7.5	350–500	6–7.5	12–15
Gentamicin	2.2	53	32	1.5–1.7	120	4–6	8–12
Netilmicin	2.1	42	ND	1.5–2.0	140	4–6	8–12
Tobramycin	2.5	58	36	1.5–1.7	120	4–6	9–12
Cephalosporins							
Cefamandole	1.0	10	8.0	—	1000	ND	ND
Cefazolin	2.2	28	27	—	500–1000	125–250	250–500
Cefoperazone	1.8	2.3	2.2	—	2000	500	1000
Cefotaxime	0.9	2.5	2.4	—	2000	250	500
Cefoxitin	0.8	20	15	—	1000	100	200
Ceftazidime	1.8	26	16	—	1000	125	250
Ceftizoxime	1.6	28	11	—	1000	125	250
Ceftriaxone	8.0	15	13	—	1000	ND	ND
Cefuroxime	1.3	18	15	—	1500	250	500
Cephalothin	0.2	3.7	ND	—	2000	250	500
Moxalactam	2.2	20	16	—	1000	ND	ND
Cephradine	0.9	12	ND	—	500	125–250	250–500
					1000 PO	NA	NA
Cephalexin	0.8	19	9	—	1000 PO	NA	NA
Penicillins							
Ampicillin	1.3	15	ND	—	500	50	100
Azlocillin	0.9	5.1	ND	—	500	250	500
Mezlocillin	1.0	4.3	ND	—	3000 IV	3000/12 h IV	ND
Piperacillin	1.2	3.9	ND	—	4000 IV	4000/12 h IV	ND
Ticarcillin	1.2	15	ND	—	2000 IV	2000/12 h IV	ND
Vancomycin and others							
Vancomycin	6.9	161	83	—	1000	15	30
Aztreonam	2.0	7.0	7.1	—	1000	250	500
Ciprofloxacin	4.0	8.0	13	—	750 PO	ND	ND
Clindamycin	2.8	2.8	ND	—	300	150	300
Erythromycin	2.1	4.0	ND	—	300	75	150
Metronidazole	7.9	7.7	11	—	500 PO/IV	ND	ND
Rifampin	4	8	ND	—	600 PO	NA	NA
Sulfamethoxazole	10	13	14	—	1600 PO	100–200	200–400
Trimethoprim	14	33	34	—	320 PO	20–40	40–80
Antifungal							
Amphotericin	360	360	ND	—	0.5	0.5	1
Flucytosine	4.2	115	ND	—	3000 PO	NA	NA
					200	50–100	100–200
Ketocanazole	2	1.8	2.4	—	400 PO	NA	NA
Miconazole	24	25	ND	—	100	50	100

* All doses are calculated for a 70 kg person who is using standard 2 L bags. The route of administration is intraperitoneal unless otherwise specified. These data should only be utilized as initial 'guidelines'. Individualized dosing is recommended when possible.
The Pharmacokinetic data and dosing recommendations presented here are based on published literature reviewed through January 1987 and personal experience. Those dosage recommendations which differ from product labelling are based on more recent experience. There is no evidence that mixing different antibiotics in dialysis fluid (except for aminoglycosides and penicillins) is deleterious for the drugs or patients. Do not use the same syringe to mix antibiotics.

ESRD = creatinine clearance at 10 mg/min, patient not on dialysis
NA = not applicable
ND = no data
IV = intravenous
PO = oral

PERITONITIS TREATMENT DECISION TREE

OVERVIEW OF AREAS COVERED

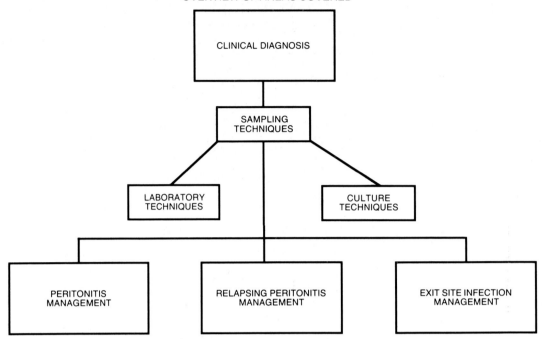

LABORATORY & CULTURE TECHNIQUES

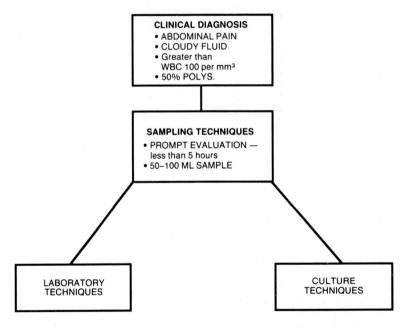

Table 12. Alternative dosing schedule (with permission of the publisher from [178]

	Dose*		
	Initial		Maintenance
	mg/kg	mg/2l bag	mg per 2l bag dosing interval
Aminoglycosides			
Amikacin	5.0–7.5	350–500	140/24 h
Gentamicin	1.5–1.7	120	40–60/24 hr
Netilmicin	1.5–2.0	140	50–70/24 hr
Tobramycin	1.5–1.7	120	40–60/24
Cephalosporins			
Cefamandole	—	1000	1000/24 hr
Cefazolin	—	500–1000	ND
Cefoperazone	—	2000	2000/12 hr
Cefotaxime	—	2000	2000/12 hr
Cefoxitin	—	1000	1000/24 hr
Ceftazidime	—	1000	1000/24 hr
Ceftizoxime	—	1000	1000/24 hr
Ceftriaxone	—	1000	1000/24 hr
Cefuroxime	—	1500	ND
Cephalothin	—	2000	NA
Moxalactam	—	1000	1000/24 hr
Cephradine	—	500	ND
		1000 PO	500/6 hr PO
Cephalexin	—	1000 PO	500/6 hr PO
Penicillins			
Ampicillin	—	500	ND
Azlocillin	—	500	ND
Mezlocillin	—	3000 IV	3000/12 hr IV
Piperacillin	—	4000 IV	4000/12 hr IV
Ticarcillin	—	2000 IV	2000/12 hr IV
Vancomycin and others			
Vancomycin	—	1000	1000/5–7 d
Aztreonam	—	1000	ND
Ciprofloxacin	—	750 PO	750/12 hr PO
Clindamycin	—	300	ND
Erythromycin	—	300	ND
Metronidazole	—	500 PO/IV	500/8 hr PO
Rifampin	—	600 PO	600/24 hr PO
Sulfamethoxazole	—	1600 PO	1600/24 hr PO
Trimethoprim	—	320 PO	320/24 hr PO
Antifungal			
Amphotericin	—	0.5	1–3/12 hr
Flucytosine	—	3000 PO	1000/24 hr PO
		200	400/24 hr
Ketocanazole	—	400 PO	400/24 Hr PO
Miconazole	—	100	ND

* Since serum levels of potentially oto- and vestibular toxicity antibiotics are relatively constant when administered in each exchange (see text), alternative dosing approaches are being developed. One such approach utilizes a longer dosing interval thereby allowing peak and trough serum levels to be achieved. In this table after the initial loading is administered intraperitoneally, the amount of antibiotic given and the time interval for maintenance dose is presented. Clinical experience with this approach is limited. All doses are calculated for a 70 kg adult who is using standard 2 l bags. The route of administration is intraperitoneal unless otherwise specified. These data should only be utilized as initial 'guidelines.' Individualized dosing is recommended when possible.

The Pharmacokinetic data and dosing recommendations presented here are based on published literature reviewed through January 1987 and personal experience. Those dosage recommendations which differ from product labelling are based on more recent experience. There is no evidence that mixing different antibiotics in dialysis fluid (except for aminoglycosides and penicillins) is deleterious for the drugs or patients. Do not use the same syringe to mix antibiotics.

ESRD = creatinine clearance 10 ml/min, patient not on dialysis
NA = not applicable
ND = no data
IV = intravenous
PO = oral

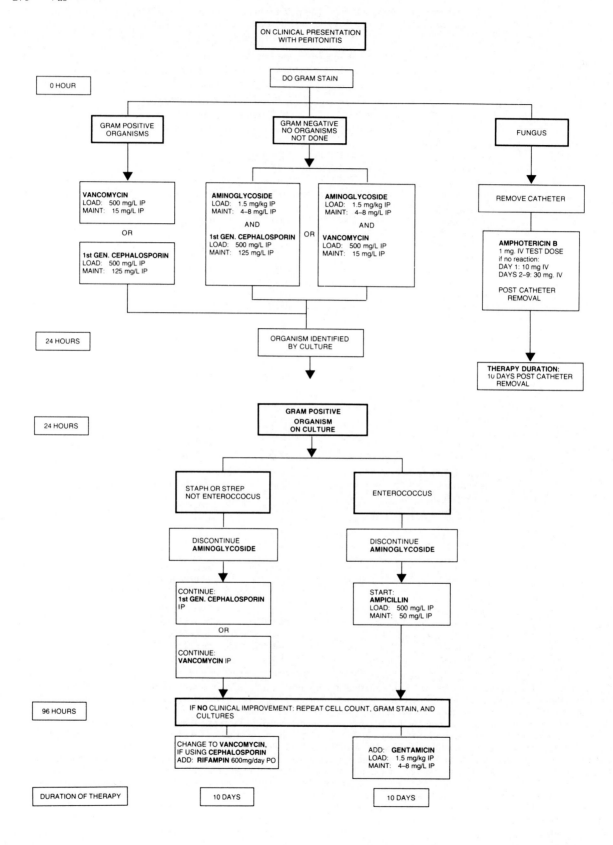

rifampin per day which if distributed to 150 mg four times a day has less toxic effect. Serious side effects of antibiotics may be seen on peritoneal dialysis patients resulting in psedomembranous enterocolitis, due to Clostridium difficile, a serious complication [111]. This necessitates the discontinuation of antibiotic therapy and the institution of oral vancomycin or neomycin or the use of cholestyramine. All efforts should be made to diagnose such condition by cultures and toxin assay so appropriate management can be instituted.

8.4. Peritoneal lavage

Peritoneal lavage has been instituted in the treatment of peritonitis following experience with this treatment in the surgical field [112]. The reason for peritoneal lavage in surgical peritonitis is explained by the need of removing detritus and faecal contamination from the peritoneal cavity. It has been shown that the effect of lavage may be to reduce peritoneal defenses and remove necessary phagocytic cells [64]. Peritoneal lavage with added iodine has been advocated [113] but the use of such treatment has not been clinically substantiated [114]. Studies show that peritoneal antibiotic treatment using the CAPD protocol is clinically efficacious and less costly than peritoneal lavage [115–118, 146].

8.5. The role of heparin

Heparin addition to the peritoneal dialysis fluid during peritonitis is important. Since the inflammatory process will result in the diapedesis of large amounts of fibrinogen into the peritoneal fluid, the inhibition of formation of fibrin is necessary. In addition, it appears that heparin will reduce subsequent adhesion of the peritoneal membrane, therefore reducing postinfectious complications [147].

8.6. Treatment protocols

Development of standard treatment protocols for peritonitis are useful for efficient treatment of patients. It is necessary since the appropriate microbiological diagnosis will not be available for 24 to 72 hours and until that time arbitrary antibiotic combinations have to be used to cover the most likely pathogens [178, 179].

At the Toronto Western Hospital, we use the following protocol: the patient is instructed at the first sign of peritonitis (pain, cloudy fluid, etc.) to drain the fluid in the abdomen immediately and put the drainage bag aside for later transportation to the laboratory. Three quick in and out 1 l flushes are then applied with very short dwell times. While the effectiveness of these flushes is not established, it appears that pain is decreased. The next one litre bag is prepared containing 1.7 mg/kg present body weight of tobramycin, 1 g/bag of cephalothin and 2000 units of heparin. The dwell time of this bag is 3 hours. This is considered the loading dose of the patient. The next exchanges for the next 2 days (exchanges 5 to 11) are 1 l volume and the dwell time is 3 hr. These bags contain appropriate maintenance doses of the same antibiotics as well as heparin (tobramycin 8 mg/l, cephalothin 250 mg/l, heparin 2000 units/l). Also, insulin doses are increased

for diabetics. In the first 24 hr (but after the initiation of antibiotic therapy) the tubing is changed to prevent reinfection of the abdominal cavity.

Appropriate changes in antibiotics are made when culture and sensitivity data are available.

If the patients' symptoms are mild, oral cephalosporins can be used for treatment on outpatient basis.

If patient reports accidental contamination but no peritonitis they are instructed to change their tubing then perform 3 flushes with one litre of peritoneal dialysis fluid after which they add tobramycin, 1.7 mg/kg body weight per 2 l bag and cephalothin 1 g per 2 l bag to the next dialysis fluid. They hold this fluid for a dwell time of 6 hours. After that they start oral cephalosporin (cephalexin 500 mg p.o. 1/2 hr before each bag exchange) for a total of 10 days.

8.7. Treatment of exit site and tunnel infections

Exit site infections are a major problem of peritoneal dialysis [226]. Their treatment is not very successful and often it requires removal of the catheter. Most commonly exit sites are infected with Staphylococcus epidermidis or Staphylococcus aureus though occasionally Pseudomonas or Proteus infections can be observed. The infected exit site is erythematous and elevated showing draining pus or serous fluid but generally not painful. For tunnel infections sometimes an abscess can be palpated under the skin along the canula tract.

In order to establish microbiological diagnosis a culture swab should be taken carefully from the depth of the exit site, not touching adjoining skin. Since the organisms present in tunnel and exit site infections are the same as skin organisms, care has to be exercised to avoid contamination with skin organisms.

Treatment of exit site infections can be attempted with local disinfectants or oral antibiotics. The use of neomycin ointment should be discourages since its effectiveness is questionable and may lead to the emergence of resistant organisms. In addition, the ointment forms a crust over the exit site making cleaning it difficult.

With daily cleaning and local care exit site infections sometimes can be cured.

If the outer cuff (double cuffed catheters) appears in the exit site or is extruded, catheter shaving [74, 119] can be attempted, though with no great success [190].

Exit site infections are frequent. The 1987 report of the National CAPD Registry of NIH shows that about 31% of the patients develop exit site infections within the first year and probably about ½ of these patients will require catheter replacement during this period [31].

8.8. Catheter removal

The most common cause for catheter removal is a persistently infected exit site or tunnel [121].

Catheter replacement can be done on these patients usually one to two weeks after catheter removal into a different site.

If the catheter has to be removed because of frequent recurrence of peritonitis with the same organism of other infectious causes, the catheter usually can be replaced after

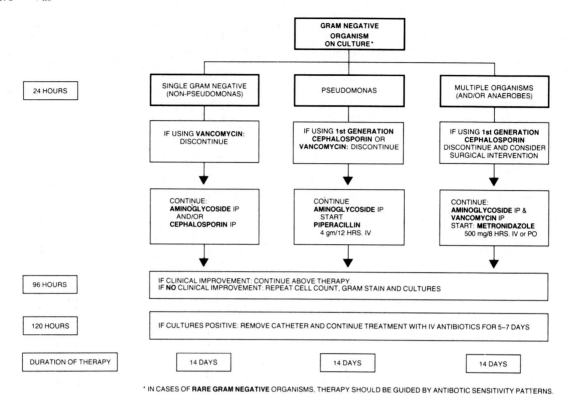

* IN CASES OF **RARE GRAM NEGATIVE** ORGANISMS, THERAPY SHOULD BE GUIDED BY ANTIBOTIC SENSITIVITY PATTERNS.

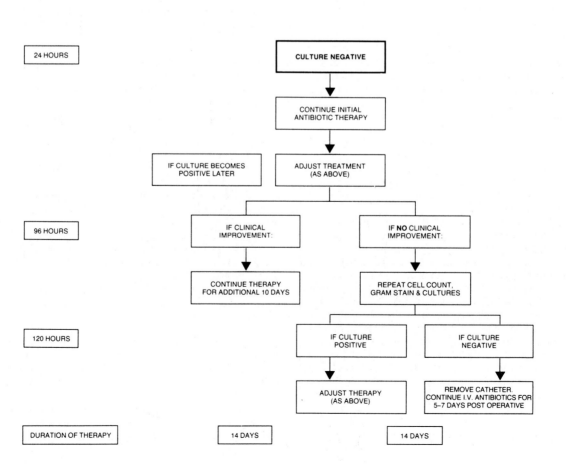

three weeks of termination of successful treatment of peritonitis. A report recommending replacement of catheters at the same time as removal [222] requires further study.

Other infectious causes for catheter removal are fungal peritonitis, tuberculous peritonitis, and faecal peritonitis which requires laparotomy. For the latter, catheter replacement can be considered after the successful treatment of peritonitis or the complete healing of the operative wound.

If peritonitis is not responding to adequate therapy and a change in appropriate antibiotics, catheter removal also should be considered.

9. COMPLICATIONS OF PERITONITIS

9.1. Intestinal perforation and diverticulitis

A small prospective study [44] from our unit has shown the role of diverticulosis; a risk factor for development of faecal peritonitis. It is an alarming complication when patients who have preexisting diverticulosis develop faecal peritonitis. Aggressive treatment, early laparotomy and sometimes surgical excision of the diverticulum will be necessary. Unfortunately, some of the surgical solutions will require colostomy which may delay the reinstitution of peritoneal dialysis.

9.2. Adhesions, sclerosing peritonitis

As a consequence of peritonitis, fibrous adhesions may develop between the peritoneal membranes [140, 141]. This is especially frequent as a consequence of Staphylococcus aureus peritonitis or faecal peritonitis.

Lysis of adhesion at implantation of the peritoneal catheter may be attempted by blunt dissection but this procedure increases the risk of producing microperforations with resulting peritonitis. An alarming condition has been described in peritoneal dialysis patients called sclerosing peritonitis [122–124]. This is really the end result of some process in which the peritoneum develops a thick fibrinous exudate making the exchange of fluid and solutes impossible. It is not clear at the present moment whether this is due to repeated injuries to the peritoneum like frequent peritonitis or due to some chemical injury.

9.3. Mortality

It is difficult to establish the accurate mortality due to peritonitis. One report puts the mortality at 2 to 3% [125]. Many of the causes of death during peritonitis are not directly attributable to the inflammation but may have been triggered by the patients hospitalization or the added stress (myocardial infarction, metabolic imbalance, etc.) [126].

10. DIFFERENTIAL DIAGNOSTIC PROBLEMS

Various diseases may mimic peritonitis or may be the initiating event which leads to peritonitis but without treatment of the cause the peritonitis will not improve.

10.1. Constipation

Constipation may lead to diffuse abdominal pain mimicking peritonitis but will not lead to cloudy fluid of positive cultures. In the absence of the latter, treatment with antibiotics should not be initiated. If the patient presents with diffuse abdominal pain but clear fluid, careful history for bowel habits and a radiographic examination without contrast material should be done for appropriate diagnosis. Constipation should be solved by mild laxatives, enema or if necessary, disimpaction.

10.2. Appendicitis

Appendicitis in a patient on peritoneal dialysis may mimic peritonitis producing even cloudy fluid with an elevated polymorphonuclear cell count due to inflammation of the bowel wall extending to the serosa [227]. Usually the early diagnosis is difficult and patients are treated for peritonitis delaying the accurate diagnosis but not resulting in cure. It is important to diagnose appendicitis in a peritoneal dialysis patient early since the delay of treatment may lead to perforation and resulting faecal peritonitis.

10.3. Pancreatitis

Acute pancreatitis or an infected pseudocyst may lead to symptoms of peritonitis. Elevated serum amylase levels are an early indication of such infection. Sometimes amylase may be measured in the peritoneal dialysis fluid though this test is not reliable.

10.4. Cholecystitis

Cholecystitis may also mimic peritonitis in dialysis patients. Early ultrasound demonstrating the presence of stones may be a diagnostic clue. Sometimes the cholecystitis may lead to perforation of the gallbladder resulting in true peritonitis. A positive blood culture with a gram negative organism may be an early sign of cholecystitis or cholangitis since positive blood cultures are nearly nonexistent during true CAPD peritonitis.

10.5. Perforated ulcer

Perforation of a gastric or duodenal ulcer may also lead to peritonitis. Usually the organisms cultured from such a peritonitis are gram positive, most commonly alpha haemolytic streptococci. Surgical management of this complication is essential.

In general the early involvement of a surgeon in the management of a patient with peritonitis is advisable [228].

11. PREVENTION OF PERITONITIS

11.1. Sterile connections

Obviously the most sensible approach to peritonitis is the prevention of infectious events which may lead to the development of the disease. The observance of strict sterile conditions during connections and disconnections, the use

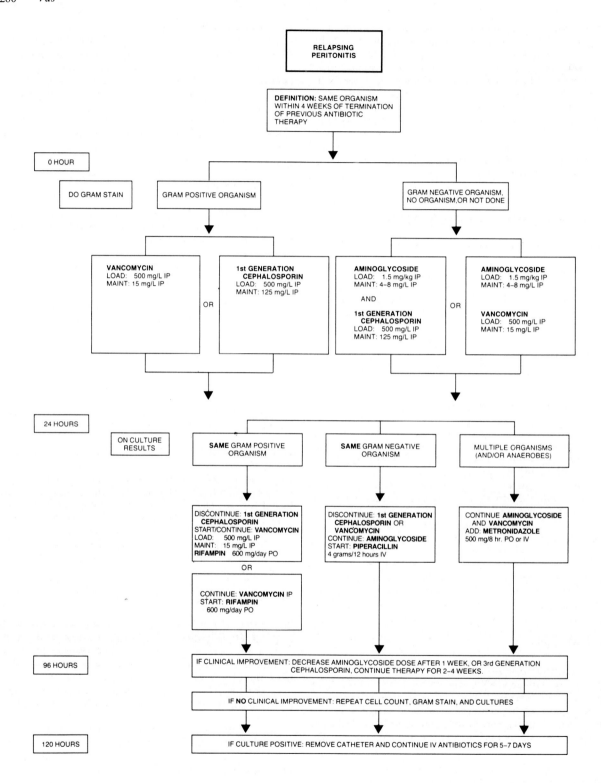

RELAPSING
PERITONITIS

DEFINITION: SAME ORGANISM
WITHIN 4 WEEKS OF TERMINATION
OF PREVIOUS ANTIBIOTIC
THERAPY

0 HOUR

DO GRAM STAIN

GRAM POSITIVE ORGANISM

GRAM NEGATIVE ORGANISM,
NO ORGANISM,OR NOT DONE

VANCOMYCIN
LOAD: 500 mg/L IP
MAINT: 15 mg/L IP

OR

**1st GENERATION
CEPHALOSPORIN**
LOAD: 500 mg/L IP
MAINT: 125 mg/L IP

AMINOGLYCOSIDE
LOAD: 1.5 mg/kg IP
MAINT: 4–8 mg/L IP

AND

**1st GENERATION
CEPHALOSPORIN**
LOAD: 500 mg/L IP
MAINT: 125 mg/L IP

OR

AMINOGLYCOSIDE
LOAD: 1.5 mg/kg IP
MAINT: 4–8 mg/L IP

VANCOMYCIN
LOAD: 500 mg/L IP
MAINT: 15 mg/L IP

24 HOURS

ON CULTURE
RESULTS

SAME GRAM POSITIVE
ORGANISM

SAME GRAM NEGATIVE
ORGANISM

MULTIPLE ORGANISMS
(AND/OR ANAEROBES)

DISCONTINUE: **1st GENERATION
CEPHALOSPORIN**
START/CONTINUE: **VANCOMYCIN**
LOAD: 500 mg/L IP
MAINT: 15 mg/L IP
RIFAMPIN   600 mg/day PO

OR

CONTINUE: **VANCOMYCIN** IP
START: **RIFAMPIN**
   600 mg/day PO

DISCONTINUE: **1st GENERATION
CEPHALOSPORIN** OR
VANCOMYCIN
CONTINUE: **AMINOGLYCOSIDE**
START: **PIPERACILLIN**
4 grams/12 hours IV

CONTINUE **AMINOGLYCOSIDE**
AND **VANCOMYCIN**
ADD: **METRONIDAZOLE**
500 mg/8 hr. PO or IV

96 HOURS

IF CLINICAL IMPROVEMENT: DECREASE AMINOGLYCOSIDE DOSE AFTER 1 WEEK, OR 3rd GENERATION
CEPHALOSPORIN, CONTINUE THERAPY FOR 2–4 WEEKS.

IF **NO** CLINICAL IMPROVEMENT: REPEAT CELL COUNT, GRAM STAIN, AND CULTURES

120 HOURS

IF CULTURE POSITIVE: REMOVE CATHETER AND CONTINUE IV ANTIBIOTICS FOR 5–7 DAYS of disinfectants on all areas exposed to possible contaminations, the wearing of appropriate face masks, scrubbing etc. is essential. The single most important prophylactic method for prevention of peritonitis is the development of appropriate training protocols and the careful training of patients [127].

11.1.1. U.V. Box and sterile weld
An ultraviolet device producing sterile connections (UV System Travenol, 230, 231) and a sterile weld device (Sterile Connection Device SCD DuPont, 232) have been reported to reduce infections. While these devices show benefits, especially in high risk populations, they do add to expense.

11.1.2. O-Z connection
For patients who have had repeated peritonitis episodes and are at high risk for developing others, a special connection has been designed. This connection maintains the spike between dialysis in a disinfectant and makes a connection in the presence of this disinfectant (Betadine). Improvement of peritonitis episodes in high risk patients can be expected [127].

11.1.3. Disinfectant in tubing
Several attempts have been reported where different types of connections were used to avoid intraluminal infections. One recent such publication advocates the use of a Y tubing which is filled and rinsed with sodium hypochlorite solution before connection. Reduction in peritonitis has been reported by this method [129].

Various other connecting devices have been reported to be useful in reducing peritonitis rates.

Most of these are replacing the tubing used for transfer of fluid after each application (0 set etc., 229). The advantage of these sets is that bag disconnections is reasonably safe and there is good patient acceptance.

11.1.4. Millipore filter
To prevent intraluminal infections a bacterial retaining device close to the peritoneal surface would be useful. To solve this problem a bacteriological filter (Peridex, Millipore Corporation) has been prepared which fits into the tubing set used for peritoneal dialysis and which incorporates a bypass valve to facilitate drainage of the fluid. Some reduction in peritonitis from use of such device may be expected [130]. This device has now been superseded by other methods.

11.1.5. Auxiliary devices for the handicapped
Several auxiliary devices have been developed for use of patients handicapped in movement or vision. The development of such devices is essential to facilitate self care in these patients.

11.2. Antibiotic prophylaxis

Previous clinical studies have examined the use of prophylactic antibiotics primarily in patients on intermittent peritoneal dialysis [131–133]. It is difficult to draw conclusions from these studies because of the small number of events and the otherwise low incidence of peritonitis in these patients. We have instituted a double blind prospective study [134] to examine the use of oral cephalexin twice daily for peritonitis prophylaxis. We have found that this approach did not decrease the number of infections. Another prospective study using oral Septra for prophylaxis was also unsuccessful [192].

Antibiotic prophylaxis to prevent wound infections during catheter implantations should be used according to the surgical protocol of each hospital. If perioperative antibiotic prophylaxis is used during surgical implantation the wound infection rate due to catheter implantations is exceedingly small.

11.3. Patient selection

It is difficult to predict which patients are going to have frequent peritonitis episodes. Analysis of patient populations and peritonitis rates do not yield significant differences for prediction [135]. It is quite obvious that the compliant patients who have reasonable intellectual capabilities to absorb training and have good family support are doing better on peritoneal dialysis and have lower peritonitis rates. There are very few absolute contraindications to peritoneal dialysis at present and it is hoped that future analysis of peritonitis episodes in large populations of peritoneal dialysis patients may result in some clues as far as these factors are concerned. Immunological assessment for increased risk of peritonitis at this time is not justified.

11.4. New catheters

The present peritoneal dialysis catheters whether they are single cuffed or double cuffed models do not show significant differences in peritonitis rates. It is hoped that new catheters will be developed in the future where the implant will form a complete integrated seal with the skin, therefore reducing exit site infections due to periluminal penetration of organisms. The role of biofilm on implanted devices will have to be explored and recommendations made.

An expert committee recently has made recommendations on peritoneal catheter implantation and the use of various catheters [186].

12. EVALUATION OF PERITONITIS RATE

Statistical evalutation of peritonitis incidents and the establishment of comparable peritonitis rates is a difficult subject. Initially, the simple ratio of peritonitis episodes over months was used. While this ratio is a useful initial evaluation it is not capable of expressing the true differences in peritonitis rates. This lies in the fact that patients enter and leave peritoneal dialysis programs at different times and stay in them for different lengths of time. Their experiences are different and therefore they are not suitable for simple statistical maneuvers.

The developed statistical approaches [136–139] are based on an actuarial approach analyzing the time elapsed till the first peritonitis episode of the patient therefore expressing the probability at different times when peritonitis develops in peritoneal dialysis patients. The probability to develop the first episode of peritonitis is approximately 45% in the first 6 month while approximately 25% of the patients

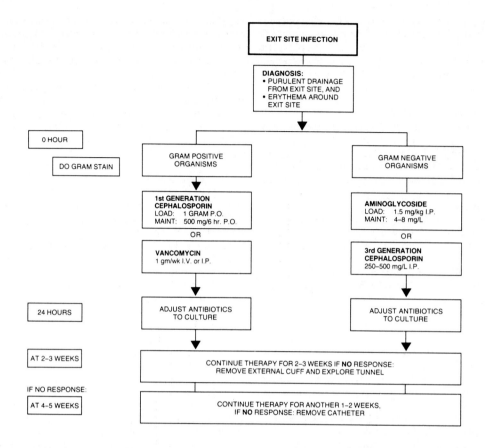

develop exit site infections during this period. Using such a statistical approach, it has been found that there are no significant differences in peritonitis rates in the two sexes. The age related incidence is not significantly different though it appears to be better in the older age groups and certain diseases (for example diabetes) do not represent any major increased risk factors. The use of statistical analysis in larger groups of patients may result in the future in information helping to reduce peritonitis [139].

Another statistical approach to evaluate peritonitis rates is based on the negative binomial probability model [231] and appears to approach peritonitis morbidity rates more closely.

13. FUTURE CONSIDERATIONS

It appears from experience acquired in the last few years that we have reached a certain plateau in the frequency of peritonitis and a peritonitis rate of one every two patient years may be acceptable. Further reduction of this peritonitis rate will require inordinately large efforts on all fronts. New developments in catheter technology and improved connections, may lead to reduction in exit site and tunnel infections, the main problem at present. Better understanding of patient selection and training programs, improved diagnostic and therapeutic methods in the management of peritonitis, the possibility of some sort of chemical, drug or immune prophylaxis of peritonitis and understanding of the infectious and immune processes are developments eagerly awaited.

REFERENCES

1. Seligman AM, Frank HA, Fine J: Treatment of experimental uremia by means of peritoneal irrigation. J Clin Invest 25: 211–219, 1946.
2. Fine J, Frank HA, Seligman AM: The treatment of acute renal failure by peritoneal irrigation. Ann Surg 124: 857–878, 1946.
3. Frank HA, Seligman AM, Fine J: Further experiences with peritoneal irrigation for acute renal failure. Ann Surg 128: 561–608, 1948.
4. Grollman A, Turner LB, McLean JA: Intermittent peritoneal lavage in nephrectomized dogs and its application to the human being. Arch Intern Med 87: 379–390, 1951.
5. Doolan PD, Murphy WP, Wiggins RA, Carter NW, Cooper WC, Watten RH, Alphen EL: An evaluation of intermittent peritoneal lavage. Am J Med 26: 831–844, 1959.
6. Weston RE, Roberts M: Clinical use of stylet-catheter for peritoneal dialysis. Arch Intern Med 115: 659–662, 1965.
7. Maxwell MH, Rockney RE, Kleeman CR, Twiss MR: Peritoneal dialysis I. Technique and applications. JAMA 170: 917–924, 1929.

8. Cohen SL, Percival A: Prolonged peritoneal dialysis in patients awaiting renal transplantation. Br Med J 1: 409–413, 1968.

9. Leigh DA: Peritoneal infections in patients on long-term peritoneal dialysis before and after human cadaveric renal transplantation. J Clin Pathol 22: 539–544, 1969.

10. Palmer RA, Quinton WE, Gray JE: Prolonged peritoneal dialysis for chronic renal failure. Lancet 1: 700–702, 1964.

11. Tenckhoff H, Schecter H: A bacteriologically safe peritoneal access device. Trans Am Soc Artif Intern Organs 14: 181–187, 1968.

12. Tenckhoff H, Curtis FK: Experience with maintenance peritoneal dialysis in the home. Trans Am Soc Artif Intern Organs 16: 90–95, 1970.

13. Brewer TE, Caldwell FT, Patterson RM, Flanigan WJ: Indwelling peritoneal (Tenckhoff) dialysis catheter. Experience with 24 patients. JAMA 219: 1011–1015, 1972.

14. Lankisch PG, Tonnis HJ, Fernandez-Redo E, Girndt J, Kramer P, Quellhorst E, Scheller F: Use of Tenckhoff catheter for peritoneal dialysis in terminal renal failure. Br Med J 4: 712–713, 1973.

15. Palmer RA: Peritoneal dialysis by indwelling catheter for chronic renal failure 1963–1968. Can Med Assoc J 105: 376–380, 1971.

16. Rae A, Pendray M: Advantages of peritoneal dialysis in chronic renal failure. JAMA 225: 937–941, 1973.

17. Devine H, Oreopoulos DG, Izatt S, Mathew R, deVeber GA: The permanent Tenckhoff catheter for chronic peritoneal dialysis. Can Med Assoc J 113: 219–221, 1975.

18. Petrie JJB, Jones EOP, Hartley LCJ, Olife KP, Clunie CJA: The use of an indwelling peritoneal catheter in the treatment of chronic renal failure. Med J Aust 2: 119–122, 1976.

19. Popovich RP, Moncrief JW, Decherd JB, Bomar JB, Pyle WK: The definition of a novel portable/wearable equilibrium peritoneal dialysis technique (abstract). Abstr Am Soc Artif Intern Organs 5: 64–68, 1976.

20. Popovich RP, Moncrief JW, Nolph KD, Ghods AJ, Twardowski ZJ, Pyle WK: Continuous ambulatory peritoneal dialysis. Ann Intern Med 88: 449–k456, 1978.

21. Oreopoulos DG, Robson M, Izatt S, Clayton S, deVeber GA: A simple and safe technique for continuous ambulatory peritoneal dialysis(Capd). Trans Am Soc Artif Intern Organs 24: 484–487, 1978.

22. Rubin J, Rodgers WA, Taylor HM, Everett ED, Prowant BF, Fruto LU, Nolph KD: Peritonitis during continuous ambulatory dialysis. Ann Intern Med 92: 7–13, 1980.

23. Oreopoulos DG: Continuous ambulatory peritoneal dialysis in Canada. Can Med Assoc J 120: 16–19, 1979.

24. Oreopoulos DG, Clayton S, Dombros N, Zellerman G, Katirtzoglou A: Experience with continuous ambulatory peritoneal dialysis (CAPD). Trans Am Soc Artif Intern Organs 25: 95–97.

25. Fenton SSA, Cattran DC, Ahlen AF, Rutledge P, Ampil M, Dadson J, Locking H, Smith D, Wilson DR: Initial experiences with continuous ambulatory peritoneal dialysis. Artif Organs 3: 206–209, 1979.

26. Oreopoulos DG, Khanna R, McCready W, Katirtzoglou A, Vas S: Continuous ambulatory peritoneal dialysis in Canada. Dial Transpl 9: 224–226, 1980.

27. Blagg Cr, Scribner BH: Long-term dialysis; current problems and future prospects. Am J Med 68: 633–635, 1980.

28. Peritoneal dialysis in chronic renal failure (editorial): Lancet 2: 303, 1978.

29. Moncrief JW: Continuous ambulatory peritoneal dialysis. Dial Transpl 8: 1077–1078, 1979.

30. Home peritoneal dialysis for end-stage renal disease. Med Lett Drugs Ther 21: 69–70.

31. National CAPD Registry of the NIH.: Characteristics of participants and selected outcome measures for the period January 1. 1981 through August 31 1986, 1987.

32. Dias-Bruxo JA, Walker PJ, Farmes CD, Chandler JT, Holt KL: Continuous cyclic peritoneal dialysis – The Nalle Clinic experience. In: Price JDE (ed), Peritoneal Dialysis. The State of the Art. Communications Media for Education, Princeton, NY pp 23–25, 1983.

33. Hau T, Ahrenholz DH, Simmons RL Secondary bacterial peritonitis: The biologic basis of treatment. In: Current problems in Surgery. Vol 16 No. 10 Year Book Medical Publ Inc Chicago, 1979.

34. Correia JP, Conn HO: Spontaneous bacterial peritonitis in cirrhosis: endemic or epidemic? Med Clin North Am 59: 963–981, 1975.

35. Conn HO, Fessel JM: Spontaneous bacterial peritonitis in cirrhosis: variations on a theme. Medicine (Balt) 50: 161–197, 1971.

36. Bar-Meir S, Conn HO: Spontaneous bacterial peritonitis induced by intraarterial vasopressin therapy. Gastroenterology 70: 418–421, 1976.

37. Conn HO: Bacterial peritonitis: spontaneous or paracentric? (editorial). Gastroenterology 77: 1145–1146, 1979.

38. Targan SR, Chow AW, Guze LB: Role of anaerobic bacteria in spontaneous peritonitis of cirrhosis. Report of two cases and review of the literature. Am J Med 62: 397–403, 1977.

39. Stephen CG, Meadows JG, Kerkering TM, Markowitz SW, Nisman RM: Spontaneous peritonitis due to Hemophilus influenzae in an adult. Gastroenterology 77: 1088–1090, 1979.

40. Hau T, Hoffman R, Simmons RL: Mechanisms of the adjuvant effect of hemoglobin in experimental peritonitis. I. In vivo inhibition of peritoneal leukocytosis. Surgery 83: 223–229, 1978.

41. Stewart WK, Anderson DC, Wilson MI: Hazard of peritoneal dialysis: contaminated fluid. Br Med J 1: 606–607, 1967.

42. Helfrick GB, Pechau BW, Alijani MR, Barnard WF, Rakowski TA, Winchester JF: The direction of catheter complications with lateral placement. Perit Dial Bull Suppl 3: No. 4 2–4, 1983.

43. Schweinburg FB, Seligman AM, Fine J: Transmural migration of intestinal bacteria. A study based on the use of radioactive Escherichia coli. N Engl J Med 242: 747–751, 1950.

44. Wu G, Khanna R, Vas S, Oreopoulos DG: Is extensive diverticulosis of the colon a contraindication to CAPD. Perit Dial Bull 3: 180–183, 1983.

45. Singh MM, Bhargawa AN, Jain KB: Tuberculous peritonitis: An evaluation of pathogenic mechanisms, diagnostic procedures and therapeutic measures. New Eng J Med 281: 1091–1094, 1969.

46. Khanna R, Oreopoulos DG, Vas SI, McCready W, Dombros N: Fungal peritonitis in patiens undergoing chronic intermittent or continuous peritoneal dialysis. Proc EDTA 17: 291–296, 1980.

47. Coward RA, Gokal R, Mallick NP: Recurrent peritonitis associated with vaginal leak. Perit Dial Bull 3: 164–165, 1983.

48. Dias-Buxo JA, Burgess P, Walker PJ: Peritoneovaginal fistula-unusual complication of peritoneal dialysis. Perit Dial Bull 3: 142–143, 1983.

49. Abrutyn E, Goodhart GL, Roos K, Anderson R, Buxton A Acinetobacter calcoaceticus outbreak associated with peritoneal dialysis. Am J Epidemiol 107: 328–335.

50. Mader JT, Reinarz JA: Peritonitis during peritoneal dialysis. The role of the preheating water bath. J Chron Dis 31: 635–664, 1978.

51. Baud JD, Ward J, Fraser DW, Peterson NJ, Silcox VA, Good RC, Ostroy PR, Kennedy J: Peritonitis due to a mycobacterium chelonei like organism associated with intermittent chronic peritoneal dialysis. J Inf Dis 145: 9–17, 1982.

52. Poisson M, Beromicide V, Falardeau C, Vega C, Morisset R: Mycobacterium chelonei peritonitis in a patient undergoing continuous ambulatory peritoneal dialysis (CAPD). Perit Dial

Bull 3: 86–88, 1983.

53. Majno G, Palade GE: Studies on inflammation. I. The effect of histamine and serotonin on vascular permeability: an electron microscopic study. J Biophys Cytol 11: 571–600, 1961.

54. Ellis H: The cause and prevention of post-operative intra-peritoneal adhesions. Surg Gynecol Obstet 133: 497–511, 1971.

55. Myhre-Jensen O, Larsen SB, Astrup T: Fibrinolytic activity in serosal and synovial membrane. Arch Pathol 88: 623–630, 1969.

56. Porter JM, McGregor FH, Mullen DC, Silver D: Fibrinolytic activity of mesothelial surfaces. Surg Forum 20: 80–82, 1969.

57. Ellis H: The aetiology of post-operative abdominal adhesions. An experimental study. Br J Surg 50: 10–16, 1962.

58. Buckman RF, Woods M, Sargent L, Gervin AS: A unifying pathogenetic mechanism in the etiology of intraperitoneal adhesions. J Surg Res 20: 1–5, 1976.

59. Gervain AS, Puckett CL, Silver D: Serosal hypofibrinolysis. A cause of post-operative adhesions. Am J Surg 125: 80–88, 1973.

60. Hau T, Payne WD, Simmons RL: Fibrinolytic activity of the peritoneum during experimental peritonitis. Surg Gynecol Obstet 148: 415–418, 1979.

61. Weinstein MP, Iannini PB, Stratton CW, Eickhoff TL: Spontaneous bacterial peritonitis. A review of 28 cases with emphasis on improved survival and factors influencing prognosis. Am J Med 64: 592–598, 1978.

62. Gilmour J, Tymiansky R, Pierratos A, Vas S, Klein M, Khanna R, Digenis D, Cuff S, Oreopoulos DG: Changes in some inflammatory proteins during peritonitis in CAPD patients. Perit Dial Bull 3: 201–204, 1983.

63. Verbough HA, Keane WF, Hoidal JR, Freiberg MR, Elliott GR, Peterson PK: Peritoneal macrophages and opsonins: Antibacterial defense in patients undergoing chronic peritoneal dialysis. J Inf Dis 147: 1018–1029, 1983.

64. Duwe A, Vas SI, Weatherhead JW: Effect of composition of peritoneal dialysis fluid on chemiluminescence, phagocytosis and bactericideal activity in vitro. Infec Immun 33: 130–135, 1981.

65. Collart F, Tielemaus C, Schandene L, Dupont E, Wybrau Y, Dratwe M: CAPD and cellular immunity: No different than hemodialysis patients. Perit Dial Bull 3: 163–164, 1983.

66. Giaccino F, Alloatti S, Guarello F, Coppo R, Pellerey M, Piccoli G: The influence of peritoneal dialysis on cellular immunity. Perit Dial Bull 2: 165–168, 1982.

67. Vas SI, Low DE, Layne S, Khanna R, Dombros N: Microbiological diagnostic approach to peritonitis in CAPD patients (1981). In: Atkins RC *et al.* (ed), Peritoneal Dialysis. Churchill Livingstone, Edinburgh, pp 269–271, 1981.

68. Vas SI: Peritoneal fluid cultures remain positive for days. Perit Dial Bull 2: 144, 1982.

69. Swartz RD, Campbell DA, Stone D, Dickinson C: Recurrent polymicrobial peritonitis from a gynecological source as a complication of CAPD. Perit Dial Bull 3: 32–33, 1983.

70. Vas SI: Microbiologic aspects of chronic ambulatory peritoneal dialysis. Kidney International 23: 83–92, 1983.

71. Dobbelstein H: Immune system in uremia. Nephron 17: 409–414, 1976.

72. Montgomery YZ, Kalmanson GR, Guze LB: Renal failure and infection. Medicine 47: 1–32, 1968.

73. Vas SI: Peritonitis during CAPD. A mixed bag. Perit Dial Bull 1: 47–49, 1981.

74. Nichols WK, Nolph KD: A technique for managing exit site and cuff infection in Tenckhoff catheters. Perit Dial Bull Suppl 3: S4–S5, 1983.

75. Khanna R, McNeely DJ, Oreopoulos DG, Vas SI, McCready W: Treating fungal infections: Fungal peritonitis in CAPD. Br Med J 280: 1147–1148, 1980.

76. Kloos WE, Schleifer KH: Simplified scheme for the routine identification of human staphylococcus species. J Clin Microbiol 1: 82–88, 1975.

77. Peter G, Locci R, Pulverer G: Adherence and growht of coagulase negative staphylococci on surfaces of intravenous catheters. J Infect Dis 146: 479–482, 1982.

78. Gregory MC, Duffy DP: Toxic shock following staphylococcal peritonitis. Clin Nephrol 20: 101–104, 1983.

79. Facklam RR: Physiological differentiation of viridans streptococci. J Clin Microbiol 5: 184–201, 1977.

80. Pierard D, Lauwers S, Monton MC, Sennesael J, Verbeelen D: Group JK Corynebacterium peritonitis in a patient undergoing continuous ambulatory peritoneal dialysis. J Clin Microbiol 18: 1011–1014, 1983.

81. Arfania D, Everett ED, Nolph K, Rubin J: Uncommon causes of peritonitis in patients undergoing peritoneal dialysis. Arch Int Med 141-61–64, 1981.

82. Kolmos HJ, Anderson KEH: Peritonitis with Pseudomonas aeruginosa in hospitalized patients treated with peritoneal dialysis. Scand J Infect Dis 11: 207–210, 1979.

83. Matthews P: Primary anaerobic peritonitis. Br Med J 2: 903–904, 1979.

84. Onderdonk AB, Bartlett JG, Louie T, Sullivan-Seigler N, Gorbach SL: Microbial synergy in experimental intra-abdominal abscess. Infect Immun 13: 33–26.

85. Simkin EP, Wright FK: Perforating injuries of the bowel complicating peritoneal catheter insertion. Lancet 1: 64–66, 1968.

86. Rubin J, Oreopoulos DG, Lio TT, Mathews R, deVeber GA: Management of peritonitis and bowel perforation during chronic peritoneal dialysis. Nephron 16: 220–225, 1976.

87. Wu G: Review of peritonitis episodes that caused interruption of CAPD. Perit Dial Bull Suppl Vol 3: S11–S13, 1983.

88. Sasaki S, Aliba T, Suenaga M, Tornura S, Yoobiyama N, Nakagawa S, Shoji T, Sasavka T, Takenchi J: Ten years survey of dialysis associated tuberculosis. Nephron 24: 141–145, 1979.

89. O'Connor J, MacCormick M: Tuberculous peritonitis in patients on CAPD: the importance of lymphocytosis in the peritoneal fluid. Perit Dial Bull 1: 106.

90. Morford DW: High index of suspicion for tuberculous peritonitis in CAPD patients. Perit Dial Bull 2: 189–190, 1982.

91. Dineen P, Hornan WP, Grafe WR: Tuberculous peritonitis: 43 years experience in diagnosis and treatment. Am Surg 184: 712–717, 1976.

92. Wolfe JHN, Behn AR, Jackson BT: Tuberculous peritonitis and role of diagnostic laparoscopy. Lancet 1: 852–853, 1978.

93. Vas SI: Editorial comment: Perit Dial Bull 2: 190, 1982.

94. Bayer AS, Blumenkrantz MY, Montgomerie JZ, Galpin JE, Coburn JW, Gruze LB: Candida peritonitis. Am J Med 61: 832–840, 1976.

95. Kerr CM, Perfect JR, Craven PC, Jorgensen JH, Drutz DJ, Shelburne JD, Gallis HA, Gutman RA: Fungal peritonitis in patients on continuous ambullatory peritoneal dialysis. Ann Int Med 99: 334–337, 1983.

96. Holdsworth SR, Atkins RC, Scott DF, Jackson R: Management of Candida peritonitis by prolonged peritoneal lavage containing 5-fluorocytosine. Clin Nephrol 4: 157–159, 1975.

97. Lrmprty KD, Jones JM: Flucytosine – miconazole treatment of Candida peritonitis: Its use during continuous ambulatory peritoneal dialysis. Arch Int Med 142: 577–578, 1982.

98. Chapman JR, Warnoch DW: Ketoconazole and fungal CAPD peritonitis. Lancet II: 510–511, 1983.

99. Pearson JG, McKinney TD, Stone WJ: Penicillium peritonitis in a CAPD patient. Perit Dial Bull 3: 20–21, 1983.

100. NIH CAPD Patient Registry Report: Characteristics of participants and selected outcome measures for the period January 1 1981 through August 31 1986, 1987.

101. Steiner R: Clinical observations on the phathogenesis of peritoneal dialysate eosinophilia. Perit Dial Bull 2: 118–119,

1982.

102. Verger C, Berry JP, Galle P, Lavergue A, Hoang C, LeCharpentier Y: Foreign material inclusions in the peritoneum of CAPD patients: a study with X-ray microanalysis. Perit Dial Bull 2: 138–139, 1982.

103. Williams P, Khanna R, Simpson H, Vas SI: Tobramycin blood levels of CAPD patients during peritonitis. Perit Dial Bull 2: 48, 1983.

104. Manuel MA, Paton TW, Cornish WR: Drugs and peritoneal dialysis. Perit Dial Bull 3: 117–125, 1983.

105. Sewell DL, Golper TA: Stability of antimicrobial agents in peritoneal dialysate. Antimicrob Agents Chemother 21: 528–529, 1982.

106. Sewell DL, Golper TA, Brown SD, Nelson E, Knower MM, Kimbrough RC: Stability of single and combination antimicrobial agents in various peritoneal dialysates in the presence of insulin and heparin. Am J Kidney Dis 3: 209–212, 1983.

107. Rubin J, Humphries J, Smith G, Bower J: Antibiotic activity in peritoneal dialysate. Am J Kidney Dis 3: 205–208, 1983.

108. Bunke CM, Aronoff GR, Luft C: Pharmacokinetics of common antibiotics used in continuous ambulatory peritoneal dialysis. Amer J Kidney Dis 3: 114–117, 1983.

109. Vas SI: Letter. Perit Dial Bull 1: 67, 1981.

110. Gokal R, Vas SI: Risk of tobramycin use in CAPD patients with peritonitis. Perit Dial Bull 2: 139–141, 1982.

111. Silva J, Fekety R: Clostridia and antimicrobial entocolitis. Am Rev Med 32: 327–333, 1981.

112. Antibiotic lavage for peritonitis. Editorial (1979) Brit Med Jour Sept 22, 1979. 691–692.

113. Stephen RL, Kablitz C, Kitahara M, Welson JA, Duffin DP, Kolff WJ: Peritoneal dialysis: peritonitis: saline iodine flush. Dial Transpl 8: 584–595, 1979.

114. Nolph KD: In: Legrain M (ed), Continuous Ambulatory Peritoneal Dialysis. Excerpta Medica, New York, p 272, 1980.

115. Digenis GE, Khanna R, Pierratos A, Vas S: Morbidity and mortality after treatment of peritonitis with prolonged exchanges and intraperitoneal antibiotics. Perit Dial Bull 2: 45–46, 1982.

116. Cantaluppi A, Scalamogna A, Guerra L, Graziani G, Ponticelli C: Treatment of peritonitis in patients on CAPD. Perit Dial Bull 2: 142, 1982.

117. DeGroc F, Rottembourg J, Jacq D, Jaslier V, N'Guyen J, Legrain M: Les peritonites au cours de la dialyse peritoneal continue ambulatoire. Traitment par lavage ou non? Etude prospective. Nephrologie (SWZ) 4: 24–27, 1983.

118. De Tremont JF, Khissi H, Thomas D, Tolain M, Lawrence G, Coevoet B, Fournier A, Orfica J: Traitement des peritonites ou dialyse peritoneal. Comparison entre lavage continue avec machine et lavage intermittent par quatre sac/jour de DPCA. Pathol Biol (Paris) 31: 544–547, 1983.

119. Helfrich GB, Winchester JF: Shaving of external cuff or peritoneal catheter. Perit Dial Bull 2: 183, 1982.

120. Digenis GE, Khanna R, Pantalony D: Eosinophylia after implantation of the peritoneal catheter. Perit Dial Bull 2: 98–99, 1982.

121. Vas SI: Indications for removal of peritoneal catheter. Perit Dial Bull 1: 145–146, 1981.

122. Gandhi VC, Humayun HM, Ing TS, Daugirdas JT, Jablokow VR, Iwantsuki S, Geis WP, Hano JE: Sclerotic thickening of the peritoneal membrane in maintenance peritoneal dialysis patients Arch Int Med 140: 1201–1203, 1980.

123. Schmidt RW, Blumenkrantz M: Peritoneal sclerosis. A sword of Democles for peritoneal dialysis. Arch Int Med 141: 1265–1267, 1981.

124. Sclerosing Peritonitis, Letters to the editor: Lancet July 9, August 13, September 3, September 24, November 5, 1983.

125. Fenton SSA: Peritonitis related deaths among CAPD patients. Perit Dial Bull Suppl Vol 3 No 3: S9–S11.

126. Wu G: Cardiovascular deaths among CAPD patients. Perit Dial Bull Suppl Vol 3 No 3: S23–S26, 1983.

127. Oreopoulos D, Vas S, Khanna R: Prevention of peritonitis during continuous ambulatory peritoneal dialysis. Perit Dial Bull Suppl Vol 3 No 3: S18–S20, 1983.

128. Hamilton RW, Disher BA, Dillingham GA, Nicholas AF: The sterile weld a new method for connection in continuous ambulatory peritoneal dialysis. Perit Dial Bull Suppl Vol 3 No 4: S8–S10, 1983.

129. Buonchristiani U, Cozzari M, Quintiliani G, Carobi C: Abatement of exogenous peritonitis using the Perugia CAPD system. Dial Transplant 12: 14–25, 1983.

130. Ash SR, Hoswell R, Heefer EM, Bloch R: Effect of the Peridex filter on peritonitis rates in a CAPD population. Perit Dial Bull 3: 89–93, 1983.

131. Eremin J, Marshall VC: The place of prophylactic antibiotic in peritoneal dialysis. Aust Ann Med 18: 264–266, 1969.

132. Sharma BK, Smith EC, Rodriguez H, Pillay UKG, Gandhi VC, Dunea G: Trial of oral neomycin during peritoneal dialysis. Am J Med Sci 262: 175–178, 1971.

133. Axelrod J, Meyers BR, Hirschman SZ, Stein R: Prophylaxis with cephalothin in peritoneal dialysis. Arch Intern 132: 368–371, 1973.

134. Low DE, Vas SI, Oreopoulos DG, Manuel RA, Saiphoo CS, Finer C, Dombros N: Randomized Clinical trial of prophylactic cephalexin in CAPD. Lancet 2: 753–754, 1980.

135. Corey PN, Steele C: Risk factors associated with time to first infection and time to failure on CAPD. Perit Dial Bull Suppl Vol 3 No 3: S-14–S-17, 1983.

136. D'Apice AJF, Atkins RC: Analysis of peritoneal dialysis data. In: Atkins RC (ed), Peritoneal Dialysis. Thomas NM, Farrell PC, Churchill Livingstone, Edinburgh, pp 440–444, 1981.

137. Randerson DH, Farrell PC: Analysis of peritonitis data in CAPD 2nd Int. Symposium in Peritoneal Dialysis, Berlin, p 52, 1981.

138. Corey P: An approach to the statistical analysis of peritonitis data from patients on CAPD. Perit Dial Bull Suppl Vol 1 No 6: S-29–S-32, 1981.

139. Pierratos A, Amair P, Corey P, Vas SI, Khanna R, Oreopoulos DG: Statistical analysis of the incidence of peritonitis in continuous ambulatory peritoneal dialysis. Perit Dial Bull 2: 32–36, 1982.

140. Ryan GB, Grobety J, Majno G: Post-operative peritoneal adhesions. A study of the mechanisms. Am J Pathol 65: 117: 117–138, 1971.

141. Mion CM, Boen ST, Scribner P: Analysis of factors responsible for the formation of adhesions during chronic peritoneal dialysis. Am J Med Sci 250: 675–679, 1965.

142. Steiner RW, Kipper S, Savoia MC, Witztum KF: Identification of peritoneal dialysis catheter tunnel infection by scanning with Indium-111 labelled leukocytes. Amm Int Med 99: 44–45, 1983.

143. Williams P, Pantalony D, Vas SI, Khanna R, Oreopoulos DG: The value of dialysate cell count in the diagnosis of peritonitis in patients on continuous ambulatory peritoneal dialysis. Perit Dial Bull 1: 59–62, 1981.

144. Kapral FA, Godwin JR, Dye ES: Formation of intraperitoneal abscesses by Staphylococcus aureus. Infec Immun 30: 204–211, 1980.

145. Karanicolas S, Oreopoulos DG, Frath Sh, Shiminer A, Manning RF, Sepp H, deVeber GA, Darby T: Epidemic of aseptic peritonitis caused by endotoxin during chronic peritoneal dialysis. N Engl J Med 296: 1336–1337, 1972.

146. Williams P, Khanna R, Vas S, Layne S, Pantalony D, Oreopoulos DG: Treatment of peritonitis in patients on CAPD: To lavage or not. Perit Dial Bull 1: 14–17, 1980.

147. O'Leary JP, Malik FS, Donahoe RR, Johnston AD: The effects of a minidose of heparin on peritonitis in rats. Surg Gynecol Obstet 148: 571–575, 1979.

148. Cotran RS, Karnowsky MJ: Ultrastructural studies on the

permeability of the mesothelium to horse radish peroxidase. J Cell Biol 37: 123–137, 1968.

149. MacCallum WG: On the mechanism of absorption of granular materials from the peritoneum. Bull Johns Hopkins Hosp 14: 105–110, 1903.

150. Casley-Smith JR: An electron microscopical study of the passage of ions through the endothelium of lymphatic and blood capillaries, and through the mesothelium. Quart J Exp Physiol 52: 105–113, 1967.

151. Courtice FC, Simmonds WJ: Physiological significance of lymph drainage of the serous cavities and lungs. Physiol Rev 34: 419–448, 1954.

152. Lorber B, Swenson RM: The bacteriology of intraabdominal infections. Surg Clin North Am 55: 1349–1354, 1975.

153. McNeely D, Vas SI, Dombros N, Oreopoulos DG: Fusarium peritonitis: an uncommon complication. Perit Dial Bull 1: 94–96, 1981.

154. Marrie TJ, Noble MA, Costerton JW: Examination of the morphology of bacteria adhering to peritoneal dialysis catheters by scanning and transmission electron microscopy. Jour Clin Microbiol 18: 1388–1398, 1983.

155. Vas SI and Low L: Microbiological diagnosis of peritonitis in patients on continuous ambulatory peritonel dialysis. J Clin Microb 21, 522–523, 1985.

156. Rubin SJ: Continuous ambulatory peritoneal dialysis: Dialysate fluid cultures. Clin Microbiol Newsl 6, 3–5, 1984.

157. Fenton P: Laboratory diagnosis in patients undergoing continuous ambulatorey peritoneal dialysis. J Clin Path 35, 1181–1184, 1982.

158. Knight KR, Polak A, Crump J and Maskell R: Laboratory diagnosis and oral treatment of CAPD patients. Lancet ii. 1301–1304, 1982.

159. Buggy BP: Culture methods for continuous ambulatory peritoneal dialysis associated peritonitis. Clin Microb Newsletter 8: 12–14, 1986.

160. Smalley DL, Baddour LM, Kraus AP: Rapid detection of Gram-negative bacterial peritonitis by the Limulus amoebocyte lysate assay. J Clin Microbiol 24: 882–883, 1986.

161. Clayman MD, Raymond A, Colen D, Moffit C, Wolf C, Neilson E: The Limulus amebocyte lysate assay. Arch Int Med 147: 337–340, 1987.

162. Oreopoulos DG, Vas SI: Peritonitis in continuous ambulatory peritoneal dialysis: Making therapeutic decisions easier. Arch Int Med 147: 818–819, 1987.

163. Heering PJ, Bach D, Henzler P, Grabensee B: Dialysis and HIV infection. Nephron 47: 158–159, 1987.

164. Berlyne GM, Rubin J, Adler AJ: Dialysis in AIDS patients. Nephron 44: 265–266, 1987.

165. Robles R, Lopex-Gomez JM, Muino A, Valderrabano F: Dialysis in AIDS patients: A new problem. (1987) Nephron 44: 375–376, 1987.

166. DeRossi A, Vertoli U, Romagnoli G, Bertoli M, Dalla Grassa O, Chieco-Bianchi L: LAV/HTLV-III and HTLV-I antibodies in hemodialysis patients. Nephron 44: 377–378, 1987.

167. Morrison AJ, Freer CV, Poole CL, Johnston DO, Westervelt F, Normansell DE, Wenzel RP: Prevalence of human lymphotropic virus type III antibodies among patients in dialysis programs at a university hospital. Ann Int Med, 104: 805–807, 1986.

168. Humphreys MH, Scoenfield PY, Aids and renal disease: The Kidney, 20: 7–12, 1987.

169. Rubin RH, Jenkins RL, Shaw BW, Shaffer D, Pearl RH, Erb S, Monaco AP, VanThiel DH: The aquired immunodeficiency syndrome and transplantation. Transplantation, 44: 1–4, 1987.

170. Olivera DBG, Winearls CG, Cohen J, Ind PW, Williams G: Severe immunosuppression in a renal transplant recipient with HTLV-III antibodies. Transplantation, 41: 260–262, 1986.

171. Favero MS: Recommended precautions for patients undergoing hemodialysis who have AIDS or non-A non-B hepatitis. Infection Control 6: 301–305, 1985.

172. Recommendations for providing dialysis treatment to patients infected with human T-lymphotropic virus type III/lymphadenopathy-associated virus. MMWR 35: 376–378, 383, 1986.

173. Harnett JD, Zeldis JB, Parfrey PS, Kennedy M, Sircar R, Steinmann TI, Guttmann RD: Hepatitis B disease in dialysis and transplant patients. Transplantation 44: 369–376, 1987.

174. Vas SI: Peritonitis of peritoneal dialysis patients: Pathogenesis and treatment. In: Easmon CSF and Jeljaszewicz J (eds), Medical Microbiology Vol 5: Academic Press London pp 21–63, 1986.

175. Guer LD, Bartlett R, Aycliffe AJ, Species identification and antibiotic sensitivity of coagulase negative staphylococci from CAPD peritonitis: J Antimic Chemother, 13: 577–583, 1984.

176. Baddour LM, Smalley DL, Kraus AP, Lamoreaux WJ, Christensen GD: Comparison of microbiologic characteristics of pathogenic and saprophytic coagulase negative staphylococci from patients on continuous ambulatory peritoneal dialysis. Diagn Microbiol Infect Dis, 5: 197–205, 1986.

177. Horsman GB, Macmillan L, Amatnieks Y, Rifkin O, Vas SI, Plasmid profile and slime analysis of coagulase negative staphylococci from CAPD patients with peritonitis: Perit Dial Bull, 6: 195–198, 1986.

178. Keane WF, Everett ED, Fine RN, Golper TA, Vas SI, Peterson PK: CAPD related peritonitis management and antibiotic therapy recommendations: Travenol peritonitis management advisory committee. Perit Dial Bull, 7: 55–68, 1987.

179. Diagnosis and management of peritonitis in continuous ambulatory peritoneal dialysis: Report of a workin party of the British Society for Antimicrobial Chemotherapy: Lancet 1987 I. 845–848, 1987.

180. Goldstein CS, Garrik RE, Polin RA, Gerdes JS, Kolski GB, Neilson EG, Douglas SD: Fibronectin and complement secration by monocytes and peritoneal macrophages in vitro from patients undergoing continuous ambulatory peritoneal dialysis. J Leucocyte Biol, 38: 457–464, 1986.

181. Khan RH, Klein M, Vas S: Fibronectin in the normal peritoneal fluids of patients on chronic ambulatory peritoneal dialysis and during peritonitis. Perit Dial Bull. 7: 69–773, 1987.

182. Holley J, Seibert D, Moss A: Peritonitis following colonoscopy and polypectomy: A need for prophylaxis? Perit Dial Bull. 7: 105, 1987.

183. Stuck A, Seiler A, Frey FJ: Peritonitis due to an intrauterine contraceptive device in a patient on CAPD. Perit Dial Bull. 7: 158–159, 1986.

184. Sombolos K, Vas S, Rifkin O, Ayomamitis A, McNamee P, Oreopoulos DG: Propionibacteria isolates and asymptomatic infections of the peritoneal effluent in CAPD patients. Nephrol Dial Transplant 1: 175–178, 1986.

185. Williams PS, Hendy MS, Ackrill P: Routine daily surveillance cultures in the management of CAPD patients. Peri Dial Bull. 7: 183–186, 1987.

186. Oreopoulos DG, Helfrich GB, Khanna R, Lum GM, Matthews R, Paulsen K, Twardowski ZJ, Vas S: Peritoneal catheters and exit site practices: Current recommendations. Perit Dial Bull. 7: 130–138, 1987.

187. Dasgupta MK, Bettcher KB, Ulan RA, Burns V, Lam K, Dossetor JB, Costerton JW: Relationship of adherent bacterial biofilms to peritonitis in chronic ambulatory peritoneal dialysis. Perit Dial Bull. 7: 168–173, 1987.

188. Holmes CJ, Evans R: Biofilm and foreign body infection – The significance to CAPD associated peritonitis. Perit Dial Bull. 6: 168–177, 1986.

189. Verger C, Chesneau AM, Thibault M, Bataille N: Biofilm on Tenckhoff catheters: A negligible source of contamination. Perit Dial Bull 6: 174–178, 1987.

190. Piraino B, Bernardini J, Peitzman A, Sorkin M: Failure of

peritoneal cuff sahaving to eradicate infection. Perit Dial Bull. 7: 179–182, 1987.

191. Piraino B, Bernardini J, Johnston J, Sorkin M: Chemical peritonitis due to intraperitoneal vancomycin (Vancoled). Peri Dial Bull. 7: 156–159, 1987.

192. Churchill DN, Oreopoulos DG, Taylor DW, Vas SI, Manuel MA, Wu G: Peritonitis in CAPD patients- A randomized clinical trial of trimethoprim-sulfamethoxazole prophylaxis. Abstr. 20th Ann Meeting of the American Society of Nephrology, p 97A, 1987.

193. Harvey DM, Sheppard KJ, Morgan AG, Fletcher J: Effect of dialysate fluids on phagocytosis and killing by normal neutrophyls. J Clin Microbiol 25: 1424–1427, 1987.

194. McGregor SJ, Brock JH, Briggs JD, Junor BJ: Bactericidal activity of peritoneal macrophages from continuous ambulatory peritoneal dialysis patients. Nephrol Dial Transplant 2: 104–108, 1987.

195. Alobaidi HM, Coles GA, Davies M, Lloyd D: Host defence in continuous ambulatory peritoneal dialysis: the effect of dialysate on phagocyte function. Nephrol Dial Transplant 1: 16–21, 1986.

196. Lewis SL, Van Epps DE: Neutrophil and monocyte alterations in chronic dialysis patients. Am J Kidney Dis 9: 381–395, 1987.

197. Lamperi S, Carozzi S: Suppressor resident peritoneal macrophages and peritonitis incidence in continuous ambulatory peritoneal dialysis. Nephron 44: 219–225, 1986.

198. Clark LA, Easmon CS: Opsonic activity of intravenous immunoglobulin preparations against Staphylococcus epidermidis. J Clin Pathol 39: 856–860, 1986.

199. Clark LA, Easmon CS: Opsonic requirements of Staphylococcus epidermidis. J Med Microbiol 22: 1–7, 1986.

200. Peterson PK, Lee D, Suh HJ, Devalon M, Nelson RD, Keane WF: Intracellular survival of Candida albicans in peritoneal macrophages from chronic peritoneal dialysis patients. Am J Kidney Dis 7: 146–152, 1986.

201. Peterson PK, Gaziano E, Suh HJ, Devalon M, Peterson L, Keane WF: Antimicrobial activities of dialysate-elicited and resident human peritoneal macrophages. Infect Immun 49: 212–218.

202. Goldstein CS, Bomalaski JS, Zurier RB, Neilson EG, Douglas SD: Analysis of peritoneal macrophages in continuous ambulatory peritoneal dialysis patients. Kidney Int 26: 733–740, 1984.

203. Wierusz-Wysocka B, Wysocki H, Michta G, Wykretowicz A, Czarnecki R, Baczyk K: Phagocytosis and neturophil bactericidal capacity in patients with uremia. Folia Haematol 111: 589–594, 1984.

204. Huttunen K, Lampainen E, Silvennoinen-Kassinen S, Tiilikainen A: The neutrophil function of uremic patients treated by hemodialysis or CAPD. Scand J Urol Nephrol 18: 167–172, 1984.

205. Maddox Y, Foegh M, Zeligs B, Zmudka M, Bellanti J, Ramwell P: A routine source of human peritoneal macrophages. Scand J Immunol 19: 23–29, 1984.

206. Cichocki T, Hanicki Z, SuLowicz W, Smolenski O, Kopec J, Zembala M: Output of peritoneal cells into peritoneal dialysate. Cytochemical and functional studies. Nephron 35: 175–182, 1983.

207. Rubin J, Lin LM, Lewis R, Cruse J, Bower JD: Host defense mechanisms in continuous ambulatory peritoneal dialysis. Clin Nephrol 20: 140–144, 1983.

208. Verbrugh HA, Keane WF, Hoidal JR, Freiberg MR, Elliott GR, Peterson PK: Peritoneal macrophages and opsonins: antibacterial defense in patients undergoing chronic peritoneal dialysis. J Infect Dis 147: 1018–1029, 1983.

209. Lamperi S, Carozzi S: Defective opsonic activity of peritoneal effluent during continuous ambulatury peritoneal dialysis (CAPD): Importance and prevention. Perit Dial Bull 6: 87–92, 1986.

210. Struijk RG, van Ketel RJ, Krediet RT, Boeschoten EW, Arisz L: Patient viral peritonitis in a continuous ambulatory peritoneal dialysis. Nephron 44: 384, 1986.

211. Goodship THJ, Heaton A, Rodger RSC. Ward MK, Wilkinson R, Kerr DNS: Factors affecting development of peritonitis in continuous ambulatory peritoneal dialysis. Br Med J 289: 1485–1486, 1984.

212. Goodman W, Gallagher N, Sherrard DJ: Peritoneal dialysis fluid as a source of hepatitis antigen. Nephron 29: 107–109, 1981.

213. Salo RJ, Salo AA, Fahlberg WJ, Ellzey JT: Hepatitis B surface antigen (HB(s)Ag) in peritoneal fluid of HB(s)Ag carriers undergoing peritoneal dialysis. J Med Virol 6: 29–35, 1980.

214. Spector D: Hepatitis B miniepidemic in a peritoneal dialysis unit. Arch Int Med 137: 1030–1031, 1977.

215. Vas SI, Oreopoulos DG: Handle with care: Hepatitis B antigen carriers in peritoneal dialysis units. Nephron 29: 105–106, 1981.

216. Eisenberg ES, Leviton I, Soeiro R: Fungal peritonitis in patients receiving peritoneal dialysis: Experience with 11 patients and review of the literature. Rev Inf Dis 8: 309–321, 1986.

217. Oh SH, Conley SB, Rose GM, Rosenblum M, Kohl S, Pickering LK: Fungal peritonitis in children undergoing peritoneal dialysis. Pediatr Inf Dis 4: 62–66, 1985.

218. Vargamezis V, Papadopoulou ZL, Liamos H, Belechri AM, Natscheh T, Vergoulas G, Antoniadou R, Kilintzis V, Papadimitriou M: Management of fungal peritonitis doring continuous ambulatory peritoneal dialysis (CAPD). Perit Dial Bull 6: 17–20, 1986.

219. Cecchin E, DeMarchi S, Panarello G, Tesio F: Chemotherapy and/or removal of the peritoneal catheter in the management of fungal peritonitis complicating CAPD? Nephron 40: 251–252, 1985.

220. Tapson JS, Mansy H, Freeman R, Wilkinson R: The high morbidity of CAPD fungal peritonitis- Description of 10 cases and review of treatment strategies. Quart J Med 61: 1047–1053, 1986.

221. Kravitz SP, Berry PL: Successful treatment of Aspergillus peritonitis in a child undergoing continuous cycling peritoneal dialysis. Arch Int Med 146: 2061–2062, 1986.

222. Paterson AD, Bishop MC, Morgan AG, Burden RP: Removal and replacement of Tenckhoff catheter at a single operation: Successful treatment of resistant peritonitis in continuous ambulatory peritoneal dialysis. Lancet ii 1245–1247, 1986.

223. Craddock CF, Edwards R, Finch RG: Pseudomonas peritonitis in continuous ambulatory peritoneal dialysis: laboratory predictors of treatment failure. J Hosp Infec 10: 179–186, 1987.

224. West TE, Welshe JJ, Krol CP, Amsterdam D: Staphylococcal peritonitis on continuous peritoneal dialysis. J Clin Microbiol 23: 809–812, 1986.

225. Peterson PK, Lee D, Suh HJ, Devalon M, Nelson RD, Keane WF: Intracellular survival of Candida albicans in peritoneal macrophages from chronic peritoneal dialysis patients. Am J Kidney Dis 7: 146–152, 1986.

226. Piraino B, Bernardini J, Sorkin M: The influence of peritoneal catheter exit site infections on peritonitis, tunnel infections and catheter loss in patients on continuous ambulatory peritoneal dialysis. Am J Kidney Dis 8: 436–440, 1986.

227. Beasley SW, Meech PR, Neale TJ, Hatfield PJ, Morrison RB: Continuous ambulatory peritoneal dialysis and acute appendicitis. NZ Med J 99: 145–146, 1986.

228. Spence PA, Mathews RE, Khanna R, Oreopoulos DG: Indications for operation when peritonitis occurs in patients on chronic ambulatory peritoneal dialysis. Surg Gynecol Obstet 161: 450–452, 1985.

229. Lempert KD, Kolb JA, Swartz RD, Campese V, Golper TA,

Winchester JF, Nolph KD, Husserl FE, Zimmerman SW, Kurtz SB: A multicenter trial to evaluate the use of the CAPD '0' set. ASAIO Trans 32: 557–559, 1986.

230. Holmes CJ, Miyake C, Kubey W: In vitro evaluation of an ultraviolet germicidal connection system for CAPD. Perit Dial Bull 3: 215–218, 1984.

231. Nolph KD: Randomized multicanter clinical trial to evaluate the effects of an ultraviolet germicidal system on peritonitis rates in continuous ambulatory peritoneal dialysis. Perit Dial Bull 5: 19–24, 1985.

232. Hamilton RW, Disher BA, Dillingham SA, Nicholas AF: The sterile weld: A new method for connections in continuous ambulatory peritoneal dialysis. Perit Dial Bull 3: (Suppl. 4) 8–10, 1983.

233. LaRocco MT, Mortensen JE, Robinson A: Mycobacterium fortuitum peritonitis in a patient undergoing chronic peritoneal dialysis. Diagn Microbiol Infect Dis 161–164, 1986.

234. Eisenberg ES, Ambalu M, Szylagi G, Aning V, Soeiro R: Colonization of skin and development of peritonitis due to coagulase negative staphylococci in patients undergoing peritoneal dialysis. J Inf Dis 156: 478–482, 1987.

15

COMPLICATIONS OTHER THAN PERITONITIS OR THOSE RELATED TO THE CATHETER AND THE FATE OF UREMIC ORGAN DYSFUNCTION IN PATIENTS RECEIVING PERITONEAL DIALYSIS

JOANNE M. BARGMAN and DIMITRIOS G. OREOPOULOS

INTRODUCTION

This chapter is divided into two sections. In the first, we will discuss the complications of peritoneal dialysis other than peritonitis and those related to the catheter, which are discussed elsewhere in this book. In the second part of this chapter, we will discuss the fate or 'unnatural history' of uremic organ dysfunction in patients receiving peritoneal dialysis. Inclusion of some topics into one or the other section has been arbitrary, since it is not clear to what extent the condition being discussed is a complication of uremia or dialysis itself.

1. COMPLICATIONS OF PERITONEAL DIALYSIS OTHER THAN PERITONITIS OR THOSE RELATED TO THE CATHETER

1.1. Hernias and genital edema

1.1.1. Hernias

The presence of two liters of fluid in the peritoneal cavity increases intra-abdominal pressure. Laplace's law dictates that the tension on the abdominal wall increases because of increased intraperitonal pressure and chamber (i.e., abdominal) radius. Pressure within the abdomen increases with higher dialysate volume and changes in posture [1, 2]. Coughing and straining in the sitting and upright positions cause the highest pressures. In addition, patients who are older and more obese generate higher intraperitoneal pressure for a given activity [2].

Increased abdominal pressure and abdominal wall tension lead to hernia formation in those with congenital or acquired defects in or around the abdomen. A host of hernias has been described in peritoneal dialysis patients (see Table 1). In many series, the most common hernia is incisional or through the catheter placement site [3, 4], whereas, in other series, inguinal [5, 6, 7, 8] or umbilical [9, 10, 11] hernias occur most frequently. Hernias are quite common and may not be detectable until some complication such as dialysate leak or bowel strangulation occurs. One review found that 11.5% of CAPD patients developed hernias during a five year follow-up. Patients with hernias tend to be older, female, multiparous, those who experienced a higher frequency of post-operative leak at the time of catheter insertion [4] and those who have undergone a previous hernia repair [3]. The mean time for development of hernia is one year and the risk increases by 20% for each year on CAPD [3].

Potential areas of weakness include the abdominal incision for catheter implantation. In our institution, we have changed from an incision through the midline to a paramedian incision through the rectus muscle. This approach has led to less perioperative leak and hernia formation [12]. Another potential area for herniation is the processus vaginalis. After the migration of the testes in fetal life, the processus vaginalis undergoes obliteration. Frequently, this does not occur, and the increased abdominal pressure during CAPD may push bowel into the processus vaginalis leading to formation of an indirect inguinal hernia. Bowel may herniate through the diaphragm at the foramen of Morgagni and present as a retrosternal air-fluid level [13].

While most hernias present as a painless swelling [4], the worrisome complications are incarceration and strangulation of bowel. Bowel incarceration can occur through almost any kind of hernia, especially a small one. It may present as a tender lump [14, 15], a bowel obstruction [4], or perforation [16]. Bowel incarceration or strangulation may mimic peritonitis [7, 15, 16] and this complication must be kept in mind in the differential diagnosis of peritonitis. The diagnosis may be particularly difficult to make if the hernia itself is not evident.

1.1.2. Genital edema
Edema of the labia majoris or scrotum and penis is a distressing complication which may occur in as many as 10% of CAPD patients [17–22]. Two mechanisms have been suggested to explain the edema [17]. Firstly, dialysate can track through the soft-tissue plane from the catheter insertion site, from a soft-tissue defect in a hernia, or from a peritoneo-fascial defect. In this case, genital edema can be associated with edema of the anterior abdominal wall [18]. Secondly, fluid can travel through a patent processus vaginalis to the labia or scrotum, where it may or may not leak into the surrounding tissues. If bowel accompanies the dialysate there will be an associated inguinal hernia. In fact, the presence of scrotal edema may suggest a clinically occult indirect inguinal hernia [19].

Diagnosing the cause of genital edema can be difficult, particularly in the presense of massive edema. In several reports abdominal scintigraphy with Technetium 99 m has been successful in identifying a patent processus vaginalis. One to five millicuries are injected into one-half to two liters of dialysate. The radioisotope can be seen to flow into the scrotum through the processus vaginalis [17, 22–24]. Alternatively, CT scanning can be useful, either plain or after addition of 100 ml of 60% diatrizoate into two liters of dialysate. Having the patient move about upright after instillation of dye may facilitate its caudal movement to the edematous tissues [21].

Treatment of genital edema includes bedrest, scrotal elevation, and the use of frequent low volume exchanges [17]. In the case of a leak, cessation of peritoneal dialysis for a week or more may allow a defect to seal. Converting the patient to night-time cycling dialysis with an empty peritoneum during the day allows dialysate to dwell under conditions of relatively low pressure and can allow closure of a leak without changing to hemodialysis. Sometimes these patients can resume CAPD [18].

Hernias warrant surgical repair. Although large ventral hernias carry little but still measurable risk of bowel incarceration [25], they are unsightly and prone to enlarge. The other types of hernias should be repaired because of the risk of incarceration and strangulation of bowel. The patient can be maintained on low volume intermittent peritoneal dialysis post-operatively to allow time for wound healing, before CAPD is recommenced. If hernias recur, other options are changing the patient to night-time peritoneal dialysis, or using low volume dialysate and more frequent exchanges.

1.2. Failure of ultrafiltration

The peritoneal membrane is a delicate structure composed of capillaries, interstitial tissue and a single layer of epithelial cells. Peritoneal biopsy after months to years of CAPD demonstrates loss of microvilli, vacuolization of mesothelial cells and their separation from underlying basement membrane. Widening of intercellular junctions is seen, as well as the deposition of inorganic foreign bodies [36].

Early experience with acute peritoneal dialysis suggested that the peritoneal membrane could be used without serious side effects. However, as experience with chronic peritoneal dialysis increased, it became apparent that the peritoneal membrane could fail. The syndrome of ultrafiltration failure began to emerge when we described a patient who was unable to continue on peritoneal dialysis after eight years of this treatment because of ultrafiltration difficulties in the face of preserved transport of solutes such as urea and creatinine [37]. Other workers reported that subgroups of long-term CAPD patients need increasing numbers of hypertonic exchanges daily to maintain salt and water

Table 1. Types of hernias reported in peritoneal dialysis patients

Inguinal [3–9, 11, 26, 27].
Catheter Insertion Sire [3, 5, 8, 14, 16, 26, 27, 29, 30, 31].
Epigastric [3, 4, 7, 32].
Umbilical [3–5, 7–11, 26, 27].
Incisional [3–5, 7, 9, 12, 27].
Ventral [5, 8, 11, 25, 26, 33].
Foramen of Morgagni [4, 13].
Richter's [15, 30].
Cystocele [4].
Enterocele [4, 34].
Spigelian [31].
Obturator [35].

balance [38].

The search for an understanding of membrane failure is complicated by the observation that in most of these cases solute transport remains intact at a time when water transport is impaired (type I ultrafiltration failure). Chief among the possible mechanisms underlying ultrafiltration failure is the inability to maintain an osmotic gradient across the peritoneal membrane due to increased permeability of the peritoneal membrane to glucose. The diffusion of glucose from the dialysate to plasma compartment rapidly dissipates its concentration gradient and hence the osmotic gradient across the peritoneal membrane for water removal. Less commonly, transport of solute is impaired to the same extent as ultrafiltration. This transport disorder (type II ultrafiltration failure) results from a reduction in the surface area available for transport and can be seen in the patient with extensive adhesions or sclerosing encapsulating peritonitis [39].

There appears to be regional variation in the incidence and prevalence of ultrafiltration failure. Centers in Europe report a relatively high incidence of this problem [40–42], whereas it does not appear to be as common in North America [43]. In one European center, over an eight year observation period, ten percent of patients on IPD and 20% on CAPD permanently lost ultrafiltration ability. Actuarial analysis suggested a risk rate for ultrafiltration failure of 10% in the first year and thirty percent in the second year of CAPD. There was no difference between men and women, nor in episodes of peritonitis. Younger patients, however, had a higher incidence of ultrafiltration loss [40]. When patients are grouped into those able and unable to ultrafilter large volumes, the low ultrafiltration group had been on CAPD almost as long as those capable of large ultrafiltration volumes. Not surprisingly, the patients with poor ultrafiltration demonstrate greater peritoneal permeability to glucose and creatinine. No difference in incidence of peritonitis was discerned between the two groups [42]. On the other hand, a prospective study of patients on CAPD found that almost as many patients had increased as decreased ultrafiltration over time. These differences were apparent within the first year of treatment. In fact, the patients who eventually showed reduction in ultrafiltration had higher peritoneal permeability to solutes at the outset [44].

To try to further define the reasons behind the regional differences in ultrafiltration failure, twenty-nine centers from France, the United States, Canada, Greece and the United Kingdom participated in a study examining ultrafiltration in their patients. The first report comprised information from twenty of the centers [45]. When patients were stratified on the basis of buffer anion in the dialysate, net ultrafiltration was strikingly higher in those using lactate-based dialysate as compared to those using acetate. The increased ultrafiltration was likely the result of preservation of the osmotic gradient across the peritoneal membrane. Indeed, patients using lactate-based buffers demonstrated higher dialysate glucose concentrations at the end of a four hour dwell, despite the diluting effect of the ultrafiltered water. Furthermore, for the majority of patients in the early study, there was no correlation of ultrafiltration with time on CAPD nor with number of episodes of peritonitis. Therefore, it appeared that the use of acetate

was associated with increased glucose permeability of the peritoneal membrane, rapid dissipation of the osmotic gradient, and compromised ultrafiltration.

However, it was not clear whether there was something unique about acetate, or whether acetate served as an 'innocent bystander' or marker for some other product in the dialysate which was responsible for the measured differences [46].

A subsequent report incorporating data from more centers showed the issue to be more complex [47]. When this larger group was substratified on the basis of the company producing the dialysate, it became apparent that lactate-based solutions from different companies did not produce comparable results. Ultrafiltration rate with one lactate brand was comparable to that seen with acetate. Because the highest rate of ultrafiltration was seen in the one lactate-based solution which was used with the greatest frequency, ultrafiltration was higher for the lactate group overall. Once again, there was no correlation between number of episodes of peritonitis and ultrafiltration volume.

The inter-company results must be interpreted with caution, however. When results from another center using lactate were added, the dichotomy in ultrafiltration between lactate and acetate reappeared. In summary, acetate must remain suspect in the ultrafiltration abnormalities reported from Europe, although it is recognized that this association is not universal [48].

It is not clear how acetate exerts its effect on transperitoneal transport. It can act as a vasodilator [49] and may have different transport kinetics across the peritoneum than lactate [50]. Animal studies suggest that acetate-based dialysate compromises ultrafiltration even in the short-term [51].

Treatment of ultrafiltration failure entails shortening dwell time to minimize diffusion of glucose. This can be done by more frequent, shorter exchanges, or leaving the peritoneal cavity empty overnight. Rapid cycler dialysis can be substituted for CAPD in the form of night-time peritoneal dialysis (CCPD or APD) or once- or twice-weekly cycler PD added to the CAPD regimen. Finally, there is preliminary evidence that the addition of the surfactant phosphatidylcholine to the peritoneal dialysate can improve ultrafiltration in those with failure of this function [52].

1.3. Sclerosing encapsulating peritonitis

This unfortunate syndrome, consisting of anorexia, nausea, vomiting, malnutrition, intermittent bowel obstruction, and decreased peritoneal transport of water and solutes, has been reported mainly from Europe [53–58], although sporadic cases have been found in the United States [59, 60]. At surgery or postmortem examination, the small intestine is bound or encapsulated by a thick fibrous layer, rendering the peritoneal surface opaque. The fibrous layer resembles a 'thick shaggy membrane' [53], 'marble' [59], 'cocoon' or a 'fruit rind' which may or may not peel off the bowel relatively easily [61]. The bowel so exposed may appear normal [61]. More recently, a different form of sclerosing peritonitis has been described where the diffuse sclerosing process extends transmurally with incorporation of the inner circular muscular layer and myenteric plexus of the small bowel in the fibrosing process [62]. Patients with this syndrome do poorly, with 50% mortality [59], probably on the basis of severe malnutrition and recurrent bowel obstruction. Those whose symptoms lead to laparotomy have a mortality rate of close to 80% [59]. The diagnosis of bowel obstruction may be delayed because the fibrosing process does not allow the bowel to distend and display the typical radiologic findings [55].

Sclerosing encapsulating peritonitis (SEP) appears to be a distinct and devastating syndrome and the name should not be used interchangeably with 'peritoneal sclerosis'. The second term should be reserved for the finding of non-encapsulating sclerosis and fibrous adhesions associated with ultrafiltration failure. The latter condition is seen in patients who have had prolonged peritoneal dialysis or recurrent episodes of peritonitis, but may be present at the initiation of dialysis (see section on ultrafiltration failure). Indeed, the lack of rigorous differentiation between these two entities may confuse any attempt to define etiological factors, particularly among different dialysis centers.

The cause of SEP is uncertain. There are numerous possibilities (see Table II). The original reports came from centers where the dialysate buffer was primarily acetate rather than lactate [53, 58]. It has been suggested that acetate may be irritating to the peritoneal membrane and perhaps initiate the fibrosing process [53, 63]. However, SEP has also been reported in patients dialyzing with lactate [60, 64], although in some cases the disease in question may be peritoneal sclerosis [60] or transmural bowel fibrosis [62].

Recurrent peritonitis or subclinical 'grumbling' peritonitis [65] has been suggested as a cause of this distressing syndrome, althoug clearly many patients have either never had peritonitis (detectable clinically) or had a relatively low incidence of peritonitis [58].

Because the incidence of SEP in a unit with a low incidence of peritonitis suggested some other cause, Shaldon and colleagues postulated that the use of a bacterial filter may be linked to the high incidence of SEP. They suggested that bacteria trapped upstream of the filter secrete pyrogen which crosses the filter and enters the peritoneal cavity where it stimulates macrophages to secrete interleukin-1 [66]. This lymphokine stimulates fibroblast proliferation and so could accelerate the fibrosing process. Once again,

Table 2. Postulated causes of sclerosing encapsulating peritonitis

Acetate-containing dialysate [53, 58, 63, 70].
Recurrent peritonitis [53, 55, 60, 70, 71].
Plastic particles [58, 72].
Formaldehyde [58, 73].
Bacterial filter causing upstream multiplication of bacteria with pyrogen release into peritoneum stimulating interleukin-1 production [66].
Multiple abdominal surgeries [60].
Unrecognized subclinical peritonitis with fastidious bacteria or fungi [65].
IP contamination with chlorhexidine in alcohol sprayed on connector [64].
Hypertonic acidic dialysate [58].
Catheter [58, 74].
Beta blockers [54, 58, 63].
High interdialytic peritoneal content of fibrinogen [61].

however, not all patients with SEP have used bacterial filters.

A retrospective analysis in one dialysis unit demonstrated that all the patients who developed SEP were members of a subgroup who sprayed their connectors at each exchange with 0.5% chlorhexidine in 70% alcohol [64]. The authors studied the effect of this antiseptic over the short term in a rat model and demonstrated inflammation in submesothelial tissues. The incidence of SEP in this unit has diminished since changing the antiseptic protocol.

The presence of the dialysis catheter in the peritoneal cavity could promote an inflammatory or foreign-body response. In this regard, a similar encapsulating peritoneal sclerosis has been described in patients with ascites in whom LeVeen shunts have been implanted [67]. Given all the patients with implanted silastic catheters, the SEP-type response is very rare. In addition, it would not explain the predilection for European centers.

Other factors include the use of beta blockers, which has been linked to peritoneal sclerosis [68, 69].

Finally, there are many potentially toxic factors related to the dialysis itself, including hypertonicity and acidity of the dialysate.

Taken in sum, there is no single factor which can be incriminated in the pathogenesis of SEP. Assuming that the published reports are describing a unique entity, it is likely that the etiology is multifactorial. The strongest association, however, seems to be with the use of acetate in the dialysis solution and most centers therefore are avoiding its use.

1.4. Respiratory complications

Early studies of pulmonary function in patients on peritoneal dialysis suggested that this process compromised pulmonary function [75]. However, the early studies were performed on subjects who were acutely ill and as such many other factors could have affected the integrity of the lungs, respiratory muscles and pleura. More recent studies on stable PD patients have confirmed that the presence of two liters of dialysate does reduce most lung volumes, including the functional residual capacity (FRC) [76–79]. These abnormalities, however, reverse at the end of a session of IPD [76], or normalize after only two weeks of CAPD [78].

It has been suggested that when the FRC decreases to less than the closing volume, small airways will collapse leading to ventilation-perfusion mismatch and arterial hypoxemia [80]. Indeed, at the outset of dialysis, the instillation of two liters of dialysate is associated with decreased FRC and an average 5 Torr fall in arterial pO_2 in the sitting position and an average 8 Torr decrease when supine. However, when re-studied a few months later, these patients showed no decrease in pO_2, despite a similar fall in FRC as at the commencement of dialysis [79]. The authors suggested that some long-term adjustment takes place, such as redistribution of blood away from the more poorly ventilated lower segnments of the lungs. Other studies have not found arterial hypoxemia [76, 78, 81], although an increased alveolar-arterial gradient for oxygen has been demonstrated in supine patients with intraperitoneal dialysate [81]. The changes in lung volumes have been found to be no more severe in patients with chronic obstructive airways disease undergoing peritoneal dialysis [78] and it has been suggested that peritoneal dialysis should not be withheld from this group [82].

The maximal inspiratory pressure in patients on peritoneal dialysis is subnormal when the peritoneal cavity is empty [77]. However, when two litres of dialysate are instilled, there is a small increase, rather than decrease, in respiratory function. It has been suggested that this change can be explained by altered diaphragmatic contractility secondary to stretch of the muscles of the diaphragm by the dialysate [77]; that is, with increased muscle fiber length, there is improved effectiveness of muscle function [83]. The intraperitoneal fluid may also increase the curvature of the diaphragm. The radius of this curve is therefore diminished. Laplace's law dictates that the diaphragm generates more pressure for a given amount of muscle tension at a lower radius. Therefore, diaphragmatic contractility may increase in the presence of intraperitoneal fluid, offsetting the effect of diminished lung volumes. Of course, there is probably an upper limit to this relationship after which the diaphragm loses efficiency and pulmonary compromise ensues [83]. This usually becomes apparent clinically with a dialysate volume of three liters.

There is evidence that the character and availability of energy substrate will alter metabolism which in turn affects ventilation. This relationship has been described in patients undergoing total parenteral nutrition, where hypercaloric glucose and amino acid solutions produce significant increases in minute ventilation, carbon dioxide excretion and oxygen consumption [84]. A theoretical treatment of substrate absorption during CAPD predicts that the absorption of glucose and, to a lesser extent, lactate, would drive intermediary metabolism, leading to increases in minute ventilation, carbon dioxide excretion and oxygen consumption [84]. (In addition, loss of bicarbonate via the peritoneal membrane would be only 8% of that lost during hemodialysis, and so there would be no tendency toward compensatory hypoventilation as seen in hemodialysis.) The increase in metabolically-driven ventilation could theoretically prove dangerous to the patient with lung disease [84]. Studies in patients on CAPD confirm increased minute volume, oxygen consumption and carbon dioxide excretion compared with controls [85]. The studies suggest that the acetate and lactate absorbed are incorporated into the Krebs cycle. Moreover, because some glucose may be metabolized in a manner not requiring oxygen but producing carbon dioxide, the respiratory quotient increases. The arterial pCO_2 does not increase, however, because the patients hyperventilate and so exhale the increased carbon dioxide produced.

1.5. Hydrothorax

Peritoneal dialysis may give rise to hydrothorax [86]. This complication can be life-threatening, leading to respiratory failure [87]. In contrast, clinical symptoms can be minimal or lacking and the diagnosis delayed until a chest x-ray is done.

Massive hydrothorax has been reported to occur in both adults and children, during acute or intermittent peritoneal dialysis and during CAPD [88, 89]. It occurs predominantly on the right side. There have been a few reports of left-sided and even bilateral hydrothorax. The pathophysiology of this condition remains poorly understood.

The majority of the reported patients are females. Sixty-seven percent of the reported patients were on chronic peritoneal dialysis, including CAPD and IPD, and the rest were undergoing acute peritoneal dialysis when this complication occurred. The interval between starting peritoneal dialysis and the onset of hydrothorax ranged between six hours to 22 months, with a median of 25.5 days. The majority of patients presented with shortness of breath. Other less common symptoms were weight gain, chest pain, abdominal pain and hypotension. Lorentz *et al.* [90] reported three infants who had increased drainage of fluid with a high glucose concentration through their chest tubes and simultaneously decreased dialysis effluent return during acute peritoneal dialysis.

Pleuroscopic examination of the right hemidiaphragm does not reveal discontinuities in its structure with this complication [89]. Congenital diaphragmatic hernia has been implicated by Khanna *et al.* [91], as this is more common on the right side. Two areas of small pleural blebs overlying two small defects in the right hemidiaphragm were observed during thoracotomy in a 65-yr-old patient who developed hydrothorax four months after instituting CAPD [92].

The negative intrathoracic pressure and positive intra-abdominal pressure generated during the descent of the diaphragm has been postulated to open up a small defect in the diaphragm. This defect could possess features of a ball valve, preventing admixture of the hydrothorax with dialysis fluid [93], but promoting unidirectional flow from peritoneal to pleural cavity in some patients. This effect may be prominent with the use of hypertonic fluid where the increased ultrafiltration volume may lead to profound increases in intra-abdominal pressure and further increases in the hydrothorax. Transdiaphragmatic lymphatic transport of ascitic fluid has been proposed as the etiology of hepatic hydrothorax [94].

Other causes of hydrothorax, such as cardiac failure, inflammatory disease, infections and malignancy should be ruled out.

Autopsy findings in a 73-yr-old CAPD patient who developed massive right-sided pleural effusions [95] demonstrated the presence of carcinoma of the liver. Haberli *et al.* observed a 3×7 cm scar with a 2 mm hole in the right hemidiaphragm of a patient at autopsy [96]. In this patient, the onset of hydrothorax occurred 4½ hr after institution of acute PD.

Grefberg *et al.* [97] demonstrated the presence of 20 defects in the diaphragm of patients with hydrothorax. The defects measured 0.5 to 1.5 mm in diameter, and some were partly covered by a thin membrane which histologically consisted of peritoneum and pleura, but lacked the tendinous part of the central tendon of the diaphragm.

Clinically, the rapid onset of hydrothorax after the institution of dialysis and its rapid resolution after cessation of PD suggests the presence of a pre-existing or congenital defect with bidirectional flow [98]. The hydrothorax that appears after several weeks or months of peritoneal dialysis is likely the result of an acquired defect secondary to increased intra-abdominal pressure. Higher pressures lead to separation of collagenous fibers, pleural bleb formation, and subsequent rupture [93].

Simultaneous estimation of protein, sugar and lactate dehydrogenase (LDH) concentrations in pleural fluid, peritoneal fluid and blood should be undertaken. The presence of a transudate (protein < 3 g/dl), high sugar concentration and low LDH in the pleural fluid compared to blood levels suggests the presence of a transdiaphragmatic leak. The intraperitoneal instillation of 2 ml of methylene blue mixed with two liters of dialysis solution and subsequent detection in the pleural fluid by thoracentesis can demonstrate a leak [99]. However, this test may be unreliable, since the dye can become diluted by the two liters of dialysate and give a false negative result [100]. As well, methylene blue can give rise to chemical peritonitis. Radioactive methods utilizing 10 uCi of ^{131}I-RISA have been reported to be effective in detecting a leak. Macro-aggregated albumin, 99mTc, sulphur colloid or human serum albumin in doses ranging from 3–5 mCi can be instilled into the peritoneal cavity with two liters of dialysis fluid. Subsequent counting of the activity of the radiosotope in the thorax is a reliable method of detecting a defect [98, 99].

1.5.1. Management and outcome
Small effusions do not need specific treatment. In the patient with respiratory failure, peritoneal dialysis should be stopped and thoracentesis performed. The patient should be changed to hemodialysis. Those who cannot tolerate hemodialysis could be treated with careful peritoneal dialysis and repeated thoracenteses as necessary [86, 87, 101]. Pleurodesis has been successful in preventing recurrence of massive hydrothorax [89, 95, 100, 102–106].

Although opinions differ as to the ideal treatment, intermittent peritoneal dialysis can be continued in many patients who are at risk for either hemodialysis, surgical treatment or pleurodesis. This can be done with low volume exchanges, although some patients can tolerate normal volumes on IPD without reaccumulating pleural fluid. In 50 patients with hydrothorax, 17 were maintained on CAPD, IPD was prescribed in 11 (interim hemodialysis in four), 18 patients were transferred to hemodialysis, two patients died from uremia or peritonitis and the outcome was unknown in the other two. Despite recurrence, patients can continue on peritoneal dialysis [89, 103, 106].

1.6. Abnormalities of lipid metabolism

The leading cause of death in patients on long-term dialysis therapy is cardiovascular disease [107, 108]. Chronic dialysis is associated with both accelerated atherosclerosis [109] and abnormalities of lipid metabolism. The latter may persist from uremia [110, 111], or appear *de novo* during dialysis. A focus of concern in patients on peritoneal dialysis is the continuous absorption of glucose from the dialysate. This glucose loading could cause increased insulin levels and altered lipid metabolism and further increase atherogenesis and the risk of serious cardiovascular events.

Numerous prevalence studies have documented increased plasma cholesterol levels in CAPD patients when compared to those on hemodialysis [112–115], although others have not found a difference [116]. Prospective studies, however, have almost uniformly reported increased cholesterol con-

centrations over the first months of CAPD [117–122] even when baseline levels were normal [117, 120, 121]. There is a trend for the cholesterol to return to more normal levels in the second year [119–121] suggesting that cholesterol metabolism adapts over time to the glucose infusion.

Plasma triglyceride values tend to be more variable in a given patient [119–121] which may make analysis more difficult. As is the case with cholesterol, prevalence studies demonstrate higher triglyceride levels in patients on CAPD when compared to hemodialysis patients [114, 115] or normals [120, 123]. Prospective analyses again demonstrate increased plasma triglyceride levels over time [117–122, 124]. Unlike cholesterol, elevated triglyceride levels seem to persist [119, 120].

Despite the increase in mean triglyceride level, not all patients develop hypertriglyceridemia during CAPD. Therefore, other factors may contribute to this abnormality. Potential contributing factors include diet,* drugs such as beta blockers or anabolic steroids, underlying conditions such as nephrotic syndrome, and genetic susceptibility to hyperlipidemia. Moreover, other studies in CAPD or hemodialysis patients have found no difference in the prevalence of hypertriglyceridemia [113], or the serum triglyceride levels at one year of therapy [121].

The mechanism of the lipid abnormalities described in the majority of the studies may relate to the glucose absorbed from the dialysate. Serum insulin levels are elevated [123, 125] and rise in parellel to plasma glucose concentration during a dialysate dwell. The insulin levels remain elevated at the end of the dwell [125]. The plasma triglyceride levels correlate with the serum insulin concentrations. In addition, disposal of an exogenous lipid load is impaired with rising insulin levels [113]. It has been suggested that the hyperinsulinemia seen in chronic renal failure, but particularly in PD, leads to increased triglyceride levels in two ways. First, increased insulin levels stimulate hepatic triglyceride synthesis. Second, in the face of peripheral insulin resistance, there is diminished activity of the insulin-inducible hormone lipoprotein lipase. This compromises the removal of the triglycerides produced [113]. A correlation of the lipid abnormalities with the total amount of glucose used in the dialysate has been reported in one [121], but not another [120] study.

The role of hyperglycemia *per se* in the pathogenesis of the lipid disorders is unclear. Fasting hyperglycemia may occasionally develop in previously non-diabetic patients on CAPD, but is an unusual event [123, 125]. The administration of insulin to non-diabetics on peritoneal dialysis results in lower levels of plasma glucose and glycosylated hemoglobin, but does not lead to changes in the concentration of cholesterol, triglyceride or other lipoproteins [126].

Studies of lipoprotein subfractions in patients before commencing dialysis have shown elevated very low density lipoprotein (VLDL) cholesterol and triglyceride [119–121]. Unfortunately, the VLDL cholesterol rises further in the first few months of dialysis and stays elevated as much as 50% over baseline [118, 120, 121]. The fate of the so-

---

* In some cases, patients commencing dialysis undergo significant changes in both eating habits and dietary prescription.

called 'protective' high density lipoprotein (HDL) cholesterol is quite interesting. Initial levels are low [119–121]. However, in patients who are not hypertriglyceridemic, the HDL cholesterol increases over the first six months of CAPD [119, 124]. Unfortunately, it appears that the HDL cholesterol levels subsequently fall over the next six months so that they return to baseline or below baseline by one year [117, 120, 124]. Loss of lipoproteins into the dialysate occurs, but this appears to be minimal compared to their synthetic rate and so plays a small role in lipid metabolism [127]. It appears that whatever metabolic adjustments occur over the first year of peritoneal dialysis to bring the total serum cholesterol back toward baseline are responsible for the downward trend seen in HDL cholesterol over the same time. Further studies are needed to more closely examine the relationship between VLDL and LDL cholesterol with HDL cholesterol to provide a clearer index of atherogenic risk. Taken in sum, though, the increased VLDL cholesterol which persists accompanied by unchanging concentrations of LDL cholesterol [118–120] factored by diminished levels of HDL cholesterol after several months on CAPD suggests an unfortunate ratio conductive to accelerated atherogenesis.

A recent elegant study of cholesterol metabolism demonstrates a defect in hemodialysis patients of cholesterol esterification in plasma [115]. This leads to a reversal of the cell-to-plasma gradient for cholesterol transport and may cause inappropriate accumulation of cholesterol in the cell. Unlike hemodialysis patients, however, these transport steps are no different in CAPD patients than in healthy controls. A drawback is that only patients without elevated lipid levels were chosen for study and so these findings do not reflect the dialysis population as a whole.

Treatment of lipid disorders in uremic patients is difficult. Certainly, careful dietary counseling, weight loss, exercise and restriction of alcohol intake are strongly recommended. Unfortunately, many patients are non-compliant and in others these measures are not sufficient. Drug therapy is problematic. Several workers have studied the effect of clofibrate in lowering triglyceride levels in uremic patients [128–130]. The major drawback is toxicity: its use in uremic patients is associated with cholelithiasis, myalgias, elevation of creatine phosphokinase levels and hyperkalemia [131–133]. In our experience, clofibrate in as low a dose as 0.5 g per week can produce severe muscle toxicity. Moreover, experience with other lipid-lowering agents in dialysis patients is preliminary or non-existent. Therefore, more therapeutic measures are needed to bring the highly prevalent lipid normalities under control in peritoneal dialysis patients, in order to reduce the worrisome incidence of atherosclerotic complications.

1.7. Cardiovascular complications

Review of dialysis registry data presented elsewhere in this book confirms the predominance of cardiovascular events in peritoneal dialysis patients. The factors contributing to cardiovascular complications are threefold. Firstly, there is the initial disease leading to renal failure, such as malignant hypertension. Secondly, the uremic state itself can contribute through ongoing hypertension and other atherogenic factors. Finally, the dialytic process can contribute to atherogenesis through, for example, the development of lipid disorders, as discussed elsewhere in this chapter.

Studies have demonstrated that patients commencing CAPD with evidence of heart disease have lower survival rates than those without. More than 80% of those dying of cardiovascular complications have evidence of ischemic or hypertensive heart disease before starting dialysis. The *de novo* incidence of ischemic heart disease in patients between ages 40 and 50 is 8.8% at the end of the first year, and 15% at the end of the second [134].

The control of blood pressure seen in patients on CAPD may lead to improvement in cardiac function. After six to 12 months on CAPD, there is a decrease in left ventricular mass in the majority in whom it was increased at the outset. Moreover, the majority also experience near-normalization of the end-diastolic dimension, left ventricular fractional shortening, and ejection fraction, as assessed by M-mode echocardiography [135]. Presumably, these changes are the welcome result of better blood pressure control.

The improvement in hypertension can also have deleterious effects. Diabetic patients have been reported to experience exacerbation of peripheral vascular disease during CAPD. Risk factors for the worsening of peripheral perfusion include smoking, previous symptoms of peripheral vascular disease, and absent limb pulses. It has been suggested that the lowered blood pressure on CAPD compromises blood flow to the ischemic limbs. Furthermore, one patient who was changed from CAPD to intermittent peritoneal dialysis had increased blood pressure and improvement in limb perfusion [136].

The elevated intra-abdominal pressure in CAPD patients can potentially lead to cardiac side effects. In cirrhotic patients, drainage of ascitic fluid produces a fall in right and left atrial pressure and a dramatic improvement in cardiac function [137]. However, no changes in right atrial pressure, pulmonary artery pressure and cardiac index are found after the infusion of three liters of dialysate [138]. The presence of two liters of dialysate did not compromise the response to postural stress in CAPD patients in another study [139]. Blood pressure may actually be a little higher with dialysate *in situ* [140], especially in the standing position [139]. However, others have reported up to a 20% decrease in cardiac index with two liters of intraperitoneal fluid [141, 142]. In summary, it appears that the presence of intraperitoneal dialysate does not exert a clinically significant effect on the cardiovascular system.

1.8. Metabolic complications

1.8.1. Disorders of water metabolism

The plasma sodium concentration reflects the relationship of extracellular water to extracellular sodium. Insofar as the renal contribution to water balance in patients with end-stage renal disease is minimal, the determinants of water balance and hence sodium concentration in these patients are oral or intravenous intake, and net flux across the peritoneum. Patients on CAPD with an intact thirst mechanism and access to water may actually demonstrate plasma sodium concentrations slightly lower than normal [143].

In hyperglycemic individuals, the increased extracellular

glucose concentration causes the osmotic flux of water from the intracellular to extracellular compartment, leading to restoration of extracellular osmolality towards normal at the cost of intracellular dehydration. Therefore, the fall in serum concentration can be predicted. Patients on hemodialysis, however, demonstrate a greater fall in serum sodium for a given rise in glucose concentration than normals. In other words, the rise in plasma tonicity is less than that predicted for the degree of hyperglycemia [144]. However, patients on CAPD or CCPD demonstrate the expected change. One explanation is that the hemodialysis patient drinks water in response to increased plasma osmolality and, in the absence of osmotic diuresis, is able to lower tonicity. In contrast, the patient on CAPD is undergoing continuous loss of water greater than sodium in the peritoneal effluent (see below) which may perpetuate the hypertonic state in the same manner as an osmotic diuresis [144].

Because the reflection coefficient for sodium is low but greater than zero, the filtrate formed is hyponatremic compared to plasma [145]. Losses in the peritoneal dialysis of more water than sodium can lead to hypernatremia if oral water intake is not correspondingly increased. Therefore, dehydration and hypernatremia are occasionally seen [146–148]. The use of dialysis solutions containing sodium at concentrations hyponatremic to plasma may be helpful and perhaps even lead to positive water balance [143].

1.8.2. Disorders of potassium metabolism

Hypokalemia is found in 10–36% of CAPD patients [149, 150]. Profound hypokalemia (serum K 1.5 mEq/l) was found in a CAPD patient with vomiting and diarrhea [151]. Ongoing losses of small amounts of potassium in the peritoneal effluent may account for the hypokalemia in some patients. However, other factors such as cellular uptake and bowel losses play a role. It is recommended that serum potassium levels be maintained at levels greater than 3.0 mEq/l in the asymptomatic patient, and greater than 3.5 mEq/l in the patient on digitalis or with a history of angina or cardiac arrhytmias [152]. Potassium supplements should be used with caution in CAPD patients because of their lack of renal reserve. Potassium chloride can be added to the peritoneal dialysate to diminish the plasma-dialysate concentration gradient for potassium and hence stop diffusional losses. In an acute setting, up to 20 mEq/l of KCl can be added to the peritoneal dialysate with minimal side effects. This dose raises plasma potassium concentration by an average 0.44 mEq/l over 2–3 hr. However, the effect of this very hyperkalemic solution on the peritoneal membrane is unknown and this therapy should not be used on a chronic basis [149].

Hyperkalemia is seen in both acute PD and CAPD patients. Hyperkalemia has been noted after acute peritoneal dialysis [153, 154]. It has been attributed to breakdown of glycogen stored during the dialysis with consequent release of potassium [153]. Patients on CAPD with hyperkalemia may benefit from dietary counselling. Other factors which affect extrarenal potassium disposal, such as insulin deficiency or use of adrenergic blocking agents, should be considered.

1.9. Acid base balance

In health, the kidneys help to maintain acid base balance via excretion of acid generated from dietary intake. Through this process, bicarbonate is regenerated and returned to the body buffer pool. As the kidneys fail, however, net acid excretion diminishes and metabolic acidosis develops. It is important, therefore, that any form of dialysis provide replenishment of buffer.

In the early years of peritoneal dialysis, bicarbonate, the obvious choice, was employed as buffer. However, bicarbonate reacts with calcium chloride leading to precipitation of calcium carbonate. Therefore, other less reactive buffers had to be used, and experience has accumulated with lactate and acetate. Dialysate containing glucose must be kept at pH 5–6 to prevent caramelization. At equimolar concentrations of acetate and lactate, acetate demonstrates higher titratable acidity. Therefore, when instilled into the peritoneal cavity, solutions containing acetate remain acid longer than lactate-based dialysate [155]. The prolonged acidity of the solution may explain reports of abdominal pain and chemical peritonitis with the use of acetate-based dialysate [155, 156]. (Other long-term effects of acetate are discussed in the sections on sclerosing peritonitis and ultrafiltration failure). Serum lactate remains low in patients receiving lactate-containing dialysate. Patients receiving equimolar amounts of acetate-containing dialysate, on the other hand, demonstrate abnormally high levels of plasma acetate [157]. This finding suggests that less lactate is absorbed or it is more efficiently metabolized than acetate. The patients receiving lactate show normal serum bicarbonate levels [157, 158] suggesting that adequate amounts of lactate are being absorbed and converted to bicarbonate. The dialysate lactate is composed of both the easily metabolized L isomer and the slowly metabolized D isomer. Both isomers are absorbed from dialysate in equal amounts. The lack of accumulation of the D isomer in blood suggests that it is, indeed, metabolized to a significant extent [50], although previous investigations have suggested otherwise [159]. The fate of absorbed D-lactate is of concern because of reports of cerebral dysfunction in patients with high blood levels of this isomer [160]. During IPD, there is a net gain in body buffer of about 80 mmol, owing to lactate absorption surpassing bicarbonate loss from plasma to dialysate. High rates of ultrafiltration mitigate this effect via both increased loss of bicarbonate and diminished absorption of lactate. Presumably, this is on the basis of convective forces [50].

Ammonium chloride loading has demonstrated that patients on CAPD tolerate an acid load better than patients receiving hemodialysis. However, this tolerance does not seem to increase with time on CAPD [161].

Use of lactate does have its drawbacks. Its use in patients with lactic acidosis may worsen the metabolic derangement [162, 163]. In this setting, specially prepared bicarbonate-based solutions are recommended [164], or the use of a proportioning system similar to that used in bicarbonate-based hemodialysis [165]. Lactate may be an inappropriate buffer in patients with hepatic failure. In this setting, lactate may not be sufficiently converted to bicarbonate, leading to acidosis and lactate accumulation [154, 166].

Patients on peritoneal dialysis may develop metabolic or respiratory alkalosis. The metabolic alkalosis can result from contraction of the extracellular fluid volume, as reported in the treatment phase of hyperglycemia [167, 168] or with the frequent use of hypertonic dialysis solutions [169]. In patients with respiratory alkalosis, the normally functioning kidneys defend against serious alkalemia by excreting bicarbonate. The CAPD patient has no such mechanism. Furthermore, the constant infusion of buffer in the patient with respiratory alkalosis can lead to serious alkalemia [170].

Respiratory alkalosis may appear during the initial stages of dialysis. In the acidotic patient commencing dialysis, the infusion of buffer will correct the extracellular acidosis. However, because the bicarbonate anion crosses the blood-brain barrier relatively slowly, the cerebrospinal fluid bathing the respiratory centre will remain relatively acid. This cerebrospinal fluid acidosis will continue to stimulate respiratory drive and maintain hyperventilation in the face of now-normal extracellular fluid pH. Therefore, respiratory alkalosis will develop as a response to the hyperventilation [153, 171]. This phenomenon poses only a minor problem in peritoneal dialysis because the conversion of lactate to bicarbinate occurs slowly enough to allow cerebrospinal fluid equilibration with extracellular fluid.

1.10. Musculoskeletal complications

1.10.1. Back pain
Patients on CAPD include a large subset who are elderly. Age is associated with an increased frequency of degenerative changes in the spine, including degenerative disc disease, facet hypertrophy, spondylolysis and spondylolisthesis. In addition, other coincident systemic diseases, including uremia, ischemic heart disease and diabetes mellitus, lead to low activity levels and poor exercise tolerance. Moreover, uremic patients may demonstrate osteoporosis with compression fractures which accentuate thoracic kyphosis and, as compensation, lumbar lordosis [172]. Multiple abdominal operations or obesity weaken the muscles of the abdomen and shift the line of gravity anteriorly. All these factors alter normal spinal mechanics and lead to abnormal posture. Furthermore, the addition of two or three liters of dialysate into the peritoneal cavity pulls the center of gravity forward even more. The further accentuation of lumbar lordosis may aggravate back strain [172] (Figure 1).

It is the patient with an antecedent longstanding history of back ailments or with evidence of back disease who shows exacerbation of back pain while on CAPD [172]. Treatment includes educating the patient in maneuvers to avoid undue strain during daily activity. In addition, exercises to improve abdominal musculature or pelvic tilts may be indicated, but obviously those exercises which increase intra-abdominal pressure, such as sit-ups, are not indicated. Using the minimum volume of dialysate needed to achieve adequate dialysis is advisable, even at the expense of more frequent exchanges. Finally, dialysis while supine with continuous cyclic peritoneal dialysis (CCPD) or automated peritoneal dialysis (APD) or a change to hemodialysis may be indicated for the patient in whom intractable back symptoms develop.

1.10.2. Tendinitis and tendon rupture
Lateral epicondylitis or 'spike elbow' has been described in CAPD. This inflammation may be caused by the repetitive insertion of the spike with a vigorous twisting and pushing motion [173]. Bilateral rupture of the tendon of the long head of the biceps muscle has also been described, and attributed to the strain of performing CAPD [174].

1.10.3. Amyloidosis
Dialysis-associated amyloidosis has been extensively described in hemodialysis patients. This syndrome consists of carpal tunnel compression due to amyloid deposition [175] and, less often, amyloid deposits in periarticular tissues leading to arthropathy and formation of juxta-articular bone cysts [176, 177]. The amyloid material in this syndrome is unique because it is composed of beta-2-microglobulin [178].

Recently, a patient on CAPD has been reported who presented with carpal tunnel syndrome and hip fracture. Tissue from the wrist was composed of amyloid, and beta-2-microglobulin was found in the deposits [179]. Therefore, it is possible that the dialysis-related amyloid has an equal predilection for the peritoneal dialysis population.

Plasma levels of beta-2-microglobulin were determined by radioimmunoassay in CAPD and in predialysis blood from hemodialysis patients. While there was a tendency for the levels to be higher in the hemodialysis patients (46.2 ± 11.1 mg/l) as compared to CAPD patients (38.2 ± 7.7. mg/l), this difference was not statiscally significant and both

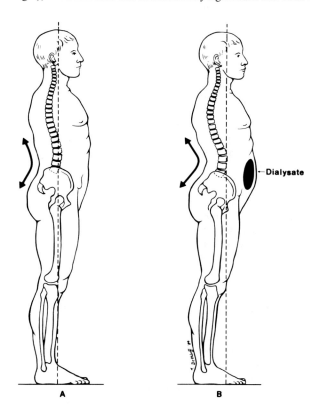

Figure 1. Normal posture (A); addition of the dialysate increases the lumbar lordosis (B).

levels were much greater than in normals (1.8 ± 0.5 mg/l). However, there appears to be no change in plasma concentration with increasing duration of dialysis [179]. Studies have confirmed elevated beta-2-microglobulin levels in CAPD as well as in hemodialysis patients [180], although others have found the levels to be actually lower in CAPD patients than in hemodialysis patients [181].

Why the dialysis-associated amyloid syndrome has been reported much more frequently in hemodialysis than in CAPD patients is not clear. If the tissue deposition simply reflects prolonged exposure to elevated plasma levels of the amyloid-forming protein, then the incidence in the two populations with similar levels of beta-2-microglobulin should be similar. What role aluminium might play in polymerization of the protein into amyloid is unclear [182]. Perhaps the kinetics of the protein are important in its transfer from plasma to extravascular tissues. Peritoneal dialysis affords ongoing clearance of this 11,815 dalton protein [183] while it has been suggested that, in addition to providing poor clearance of this protein, the hemodialysis membrane may actually cause stimulation of beta-2-microglobulin production on an immune basis [184]. Perhaps rapid changes in beta-2-microglobulin concentration during the hemodialysis procedure are responsible for a greater propensity to tissue deposition. Alternatively, it may be that this syndrome is as prevalent in the peritoneal dialysis population, but has not been looked for with the same degree of vigilance. It is intriguing, however, that improvement in the hemodialysis-associated amyloid syndrome has been reported by changing the patients to CAPD [185].

1.11. Kidney stones and oxalate metabolism

The development of kidney stones in patients on CAPD is not a rare occurence. In one survey [186], ten of 186 CAPD patients (5.4%) passed renal calculi after six to nine months on CAPD. Half of these stones were composed of calcium oxalate monohydrate and the rest were made of protein matrix alone or calcium apatite. Metabolic investigation of CAPD patients has demonstrated that, while the total excretion of calcium and oxalate is necessarily diminished, the concentration of oxalate is significantly elevated compared to normals and the ionic calcium concentration in the urine is lower than normal. However, the calcium oxalate activity product is in the 'labile' region and varies according to the urinary ionic calcium concentration. This dependence upon urinary calcium is different from normals, where the calcium oxalate activity product depends upon the concentration of both urinary oxalate and calcium. Therefore, although the urine ionic calcium concentration is low in renal failure, relative increases in this level will significantly influence the activity product and lead to crystallization. The administration of 1,25-dihydroxyvitamin D_3 correlates with the urine ionic calcium concentration [186] and could be considered a risk factor for stone formation. With the move from aluminum-containing to calcium-containing phosphate binders, it will be interesting to see whether the incidence of calcium-containing stones increases in CAPD patients.

1.11.1. Hyperoxalemia
As alluded to above, the total excretion of oxalate decreases

in renal failure, leading to accumulation of oxalate in the blood and consequent hyperoxalemia. The hyperoxalemia may result in precipitation of calcium oxalate in the body organs such as heart and kidney [187]. In CAPD, plasma oxalate levels are three to five times higher than normal [188] and are equivalent to predialysis levels in hemodialysis patients [189]. Because of its low molecular weight (90 daltons), it is rapidly cleared by hemodialysis and post-dialysis levels are 40% lower. On the other hand, the amount cleared by CAPD is about 300 μmol/day, similar to the amount synthesized daily. Therefore, CAPD may maintain a steady state plasma oxalate concentration, but at levels higher than normal.

There is a correlation between plasma oxalate concentration and urea nitrogen appearance rate, suggesting that dietary protein is an important source of oxalate in CAPD patients not taking ascorbic acid [189]. Patients with renal failure taking excessive vitamin C supplements may develop hyperoxalemia and it is recommended that patients on hemodialysis or peritoneal dialysis take only enough ascorbic acid to replace losses. The daily dose should not exceed 100 mg [188].

1.12. Hemoperitoneum

The appearance of blood-tinged peritoneal dialysate is a common finding in CAPD patients [150]. It is usually benign and disappears spontaneously. As little as 2 mls of blood can render one liter of dialysate noticeably blood-tinged [190] and so small bleeds in the peritoneal cavity are apparent in this population, whereas, of course, they would rarely come to medical attention in patients not on peritoneal dialysis. For example, peritoneal bleeding has been noted after extracorporeal lithotripsy in a CAPD patient [191].

The association of hemoperitoneum with menstruation has been noted [150, 192–194]. Blood can appear in the peritoneal cavity via two mechanisms: (1) the shedding of ectopic endometrial tissue, i.e., endometriosis, into the peritoneum simultaneous with the shedding of the uterine endometrium, or (2) the movement of the shed uterine tissue and blood both out of the cervix and in 'retrograde' fashion through the fallopian tubes into the peritoneal cavity. Surveys of menstruating women have found that the majority experience hemoperitoneum [192, 194]. The peritoneal bleeding may start a few days prior to the appearance of menses [192]. Indeed, it has been observed that the pattern of menstrual pain parallels the timing of peritoneal bleeding and it has been suggested that peritoneal blood may be an important cause of dysmenorrhea [192]. Hemoperitoneum may also occur at mid-cycle, associated with ovulation [194]. The ovulatory bleeding can be suppressed with anovulant medication. The related formation of ovarian cysts and their rupture may also cause hemoperitoneum [194]. No evidence of endometriosis has been found on laparotomy in CAPD patients [192]. An association between bloody dialysate and staphylococcal epidermidis peritonitis suggests that the bloody dialysate may provide a rich growth medium for intraperitoneal bacteria. Moreover, the retrograde movement of blood from the uterine cavity through the fallopian tubes may passively carry bacteria residing in these structures into the peritoneal cavity and lead to peritonitis [193, 195].

There are non-gynecologic causes of hemoperitoneum. In peritoneal dialysis patients, hemoperitoneum has been observed in association with cholecystitis, colonoscopy [190] and bleeding bowel adhesions [196]. Ischemic bowel is another important cause. In these 'surgical' causes of hemoperitoneum, the outcome is not nearly so benign. Bleeding may be brisk or even fatal [196]. Previous intra-abdominal or pelvic irradiation may render these tissues particularly friable and prone to hemorrhage. Placing a peritoneal catheter in patients with previous abdominal or pelvic irradiation should be weighed against the potential risk for tissue trauma and bleeding [197].

1.13. Chyloperitoneum

An interesting and unusual complication of peritoneal dialysis is the leakage of intestinal chyle into peritoneal fluid. This phenomenon is more commonly seen after intra-abdominal trauma or in association with intraperitoneal neoplasm [198, 199]. However, chyloperitoneum was reported in a 63-yr-old male on IPD 4 months after Tenckhoff catheter insertion [200] and in a 8-yr-old girl receiving CAPD 3 to 4 days after undergoing medical insertion of a Tenckhoff catheter [201]. The diagnosis was suggested by the white, milky appearance of the dialysate in the absence of infection. Lipoprotein electrophoresis identified high density lipoproteins and chylomicrons in the young girl. In the man, it was noted that the dialysis fluid separated into two layers upon standing and the supernatant layer stained positively for fat with Sudan III and dissolved in ether. The triglyceride level of the dialysate was greater than the plasma triglyceride level, which is characteristic of intestinal lymph [199]. Both groups of authors postulated a disruption of the abdominal lymph flow from bowel to thoracic duct. In the acute case, because the chyloperitoneum occurred so soon after catheter insertion, it was suggested that the catheter or the trocar may have severed a major lymph vessel [201]. In the case where the chyloperitoneum did not occur until 4 months after catheter insertion, the etiology is less clear. The catheter could still have eventually severed a lymphatic vessel. Alternatively, the authors speculated that the patients's previous multiple episodes of peritonitis could have resulted in the formation of peritoneal adhesions, leading to lymphatic obstruction and chyloperitoneum [200].

While it is not frequently reported, chyloperitoneum should be kept in mind in the differential diagnosis of 'culture-negative' peritonitis.

2. THE FATE OR 'UNNATURAL HISTORY' OF UREMIC ORGAN DYSFUNCTION IN PATIENTS RECEIVING PERITONEAL DIALYSIS

2.1. Hematologic disorders

2.1.1. Anemia and red cell metabolism
It is an almost consistent observation that there is improvement in the anemia of chronic renal failure when patients are placed on CAPD or changed from hemodialysis or IPD to CAPD [202–212]. One patient has even developed overt polycythemia on CAPD and then became anemic when changed to hemodialysis [213]. Most of these studies have found that the improvement in anemia occurs within the first 6 months of CAPD [205, 207, 210], but can be followed by a subsequent decline in hemoglobin concentration to a new steady-state level [206]. Unlike the rapid rise in hematocrit more commonly reported, others [209] have found the increase to be gradual and still ongoing at one year, while one study could not demonstrate any change in the hematocrit over time in patients on CAPD [214].

Increased hemoglobin concentration may result from increased red cell mass, decreased plasma volume, or both. Increased red cell mass in patients placed on CAPD could be the result of improved erythropoiesis, possibly as a result of better removal of uremic toxins functioning as erythropoietic inhibitors. Alternatively, an increased red cell mass could be due to improved red cell metabolism leading to less hemolysis and prolonged red cell survival. Finally, better control of extracellular fluid colume by more constant ultrafiltration in CAPD as compared to intermittent PD or hemodialysis could lead to increased hematocrit solely on the basis of hemoconcentration.

Most studies have found the increased hemoglobin concentration to be the result of increased red cell mass [202, 205, 210, 212] associated with a significant [202, 205] or insignificant [210, 212] change in plasma volume. Only one recent study [204] found no increase in red cell mass, and the increased hematocrit correlated with decreased plasma volume. However, the method of measurement of red cell mass was different than in the other studies where different results were obtained.

The increased red cell mass may result from improved erythropoiesis or improved red cell survival. There is no evidence for increased erythropoietin secretion as a cause for the improved erythropoiesis [202, 206, 208, 210]. It may be that CAPD, compared to IPD or hemodialysis, affords more efficient removal of inhibitors of erythropoiesis in the 'middle molecule' range. The uremic toxins inhibit the earliest precursors in the erythroid cell line, the burst-forming units (BFU-E), and colony-forming units (CFU-E). Adding sera from either hemodialysis or CAPD patients leads to inhibition of CFU-E formation [208]. The degree of inhibition correlates in a negative fashion with the hematocrit, suggesting that it is this inhibition of erythropoiesis which is mainly responsible for the anemia of dialysis patients. In contrast, Summerfield [215] found that whereas plasma from uremic non-dialyzed patients inhibited BFU-E and CFU-E activity, sera from patients on CAPD or hemodialysis did not have this effect. Another study demonstrated improvement in BFU-E activity with CAPD [206]. After starting CAPD, sera from patients causes progressive increases in proliferation of CFU-E [207]. These studies, taken together, suggest that the increased hematocrit in patients undergoing CAPD results from increased erythropoiesis secondary to the removal of inhibitors of this process at the stem cell level.

Another potential contribution to the improvement of anemia in CAPD patients comes from increased red cell longevity. Increased red cell survival during CAPD has been demonstrated in several studies [202, 212, 214]. The mean red cell half-life in the populations stdied has changed from below normal to within the lower end of the normal range

(25–26 days) [212, 214], while only one study found the mean red cell survival on CAPD to remain well below normal (20 days) [216]. In this report, the study interval was only 2 weeks, which may have led to a spuriously low value [217].

If the greater half-life of red cells on CAPD is real, the improvement could be the result of better red cell metabolism leading to increased resistance to oxidative stress and consequent hemolysis. Unlike patients on hemodialysis, patients on CAPD demonstrate normal activity of the pentose phosphate shunt, hexose monophosphate shunt and glucose-6-phosphate dehydrogenase [216, 218]. This normal activity provides greater resistance to oxidant stress. Whereas vitamin E in the red cell is recruited as an anti-oxidant in hemodialysis patients, leading to diminished erythrocyte levels of this vitamin, the red cell vitamin E levels in CAPD are normal or even greater than normal. Moreover, there is less evidence of peroxidation of polyunsaturated fatty acids in the red cell membrane, a marker of oxidant stress, in CAPD patients compared to the hemodialysis population [218].

In addition to improved anemia, there is evidence that patients on CAPD have an advantage with respect to tissue oxygenation. The hemoglobin-oxygen dissociation curve has been demonstrated to be shifted to the right; that is, for a given partial pressure of oxygen, there is increased oxygen delivery to the tissues [219]. The shift is not the result of increased erythrocyte 2,3-diphosphoglycerate (2,3-DPG) as this level is normal [219] or even decreased [202]. Usually anemia stimulates 2,3-DPG production by red cells. It may be that the mild metabolic and erythrocyte acidosis, in combination with lower phosphate levels in CAPD, dampens production of 2,3-DPG [219]. Another explanation may be decreased activity of the red cell enzyme phosphofructokinase. There is a decrease in phosphofructokinase and products past this step in the glycolytic pathway, including 2,3-DPG [202]. Others, however, have not been able to demonstrate a shift in the hemoglobin-oxygen dissociation curve [202], except in patients recently transferred to CAPD from hemodialysis [220].

There is a progressive decline in serum ferritin concentration in the first months of CAPD [205, 206, 210, 211]. This fall is consistent with improved erythropoiesis and iron utilization. Ferritin losses into the dialysate are negligible [211] and do not account for the falling levels. The administration or iron supplements may mitigate this fall [206]. There is a significant correlation between stainable iron on bone marrow specimens and serum ferritin. All but one patient in a cohort of CAPD patients with adequate stores of iron had serum ferritin levels greater than 96 ng/ml, and all patients with iron deficiency had serum ferritin levels less than 70 ng/ml [221]. Others, however, suggest that serum ferritin levels may not be a reliable marker of iron deficiency in CAPD patients [222].

No change over time in vitamin B_{12} levels has been shown in patients on CAPD [210], whereas a downward trend in serum but not red blood cell folate levels has been found [210, 223].

Anemia and neutropenia associated with copper deficiency has been reported in a CAPD patient. It was postulated but not proven that the loss of ceruloplasmin-bound copper in the dialysate led to the copper deficiency

and hematologic abnormalities [224].

2.1.2. Eosinophilia

Three studies have examined blood eosinophilia in patients on peritoneal dialysis [225–227]. In a group of mostly IPD patients, more than half had at least one episode of eosinophilia over a mean observation period of 14 months. No patient had sustained eosinophilia. The increased eosinophil count was associated with a high total white blood count, peritoneal catheter insertion, and resolving peritonitis [226]. The authors suggested that antibiotics or tubing changes could play a role in the eosinophilia associated with resolving peritonitis. Indeed, eosinophilia correlated with increased tubing changes in CCPD and CAPD patients also [227]. It is likely, however, that more blood counts are performed around the catheter insertion and peritonitis periods and so the statistical chance of detecting eosinophilia is simply increased. However, the eosinophilia may be a reaction to the dialysis catheter [225]. Alternatively, the eosinophilia may be related to abnormal eosinophil kinetics in uremia, or occur secondary to abnormalities in other immune functions such as T-cell function, or result from exposure to allergens such as ethylene oxide used for tubing sterilization [226, 227]. Interestingly, blood eosinophilia predicted eosinophilia of the peritoneal effluent (> 10% of peritoneal white count), but not vice versa.

2.1.3. Iron overload

For peritoneal dialysis patients suffering from iron overload, desferoxamine has been shown to be effective in removing iron. Just over half of the desferoxamine instilled in the peritoneal cavity is absorbed during a typical dwell time [228]. The intraperitoneal administration of the chelator in a concentration of 250 mg/l leads to removal of iron complexed to desferoxamine. The amount of iron removed is proportional to the number of desferoxamine infusions given. For example, giving 1250 mg of desferoxamine daily caused removal of 99 mg of elemental iron per week. Intravenous infusion of identical amounts of chelator caused removal of 50 mg of iron per week on hemodialysis and 78 mg per week on CAPD [228]. The authors postulated that the iron-chelator complex, with a molecular weight of 617, which falls into the 'middle molecule' range, is removed more efficiently by CAPD than hemodialysis. Other investigators have confirmed the efficient iron removal in peritoneal dialysis patients using either intraperitoneal desferoxamine [229, 230], or desferoxamine by the intramuscular or subcutaneous route [229]. Intravenous administration of desferoxamine can also lead to sizable losses of iron (and aluminum) in the stool [231]. The iron loss by this route is the result of biliary excretion of desferoxamine metabolites which chelate hepatic iron. Therefore, the authors postulate that the stool iron and peritoneal dialysate iron losses may originate from different (i.e., hepatic and non-hepatic) pools [231]. There has been no evidence of long-term toxicity of desferoxamine in peritoneal dialysis patients. However, the use of high doses (2 grams a day IP for 3 days) has been associated with an acute reaction consisting of gastrointestinal symptoms, shivering, vertigo and headaches [232]. It is recommended that lower doses be used, such as 500 mg by intraperitoneal route daily.

2.1.4. Platelets, coagulation and bleeding

Peritoneal dialysis and hemodialysis can improve the platelet dysfunction and prolonged bleeding time associated with uremia [233]. The improvement has been attributed to the removal of uremic toxins [234], although more specific mechanisms are not well-defined. For example, the improvement in the platelet release reaction seen after dialysis correlates with decreases in plasma guanidinosuccinic acid and phenol concentration, which have been postulated to inhibit this reaction [235].

The bleeding time in 11 uremic patients, 8 of whom had been previously maintained on hemodialysis, improved from a mean of 11.2 minutes to 5.8 minutes after an average of 3 months on CAPD [236]. Moreover, bleeding time normalized in six out of seven patients in whom it was prolonged prior to CAPD. Platelet aggregation as induced by ristocetin and adrenaline (but not collagen) improved. There was a significant increase in the platelet count from 195 000 to 311 000 $\times$ 10^6/l over the same period. The improved bleeding time, however, did not correlate with the increased platelet count. The improvement in platelet function seen in presumably well-dialyzed hemodialysis patients upon their transfer to CAPD was ascribed to better removal of middle molecular weight platelet toxins or to the absence of exposure to toxic factors during hemodialysis. These factors include the dialysis membrane and routine heparinization [236]. Peritoneal dialysis also leads to improvement in the biochemical aspect of platelet function, including thromboxane and malondialdehyde production in response to arachidonic acid [237].

CAPD not only corrects the bleeding diathesis of uremia, but may actually produce a hypercoagulable state. Patients on peritoneal dialysis have a higher prevalence of thrombocytosis [238]. Moreover, the platelet count increases with increasing duration of PD. The higher platelet counts are associated with lower hematocrit and ferritin levels [238]. Albumin has been demonstrated to inhibit collagen and ADP-induced platelet aggregation [239] and the platelets in CAPD patients may be hyperaggregable as a result of decreased albumin concentration [240]. Indeed, many CAPD patients with hypoalbuminemia have platelet aggregation responses greater than controls. The authors suggest that the low serum albumin levels leave more arachidonic acid unbound and hence available for uptake into platelets. Once taken into platelets, the arachidonic acid is metabolized to thromboxane A_2 which enhances platelet aggregation.

Intermittent peritoneal dialysis causes a significant increase in plasma antithrombin III levels post-dialysis, which may protect against thrombotic events. The elevation of antithrombin III may be the result of removal of a dialyzable substance which suppresses its production or release by liver as well as endothelial cells [241]. The losses of antithrombin III into dialysate (during CAPD) are of the same magnitude as urinary losses in nephrotic syndrome [242]. However, the plasma levels of antithrombin III are higher in patients on CAPD than in nephrotic patients [242].

Patients on CAPD demonstrate increased plasma levels of both fibrinogen and fibrin degradation products (FDP) when compared to normals [242]. The increased fibrinogen may be a non-specific response by the liver to inflammation or protein loss in the dialysate. The half-life of fibrinogen is reduced, consistent with increased FDP levels, suggesting activation of the coagulation pathway. The loss of fibrinogen into the dialysate is minimal and does not account for the decreased half-life. To further aggravate the hypercoagulable state, fibrinolysis may be markedly impaired, particularly in patients on intermittent peritoneal dialysis. This deterioration in fibrinolytic activity is attributed to poor removal of low MW inhibitors of fibrinolysis and relatively efficient removal of high MW activators of fibrinolysis. In fact, dialysis effluent produces areas of lysis on fibrin plates [243]. Therefore, increased numbers of platelets, platelet aggregation which may be greater than normal, dialysate loss of antithrombin III, and impaired fibrinolysis may contribute to hypercoagulability in peritoneal dialysis patients.

2.2. Gastrointestinal function

2.2.1. Pancreas

Patients on peritoneal dialysis may be at special risk for the development of pancreatitis. Peritoneal dialysate can gain access to the lesser sac of the peritoneal cavity via the epiploic foramen. The posterior surface of the lesser sac is also the anterior surface of the pancreas. Therefore, any factor in the dialysate can potentially irritate the pancreas. Proposed irritants include high glucose concentration, toxic byproducts of the dialysate, bags, or tubing [244], acidic dialysate [245] and, of course, infected dialysate as seen in peritonitis [245, 246]. Rechallenge with peritoneal dialysate after its discontinuation has lead to recurrence of pancreatitis [247]. In addition, there may be a predilection for pseudocyst formation [245]. Patients on CAPD may face additional risk of pancreatitis because of the high prevalence of hypertriglyceridemia [248].

Diagnosis of pancreatitis may be difficult. It should be considered in cases of 'culture-negative' peritonitis, or if the abdominal pain associated with peritonitis fails to resolve or localizes in the upper abdomen. Hiccoughs may be present [249]. The serum amylase levels will rise with pancreatitis. However, because patients with chronic renal failure may have elevated amylase levels, there is overlap between the elevated levels seen in patients with renal failure and pancreatitis and those with renal failure alone [245]. Serum lipase levels may also increase [247], but both the amylase and lipase levels may be normal [246]. Hypoglycemia and glucose intolerance can develop as in non-uremic patients [244, 246]. Ultrasound and CT scanning may demonstrate an engorged, edematous pancreas [244, 247], or pseudocyst formation. Unfortunately, these studies are also frequently normal [244, 245]. Overall, the mortality is high with the condition, not least because of the difficulty in making the diagnosis in patients receiving peritoneal dialysis.

2.2.2. Hepatobiliary system

There are few reported hepatic complications in peritoneal dialysis. We recently described a unique hepatic lesion in CAPD patients receiving intraperitoneal insulin [249]. A layer of fat is deposited just under the hepatic capsule exposed to the peritoneal cavity. The thickness of this fatty layer correlates with the degree of obesity, as well as the dose of intraperitoneal insulin. We proposed that insulin in the peritoneal dialysate causes locally increased concentration of this hormone at the capsule and subcapsular hepatocytes. In the face of insulin deficiency, free fatty acids are delivered to the liver where they are re-esterified in the presence of high insulin concentrations under the hepatic capsule. There is no apparent hepatic dysfunction with this lesion, although, in one case, steatonecrosis was present. A survey of CAPD patients has demonstrated only transient and mild elevation of hepatic enzymes usually associated with a known cause such as use of hepatotoxic drugs [250].

The liver is at risk for abscess formation in the face of bacterial peritonitis and this diagnosis should be considered in cases of persistent peritonitis. Ultrasound may be normal and exploratory laparotomy warranted [251]. Non A, non-B hepatitis is a risk in patients on PD receiving blood transfusions [252].

A survey of 114 CAPD patients [253] has shown a high incidence of gallstones. Using ultrasound screening, 23% of patients had evidence of gallstones or a previous cholecystectomy. Eight patients needed cholecystectomy while on CAPD, usually for acute cholecystitis. The surgery proceeded uneventfully and 5 of the 8 needed hemodialysis during prolonged post-operative drainage. Eventually, all 8 patients were able to return to CAPD. Cholecystitis may be associated with peritonitis [253] or hemoperitoneum [190].

2.2.3. Colonic complications
There have been infrequent reports of ischemic colitis or necrotizing enteritis as complications of IPD [254] and CAPD [53, 255]. Hypotension with consequent bowel hypoperfusion is the probable etiology, as it is in patients with ischemic colitis not on peritoneal dialysis. However,

the development of ischemic bowel in a 6-yr-old child on IPD with marked improvement upon transfer to hemodialysis suggests that peritoneal dialysis itself may play a role in the bowel lesion [254]. What role the increased abdominal pressure or use of hypertonic solutions in PD might play in contributing to the development of ischemic colitis is unclear. Marked GI bleeding from dilated submucosal vessels in the bowel associated with the use of hypertonic dextrose solutions has been reported. When on hemodialysis no such bleeding occurred. It was suggested that peritoneal dialysis provoked mesenteric vasodilatation which increased the calibre of the submucosal vessels and led to the bleeding [256].

2.3. Endocrine function

2.3.1. Thyroid function
Many authors have described the association of abnormal thyroid tests and uremia [257, 258]. The etiology of the abnormalities of thyroid function is complex, and likely results from a combination of factors, which include abnormal protein metabolism, altered peripheral conversion of T4 and hypothalamic-pituitary abnormalities. More recently, thyroid function has been examined in peritoneal dialysis patients, with particular emphasis on those undergoing CAPD. The results have been quite varied (see Table 3).

In almost all the studies, total T4 and T3 measurements are decreased, compared to controls. However, decreased total hormone measurement results from either decreased hormone production (or increased hormone catabolism), or a diminished amount of carrier protein. Therefore, it is important to examine concentrations of free hormone

Table 3. Summary of results of thyroid function tests in peritoneal dialysis. For description, see text. TBG, thyroid-binding globulin

Ref.	Total T4	Total T3	Free T4	Free T3	T3 Resin uptake	Reverse T3	TSH	TRH stimulation	Other
259	↓	↓	↑	normal		↑	↑		
260	↓	↓	↑	normal		↑	↑	delayed TSH response	TBG normal
261	↓	↓	depends on assay used			low normal	normal		
262	↓	↓	normal		↑	↑	↑		↓TBG
263	↓	↓	normal				↑ at start, returns to normal		T4 not detectable in dialysate
264	↓	↓↓	↓				↑	blunted response	
265	normal	↓	↓				normal	blunted response	
266	normal	↓				normal	normal		30% of normal T4 production lost in dialysate
267	↓	low normal					high normal		
271								blunted and delayed TSH response	
272	↓ in 2/12			↓ in 2/12	normal		normal		

which would not be significantly influenced by carrier protein production or loss. Studies looking at free hormone concentration have shown the T3 levels to be the same as normals [259, 260]. However, the free T4 concentration has been found to be either increased [259–261], the same [262, 263] or decreased [264, 265] when compared with controls. Indeed, Thysen *et al.* [261] showed that free T4 measurements in the same population of patients were either higher or lower than normal, depending on which assay was used.

In many cases of non-thyroidal illness, there is an increased peripheral conversion of thyroxine to 'reverse' T3 and this has recently been demonstrated in the CAPD population [259, 260, 262]. Another potential source of alteration in thyroid function in CAPD patients may involve loss of thyroxine into the dialysate. Gavin *et al.* [266] found that dialysate thyroxine loss averaged about 29 μg a day, which amounted to 30% of the normal production rate. On the other hand, Selgas *et al.* [263] could not detect any thyroxine in the dialysate. However, if CAPD does cause ongoing loss of thyroxine, this could 'drive' the pituitary to compensate with increased production of thyroid-stimulating hormone. Many of the recent studies have found that TSH levels are either elevated, or in the upper range of normal, compared to controls [259, 260, 262, 264, 267]. A retrospective analysis of 104 CAPD patients at the Toronto Western Hospital [268] showed that the mean thyroid-stimulating hormone level increased significantly during the course of CAPD. Therefore, it is intriguing to postulate that ongoing losses of thyroxine in the dialysate lead to a state of 'compensated hypothyroidism' with increased pituitary output of thyroid-stimulating hormone.

It has previously been reported in patients with nephrotic syndrome that urinary losses of thyroid-binding globulin can contribute to low total T4 levels [269]. In the same way, it has been postulated that there may be a loss of this binding globulin in the peritoneal dialysate. However, this has been recenlty investigated by Inaba *et al.* [267] who found that the loss of thyroid-binding globulin in the peritoneal dialysate amounted to only about one-sixth of the daily production of this protein and was easily compensated. There were no differences in thyroid-binding globulin levels between CAPD patients and controls. This result was confirmed by other investigators [260]. To account for the low total T4 in the face of normal TBG levels, a role for desialyated TBG has been postulated in CAPD patients. This moiety binds T4 with about only one-tenth the affinity of the normal TBG [270], but reacts fully in a TBG assay. This, however. remains to be proven.

The TRH stimulation test, which involves the injection of thyrotropin-releasing hormone, has been used as a measure of pituitary function. In patients on CAPD, the TRH stimulation test has uniformly shown a delayed TSH output from the pituitary, and diminished maximum TSH levels [260, 264, 265, 271]. This suggests that, in addition to the other factors mentioned, there is an alteration in the hypothalamic-pituitary axis leading to submaximal pituitary response to TRH stimulation.

Finally, it has been suggested that the use of Poviodine during the intraperitoneal installation of catheters or for exit site care has led to a significant iodine load in the CAPD population, leading to hypothyroidism via the Wolf-Chaikoff effect. Two patients on CAPD have been described who developed hypothyroidism soon after starting CAPD and this was associated with increased iodine levels [266]. One patient remained hypothyroid with the withdrawal of the iodine, but the other patient showed a return to euthyroid status after withdrawal of Poviodine and consequent fall in serum iodine levels. However, Gardner *et al.* [272] could not show any correlation between plasma iodine and thyroid function tests, although there was a significant correlation between plasma iodine and TSH levels in hemodialysis, but not CAPD patients.

In summary, although there is variability in the results, the consensus is that in CAPD patients there is a decrease in total T4 and total T3, probably related to changes in thyroid-binding globulin or an altered affinity between thyroxine and its binding globulin. Results of free T4 are variable, depending on the assay used. There is an increased circulating amount of reverse T3. Finally, the TSH is at the high normal or elevated range and this is associated with a blunted response to TRH stimulation. It is suggested, although not proven, that TSH may be stimulated by ongoing losses of thyroxine in the dialysate.

2.3.2. Pituitary function

Prolactin. Serum levels of prolactin are elevated in CAPD patients [273–275] and hyperprolactinemia has been identified as one of the many causes of infertility and sexual dysfunction that occurs in uremia (reviewed in 275). In a recent survey, 73% of CAPD patients had an elevated serum prolactin level which was not significantly different from the prevalence in hemodialysis [275]. In assessing prolactin levels, it is important to consider whether the patient is on any medications, such as alphamethyldopa, metoclopramide, or antipsychotic agents, which may affect its metabolism [275]. Despite elevated basal levels of prolactin, the normal rise in plasma levels seen with insulin-induced hypoglycemia or TRH is blunted, suggesting other disorders in regulation of pituitary secretion of this hormone [274].

Growth hormone. Basal levels of growth hormone are not significantly different between CAPD patients and hemodialysis patients [276]. The growth hormone response to insulin-induced hypoglycemia is greater in hemodialysis patients than those on CAPD. Indeed, seven of ten CAPD patients had impaired response to hypoglycemia. It has been suggested that clearance of growth hormone may be greater in CAPD patients or, alternatively, elevated somatostatin levels may inhibit the growth hormone response [276]. On the other hand, perhaps as a response to continuous glucose loading, the paradoxical rise in growth hormone seen in response to glucose in uremic patients is corrected in CAPD patients [277].

Gonadotrophins. Studies have found levels of follicle-stimulating hormone (FSH) and luteinizing hormone (LH) to be elevated in both CAPD and hemodialysis patients when compared to normals [274, 278]. However, there is no difference in these levels between the two dialysis groups. Elevated levels of gonadotrophins could be the result of primary gonadal failure with diminished feedback of sex hormones to the pituitary, or the result of some intrinsic pituitary dysfunction. The fact that injection of the hypothalamic luteinizing releasing hormone (LRH) leads to a normal increment in pituitary secretion of FSH and LH suggests that primary gonadal dysfunction is responsible for elevated levels of gonadotrophins [278]. Studies in male CAPD patients have found serum testosterone levels to be less than normal [278], although another survey found no decrease in mean testosterone levels in CAPD patients [274]. However, both studies found testosterone levels to be higher in men receiving CAPD than in men on hemodialysis [274, 278]. Less than 0.1% of daily testosterone production is lost into the dialysate [278].

Although plasma levels of testosterone are higher in CAPD versus hemodialysis patients, the incidence of impotence is the same. A survey of impotence in males on dialysis showed those with impotence to have higher FSH levels, suggestive of primary gonadal dysfunction. However, sexual dysfunction is not reliably corrected with the administration of exogenous testosterone. Impotence on the basis of vascular insufficiency could be implicated in only six percent of patients [274]. It is clear that the causes of sexual dysfunction in patients on dialysis are many. These include disorders in gonadal function, prolactin secretion, medications, other unspecified uremic toxins and the anemia, fatigue and malaise found in many of these patients.

Reproductive function. Chronic renal failure is frequently associated with menstrual irregularities, anovulatory cycles and ovarian cystic disease [279]. These abnormalities are not easily reversible during chronic hemodialysis. If it does resume, menstruation is irregular and complicated by memenometrorrhagia and anovulatory cycles [280, 281]. Cycles are associated with an abnormal luteal phase and inadequate progesterone production [282]. Pregnancy has been described in hemodialysis patients [282–288], but is a rare event.

Many women on CAPD have normal menstruation with ovulatory cycles [289], and some have become pregnant [290–292]. One survey found that 86% of women on CAPD, as opposed to 25% of women on hemodialysis, had regular menses. Moreover, upon transfer to CAPD, two amenorrheic women resumed regular menstruation. Vaginal smears show evidence of estrogen effect [293].

Similar to the studies in males, gonadal dysfunction has been demonstrated in uremic women which does not respond to gonadotrophins [294]. Once again, many factors may be involved, including hypothalamic dysfunction [294, 295], and elevated prolactin levels [279, 295, 296].

2.4. Renin, angiotensin, aldosterone and blood pressure

In many patients, hypertension becomes more easily treatable upon commencing CAPD [297–299]. Most of the hypotensive response occurs in the first weeks on CAPD, but a further fall in blood pressure occurs during the first year [297, 299]. Presumably, the improved blood pressure is to a large extent the result of correction of hypervolemia in the end-stage renal failure patient. Therefore, the mechanism of improvement of hypertension is no different than that seen in hemodialysis patients who achieve good control of salt and water balance [299].

A prospective study of patients during the first six months of CAPD showed a significant increase in plasma renin activity during the study period [298]. Other investigators have confirmed elevated levels of plasma renin activity and active renin in CAPD patients, and these values are significantly higher than those on hemodialysis [300]. There is a parallel increase in plasma aldosterone which correlates with the rise in plasma renin activity [298]. Plasma aldosterone and 18-hydroxycorticosterone levels are higher in CAPD than hemodialysis patients [300]. Despite the observation of large daily losses of renin substrate into the peritoneal effluent [301], no change in the level of serum renin substrate over time has been discerned [298]. Studies after one year of CAPD demonstrate diminished pressor response to infusion of angiotensin II [298]. These findings can be reconciled by postulating ongoing salt and water removal with CAPD, leading to euvolemia or hypovolemia with its consequent normalization of blood pressure and stimulation of the renin-angiotensin-aldosterone axis. The diminished pressor response to angiotensin II is probably a non-specific result of ongoing stimulation of this system by salt and water removal similar to that seen in, for example, Bartter's syndrome [302]. Alternatively, it has been suggested that the diminished sensitivity of the vascular tree to vasoconstrictors could contribute to improved blood pressure control [298].

Some patients on CAPD develop symptomatic orthostatic hypotension. This effect may result from excessive removal of salt and water and consequent hypovolemia. Furthermore, during the first few months of CAPD, patients often experience a return of appetite and increased food intake. Failure to adjust the 'dry weight' upwards to keep pace with the increased body mass may result in extracellular fluid volume depletion. Diminished plasma oncotic pressure can result in contraction of the plasma volume in the face of extracellular fluid volume overload and edema. Diminished plasma volume may contribute to orthostatic symptoms in a subset of patients. As discussed elsewhere in this chapter, autonomic neuropathy can prevent a normal baroreceptor-mediated response to orthostatic hypotension.

We have treated patients with oral sodium loading, in doses ranging between 85 to 170 millimoles per day. Dialysate is chosen to keep the body weight unchanged. On this regimen, blood pressure increases to more tolerable levels. Plasma norepinephrine levels increase, as does the pressor reactivity to the infused norepinephrine. We suggested that the increased blood pressure was the result of shift of water from the intracellular to extracellular fluid compartments secondary to the osmotic load of solute (sodium) limited mostly to the extracellular space. What role the increased norepinephrine levels and augmented vascular sensitivity to norepinephrine plays is unclear [303].

Besides salt loading, other strategies to treat orthostatic hypotension include increasing the dry weight, changing to an intermittent dialysis regimen and, of course, careful assessment of the patient's medications to ensure that none of the drugs are contributing towards the hypotensive response.

2.5. Renal osteodystrophy

Renal osteodystrophy becomes established early in the

course of renal failure and its incidence and severity increases with the progression of uremia [304, 305]. The prolongation of life in patients with end-stage renal disease by chronic dialysis allows renal osteodystrophy more time to evolve. In addition, the disease process may change in response to dialysis-related factors, such as concentration of calcium or aluminum content of the dialysate.

While we know much about the evolution of renal osteodystrophy in patients undergoing chronic hemodialysis [305], studies of this disease in patients undergoing continuous ambulatory peritoneal dialysis have been of short duration and have provided conflicting results [306–308].

In 1980 we described the evolution of renal osteodystrophy in our patients on short-term CAPD; at that time we had studied 28 patients on CAPD for 6–23 months. The radiologically-diagnosed osteitis fibrosa element of renal osteodystrophy progressed in these CAPD patients, whereas osteomalacia seemed to improve. At that time we did no studies of bone histology. The mean plasma iPTH level, which remained high, was accompanied by high levels of serum alkaline phosphatase. Arterial calcifications did not progress [307].

A more recent study [309] updated the status of renal osteodystrophy in 27 patients at our hospital maintained on CAPD for over three years. Ten men and 17 women with a mean age of 49.5 years had been on CAPD for a mean of 45 months. Dialysate calcium was 6 mg%. For all the patients oral dietary calcium intake was low (500 mg/day). Al $(OH)_3$, vitamin D and/or $1,25(OH)_2D_3$ were prescribed to maintain serum calcium and phosphorus at normal levels. Patients were divided into two groups according to the radiological findings at the beginning of treatment. Group A (10 patients) included those who had no subperiosteal resorption, and Group B (17 patients) those with subperiosteal resorption at the initiation of CAPD. In Group A, the subperiosteal resorption grade remained normal in eight patients and progressed in two. In Group B, subperiosteal resorption remained unchanged or increased in 14, while it improved in the remaining three.

Two patients with no subperiosteal resorption (Group A) showed severe osteomalacia, with positive aluminum staining on bone biopsy. In two Group B patients, bone biopsy showed severe osteitis fibrosa, with negative aluminum staining. Of the 27 patients, five developed spontaneous fractures; these, however, healed with callus formation after adjustments in treatment. This study again confirmed the earlier observation that hyperparathyroidism persists in patients on long-term CAPD; this may be attributed to a low dialysate calcium and low oral calcium intake.

This was the first long-term study of renal osteodystrophy in CAPD patients. Most of the patients (17/27) had evidence of subperiosteal resorption at the beginning of CAPD and a similar number had abnormal subperiosteal resorption at the end of the study. There was good correlation between the mean level of iPTH and the severity of subperiosteal resorption – the iPTH being nearly normal in those with normal grades of subperiosteal resorption (Group A) throughout the study. However, osteomalacia was the main finding in the biopsies of two of these patients, both of whom had developed spontaneous fractures before biopsy examination; at the same time, both showed decreased bone-mineral mass and density in the radius. Generally, the dietary calcium of our patients was low, mainly because we were prescribing a low phosphorus diet which, by necessity, is low in calcium as well. Dietary calcium was the lowest in Group A2, who was receiving the highest mean amounts of vitamin D and $1,25(OH)_2D_3$, and who also had high plasma levels of iPTH and markedly increased subperiosteal resorption. It seems that, in the presence of low dietary calcium intake, high doses of $1,25(OH)_2D_3$ may increase serum calcium by increasing bone resorption. If this is correct, we may have to give supplemental calcium to these patients; however, the risk of severe constipation is high when calcium supplements are administered along with aluminum-containing phosphate binders.

A review of the literature on the effect of CAPD on the various biochemical, radiological and histological parameters of renal osteodystrophy shows various responses not only among various units, but also among patients within the same unit. These differences are the result of varying duration of CAPD in the patients studied and the heterogeneous protocols of calcium and vitamin D supplementation. The following is an attempt to summarize those observations agreed upon by most authors on this subject.

2.5.1. Biochemistry

Serum ionic or total calcium concentration (corrected for protein) is initially low, and normalizes after initiation of CAPD and remains within normal levels [310]. Serum phosphorus is easily controlled and patients on CAPD require smaller amounts of antacids [$CaCO_3$ or $Al(OH)_3$)] than hemodialysis patients [311–313].

Serum iPTH falls with time on CAPD [310, 313–315], except in those with autonomous hyperparathyroidism where PTH levels remain elevated and parathyroidectomy may be indicated. Despite this trend for improvement, PTH reaches normal levels in only a few patients and remains above the normal range in most [310].

Although up to 14% of the PTH produced daily is removed by CAPD, this is not sufficient by itself to control hyperparathyroidism. To control the elevated PTH levels in these patients, the serum calcium levels have to be maintained at high normal or slightly above-normal levels.

Most investigators have observed a gradual decline in serum $25(OH)D_3$ levels, probably due to the permeability of the peritoneal membrane to middle-sized proteins [316–318].

2.5.2. Radiology

Subperiosteal resorption of hyperparathyroidism has been reported to improve in some patients, but progress in others [309, 313, 315, 319].

Bone mineral content that is normal at the start of dialysis may decrease after one year of CAPD [314]. Spontaneous fractures may develop in a small number of patients, but usually heal with callus formation after adjustment of treatment.

Small vessel calcifications may develop or progress and have been found in 45% of non-diabetics on CAPD for over two years and 100% of diabetics [320]. Similar but less prevalent findings were reported by Cassidy *et al.* [321]

who observed small vessel calcifications developing in 20% of their patients, large vessel calcifications in 24% and soft-tissue calcification in 22%, while Zecchelli *et al.* [313] observed *de novo* appearance of vascular calcifications in only 2/17 patients on CAPD.

2.5.6. Histology

Osteitis fibrosa on bone bipsy seems to improve with CAPD [310, 313, 317, 321]. Similarly, osteomalacia improves with treatment, especially after administration of calcium and vitamin D supplements [310, 321, 322]. A reduction in the cancellous bone has been reported in some CAPD patients [314].

2.6. Aluminum, osteomalacia and CAPD

Increasing evidence has linked aluminum overload with osteomalacia [323–325]. Excess amounts may be deposited along unmineralized osteoid seams in patients with end-stage renal disease suffering from osteomalacia [323–325]. Accumulating evidence suggests that aluminum is causally related to this condition, although it is possible that aluminum is deposited secondary to some other tissue injury.

Aluminum overload may develop in patients with end-stage renal disease because of chronic ingestion of aluminum-containing antacids [326], or in patients on hemodialysis following exposure to dialysate containing substantial amounts of aluminum [327, 328].

At the 1983 meetings of the American Society of Nephrology, several speakers addressed the question of aluminum-associated osteomalacia in patients with end-stage renal disease: the significant points can be summarized as follows:

1) Normal aluminum levels are less than 10 mcg/l.

2) Most dialysis patients who develop aluminum-associated osteomalacia have levels in excess of 100 mcg/l.

3) Most dialysis patients who do not develop aluminum-associated osteomalacia have levels less than 50 mcg/l.

4) The risk of developing aluminum-associated osteomalacia can be estimated by measuring the increment in serum aluminum levels following the administration of desferoxamine [329, 330].

5) The incidence of aluminum-associated osteomalacia is high in hemodialysis patients. In a series of bone biopsies done on 131 unselected hemodialysis patients, 31 had osteomalacia. Twenty-nine of the latter had aluminum-associated osteomalacia and average serum aluminum levels of 170 mcg/l [331].

6) Aluminum-associated osteomalacia is a treatable disease; desferoxamine results in significant removal of excess aluminum stores and clinical improvement in the osteomalacia [324, 325].

The level of aluminum in commercial CAPD solutions is well below 20 mcg/l. Thus, CAPD patients are not exposed to dialysate containing significant quantities of aluminum. Furthermore, because of better phosphate control on CAPD, these patients usually require less phosphate binders than patients on hemodialysis. Therefore, CAPD patients are probably at less risk of developing aluminum-associated osteomalacia.

CAPD appears to remove aluminum more efficiently than hemodialysis [323]. In renal failure patients with aluminum levels greater than 100 mcg/l, CAPD removed 206 mcg of aluminum per day *versus* only 70–100 mcg during a four hour hemodialysis. Most of the aluminum in the circulation is bound to a low-molecular-weight protein (MW about 10 000). Thus, one would not expect significant aluminum removal during hemodialysis, whereas one would anticipate greater removal rates during CAPD.

Thus, the status of aluminum toxicity in patients on CAPD can be summarized as follows:

1) Aluminum has been strongly associated with osteomalacia in patients with end-stage renal disease.

2) The aluminum can be absorbed from the dialysis solution or from orally-administered aluminum hydroxide.

3) Since the concentrations in peritoneal dialysate are less than 20 mcg/l, there should be no significant aluminum absorption from that source.

4) CAPD patients are less likely to develop osteomalacia because the dialysate aluminum content is low and these patients tend to require lower doses of phosphate binders.

5) At the present time, the true incidence of osteomalacia or aluminum-related osteomalacia in patients on CAPD is unknown.

2.7. Treatment

Dialysate formulations should include calcium at a concentration of 1.75 mmol/l. For phosphate control, use of $CaCO_3$ at doses of 3–6 g/day seems to be adequate in most patients. If not, or if hypercalcemia develops, then small doses of $Al(OH)_3$ can be used. Large doses of the latter over long periods should be avoided, without monitoring of serum aluminum levels. Most CAPD patients have low or undetectable levels of $1,25(OH)_2D_3$ and, therefore, should be supplemented with this vitamin. We also feel that even though $1,25(OH)_2D_3$ is the active metabolite of vitamin D, these patients should receive adequate amounts of vitamin D_3, and maintain their serum $25(OH)D_3$ levels within the normal range.

2.8. Neurologic function

2.8.1. Peripheral nervous system

Preliminary reports initially suggested that peripheral neuropathy in patients on peritoneal dialysis was less severe than in patients on hemodialysis [332]. In contrast, we reported that peripheral neuropathy was more frequent in peritoneal dialysis than in hemodialysis patients [333]. A review of the literature at that time suggested that the different observations could be explained by pre-existing differences in the populations under study and different treatment regimens. From his review, Blumenkrantz concluded that nerve-conduction velocities do not change over time in either hemodialysis or peritoneal dialysis patients, except in those who are underdialyzed or severely malnourished [334].

Long-term studies of patients on CAPD would tend to support these observations. Patients on CAPD for one year or more show no significant change in motor nerve-conduction velocity [335]. In patients on CAPD for three years or longer, there is no significant change in motor or sensory nerve-conduction velocity in either diabetics or non-diabetics except for the ulnar nerve, where the motor nerve-conduction velocity decreased from a mean of 50.0 m/sec to 46.9 m/sec (p<0.02) by the end of the study [336]. In contrast, motor nerve-conduction velocity fell by about 5% in both CAPD and hemodialysis patients in another study after a mean follow-up of 30 months. Indeed, none of the 43 patients in this study demonstrated any improvement with time. Sensitivity to a vibratory stimulus decreased over time in CAPD but not in hemodialysis patients. Despite the results of these electrophysiologic tests, on clinical examination there was overall deterioration in the hemodialysis but not in the CAPD population [337].

There may be problems with interpretation of these studies. Results may vary depending on the mix of diabetics and non-diabetics, or males and females. There may have been selection bias in placing patients in one dialysis modality versus another. Finally, patients with worsening neuropathy as a reflection of deteriorating status may 'die out' over the course of the studies, leaving behind the patient with well-preserved peripheral nerve function.

2.8.2. Autonomic nervous system

Autonomic neuropathy has been proposed as a cause of hemodialysis-related hypotension [338]. However, hypotension in patients on CAPD has been attributed to salt and water removal and impaired vascular reactivity secondary to the resultant salt depletion [303]. If CAPD patients also have autonomic insufficiency, however, hypotension could result from this disturbance alone. Recent studies have demonstrated impaired Valsalva responses in non-diabetics on CAPD [339, 340]. In addition, other tests of autonomic function such as the diving reflex [339], deep breathing or prolonged standing [340] have also shown abnormal results. Not surprisingly, diabetics on CAPD demonstrated impaired responses to all autonomic tests [339]. Overall, it appears that the non-diabetic CAPD patients have normal sympathetic but impaired parasympathetic function, whereas the diabetic patients have evidence of both parasympathetic and sympathetic insufficiency [339]. On the other hand, the results in non-diabetics have been interpreted as being similar to those found in animals who have undergone partial baroreceptor deafferentiation, a sympathetic lesion [340]. Taken in sum, it appears that both non-diabetics and diabetics on CAPD demonstrate abnormalities in autonomic nervous system function, which could compromise maintenance of blood pressure under conditions of salt and water depletion.

2.8.3. Organic brain syndromes

The differential diagnosis of a confusional state in the peritoneal dialysis patient is extensive. Possibilities include uremia, abnormally high or low blood glucose concentrations, altered electrolyte concentrations, drug toxicity and aluminum intoxication with its dementing encephalopathy [341]. With the increasing use of calcium carbonate as an oral phosphate binder, hypercalcemia will likely become more prevalent. This diagnosis should be considered in the hospitalized patient receiving oral calcium. The non-compliant CAPD patient may be prescribed increasing doses of calcium carbonate to control hyperphosphatemia. When this patient actually receives this medication as prescribed in hospital, hypercalcemia may develop.

Dialysis dementia or dialysis encephalopathy is characterized by progressive neurological impairment, dysarthria, dyspraxia, dysphasia, mutism and myoclonus [341]. The syndrome is associated with 'fracturing osteomalacia' and microcytic anemia. The EEG shows paroxysmal slowing, diffuse rhythmical bursts, and diphasic or triphasic spiked delta waves. It has been suggested that aluminum intoxication is the cause of this syndrome [342]. Potential sources of aluminum include that in water used for hemodialysis and aluminum-containing antacids used as phosphate binders.

While this unfortunate syndrome is usually confined to chronic hemodialysis patients, dialysis dementia has also been described in patients on peritoneal dialysis [343, 344]. Indeed, higher aluminum levels have been found in sera of patients on IPD than in sera of patients on hemodialysis [345]. The explanation may relate to the acidic pH of peritoneal dialysate, which increases solubility and transport rate of Al across a membrane [341]. Therefore, for a given Al contamination of dialysate, more will potentially cross the peritoneal membrane during the early dialysate dwell while the peritoneal fluid is still acidic. Given the sporadic nature of this syndrome, however, it is clear that other factors must be involved in its pathogenesis.

The dialysis disequilibrium syndrome refers to the clinical signs and symptoms observed mainly in hemodialyzed patients. Cerebral edema develops in response to the osmotic gradient established following the rapid removal of urea and other soutes from the extracellular compartment during dialysis [346–348]. Symptoms and signs include headache, confusion, vomiting, hypertension, convulsions and coma. This syndrome has rarely been reported in patients treated with peritoneal dialysis [154, 349, 350], probably because the removal of small solutes across the peritoneal membrane occurs more slowly than by hemodialysis.

A recent report detailed features of Wernicke's encephalopathy in peritoneal dialysis patients. In all cases, the diagnosis was made only on postmortem examination of the brain. In life the neurological symptoms and signs, including nystagmus, confusion, memory loss and obtundation, were ascribed to other causes such as disequilibrium and uremic encephalopathy. The authors suggest that a combination of defective transketolase binding, poor diet and other insults such as sepsis may lead to the encephalopathy [351]. This diagnosis may be particularly applicable to PD patients, because glucose loads increase thiamine requirements and may precipitate a deficiency state. In addition, losses of the water-soluble vitamin into the dialysate may cause thiamine depletion.

Tests of cognition and neuropsychiatric function have led to differing results. Manual dexterity has been shown to decline in peritoneal dialysis patients [352]. Performance testing, however, showed no differences in cognitive function between matched peritoneal dialysis and hemodialysis patients [353].

When compared to a non-dialysis population referred for psychometric testing, however, CAPD patients were more likely to demonstrate cognitive impairment [354]. Moreover, a poor score at the outset of CAPD was associated with a poor treatment outcome or death. After one year, however, there was improvement so that 60% of patients were essentially non-impaired compared with only 30%-pre-CAPD. Once again, these findings must be interpreted with the consideration that deaths and treatment dropout will skew the data.

Despite the regression of uremic symptoms with dialysis, many patients complain of fatigue. It is not clear what the etiology of this complaint is, although it is probably multifactorial. There is no difference in age or sex of patients suffering from fatigue. Interestingly, patients whose under-lying disease is systemic lupus erythematosus seem to be more fatigued [355]. A survey demonstrated that only 14% of CAPD patients complained of severe fatigue compared to 26% of hemodialysis patients. Morning fatigue correlated well with depression on psychological testing [355]. Finally, fatigue may be in part related to sleep disturbances. CAPD patients may experience nocturnal myoclonus which can interrupt sleep. Moreover, factors lost in the peritoneal dialysate may be sleep-promoting and so the dialysis itself may contribute to sleep disturbances and daytime fatigue [356]. The dramatic improvement in fatigue seen in he-modialysis patients receiving erythropoietin suggests that anemia contributes importantly to this complaint [351].

2.9. Immune function

Uremic patients have subnormal immune responsiveness and frequently demonstrate ongoing defects in immuno-competence, even after the institution of hemodialysis [358, 359].

The abnormal immune reactivity persists, despite being well-dialyzed with respect to small solute removal. It is likely, therefore, that retained middle molecules may be responsible for the ongoing alteration in immune function. Because CAPD leads to increased clearance of these larger molecules, immune function may be more normal compared to that in patients undergoing hemodialysis. The obser-vation of flares in patients with previously quiescent sy-stemic lupus erythematosus upon commencing CAPD or changing from hemodialysis to CAPD supports this con-tention [360].

The number of T cells (E-rosette-forming cells) in uremic patients may be less than normal. However, upon starting CAPD, the number of these cells increases to normal in the majority after a few months [361, 362], whereas a similar change is not observed in patients on hemodialysis or hemofiltration [361]. Interestingly, peritoneal dialysis ef-fluent inhibits E-rosette formation of normal lymphocytes. The inhibitory factor has a molecular weight of less than 500 daltons [362]. Other studies have not confirmed nor-malization of the number of T lymphocytes in CAPD patients [363, 364]. The ratio of 'helper/inducer' T lym-phocytes to 'suppressor/cytotoxic' lymphocytes [CD4/ CD8] in these patients is normal [362, 365], although a trend toward an increased ratio as the result of increased CD4(+) lymphocytes [363] and decreased CD8(+) lympho-cytes [363, 366] has been described. It is not clear to what extent therapy with 1,25–dihydroxyvitamin D_3, a vitamin shown to alter CD4:CD8 ratios, may have played in these observations [367].

The *in vitro* proliferative response to the non-specific mitogens, phytohemagglutinin and concanavalin A is less than [366] or the same as [368] that in non-uremic controls, and better than the response seen in hemodialysis patients [366, 368]. Furthermore, while these responses diminish over time in patients on hemodialysis, they stay the same or improve on CAPD [363, 366]. The mixed lymphocyte response in CAPD patients is also subnormal but better than that seen in hemodialysis patients.

Other tests of T-cell function have revealed that the delayed hypersensitivity response to intradermal antigens such as PPD and DNCB is better in CAPD compared to hemodialysis patients [365] and patients will lose their skin anergy over time on CAPD but not on hemodialysis or hemofiltration [361]. A local xenogeneic graft-versus-host reaction improved over time in non-diabetic patients on CAPD [364].

There is less data on circulating B lymphocytes. B-cell numbers have been found to be normal [361] or less than normal and decrease further with time on CAPD [363]. There is no parallel fall in serum immunoglobulin con-centration [361, 363]. The level of circulating immune complexes as measured by the C1q binding assay is increased in CAPD patients when compared to controls, but less than the levels found in hemodialysis subjects [369]. It has been suggested that the uremic individual is unable to eliminate antigens. The persistence of these antigens leads to antibody formation and the development of the immune complexes. The clinical significance of these complexes is unclear.

In summary, studies of T-cell function have suggested greater responsiveness in patients on CAPD as compared to patients on hemodialysis. This improved T-cell function may explain why the incidence of neoplasm in CAPD patients is the same as in non-uremic patients. It is not clear whether patients on CAPD have a lower incidence of infections than those on hemodialysis. Finally, despite the greater T-cell responsiveness, the incidence of allograft acceptance seems no different than that seen in hemodialysis patients (see section on Transplantation). Perhaps the immunosuppressive therapy in the post-transplant period negates the intrinsic differences in immune responsiveness with these two modes of dialysis therapy.

2.10. Cancer

Uremia and dialysis can be considered immunosuppressed states (see Section 2.9.). One important immune function is tumor surveillance. Patients who are immunocompro-mised have an incidence of cancer which is greater than that of the general population [379]. Previous studies have suggested that patients on hemodialysis have an increased incidence of tumor formation, presumably on the basis of impaired tumor surveillance [371].

A recent review studied 328 CAPD patients at our institution [372]. The mean duration of CAPD was 19 months. Epitheliomas of the skin were not included because of their higher detection rate in closely scrutinized patient populations. Nine patients developed cancer during dialysis, after a mean duration of 21 months. One third of these patients had received immunosuppressive drugs. If all nine patients are considered, there was a trend that was not statistically significant for a higher incidence of cancer in patients on CAPD when compared to the general popu-lation matched for age, sex and duration of follow up. However, if the three patients who received the immuno-suppressive medications are excluded from the analysis, there was no difference between the CAPD and general populations in the incidence of cancer. This negative finding may be a function of the relative small number of patients surveyed. On the other hand, it may reflect better immunocompetence in this population, as manifested by heightened tumor surveillance, when compared to patients on hemodialysis or chronic renal failure not receiving dialysis.

2.11. Transplantation

There are a number of theoretical risks associated with renal transplantation in the patient on peritoneal dialysis. As reviewed in this chapter and elsewhere [373], the patient on CAPD may be more immunocompetent than the patient receiving hemodialysis. This more normal immune response may predispose the patient to rejection of the renal allograft. Furthermore, the peritoneal dialysis patient may face special risks while receiving immunosuppressive therapy post-transplant. Previous episodes of peritonitis could leave a nucleus of infection which could develop into overwhelming sepsis. The development of peritonitis might pose a life-threatening complication in patients receiving immunosuppressive therapy [374]. Finally, if the patient needs peritoneal dialysis post-operatively, the operative site could interfere with the performance of dialysis, especially if the integrity of the peritoneum has been disrupted during surgery.

Two reports have lead to concern. A significant increase in the helper to suppressor T lymphocyte ratio in patients on long-term CAPD was associated with an increased incidence of graft rejection when compared to hemodialysis patients [375]. Similarly, another study found decreased graft survival in patients previously receiving CAPD when compared to those on hemodialysis. This decreased survival was quite apparent as early as one month post-transplant. The peritoneal dialysis patients had a higher ratio of circulating T lymphocytes of the 'helper/inducer' subtype and did not display the T-cell lymphopenia found in the hemodialysis patients [376]. Furthermore, unlike hemodialysis patients, CAPD patients did not benefit from pre-transplant blood transfusions [376]. Although the implication is that the greater number of circulating T lymphocytes are responsible for graft rejection, it has not been shown that the ratio of helper to suppressor T lymphocytes bears any consistent relationship to graft outcome [373].

A number of centers have examined the graft and patient survival data of their hemodialysis and peritoneal dialysis populations. Graft survival has not been different between the two [374, 377–384) for one year and up to two years [374, 378]. Patients on long-term and short-term PD have the same graft survival [378, 380]. One study showed a trend to lower one year graft survival in PD patients [385], but the difference was not statistically significant. Patient survival has not been shown to be different [377, 379, 380, 382], although a different study demonstrated a trend to diminished patient survival which did not reach statistical significance [381]. Unfortunately, many of these studies consisted of small numbers of peritoneal dialysis patients, limiting the statistical power of the analyses. However, there does not seem to be any convincing evidence that CAPD patients have a higher rate of graft rejection compared to patients on hemodialysis.

In terms of septic complications related to the peritoneal dialysis, there are no reports of occult residual infection from previous peritonitis developing into generalized sepsis with the administration of immunosuppressive drugs. The incidence of peritonitis in the post-transplant period does seem to be sizable, especially if the patient needs to resume peritoneal dialysis [380, 383], but peritonitis seems to be easily managed with antibiotics, lavage, and catheter removal if necessary [374, 378, 386], although in one patient it led to death from sepsis [381]. The simultaneous administration of cytotoxic agents in patients with peritonitis does not seem to lead to resistance to the usual methods of treatment.

Most centers electively remove the peritoneal dialysis catheter about two to three months post-transplant [377, 378, 380, 386, 387] although some remove it at the time of transplant and hemodialyze the patient as needed thereafter [385]. Because of the risk of bowel perforation, an unused catheter should be flushed weekly and removed no later than two months after transplant.

Mechanical problems in relationship to the transplant appear to be manageable. The exit site of the catheter may be close to the transplant bed, and initial implantation of catheters at the outset of dialysis should be done with this potential problem in mind. If the peritoneum has not been cut during surgery, peritoneal dialysis can usually be performed if necessary post-operatively. There have been reports of drainage of dialysate through the transplant site [381, 383] and through the incision of a transplant nephrectomy [382]. This complication can be managed by temporarily stopping the dialysis and providing antibiotic coverage.

Post-transplant ascites has been reported in children [388] and adults [389] who were previously on CAPD. In adults the ascites has lasted up to 50 days, but ultimately resolves on its own [389].

In summary, with the exception of two reports, graft survival in patients on CAPD appears to be comparable to that in patients on hemodialysis. There is a risk of peritonitis in the post transplant period in those who need to continue peritoneal dialysis, but in most cases this complication is manageable in the same way as peritonitis in CAPD patients not undergoing transplantation.

2.12. Acquired cystic disease of the kidneys

Patients on long-term hemodialysis can develop multiple renal cysts [390]. The reason for the formation of cysts is not well understood. As with other disorders affecting hemodialysis patients, the etiology may relate to toxins encountered in the extracorporeal circuit. However, the finding of cysts in uremic patients who had not yet started dialysis [391] suggests that the uremic state itself may lead to renal cyst formation, perhaps by the retention of certain cyst-producing toxins.

There have been few reports of acquired cystic disease of the kidney in peritoneal dialysis patients. One patient who had been treated exclusively with CAPD for 18 months demonstrated many small cysts throughout both the renal cortex and medulla on postmortem examination. These cysts were histologically identical to those seen in hemodialysis patients [392].

In a survey of 8 patients who had been on CAPD for more than three years, 6 had renal cysts (but, one had been on hemodialysis for seven years before CAPD.) There was an association between the number of cysts and the length of time on CAPD [393]. Therefore, uremia itself or exposure to toxins may make CAPD patients prone to the development of cystic disease of the kidneys. This could be significant because of the potential complication in these cysts of retroperitoneal hemorrhage or malignant transformation [390, 394].

REFERENCES

1. Gotloib L, Mines M, Garmizo L et al.: Hemodynamic effects of increasing intra-abdominal pressure in peritoneal dialysis. Perit Dial Bull 1(4): 41–43, 1981.
2. Twardowski Z, Khanna R, Nolph K et al.: Intraabdominal pressures during natural activities in patients treated with continuous ambulatory peritoneal dialysis. Nephron 44: 129–135, 1986.
3. O'Connor J, Rigby R, Hardie I et al.: Abdominal hernias complicating continuous ambulatory peritoneal dialysis. Am J Nephrol 6: 271–274, 1986.
4. Digenis G, Khanna R, Mathews R et al.: Abdominal hernias in patients undergoing continuous ambulatory peritoneal dialysis. Perit Dial Bull 2(3): 115–117, 1982.
5. Rubin J, Raju S, Teal N et al.: Abdominal hernia in patients undergoing continuous ambulatory peritoneal dialysis. Arch Intern Med 142: 1453–1455, 1982.
6. Kauffman H, Adams M: Indirect inguinal hernia in patients undergoing peritoneal dialysis. Surgery 99(2): 254–255, 1986.
7. Engeset J, Youngson G: Ambulatory peritoneal dialysis and hernial complications. Surg Clin North Am 64(2): 385–392, 1984.
8. Rocco M, Stone W: Abdominal hernias in chronic peritoneal dialysis patients: A review. Perit Dial Bull 5(3): 171–174, 1985.
9. Tzamaloukas A, Bevan M, Cox B et al.: Clinical associations and effects of hernias in CAPD patients (abst). Perit Dial Bull Suppl 6(4): S21, 1986.
10. Wise M, Manos J, Gokal R: Small umbilical hernias in patients on CAPD (letter). Perit Dial Bull 4(4): 270–271, 1984.
11. Wetherington G, Leapman S, Robison R et al.: Abdominal wall and inguinal hernias in continuous ambulatory peritoneal dialysis patients. Am J Surg 150: 357–360, 1985.
12. Spence P, Mathews R, Khanna R et al.: Improved results with a paramedian technique for the insertion of peritoneal dialysis catheters. Surg Gynecol Obstet 161: 585–587, 1985.
13. Ramos J, Burke D, Veitch P: Hernia of Morgagni in patients on continuous ambulatory peritoneal dialysis (letter). Lancet 1: 161–162, 1982.
14. Griffin P, Coles G: Strangulated hernias through Tenckhoff cannula sites. Br Med J 284: 1837, 1982.
15. Power D, Edward N, Catto G et al.: Richter's hernia: an unrecognised complication of chronic ambulatory peritoneal dialysis. Br Med J 283: 528, 1981.
16. Shohat J, Shapira Z, Shmueli D et al.: Intestinal incarceration in occult abdominal wall herniae in continuous ambulatory peritoneal dialysis. Isr J Med Sci 21: 985–987, 1985
17. Kopecky R, Funk M, Kreitzer P: Localized genital edema in patients undergoing continuous ambulatory peritoneal dialysis. J Urol 134: 880–884, 1985.
18. Beaman M, Feehally J, Smith B et al.: Anterior abdominal wall leakage in CAPD patients; management by intermittent peritoneal dialysis (letter). Perit Dial Bull 5(1): 81–82, 1985.
19. Cooper J, Nicholls A, Simms J et al.: Genital oedema in patients treated by continuous ambulatory peritoneal dialysis: an unusual presentation of inguinal hernia. Br Med J 286: 1923–1924, 1983.
20. Orfei R, Seybold K, Blumberg A: Genital edema in patients undergoing continuous ambulatory peritoneal dialysis (CAPD). Perit Dial Bull 4(4): 251–252, 1984.
21. Twardowski Z, Tully R, Nichols W et al.: Computerized tomography CT in the diagnosis of subcutaneous leak sites during continuous ambulatory peritoneal dialysis (CAPD). Perit Dial Bull 4(3): 163–166, 1984.
22. Schurgers M, Boelaert J, Daneels R et al.: Open processus vaginalis. Perit Dial Bull 3(1): 30–31, 1983.
23. Mandel P, Faegenburg D, Imbriano L: The use of technetium-99m sulfur colloid in the detection of patent processus vaginalis in patients on continuous ambulatory peritoneal dialysis. Clin Nucl Med 10(8): 553–555, 1985.
24. Dubin L, Froelich J: Evaluation of scrotal edema in a patient on peritoneal dialysis. Clin Nucl Med 10(3): 173–174, 1985.
25. Moffat F, Deitel M, Thompson D: Abdominal surgery in patients undergoing long-term peritoneal dialysis. Surgery 92(2): 598-604, 1982.
26. Gloor H, Nichols W, Sorkin M et al.: Peritoneal access and related complications in continuous ambulatory peritoneal dialysis. Am J Med 74: 593–598, 1983.
27. Chan M, Baillod R, Tanner A et al.: Abdominal hernias in patients receiving continuous ambulatory peritoneal dialysis (letter). Br Med J 283: 826, 1981.
28. Jorkasky D, Goldfarb S: Abdominal wall hernia complicating chronic ambulatory peritoneal dialysis. Am J Nephrol 2: 323–324, 1982.
29. Shenouda A, Puckett W, Burns R et al.: Acute intestinal obstruction complicating CAPD (letter). Perit Dial Bull 2(1): 49, 1982.
30. Madden M, Beirne G, Zimmerman S et al.: Acute bowel obstruction: an unusual complication of chronic peritoneal dialysis. Am J Kidney Dis 1(4): 219–221, 1982.
31. Francis D, Schofield I, Veitch P: Abdominal hernias in patients treated with continuous ambulatory peritoneal dialysis. Br J Surg 69: 409, 1982.
32. Barone J, Buzzeo L: Incarcerated epigastric hernia in a CAPD patient with diastasis of the rectus muscles (letter). Perit Dial Bull 2(3): 144–145, 1982.
33. Nelson H, Lindner M, Schuman E et al.: Abdominal wall hernias as a complication of peritoneal dialysis. Surg Gynecol & Obstet 157: 541–544, 1983.
34. Nassberger L: Enterocele due to continuous ambulatory peritoneal dialysis (CAPD). Acta Obstet Gynecol Scand 63: 283, 1984.
35. Lee A, Waffle C, Trebbin W et al.: Clostridial myonecrosis. Origin from an obturator hernia in a dialysis patient. J Am Med Assoc 246: 1232–1233, 1983.
36. DiPaolo N, Sacchi G, DeMia M et al.: Morphology of the peritoneal membrane during continuous ambulatory peritoneal dialysis. Nephron 44: 204–211, 1986.
37. Oreopoulos D, Gotloib L, Calderaro V et al.: For how long

ACKNOWLEDGEMENTS

The authors wish to thank M.C. Miller for typing and editorial assistance, Drs. G. Abraham and A. Shoker for their help in the section on hydrothorax, and Dr. E. Silverman for helpful discussions.

can peritoneal dialysis be continued? Can Med Assoc J 124: 12–13, 1981.

38. Faller B, Marichal J: Loss of ultrafiltration in continuous ambulatory peritoneal dialysis: clinical data. In: Gahl G, Kessel M, Nolph K (eds), Advances in Peritoneal Dialysis. Excerpta Medica: pp 227–232, 1981.

39. Wu G, Oreopoulos D: Diminished peritoneal ultrafiltration and solute permeability. In: Daugirdas J, Ing T (eds), Handbook of Dialysis. Little, Brown: pp 244–251, 1988.

40. Slingeneyer A, Canaud B, Mion C: Permanent loss of ultrafiltration capacity of the peritoneum in long-term peritoneal dialysis: an epidemiological study. Nephron 33: 133–138, 1983.

41. Faller B, Marichal J–F: Loss of ultrafiltration in continuous ambulatory peritoneal dialysis: a role for acetate. Perit Dial Bull 4(1): 10–13, 1984.

42. Krediet R, Boeschoten E, Zuyderhoudt F et al.: Peritoneal transport characteristics of water, low-molecular weight solutes and proteins during long-term continuous ambulatory peritoneal dialysis. Perit Dial Bull 6(2): 61–65, 1986.

43. Manual M, The University of Toronto Collaborative Dialysis Group: Failure of ultrafiltration in patients on CAPD. Perit Dial Bull. Suppl. 3(3): S38–S40, 1983.

44. Wideroe T-E, Smeby L, Mjaland S et al.: Long-term changes in transperitoneal water transport during continuous ambulatory peritoneal dialysis. Nephron 38: 238–247, 1984.

45. Nolph K, Ryan L, Moore H et al.: Factors affecting ultrafiltration in continuous ambulatory peritoneal dialysis. First report of an international cooperative study. Perit Dial Bull 4(1): 14–19, 1984.

46. Nolph K, Legrain M, Mion C et al.: Loss of peritoneal ultrafiltration: an international detective story. Perit Dial Bull 4(3): 128, 1984.

47. Nolph K, Ryan L, Moore H et al.: A survey of ultrafiltration in continuous ambulatory peritoneal dialysis. An international cooperative study – second report. Perit Dial Bull 4(3): 137–142, 1984.

48. Katirtzoglou A, Digenis G, Kontesis P et al.: Is peritoneal ultrafiltration influenced by acetate or lactate buffers? In: Maher J, Winchester J, (eds), Frontiers in Peritoneal Dialysis. Field, Rich and Associates, Inc: pp 270–273, 1986.

49. Liang C, Lowenstein J: Metabolic control of the circulation. J Clin Invest 62: 1029–1038, 1978.

50. Richardson R, Roscoe J: Bicarbonate, L-Lactate and D-Lactate balance in intermittent peritoneal dialysis. Perit Dial Bull 6(4): 178–185, 1986.

51. Kwong M, Wu G, Rodella H et al.: Effect of the peritoneal dialysate buffer on ultrafiltration: studies in normal rabbits. Perit Dial Bull 5(3): 182–185, 1985.

52. DiPaolo N, Buoncristiani U, Gaggiotti E et al.: Improvement of impaired ultrafiltration after addition of phosphatidylcholine in patients on CAPD (letter). Perit Dial Bull 6(1): 44–45, 1986.

53. Rottembourg J, Gahl G, Poignet J et al.: Severe abdominal complications in patients undergoing continuous ambulatory peritoneal dialysis. Eur Dial Transpl Assoc Proc 20: 236–242, 1983.

54. Grefberg N, Nilsson P, Andreen T: Sclerosing obstructive peritonitis, beta-blockers, and continuous ambulatory peritoneal dialysis (letter). Lancet 2: 733–734, 1983.

55. Bradley J, McWhinnie D, Hamilton D et al.: Sclerosing obstructive peritonitis after continuous ambulatory peritoneal dialysis (letter). Lancet 2: 113–114, 1983.

56. Hauglustaine D, Monballyu J, Van Meerbeek J et al.: Sclerosing obstructive peritonitis, beta-blockers, and continuous ambulatory peritoneal dialysis (letter). Lancet 2: 734, 1983.

57. Verger C, Celicout B, Larpent L et al.: Sclerosing encapsulating peritonitis during continuous ambulatory peritoneal dialysis. La Presse Medicale 15(28): 1311–1314, 1986.

58. Slingeneyer A, Mion C, Mourad G et al.: Progressive sclerosing peritonitis: a late and severe complication of maintenance peritoneal dialysis. Trans Am Soc Artif Intern Organs 29: 633–640, 1983.

59. Pusateri R, Ross R, Marshall R et al.: Sclerosing encapsulating peritonitis: report of a case with small bowel obstruction managed by long-term home parenteral hyperalimentation, and a review of the literature. Am J Kidney Dis 8(1): 56–60, 1986.

60. Daugirdas J, Gandhi V, McShane A et al.: Peritoneal sclerosis in continuous ambulatory peritoneal dialysis patients dialyzed exclusively with lactate-buffered dialysate. Int J Artif Organs 9(6): 413–416, 1986.

61. Ing T, Daugirdas J, Gandhi V: Peritoneal sclerosis in peritoneal dialysis patients. Am J Nephrol 4: 173–176, 1984.

62. Hauglustaine D, Van Meerbeek J, Monballyu J et al.: Sclerosing peritonitis with mural bowel fibrosis in a patient on long-term CAPD. Clin Nephrol 22(3): 158–162, 1984.

63. Oreopoulos D, Khanna R, Wu G: Sclerosing obstructive peritonitis after CAPD (letter). Lancet 2: 409, 1983.

64. Junor B, Briggs J, Forwell M et al.: Sclerosing peritonitis – The contribution of chlorhexidine in alcohol. Perit Dial Bull 5(2): 101–104, 1985.

65. Ing T, Daugirda J, Gandhi V et al.: Sclerosing peritonitis after peritoneal dialysis (letter). Lancet 2: 1080, 1983.

66. Shaldon S, Koch K, Quellhorst E et al.: Pathogenesis of sclerosing peritonitis in CAPD. Trans Am Soc Artif Intern Organs 30: 193–194, 1984.

67. Greenlee H, Stanley M, Reinhardt G et al.: Small bowel obstruction from compression and kinking of intestine by thickened peritoneum in cirrhotics with ascites treated with LeVeen shunt. Gastroenterol 76: 1282–1285, 1979.

68. Brown P, Baddeley H, Read A et al.: Sclerosing peritonitis, an unusual reaction of a B-adrenergic-blocking drug (practolol). Lancet 2: 1477–1481, 1974.

69. Clark C, Terris R: Sclerosing peritonitis associated with metoprolol. Lancet 1: 937, 1983.

70. Sabatier J, Genin C, Berthoux F: Sclerosing obstructive peritonitis after continuous ambulatory peritoneal dialysis in 3 patients (letter). Clin Nephrol 23(5): 266, 1985.

71. Gandhi V, Humayun H, Ing T et al.: Sclerotic thickening of the peritoneal membrane in maintenance peritoneal dialysis patients. Arch Intern Med 140: 1201–1203, 1980.

72. Lasker N, Burke J, Patchefsky A et al.: Peritoneal reactions to particulate matter in peritoneal dialysis solutions. Trans Am Soc Artif Intern Organs 21: 342–345, 1975.

73. Backenroth-Maayan R, Longnecker R, Kambasos D: Failure of the peritoneal membrane during chronic intermittent peritoneal dialysis. In: Gahl G, Kessel M, Nolph K (eds): Advances in Peritoneal Dialysis. Proceedings of the Second International Symposium on Peritoneal Dialysis. Berlin, 1981, International Congress Series 567. Excerpta Medica, Amsterdam: pp 208–213, 1981.

74. Novello A, Port F: Sclerosing encapsulating peritonitis (editorial). Int J Artif Organs 9(6): 393–396, 1986.

75. Berlyne G, Lee H, Ralston A et al.: Pulmonary complications of peritoneal dialysis. Lancet 2: 75–78, 1966.

76. Ahluwalia M, Ishikawa S, Gellman M et al.: Pulmonary functions during peritoneal dialysis. Clin Nephrol 18(5): 251–256, 1982.

77. Gomez-Fernandez P, Sanchez Agudo L, Calatrava J et al.: Respiratory muscle weakness in uremic patients under continuous ambulatory peritoneal dialysis. Nephron 36: 219–223, 1984.

78. Singh S, Dale A, Morgan B et al.: Serial studies of pulmonary function in continuous ambulatory peritoneal dialysis. Chest 86(6): 874–877, 1984.

79. Taveira da Silva A, Davis W, Winchester J et al.: Peritonitis, dialysate infusion and lung function in continuous ambulatory

peritoneal dialysis (CAPD). Clin Nephrol 24(2): 79–83, 1985.

80. Freedman S, Maberly D: Gas exchange in renal failure (letter). Br Med J 3: 48, 1971.

81. Blumberg A, Keller R, Marti H: Oxygen affinity of erythrocytes and pulmonary gas exchange in patients on continuous ambulatory peritoneal dialysis. Nephron 38: 248–252, 1984.

82. Oreopoulos D, Rebuck A: Risks and benefits of peritoneal dialysis. Chest 88(4): 6742, 1985.

83. Rebuck A: Peritoneal dialysis and the mechanics of the diaphragm (editorial). Perit Dial Bull 2(3): 109–110, 1982.

84. Eiser A: Pulmonary gas exchange during hemodialysis and peritoneal dialysis: interaction between respiration and metabolism. Am J Kidney Dis 6(3): 131–142, 1985.

85. Fabris A, Biasioli S, Chiaramonte C et al.: Buffer metabolism in continuous ambulatory peritoneal dialysis (CAPD): relationship with respiratory dynamics. Trans Am Soc Artif Intern Organs 28:L 270–275, 1982.

86. Maher J, Schreiner G: Hazards and complications of dialysis. N Eng J Med 273: 370–377, 1965.

87. Edwards S, Unger A: Acute hydrothorax: a new complication of peritoneal dialysis. J Am Med Assoc 199: 189–191, 1967.

88. Bunchman T, Wood E, Lynch R: Hydrothorax as a complication of peritoneal dialysis. Perit Dial Bull 7(4): 237–239, 1987.

89. Scheldewaert R, Bogaerts Y, Pauwels R et al.: Management of a massive hydrothorax in a CAPD patient: A case report and a review of the literature. Perit Dial Bull 2: 69–72, 1982.

90. Lorentz, W: Acute hydrothorax during peritoneal dialysis. J Pediatr 94: 417, 1979.

91. Khanna R: Questions and answers. Perit Dial Bull 1: 17, 1980.

92. Pattison C, Rodger R, Adu D et al.: Surgical treatment of hydrothorax complicating CAPD. Clin Nephrol 21: 191–193, 1984.

93. Lieberman F, Hindemura R, Peters R et al.: Pathogenesis and treatment of hydrothorax complicating cirrhosis with ascites. Ann Intern Med 64: 341–351, 1966.

94. Johnston R, Loo R: Hepatic hydrothorax. Studies to determine the source of fluid and report of thirteen cases. Ann Intern Med 61: 385–401, 1964.

95. Karpiak D, Rose I, Patch J: Treatment of pleuroperitoneal fistula by obliteration of the pleural space (letter). Perit Dial Bull 4: 108–109, 1984.

96. Haberli R, Stucki R: Akuter hydrothorax als komplikation bei peritoneal dialyse. Praxis 1: 13, 1971.

97. Grefberg N, Danielson B, Benson L et al.: Right-sided hydrothorax complicating peritoneal dialysis. Nephron 34: 130–134, 1983.

98. Gibbons G, Baumert J: Unilateral hydrothorax complicating peritoneal dialysis. Use of radionuclide imaging. Clin Nucl Med 3: 83–84, 1983.

99. Kennedy J: Procedures used to demonstrate a pleuroperitoneal communication: a review. Perit Dial Bull 5: 168–170, 1985.

100. Benz R, Schleifer C: Hydrothorax in CAPD. Successful treatment with intraperitoneal tetracycline and a review of the literature. Am J Kidney Dis 2: 136–140, 1985.

101. Rudnick M, Coyle J, Beck L et al.: Acute massive hydrothorax complicating peritoneal dialysis: report of two cases and a review of the literature. Clin Nephrol 12: 38–44, 1979.

102. Vlachojannis J, Boettcher I, Brand L et al.: A new treatment for unilateral recurrent hydrothorax during CAPD. Perit Dial Bull 5: 180–181, 1985.

103. Finn R, Jowett E: Acute hydrothorax complicating peritoneal dialysis. Br Med J 2: 94, 1970.

104. Rodriguez-Perez J, Palop L, Plaza C et al.: Diagnosis and treatment of massive hydrothorax in CAPD (Abstr.). Perit Dial Bull 4: S49, 1984.

105. Posen G, Sachs H: Treatment of recurrent pleural effusions in dialysis patients by talc insufflation (Abstr.). Am Soc Artif Intern Organs, 25th Annual Meeting, New York: pp 75, 1979.

106. Adam W, Arkies L, Gill G et al.: Hydrothorax with peritoneal dialysis: radionuclide detection of a pleuro-peritoneal connection. Austr NZ J Med 10: 330–332, 1980.

107. Lowrie E, Lazarus J, Mocelin A: Survival of patients undergoing chronic hemodialysis and renal transplantation. N Eng J Med 288: 863–867, 1973.

108. Haire H, Sherrard D, Scardapan D: Smoking, hypertension and mortality in a maintenance dialysis population. Cardiovasc Med 3: 1163–1168, 1978.

109. Lindnew A, Charra B, Sherrard D et al.: Accelerated atherosclerosis in prolonged maintenance hemodialysis. N Eng J Med 290: 697–701, 1974.

110. Bagdale J, Porte D Jr, Bierman E: A metabolic consequence of chronic renal failure. N Eng J Med 279: 181–185, 1968.

111. Novarini A, Zuliani U, Bandini L et al.: Observations on lipid metabolism in chronic renal failure during conservative and hemodialysis therapy. Eur J Clin Invest 6: 473, 1976.

112. Cattran D, Fenton S, Wilson D et al.: Defective triglyceride removal in lipemia associated with peritoneal dialysis and hemodialysis. Ann Intern Med 85: 29–33, 1976.

113. Chan M, Varghese Z, Persaud J et al.: Hyperlipidemia in patients on maintenance hemo- and peritoneal dialysis: the relative pathogenetic roles of triglyceride production and triglyceride removal. Clin Nephrol 17(4): 183–190, 1982.

114. Sniderman A, Cianflone K, Hutchinson T et al.: Increased prevalence of hyperapobetalipoproteinemia in patients treated with continuous ambulatory peritoneal dialysis (Abstr.). Perit Dial Bull Suppl 6(4): S20, 1986.

115. Dieplinger H, Schoenfeld P, Fielding C: Plasma cholesterol metabolism in end-stage renal disease. J Clin Invest 77: 1071–1083, 1986.

116. Oreopoulos D, Khanna R, McCready W et al.: Continuous ambulatory peritoneal dialysis in Canada. Dial and Transplant 9: 224–226, 1980.

117. Cantaluppi A, Scalamogna A, Guerra L et al.: Plasma lipid and lipoprotein levels in patients treated with CAPD (letter). Perit Dial Bull 2(2): 99, 1982.

118. Keusch G, Bammatter F, Mordasini R et al.: Effect of continuous ambulatory peritoneal dialysis on lipoprotein metabolism (Abstr.). Kidney Int 20: 140, 1981.

119. Khanna R, Breckenridge C, Roncari D et al.: Lipid abnormalities in patients undergoing continuous ambulatory peritoneal dialysis. Perit Dial Bull Suppl 3(1): 513–515, 1983.

120. Ramos J, Heaton A, McGurk J et al.: Sequential changes in serum lipids and their subfractions in patients receiving continuous ambulatory peritoneal dialysis. Nephron 35: 20–23, 1983.

121. Lindholm B, Norbeck H: Serum lipids and lipoproteins during continuous ambulatory peritoneal dialysis. Acta Med Scand 220: 143–151, 1986.

122. Young G, Hobson S, Young S et al.: Adverse effects of hypertonic dialysis fluid during CAPD (letter). Lancet 2: 1421, 1983.

123. Bories P, Slingeneyer A, Solera M et al.: Lipoprotein disorders in chronic ambulatory peritoneal dialysis (Abstr.). Kidney Int 20: 427, 1981.

124. Triolo G, Boggio-Bertinet D, Salomone M et al.: Changes in serum lipids with prolonged CAPD (letter). Perit Dial Bull 2(4): 192–193, 1982.

125. Heaton A, Johnston D, Burrin J et al.: Carbohydrate and lipid metabolism during continuous ambulatory peritoneal dialysis (CAPD): the effect of a single dialysis cycle. Clin Sci 65: 539–545, 1983.

126. Beardsworth S, Goldsmith H, Stanbridge B: Intraperitoneal insulin cannot correct the hyperlipidemia of CAPD. Perit Dial Bull 3(3): 126–127, 1983.

127. Breckenridge W, Roncari D, Khanna R et al.: The influence

of continuous ambulatory peritoneal dialysis on plasma lipoproteins. Atherosclerosis 45: 249–258, 1982.

128. DiGuilio S, Boulu R, Druecke T *et al.*: Clofibrate treatment of hyperlipidemia in chronic renal failure. Clin Nephrol 3: 304, 1977.

129. Goldberg A, Brunzell J, Holmes J *et al.*: Clofibrate: effective treatment for uremic hypertriglyceridemia. Kidney Int 8: 412, 1975.

130. Kurokawa K: Clofibrate in hemodialysed patients (letter). N Eng J Med 296: 942, 1977.

131. Bridgman J, Rosen S, Thoyer J: Complications during clofibrate treatment of nephrotic syndrome hyperlipoproteinemia. Lancet 2: 506, 1972.

132. Pierides A, Alvarez-Ude F, Kerr D: Clofibrate induced muscle damage in patients with chronic renal failure. Lancet 2: 1279, 1975.

133. Kijima Y, Sasaoka T, Kanayama M *et al.*: Untoward effects of clofibrate in hemodialysis patients (letter). N Eng J Med 296: 515, 1977.

134. Wu G and the University of Toronto Collaborative Dialysis Group. Cardiovascular deaths among CAPD patients. Perit Dial Bull Supp 3(3): S26–S28, 1983.

135. Leenen F, Smith D, Khanna R *et al.*: Changes in left ventricular anatomy and function on CAPD. Perit Dial Bull Supp, 3(3): S26–S28, 1983.

136. Brown P, Johnston K, Fenton S *et al.*: Symptomatic exacerbation of peripheral vascular disease with chronic ambulatory peritoneal dialysis. Clin Nephrol 16(5): 258–261, 1981.

137. Guazzi M, Polese A, Magrini F *et al.*: Negative influences of ascites on cardiac function of cirrhotic patients. Am J Med 59: 165–170, 1975.

138. Schurig R, Gahl G, Schartl M *et al.*: Central and peripheral hemodynamics in long term peritoneal dialysis patients. Proc Eur Dial Transpl Assoc 16: 165–169, 1979.

139. Kong C, Raval U, Thompson F: Effect of 2 liters of intraperitoneal dialysate on the cardiovascular system. Clin Nephrol 26(3): 134–139, 1986.

140. Fleming S, Powell J, Baker L et al: Influence of intraperitoneal dialyzate on blood pressure during continuous ambulatory peritoneal dialysis. Clin Nephrol 19(3): 132–133, 1983.

141. Swartz C, Onesti G, Mailloux L *et al.*: The acute hemodynamic and pulmonary perfusion effects of peritoneal dialysis. Trans Am Soc Artif Intern Organs 15: 367–372, 1969.

142. Acquatella H, Perez-Rozas M, Burger B *et al.*: Left ventricular function in uremia: A hemodynamic and echocardiographic study. Nephron 22: 160–174, 1978.

143. Lindholm B, Alvestrand A, Hultman E *et al.*: Muscle water and electrolytes in patients undergoing continuous ambulatory peritoneal dialysis. Acta Med Scand 219: 323–330, 1986.

144. Tzamaloukas A and Avasthi P: Effect of hyperglycemia on serum sodium concentration and tonicity in outpatients on chronic dialysis. Am J Kidney Dis 7(6): 477–482, 1986.

145. Nolph K, Hano J, Teschan P: Peritoneal sodium transport during hypertonic peritoneal dialysis. Ann Intern Med 70: 931–941, 1969.

146. Swales J: Sodium uptake in peritoneal dialysis. Br Med J 3: 345–347, 1967.

147. Boyer J, Gill G, Epstein F: Hyperglycemia and hyperosmolality complicating peritoneal dialysis. Ann Intern Med 67: 568–572, 1967.

148. Miller R, Tassistio C: Peritoneal dialysis. N Eng J Med 281: 945–949, 1969.

149. Spital A, Sterns R: Potassium supplementation via the dialysate in continuous ambulatory peritoneal dialysis. Am J Kidney Dis 6(3): 173–176, 1985.

150. Oreopoulos D, Khanna R, Williams P *et al.*: Continuous ambulatory peritoneal dialysis – 1981. Nephron 30: 293–303, 1982.

151. Rostand S: Profound hypokalemia in continuous ambulatory peritoneal dialysis. Arch Intern Med 143: 377–378, 1983.

152. Bargman J, Jamison R: Disorders of potassium homeostasis. In: Sutton R, Dirks J (eds): Diuretics: Physiology Pharmacology & Clinical Use. W B Saunders Co: pp 296–319, 1986.

153. Boen S: Peritoneal dialysis in clinical medicine. Charles C Thomas: Springfield Illinois, 1964.

154. Vaamonde C, Michael V, Metzger R *et al.*: Complications of acute peritoneal dialysis. J Chron Dis 28: 637-659, 1975.

155. Pedersen F, Ryttov N, Deleuran P *et al.*: Acetate versus lactate in peritoneal dialysis solutions. Nephron 39: 55–58, 1985.

156. Ahlmen J, Stelin G: Abdominal pains during CAPD with acetate buffered dialysate (letter). Lancet 2: 1247, 1983.

157. LaGreca G, Biasioli S, Chiaramonte S *et al.*: Acid-base balance on peritoneal dialysis. Clin Nephrol 16(1): 1–7, 1981.

158. Nissenson A: Acid-base homeostasis in peritoneal dialysis patients. Int J Artif Organs 7(4): 175–176, 1984.

159. Rubin J, Adair C, Johnson B *et al.*: Stereospecific lactate absorption during peritoneal dialysis. Nephron 31: 224-228, 1982.

160. Veech R, Fowler R: Cerebral dysfunction and respiratory alkalosis during peritoneal dialysis with D-lactate-containing dialysis fluids (letter). Am J Med 82: 572–573, 1987.

161. Singh S, Hong C, Dale A *et al.*: Comparison of buffering capacity in patients on hemodialysis and continuous ambulatory peritoneal dialysis. Nephron 42: 29–33, 1986.

162. Naparstek Y, Friedlaender M, Rubinger D *et al.*: Lactic acidosis and peritoneal dialysis. Isr J Med Sci 18: 513–514, 1982.

163. Conte F, Tommasi A, Battini G *et al.*: Lactic acidosis coma in continuous ambulatory peritoneal dialysis (letter). Nephron 43: 148, 1986.

164. Foulks C, Wright L: Successful repletion of bicarbonate stores in ongoing lactic acidosis: a role for bicarbonate-buffered peritoneal dialysis. Southern Med J 74(9): 1162–1163, 1981.

165. Feriani M, Biasioli S, Borin D *et al.*: Bicarbonate buffer for CAPD solution. Trans Am Soc Artif Intern Organs 31: 668–672, 1985.

166. Lee H, Hill L, Hewill V *et al.*: Lactic acidemia in peritoneal dialysis. Proc Eur Dial Transpl Assoc 4: 150–155, 1967.

167. Tzamaloukas A: 'Contraction' alkalosis during treatment of hyperglycemia in CAPD patients. Perit Dial Bull 3(4): 196–199, 1983.

168. Garella S, Contraction alkalosis in patients on CAPD (letter). Perit Dial Bull 4(3): 187–188, 1984.

169. Gault M, Ferguson E, Sidhu J *et al.*: Fluid and electrolyte complications of peritoneal dialysis. Ann Intern Med 75: 253–262, 1971.

170. Kenamond T, Graves J, Lempert K *et al.*: Severe recurrent alkalemia in a patient undergoing continuous cyclic peritoneal dialysis. Am J Med 81: 548–550, 1986.

171. Posner J, Plum F: Spinal fluid pH and neurological symptoms in systemic acidosis. N Eng J Med 277: 605–613, 1967.

172. Hamodraka-Mailis A: Pathogenesis and treatment of back pain in peritoneal dialysis patients. Perit Dial Bull Supp 3(3): S41–S43, 1983.

173. Baum J, Cestero R, Jain V: Peritoneal-dialysis-spike elbow (letter). N Eng J Med 308 (25): 1541, 1983.

174. Lustig S, Morduchowicz G, Rosenfeld J *et al.*: Bilateral rupture of the tendon of the long head of the biceps muscle in continuous ambulatory peritoneal dialysis (letter). Perit Dial Bull 6(1): 42–43, 1986.

175. Kenzora J: Dialysis carpal tunnel syndrome. Orthopaedics 1: 195–203, 1978.

176. Clanet M, Mansat M, Durroux K *et al.*: Syndrome du canal carpien, tenosynovite amyloide et hemodialyse periodique. Rev Neurol (Paris) 10: 613–624, 1981.

177. Bardin T, Zingraff J, Shirahama T *et al.*: Hemodialysis-associated amyloidosis and beta-2 microglubulin. Am J Med 83: 419–424, 1987.

178. Gejyo F, Yamada T, Odani S *et al.*: A new form of amyloid protein associated with hemodialysis was identified as beta-2-microglobulin. Biochem Biophys Res Comm 129: 701–706, 1985.

179. Gagnon R, Somerville P, Kaye M: Beta-2-Microglobulin serum levels in patients on long-term dialysis. Perit Dial Bull 7(1): 29–31, 1987.

180. Ballardie F, Kerr D, Tennent G *et al.*: Haemodialysis versus CAPD: equal predisposition to amyloidosis? (letter). Lancet 1: 795–796, 1986.

181. DiRaimondo C, Stone W: Beta-2-microglobulin in peritoneal dialysis patients (Abstr.). Kidney Int 31: 197, 1987.

182. DiRaimondo C, Stone W: A B-2-microglobulin amyloidosis. Int J Art Organs 10(5): 281–283, 1987.

183. Lillo-Ferez M, Dupommereulle C, Prieur P *et al.*: B2-microglobulin clearance by chronic intermittent peritoneal dialysis (CIPD). Perit Dial Bull 6(4): 215–216, 1986.

184. Chanard J, Lavaud S, Toupance O *et al.*: B2-microglobulin-associated amyloidosis in chronic hemodialysis patients. Lancet 1: 1212, 1986.

185. Laurent G, Charra B, Calemard E *et al.*: Amelioration par la dialyse peritoneale continue ambulatoire des douleurs abarticulaires accompagnant le syndrome du canal carpien des hemodialyses (letter). La Presse Medicale 14(41): 2105–2106, 1985.

186. Oren A, Husdan H, Cheng P-T *et al.*: Calcium oxalate kidney stones in patients on continuous ambulatory peritoneal dialysis. Kidney Int 25: 534–538, 1984.

187. Salyer W, Hutchins G: Cardiac lesions in secondary oxalosis. Arch Intern Med 134: 250–252, 1974.

188. Mitwalli A, Oreopoulos D: Hyperoxaluria and hyperoxalemia: one more concern for the nephrologist (editorial). Int J Artif Organs 8(2): 71–74, 1985.

189. Yamauchi A, Fujii M, Shirai D *et al.*: Plasma concentration and peritoneal clearance of oxalate in patients on continuous ambulatory peritoneal dialysis (CAPD). Clin Nephrol 25(4): 181–185, 1986.

190. Nace G, George A Jr., Stone W: Hemoperitoneum: a red flag in CAPD. Perit Dial Bull 5(1): 42–44, 1985.

191. Husserl F, Tapia N: Peritoneal bleeding in a CAPD patient after extracorporeal lithotripsy (letter). Perit Dial Bull 7(4): 262, 1987.

192. Blumenkrantz M, Gallagher N, Bashore R *et al.*: Retrograde menstruation in women undergoing chronic peritoneal dialysis. Obstet Gynecol 57: 667–670, 1981.

193. Coronel F, Maranjo P, Torrente J *et al.*: The risk of retrograde menstruation in CAPD patients (letter). Perit Dial Bull 4(3): 190–191, 1984.

194. Harnett J, Gill D, Corbett L *et al.*: Recurrent hemoperitoneum in women receiving continuous ambulatory peritoneal dialysis. Ann Intern Med 107: 341–343, 1987.

195. Coward R, Gokal R, Wise M *et al.*: Peritonitis associated with vaginal leakage of dialysis fluid in continuous ambulatory peritoneal dialysis. Br Med J 284: 1529, 1982.

196. Modi K, Henderson M: Fatal massive hemoperitoneum after cessation of CAPD (letter). Clin Nephrol 27(1): 47, 1987.

197. Hassell L, Moore J Jr., Conklin J: Hemoperitoneum during continuous ambulatory peritoneal dialysis: a possible complication of radiation induced peritoneal injury. Clin Nephrol 21(4): 241–243, 1984.

198. Vasko J, Tapper R: The surgical significance of chylous ascites. Arch Surg 95: 355–368, 1967.

199. Kelley M Jr., Butt H: Chylous ascites: an analysis of etiology. Gastroenterol 39: 161–170, 1960.

200. Humayun H, Daugirdas J, Ing T *et al.*: Chylous ascites in a patient treated with intermittent peritoneal dialysis. Artif Organs 8(3): 358–360, 1984.

201. Pomeranz A, Reichenberg Y, Schurr D *et al.*: Chyloperitoneum: a rare complication of peritoneal dialysis. Perit Dial Bull 4(1): 35–37, 1984.

202. Summerfield G, Bellingham A, Manlove L *et al.*: Erythrocyte metabolism in patients on haemodialysis and continuous ambulatory peritoneal dialysis. Clin Sci 62: 479–488, 1982.

203. Cantaluppi A, Scalamogna A, Castelnovo C *et al.*: Anemia in CAPD and haemodialysis (letter). Lancet 2: 1489, 1983.

204. Mehta B, Mogridge C, Bell JD: Changes in red cell mass, plasma volume and hematocrit in patients on CAPD. Trans Am Soc Artif Intern Organs 29: 50–52, 1983.

205. De Paepe M, Schelstraete K, Ringoir S *et al.*: Influence of continuous ambulatory peritoneal dialysis on the anemia of endstage renal disease. Kidney Int 23: 744–748, 1983.

206. Lamperi S, Carozzi S, Icardi A: In Vitro and In Vivo studies of erythropoiesis during continuous ambulatory peritoneal dialysis. Perit Dial Bull 3(2): 94-96, 1983.

207. Wideroe T-E, Sanengen T, Halvorsen S: Erythropoietin and uremic toxicity during continuous ambulatory peritoneal dialysus. Kidney Int 24: S208–S217, 1983.

208. McGonigle R, Husserl F, Wallin J *et al.*: Hemodialysis and continuous ambulatory peritoneal dialysis effects on erythropoiesis in renal failure. Kidney Int 25: 430–436, 1984.

209. Steiner R: Characteristics of the hematocrit response to continuous ambulatory peritoneal dialysis. Arch Intern Med 144: 728–732, 1984.

210. Saltissi D, Coles G, Napier J *et al.*: The hematological response to continuous ambulatory peritoneal dialysis. Clin Nephrol 22(1): 21–27, 1984.

211. Movilli E, Natale C, Cancarini G *et al.*: Improvement of iron utilization and anemia in uremic patients switched from hemodialysis to continuous ambulatory peritoneal dialysis. Perit Dial Bull 6(3): 147–149, 1986.

212. Lameire N, Matthys E, De Paepe M, *et al.*: Red-cell survival in patients on continuous ambulatory peritoneal dialysis. Perit Dial Bull 6(2): 65–68, 1984.

213. Ragnaud J, Vallot C, Wone C: Un cas de polyglobulie chez un unsuffisant renal chronique traite par dialyse peritoneale continue ambulatoire. La Presse Medicale 13(23): 1458–1459, 1984.

214. Salahudeen A, Keavey P, Hawkins T *et al.*: Is anaemia during continuous ambulatory peritoneal dialysis really better than during haemodialysis? Lancet 2: 1046–1048, 1983.

215. Summerfield G, Bellingham A: The effects of therapeutic dialysis and renal transplantation on uraemic serum inhibitors of erythropoiesis in vitro. Br J Haematol 58: 295–304, 1984.

216. Hefti J, Blumberg A, Marti H: Red cell survival and red cell enzymes in patients on continuous peritoneal dialysis (CAPD). Clin Nephrol 19(5): 232–235, 1983.

217. Salahudeen A, Keavey P, Hawkins T *et al.*: Red cell survival and erythrocyte iron utilization in patients on continuous ambulatory peritoneal dialysis (CAPD) (letter). Clin Nephrol 21(4): 247–248, 1984.

218. Taccone-Gallucci M, Giardini O, Lubrano R *et al.*: Red blood cell membrane lipid peroxidation in continuous ambulatory peritoneal dialysis patients. Am J Nephrol 6: 92–95, 1986.

219. Agrafiotis A, Camus F, Rottembourg J *et al.*: Erythrocyte organic phosphates and whole blood oxygen affinity in patients on continuous ambulatory peritoneal dialysis. Eur J Clin Invest 12: 463–465, 1982.

220. Spinowitz B, Sherwood J, Galler M *et al.*: Anemia and oxygen affinity in patients on continuous ambulatory peritoneal dialysis. Perit Dial Bull Suppl 3(1): S33–S35, 1983.

221. Blumberg A, Marti H, Graber C: Serum ferritin and bone marrow iron in patients undergoing continuous ambulatory peritoneal dialysis. J Am Med Assoc 250(24): 3317–3319, 1983.

222. Winearls C, Savage C, Oliviera D *et al.*: Anaemia in CAPD and haemodialysis (letter). Lancet 2: 1488, 1983.

223. Sombolos K, Vas M, McNamee P: Folic acid status in CAPD patients (letter). Perit Dial Bull 6(2): 104, 1986.

224. Becton D, Schultz W, Kinney T: Severe neutropenia caused

by copper deficiency in a child receiving continuous ambulatory peritoneal dialysis. J Pediatr 108(5): 735–737, 1986.

225. Digenis G, Khanna R, Pantalony D: Eosinophilia after implantation of the peritoneal catheter (letter). Perit Dial Bull 2(3): 98–99, 1982.

226. Chandran P, Humayun H, Daugirdas J et al.: Blood eosinophilia in patients undergoing maintenance peritoneal dialysis. Arch Intern Med 145: 114–116, 1985.

227. Backenroth R, Spinowitz B, Galler M et al.: Comparison of eosinophilia in patients undergoing peritoneal dialysis and hemodialysis. Am J Kidney Dis 8(3): 186–191, 1986.

228. Falk R, Mattern W, Lamanna R et al.: Iron removal during continuous ambulatory peritoneal dialysis using deferoxamine. Kidney Int 24: 110–112, 1983.

229. Stanbaugh G Jr, Holmes A, Gillit D et al.: Iron chelation therapy in CAPD: a new and effective treatment of iron overload disease in ESRD patients. Perit Dial Bull 3(2): 99–101, 1983.

230. Agar J, Farrance I, Hocking D: Iron chelation therapy in CAPD for chronic iron overload (letter). Perit Dial Bull 6(3): 159, 1986.

231. McCarthy J, Kurtz S, Mussman G: Deferoxamine-enhanced fecal losses of aluminum and iron in a patient undergoing continuous ambulatory peritoneal dialysis. Am J Med 82: 367–370, 1987.

232. Benevent D, Ozanne P, Lagarde C: Desferrioxamine overdosage in CAPD (letter). Perit Dial Bull 6(3): 161–162, 1986.

233. Stewart J, Castaldi P: Uremic bleeding: a reversible platelet defect corrected by dialysis. Q J Med 36: 409–423, 1967.

234. Horowitz H: Uremic toxins and platelet function. Arch Int Med 126: 823, 1970.

235. Rabiner S, Hrodek O: Platelet factor 3 in normal subjects and patients with renal failure. J Clin Invest 47: 901–911, 1968.

236. Arends J, Krediet R, Boeschoten E et al.: Improvement of bleeding time, platelet aggregation and platelet count during CAPD treatment. Proc Eur Dial Trans Assoc 18: 280–285, 1981.

237. Martinez-Brotons F, Sarrias X, Reynaldo C et al.: Platelet function in chronic uremia: effect of hemodialysis, peritoneal dialysis and renal allograft (Abstr.). Thromb Haemost 54: 11, 1985.

238. Zimmerman, S: Chronic peritoneal dialysis is associated with progressive thrombocytosis. Perit Dial Bull 6(2): 71–73, 1986.

239. Yoshida N, Aoki N: Release of arachidonic acid from human platelets: a key role for the potentiation of platelet aggregability in normal subjects as well as those with the nephrotic syndrome. Blood 52: 969–975, 1978.

240. Sloand E, Bern M, Kaldany A: Effect on platelet function of hypoalbuminemia in peritoneal dialysis. Thrombosis Res 44: 419–425, 1986.

241. Woo K, Wei S, Lee E et al.: Effects of hemodialysis and peritoneal dialysis on antithrombin III and platelets. Nephron 40: 25–28, 1985.

242. Bertoli M, Gasparotto M, Vertolli U et al.: Does hypercoagulability exist in CAPD patients? Perit Dial Bull 4(4): 237–239, 1984.

243. Canavese C, Stratta P, Pacitti A et al.: Impaired fibrinolysis in uremia: partial and variable correction by four different dialysis regimes. Clin Nephrol 17(2): 82–89, 1982.

244. Caruana R, Wolfman N, Karstaedt N et al.: Pancreatitis: an important cause of abdominal symptoms in patients on peritoneal dialysis. Am J Kidney Dis 7(2): 135–140, 1986.

245. Rutsky E, Robards M, Van Dyke J et al.: Acute pancreatitis in patients with end-stage renal disease without transplantation. Arch Intern Med 146: 1741–1745, 1986.

246. Singh S, Wadhwa N: Peritonitis, pancreatitis and infected pseudocyst in a continuous ambulatory peritoneal dialysis patient. Am J Kidney Dis 9(1): 84–86, 1987.

247. Flynn C, Chandran P, Shadur C: Recurrent pancreatitis in a patient on CAPD (letter). Perit Dial Bull 6(2): 106, 1986.

248. de Boer B, Agar J: The role of hyperlipidemia in the etiology of pancreatitis in CAPD (letter). Perit Dial Bull 7(4): 264, 1987.

249. Pitrone F, Pelligrino E, Mileto G et al.: May pancreatitis represent a CAPD complication? Report of two cases with a rapidly evolution to death (letter). Int J Artif Organs 8(4): 235–236, 1985.

250. Heathcote J, Thomas D, deVeber G et al.: Liver dysfunction in patients treated for end stage renal failure (Abstr.). Hepatology 2(5): 747, 1982.

251. Luciani L, Gentile M, Scarduelli B et al.: Multiple hepatic abscesses complicating continuous ambulatory peritoneal dialysis. Br Med J 285: 543, 1982.

252. Seaworth B, Garrett L, Stead W et al.: Non-A, non-B hepatitis and chronic dialysis – another dilemma. Am J Nephrol 4: 235–239, 1984.

253. Nelson W, Khanna R, Mathews R et al.: Gallbladder stones, cholecystitis and cholecystectomy in patients on continuous ambulatory peritoneal dialysis. Perit Dial Bull 4(4): 245–248, 1984.

254. Koren G, Aladjem M, Militiano J et al.: Ischemic colitis in chronic intermittent peritoneal dialysis. Nephron 36: 272–274, 1984.

255. Wehling M, Jenni R, Steurer J et al.: Ischemic colitis in a patient undergoing continuous ambulatory peritoneal dialysis. Perit Dial Bull 2(3): 123–124, 1982.

256. Tomson C, Morgan A: Bleeding from small intestinal telangiectases complicating CAPD (letter). Perit Dial Bull 5(4): 258, 1985.

257. Ramirez G, Jubiz W, Gutch C et al.: Thyroid abnormalities and renal failure – a study of fifty-three patients on chronic hemodialysis. Ann Intern Med 79: 500–504, 1973.

258. Lim V, Fang V, Katz A et al.: Thyroid dysfunction in chronic renal failure. J Clin Invest 60: 522–534, 1977.

259. Giordano C, De Santo N, Carella C et al.: Thyroidal status in uremia – effects of hemodialysis and CAPD. Int J Artif Organs 5(6): 339–334, 1982.

260. Giordano C, De Santo N, Carella C et al.: TSH response to TRH in hemodialysis and CAPD patients. Int J Artif Organs 7(1): 7–10, 1984.

261. Thysen B, Gatz M, Freeman R et al.: Serum thyroid hormone levels in patients on continuous ambulatory peritoneal dialysis and regular hemodialysis. Nephron 33: 49–52, 1983.

262. Perez A, Arreola F, Paniagua R et al.: Serum thyroid hormones in the patient under intermittent peritoneal dialysis. Arch Invest Med (Mex) 16: 255–260, 1985.

263. Selgas R, Albero R, Beberide J et al.: Evaluation of thyroid function in patients treated with continuous ambulatory peritoneal dialysis (CAPD). Perit Dial Bull 3(1): 25–29, 1983.

264. Semple C, Beastall G, Henderson I et al.: Thyroid function and continuous ambulatory peritoneal dialysis. Nephron 32: 249–252, 1982.

265. Goodwin F, Ross R: Alteration of pituitary-thyroid function in patients treated with haemodialysis (HD) and chronic ambulatory peritoneal dialysis (CAPD) (Abstr.). Clin Sci 65: 14, 1984.

266. Gavin L, Eitan N, Cavalieri R et al.: Hypothyroidism induced by continuous ambulatory peritoneal dialysis. Western J Med 138(4): 562–565, 1983.

267. Inaba M, Nishizawa Y, Nishitani H et al.: Concentrations of thyroxine-binding globulin in sera and peritoneal dialysates in patients on chronic peritoneal ambulatory dialysis. Nephron 42: 58–61, 1986.

268. Walker F, From G, Khanna R et al.: Study of thyroid function in patients on CAPD (Abstr.). 15th Ann Meeting, Am Soc Nephrol, 1982.

269. Wahner H, Wasler A: Measurements of thyroxine-plasma

protein interactions. Med Clin N Am 56: 849–860, 1972.

270. Reilly C, Wellby M: Slow thyroxine binding globulin in the pathogenesis of increased dialysable fraction of thyroxine in nonthyroidal illness. J Clin Endocr Metab 57: 15–18, 1983.

271. Boero R, Quarello F, Belardi P et al.: Blunted response to TRH stimulation in CAPD patients (letter). Perit Dial Bull 3(4): 213, 1983.

272. Gardner D, Mars D, Thomas R et al.: Iodine retention and thyroid dysfunction in patients on hemodialysis and continuous ambulatory peritoneal dialysis. Am J Kidney Dis 7(6): 471-476, 1986.

273. Nicoletti I, Buoncristiani U, Filipponi P et al.: Prolactin and growth hormone dynamics in chronic renal failure: Effect of hemodialysis, peritoneal dialysis and kidney transplantation. IRCD Med Sci Biochem 9: 879–880, 1981.

274. Rodger R, Fletcher K, Dewar J et al.: Prevalence and pathogenesis of impotence in one hundred uremic men. Uremia Invest 8(2):L 89–96, 1984–85.

275. Hou S, Grossman S, Molitch M: Hyperprolactinemia in patients with renal insufficiency and chronic renal failure requiring hemodialysis or chronic ambulatory peritoneal dialysis. Am J Kidney Dis 6(4): 245–249, 1985.

276. Rodger R, Dewar J, Turner S et al.: Anterior pituitary dysfunction in patients with chronic renal failure treated by hemodialysis or continuous ambulatory peritoneal dialysis. Nephron 43: 169–172, 1986.

277. Von Baeyer H, Gahl G, Riedinger Borozak R et al.: Adaption of CAPD patients to the continuous ambulatory peritoneal energy uptake. Kidney int 23: 29–34, 1983.

278. Semple C, Beastall G, Henderson I et al.: The pituitary-testicular axis of uraemic subjects on haemodialysis and continuous ambulatory peritoneal dialysis. Acta Endocrinologica 101: 464–467, 1982.

279. Gomez F, De La Gueva R, Wauters J et al.: Endocrine abnormalities in patients undergoing long-term hemodialysis. Am J Med 68: 322–350, 1980.

280. Rice G: Hypermenorrhea in the young hemodialysis patient. Am J Obstet Gynecol 116: 539–543, 1973.

281. Goodwin N, Valenti C, Hall J et al.: Effects of uremia and chronic hemodialysis on the reproductive cycle. Am J Obstet Gynecol 100: 528–535, 1968.

282. Pepperell R, Adam W, Dawborn J: Hemodialysis in the management of chronic renal failure during pregnancy. Austr NZ Obstet Gynaecol 10: 180–186, 1970.

283. Unzelman R, Alderfer G, Chojnacki R: Pregnancy and chronic hemodialysis. Trans Am Soc Artif Intern Organs 19: 144–149, 1973.

284. Sheriff M, Hardman M, Lamont C et al.: Successful pregnancy in a 44-year old hemodialysis patient. Br J Obstet Gynaecol 5: 386–389, 1978.

285. Kobayashi H, Matsumoto Y, Otsubo O et al.: Successful pregnancy in a patient undergoing chronic hemodialysis. Obstet Gynaecol 57: 382–386, 1981.

286. Ackrill P, Goodwin F, Marsh F et al.: Successful pregnancy in a patient on regular dialysis. Br Med J 2: 172–174, 1975.

287. Wing A, Brunner F, Brynger H et al.: Combined report on regular dialysis and transplantation in Europe VIII. Proc Eur Dial Trans Assoc 15: 4–76, 1978.

288. Brunner F, Brynger H, Chantler C et al.: Combined report on regular dialysis and transplantation in Europe IX. Proc Eur Dial Trans Assoc 16: 2–73, 1979.

289. Winchester J, Foegh M, Kloberdanz N et al.: Return of menstruation and improvement in sexual function as a result of CAPD (Abstr.). Int Symp Perit Dial, Berlin, 75, 1981.

290. Rubin J: Can a female patient on CAPD become pregnant? Perit Dial Bull 1: 44, 1981.

291. Cattran D, Benzie R: Pregnancy in a CAPD patient. Perit Dial Bull 3: 3–16, 1983.

292. Kioko E, Shaw K, Clarke A et al.: Successful pregnancy in

a diabetic patient treated with CAPD. Diabetes Care 6: 298–300, 1983.

293. Galler M, Spinowitz B, Charyton C et al.: Reproductive function in dialysis patients: CAPD vs. hemodialysis. Perit Dial Bull Suppl 3(1): S30-S32, 1983.

294. Lim V, Henriquez C, Sievertsen G et al.: Ovarian function in chronic renal failure: evidence suggesting hypothalamic anovulation. Ann Intern Med 93: 21–27, 1980.

295. Lim V, Kathpalia S, Frohman L: Hyperprolactinemia and impaired pituitary response to suppression and stimulation in chronic renal failure: reversal after transplantation. J Clin Endocrinol Metab 48: 101–107, 1979.

296. Peces R, Horcajada C, Lopez-Novos J et al.: Hyperprolactinemia in chronic renal failure: impaired responsiveness to stimulation and suppression. Nephron 28: 11–16, 1981.

297. Khanna R, Oreopoulos D, Dombros N et al.: Continuous ambulatory peritoneal dialysis (CAPD) after three years: still a promising treatment. Perit Dial Bull 1: 24–34, 1981.

298. Glasson P, Favre H, Vallotton M: Response of blood pressure and the renin-angiotensin-aldosterone system to chronic ambulatory peritoneal dialysis in hypertensive endstage renal failure. Clin Sci 63: 207S–209S, 1982.

299. Young M: Anti-hypertensive drug requirements in continuous ambulatory peritoneal dialysis. Perit Dial Bull 4(2): 85–88, 1984.

300. Zager P, Spalding C, Frey H: Plasma levels of adrenocortical steroids in CAPD and hemodialysis patients. Perit Dial Bull Suppl 4(3): S88-S91, 1984.

301. Osmond D, Loh A, Dombros N et al.: Effects of CAPD on the renin-angiotensin system (Abstr.). Clin Res 26: 870, 1978.

302. Sasaki H, Okumura M, Tkeda M et al.: Hypotensive response to angiotensin II analog in Bartter's syndrome. N Eng J Med 294: 611, 1976.

303. Leenen F, Shah P, Boer W et al.: Hypotension on CAPD: an approach to treatment. Perit Dial Bull Supp 3(3): S33-S35, 1983.

304. Avioli L, Teitelbaum S: The renal osteodystrophies. In: Early L et al. (eds): Diseases of the Kidney. Little Brown and Co Boston: pp 307–310, 1979.

305. Coburn J: Renal osteodystrophy. Kidney Int 17: 677–693, 1980.

306. Gokal R, Ellis H, Ramos J et al.: Improvement in secondary hyperparathyroidism in patients on CAPD. In: Gahl G et al. (eds): Advances in Peritoneal Dialysis. Excerpta Medica, Amsterdam, 1981: pp 461–466.

307. Calderaro V, Oreopoulos D, Meema H et al.: The evolution of renal osteodystrophy in patients undergoing CAPD. Proc Eur Dial Transpl Assoc 17: 533–542, 1980.

308. Nolph K, Sorkin M, Arjanin D et al.: CAPD–three years experience at a single center. Ann Intern Med 92: 609–612, 1980.

309. Digenis G, Khanna R, Pierratos A et al.: Renal osteodystrophy in patients maintained on CAPD for more than three years. Perit Dial Bull 3: 81–86, 1983.

310. Rahman R, Heaton A, Goodship T et al.: Renal osteodystrophy in patients on continuous ambulatory peritoneal dialysis: a five-year study. Perit Dial Bull 7: 20–26, 1987.

311. Buccianti G, Bianchi M, Valenti G. Progress of renal osteodystrophy during continuous ambulatory peritoneal dialysis. Clin Nephrol 22: 279–283, 1984.

312. Cannata J, Briggs J, Fell G et al.: Comparison of control of serum phosphate levels during continuous ambulatory peritoneal dialysis. Perit Dial Bull 3: 97–98, 1983.

313. Zucchelli P, Catizone L, Casanova S et al.: Renal osteodystrophy in CAPD patients. Mineral Electr Metabol 9: 82–86, 1983.

314. Loschiava C, Fabris A, Adami S et al.: Effects of continuous ambulatory peritoneal dialysis (CAPD) on renal osteodystro-

phy. Perit Dial Bull 5: 53-55, 1985.

315. Nilsson P, Danielson B, Grefberg N *et al.*: Secondary hyperparathyroidism in diabetic and nondiabetic patients on long-term continuous ambulatory peritoneal dialysis (CAPD). Scand J Urol Nephrol 19: 59-65, 1985.

316. Shany S, Rapoport J, Goliforsky M *et al.*: Losses of 1,25- and 24,25-dihydroxycholecalciferol in the peritoneal fluid of patients treated with continuous ambulatory peritoneal dialysis. Nephron 36: 111-113, 1984.

317. Gokal R, Ramos J, Ellis H *et al.*: Histological renal osteodystrophy, and 25 hydroxycholecalciferol and aluminum levels in patients on continuous ambulatory peritoneal dialysis. Kidney Int 23: 15-21, 1983.

318. Alony Y, Shany S, Chaimovitz C: Losses of 25-hydroxyvitamin D in peritoneal fluid: possible mechanism for bone disease in uremic patients treated with chronic ambulatory peritoneal dialysis. Mineral Electr Metabol 9: 82-86, 1983.

319. El Shahat Y, Issad B, Jacobs C *et al.*: Evolution of renal osteodystrophy (RO) in patients treated with CAPD. Mineral Electr Metabol 6: 265, 1981.

320. Meema H, Oreopoulos D: Arterial calcifications in patients undergoing chronic peritoneal dialysis: incidence, progression and regression. Perit Dial Bull 5: 241-247, 1985.

321. Cassidy M, Owen J, Ellis H *et al.*: Renal osteodystrophy and metastatic calcification in long-term continuous ambulatory peritoneal dialysis. Q J Med (New series) 54: 29-48, 1985.

322. Delmez J, Fallon M, Bergfeld M *et al.*: Continuous ambulatory peritoneal dialysis and bone. Kidney Int 30: 379-384, 1986.

323. Hercz G, Milliner D, Shinaberger J *et al.*: Aluminum metabolism and removal during CAPD (Abstr.). Am Soc of Neph 16: 120, 1983.

324. Pierides A, Van Den Berg C, Pierce-Myli M *et al.*: Resolution of aluminum osteomalacia with IV desferoxamine followed by vitamin D (Abstr.) Am Soc Neph: 1983.

325. Nebeker H, Milling D, Ott S *et al.*: Aluminum related osteomalacia. Chemical response to desferrioxamine (Abstr.). Am Soc Neph: 1983.

326. Kaehney W, Hegg A, Alfrey A: Gastrointestinal absorption of aluminum containing antacids. N Eng J Med 296: 1389, 1977.

327. Pascoe M, Gregory M: Dialysis encephalopathy: aluminum concentrations in dialysate and brain. Kidney Int 16: 90, 1979.

328. Pierides A, Edwards W, Cullum W *et al.*: Hemodialysis encephalopathy with osteomalacic fractures and muscle weakness. Kidney Int 18: 115, 1980.

329. Milliner D, Nebeker H, Ott S *et al.*: Desferrioxamine infusion test for diagnosis of aluminum osteomalacia (Abstr.). Am Soc Neph: 1983.

330. Simon P, Meyrier A, Allain P: Evaluation of aluminum tissue storage by a desferrioxamine test in chronic hemodialysis patients (Abstr.). Am Soc Neph: 1983.

331. Llach F, Felsenfeld A, Coleman M *et al.*: Renal osteodystrophy in 131 unselected hemodialysis patients (Abstr.). Am Soc Neph 16: 50, 1983.

332. Fernandez E, Quellhorst E, Meitzsch G: Treatment of chronic uremia. A comparison of intermittent peritoneal dialysis and hemodialysis (Abstr.). 13th Congr Eur Dial Trans Assoc: 1367, 1976.

333. Oreopoulos D, Blair G, Meema H *et al.*: Overall experience with peritoneal dialysis. Dial Transpl 7: 783-787, 1978.

334. Blumenkrantz M, Lindsay R: Comparison of hemodialysis and peritoneal dialysis: a review of the literature. Contr Nephrol (Karger) 17: 20-29, 1979.

335. Sunderrajan S, Nolph K: Longitudinal study of nerve conduction velocities during continuous ambulatory peritoneal dialysis. Perit Dial Bull 5(1): 45-48, 1985.

336. Kim D, Blair G, Wu G *et al.*: Electrophysiological studies

337. Tegner R, Lindholm B: Uremic polyneuropathy: different effects of hemodialysis and continuous ambulatory peritoneal dialysis. Acta Med Scand 218: 409-416, 1985.

338. Kersch E, Kronfield S, Unger A *et al.*: Autonomic insufficiency in uremia as a cause of hemodialysis-induced hypotension. N Eng J Med 290: 650-653, 1974.

339. Zucchelli P, Chiarini C, Esposti E *et al.*: Influence of continuous ambulatory peritoneal dialysis on the autonomic nervous system. Kidney Int 23: 46-50, 1983.

340. Mallamaci F, Zoccali C, Ciccarelli M *et al.*: Autonomic function in uremic patients treated by hemodialysis or CAPD and in transplant patients. Clin Nephrol 25(4): 175-180, 1986.

341. Sideman S, Manor D: The dialysis dementia syndrome and aluminum intoxication (editorial). Nephron 31: 1-10, 1982.

342. Dunea G, Mahurkar S, Mamdani B *et al.*: Role of aluminum in dialysis dementia. Ann Intern Med 88: 502, 1978.

343. Smith D, Lewis J, Burks J *et al.*: Dialysis encephalopathy in peritoneal dialysis. J Am Med Assoc 244: 365-366, 1980.

344. Oreopoulos D: Chronic peritoneal dialysis. Clin Nephrol 9: 165, 1978.

345. Gilli P, Farinelli A, Fagioli F *et al.*: Serum aluminum levels in patients on peritoneal dialysis. Lancet 2: 742-743, 1980.

346. Sitpria V, Holmes J: Preliminary observation on intracranial pressure and intraocular pressure during hemodialysis. Trans Am Soc Artif Intern Organs 10: 340-344, 1964.

347. Dossetor J, Oh J, Dayes L *et al.*: Urea and water changes with rapid hemodialysis of uremic dogs. Trans Am Soc Artif Intern Organs 10: 323-327, 1964.

348. Kennedy A, Linton A, Lake R *et al.*: Electroencephalographic changes during hemodialysis. Lancet 1: 408-411, 1963.

349. Maher J, Schreiner G: Hazards and complications of dialysis. N Eng J Med 273: 370-377, 1965.

350. Nienhuis L: Clinical peritoneal dialysis. Arch Surg 93: 643-653, 1966.

351. Jagadha V, Deck J, Halliday W *et al.*: Wernicke's encephalopathy in patients on peritoneal dialysis or hemodialysis. Ann Neurol 21: 78-84, 1987.

352. Colotla V, Campbell E, Oreopoulos D *et al.*: Neuropsychological comparison of patients on home peritoneal dialysis (HPD) and on home hemodialysis (HHD) (Abstr.). Am Soc Neph: p 28, 1975.

353. Roxe D: Comparisons of maintenance peritoneal and hemodialysis. Dial Transpl 7: 800-802, 1978.

354. Kenney F: Neurotoxicity, cognitive function and the outcome of CAPD. Perit Dial Bull Supp 3(3): S43-S47, 1983.

355. Cardenas D, Kutner W: The problem of fatigue in dialysis patients. Nephron 30: 336-340, 1982.

356. Moldofsky H, Krueger J, Walter J *et al.*: Sleep-promoting material extracted from peritoneal dialysate of patients with end-stage renal disease and insomnia. Perit Dial Bull 5(3): 189-193, 1985.

357. Eschbach J, Egrie J, Downing M *et al.*: Correction of the anemia of end-stage renal disease with recombinant human erythropoietin. N Eng J Med 316: 73-78, 1987.

358. Raskova J, Ghobrial I, Czerwinski D *et al.*: B-cell activation and immunoregulation in end-stage renal disease patients receiving hemodialysis. Arch Intern Med 147: 89-93, 1987.

359. Kurz P, Kohler H, Meuer S *et al.*: Impaired cellular immune responses in chronic renal failure: evidence for a T cell defect. Kidney Int 29: 1209-1214, 1986.

360. Wu G, Gelbart D, Hasbargen J *et al.*: Reactivation of systemic lupus in three patients undergoing CAPD. Perit Dial Bull 6(1): 6-9, 1986.

361. Giacchino F, Alloatti S, Quarello F *et al.*: The influence of peritoneal dialysis on cellular immunity. Perit Dial Bull 2(4): 165-168, 1982.

362. Giagrande A, Cantu P, Limido A *et al.*: Continuous am-

bulatory peritoneal dialysis and cellular immunity. Proc Eur Dial Trans Assoc 19: 372–379, 1982.

363. Webb D, Smith C, Lee G *et al.*: Does continuous ambulatory peritoneal dialysis alter immune function? (Abstr.). Clin Sci 66: 14, 1984.

364. Shohat B, Boner G, Waller A *et al.*: Cell-mediated immunity in uremic patients prior to and after 6 months' treatment with continuous ambulatory peritoneal dialysis. Isr J Med Sci 22: 551–555, 1986.

365. Giacchino F, Pozzato M, Formica M *et al.*: Improved cell-mediated immunity in CAPD patients as compared to those on hemodialysis. Perit Dial Bull 4(4): 209–212, 1984.

366. Collart F, Tielemans C, Schandene L *et al.*: CAPD and cellular immunity: no different than that in hemodialysis patients (letter). Perit Dial Bull 3(3): 163–164, 1983.

367. Bargman J, Kuzniak S, Klein M: Changes in immune function induced by 1,25–dihydroxyvitamin D3 (Abstr.). Kidney Int 31: 342, 1987.

368. Langhoff E, Ladefoged J: Improved lymphocyte transformation in vitro of patients on continuous ambulatory peritoneal dialysis. Proc Eur Dial Trans Assoc 20: 230–235, 1983.

369. Perez G, Glasson P, Havre H *et al.*: Circulating immune complexes in regularly dialyzed patients with chronic renal failure. Am J Nephrol 4: 215–221, 1984.

370. Penn I: Malignancies associated with immunosuppressive or cytotoxic therapy. Surgery 83: 492–496, 1978.

371. Lindner A, Farewell Y, Sherrard D: High incidence of neoplasia in uremic patients receiving long-term dialysis. Nephron 27: 292–296, 1981.

372. Digenis G, Pierratos A, Ayiomamitis A *et al.*: Cancer in patients on CAPD. Perit Dial Bull 6(3): 122–124, 1986.

373. Cardella C: Peritoneal dialysis and renal transplantation (editorial). Perit Dial Bull 5(3): 149–151, 1985.

374. Gokal R, Ramos J, Veitch P *et al.*: Renal transplantation in patients on CAPD. Dial and Trans 11(2): 125, 155, 1982.

375. Gelfand M, Kois J, Quillin B *et al.*: CAPD yields inferior transplant results compared to hemodialysis (Abstr.). Perit Dial Bull 4: 526, 1984.

376. Guillou P, Will E, Davison A *et al.*: CAPD – a risk factor in renal transplantation? Br J Surg 71: 878–880, 1984.

377. Shapira Z, Shmueli D, Yussim A *et al.*: Kidney transplantation in patients on continuous ambulatory peritoneal dialysis. Proc Eur Dial Trans Assoc 21: 932–935, 1984.

378. Evangelista J, Bennett-Jones D, Cameron J *et al.*: Renal transplantation in patients treated with haemodialysis and short term and long term continuous ambulatory peritoneal dialysis. Br Med J 291: 1004–1007, 1985.

379. Donnelly P, Lennard T, Proud G *et al.*: Continuous ambulatory peritoneal dialysis and renal transplantation: a five year experience. Br Med J 291: 1001–1004, 1985.

380. Tsakiris D, Bramwell S, Briggs J *et al.*: Transplantation in patients undergoing CAPD. Perit Dial Bull 5(3): 161–164, 1985.

381. Diaz-Buxo J, Walker P, Burgess W *et al.*: The influence of peritoneal dialysis on the outcome of transplantation. Int J Artif Organs 9(5): 359–362, 1986.

382. Glass N, Miller D, Sollinger H *et al.*: Renal transplantation in patients on peritoneal dialysis. Perit Dial Bull 5(3): 157–160, 1985.

383. Rubin J, Kirchner K, Raju S *et al.*: CAPD patients as renal transplant patients. Am J Med Sci 294(3): 175–180, 1987.

384. Cardella C: Renal transplantation in patients on peritoneal dialysis. Perit Dial Bull 1(3): 12–14, 1980.

385. Steinmuller D, Novick A, Braun W *et al.*: Renal transplantation of patients on chronic peritoneal dialysis. Am J Kid Dis 3(6): 436–439, 1984.

386. Rigby R, Petrie J: Transplantation in patients on continuous ambulatory peritoneal dialysis (letter). Transplantation 37(5): 533, 1984.

387. Ryckelynck J-P, Verger C, Pierre D *et al.*: Early post transplantation infections in CAPD patients. Perit Dial Bull 4(1): 40-41, 1984.

388. Stephanidis C, Balfe J, Arbus G *et al.*: Renal transplantation in children treated with continuous ambulatory peritoneal dialysis. Perit Dial Bull 3(1): 5–8, 1983.

389. Dutton S: Transient post-transplant ascites in CAPD patients (letter). Perit Dial Bull 3(3): 164, 1983.

390. Dunnill M, Millard P, Oliver D: Acquired cystic disease of the kidney. Lancet 2: 1063, 1977.

391. Mickisch O, Bommer J, Bachmann S *et al.*: Multicystic transformation of kidneys in chronic renal failure. Nephron 38: 93–99, 1984.

392. Purandare V, Ing T, Daugirdas J *et al.*: Renal cysts in a CAPD patient (letter). Artif Organs 8(4): 501, 1984.

393. Beardsworth S, Goldsmith H, Ahmad R *et al.*: Acquisition of renal cysts during peritoneal dialysis (letter). Lancet 2: 1482, 1984.

394. Ishikawa I, Siato Y, Onouchi Z *et al.*: Development of acquired cystic disease and adenocarcinoma of the kidney in glomerulonephritic chronic hemodialysis patients. Clin Nephrol 14: 1–6, 1980.

16

PERITONEAL DIALYSIS ACCESS

RAMESH KHANNA and ZBYLUT J. TWARDOWSKI

1. INTRODUCTION

Access to the peritoneal cavity using an indwelling permanent and trouble free catheter is the key factor in the success of long term peritoneal dialysis. With the introduction of continuous ambulatory peritoneal dialysis, an increasing proportion of patients with end-stage renal disease are being managed at home and for this an easy and safe access to the peritoneal cavity is essential. Since Palmer *et al.* [1–2] introduced an indwelling silicone rubber peritoneal catheter in 1964, several modifications have been made to the original design directed chiefly towards improved anchoring to subcutaneous tissues and decreasing free movement inside the peritoneal cavity. The Tenckhoff version of the silicone catheter is still the most widely used catheter [3]. Catheter related complications such as catheter

tip migration, dialysis solution leak, and exit site infection are frequently encounterd with the use of Tenckhoff's catheter often related to improper placement and post placement care. Overall one year survival of the peritoneal catheter is 60–70% [4]. Catheter exit site and tunnel infections are frequent in patients on CAPD and are the cause of increased morbidity, prolonged antibiotic therapy, recurrent peritonitis, and catheter failure. According to the National CAPD Registry 12.4% of catheters are removed because of exit or tunnel infection [4].

2. HISTORY OF CATHETER DEVELOPMENT

In the early years of peritoneal dialysis, the access was not specifically designed for peritoneal dialysis; rather, equipment used for other purposes was adapted. In 1923 Ganter [5] carried out peritoneal dialysis in anuric rabbits and subsequently for the first time in humans. Ganter [5] used a metal trocar to gain access to the peritoneal cavity. Rosenak and Siwon [6] inserted a surgical drain made of a glass cannula with multiple side holes to infuse and drain dialysis solution. Desider Engel [7] from Prague used a glass catheter with a mushroom like opening inside the peritoneal cavity to maximize fluid distribution. Wear, Sisk and Trinkle [8] used a regular gallbladder trocar for the inflow and a trocar with numerous side holes for outflow. Reid, Penfold and Jones [9] used a Foley catheter. Fine, Frank and Saligman [10] in 1946 used a rubber catheter threaded on a perforated small stainless steel tube as an inlet tube and a stainless sumpdrain as an outlet tube.

Although, these devices allowed for adequate in-and-out flow, several problems were recognized. Major problems in those days were leakage, infection and catheter occlusion by clot or omental fat sucked into the catheter lumen. Some unusual problems that we do not see these days were: rigidity of tube with resulting pressure to viscera, constant suction of contaminated air in to the peritoneal cavity, and difficulties of proper aseptic fixation of the tube to abdominal wall.

Stephen Rosenak [11], a Hungarian doctor who got interested in the technique of dialysis during his medical student days, recognized these draw backs and in 1947 while working at the Mt. Sinai Hospital, N.Y. for the first time developed an access specifically meant for peritoneal dialysis. His access consisted of an upper rigid tube with an interchangeable lower, spiral, flexible, stainless steel coil extension. A straight inner tube extended from the outlet to the upper part of a flexible tube. This inner tube was connected to suction through a rubber tubing. This device permitted continuous inflow through the outer tube and outflow through the inner tube. There was an adjustable tie plate for fixation of the tube to skin. This device overcame some of the problems but dit not become popular because of inadequate drainage, and metal tube was very irritating to the peritoneum.

The next major progress was made during the 50's when Derot *et al.* [12] and Legrain and Merrill [13] used PVC tubes and Maxwell, Reckney, Kleeman, and Twiss [14] from UCLA introduced a semirigid nylon catheter with multiple tiny side perforations, slightly curved at the distal end with a solid rounded tip. The small perforations prevented omentum from entering the lumen during drainage. Around same time, Paul Doolan [15] from the US Naval Hospital, with the help of William Murphy, then President of Cordis Corporation manufactured a PVC catheter with multiple small holes between the raised ridges to prevent the omentum from being sucked during drainage. Doolan has also been credited with using IP insulin for blood sugar control during PD [15]. Both Maxwell's and Doolan's catheters were inserted into the peritoneal cavity with the help of a trocar used for abdominal paracentesis. Smooth nylon and PVC materials were less irritating to the peritoneum. Drainage improved considerably. But, pericatheter dialysis solution leaks and infections still persisted at a very high rate.

A year later, Weston and Roberts [16] invented the stylet catheter. This nylon rigid catheter could be inserted without the use of a trocar. A sharp stainless steel stylet inserted through the catheter was used to penetrate the abdominal wall. The catheter fitted snugly in the hole created by the stylet and prevented dialysis solution leak. Prototypes of this catheters are still being used in many centers for acute peritoneal dialysis.

In 1962, Dr. Scribner from the Seattle wrote and invited Dr. Boen from the Netherlands to come to Seattle to work in peritoneal dialysis research. At that time the Seattle group had only a limited capacity for hemodialysis, and Dr. Scribner foresaw that peritoneal dialysis promised to be a good alternative for handling a larger number of patients.

With the help of chief technician, George Shilipetar, Dr. Boen in 1962 developed a 'fluid factory' in Seattle and designed an automatic machine for dialysis solution delivery [17]. The first patient Dr. Boen treated was a patient unsuitable for hemodialysis. He implanted an indwelling peritoneal button in the abdominal wall. This button was a teflon modification of a plastic device. Through this button a long catheter was inserted inside the peritoneal cavity. After each dialysis, the catheter was removed and the button was capped. This patient had frequent episodes of peritonitis. Nevertheless, the patient survived for seven months and eventually died of peritonitis. Others also developed conduits for dialysis [18, 19].

Because of frequent infections, Boen in 1963, developed the intermittent puncture technique [20]. He would insert a small nylon catheter into the abdomen, perform dialysis and then remove it. A new puncture and a new catheter was used each time the patient was dialyzed.

In 1965, Henry Tenckhoff, at the University of Washington, was beginning to treat patients on chronic peritoneal dialysis [21]. After the initial few dialyses in the hospital, ESRD patients would be trained for home dialysis. On the weekends Tenckhoff would go to patient's home, insert the catheter and begin the dialysis. After the appropriate time on dialysis with a machine, the patient would remove the catheter and cover the exit wound with a bandage. This method was used over a 3½ yr period during which 380 catheter punctures were performed. Although, with this technique, the complications were very low, it was not a practical proposition.

Jacob and Deane [22] in 1967 invented a teflon rod to keep the catheter hole patent between dialyses. Using this prosthesis, Oreopoulos in Toronto maintained a patient on chronic dialysis for a period of one year [23]. Other subcutaneous access devices were designed and used with success [24, 25].

About this time, Russell Palmer [1], a physician at the Canadian Army Medical Corps was developing a peritoneal access which would be safe and easy to insert. With the help of Wayne Quinton, Palmer developed catheters made of polyethylene, polypropylene and nylon. These catheters were relatively rigid and hence did not always make a good seal at the exit site. Also, these materials posed difficulties in creating a subcutaneous tunnel. He was looking for a catheter material which would be more biocompatible and less irritating to the peritoneum. The observations of Frank Gutch [26] in both acute and chronic patients pointed out the remarkable compatibility of silastic with the peritoneal membrane. He found considerably lower protein losses in patients using silastic material compared to PVC. This

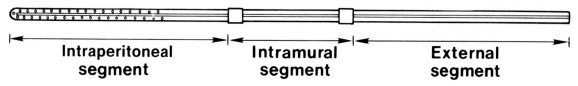

Intraperitoneal segment   **Intramural segment**   **External segment**

Fig. 1. Diagram of Tenckhoff catheter showing various segments.

finding lead Palmar and Quinton [1, 2] to develop the first permanent silicone catheter. This catheter had a long intramural segment. The intraperitoneal segment was coiled and had lead at the tip to prevent catheter migration. Halfway along the tube was a triflanged step for fixing the tube in the deep fascia and peritoneum. This catheter sealed properly at the exit site and because of the long subcutaneous tunnel, prevented the migration of bacteria to the peritoneal cavity. Autopsy of the first patient who received Palmar's catheter showed that the catheter was in good position and there was no infection around the exit site. McDonald *et al.* [27] incorporated a teflon velour skirt in the subcutaneous tissue and a dacron-weaveknit sleeve from the skirt down to the peritoneum.

Henry Tenckhoff [3] modified Palmer's catheter in several ways to adapt it for chronic use (Figure 1). For better mechanical fixation of the catheter to the abdominal wall tissue, he bonded felt Dacron® cuffs to the catheter. He used medical adhesives as bonding material. He reasoned that a Dacron® felt cuff besides functioning as a stabilizer also created a barrier against bacterial invasion of the peritoneal cavity. He used large numbers of both single and double cuff catheters with success. To simplify the implantation procedure, he shortened the intramural tunnel segment. Intra-peritoneal segment was kept open ended and the size of side holes was optimized to 0.5 mm to prevent tissue incarceration. For bedside insertion of the catheter, he developed, at the University Medical Instrument Shop, the first trocar which was later patented (Figure 2).

Twenty years later, even today, Tenckhoff's catheter in its original form is still the most widely used catheter type. Some of the recommendations for catheter insertion such as cephalad tilting of the trocar for pelvic placement, placement of the subcutaneous cuff immediately beneath the skin, and an arc shaped subcutaneous tunnel are still considered important steps in the successful implantation

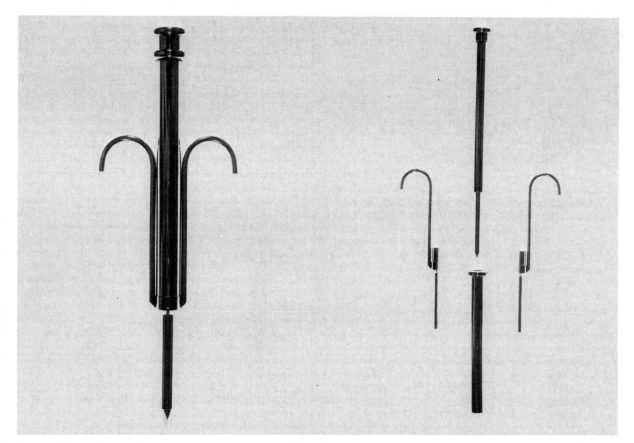

Figure 2. The bedside Tenckhoff catheter insertion trocar, fully assembled and with parts seperated.

of the catheter [28].

In CAPD patients the use of the straight intraabdominal portion of the Tenckhoff catheter was associated with a high incidence of catheter tip displacement and one way obstruction. To prevent such complications several modified catheters were used in the subsequent years [29–31]. This chapter will describe in detail some of those catheters which are in current use, their insertion technique and their long-term results.

3. BACKGROUND OF NEW CATHETER DESIGNS

3.1. Catheter skin-exit direction

Tenckhoff in 1968 recommended creating an arc tunnel with the skin-exit pointing downward [3]. In subsequent years, probably because of a high incidence of superficial cuff extrusion, little attention has been paid to his recommendation. In a retrospective analysis of our catheter experience [32], we found that catheters with a downward directed skin-exit tended to be infected less often and when infected, were significantly less resistant to treatment than exit holes pointing in other directions. A tunnel with an exit hole pointing upward is prone to contamination by down flowing sweat, water, and dirt on the skin surface (Figure 3). Whenever such an exit is infected, it tends to be resistant to treatment because of poor pus drainage to outside, and tends to penetrate deep down into the tunnel. The rationale of gravity helping prevent infection and facilitate treatment when it occurs has analogies in several other clinical conditions: periodontitis, which may be considered as a biologically occurring 'foreign' body exit site infection, more often affects the lower incisors because their 'exits' are directed upward [33]. All body cavities in humans drain by gravity through a favorably positioned exit except the maxillary sinus which has its exit, the ostium maxillare located at the top of the cavity in the upright position, a most unfavorable site for free drainage [34]. Because of this reason, recurrent chronic maxillary sinus infection is frequent in humans and is resistant to treatment. Sub-

clavian catheters, which have a downward directed tunnel, are less frequently infected at the exit site than those of peritoneal catheters [35, 36]. Thus, for chronic peritoneal dialysis, if the catheter skin-exit is directed downward, it would be exposed to less contamination, drain pus better and facilitate drainage of necrotic tussue in the immediate post-implantation period.

3.1. Sinus tract length

In a completely healed tunnel, the term sinus tract refers to that part of the tunnel from the skin exit to the margin of the nearest cuff (Figure 4). Contrary to the observation in animals, we found in humans that the sinus tract is covered by a continuous layer of skin epidermis only for about 4-5 mm from the skin margin and rest of the tract is covered by a foreign body reaction tissue. The epidermis covering the sinus tract undergoes a turnover probably similar to the normal epidermis with cell maturation and desquamation. Desquamated epidermal cells and the dead inflammatory cells, if not expelled, create a favorable milieu for bacterial growth. With a long sinus tract, the drainage may not be the most efficient, and predispose to a higher incidence of infection [37–39]. Therefore, the sinus tract length should be as short as possible, preferably the length of the epidermal layer.

Tenckhoff recommended that the subcutaneous Dacron® felt cuff should be placed immediately beneath the skin exit [28]. Such a location of the cuff, however, predisposes to its extrusion [40], and thus, the wisdom of using a superficial cuff is questioned. There are at least three forces, the resilience force of silastic, the forces created because of external manipulation, and the vector force of maturing epidermal cells, which tend to extrude the cuff from its subcutaneous location. Resilience forces of a straight silastic catheter inserted in an arc shape gradually push the superficial cuff through the skin-exit, especially when the deep cuff is firmly anchored to the peritoneal tissue and posterior rectus fascia. With a short subbcutaneous tunnel, such extrusion would be much more frequent [28]. Pulling, twisting, and tugging forces applied unintentionally on the

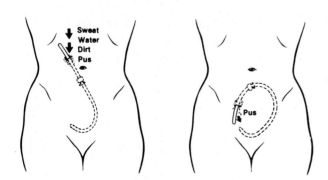

**UPWARD AND DOWNWARD TUNNEL DIRECTION–
EXIT SITE INFECTION**

Figure 3. (Left) Exit site contamination with cranial tunnel direction and (Right) fecilitated plus drainage with tunnel directed downward.

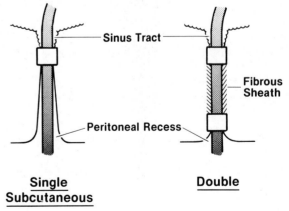

Figure 4. Diagram showing tissue structures in relation to catheter cuff position.

catheter during its daily use may cause tear and recurrent trauma resulting in displacement and external extrusion. A vector force, directed to exterior, created by maturing epidermal basal cells in the sinus tract tends to extrude the implant [37]. The rate of implant migration due to this vector force has been calculated at 1 mm/month in the miniature pigs [37]. This concept was challenged by Tenckhoff, who observed cuff extrusion as an early phenomenon (within weeks or months). He argued that late extrusion would be more common if vector force were to play a major role [41]. Contrary to Tenckhoff's experience with patients on intermittent peritoneal dialysis, cuff extrusion has been seen as late as 4–5 years after successful CAPD treatment. This rather slow process of cuff extrusion in humans may in part be due to a lower epidermal turnover rate compared to animals [42] and may in part be due to the non attachment of the epidermal cell layer to the cuff. The resilience of the straight silastic catheter implanted in an arcuate tunnel undoubtedly plays a major role in cuff extrusion but pulling and tugging forces applied on catheter during its daily usage also contribute significantly to this complication.

Thus, in order to promote epidermal growth as close to the collagen in the vicinity of cuff as possible, the sinus tract needs to be no longer than 5–6 mm; yet, to avoid cuff extrusion a longer sinus tract length may be needed. As a compromise we feel that the cuff should be implanted approximately 1 cm from the exit. Resilience forces could be eliminated with a molded bent catheter as in the Swan Neck catheters to be discussed later.

The exit should be kept clean of desquamated cells. Using soap and water some patients are able to maintain perfectly clean exits. The importance of a clean exit is supported by the experience with periodontitis, which usually is a sequela of poor oral hygiene. Interestingly, deep gingival sulci (>3 mm) in some individuals are difficult to clean and are more susceptible to infection [43].

3.3. Material for the external cuff

The external cuff should support attachment with collagen fibers to provide a strong anchorage [37]. Living materials like cementum with which periodontal ligament creates a strong bond [44], are unlikely to be used in the near future for the external cuff. Nonliving materials such as Dacron® have been used with success to provide a strong bond between it and collagen. Poirier, *et al.* [45] evaluated collagen attachment to various materials on their elaborate external seal for a percutaneous energy transmission system. The seal is composed of a semirigid polyurethane skirt positioned at the subdermal level and a hollow collar protruding through the skin. The polyurethane was covered with sintered titanium spheres, porous polytetrafluoroetheylene, or Dacron® velour. In experiments on miniature pigs, the Dacron® velour, especially when wetted with saline before implantation, provided the strongest collagen attachment with an excellent inhibition of epidermal down growth. These observations led Daly and coworkers [46] to hypothesize (and later obtain support by histopathological evaluation in animals [38]) that epidermal downgrowth around a percutaneous device may be prevented by encouraging collagen extension into the device. Our observation of catheter cuffs removed from long-term CAPD

patients indicated a profuse collagen tissue ingrowth between the Dacron® felt cuff fibers providing a strong bondage between the two. Paradoxical to these observations, the use of a polytetrafluoroethylene covered right angled catheter by Ogden *et al.* [47] resulted in a very high rate of chronic exit site infections. These catheters were provided with a subcutaneous flange covered with expanded polytetrafluoroethylene and a cuff of the same material. Ten of 17 catheters developed chronic exit site infection and 7 of them had to be removed when antibiotics failed to eradicate infections. Thus, it seems saline wetted Dacron® velour and polyurethane are the best materials for the cuff at present.

3.4. Role of the catheter cuff in the tunnel

Catheters with no cuffs create a fistulous tract between peritoneum and the exterior. Fistulous communication predisposes to penetration of bacteria into the peritoneal cavity and such a practice was abandoned after the introduction of cuffed Tenckhoff catheters. Single (only external) cuff catheters were used by Tenckhoff for management of acute renal failure. In patients undergoing chronic intermittent peritoneal dialysis, such single cuff catheters and double cuff catheters yielded similar results [28]. However, in patients on continuous ambulatory peritoneal dialysis, a major problem of single subcutaneous cuff catheters was the tendency to develop pseudoherniae through the long peritoneal recess, due to constant high intraabdominal pressure. Another type of single cuff catheter, provided with only a deep cuff at the peritoneal level, came to be used extensively because double cuff catheters were associated with a high incidence of external cuff extrusion and had questionable value in preventing exit site infections. A prospective randomized study showed exit site infection rate to be similar with single and double cuff catheters [48]; however, in a retrospective survey of catheters, in 395 patients, the tunnel infections were almost 3 times more frequent with single cuff than with double cuff catheters [40]. Also, in our experience the exit infections tended to be more frequent and were significantly more resistant to treatment with single cuff catheters compared to double cuff ones [32]. The discrepancy in the results reported may in part be due to the difference in the length of the sinus tract with different implantation techniques. A single deep cuff catheter when inserted is expected to have a longer sinus tract. If sinus tract lengths are similar, the incidence of exit infections is expected to be similar irrespective of which cuff limits the tract. Moreover, conflicting survival results have been reported with double cuff catheters compared to single cuff catheters in CAPD patients [48, 49]. Thus, it appears, for better anchorage, longer survival, and may be to restrict the migration of bacteria deep into the tunnel, a double cuff catheter may have advantages over a single cuff catheter.

3.5. Catheter tip migration

One way or two way catheter obstruction is usually the result of catheter wrapping by the omentum. The optimum conditions for free drainage of dialysis solution are created when the catheter tip is positioned in the true pelvis. In the upright position, the pelvis is the most dependent part of the peritoneal cavity. Moreover, in the majority, the omentum does not reach all the way to the true pelvis. Therefore, Tenckhoff recommended a caudal direction of the intraperitoneal catheter segment with pelvic placement to prevent catheter tip migration out of the true pelvis [28]. For the intraperitoneal catheter segment to remain within the deep pelvis, the intramural segment should be directed towards the pelvic cavity. In support of this observation, we found that when a catheter was implanted with a straight tunnel with the external skin exit directed downward and the intraperitoneal entrance directed upward (either pointing to liver or spleen), even if the catheter tip was placed in the true pelvis, it migrated to the upper abdomen significantly more frequently compared to the opposite tunnel direction [32]. This migration is the result of silastic resilience forces influencing the intraperitoneal segment of the catheter (Figure 5). Therefore, to avoid unfavorable influence of resilience forces on the intra-abdominal catheter segment, the catheter should be molded in the shape it is to be implanted in the body.

3.6. Tissue reaction to a skin-penetrating foreign body and factors that cause early infection and delay healing

The tissue reaction begins immediately after a break in the integument occurs. Bleeding from capillaries and body fluids form a coagulum of clot and cellular debris. Polymorphonuclear leukocytes phagocytize local bacteria and together with the coagulum form a scab. Healing of the wound starts with the production, beneath the scab, of granulation tissue composed of new vessels and fibroblasts. Upon this tissue, there is a peripheral ingrowth of new epithelial cells. These cells stop spreading over the granulation tissue only if they meet cells from the opposite shore (marsupialization) or encounter collagen fibers attached to the foreign body, (Dacron® Cuff in the case of peritoneal catheter) thus, creating a sinus tract [37], an interrelationship similar to that seen between tooth and gingival epithelium. The tooth is the only natural 'foreign' body

penetrating through epithelium in humans. The peridontal membrane (alveolar periosteum), a vascular fibrous tissue, is firmly attached to the cementum (substantia ossea) of tooth. Squamous epithelium covering the gum penetrates only to the level of attachment between the peridontal membrane and the cementum. The resulting gingival sulcus is only 1–3 mm deep [50]. However, the collagen fibers do not attach to the smooth surface of the silicone rubber, the material from which peritoneal dialysis catheters are made, but they attach to the rough surface of Dacron® and nylon velour or porous polytetrafluoroethylene [38]. Our recent observation of sinus tracts removed several years after catheter insertion indicate that epidermal downgrowth stops several millimeter from the exit, inhibited by collagen fibers of the foreign body reaction tissue.

Part of the coagulum is absorbed and part of it, along with necrotic tissue is gradually drained from the sinus tract. The tract should be wide enough to allow free drainage of necrotic tissue and prevent skin sloughing due to pressure necrosis. On the other hand, too large a tract prolongs healing because of the volume of repair needed and excessive movements of tubing. Mechanical stresses slow the healing process [39]. Thus, to promote unhindered healing, the catheter should be firmly anchored at the cuff and well immobilized outside the tunnel, especially during the break-in period.

Antibiotic penetration into the coagulum is poor, therefore, antibiotics should be present in sufficient concentration in the blood and tissue fluids before the coagulum is formed. This may be achieved if antibiotics are given prior to implantation. Recently, antibiotic impregnated catheters have been introduced to the market [51], although their efficacy has not been proven.

Epidermal cells grow over the granulation tissue beneath the scab. If the scab is forcibly removed during cleansing, the epidermal layer is broken, thus prolonging the process of epidermization. The healing process is complete when the epidermis reaches its final depth and the granulation tissue is replaced by the foreign body reaction tissue.

4. FREQUENTLY USED CATHETERS

4.1. Straight and curled Tenckhoff catheters

The catheter consists of a length of a silicone rubber tube with a 2.6 mm internal diameter and a 5 mm external diameter. The cuff is made of Dacron® felt and is 1 cm long. The double cuff catheter has three segments: external, intramural and intraperitoneal (Figure 1). The length of the intramural segment may vary between 5 and 7 cm. The length of the intraperitoneal segment can vary between 11 and 15 cm. in both single and double cuff catheters. The intraperitoneal and intramural segments in pediatric double cuff catheters are 7 and 2 cm long. The intraperitoneal segment has multiple 0.5 mm perforations in the terminal 3 to 9 cm portion. The curled Tenckhoff catheter differs from the straight in having a longer perforated section which is molded to assume a coiled shape. The length of the coiled section is 18.5 cm. The coil is supposed to prevent migration and to reduce the force of the inflowing stream thereby diminishing inflow discomfort. The variety of catheter

CATHETER TIP MIGRATION

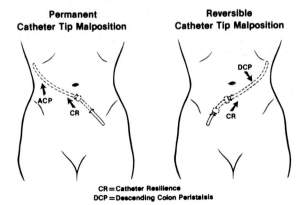

Figure 5. Straight catheter insertion: Catheter tip migration out of true pelvis with external exit directed downward and intraperitoneal entrance directed upward either pointing to liver or spleen. Note the tendency of catheter to assume its original shape.

lengths permits one to choose an appropriate catheter for every patient size.

4.2. The Toronto Western Hospital Catheter

The Toronto Western Hospital Catheter was designed by Oreopoulos and Zellerman in 1976 [31]. Its main distinguishing feature is two flat silicone rubber discs on the intra-abdominal segment of the catheter (Figure 6).

These flat discs prevent the free movement of catheter tip within the peritoneal cavity and thereby help the catheter remain in the minor pelvis. A prospective controlled study [31] in 1976 showed a lower incidence of catheter tip dislodgement from the pelvis with The Toronto Western Hospital Catheters (7%), when compared with the Tenckhoff Catheters (33%). Other complications encountered with the Toronto Western Catheter were the cramping rectal and abdominal pain which lasted for two to six weeks in 33% of the patients. The major disadvantage recognised with the use of the Toronto Western Catheter was the need for surgical implantation and removal.

Whereas the basic design of the intra-abdominal segment of the Toronto Western Catheter remains unchanged, further modifications have been made since 1976. The intra-abdominal segment was shortened to eliminate the rectal pain experienced by some patients in the initial study (Toronto Western Hospital Type 1 Catheter). Further alterations were made at the level of peritoneal Dacron® cuff to reduce the incidence of early and late dialysate leaks and the risk of incisional hernias. These modifications included the addition of a Dacron® disc, one centimeter in diameter, on the base of the peritoneal cuff, which at the time of insertion is placed between the peritoneum and fascia,, to seal the peritoneal hole, and a silastic ring one millimeter distal to the Dacron® disc to provide a groove (C in figure 6) between them, in which the surgeon ties the peritoneum tightly (Toronto Western Hospital, Type 2 Catheter).

In 1981 Ponce *et al.* [52] reported an experience with the two most frequently used Toronto Western Hospital Catheters (Type 1 and 2) and compared them with the straight Tenckhoff Catheters implanted either medically or surgically (94 Toronto Western Hospital, Type 1 Catheters, 83 Toronto Western Hospital, Type 2 Catheters and 90 straight Tenckhoff Catheters). Cumulative catheter survival rates at the end of the first and second years were significantly better (p < 0.05) for Toronto Western Hospital Type 2 Catheters compared to the Straight Tenckhoff Catheters inserted medically. No significant differences were observed between the other groups. The data on catheter survival among various subgroups showed a trend to lower

survival of catheters in patients older then 60 years and diabetics, compared to younger patients and non diabetics respectively. Considered together, all first time catheters had significantly better one year survival than all the second or subsequent catheters.

A significant complication, observed among all catheters, was early dialysate leak which occurred at a rate ranging from 18 to 32%. Patients older than 60 years had a higher incidence of leakage (42.3%) than younger patients (26.9%) (p < 0.01). Also women had a higher incidence of leakage (36.2%) than men (18.6%) (p < 0.01), and leakage was more common among second or subsequent catheters (42.7%) than in first catheters (26.9%) (p < 0.01).

Immediate post operative complications related to the catheter were: perioperative pain (1–6%), infection (1–5%) and poor drainage (11–22%), cuff extrusion (1–7%) and late one way obstruction (9–16%). In all four groups, the major cause of catheter failure and consequent removal was one way obstruction due to dislodgement of the catheter from the pelvis and encasement by omentum, or two way obstruction.

In an effort to reduce the frequency of dialysate leak, the catheter implantation technique was modified in such a way that the catheters passed through the rectus muscle rather than through the midline and the 1st post-operative dialysis was delayed for at least 24 hr after implantation of the catheter instead of starting immediately. This approach practically eliminated the complication of dialysate leak.

In this chapter we will describe in detail the catheter design, insertion technique, post-operative care of the catheter, and complications observed with Toronto Western Type II catheters.

4.2.1. Catheter design

The Toronto Western Hospital Catheters are made of medical grade silicone rubber, thus making them soft, flexible, and atraumatic to bowel. The silicone rubber is nonimmunogenic, induces no tissue reaction and is not water wettable. These catheters are available with a barium impregnated radio-opaque stripe to assist in the radiological localization of the intraabdominal section. Adult Toronto Western Catheters are 41 cm long whereas pediatric catheters are 35 cm long (Figure 6). The extraabdominal section (segment F in Figure 6) of the catheter is about 20 cm long, and is identical in design to the Tenckhoff catheter. This long length of the extraabdominal section allows easy handling and reserves enough length to permit trimming if a catheter split occurs at the connector site during its long use. The subcutaneous and transmural segment (segment E in Figure 6) is about 2 cm long. A

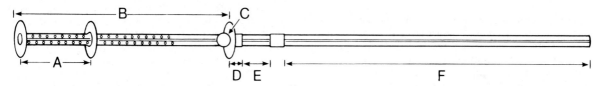

Figure 6. Diagram of Toronto Western Hospital catheter showing various segments. A = distance between two discs; B = intraperitoneal segment; C = groove between the Dacron disc and silastic disc; D = Dacron disc and cuff; E = intramural segment; F = external segment.

Dacron® felt cuff 1 cm wide is bonded to the catheter by the manufacturer (Accurate Surgical Instruments Corporation, 588 Richmond St. W., Toronto, Ontario, Canada M5V 1Y9) at the junction of extra-abdominal section and subcutaneous part. Except for the absence of a subcutaneous cuff, the Toronto Western II single cuff catheter is identical in design to the Toronto Western II double cuff catheter. The short intramural section of the catheter that passes through the abdominal wall muscles has several functions. It provides a mechanical anchorage, a water tight peritoneal seal and a further bacterial seal. In order to maximize the efficiency of this segment, the end of the intramural segment in Toronto Western II Catheters is provided with another Dacron® felt cuff (D in Figure 6) identical to subcutaneous cuff, and a Dacron® disc one cm in diameter at the base of this cuff. One mm distal to the Dacron® disc an elastic ring or bubble is provided to create a groove (C in Figure 6) on which peritoneum is tightly tied. The fibrous tissue ingrowth bonds the catheter firmly to muscle and fascia to prevent its displacement. When the cuff is routed obliquely to the tissues, this bond will stabilize the intra-peritoneal segment (B in Figure 6) of the catheter in a direction pointing towards the pelvis. At the level of the dacron cuff, tissue fibrosis in and around the peritoneum forms an effective seal preventing fluid leak from occurring. This design affords a good barrier against early or late dialysate leaks and later incision hernias.

The intraperitoneal segment of this catheter is 15 cm long and is designed to provide an unrestricted flow of dialysis solution to and from the peritoneal cavity. When the peritoneal cavity is full of dialysis solution, the freely mobile small intestine and the active omentum tend to float over the fluid sump. During the drainage, typically fluid runs out at a rate of 200 ml/min, thus creating a negative suction due to a siphon effect the force of which is determined by the difference in the height between the catheter tip and the empty dialysis bag. This force tends to pull the abdominal contents towards the catheter tip and side holes tending to occlude and prevent free drainage of dialysis solution. When the catheter tip is placed deep in the true pelvis, omentum is unable to reach the side holes and tip, thus allowing free fluid flow without being obstructed by the intra-abdominal contents. With the object of stabilizing the catheter tip deep in the true pelvis, Toronto Western Catheters are provided with two flat silicone rubber disks which are 1 mm thick and 28 mm in diameter and 5 cm apart on the intra-abdominal portion of the catheter. Because of their shape and design, two discs prevent the free mobility of intra-abdominal section of catheter in the peritoneal cavity.

4.3. Swan Neck catheters

The distinguishing feature of Swan Neck peritoneal dialysis catheters is the molded bend between the two cuffs (Figure 7). As a result of this design, the catheter can be placed in an arcuate tunnel in an unstressed condition with both external and internal segments of the tunnel directed downward [53]. A permanent bend between cuffs eliminates the silastic resilience force or the 'shape memory' which tends to extrude the external cuff. As reported previously, Swan Neck catheter prototypes made from 80-degree arc angle

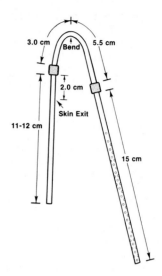

DOUBLE CUFF TENCKHOFF CATHETER WITH BENT SUBCUTANEUS SEGMENT (T-T)

Figure 7. Swan Neck Tenckhoff Catheter. The intercuff distance in Missori-2 catheter is 5 cm, in Missouri-3 is 3 cm. The Swan Neck Tenckhoff catheter is not provided with flange or bead. The Swan Neck Toronto catheter is provided with intraperitoneal discs. Stencils for each catheter is provided by the manufacturer. (Reproduced with permission, ref 53).

tubing and provided with 8.5 cm spaced cuffs, decreased catheter migration and leak rates but, due to an insufficient bend and too long a distance between cuffs, did not eliminate resilience forces completely resulting in external cuff extrusions [54, 55]. Based on this observation the catheters were modified; the new catheters, Swan Neck 2, were made from 170-degree arc angle tubing and the distance between cuffs was shortened to 5 cm.

4.3.1. Swan Neck-2 Missouri, Toronto, and Tenckhoff catheters

The Swan Neck catheters are available in three basic designs: the Missouri, the Toronto and the Tenckhoff catheters. The Toronto type of the Swan Neck catheter, a modification of the Toronto Western Hosptial (TWH) catheter [31, 56, 57] has a flange and bead circumferentially surrounding the catheter just below the internal cuff. Unlike the TWH catheter, the flange and bead are slanted approximately 45° relative to the axis of the catheter. When the slanted flange is positioned flat against the posterior rectus sheath, the desired direction of the catheter is maintained within the abdominal wall with the intraperitoneal portion pointing in the desired caudal direction within the peritoneal cavity. Like TWH catheters these catheters are also provided with two intraperitoneal discs. The Missouri catheter is identical to the Swan Neck Toronto catheter with the exception that it is not provided with the intraperitoneal discs. The Tenckhoff type of the Swan Neck peritoneal dialysis catheter is provided with two dacron cuffs. It differs from the double cuff Tenckhoff catheter only by being permanently bent between cuffs (Figure 7). This type of catheter may be inserted at the bedside and does not require surgical insertion; however, a subcutaneous tunnel has to be created in the same way as for other Swan Neck catheters (see below).

4.3.1.1. Swan Neck-3 catheter For a lean person with a thin subcutaneous tissue layer, the distance between the cuffs is shortened (Swan Neck-3 catheter). This catheter, otherwise is identical to the Swan Neck-2 catheter.

4.3.1.2. Other Swan Neck catheters The Swan Neck catheters with the modified intraperitoneal segment designs are also available. The catheters with longer intraperitoneal segment (22 cm) are suitable for patients who are tall or require the exit site placed above the belt line. The Swan Neck coiled catheters have a coiled intraperitoneal segment.

4.3.2. Radiopaque stripe
The slanted flange and bead, and bent tunnel segment require that the Swan Neck Missouri and Toronto catheters for right and left tunnels be mirror images of each other. To facilitate recognition of right and left Toronto and Missouri catheters, each tubing has a radiopaque stripe in front of the catheter (Figures 7). The stripe is also useful during insertion and post-implantation care, facilitating recognition of catheter twisting. Because of this last feature Tenckhoff type catheters are also provided with the stripe. Right and left Swan Neck Tenckhoff catheters differ only with respect to the position of the stripe. Unlike Swan Neck Toronto and Missouri catheters the Swan Neck Tenckhoff catheter intended for right or left tunnel may be implanted with an opposite tunnel. In this case the stripe should be kept in back of the catheter. Nevertheless, to retain uniformity of the stripe position it is recommended that Swan Neck Tenckhoff catheters be inserted with the corresponding tunnel direction (right tunnel with right catheter, left tunnel with left catheter).

4.3.3. Stencil
The catheter must be implanted with its shape undistorted. If catheters are not implanted properly, no advantage will result from its use, rather worse results may be expected. For instance, if the right Missouri catheter were to be implanted with the left tunnel, the catheter tip would almost inevitably migrate out of true pelvis because of unfavorable resilience forces. If the tunnel is too short, the external cuff will inevitably extrude out of the skin exit or the catheter will kink in the tunnel causing obstruction.

To facilitate the creation of a proper tunnel during surgery, stencils have been developed for skin markings before surgery. Stencils reproduce exactly the shapes of Swan Neck catheters.

4.4. Lifecath® column disc catheter

The column disc catheter was developed by Ash *et al.* [58] in 1980 (Figure 8). Problems of slow outflow and one-way obstruction with the Tenckhoff catheter and its modification led Ash and co-workers to design a catheter that minimized omental involvement, prevented catheter migration and decreased fluid inlet velocity. They evaluated a catheter that could be anchored against the abdominal wall in the lower abdomen, in order to optimally drain the patient in the upright position. The intra-abdominal end of the catheter was attached to a head made of two parallel discs 5.1 cm in diameter of silicone elastomer separated by 40 short pillars 6 mm long, and anchored against the abdominal wall by a Dacron® felt sleeve. Fixed to the anterior abdominal wall, the column disc catheter cannot drift down into the abdomen between bowel loops as can other catheters. Another Dacron® felt sleeve served to stabilize the catheter and prevent exit site infection. They tested their catheter both in normal and uremic dogs ([58], as well as in uremic patients [58]. Fluid inflow and outflow occur at the periphery of the large disc. Because of the large area of the disc, fluid inflow and outflow velocities are very low,

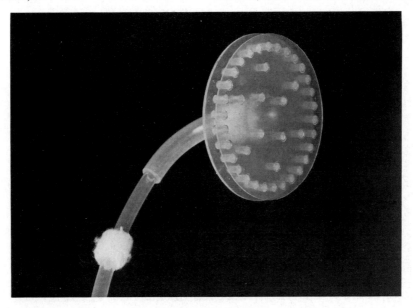

Figure 8. Lifecath® column disc catheter.

resulting in less attraction of omentum toward the catheter. With the column disc catheter, outflow rate was equal to inflow rate throughout the drainage cycle. For a 2 l exchange, the abdomen could be drained completely within 300 sec.

4.5. Polyurethane percutaneous access device

This device is constructed from porous polyurethane [38]. It is designed to encourage infiltration of dermal fibroblasts, and to promote deposition of collagen into interstices of the intercommunicating pores. The presence of the collagen around the circumference of the device ideally inhibits epidermal migration while anchoring the device firmly in place. A natural barrier to opportunistic organism is formed that ideally reduces the risk of infection. The access consists of a small cylinder measuring approximately one cm in diameter which protrudes through the skin (Figure 9). This is attached to a thin disc approximately 2.5 cm in diameter which is positioned in a subdermal/subcutaneous plane. The surface of both these components are textured in such a way to encourage tissue ingrowth. A 12 F polyurethane tube passes through the access device. The tubing is identical to that found in the standard peritoneal dialysis catheters except that it is bent at a right angle as it enters and exits the access device and allows the disc to lie flat in the subdermal plane. An implantable cuff is also provided with the catheter for interfacing with the peritoneum. The cuff is supplied separately to facilitate the insertion of the device. By placing the cuff on the catheter after the access portion of the device is implanted, it can be positioned to account for differences in abdominal wall thickness.

5. CATHETER INSERTION

Several techniques of catheter insertion are being currently practiced. In this chapter, we will describe in detail those techniques which are used extensively by many centers. The relative merits and demerits of these techniques are summarized in Table 1.

5.1. Bedside catheter insertion techniques

5.1.1. Pre-insertion patient assessment and preparation
When the need to start peritoneal dialysis is urgent, one may elect to access the peritoneal cavity through a rigid or Tenckhoff catheter. Both these catheters could be inserted at the bedside, with very minimal preparation. Equipment required for paracentesis is all that is needed. Bedside insertion should not be offered to patients who are extremely obese, or have had previous abdominal surgery, since abdominal adhesions increase the risk of inadvertent viscus perforation. In addition, this approach should not be done in children except by an experienced pediatric nephrologist or nephrologist with a pediatrician in attendance. If a nephrologist implants the catheter a surgeon should be on stand by, in case of complications. The patient should

Table 1. Advantages and disadvantages of different catheter insertion techniques

Advantages	
Bedside Insertion	*Surgical Insertion*
Quick and convenient	Good hemostasis
Smaller incision	Low risk of viscus perforation
Immediate use possible	Direct vision of peritoneum
Lower cost	possible
Disadvantages	
High incidence of bleeding, dialysis solution leak, poor flow, and viscus perforation	Delay in set up time
	Larger incision
	Late hernias
	Risk of general anesthesia
	Higher cost

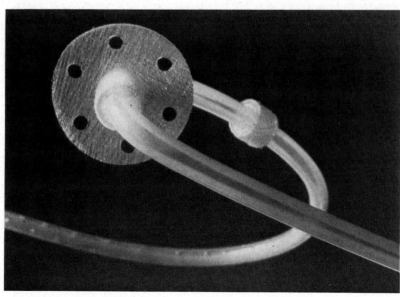

Figure 9. Polyurethane percutaneous access device.

receive preoperative sedation and have nothing to eat or drink at least 12 hours prior to the procedure.

All observers and persons in the immediate area, including the patient, should wear surgical masks. Those patients who experience discomfort while completely supine should raise their heads slightly. If the patient is conscious, it may be useful to familiarize him with the Valsalva maneuver. The 'surgeon' and 'surgical assistant(s)' should 'scrub, gown and glove'. A 'circulating' nurse should be present to assist.

5.1.2. Anesthesia
Premedication should be given if the patient is very restless. Heavy sedation should be avoided to retain the patient's co-operation during catheter insertion. After confirming that the bladder and rectum have been emptied, the skin of the lower abdomen is shaved and prepared with povidine. The insertion site is 'frozen' with a subcutaneous infiltration of 1 or 2% Lidocaine without epinephrine. The anesthetized area should include 2–3 cm around the intial skin incision in the midline 2–3 cm inferior to the umbilicus. Infiltration is extended in the arcuate direction of the desired subcutaneous tunnel and exit site. At the insertion site anesthesia is extended downward with a larger needle and the deeper tissues are infiltrated as well.

5.1.3. Rigid catheter insertion
The two most widely used rigid catheters in North America are the Stylocath (Abbott Laboratories, North Chicago, Illinois) and the Trocath (Baxter Healthcare System).

Taking all sterile precautions, a small stab wound (2–3 mm) is made in the midline under local anesthesia, 2–3 cm below the umbilicus. The stab wound should be small so that the abdominal wall holds the catheter firmly and thus, minimizes dialysis solution leak.

With the stylet in place, the catheter is forced through the abdominal wall by a short thrust or preferably with a rotary motion. The operator will recognize the loss or resistance as a 'pop' as soon as the peritoneal cavity is entered. While the catheter is being thrust through the abdominal wall, its tip is directed towards the coccyx. Because successful perforation of the abdominal wall for introduction of the catheter requires a sensitive 'feel' for the pressure applied, infusion of 2–3 l of dialysate will distend the abdomen which in turn will facilitate this maneuver. Some infuse 2 l of dialysis fluid via a small gauge needle prior to stylet puncture. A co-operative patient can also assist successful perforation by voluntarily contracting the abdominal musculature.

Once the peritoneal cavity has been entered the stylet is withdrawn a few cm and the catheter is advanced deep into the pelvis. If the operator encounters resistance while the catheter is being advanced or if the patient complains of pain, the advance in this direction should be stopped and another direction tried. If this is still not possible, he may infuse two or three liters of dialysis solution into the peritoneal cavity if this has not been done. It can be via the catheter if the holes in the distal end are in the cavity. This infusion accomplishes two important objectives: first, it facilitates recognition of the 'true' intraperitoneal space; second, dialysis solution in the peritoneal cavity reduces the likelihood of viscus perforation by moving the intraabdominal contents away from the advancing catheter.

After one or two good in-and-out exchanges, the catheter is firmly secured to the skin with the aid of a metal disc.

5.1.4. Tenckhoff catheter insertion
Because of the high frequency of dialysis solution leak, and poor drainage necessitating frequent catheter manipulation and resultant peritonitis with the use of rigid catheters, some centers prefer to insert single or double cuff Tenckhoff catheter at the bedside.

While inserting the catheter at the bedside a sterile procedure must be strictly followed. A 2–3 cm incision is made in the skin at the insertion site (e.g. the midline 2 cm inferior to the umbilicus). This places the site of entry at the linea alba, a point of minimal vascularity and tissue resistance. The lateral margins of either rectus muscle are alternative sites because they are also relatively avascular.

Through the skin incision, the wound is extended to the linea alba with blunt dissection using a curved hemostat. At this time an 'anchoring' suture is inserted in the fascia. The peritoneal cavity is entered with a 'priming needle', (a 'catheter over a needle', venicath-type needle or a stylet peritoneal catheter via stylet or trocar) into the superior aspect of the wound and through the linea alba. One must take care to ensure 'intraperitoneal' placement. If the parietal peritoneal membrane is separated from the peritoneal tissue, this will result in 'pre-peritoneal' infusion of dialysis fluid and make impossible any further 'intraperitoneal' infusion of dialysis fluid by this method. Furthermore the expansion of the preperitoneal 'pocket' is extremely painful. When dialysis solution infusion produces pain, the operator should suspect preperitoneal instillation; however, the heavily sedated patient may not be able to voice objection. At this time poor dialysis solution inflow may also indicate hole outlets are lodged in a preperitoneal position, although one should also expect a moderate restriction of flow, given the relatively small lumen of the access catheter.

Following sterile connection of the administration tubing, 2–3 l of dialysis solution are infused into the peritoneal cavity, until the patient feels distended. While solution is being instilled to the desired volume, the Tenckhoff catheter should be 'prepared' by wetting it with a small volume of normal saline or solution containing antibiotics. Air from the cuffs is removed by squeezing. A wetted obturator is inserted into the catheter, thus straightening and 'stiffening' it to permit introduction of the catheter into the Tenckhoff trocar, and beyond it into its correct intra-abdominal position.

It is useful to start perforation of the linea alba with a smaller trocar or dilator rather than a needle, thereby facilitating introduction of the larger Tenckhoff trocar. With firm but gentle pressure and a twisting action, the trocar with its pointed obturator in place (Figure 2) is pushed into the peritoneal cavity via the small perforation. Immediately, after the resistance ceases (indicating entrance into the peritoneal cavity), the obturator is removed. Then the true intraperitoneal placement should be recognized by the 'welling-up' of dialysis solution into the barrel of the trocar. If the operator has instilled enough dialysis solution during the priming procedure, he should insert the trocar until its wider portion comes to rest on the linea alba. This portion should not enter the peritoneal cavity, thus keeping the perforation at the desired diameter. This larger barrel is designed to accept not only the Tenckhoff catheter, but also allows for the passage of the Dacron® cuffs.

Proper placement of the catheter in the pelvis will greatly facilitate siphon drainage. During this phase of insertion certain details, although they may seem trivial, if not attended to with care, may produce unfavorable results. For example, as the catheter is introduced into the trocar on its way to the abdominal cavity, the tip should be passed smoothly beyond the trocar. Careful, gentle, and angular movement of the trocar (adjusting its intra-abdominal position and relationship to abdominal contents) may be needed to achieve easy passage of the catheter deep into pelvis. Although, at times, it may appear to be the course of 'least resistance' to insert the catheter at an angle horizontal to the abdominal wall and likewise to the intra-abdominal contents, such a manuever usually achieves only a temporary pelvic placement of the drainage segment. Placement of the catheter 'atop' abdominal contents is a frequent cause of early, postoperative migrations into non-functioning positions.

Once the catheter has completed its 'internal' course, the detachable trocar barrel should be removed leaving the split side-pieces in situ for easier manipulation until the final positioning is satisfactory. At this point, the catheter obturator should be removed while the operator holds the catheter firmly in place. Once the desired depth of placement is achieved. the remaining catheter is 'fed' into the peritoneal cavity while slowly withdrawing the obturator until the preperitoneal (inner or deep) Dacron® 'cuff' comes to rest on the rectus fascia and preperitoneal tissue. Then the trocar is separated into its two longitudinal sections and withdrawn, leaving the catheter cuff in proper position. The ideal location for the internal cuff is at the pre peritoneal level. However, if the catheter is intended for a short-term use until patient recovers from an acute renal failure event, the location of deep cuff at the pre-peritoneal level is not that critical as in the case of chronic long-term use.

Catheter patency is tested in the same manner described in the surgical procedure. When the function is deemed satisfactory, the catheter is secured in place to the posterior rectus fascia with an anchoring suture before preparing for the creation of the subcutaneous 'tunnel' toward the proposed exit site.

After choosing the catheter exit-site, a 'stab' wound (not an incision) is made using a blade, taking care to penetrate only the skin. The opening should be just the size of the catheter. Choose a site that will permit the creation of a tunnel of an appropriate length and shape of the catheter. Care is taken to ensure that the subcutaneous cuff is at least 2 cm below the skin. A subcutaneous tunnel is created using a malleable uterine sound or the Faller guide, being careful to manipulate the catheter gently. For the Swan Neck Tenckhoff catheter, the tunnel must follow the skin marking made prior to the insertion. The outer cuff should be positioned approximately 1 cm from the skin exit. The recommended method for tunnel creation for the Swan Neck Tenckhoff catheter is to make a superior subcutaneous pocket as described for surgical insertion (see below). The titanium connector is then inserted into the end of the catheter. The skin of the insertion wound is sutured, and

appropriate surgical dressings applied. Dressings are applied for at least one week while leaving an accessible length of catheter to permit the catheter to be handled without disturbing the dressings.

5.1.5. Complications related to bedside insertion (Table 2)

After catheter implantation bloody effluent appears after the first exchange in approximately 30% of cases [59, 60]. This bleeding (usually minor) comes from the small vessels in the abdominal wall. After three to four exchanges, bleeding usually stops unless the procedure has damaged a major vessel or the patient has a bleeding disorder. Pressure applied over the catheter insertion site usually controls minor bleeding. Occasionally, a transfusion of fresh blood will stop the bleeding. If the bleeding is copious, it may obstruct the catheter; in this event, it is a common practice to add 1000 units of heparin to each liter of dialysate to minimize the risk of obstruction.

Dialysis solution leak is encountered in 14% to 36% of patients after rigid catheter insertion [59–61]. Frequent manipulation of the catheter to improve drainage increases the risk of dialysis solution leak from the catheter-exit site. Such leaks may also occur when the catheter is not properly secured to the skin. The risk of external leak is higher in elderly or debilitated patient who have lax abdominal wall. The presence of a large intra-abdominal mass, such as a polycystic kidney(s) may raise the intra-abdominal pressure to high levels and promote an external dialysis solution leak after the standard 2 l volume has been instilled.

Fluid may extravasate into the abdominal wall, particularly in patients who have had a previous abdominal operation or multiple catheter insertion. This complication usually results from tears in the peritoneum or represents an infusion of dialysate into the potential space between the layers of abdominal wall. Uncommonly dialysis fluid may enter the pleural cavity [62–63]. In such cases, peritoneal dialysis is usually discontinued and the patients are switched to hemodialysis. Acute hydrothorax results from either a traumatic or a congenital defect in the diaphragm.

Inadequate drainage is frequent during initial dialysis, and may be due to one or more of the following factor; loss of siphon effect, one-way obstruction, and/or incorrect placement of the catheter.

One-way (outflow) catheter obstruction may have multiple causes. Fibrin or blood clots may be trapped in the catheter and block the terminal holes, especially when dialysis is complicated by major hemorrhage or peritonitis. Poor outflow may also reflect extrinsic pressure on the catheter from adjacent organs such as a sigmoid colon full

Table 2. Complications of bedside catheter insertion

1. Bleeding
2. Dialysis solution leak
3. Poor drainage
4. Extra-peritoneal space penetration
5. Viscus perforation
6. Peritonitis
7. Abdominal pain
8. Loss of rigid catheter in the peritoneum

of feces or a distended bladder. Omental wrapping is likely if the catheter is misplaced into the upper abdomen.

Occasionally, accidental penetration of the extra-peritoneal space by the catheter may cause poor drainage. In such a situation, continued infusion produces further dissection, and the fluid may become trapped and is no longer available for drainage. Loculation of fluid, another cause of poor drainage, is encountered in patients who have had previous intra-abdominal operations or peritonitis. Such loculation not only diminishes the surface area available for dialysis but may seriously reduce ultrafiltration capacity. The incidence of this complication is low, varying between 0.5% and 1.3% [61, 74, 75].

Perforation or laceration of internal organs during bedside insertion of catheter has been frequently reported. Lacerated or perforated organs include the bowel, bladder, liver, a polycystic kidney, aorta, mesenteric artery and hernia sac [61, 76–86]. Abdominal distention due to paralytic ileus or bowel obstruction may predispose the patient to bowel perforation. Those who are unconscious, cachectic or heavily sedated are also at high risk. Clinical evidence of bowel perforation includes sudden, sharp or severe abdominal pain followed by watery diarrhea, and poor drainage of dialysis solution, which may be cloudy, foul-smelling or mixed with fecal material. Such a situation requires prompt removal of the catheter, and allowing the perforation to seal off completely in about 12–24 hr.

The incidence of peritonitis when the stylet catheter was used, was 2.5% of all the dialyses and 1.2% when the Tenckhoff catheter was used [87]. The incidence of peritonitis almost doubled when the duration of dialysis was longer than 60 hr. The treatment of peritonitis is described in detail in the peritonitis chapter later in this book.

Abdominal pain may be encountered in as many as 56–75% of patients with the first use of the catheter [59]. There are many causes of abdominal pain, but catheter related pain occurs when it impinges on any of the viscera. Pain may occur during inflow and outflow of dialysis solution and also when the solution is dwelling. Outflow pain is due to entrapment of omentum in the catheter during the siphoning action of fluid drainage. Irrigation of the catheter with saline generally relieves this pain. Constant pain during the dialysis indicates pressure effects on intra-abdominal organs and often produces continuous rectal or low back pain. This complaint calls for an adjustment in catheter position.

Loss of a part or all of the rigid catheter has been reported following its manipulation with the trocar in place [59, 77, 79, 87, 88]. Its distal end may be amputated after intraabdominal kinking of the catheter, followed by manipulation. However, the presence of broken catheters within the abdominal cavity may not cause symptoms or ill effects. During laparoscopy, broken catheters have been found lying freely in the peritoneal cavity without causing a peritoneal reaction or have been found walled off by mesentery without an inflammatory reaction. On routine postmortem examination, Stein [89] discovered such a catheter in a patient who had had previous peritoneal dialysis. Exploration to retrieve the catheter may be unecessary because laparotomy could be more hazardous than leaving the catheter in a severely ill patient. The incidence of catheter loss into the peritoneal cavity has been greatly reduced since the intro-

duction of a design which incorporates a metal disc with a central hole; this not only allows the catheter to pass through the wall but also holds the catheter snugly to the skin of the abdominal wall.

5.2. PERITONEOSCOPIC INSERTION TECHNIQUE

The use of peritoneoscopy for peritoneal catheter placement is still relatively new and is being used extensively by Ash at Lafayette, Indiana. The technique recommended by Ash [90] is as follows: The necessary equipment (y-TEC) is manufactured by Medigroup, North Aurora, ILL., and distributed by the Quinton Instrument Co., Seattle, Wash. The abdomen is not prefilled with dialysis solution. The abdominal wall is first penetrated often directly through the rectus muscle by a 2.2-mm minitrocar housed in a metal cannula (Figure 10). The cannula is in turn surrounded by a thin plastic quill cylinder. The plastic cylinder is manufactured with a longitudinal slit to allow it to expand during catheter insertion. After penetration of the abdominal wall, the minitrocar is removed from the cannula and replaced with a small 2.2-mm Needlescope. When fully inserted, the sighted tip of the Needlescope is located exactly at the tip of the cannula. The intraperitoneal (IP) location of the cannula tip is thus confirmed under direct vision. The Needlescope is removed, and the abdomen is filled with air via the cannula. Room air is used, sterilized by passing it through a microporous filter. The air is infused using a steam-sterilized blood pressure cuff bulb (do not use ethylene oxide to sterilize the bulb). The Needlescope is now reinserted into the cannula, and the Needlescope and cannula are advanced together down into the abdomen under direct vision. The presence of omentum and adhesions can now be identified and those structures avoided. The Needlescope and cannula are advanced until the cannula tip is located in the clear space in which it is desired to locate the Tenckhoff catheter tip. At this point, the Needlescope and cannula are both removed, leaving only the

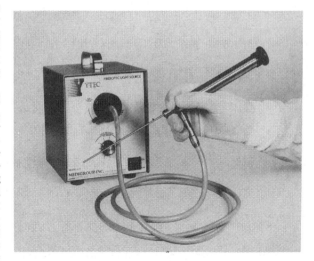

Figure 10. Y-Tec® scope for insertion of tenckhoff catheter. (This figure was kindly provided by John A. Navis of Medigroup, Inc. North Aurora, Illinois).

plastic quill catheter guide in place. Although the diameter of the longitudinally slit quill catheter guide is only 2.2 mm, dilation to 6 mm is performed using two dilators of graded diameter. An obturator is inserted into the Tenckhoff catheter to stiffen it, stopping short of the catheter tip to leave the latter soft and flexible. The Tenckhoff catheter plus obturator are then inserted into the abdomen through the dilated quill catheter guide, until the cuff is firmly seated against the abdominal musculature (for the curled Tenckhoff, the catheter is advanced into the abdomen while holding the obturator in place).

The plastic quill catheter guide is carefully removed, leaving the catheter and obturator in place. At this point a hemostat can be used to dilate the abdominal wall and to bury the deep cuff into the musculature. This is done by grasping the catheter just below the cuff with the hemostat tip and advancing the hemostat into the musculature. The hemostat is then spread, creating a space in the musculature for the cuff. The obturator is removed. A very small skin exit site incision is made and the Tunnelor tool is pushed out through the skin exit site. The other end of the tool is attached to the proximal end of the catheter, which is then pulled out through the skin exit site.

5.3. Catheter insertion through a guide wire

This technique can be used for insertion of a straight or a curled Tenckhoff catheter. The necessary equipment can be obtained through Cook Co, Bloomington, Indiana.

The preinsertion patient preparation is similar to the one described for rigid catheter insertion.

Prefilling the abdomen with dialysis solution is very essential for this technique of catheter insertion. The guidewire is inserted through the same needle or tubing that was used to fill the abdomen. A dilator, covered in a longitudinally perforated sheath, is then inserted over the guidewire. After the dilator-sheath is inserted, the dilator is removed, leaving the sheath in place. The Tenckhoff catheter, stiffened by a soft, partially inserted obturator, is then directed down into the sheath. As the cuff advances, the sheath is split by pulling tabs on its opposing sides. Splitting the sheath allows the cuff to advance to a position next to the abdominal wall. By further splitting and re-traction, the sheath is removed from its position around the catheter. The subcutaneous tunnel is then created as in surgical placement. With this technique, the incidence of early leak is very low. However, high risks of viscus perforation and improper placement of catheter are the drawbacks of this technique.

5.4. Surgical insertion of catheters for chronic dialysis

5.4.1. Preinsertion catheter preparation (Table 3)
Some catheters usually are delivered from the manufacturer in non sterile plastic bags. The catheters should never be touched with bare hands to avoid contamination. The catheters are carefully withdrawn from the package, washed, drip dried, and further dried on lint free towels, inserted into labeled peel packs, and then steam sterilized at 270°F (132 °C) and 30 PSI (2.11 kg/cm^2) for a full cycle at 40 mins.

Immediately before implantation the catheter is removed from the sterile peel pack and immersed in sterile saline. Both Dacron® cuffs and the flange are gently squeezed to remove air. When air is removed the catheter sinks. Thoroughly wetted cuffs provide markedly better tissue ingrowth compared to unwetted, air containing cuffs.

5.4.2. Preinsertion patient preparation (Table 3)
Usually one day prior to surgery, abdominal hair should be removed with an electric shaver. The belt line of the patient is identified, preferably in the sitting and/or standing position, with slacks and belt as usually worn. Depending on the size and shape of the abdomen, presence of previous scars, and taking into account the patient's preference, the tunnel site is marked on the skin using a stencil (available with the Swan Neck Missouri Catheter) in such a way that the exit hole will be created at least 2 cm from the belt line, the catheter will not be subjected to excessive motion with patient's activities, and no pressure will be exerted on the tunnel when patient bends forward. Skin markings may be made with any good surgical marker. For those who have a belt line below the umbilicus, there may not be enough space for catheter insertion below the belt line. Therefore, in such cases stencil marking for catheter insertion may be preferred above the belt line. In patients requiring high cathter insertion, it is necessary to use a catheter with a long intraperitoneal segment (approximately 20 cm). For those who have a belt line above the umbilicus, stencil markings are made below the belt line. In obese people with pendulous abdomens, it is necessary to insert the catheter above the skin fold; otherwise the intraperitoneal segment would be pulled out of the true pelvis with the patient in the vertical position when the skin fold sags.

A gram of vancomycin within 24 hr prior to surgery and a first generation cephalosporin one or two hours prior to surgery is given by slow intravenous infusion. Prior to operation the patient should empty the bladder. Tap water enemas may be required in constipated patients. General anesthesia is avoided, if possible, because vomiting and constipation are a frequent occurrence during the post-operative period. Also during this period, voluntary coughing is required for pulmonary atelectasis prevention; coughing, vomiting and straining markedly increase intra-abdominal pressure [91] and may increase the risk of dialysis solution leak. With the simultaneous administration of a sedative and a local anesthetic agent, adequate patient relaxation could be obtained for catheter insertion.

5.4.3. Surgical technique
The paramedian approach through rectus muscle, currently used in our center, will be described. The surgical preparation of the abdominal wall consists of a threefold scrub

Table 3. Catheter pre-insertion check-list

---

1. Procure appropriate sterilized catheter
2. Prepare abdominal skin (remove hair and surgical prep)
3. Identify site of catheter insertion with respect to belt-line and mark with a stencil
4. Prophylactic antibiotic
5. Empty bladder and rectum

---

with Betadine® suds, and threefold paintings with Betadine® alcohol solution. Skin markings are reinforced for better visualization. Finally, the abdomen is covered with a sterile, transparent surgical tape. The skin and subcutaneous tissue of the tunnel are anesthetized with 1% lidocaine. A 3–4 cm lateral paramedian transverse incision is made through the tape, skin, and the subcutaneous tissue. A perfect hemostasis, preferably using cauterization, is mandatory. Then an incision is made in the anterior rectus sheath and the rectus muscle fibers are dissected bluntly in the direction of the fibers down to the posterior rectus sheath. More anesthesia may be required during muscle fiber dissection. A purse string suture is placed through the posterior rectus sheath, transversalis fascia, and the peritoneum. A 5 mm incision reaching the peritoneal cavity is made with a scalpel. Care is used to protect the viscera from injury during this maneuver. The catheter is threaded on a wetted stiffening stylet and introduced deep into the true pelvis. Only a straight stiffening stylet is used because a curved one tends to pull the catheter tip into the upper abdomen during its removal. The patient may feel some pressure on the bladder or rectum. The radiopaque stripe on the catheter is kept facing up. The stylet is removed, and then a 50 ml syringe containing sterile saline is attached to the catheter and the saline is injected into the peritoneal cavity. If the solution flows freely the internal cuff (in the case of Tenckhoff catheters) is brought into the field and the peritoneum is closed tightly with absorbable suture under direct vision. At this point, the cuff is laid longitudinally, parallel to the rectus muscle, and a stab wound is made in the anterior rectus fascia 3 cm cephalad to the transverse skin incision. The external segment of the catheter is brought through the fascia and the cuff is positioned deep in the rectus muscle. In the case of the Swan Neck Missouri catheter and Toronto Western Hospital catheter, the bead is placed in the peritoneal cavity, the flange on the posterior rectus sheath and the purse string suture is tightened between them. The flange is sewn to the posterior rectus sheath with four sutures at twelve, nine, six, and three o'clock positions.

5.4.4. Creation of a subcutaneous tunnel

The catheter tunnel extending from the cuff to the skin exit should have a diameter close to that of catheter tubing. If the tunnel is too tight, it will not allow free drainage of necrotic tissue and may cause pressure necrosis with skin sloughing. On the other hand, a large tunnel prolongs healing relative to the volume of tissue repair required and allows movement of the catheter within the tunnel. This mechanical stress further delays the healing process. Thus, the last portion of the tunnel (from external cuff to the exit) should be made with a trocar of external diameter similar to that of the catheter tubing.

For Tenckhoff and Toronto Western Hospital catheters, a subcutaneous tunnel is then made with a 'tunneller' or other instrument, taking care to prevent excessive angulation or bleeding. The tunnel should be next to the abdominal wall musculature, deep to the subcutaneous tissue. The external cuff should be at least 1 cm from the skin exit-site, which should be determined during tunnelling.

For Swan Neck catheters, a superior subcutaneous packet is made to the level of skin markings to accommodate the bent portion of the catheter. The area between the subcutaneous pocket and the skin exit is anesthetized and the pocket is extended by blunt probing with the hemostat up to the point where the external cuff will lodge. A small stab wound is made in the anterior rectus sheath above the transverse incision. The catheter is grasped with the hemostat and pulled through the wound. The transverse incision in the anterior rectus sheath is sutured. The bent portion of the catheter is positioned carefully in the subcutaneous pocket. A trocar is attached to the catheter and directed through the exit site. The external cuff is positioned about 1 cm from the skin surface. Care is taken to keep the radio-opaque stripe facing anteriorly.

5.4.5. Catheter patency testing and post-operative care

A titanium adapter is attached to the catheter and a sterile extension tube is connected to the adapter. A one liter bag of sterile saline containing 1000 units of heparin is spiked via the extension tubing and the solution is infused and drained immediately. At least 200 ml of solution should drain within one minute. If good flow is obtained the skin incisioin is closed with absorbable subcuticular sutures. The operative site is covered with several layers of gauze dressings and secured with microfoam surgical tape. Care is taken to keep the radio-opaque stripe facing front.

The position of the intra-peritoneal catheter segment is checked by a plain X-ray of the abdomen and the patient is sent to the ward. The catheter is anchored with several layers of microfoam tape and dressings which should be left in place for a week. Additional in-and-out one liter exchanges are performed to check the patency of the catheter, and remove residual blood from the peritoneal cavity, if present. The exchanges are continued until the dialysis solution return is clear. If the position of the intraperitoneal catheter segment is not in the true pelvis, and even if the catheter is not functioning, no immediate correction of the position is attempted. Due to favorable resilience forces with the Swan Neck catheters, the intra-peritoneal catheter segment translocates spontaneously into the true pelvis within few days. Failure to translocate would require surgical catheter repositioning. Drainage is usually slow (< 150 ml/min) if the catheter tip is not in the true pelvis. If the catheter tip is in the true pelvis but is non functional even after 2–3 days, the omental wrapping is most likely and for correction omentectomy is required. Analgesics with constipating side effects (opiates) should be avoided in the postoperative period.

5.5. Insertion technique for the Lifecath® column disc catheter

The same general technique described above is followed for insertion except for a few modifications. The peritoneal incision is larger (1.5 cm), and the catheter is inserted in to the peritoneal cavity by folding the column disc section in half. After placing traction on the catheter, the peritoneum is closed between the column disc and deep cuff.

5.6. Insertion technique (92) for polyurethane percutaneous access device

The site selected for the skin button is marked with a

template that describes the point for the terminal and the circumference of the subdermal skirt. A circular coring knife is positioned over the central marking, and a core of tissue approximately 7 mm deep is removed. A # 11 blade is used to initiate dissection of a subdermal pocket for the skirt. This dissection is carried out radially from the margin of the core. The remainder of the subdermal pocket is created using sharp scissors. A transverse incision approximately 2 in long is made inferior to the exit site of the catheter and is carried down to the level of the peritoneum. The subcutaneous tissue at the dorsal margin of the incision is then dissected from the underlying fascia to create a plane superficial to skeletal muscle. This dissection is carried out to a level directly beneath the circular incision made by the coring knife. The floor of the superficial dermal plane is incised transversely so that the two planes communicated. This dissection creates a path for the retrograde insertion of the device. A tunnel is then made for the catheter. The initial tunnel is in the subdermal plane. It then gently curves deeper as it leaves the margin of the skirt and exits in the subcutaneous tissue at the inferior incision above the level of the second plane of dissection. The system is inserted in a retrograde fashion and the internal conduit then placed in the abdomen through a stab wound incision. The peritoneum is closed around it. All layers are closed with absorbable sutures. The position of a fully inserted catheter is diagrammatically shown in Figure 11. The patency is checked in the operating theater and left unused for a period of two weeks. A nonstick dressing is applied over the incision and the catheter exit site is protected with a transparent dressing. During the period of nonuse, the catheters are flushed with heparinized solution two to three times a week in an attempt to decrease the likelihood of obstruction due to fibrin accumulation within the device. The implant sites are visually examined on a routine basis for any evidence of sinus formation or infection arouns the terminal of the device.

5.7. Catheter insertion in children

Differences in size and nutritional status of children must be considered when choosing a peritoneal catheter. In general, adult catheters are used for children over 30 kg body weight, and pediatric versions for those between 10–30 kg. The neonatal catheter is reserved for infants less than 10 kg.

The catheter is usually inserted through a midline subumbilical incision. For peritoneal closure, slowly absorbable vicryl suture is used. The catheter is tunnelled subcutaneously for at least 5 cm, usually in a superiolateral direction.

5.8. Early insertion related complications (Table 4)

With surgical insertion the post-operative bleeding and risk of perforating an internal organ is considerably reduced and in the experienced hand the incidence is extremely low.

Dialysis solution leak around the catheter insertion site is primarily due either to inadequate fixation of catheter to the surrounding tissue or subjecting the insertion site to a too high an intraabdominal pressure, before it is well healed. Midline catheter insertion is associated with more dialysis solution leak than with lateral paramedian technique [52]. Conditions which cause delayed wound healing

Table 4. Complications of surgical catheter insertion

Early complications	Late complications
1. Dialysis solution leak	1. Exit-site infection
2. Poor drainage	2. Dialysis solution leak
3. Catheter tip migration	3. Cuff erosion
4. Omental 'capture' of catheter	4. Poor outflow (rare)
5. Catheter kink	5. Peritonitis
6. Poor inflow	

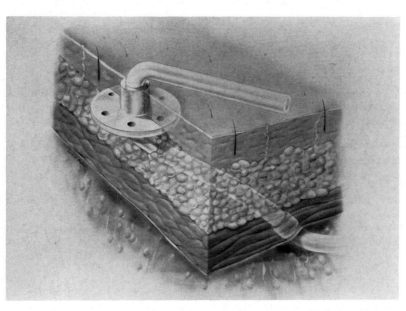

Figure 11. Position of percutaneous access device and catheter after insertion. (This figure was kindly provided by Dasse KA.)

such as obesity, poor nutritional state, and steroid therapy may increase the risk of leak if sufficient additional time is not allowed for tissue healing [56]. In addition to overt fluid leak at the insertion site and/or exit site, leak may manifest as a subcutaneous swelling, edema, weight gain and diminished drainage volume. When dialysis solution leak is detected, the immediate step to follow is to stop the peritoneal dialysis temporarily and follow the break-in procedure recommended later in this chapter. Peritoneal dialysis in the supine position for up to 2 weeks may be considered if hemodialysis is not an alternative. Intraperitoneal pressure in the supine position is considerably lower for the same amount of volume compared to upright position. Persistent leak despite an adequate resting period requires catheter replacement.

Dialysis solution leak may occur through any of the weak areas in the abdomen such as an old scar, patent processus vaginalis, congenital weakness in the diaphragm etc. In these instances the catheter per se is not the cause of the leak. Management of such problem requires localization of the site of leak with help of contrast infused CT scan and surgical repair when feasible [93].

Slow or poor drainage is usually the first sign of catheter out flow obstruction. Obstruction early during the post operative period may be due to a blood clot and/or fibrin, which may resolve after a few days. If fibrin is the cause of poor outflow, heparin in the amount 500–1000 units/liter of dialysis solution may be used to improve the flow. A cannulogram done with the aid of contrast material may aid in the diagnosis of this condition. Clot removal with the 'Italian corkscrew' or its dissolution with streptokinase [94, 95] or urokinase [96] should restore the flow immediately. Streptokinase is the cheaper of the two thrombolytic agents but has a risk of inducing anaphylactic reaction. Therefore, intraperitoneal streptokinase infusion should always be preceded by a scratch test followed by an intradermal test [97]. For infusion 750 000 IU of streptokinase is reconstituted and then diluted with 100 ml of 0.9 saline. The entire volume is then injected into the peritoneal catheter and left clamped for two hours. If on first injection obstruction is not relieved, a second injection of a similar amount of streptokinase may be infused. Urokinse, 5000 IU is used in 40 ml of 0.9% saline in the manner described for streptokinase [96]. Injection may be repeated for refractory obstruction. Catheter kinking either in the intramural or intraperitoneal segment is another common cause of poor outflow. Repositioning the catheter will restore flow immediately.

Catheter tip migration is another important cause of poor drainage. This problem is discussed in more detail earlier in this chapter. We have observed that when an intraperitoneal segment migrates under the liver instead of remaining in the deep pelvis, it is unlikely to return spontaneously back to the deep pelvis because of the ascending colon peristalsis propagating in an unfavorable direction. The reverse is the case when the intraperitoneal segment migrates under the spleen in the proximity of descending colon. The downward propagating peritstalsis of the descending colon may eventually restore the position of the catheter back to the deep pelvis. Therefore, we tend to aggressively replace a nonfunctioning catheter tip under the liver, where as splenic migration is managed conservatively in the hope of

eventual spontaneous restoration. Improving bowel motility with laxatives may aid in restoring catheter position in some patients. Irrespective of the position, refractory catheter migration requires catheter replacement.

'Capture' of the catheter by active omentum may also cause outflow obstruction. Obstruction from this cause, in the absence of peritonitis, when it occurs is usually a postoperative event (related to new catheter). We have never seen an obstruction (in the absence of peritonitis) due to omental 'capture' as a late event. We believe that foreign body silastic is more prone to attract omentum very early. In due course of time, with repeated use, a proteinaceous biofilm catheter coating may make the silastic less attractive to omental tissue. When such complications do occur, it may be necessary to relocate or replace the catheter, with or without omentectomy. Relocation or replacement of the catheter is done surgically or under a peritoneoscopic guidance. Whether early in the post insertion period or later in the course of catheter usage, one may need to reposition the intraperitoneal segment of a non-functioning catheter due to obstruction or malposition. This can be done if one follows the same steps as in initial insertion. However, the operative area is smaller because only the insertion site needs to be exposed. The exit site, being difficult to 'prep', is not included in the operative field. One must exercise caution to avoid puncturing the non-self-sealing silastic tubing when infiltrating the operative area with local anesthetic. If this should happen, the entire catheter must be replaced. Relocating the catheter can also be achieved by inserting and manipulating a bent obturator, without needing to open the peritoneal cavity.

Inflow obstruction is typically due to catheter kinking or clotting. To remove the clot, the methods described for correcting outflow obstruction should be tried. To relieve kinking of the catheter, exploration is necessary.

6. CATHETER BREAK-IN AND CATHETER CARE

The break-in period for a peritoneal catheter is that which immediately follows catheter insertion. In order to achieve optimum long-term catheter function and low rates of complications, strict adherence to break-in procedure is essential. The purpose of the different steps suggested in the break-in procedure is to allow sufficient time for the incision to heal before standard CAPD is begun and at the same time care is taken to maintain the catheter patency. During the healing period undue stress exerted on the incision by the high intraabdominal pressure with two liters of dialysis solution (especially in the upright position) may traumatize the healing tissue and predispose to dialysis solution leak. Leaks not only delay ingrowth of fibrous tissue into the cuffs, but also provide a medium for bactrial growth, thus increasing the risk of peritonitis and exit site infection. It is desirable therefore, to delay continuous ambulatory peritoneal dialysis for at least 10–15 days after catheter implantation.

Catheters inserted at the bedside usually require no break-in period although some physicians use reduced volume (500 ml, then 1000 ml) for the initial four to eight exchanges before proceeding to the normal 2000-ml exchange volume (in patients with small abdomens or with respiratory embarrassment, a reduced exchange volumes may be required indefinitely).

When a catheter is inserted in an ESRD patient for long term use, and if he needs acute dialysis, the catheter may be used for dialysis with the patient in the supine position because the intraabdominal pressure during filling in the supine position is limited and leakage is not usually a problem. Peritoneal dialysis in the supine position is started usually immediately after in and out exchanges are completed. One liter of dialysis solution is used for the first supine peritoneal dialysis. Usual cycler settings are: 10 min inflow, 10 min dwell and 12 min outflow. The outflow time may be prolonged to 15 min in case of slow drainage. Each liter of dialysis solution contains 1000 units of heparin. In spite of clear dialysate in post-implantation washouts, the dialysate is usually blood tinged during the first cycler dialysis. Some set the exchange volume at 500 ml for the first four exchanges, 1000 ml for the next four, then proceed to the desired exchange volume if tolerated. Heparin 500 units/liter is added to each dialysis solution bag for at least the first 72 hours. Several sittings of supine dialysis may be given until the incision is well healed and ready to commence standard CAPD.

When a catheter is replaced in a patient who is already on CAPD, it may be tempting to modify the break-in procedure to allow CAPD with lower volumes per exchange. However, such a practice may expose the patient to risk of a leak and delayed wound healing. It is our policy to provide them peritoneal dialysis only in the supine position with a cycler until the incision is well healed. Alternatively, hemodialysis is provided using a subclavian catheter as an access until standard CAPD can be resumed.

When a catheter is inserted at the time of another abdominal surgery, such as hernia repair, cholecystectomy etc., no change in break-in procedure is recommended except that standard CAPD may be delayed longer than 15 days depending upon the recommendation of the surgeon.

6.1. Subsequent catheter care

The surgical dressing placed at the time of insertion is removed after one week. Care is taken to avoid catheter pulling or twisting. The exit and skin surrounding the catherter are cleansed with povidone iodine scrub, rinsed with sterile water, patted dry with sterile gauze, covered with several layers of gauze dressings, and secured with microfoam surgical tape. Weekly dressing changes are continued until the healing process is completed. There are no data in humans with respect to the time needed for firm fibrous tissue ingrowth into the cuff and completion of epidermal growth into the sinus tract. We assume that it may take up to 6 weeks. The patient may shower only before the dressing change and otherwise must take sponge baths.

Protection of the catheter from mechanical stress seems to be extremely important, especially during break-in. The catheters should be anchored in such a way that the patient movements are only minimally transmitted to the exit. The method of catheter immobilization is individualized, depending on exit location and shape of abdomen. We think that better exit protection prevents infections in most

patients.

Special care of the exit site, after the healing process is completed, is essential to prevent infection. Routine exit-site care includes: 1) examining the exit site and tunnel for signs of infection, 2) cleaning the skin to remove dirt and decrease bacteria, and 3) securing the catheter to avoid tension and tugging movements. Routine exit site care should be done daily and any time the exit site is red or dirty. Several methods of exit site care are currently practiced. The three commonly used methods are a) daily cleaning and leaving the exit site exposed, b) daily cleaning and topical application of povidone iodine, or c) daily cleaning, topical application of povidone iodine, and covering the exit site with a sterile gauze. The results of a prospective study [98] indicate that cleaning with soap and water is the least expensive and tends to prevent infections better than povidone-iodine painting and hydrogen peroxide cleaning.

Following a satisfactory healing (6–8 weeks after implantation) the patient may swim in the ocean or private swimming pools preferably covering the exit site with a colostomy bag with the catheter spike and dialysate bag or capped spike within the same colostomy bag. One should discourage swimming in other surface waters such as rivers, lakes, jacuzzi, public pools, hot tubs, and skin diving. Following swimming the patient should have a shower to clean the exit site and then cover it with a sterile dry dressing. The patient should avoid tub-bathing but is allowed shower baths.

7. LATE CATHETER COMPLICATIONS (TABLE 4)

7.1. Exit site infection

The exit site is that part of the skin surrounding the catheter. The tunnel is the pathway of the catheter from the skin through the underlying fat and muscle to the peritoneal cavity. A non-infected exit site should be clean, dry, and scab and crust free. A normal exit site is painless and not red. Scabs are found following trauma to exit sites when serous discharge dries. This usually falls off after healing. Crust, on the other hand, is dried drainage or debris at the exit site, usually due to infection. It should be gently removed during the cleaning.

Problems of exit site include inflammation and infection. Inflammatiuon is said to have occurred when there is redness around the exit site. If, in addition to redness, tenderness, pain, hardness, swelling or purulent drainage is present, infection is said to have occurred. Therapy of exit site infection should include daily frequent exit site care. Any one of the methods of exit site care described above would be satisfactory. If the infection is sever, care of the exit site more than once a day may be necessary. Systemic antibiotics are indicated if exit site care does not alleviate the infection. Choice of antibiotic would depend on the organism isolated from the exit site and its sensitivity. Antibiotics are given intravenously or intraperitoneally when patients are unable to take oral antibiotics. Topical application of antibiotics include local spraying of powder, or injection in and around the exit site. In the majority of cases, the above measures would be adequate to control exit site infection. However, in a minority of patients, the infection may be resistant to therapy. With repeated courses of antibiotics followed by long-term maintenance therapy, if the infection persists, the next step would be to remove the subcutaneous dacron cuff if it is a double-cuffed catheter. Shaving the superficial cuff is a minor but delicate procedure. It can be done at the bedside or in an operating room. With appropriate antibiotic coverage and local anaesthesia, the subcutaneous dacron cuff, if it is not already extruded, is exposed through a small incision. With the help of fine scissors and/or scalpel blade, the dacron felt is shaved off the catheter, taking care not to puncture the catheter during the procedure. It is important that the remaining catheter surface be smooth after cuff removal. If it is rough, it may cause irritation and inflammation of the skin due to constant friction and pulling movements at the exit site. As a last measure, the catheter may have to be removed if exit site infection persists. When a catheter is removed because of persistent skin exit infection, ideally it should not be replaced by a new catheter at the same time but after one or two weeks. A new catheter is inserted at a site opposite to the removed one. In this way, infection of the new catheter will be avoided. In the mean time, the patient may have to be maintained on hemodialysis through a subclavian catheter. If for some reason hemodialysis is not feasible, the catheter may be replaced after three of four days under the cover of an appropriate antibiotic.

The subcutaneous peritoneal cuff is intended to prevent periluminal propagation of organisms and their entry to the peritoneujm, but it remains to be established whether it achieves this purpose. A prospective clinical study was undertaken to compare single and double cuff Toronto Catheters with respect to their influence on exit site infection [49]. From February 1983 to January 1984, alternate patients were assigned to receive a single cuff or a double cuff catheter. All catheters where implanted through the paramedian approach by the same surgeon. Thirty seven patients received a single cuff, and 38 patients received a double cuff catheter. For the first two weeks after the catheter insertion, all CAPD patients practiced IPD to prevent leakage of dialysis solution. The exit site of IPD patients was covered with a sterile gauze dressing which was changed twice a week, the exit site of those on CAPD remained exposed and they had a daily shower. All patients were assessed monthly. The diagnosis of exit site infection was made if the skin around the site was red or covered with crust. For an average follow-up of six months no significant differences were observed between the two groups with regards to either early or late catheter related complications including exit site infection. This study did not demonstrate that the double cuff peritoneal catheter had any significant advantage over the single cuff. Both the incidence of exit site infection and the response of the exit site infection to medical therapy were similar. There are several disadvantages to having a subcutaneous cuff. Even if placed 2 cm from the exit site, there is no guarantee that cuff extrusion and cuff infection will not occur. It is possible that the presence of a second cuff may contribute to the high incidence of infection seen in patients with double cuff catheters. However, exit site infections are not observed exclusively in those with double cuff catheters. Until a definitive study showing advantages of one type of catheter over the other is shown, we recommend the use of double cuff catheters. Exit site infection with drainage or redness with other signs of inflammation should be treated by local therapy and systemic antibiotics. If the exit site infection does not clear within a reasonable time of medical therapy one should consider replacing the catheter.

There is no evidence to support the use of prophylactic antibiotics to reduce the incidence or frequency of exit site tunnel infections [99, 100]. Their use is not recommended.

7.2. Dialysis solution leak

Dialysis solution leak may occur months or even years after starting CAPD. Management of late leak is similar to the one described for early leak. However, most cases of late leak are refractory to conservative therapy and require surgical repair.

7.3. Cuff extrusion

The main cause of cuff extrusion is placement of the external segment of the catheter in any shape other than its natural design. Due to the resilience force of the silastic, slowly, the catheter tends to assume its original shape. During this process, the external cuff usually extrudes. If the cuff is not infected, it is left alone. However, cuff or catheter may have to be removed for reasons of tissue trauma or infection. Infection is another cause of cuff extrusion. This aspect has been discussed in the section of exit-site infection.

7.4. Indications for catheter removal

The need for catheter removal occurs under various conditions. These may be broadly categorized under two headings: catheter malfunction and complicating medical conditions with a functioning catheter.

7.4.1. Poor functioning or non-functioning catheter
This may be seen under the following conditions. 1) intraluminal obstruction with blood or fibrin clot or omental tissue incarceration. The decision to remove the catheter is usually made only when conservative measures to dislodge the obstruction have failed, 2) catheter tip migration out of the pelvis with poor drainage, 3) a catheter kink along its course, 4) catheter tip caught in adhesions following severe peritonitis. In these situations, there usually are both inflow and outflow draining problems.

7.4.2. Functioning catheter with a complication
Under the following conditions catheters may have to be removed: 1) recurrent peritonitis with no identifiable cause, 2) peritonitis due to exit site and/or tunnel infection, 3) catheter with persistent exit site infection, 4) tunnel infection and abscess, 5) late recurrent dialysate leak through the exit or into the layers of the abdominal wall, 6) unusual peritonitis i.e. tuberculosis, fungal, etc. 7) bowel perforation with multiple organism peritonitis, 8) refractory peritonitis of other causes, 9) severe abdominal pain either due to catheter impinging on internal organs or during solution inflow, 10) catheter cuff erosion with infection, and 11) accidental break in the continuity of the catheter.

7.4.3. Functioning catheter that is no longer needed
This situation is encountered after a successful renal transplantation or peritoneal dialysis is discontinued because dialysis is no longer needed or the patient transfers to another form of dialysis.

8. LONG-TERM RESULTS

8.1. Tenckhoff catheters

Slingeneyer *et al.* [101] reported their experience with 315 straight Tenckhoff catheters in 247 patients maintained on IPD and CAPD between September 1973 and September 1980. The cumulative duration of treatment was 410 patient-years of treatment. They observed the following catheter complications: bleeding into the subcutaneous tissue or peritoneum 1.9%, dialysate leak in 3.5%, and skin exit site infection in 10.5%. Skin exit site infection was more frequent in diabetic than in non-diabetic patients. They reported a 5.3% incidence of one-way obstruction requiring either catheter revision or replacement. Subcutaneous cuff extrusion necessitating cuff repositioning or catheter replacement occurred in 2.2%. Fifteen patients (4.7%) had persistent localized abdominal pain resulting in either replacement or revision (10 catheters). Incisional hernias were observed in five patients. Cumulative catheter survival was 79.9% at one year and 69.6% at two years. From this large experience they concluded that, despite limitations due to exit site infections and one-way obstruction, the Tenckhoff catheter provides adequate access for peritoneal dialysis. Most of Slingeneyer's patients were on IPD treatment. During intermittent peritoneal dialysis, the peritoneal cavity is empty most of the time, whereas during CAPD, this cavity is full nearly all the time. Therefore, catheter tip displacement is seen more frequently in CAPD.

Rubin *et al.* [102] prospectively evaluated the complications encountered with the Tenckhoff catheter in CAPD patients between August 1981 and May 1983. They inserted 97 single cuff catheters into 90 patients, and 118 double-cuff catheters into 92 patients. Within 40 days of insertion of the single-cuff catheters, 25% had an associated complication that did not require catheter removal for correction, and 19% had a complication that required catheter removal. With the double-cuff catheters, 24% had an associated complication that did not require catheter removal, while 28% had catheter-related problems that required removal. In their long-term patients, the primary reason for catheter removal was failure of peritonitis to resolve. The catheter life span was 38% at 22 months for both single- and double-cuff catheters. Collectively, for both single- and double-cuff Tenckhoff catheters, they reported an exit site infection rate of 5.1%, an obstruction rate of 21.3%, and a leak rate of 9.3%.

Rottembourg *et al.* [103] described their large experience with curled Tenckhoff catheters. Between August 1978 and January 1980, they inserted 48 straight Tenckhoff catheters; these they compared with 95 curled catheters inserted between February 1980 and April 1983. The most important difference between the two groups was the incidence of outflow obstruction: of the straight Tenckhoff catheters, 41.6% became dislodged and 85% of these had to be

replaced; on the other hand only 10% of the curled catheters became dislodged and, of these, only 20% had to be replaced. Except for peri-operative pain, which is higher with the curled catheters, the frequency of other complications such as infection, dialysate leakage, exit site and tunnel infection and cuff extrusion, were similar in the two groups. For the straight Tenckhoff catheters, the cumulative catheter survival was 65% at one year and 60% at two years; for the curled catheters, these rates were 83% at one year and 78% at two years.

8.2. Experience with the Toronto Western Hospital catheter

During the period between January 1, 1981, and December 31, 1985, 312 Toronto Western Hospital catheters (in 80 diabetic, 232 non-diabetic patients) and 32 Tenckhoff catheters were implanted at the Toronto Western Hospital. In calculating the cumulative survival, all catheters removed because of outflow obstruction, skin exit infection or persistent peritonitis were considered as end events. Functioning catheters in patients who died or were transplanted were considered as lost to follow-up. For Toronto Western Catheters the cumulative catheter survival rates at the end of 6, 12 and 24 months were 84, 70 and 51% respectively. For the Tenckhoff catheters the survival rates at the end of 6, 12 and 24 months were 63, 52 and 47% respectively. The survival of Toronto Western catheters was marginally better than that of Tenckhoff catheters. Of the 312 Toronto Western catheters, 150 were single cuff and the remaining 162 were double cuff catheters. At 24 months, single cuff catheters had a significantly longer probability of survival (p < 0.04) when compared to that of double cuff catheters. The survival of catheters implanted in diabetic and non-diabetic patients were not significantly different.

The national CAPD Registry of the National Institute of Health reported in 1987 the results of a survey that attempted to determine the natural history of implanted peritoneal catheters and to estimate the survival distribution of different types of catheters [3]. The survey also estimated frequency of catheter complications as well as reasons for catheter removal. Standard straight (n=957, 64%) and curled (n=330, 22%) Tenckhoff catheters, and Toronto Western Hospital catheters (n=94, 6%) comprised the majority of the catheters reported for the survey. The survey did not clearly show major differences in catheter survival among various types of catheters. The probability of catheter survival at 6, 12, 18, 24, and 36 months for double cuff standard straight Tenckhoff catheter was 80, 70, 60, 51, and 33%, for standard curled Tenckhoff catheters was 85, 69, 51, 43, and 34%, and for double cuff Toronto Western catheter was 80, 70, 60, 51, and 33% respectively. Among the different catheters studied, patients using the Toronto Western Hospital catheter were more likely to claim peritonitis as a reason for catheter removal than patients using a standard type catheter. However no patients using a Toronto Western Hospital catheter claimed failure to drain as a reason contributing to catheter failure while a range of 5%–8% was claimed for the other types of catheters. Exit site infection requiring catheter removal accounted for no more than 8% of patients using any type of catheter. This survey also found exit site infection and peritonitis to be disproportionately distributed among the cuff types. Exit site infections were reported in proportionately more patients using a single subcutaneously placed cuff (13%) than for patients using a double cuff (7%). However peritonitis as a contributing cause for catheter removal, was claimed in proportionately fewer patients using a single cuff.

Grefberg from Sweden [104] in 1984 reported his comparative experience with the Tenckhoff and Toronto Western Hospital catheters. Catheters were randomly selected and both were surgically inserted. 59 Tenckhoff catheters were observed for 592 treatment months and 24 Toronto Western catheters for 220 treatment months. At 18 months, the cululative life span of both catheters were similar at 80%. With regards to complications, 11 of the 59 Tenckhoff catheters became obstructed as opposed to one of 24 Toronto Western catheters. Swedish workers believe this high incidence of Tenckhoff catheter blockage was due to inexperience and that this complication would disappear with experience. With regard to exit site infection, tunnel abscess and dialysis leak, there was no difference between the two groups. Despite the obvious advantages of Toronto Western Catheters, they abandoned its use because laparotomy was needed whenever the catheter was removed, and the bowel was perforated during the removal of two Toronto Western catheters.

More recently Hogg, *et al.* [105] used the Toronto Western catheter with considerable success in children on long term CAPD. Six of the Toronto Western catheters were inserted in children who previously had either obstruction or leakage with one to four Tenckhoff catheters. Overall, they used 15 Toronto Western Hospital catheters in 12 children and compared the results with those of 23 Tenckhoff catheters in 9 children. The rate of obstruction with Toronto Western catheters (7%) was much lower than that with Tenckhoff catheters (45%).

A retrospective analysis of single and double cuff Tenckhoff catheters and Toronto Western Hospital catheters by Flanigan *et al.* [106] showed that drainage failure occurred less frequently with Toronto catheters (9.4%) compared to single cuff (11.3) and double cuff (20.6) Tenckhoff catheters. However, in contrast to the experience of most centers with the use of Toronto Western Hospital catheters, Flanigan *et al.* observed a significantly lower survival for Toronto Western Hospital type I catheters. They attributed the lower survival of Toronto catheters to a higher incidence of unresponsive peritonitis in their patients using such catheters.

8.3. Experience with Swan Neck Missouri-2 catheters

At the University of Missouri, Columbia, between April 1, 1986 and April 30, 1987, exclusively 23 Swan Neck Missouri-2 catheters were implanted and cared for by the technique described above. Survival and complications were monitored prospectively. The prospectively collected data with the Swan Neck Missouri-2 catheters, the Swan Neck catheter prototypes (used between August 1985 and March 1986), and retrospectively collected data with Tenckhoff and Toronto Western Hospital catheters were compared [107].

One year catheter survival tended to be higher for Missouri-2 catheters compared to other types. Up to one year follow up, cuff extrusion, a major problem with the Swan Neck prototype catheters, dit not occur with Missouri-2 catheters, and the improvement was significantly better than with the Swan Neck prototypes and other catheters. Leaks and tip migrations occurred infrequently with both Swan Neck Missouri-2 and prototype catheters. Only one Missouri-2 catheter was permanently obstructed; however, the catheter was wrapped by very active omentum in the true pelvis, not in the upper abdomen. This catheter was replaced by a second catheter which also was wrapped by the omentum in the true pelvis. Finally, function of this catheter was restored only after omentectomy. Obstruction due to omental wrapping is unavoidable in patients with long, aggressive omentums reaching to the true pelvis and require omentectomy. Fortunately, according to our experience, less than 3% of patients, usually lean, young men, present such a problem.

Although not significantly different from other catheters because of low numbers, exit site infections tended to be less frequent with Missouri-2 catheters. Significantly, no tunnel infection was seen with Missouri-2 catheters. Despite the short observation, the results with the Swan Neck Missouri 2 catheters are very encouraging. Four major catheter complications were virtually eliminated: external cuff extrusion, catheter tip migration, pericatheter leaks, and tunnel infections. Low complication rates with Swan Neck catheters have been confirmed by others [108].

8.4. Experience with column disc catheter

A multicenter experience reported using 89 column disc catheters [109]. Twenty catheters were placed in patients with previous failures of Tenckhoff catheters. Outflow failure was the most common cause of early failure and was less frequent after one month. Subcutaneous leak and herniation occurred rarely. Life table analysis revealed that compared to Tenckhoff catheters, the column disc catheter is more likely to fail in the early months but over the long-term is much less likely to fail.

8.5. Preliminary experience with polyurethane percutaneous access device

Dasse and co-workers [110] reported their preliminary experience with the use of polyurethane percutaneous access devices in nineteen patients for up to 8 months. Three of the 19 devices were implanted without an internal peritoneal cuff, two of which experienced pericatheter leakage and compromised healing. In contrast, excellent tissue ingrowth and healing has been observed in the remaining 16 patients which used a peritoneal cuff. One patient experienced an episode of peritonitis. Two of the 16 catheters with a peritoneal cuff experienced transient cellulitis which subsequently healed. Their preliminary results indicate that this device may have the potential to reduce the incidence of exit-site infection.

REFERENCES

1. Palmer RA, Maybee TK, Henry EW, Eden J: Peritoneal dialysis in acute and chronic renal failure. Can Med Assoc J 88: 920–927, 1963.
2. Palmer RA, Newell JE, Gray EF, Quinton WE: Treatment of chronic renal failure by prolonged peritoneal dialysis. N Engl J Med 274: 248–254, 1966.
3. Tenckhoff H, Schechter H.: A bacteriologically safe peritoneal access device. Trans Am Soc Art Intern Organs 14: 181–186, 1968.
4. Lindblad AS, Novak JW, Stablein DM, Cutler SJ, Nolph KD: Report of the National CAPD Registry of the National Institutes of Health. A publication of the National CAPD Registry of the National Institute of Diabetes and Digestive and Kidney Diseases. pp 10–01 10–16, 1987.
5. Ganter G: Ueber die Beseitigung giftiger Stoffe aus dem Blute durch Dialyse. Munch Med Wschr 70: 1478–1480, 1923.
6. Rosenak S, Siwon P: Experimentelle Untersuchungen uber die peritoneale Ausscheidung harnpflichtiger Substanzen aus dem Blute. Mitt a.d. Grenzged Med u. Chir 39: 391–408, 1925.
7. Engel D, Kerkes A: Beitrage zum permeabilitats Problem: Entgiftungsstudien mittels des lebenden Peritoneums als 'Dialysator'. Ztschr. f. D. ges. Exp Med 55: 574–601, 1927.
8. Wear JB, Sisk IR, Trinkle AJ: Peritoneal lavage in the treatment of uremia. J Urol 39: 53–62, 1938.
9. Reid R, Penfold JB, Jones RN: Anuria treated by renal decapsulation and peritoneal dialysis. Lancet 2: 749–753, 1946.
10. Fine J, Frank HA, Seligman AM: The treatment of acute renal failure by peritoneal irrigation. Ann Surg 124: 857–878, 1946.
11. Rosenak SS, Oppenheimer GD: An improved drain for peritoneal lavage. Surgery 23: 832–833, 1948.
12. Derot M, Tanzet P, Roussilon J, Bernier JJ: La dialyse peritoneale dans le traitement de luremie aigue. J Urol 55: 113–121, 1949.
13. Legrain M, Merrill JP: Short term continuous transperitoneal dialysis. New Eng J Med 248: 125–129, 1953.
14. Maxwell MH, Rockney RE, Kleeman CR, Twiss MR: Peritoneal dialysis. JAMA 170: 917–924, 1959.
15. Doolan PD, Murphy WP, Wiggins RA, Carter NW, Cooper WC, Watten RH, Alpen EL: An evaluation of intermittent peritoneal lavage. Am J Med 26: 831–844, 1959.
16. Weston RE, Roberts M: Clinical use of stylet catheter for peritoneal dialysis. Arch Int Med 115: 659–662, 1965.
17. Boen ST, Mulinari AS, Dillard DH, Scribner BH: Periodic peritoneal dialysis in the management of chronic uremia. Trans Amer Soc Artif Intern Organs 8: 256–265, 1962.
18. Merrill JP, Sabbaga E, Henderson L, Welzant W, Crane C: The use of an inlying plastic conduit for chronic peritoneal irrigation. Trans Am Soc Artif Intern Organs 8: 252–255, 1962.
19. Barry KG, Shambaugh GE, Goler D: A new flexible cannula and seal to provide prolonged access for peritoneal drainage and other procedures. J Urol 90: 125–128, 1963.
20. Boen ST, Mion CM, Curtis FK, Shilipetar G: Periodic peritoneal dialysis using the repeated puncture technique and an automated cycling machine. Trans Am Soc Artif Intern Organs 10: 409–413, 1964.
21. Tenckhoff H, Schechter H, Boen ST: One years experience with home peritoneal dialysis. Trans Am Soc Art Intern Organs 11:11–14, 1965.
22. Jacob GB, Deane N: Repeated peritoneal dialysis by the catheter replacement method: description of technique and a replaceable prosthesis for chronic access to the peritoneal cavity. Proc Eur Dial Transpl Assoc 4: 136–140, 1967.
23. Bigelow P, Oreopoulos DG, DeVeber GA: Use of Deane prosthesis in patients on long term peritoneal dialysis Can Med J 109: 999–1001, 1973.
24. Mallette WG, McPhaul JJ, Bledsoe F, McIntosh DA, Koegel E: A clinically successfull subcutaneous peritoneal access button for repeated peritoneal dialysis. Trans Amer Soc Artif Intern Organs 10: 396–398, 1964.
25. Gotloib L, Nisencorn J, Garmizo AL, Galili N, Servadio C, Sudarsky M: Subcutaneous intraperitoneal prosthesis for maintenance peritoneal dialysis. Lancet 1: 1318–1319, 1975.
26. Gutch CF: Peritoneal dialysis. Trans Am Soc Artif Int Organs 10: 4006–408, 1964.
27. McDonald HP, Gerber N, Mishra D, Wolin L, Peng B, Waterhouse K: Subcutaneous dacron and teflon cloth adjuncts for silastic arteriovenous shunts and peritoneal dialysis catheters. Trans Am Soc Art Intern Organs 14: 176–180, 1968.
28. Tenckhoff H: Home peritoneal dialysis. In: Shaul G, Massry AL, Sellers, (eds), Clinical Aspects of Uremia and Dialysis. CC Thomas, Publ., Springfield, IL. 1976; pp 583–615.
29. Goldberg EM, Hill W, Kabins S, Levin B: Peritoneal dialysis. Dial Transpl 4: 50–56, 1975.
30. Stephen RL, Atkin-Thor E, Kolff WJ: Recirculating peritoneal dialysis with subcutaneous catheter. Trans Am Soc Artif Intern Organs 22: 575–584, 1976.
31. Oreopoulos DG, Izatt S, Zellerman G, Karanicolas S, Mathews RE: A prospective study of the effectiveness of three permanent peritoneal catheters. Proc Clin Dial Transplant Forum 6: 96–100, 1976.
32. Twardowski ZJ, Nolph KD, Khanna R, Prowant BF, Ryan LP, Nichols WK: The need for a 'Swan Neck' permanently bent, arcuate peritoneal dialysis catheter. Perit Dial Bull 5: 219–223.
33. Bossert WA, Marks HH: Prevalence and characteristics of peridontal disease of 12 800 persons under periodic dental observation. J Am Dent Assoc 52: 429–442, 1956.
34. Hajek M: Pathology and Treatment of the Inflammatory Diseases of the Nasal Accessory Sinuses. Translated and edited by Heitger JD, and Hansel FK, Fifth edition, C.V. Mosby Company, St. Louis, pg 100, 1926.
35. So SKS, Mahan JD, Jr, Mauer SM, Sutherland DER, Nevins TE: Hickman catheter for pediatric hemodialysis: a 3-year experience. Trans Amer Soc Artif Intern Organs 30: 619–623, 1984.
36. Raaf JH: Results from use of 826 vascular access devices in cancer patients. Cancer 55: 1312–1321, 1985.
37. Hall CW, Adams IM, Ghidoni JJ: Development of skin interfacing cannula. Trans Amer Soc Artif Intern Organs 21: 281–287, 1975.
38. Daly BDT, Dasse KA, Haudenschild CC, Clay W, Szycher M, Ober NS, Cleveland RJ: Percutaneous energy transmission systems: long-term survival. Trans Amer Soc Artif Intern Organs 29: 526–530, 1983.
39. Kantrowitz A, Freed PS, Ciarkowski AA, Hayashi I, Vaughan FL, VeShancey JI, Gray RH, Brabec RK, Bernstein IA: Development of a percutaneous access device. Trans Amer Soc Artif Intern Organs 26: 444–449, 1980.
40. Smith C: CAPD: One cuff vs two cuff catheters in referance to incidence of infection. In: Frontiers in Peritoneal Dialysis. Proceedings of the III International symposium on Peritoneal Dialysis, Washington D.C., 1984, Edited by Maher JF, Winchester JF, Published by Field, Rich and Associates, Inc. New York pp 181–186, 1986.
41. Tenckhoff H: Discussion for manuscript # 36. Trans Amer Soc Artif Intern Organs 21: 288, 1975.
42. Wright NA: The cell proliferation kinetics of the epidermis. In: IA Goldsmith (ed) Biochemistry and Physiology of the skin, Oxford University Press, New York and Oxford, 1983; pp 203–229.
43. Schluger S, Yuodelis RA, Page RC: Periodontal disease. Philadelphia, Lea & Febiger, p 2, 1978.

44. Schroeder HE, Page RC: The normal periodontium. In: Schluger S, Youdelis RA, Page RC (eds) Periodontal Disease, Lea & Febiger, Philadelphia 1978; pp 7–55.

45. Poirier VL, Daly BDT, Dasse KA, Haudenschild CC, Fine RE: Elimination of tunnel infection. In: Maher JF, Winchester JF (eds), Frontiers in Peritoneal Dialysis. Proceedings of the III International Symposium on Peritoneal Dialysis. Washington, D.C., 1984. Published by Field, Rich & Assoc., Inc., New York, NY 1986; pp 210–217.

46. Daly BDT, Szycher M, Dasse KA: Percutaneous energy transmission system: factors influencing long-term implantation. Trans Am Society Astif Intern Organs 227: 147–150, 1981.

47. Ogden DA, Benavente G, Wheeler D, Zukoski CF: Experience with the Right Angle GORE-TEX® peritoneal dialysis catheter. In: Khanna R *et al.* (ed), Advances in Continuous Ambulatory Peritoneal Dialysis, Peritoneal Dialysis Bulletin, Inc., Toronto, pp 155–159, 1986.

48. Kim D, Burke D, Izatt S, Mathews R, Wu G, Khanna R, Vas S, Oreopoulos DG: Single or double cuff peritoneal catheters? a prospective comparison. Trans Am Soc Artif Intern Organs 30: 232–235, 1984.

49. Diaz-Buxo JA, Geissinger WT: Single cuff versus double cuff Tenckhoff catheter. Perit. Dial. Bull., 4(Suppl 3): S100–S102, 1984.

50. Goldman HM, Cohen DW: Periodontal Therapy The C.V. Mosby Company, St. Louis, Toronto, London, p. 1, 1980.

51. Trooskin SZ, Harvey RA, Donetz AP, Greco RS: Application of antibiotic bonding to CAPD catheters. In: Maher JF, Winchester JF (eds) Frontiers in Peritoneal Dialysis. Rich and Associates, New York, 1985, 157–160.

52. Ponce SP, Pierratos A, Izatt S, Mathews R, Khanna R, Zellerman G, Oreopoulos DG: Comparison of the survival and complications of three permanent peritoneal dialysis catheters. Perit Dial Bull 2: 82–85, 1982.

53. Twardowski ZJ, Nichols WK, Khanna R, Nolph KD: Swan Neck peritoneal dialysis catheters Design, features, sterilizing, insertion and break-in. Instruction manual published by: Accurate Surgical Instruments Corp. 588–590 Richmond St. W., Toronto, Ontario, Canada M5V 1Y9, 1986.

54. Twardowski ZJ, Khanna R, Nolph KD, Nichols WK, Ryan LP: Preliminary experience with the Swan Neck peritoneal dialysis catheter. Trans Am Soc Artif Intern Organs 32: 64–67, 1986.

55. Twardowski ZJ, Prowant BF: Can new catheter design eliminate exit site and tunnel infections? Perspectives in Peritoneal Dialysis 4 (No. 2): 5–9, 1986.

56. Khanna R, Izatt S, Burke D, Mathews R, Vas S, Oreopoulos DG: Experience with the Toronto Western Hospital permanent peritoneal catheter. Perit Dial Bull 4: 95–98, 1984.

57. Spence PA, Mathews R, Khanna R, Oreopoulos DG: Improved results with a paramedian technique for the insertion of peritoneal dialysis catheters. Surg Gyn Obst 161: 585–587, 1985.

58. Ash SR, Johnson H, Hartman J, Granger J, Koszuta J, Sell L, Dhein C, Blevins W, Thornhill JA: The column disc peritoneal catheter. A peritoneal access device with improved drainage. ASAIO J 3: 109–115, 1980.

59. Vaamonde CA, Michael VF, Metzger RA, Carrol KE: Complications of acute peritoneal dialysis. J Chron Dis 28: 637–659, 1975.

60. Valk TW, Swartz RD, Hsu CH: Peritoneal dialysis in acute renal failure: analysis of outcome and complications. Dial Transpl 9: 64, 1980.

61. Maher JF, Schreiner GE: Hazards and complications of dialysis. N Engl J Med 273: 370, 1965.

62. Anderson G, Bergquist-Poppen M, Bergstrom J, Collste LG, Huttman E: Glucose absorption from the dialysis fluid during peritoneal dialysis. Scand J. Urol Nephrol 5: 77, 1971.

63. Firmat J, Zucchini A: Peritoneal dialysis in acute renal failure. Contrib Nephrol (Krager, Basel) 17: 33–338, 1979.

64. Edward SR, Unger AM: Acute hydrothorax: a new complication of peritoneal dialysis. JAMA 199: 853–855, 1967.

65. Finn R, Jowett EW: Acute hydrothorax: complication of peritoneal dialysis. Br Med J 2: 94, 1970.

66. Holm J, Lieden B, Lindgrist B: Unilateral effusion – a rare complication of peritoneal dialysis. Scand J Urol Nephrol 5: 84–85, 1971.

67. Haberli R, Stucki P: Akuter hydro-thorax als komplikation bei peritoneal dialyse. Praxis 60: 13–14, 1971.

68. Fehmirling E, Christensen E: Hydrothorax under peritoneal dialyse. Ugeskr Laeg 137: 1650b–1651, 1975.

69. Alquier P, Achard J, Bonhome R: Hydrothorax aign au loure de dialyses peritoneales. La Nouv Presse Med 4: 192, 1975.

70. Rudnick MR, Coyle JF, Beck H, McCurdy DK: Acute massive hydrothorax complicating peritoneal dialysis, report of 2 cases and a review of the literature. Clin Nephrol 12: 38–44, 1980.

71. Milutinovic J, Shyong W, Lindholme DD, Leroy N: Acute massive unilateral hydrothorax as result of complications of peritoneal dialysis. South Med J 78: 827, 1980.

72. Grefberg N, Danielson BG, Benson L, Pitkanen P: Right sided hydrothorax complicating peritoneal dialysis. Nephron 34: 130–134, 1983.

73. Kennedy JM: Procedures used to demonstrate a pleuroperitoneal communication: A review. Perit Dial Bull 5: 168–170, 1985.

74. Ribot S, Jacobs MG, frankel HJ, Bernstein A: Complications of peritoneal dialysis. Am J Med Sci 252: 505, 1966.

75. Mion CM, Boen ST: Analysis of factors responsible for the formation of adhesions during chronic peritoneal dialysis. Am J Med Sci 250: 675–679, 1965.

76. Matalon R, Levine S, Eisinger RP: Hazards in routine use of peritoneal dialysis. NY State J Med 71: 219–224, 1971.

77. Henderson LW: Peritoneal dialysis. Clinical aspects of uremia and dialysis. In: Massry SG, Sellers AL (eds), Charles C. Thomas, Springfield, IL, p 574, 1976.

78. Simkin EP, Wright FK: Perforating injuries of the bowel complicating peritoneal catheter insertion. Lancet 1: 61–67, 1968.

79. Chugh KS, Bhattacharya K, Amaresan MS, SHarma BK, Bansal VK: Peritoneal dialysis: our experience based on 550 dialyses. J Assoc Physicians India 20: 215–221, 1972.

80. Nienhuis LI: Clinical peritoneal dialysis. Arch Surg 93: 643–653, 1966.

81. Pauli HG, Billikofer E, Vorburger C: Clinical experience with peritoneal dialysis. Helv Med Acta 33: 51–58, 1966.

82. Krebes RA, Burtiss BB: Bowel perforation. JAMA 198: 486–487, 1966.

83. Denovales EL, Avendano LN: Risks of peritoneal catheter insertion (letter). Lancet 1: 473, 1968.

84. Dunea G: Peritoneal dialysis and hemodialysis. Med Clin North Am 55: 155–175, 1971.

85. Rigalosi RS, Maher JF, Schriener GE: Intestinal perforation during peritoneal dialysis. Ann Intern Med 70: 1013–1015, 1964.

86. Edwards DH, Gardner RD, Williams DG: Rupture of a hernial sac: A complication of peritoneal dialysis. J Urol 108: 255, 1972.

87. Goldsmith HJ, Edwards EC, Moorhead PJ, *et al.*: Difficulties encountered in intermittent dialysis for chronic renal failure. Br J Urol 38: 625–634, 1966.

88. Smith E, Chamberlain MJ: Complications of peritoneal dialysis. Br Med J 1: 126–127, 1965.

89. Stein MF Jr: Intraperitoneal loss of dialysis catheter. Ann Intern Med 71: 869–870, 1969.

90. Ash SR, Daugirdas JT: Peritoneal Access devices. In: Handbook of Dialysis. In: JT Daugirdas, TS Ing (eds)), Little Brown

and Company, Boston Publishers, 194–218, 1988.

91. Twardowski ZJ, Khanna R, Nolph KD, Scalamogna A, Metzler MH, Schneider TW, Prowant BF, Ryan LP: Intraabdominal pressure during natural activities in patients treated with continuous ambulatory peritoneal dialysis. Nephron 44: 129–135, 1986.

92. Daly BDT, Dasse KA, Gould KE: A new percutaneous access device for peritoneal dialysis. Trans Am Society Artif Intern Organs 32: 664–671, 1987.

93. Twardowski ZJ, Tully RJ, Nichols WK, Sunderjan S: Computerized tomography in the diagnosis of subcutaneous leak sites during CAPD. Perit Dial Bull 4: 163–166, 1984.

94. Block RA, Taylor B, Grederick G: Intraperitoneal infusion of streptokinase in the treatment of recurrent peritonitis. Perit Dial Bull 3: 162–163, 1983.

95. Scalamogna A, Castelnova C, Cantaluppi A: Intraperitoneal infusion of streptokinase in the treatment of a total peritoneal catheter obstruction. Perit Dial Bull 6: 41, 1986.

96. Benevent D, Peryonnet P, Brignon P: Urokinase infusion for obstructed catheters and peritonitis. Perit Dial Bull 5: 77, 1985.

97. Dykewicz MS: Identification of patients at risk for anaphylaxis due to streptokinase. Arch Inter Med 146: 305, 1986.

98. Prowant BF, Schmidt IM, Twardowski ZJ, Griebel SK, Ryan LP, Satalowich RJ, Burrows LM: A randomized prospective evaluation of three peritoneal exit site procedures. (Abstract) IV Congress of International Society for Peritoneal Dialysis, Venice, Italy, Perit Dial Bull S7: 70, 1987.

99. Low DE, Vas SI, Oreopoulos DG, Manuel RA, Saiphoo CS, FIner C, Dombros N: Randomized clinical trial of prophylactic cephalexin in CAPD. Lancet 2: 753–754, 1980.

100. Churchill DN, Oreopoulos DG, Taylor DW, Vas SI, Manuel MA, Wu G: Peritonitis in CAPD patients – a randomized clinical trial of trimethoprim-sulfamethoxazole prophylaxis. (Abstr.) 20th Ann Meeting of the American Society of Nephrology, p. 97A.

101. Slingeneyer A, Balmes M, Mion C: Surgical implantation of the Tenckhoff catheter in peritoneal dialysis. In: LaGreca G, Biasioli S, Roneco C (eds) Wichtig Editore, Milano, 1983, pp 133–136.

102. Rubin J, Adair C: Peritoneal access using the Tenckhoff catheter. Perspective in peritoneal Dialysis. 1: 2–3, 1983.

103. Rottembourg J, De Groc F: Peritoneal access using the curled Tenckhoff catheter. Perspectives in Peritoneal Dialysis. 1: 7–9, 1983.

104. Grefberg N: Clinical aspects of CAPD. Scand J Urol and Nephrology S72: 7–38, 1983.

105. Hogg RJ, Coln D, Chang J, Arant BS, Houser M: The Toronto Western Hospital catheter in a pediatric dialysis program. Am J Kidney Disease 3: 219–223, 1983.

106. Flanigan MJ, Ngheim DD, Schulak JA, Ullrich GE, Freeman RM: The use and complications of three peritoneal dialysis catheter designs: a retrospective analysis. Trans Am Soc Artif Intern Organs 33: 33–38, 1987.

107. Twardowski ZJ, Khanna R, Nichols WK, Nolph KD, Prowant BF, Ryan LP, Russ J (in press) One year experience with Swan Neck Missouri-2 catheter. Proceedings of the IVth Congress of the International Society for Peritoneal Dialysis. Venice, Italy, June 29 July 2, 1987.

108. Bozkurt F, Keller E, Schollmeyer P: Swan Neck peritoneal dialysis catheter can reduce complications in CAPD patients. Abstracts of the IVth Congress of the International Society for Peritoneal Dialysis. Venice, Italy, June 29 July 2, 1987. Peritoneal Dialysis Bulletin, Supplement, 7 (No 2): S9, 1987.

109. Ash SR, Slingeneyer A, Scchardin KE: Peritoneal access using the column-disc catheter. Perspective in Peritoneal Dialysis. 1: 9–11, 1983.

110. Dasse KA, Dally BDT, Bousquet G King D Smith T, Mondou R, Poirier VL: A polyurethane percutaneous access device for peritoneal dialysis. Proceedings of the 8th International CAPD Converence, Kansas City, Khanna R et al. (eds), 245–252, 1988.

17

PERITONEAL DIALYSIS IN CHILDREN

STEVEN R. ALEXANDER

1. INTRODUCTION

When this chapter was prepared for the Second Edition of Peritoneal Dialysis nearly four years ago, pediatric nephrologists were just awakening to a new era in the treatment of infants and children who suffered from chronic renal failure. The 1976 discovery of continuous ambulatory peritoneal dialysis (CAPD) by Popovich and Moncrief and their associates [1], was followed by a 'renaissance' of interest in this most venerable of renal replacement therapies. Pediatric nephrologists were quick to recognize the potential advantages offered by CAPD to their young patients, perhaps in part because peritoneal dialysis was a familiar modality. For nearly thirty years, peritoneal dialysis has been widely considered to be the dialytic treatment of choice for acute renal failure in infants and young children, primarily because the technique is intrinsically simple, safe and easily adapted for use in patients of all ages and sizes. The early promise of CAPD for pediatric patients was that the familiar simplicity and safety

of acute peritoneal dialysis could now be combined with several obviously advantageous (for children) chronic dialysis features: near steady-state biochemical and fluid control, no dysequilibrium syndrome, greatly reduced dietary restrictions, and freedom from repeated needle punctures. Even more important, CAPD promised to allow children of all ages to routinely receive dialysis in their homes, and thus to have more normal childhoods. Finally, CAPD promised to make it possible to offer treatment to very young infants, a patient group which previously was not considered suitable for renal replacement therapy.

In large measure, these promises have been fulfilled. CAPD and its mechanized cousin CCPD (continuous cycling peritoneal dialysis) have become the dialysis treatment modalities of choice for the majority of children with end-stage renal disease (ESRD) in many pediatric dialysis centers in North America and Western Europe. CAPD and CCPD have not only been shown to be safe and effective renal replacement therapies in children, but both have been shown to be entirely compatible with renal transplantation [3, 4, 5]. The latter finding was essential to the continued use of these chronic peritoneal dialysis techniques in children for whom renal transplantation is without question the optimum form of therapy [2].

This chapter will attempt to review what is known about the use of both acute and chronic peritoneal dialysis in pediatric patients through the end of 1987. Clinical and technical considerations will be emphasized throughout, and occasionally specific advice will be given which reflects only the author's current approach to a particular clinical problem. The goal of this chapter remains the same as it was in the previous edition of this text: to provide some practical assistance to those who are actively involved in the treatment of infants and children with peritoneal dialysis.

2. NOTES ON THE PEDIATRIC HISTORY OF PERITONEAL DIALYSIS

The peritoneal cavity has been used in the treatment of children's disorders for at least seventy years. In 1918, Blackfan and Maxcy described the successful treatment of severely dehydrated infants with intraperitoneal saline injections [6], a technique which is still used today in rural areas of some developing countries.

The first two reports of the use of the peritoneum to treat children with renal failure appeared in 1948 and 1949 [7, 8], at a time when worldwide clinical experience with peritoneal dialysis did not total 100 patients [9]. These initial pediatric reports are of more than historic interest; they both describe in striking detail many of the problems which have continued to complicate the use of peritoneal dialysis in children for forty years.

Writing in the premier issue of the journal, *Pediatrics,** two Houston physicians, Allan Bloxsom and Norborne Powell reported on their use of continuous peritoneal irrigation to treat an oliguric 10 yr old boy with acute post-streptococcal glomerulonephritis [7]. Bloxsum and Powell modeled their technique on methods first described by Fine and associates in 1946 [10]. Two irrigating tubes (# 30 Fr. mushroom catheters) were surgically inserted into the peritoneal cavity through a high McBurney incision above each iliac crest. The irrigating solution was then dripped continuously at 10 cc per minute into one catheter while the other catheter drained by gravity into a sterile flask. The solution was only slightly hypertonic, containing, perhaps by an oversight, only 1.5 g of dextrose per liter. In addition to sodium chloride, the irrigating solution contained physiologic amounts of potassium, calcium, magnesium, and phosphate. Sodium bicarbonate, sodium sulfadiazene, penicillin (only 5000 units/l) and heparin were added to each autoclaved one-liter flask as it was put into use. Peritoneal irrigation was continued for four days, during which the patient became fluid overloaded, devel-

oping congestive heart failure. The drainage catheter often became obstructed; at first the problem was resolved by reversing the direction of flow of the irrigation system. By the third day, suction was required to achieve drainage; by the fourth day neither catheter would drain and irrigating fluid was leaking freely around the outflow catheter. Peritoneal fluid cultures from the final day of treatment were positive for staphylococci, streptococci and gram negative bacilli. Fortunately, the boy began a spontaneous diuresis on the third day of treatment which led to his eventual complete recovery. In fact, the only obvious benefit the child received from peritoneal irrigation was an initial improvement in the blood pressure from 186/130 mm Hg to 148/105 mm Hg after 24 hr of treatment. The BUN did not fall substantially from its peak at 150 mg/dl until urine output exceeded one l/24 hr [7].

During the following year, Swan and Gordon in Denver described a more successful experience with a similar system of continuous peritoneal lavage, which they used to treat three acutely anuric children, 9 months, 3 yr and 8 yr of age [8]. Rigid operating room suction tips covered by metal sheaths with multiple perforations were used for peritoneal access, one surgically implanted into the upper abdomen, the other into the pelvis. Large volumes of dialysate flowed continuously by gravity from 20-l carboys into one catheter and drained by water suction out of the other catheter. An average of 33 l of fluid was used each day, with the child's fluid balance maintained by adjusting the dextrose content of the dialysate between 2 and 4 gm%. Dialysate temperature was regulated by varying the number of 60-W light bulbs in a box placed over the inflow water bath.

The two older children regained normal renal function after 9 and 12 days of continuous peritoneal lavage. The 9 months old infant was sustained for 28 days before she succumbed to obscure complications. Peritonitis occurred only once and responded to intraperitoneal antibiotics. Removal of urea and maintenance of fluid balance were excellent in all three children, although obviously herculean efforts were required to deliver this therapy.

In 1949, continuous peritoneal lavage was simply too time-consuming, technically difficult and expensive to become widely used. However, despite its many problems, the work of Swan and Gordon should be credited as the first to conclusively demonstrate the life-saving potential of peritoneal dialysis when used to treat acute renal failure in children of almost any age.

It was more than a decade before the use of peritoneal dialysis in children was again reported. During the 1950's the development of disposable nylon catheters and commercially prepared dialysis solutions made intermittent peritoneal dialysis a practical short-term treatment for acute renal failure in adults [11]. Successful adaptation of this technique for use in infants and children with acute renal failure was reported in 1961 by Segar and associates in Indianapolis [12] and in 1962 by Etteldorf and associates in Memphis [13]. Both of these groups also documented the effectiveness of peritoneal dialysis as a treatment for certain intoxications (boric acid and salicylate) common in infants and small children in the early 1960s [14, 15]. Subsequent reports from many parts of the world served to establish peritoneal dialysis as the most frequently employed dialytic technique in the treatment of acute renal

---

* A sense of the historic context in which the Bloxsum and Powell paper appeared is gained by noting that this first pediatric peritoneal dialysis report was flanked by articles on combined DPT immunization and the natural history of poliomyelitis, and immediately preceded by a case report describing an infant who had died from acute renal failure caused by an occult obstruction of the urethra.

failure in pediatric patients [16, 17, 18, 19, 20, 21, 22].

The manual peritoneal dialysis technique used throughout the 1960s required re-insertion of the dialysis catheter for each treatment; this fact alone made prolonged use of peritoneal dialysis in infants and small children with ESRD essentially impossible. Except for an isolated case report involving a 19 year old boy [23], the only published pediatric series from this period was that of Feldman, Baliah and Drummond, who described their generally successful results in 7 children maintained on intermittent peritoneal dialysis (IPD) in Montreal for 1.5 to 8 months while awaiting transplantation [24]. None of these children required dialysis more often than once every 7 to 12 days.

The development of a permanent peritoneal catheter, begun by Palmer and associates [25, 26] in the early 1960s and completed by Tenckhoff and Schechter in 1968 [27], made long-term IPD an acceptable form of treatment for pediatric patients. In Seattle, Tenckhoff and associates [28] combined permanent peritoneal catheters with an automated dialysate delivery system (first proposed by Boen and associates, [29]) which could be used in the home. This work culminated in the establishment in Seattle of the first pediatric home chronic peritoneal dialysis program [30]. Throughout the next decade the Seattle group made steady progress in the development of long-term automated peritoneal dialysis techniques suitable for use in children [31].

Additional limited experience with chronic IPD was reported from several other centers [32, 33, 34, 35] but enthusiasm for the technique among pediatric nephrologists was never great. Chronic IPD seemed to involve most of the undesirable features of chronic hemodialysis (eg.: dietary restrictions, fluid limits, immobility during treatments, complex machinery requiring extensive parental or nursing staff supervision), without providing the one great advantage of hemodialysis – efficiency.

The description of CAPD by Popovich, Moncrief and their associates in 1976 [1] heralded a new area in the use of peritoneal dialysis in children with ESRD. CAPD was first used in a child in 1978 in Toronto [36, 37]. Subsequent experience was soon reported from growing pediatric CAPD programs in the United States [38, 39, 40, 41] and Europe [42, 43]. In the United States, early efforts to adapt CAPD for pediatric patients were hampered by the commercial availability of dialysate only in 2000 ml plastic containers. Parents were taught to discard most of the fluid from the 2-l container before infusing the remainder [40], or to prepare small volume bags at home by filling blood bank transfer packs [38]. Hospital pharmacies were also used to periodically prepare and ship supplies of small volume dialysate containers to individual patients [44, 45]. These wasteful, expensive and potentially risky methods would finally be abandoned for most children in July, 1980 when dialysate in 500 ml and 1000 ml plastic containers became commercially available in the United States [46]. Subsequent addition of 250 ml, 750 ml and 1500 ml containers completed a range of standardized dialysate volumes which will accomodate most pediatric patients. For the rare infant for whom no standard size is appropriate, customized patient-specific CAPD exchange volumes can be obtained from the manufacturer on a prescription basis.*

The next step in the development of continuous peritoneal dialysis for children was the addition of continuous cycling peritoneal dialysis (CCPD), first described by Buoncristiani and Diaz-Buxo and their associates [47, 48], and first used in a child in 1981 by Price and Suki [49]. CCPD has subsequently grown in popularity among many pediatric dialysis programs in North America [50], perhaps because the technique offers freedom from the more intrusive daytime exchange regimen required by CAPD. Further modifications of the CCPD regimen have been proposed which include elimination of all or most of the long daytime dwell, [50, 51]. Despite concerns that a return to an *intermittent* cycling peritoneal dialysis (ICPD) regimen might undermine important physiologic advantages associated with *continuous* peritoneal dialysis for children [52], it is in this area that the most active growth in chronic peritoneal dialysis for pediatric patients is likely to take place during the next few years.

3. PERITONEAL DIALYSIS KINETICS IN CHILDREN

Peritoneal transport kinetics have been extensively studied in adults (see Chapter 6), but relatively few studies have been done with pediatric subjects. An entertaining and enlightening review of this subject was recently published by Morgenstern and Baluarte [53]. These authors noted the aversion with which most clinicians greet efforts to mathematically describe transperitoneal solute and fluid movement, but they also called attention to the special importance of an understanding of peritoneal kinetics in children. The current practice of peritoneal dialysis in children has evolved almost entirely from empiric and serendipitous observations. Optimum dialysis mechanics (i.e., exchange volume, dwell time and dialysate composition) have yet to be determined for children, and almost nothing is known about how these mechanics should be altered in various clinical situations to reflect differences in patient age or size. Certainly the lack of an adequate scientific basis for a treatment as widely used in children as peritoneal dialysis is reason enough to study peritoneal transport kinetics. In addition, Morgenstern and Baluarte warn that as more children become difficult to transplant and thus require long-term dialysis, the ability to measure small changes in peritoneal membrane function will become an essential component of therapy. It is from such studies of peritoneal kinetics that we will learn how to best protect and preserve peritoneal membrane function in these children [53].

If peritoneal transport were similar in children and adults, differing only by a 'scaling' factor reflecting relative size (e.g., body weight, height or surface area) then the many observations made in studies of adults could be applied directly to children. Only the appropriate scaling method would be needed. There exists, however, a well-entrenched (if poorly documented) perception that the peritoneum of the child functions differently (i.e., 'more efficiently') than that of the adult (e.g., see ref. 20), and that peritoneal kinetics change as a consequence of normal growth and development. The origin of this concept can be traced to comparative measurements of peritoneal surface area performed over 100 yr ago.

---

* Baxter Laboratories, Deerfield, Illinois 60015.

In a paper read before the Siberian Branch of the Russian Geographic Society in 1884, Putiloff presented the first comparative data on the peritoneal surface area of infants and adults [54]. Using direct oiled paper tracings of peritoneal contents, Putiloff determined that the peritoneal surface area of an infant weighing 2.9 kg was 0.15 m^2, compared to 2.08 m^2 for an adult assumed to weigh 70 kg. Thus the infant had a peritoneal surface area almost twice that of the adult when scaled for weight (522 cm^2/kg vs 285 cm^2/kg). These results were reminiscent of even earlier observations by Wegner that in adults peritoneal surface area and skin surface area were approximately equivalent [55]. Since the ratio of body surface area to weight is greater in infants, it seems logical that the infant should also have a greater peritoneal surface area to weight ratio.

The clinical implications of these anatomic relationships were addressed in 1966 by Esperanca and Collins, who measured peritoneal surface areas during autopsies performed on six neonates and six adults [56]. Their measurements confirmed Putiloff's: the six infants' mean peritoneal surface area per kg of body weight was roughly twice that of the adults. When standard body surface area nomograms [57] were used with the measurements of Esperanca and Collins, no significant difference was found between the ratios of peritoneal surface area to body surface area in adults and infants, thus supporting Wegner's observations that body and peritoneal surface areas are closely related [53].

Based on their findings of a two-fold greater peritoneal surface area when scaled for weight in infants, (and making the unfounded, but reasonable assumption that peritoneal surface area and membrane function were directly related), Esperanca and Collins postulated that '... peritoneal dialysis should be twice as efficient in the infant' [56]. Peritoneal urea clearance studies on uremic puppies and adult dogs performed by these same investigators seemed to support their hypothesis. When scaled for body weight, urea clearance observed in puppies was nearly three times greater than that of adult animals. However, Esperanca and Collins used markedly different dialysate flow rates in the two study groups; puppies received 128 cc/kg/hr and adult dogs only 42 cc/kg/hr. Since urea clearance is proportional to dialysate flow rate in these ranges (see Chapter 6), the observed difference in clearance is not surprising.

A final study performed in an 11-day old infant by Esperanca and Collins offers similar problems in interpretation [56]. Peritoneal urea clearance in the infant was measured at nearly 50 cc/min/kg, 'roughly twice what is usually accomplished in adult practice...' [56], but exchange volumes used in the infant were 85 cc/kg compared to the usual 30 cc/kg used in adults.

Although the studies of Esperanca and Collins failed to demonstrate any greater efficiency of the infant peritoneum, they served to emphasize the vital importance of keeping dialysis mechanics constant when performing comparative studies of peritoneal kinetics. The 'rules' for such studies have recently been stated by Gruskin and associates [58]:

1) Constant inflow, dwell and outflow times.
2) Identical exchange volumes per unit weight (or height or body surface area).
3) Identical dialysate composition.
4) Results must be adjusted for body size.

Failure to abide by these rules has been a problem in some studies of peritoneal kinetics in children where differences in dialysis mechanics have made comparisons of such studies difficult and potentially misleading.

There are other factors peculiar to pediatric patients which might influence interpretation of peritoneal kinetics data. Age-related differences in solute distribution volumes and generation rates relative to body size should also be considered. For example, total body water in the neonate approaches 70% of body weight [59], compared to the adult's 50% +/- 5%. Thus more grams of urea per unit body weight must be removed from the neonate to produce an equivalent decline in BUN. Solute generation rate is usually thought to be proportional to metabolic rate; relative to body weight, metabolic rate is highest in infants and declines with advancing age [60]. It could be argued that higher solute generation rates and larger solute pools make greater peritoneal membrane efficiency a necessity for the very young. These concerns may be mitigated by the beneficial effects of growth on dialysis requirements. Vigorous growth in infants has been likened to a 'third kidney' [61]; it seems logical that vigorously growing infants would generate less solute for removal than infants who are growing poorly, but these relationships have not been studied systematically.

Is the peritoneum of the child 'more efficient' than that of the adult? Is peritoneal mass transfer an age-related phenomenon? These questions have not been adequately studied, a deficiency which may reflect the difficulties involved in such studies rather than a lack of interest or insufficient numbers of potential study subjects.

The available information on peritoneal kinetics in children can be organized according to the transport properties of the peritoneal membrane: effective membrane surface area; permeability (both diffusive and convective) to solutes; fluid transfer (i.e., ultrafiltration); peritoneal capillary blood flow; peritoneal lymphatic absorption [62, 63].

3.1. Effective membrane surface area and permeability

Studies in adults have shown that not all of the peritoneal membrane participates equally in mass transfer, with major exchange sites located in mesentary, omentum, intestinal serosa and parietal peritoneum [58]. Effective peritoneal surface area might be greater in the infant, reflecting the infant's larger surface area to body weight ratio. Major transport sites have not been determined in the young and it is not known if the relative proportion of effective peritoneal surface area changes with growth.

It must be remembered that effective peritoneal surface area can only be estimated indirectly from such measurements of peritoneal function as the dialysance (D) and the mass-transfer area co-efficient (MTAC). Dialysance and MTAC calculations do not normally allow separation of the contributions to mass transfer of effective peritoneal surface area and membrane permeability. A more complete discussion of the derivations of D and the MTAC can be found in Chapter 6.

The most complete studies of peritoneal transport in young animals are those of Elzouki and associates who determined peritoneal dialysance values for urea (D$_u$) and inulin (D_i) in six puppies less than one month of age and five adult dogs [64]. D_u and D_i per kilogram of body weight were 1.66-fold and 2.8-fold greater, respectively, in the puppies than in the adult animals. By simultaneously determining D_u and D_i, Elzouki and associates could calculate a dialysance ratio (D_r) which they considered an index of membrane permeability independent of effective surface area [65]. D_r was greater in the puppies, suggesting that membrane permeability was greater in the younger animals. To date, these studies in dogs have not been confirmed by studies of peritoneal solute transport in humans.

Gruskin and associates examined time-related changes in dialysate-to-blood concentration ratios for seven different solutes in nine children, 4 months to 18.5 yr of age [66]. By rigidly controlling dialysis mechanics in these studies, Gruskin demonstrated the perterbations created by even minor alterations in exchange volume and dwell time. Dialysate-to-blood concentration ratios measured sequentially during an exchange were used to construct diffusion curves for each solute. These diffusion curves were found to be fundamentally similar to adult reference curves, and there were no demonstrable differences in diffusion curves observed among children of widely divergent ages and sizes as long as dialysis mechanics were held constant relative to body weight. Mean peritoneal urea and creatinine clearances scaled for weight were no different in infants 4 months to 2 yr of age compared to older children, and all were within the range of values reported for adults. Gruskin and associates concluded that apparent age-related differences in dialysis efficiency observed in previous studies were probably attributable to differences in dialysis mechanics [66].

Only two studies (involving a total of 12 children) have measured MTACs in pediatric patients [67, 68]. Popovich and associates studied 4 children 17 months to 6 yr of age [67]; no significant difference was found between mean MTACs for urea, creatinine, uric acid and glucose measured in the 4 children compared to adult reference values, when scaled for body weight.

Morgenstern and associates, in a similarly constructed study of 8 children 1.5 to 18 yr of age, also found that MTACs for urea, creatinine, uric acid and glucose were similar to adult reference values [68]. Morgenstern also determined the MTAC for total protein which was significantly greater than adult values, supporting prior observations of increased protein losses in younger children treated with CAPD [44, 51].

The Popovich and Morgenstern MTAC studies are not as conclusive as the preceding paragraphs may suggest. Different scaling factors were used and correlation with adult reference values was different depending on whether results were scaled for weight or body surface area. Results obtained in one study in the youngest patient, a 17 month old girl, gave substantially different results for 3 of the 4 solutes studied [67].

Morgenstern and associates further analyzed their MTAC data from these children in a later report which addressed convective transport [69]. Reflection coefficients for urea, creatinine, uric acid and glucose were no different in their 8 pediatric subjects compared to adult reference values. A significantly lower reflection coefficient for total protein

was observed, consistent with the higher MTAC for protein described in those children in a previous report [68].

Although the data are sparse, it seems reasonable to propose that, with appropriate size adjustments, effective membrane surface area and permeability for most small solutes are no different in children and adults. Peritoneal transport of protein may indeed be 'more efficient' in the child, and while this may contribute to a lower BUN, it could hardly be considered a desirable characteristic. Obviously more work is needed in this area, including detailed studies in young infants ($<$ 6 months of age) for whom very little data are currently available.

3.2. Ultrafiltration

Clinical experience suggests that adequate ultrafiltration may be difficult to achive in some infants and young children. Early studies have shown that younger children experience a more rapid decline in dialysate dextrose concentration and osmolality compared to older children and adult reference values [70, 71]. However, the limited available MTAC data do not support a major difference in maximum ultrafiltration rates achieved by children compared to adults [67, 68, 69]. Ultrafiltration in very young infants has been shown to be exquisitely sensitive to exchange volume [72].

3.3. Peritoneal capillary blood flow

There are no data available on peritoneal blood flow in children, but a difference in blood flow is unlikely to be a factor in differential membrane function. Peritoneal blood flow is great enough in adults under most circumstances to exceed requirements for maximum observed peritoneal mass transfer [62].

3.4. Lymphatic absorption

The potential importance of peritoneal lymphatic absorption to net solute and fluid transport has only recently been appreciated [63]. Early data available on lymphatic absorption in pediatric patients suggests that children have a relatively higher lymphatic absorption of intraperitoneal fluid than adults accounting for relatively lower net ultrafiltration [63A].

In summary, limited studies have failed to define differences in peritoneal mass transfer of small solutes in children compared to adults when scaled for body weight in some studies and for body surface area in others. Protein transport is greater in children. Much more work will be required before peritoneal dialysis kinetics in children can be confidently characterized. For the present, optimum dialysis mechanics for pediatric patients must remain an empiric exercise.

4. PERITONEAL DIALYSIS FOR ACUTE RENAL FAILURE

4.1. Incidence and etiology

In developing countries, acute renal failure (ARF) is a common pediatric disorder, occurring most often as a complication of infectious diarrhea, dehydration, bronchopneumonia, and sepsis [73]. In North America and Western

Europe, ARF is more likely to be encountered in neonates who have survived perinatal disasters of one sort or another, in infants and young children who undergo surgery for complex congenital heart disease and in children with the hemolytic uremic syndrome [74]. Independent prospective studies conducted in two large children's hospitals in the United States found that 6 to 8% of all neonates admitted to the Newborn ICU develop ARF [75, 76]. Other studies have found that ARF occurs in 8 to 10.5% of infants who undergo open heart surgery during the first year of life [77, 78]. In many parts of North America, the most common cause of ARF in children between 6 months and 5 yr of age is the hemolytic uremic syndrome [79]. Much of the experience using peritoneal dialysis to treat ARF in pediatric patients had been gained from the treatment of these high risk groups.

4.2. Diagnosis

The diagnostic approach to ARF in children is similar to that used in adults and has been reviewed in detail elsewhere [80]. Oliguric ARF occurs when urine flow is <1 cc/kg/hr and serum creatinine is elevated. The first order of business in such situations is the identification of those patients in whom it is possible to restore normal urine flow by correcting renal hypoperfusion, either by administering an intravenous fluid challenge or a cardiotropic agent such as dopamine. Clinical judgment will often separate patients with ARF from those whose oliguria and azotemia are due to hypovolemia or cardiac failure, but occasionally the use of urinary chemistries can be helpful.

Table 1 lists representative values for various indices of renal function obtained from studies of urine chemistries performed in adult patients and neonates [81, 82, 83, 84, 133]. The most useful of these indices are the renal failure index (RFI) and the fractional excretion of sodium (FE_{Na}). Note that RFI and FE_{Na} are higher in neonates, reflecting the relative inability of the neonate to conserve urinary sodium in response to renal hypoperfusion [85, 86].

The use of urinary diagnostic indices in azotemic older infants and children has not been systematically studied. For most clinical purposes, adult reference values appear to be adequate in pediatric patients beyond the neonatal period [74, 80].

4.3. Indications for peritoneal dialysis

The conservative management of ARF in infants and children employs basically the same approach to therapy as is used in adult patients [80, 87]. Meticulous attention to every detail of fluid and electrolyte therapy is essential in these small patients in whom relatively minor errors can have grave consequences. Dietary restrictions, phosphate binders, diuretics, bicarbonate, calcium, anti-hypertensive medications and sodium-potassium exchange resins can all play a role in forestalling or evading dialysis in some children who continue to have sufficient urine output. However, several factors are at work in children which tend to defeat even the best laid conservative management plans. Children have higher metabolic rates and can thus generate harmful solutes more rapidly. In the oliguric child, it is difficult to meet the relatively greater caloric requirements and still abide by the stringent limitations on allowable fluid intake. The major catabolic activity seen in children with hemolytic uremic syndrome, and in infants who have undergone major surgery or survived multiple perinatal insults often results in accumulation of potassium, phosphate, urea and other solutes in the extracellular fluid which can reach harmful levels at surprisingly rapid rates. Consequently, dialysis tends to be used more frequently and sooner in pediatric

Table 1. Urinary diagnostic indices in adults and neonates

Diagnostic indices	Prerenal azotemia		Oliguric acute renal failure		Non-oliguric acute renal failure	
	Adult[c]	Neonate[a,d]	Adult[c]	Neonate[a,d]	Adult[c]	Neonate[a]
U_{Osm}[e]	518 ± 35		369 ± 20		343 + 17	
U_{Na}[f]		31 ± 19		63 ± 34		
U/P$_{urea}$	18 ± 7	30 ± 18	3 ± 0.5	6 ± 3	7 ± 1	
U/P$_{creatinine}$	45 ± 6	29 ± 16	17 ± 2	10 ± 4	17 ± 2	q ± 2
RFI	<1	<2.5	>1	>2.5	>1	>2.5
	(0.6)[b]	(1.9)	(10)	(11)	(4)	(9)
FE_{Na}(%)	<1	<2.5	>1	>2.5	>1	>2.5
	(0.4)[b]	(1.4)	(7)	(5.8)	(3)	(6)

From refs. 81, 82, 83, 84, 133.

[a] Not valid for infants less than 32 weeks gestational age.

[b] Value in parenthesis is the average index in each category calculated from data in the references. Generalizations useful in clinical practice are given above each calculated index.

[c] Mean ± 1 SEM

[d] Mean ± 1 SD

[e] mOsm/kgH$_2$O

[f] mEq/L

$$FE_{Na} = \text{fractional excretion of filtered sodium} = \frac{(U/P)Na}{(U/P)\text{ creatinine}} \times 100.$$

$$RFI = \text{renal failure index} = \frac{(U)Na}{(U/P)\text{ creatinine}}$$

Table 2. Indications for dialysis in acute renal failure in children[a]

Hyperkalemia (serum $K^+ > 7.0$ mEq/l).
Intractable acidosis.
Fluid overload – usually with hypertension, congestive heart failure, or pulmonary edema.
Severe azotemia (BUN > 150 mg/dl).
Symptomatic uremia (encephalopathy, pericarditis, intractable vomiting, hemorrhage).
Hyponatremia, hypocalcemia, hyperphosphatemia (severe, symptomatic).
Fluid removal – for optimal nutrition, transfusions, infusions of cardiac drugs, etc.

[a] Please see text for qualifying comments; each case must be individualized.

patients, especially in neonates and young children [88].

Widely accepted indications for dialysis in children are listed in Table 2 [22, 74, 80, 88]. Such a list fails to properly emphasize the need to consider the rate at which conditions are approaching dialysis criteria. A marginally acceptable clinical situation should not be tolerated for long in children when the prompt institution of peritoneal dialysis will reliably provide better control of fluid and electrolyte disturbances. The convenience, simplicity and relative safety of peritoneal dialysis allow the nephrologist to begin dialysis in the child as soon as it is needed, and without undue alarm over possible complications associated with the procedure itself.

4.4. Contraindications to peritoneal dialysis in children with ARF

Contraindications to peritoneal dialysis are few, and all relate to the lack of an adequate or intact peritoneal cavity. Neonates with omphalocele, diaphragmatic hernia or gastroschisis cannot be treated with peritoneal dialysis. Recent abdominal surgery is not an absolute contraindication as long as there are no draining abdominal wounds. Children with vesicostomies and other urinary diversions, bilateral polycystic kidneys, colostomies, gastrostomies, prune-belly syndrome, and recent bowel surgery have all been successfully treated with peritoneal dialysis in our center and in others [46, 89]. We routinely use peritoneal dialysis to treat ARF associated with renal transplantation if the allograft has been placed in an extraperitoneal location. Extensive intra-abdominal adhesions may prevent successful dialysis in some patients. At one time we attempted to lyse such adhesions in order to create an adequate cavity for exchange of dialysate in children for whom CAPD was prescribed. This procedure had only short term success and in two children resulted in extensive intra-peritoneal hemorrhage which persisted for several days following adhesion lysis. The presence of a ventriculo-peritoneal shunt in hydrocephalic children may be another relative contraindication to peritoneal dialysis.

4.5. Mortality rates and the influence of early dialysis

Nearly one half of all acute renal failure victims will die,

death coming usually within a few days to weeks of the onset of ARF. Almost as if in defiance of advancing dialysis technology, a mortality rate of > or = 50% recurs with sobering regularity in series after series of adult and pediatric patients published since 1970 [75, 76, 77, 78, 82, 83, 90]. Mortality rates among infants and children tend to vary according to patient age and etiology of ARF. This fact, more than any real difference in management, is probably responsible for the occasional series in which an unusually high or low mortality rate is reported [22, 77, 91].

Early use of dialysis has been advocated as a means by which mortality rates might be reduced among selected patient groups. With early dialysis comes control of biochemical and fluid status and maximum nutritional support; the logic inherent in such an approach is compelling and tends to obscure the paucity of objective data on the subject.

In 1975 Chesney and associates observed a 65% mortality rate among 19 infants less than one year of age who developed ARF following major cardiac surgery [77]. Only 6 of the 19 oliguric infants received peritoneal dialysis and this only after protracted periods of conservative management. Rigden and associates reported the results of a much more aggressive approach to the use of peritoneal dialysis in 24 children who also developed ARF as a complication of cardiac surgery [78]. For Rigden, any one of the following criteria was considered sufficient indication for dialysis: potassium > or = 6.0 mEq/l; BUN > or = 240 mg/dl; oliguria (urine output < 1.0 cc/kg/hr) present for 4 hr and resistant to volume expansion, dopamine and furosemide; fluid overload with pulmonary edema and increased atrial pressures. Nine of the 16 infants who were less than one year of age died, for a mortality rate of 56%, an insignificant difference from the mortality rate observed by Chesney and associates in less aggressively dialyzed infants.

Book and associates reported somewhat better results in a smaller group of infants who developed ARF following cardiac surgery [92]. Peritoneal dialysis was begun as soon as urine output of less than 1.0 cc/kg/hr was found to be resistant to volume expansion, and/or dopamine infusion. There were two deaths among the 7 infants less than one year of age, for a mortality rate of 28.5%.

Comparisons among these reports are difficult due to the small numbers of patients and the inability to control for such variables as cardiac diagnosis and intra-operative events. A more carefully controlled study of the early use of peritoneal dialysis in oliguric infants following major cardiac surgery is needed.

4.6. Technical considerations

4.6.1. Catheters: temporary vs permanent
Nephrologists have traditionally relied on percutaneously placed, polyethylene catheters for peritoneal dialysis in the acute setting. Surgical placement of Tenckhoff silicone rubber catheters in children with ARF has recently become increasingly popular [93]. The choice between a percutaneously placed temporary catheter and the Tecnkhoff catheter placed under direct vision is usually somewhat arbitrary, and reflects local practice rather than any actual comparison of the relative merits of the two approaches.

It is generally believed that temporary catheters should

not be left in place for more than 72 hr. This tenet of practice is based on early observations of an increased incidence of peritonitis in children associated with the use of temporary catheters for longer periods [21]. While it may be reasonable on occasion to extend the life of a well-functioning temporary catheter beyond 3 days, a percutaneously placed catheter left in place beyond 5 days invites infection.

Surgical placement of a Tenckhoff catheter in the setting of ARF has the obvious advantage of assurance of good immediate function. This advantage must be weighed in the individual patient against the risks and delays which are associated with a procedure which requires general anesthesia in the operating room. For unstable infants in ICUs, surgical catheter placement at the bedside using local anesthesia is readily accomplished in most centers [94, 95].

4.6.2. Temporary catheters
The most widely used percutaneous catheter is the Trocath (R) * which comes in adult, pediatric, and infant sizes. For small neonates weighing < 2.5 kg, a standard 14 ga intravenous catheter may be used [94, 95, 96, 97], although the pediatric size Trocath has been used successfully in infants weighing as little as 800 grams [98]. For these tiny babies the fenestrated distal segment of the Trocath is trimmed to a length of only 2 cm to ensure that all fenestrations reside within the peritoneal cavity after insertion.

4.6.3. Percutaneous catheter placement technique
Percutaneous catheter placement in children is a simple procedure which, despite its simplicity, can have the sort of life-threatening complications one might expect to be associated with penetrating abdominal trauma. The bladder is first emptied with a small urinary catheter which is then removed to reduce infection risks. Precise urine output determinations are no longer particularly important once the oliguric child begins peritoneal dialysis.

Adequate sedation of older infants and children is important. Adults can be instructed to valsalva at the moment of trocar insertion, but children are rarely able to cooperate to this degree. The practice of using the '...vocally induced abdominal wall tone...' [99] of the child is cruel and unnecessary. Children old enough to describe it, remember percutaneous catheter placement under local anesthesia as a terrifying and painful experience. In conscious children we use standard pediatric doses of meperidine and hydroxyzine hydrochloride for preoperative sedation. Small doses of ketamine can then be used if needed to keep the child asleep throughout the procedure. Good sedation may increase the intraperitoneal priming volume required to safely perforate the relaxed child's peritoneum. Careful attention must be given to cardiorespiratory status throughout the procedure to prevent respiratory embarrassment caused by a large priming volume.

We prefer to use a 16 ga. polyethylene over-the-needle catheter (Intracath)* for infusion of dialysate to distend the abdomen. It may be helpful to have an assistant grasp the skin on either side of the Intracath insertion point,

---

* Quinton Instrument Company, Seattle, Washington.
** Deseret Medical Inc., Sandy, Utah.

stretching the skin taught to provide resistance. Attaching the Intracath to the dialysate inflow line, the nephrologist inserts the Intracath below the skin at a point in the midline several cm. below the umbilicus; the assistant now opens the clamp on the dialysate inflow line. By watching the drip chamber in the inflow line, dialysate can be seen to pass drip by drip into the subcutaneous tissue. The Intracath is now advanced until a steady stream of dialysate is observed in the drip chamber, demonstrating free flow of dialysate into the peritoneal cavity. The Intracath is then advanced a bit farther, the inflow line detached, the needle withdrawn, the line reattached and the remaining plastic catheter advanced until it is well within the peritoneal cavity. At least 30 cc/kg of *warmed* dialysate is infused, while close attention is given to the vital signs of the child. Neonates may require additional ventilatory and/or circulatory support at this stage. The abdomen should be well distended to provide peritoneal resistance to insertion of the dialysis catheter and trocar. A priming volume of up to 50 cc/ kg may be required, the actual limit in each case determined by the point at which respiratory fluctuations in the inflow stream become apparent.

A pre-trimmed pediatric Trocath is inserted after a small stab wound has opened a path through skin and subcutaneous tissue. Insertion is at a point no more than one third of the way down from the umbilicus to the symphysis, in the midline. We estimate ideal intraperitoneal catheter length to be 1 cm less than the distance from xyphoid to umbilicus and trim the catheter accordingly. This insures that the first fenestrations will reside at least 3 cm inside the peritoneal cavity. In general, short catheters perform better than long ones. The cut edges of the catheter should be beveled with iris scissors.

When good in-and-out dialysate flow has been demonstrated the extra-abdominal portion of the catheter is trimmed so that only 4 to 6 cm extend above the abdominal wall. The catheter is secured with a silk pursestring suture and water-resistant tape.

Poor catheter function is a common problem with percutaneous catheters, and is usually due to omental envelopment or obstruction. When this occurs it is probably best to replace the temporary catheter with a surgically placed Tenckhoff catheter.

4.6.4. Tenckhoff catheters for ARF
Standard straight and curled Tenckhoff catheters may be used to treat ARF. In our program there is no difference in the technique used to place Tenckhoff catheters whether the patient is thought to have acute or chronic renal failure. This subject will be covered in the section on chronic dialysis later in this chapter.

4.6.5. Dialysate
Dialysate is available from a growing number of manufacturers in standard dextrose concentrations of 1.5, 2.5 and 4.25%. All of these solutions may be helpful in the treatment of children with ARF; we usually begin with the 2.5% dextrose solution to obtain better ultrafiltration at the outset when fluid overload is frequently a concern.

Some critically ill infants are unable to tolerate the lactate which is absorbed from standard dialysis solutions [100]. Such babies are often hypoxic and hypotensive, and they

Table 3. Peritoneal dialysis solution containing bicarbonate[a]

	ml	Na^+ (mEq)	Cl^- (mEq)	Mg^{++} (mEq)	$SO_4^=$ (mEq)	HCO_3^- (mEq)	Hydrous dextrose (g)
NaCl (0.45%)	896.0	69	69				
NaCl (2.5 mEq/ml)	12.0	30	30				
NaHCO$_3$ (1.0 mEq/ml)	40.0	40				40	
MgSO$_4$ (10%)	1.8			1.5	1.5		
D$_{50}$W	50.0						25
Total	999.8	139	99	1.5	1.5	40	25

Calculated osmolality = 423 mOsm/kg H$_2$O.
[a] Modified from ref. 100.

usually have an ongoing metabolic acidosis due in part to accumulation of endogenous lactic acid. Additional lactate absorbed from the dialysate can result in further decompensation as metabolic acidosis becomes worse. These babies should be treated at the outset with a dialysate which has been re-formulated to contain bicarbonate instead of lactate. A typical bicarbonate reformulation is shown in Table 3. Note that calcium must be given intravenously when bicarbonate-containing dialysis solutions are used.

4.6.6. Dialysis mechanics

Exchange volumes used in children routinely range from 35 to 45 cc/kg, although somewhat smaller volumes may be advisable during the first 24 to 48 hr following surgical catheter placement to reduce the likelihood of dialysate leakage. Respiratory embarrassment and hydrothorax have been associated with the use of exchange volumes approaching 50 cc/kg [88, 101]. Exchange volumes < 25 cc/kg have been associated with poor ultrafiltration in infants [72].

Initial stabilization on peritoneal dialysis often requires 24 to 48 hr of frequent exchanges (30 to 60 min each, depending on catheter function) in order to remove accumulated solutes and excess body fluid. This period corresponds to a traditional intermittent peritoneal dialysis regimen. Once the child has been stabilized, if a Tenckhoff catheter is in place, dialysis may be continued indefinitely. By gradually extending dwell periods while slowly increasing exchange volumes, a typical maintenance CAPD or CCPD regimen may be reached in a few days, (e.g, for CAPD: 35-40 cc/kg/exchange, 4-5 exchanges/24 hr; for CCPD: similar volumes, 5-6 exchanges/24 hr).

Familiarity with prolonged dwell periods in the treatment of ESRD with CAPD and CCPD has led to adaptation of the standard CAPD and CCPD regimens for use in the treatment of ARF. In 1980 Poser and Luisello first described their use of continuous, prolonged dwell peritoneal dialysis to treat 20 adults wth oliguric ARF [102]. Abbad and Ploos van Amstel have reported their success with a CAPD-type dialysis regimen in the treatment of 5 anuric infants, 3 weeks to about 3 years of age [103]. In all 5 infants, ARF was due to hemolytic uremic syndrome. CAPD was continued in these children for 10 to 33 days. After a brief initial stabilization period using IPD, the infants improved rapidly on CAPD, despite continued anuria. They received unlimited diets averaging 2.1 g of protein/kg and 81 kcal/kg per day. Four of five infants developed peritonitis, but all responded to intraperitoneal antibiotics. All five infants eventually regained normal renal function.

Continuous, prolonged dwell peritoneal dialysis, either CAPD or CCPD, has become the standard approach to peritoneal dialysis for ARF in our center, once the child has been stabilized with an appropriate period of shorter exchanges to correct fluid and electrolyte disturbances and to lower the BUN. The steady-state biochemical and fluid control achievable with continuous, prolonged dwell peritoneal dialysis may be of particular benefit to infants and small children, whose cardiovascular status may be precarious. There have been no controlled comparisons of CAPD/CCPD vs traditional IPD for ARF in pediatric patients.

4.6.7. Specialized equipment

Most of the peritoneal dialysis equipment used to treat children with ARF is readily available. Automated systems designed for CCPD have become standard equipment in children's hospitals with active acute and chronic dialysis services. Opas has recently described the use of these systems in pediatric patients [104].

Manual dialysis systems are frequently employed in newborn and pediatric intensive care units. When exchange volume is small, placement of a volumetric measuring device (Volutrol, Buretrol, etc.) in both unfusion and outflow circuits facilitates monitoring of delivered and drained volumes. Standard peritoneal dialysis Y-tubing may be used in older children, but for infants whose exchange volumes are often < 100 cc, Y-tubing sets have too much dead space. We usually patch together a peritoneal dialysis circuit using standard IV extension tubing and a 3-way stopcock. A complete and disposable peritoneal dialysis tubing circuit designed for use in infants is now available.*

We have also used a manual system known as the 'octopus' for children whose exchange volumes match the standard commercially available dialysate bags [e.g., 250, 500, 750, 1000 ccs, etc.]. The octopus consists of a multiple pronged manifold and tubing set used for automated cycler dialysis. Five-prong and 12-prong sets are available. Each

---

* Gesco Dialy-nate Set, Gesco International, San Antonio, Texas.

day the dialysis nurse spikes all of the day's exchanges in a single procedure, leaving the fresh dialysate bags hanging from an IV pole at the bedside. Individual exchanges are then performed by the ICU or floor nurse, who simply opens and closes clamps on the tubing leading first to the empty drain bag, then from the fresh dialysate bag. Entry into the system fluid path is thus restricted to the dialysis nursing staff. The octopus system may be of benefit when ICU and floor nursing staffs are unfamiliar with the CAPD exchange procedure, and when automated cyclers are not available.

Dialysate must always be warmed to approximately 37 degrees centigrade before it is infused into the child. Adults may complain of discomfort during the inflow of dialysate at room temperature; the small infant may become frankly hypotensive as cool dialysate rapidly lowers body temperature. We have used water-filled heating pads wrapped around the bag of fresh dialysate and blood transfusion warming coils placed in the inflow circuit. Microwave heating may be used for single exchange bags, but is impractical when more than one exchange is to be drawn from the same bag.

4.6.8. Complications

Peritonitis is the most frequent serious complication of acute peritoneal dialysis. In one large series, the incidence of infection was found to be directly proportional to length of time on dialysis [21], but in another series peritonitis was an infrequent event [22]. Most authorities warn against prophylactic antibiotics and urge instead meticulous technique and a high index of suspicion [22].

Intraperitoneal hemorrhage at the time of percutaneous catheter insertion has been reported to occur in up to 5% of children [21, 77]. Adequate abdominal distension at the time of trocar insertion is essential to minimize the risk of trauma to the viscera. If percutaneous placement is not going well, it is probably advisable to arrange for surgical catheter placement rather than risk repeated abdominal punctures.

Potentially serious metabolic derangements can occur in small infants on peritoneal dialysis. Leumann and associates described 6 neonates with ARF who developed the following complications during acute peritoneal dialysis: hypophosphatemia, hypercalcemia, hypomagnesemia, hyponatremia, hyperglycemia and hypoproteinemia [94]. Hypokalemia was avoided by adding KCl to the dialysate in physiologic concentrations (4 mEq/l). Frequent laboratory studies may be needed during stabilization to minimize the risk of serious metabolic complications. Once initial stabilization has been accomplished the use of a CAPD-like regimen should reduce the likelihood of most of these complications, although hyponatremia may still be a problem for some infants [105].

5. PERITONEAL DIALYSIS FOR END-STAGE RENAL DISEASE IN CHILDREN

5.1. Intermittent peritoneal dialysis (IPD)

Reported experience with chronic IPD in children is limited to four series published since 1973 [30, 32, 33, 35]. Potter and associates summarized this experience in 1981, sug-

gesting that additional reports were unlikely because CAPD had begun to supercede IPD in most pediatric dialysis programs [35]. When this chapter was first written four yrs ago, I shared Dr. Potter's view. Compared to CAPD, IPD is not very appealing. CAPD is simpler and provides greater weekly clearances of small and middle molecular weight solutes compared to the standard 40 hr per week of IPD [106]. To obtain comparable dialysis, children would be required to spend more than 40 hrs per week attached to the IPD machinery, and this seemed unlikely. The inherent inferiority of chronic IPD compared to CAPD and CCPD led me to predict four years ago that in a very few years IPD would be used exclusively in the treatment of acute renal failure in hospitalized children.

Such reports of the demise of chronic IPD were obviously premature. As CCPD has evolved, the elimination of the daytime dwell has resurrected a form of chronic IPD which has been called 'nightly IPD' or 'intermittent cycling peritoneal dialysis' (ICPD [51]). Children treated in this manner spend as many as 70 hrs per week attached to their cycling machinery; since they also spend their waking hrs detached from the machinery and free of the need for CAPD exchanges, ICPD is understandably attractive. ICPD has not been studied adequately, and comparisons with standard CCPD and CAPD are needed. *Dis*continuous peritoneal dialysis carries theoretical disadvantages compared to *continuous* methods which may or may not be clinically important in children.

5.2. Continuous ambulatory peritoneal dialysis (CAPD) and continuous cycling peritoneal dialysis (CCPD)

In the nine years which have elapsed since the first child was treated with CAPD (in 1978), the impact of this new therapy on the care of infants and children with ESRD has been extensive. Steady growth in the number of children treated with CAPD has occurred in North America and Western Europe. Data from the European Dialysis and Transplant Association (EDTA) Registry show that the percentage of children beginning renal replacement therapy whose first method of treatment was CAPD rose from 8.3% of 436 children in 1980 to 17.7% of 492 children who began dialysis in 1984 [107]. When children switched to CAPD from another modality are added to those children for whom CAPD was the first treatment, the total contribution of CAPD to pediatric dialysis therapy in the 32 member countries of the EDTA rose from less than 4% in 1980 to 17.6% in 1984. In some countries the contribution of CAPD was much greater; in the United Kingdom, Switzerland, and Sweden, CAPD contributed more than 50% of all dialysis therapy for children in 1984 [107].

Similar data giving the proportional contribution of CAPD to total pediatric ESRD therapy are not available for the United States where no nationwide ESRD patient data system exists. The National CAPD Registry has collected data on children treated with CAPD in the United States since 1981. Because participation in the National CAPD registry is voluntary, data from the Registry on pediatric patients may not be an accurate reflection of the U.S. pediatric CAPD/CCPD patient population as a whole. Between March, 1982 and August, 1986 the number of pediatric patients followed by the Registry increased from

256 to 962 [108, 109].

5.3. Advantages of CAPD

It is not surprising that CAPD has become a popular pediatric dialysis technique. Because CAPD proceeds continuously, body fluid composition and volume change slowly, resulting in what can be considered a near 'steady state'. The dysequilibrium syndrome experienced by many children during hemodialysis does not occur in children on CAPD. Very few dietary restrictions are imposed on the pediatric CAPD patient; most children may be encouraged to eat an essentially unlimited diet, relatively high in protein with generous fluid and sodium allowances. The simplicity and safety of CAPD allow it to be performed at home by all but the most disturbed families, thereby returning the child with ESRD to regular school attendance and allowing family vacations and other normal childhood activities. CAPD avoids the many difficulties associated with maintenance of vascular access in children and eliminates the need for frequent painful dialysis needle punctures.

These features offer obvious theoretical advantages over hemodialysis for most children. However, there have been no controlled prospective studies comparing the two modalities. The best available information has been compiled by Potter and his associates in San Francisco who have collected data on 80 children treated concurrently in their center between 1979 and 1986 (55 with CAPD, 25 with hemodialysis) [110, 111]. Acknowledging that the two study populations were not comparable, Potter and associates noted higher hematocrits, lower blood pressures, higher serum carbon dioxide levels, lower serum albumin levels, more dialysis-related complications and better linear growth in the patients treated with CAPD. All differences were statistically significant except for linear growth.

It is possible to extract comparisons of selected parameters from a few other reports describing children treated with hemodialysis and either CAPD or CCPD [41, 112, 113, 114, 115, 116]. Firm conclusions regarding relative advantages of one modality over another in children must await more carefully controlled comparative studies which include assessments of psychosocial and quality of life issues as well as more objective parameters of dialysis effectiveness and safety.

5.4. Patient selection

It may be generally stated that CAPD and CCPD can be performed in any child whose peritoneal cavity is intact and will admit an adequate volume of dialysate. Thus, omphalocele, gastroschisis and diaphragmatic hernia constitute the only absolute contraindications to CAPD. Draining abdominal wounds and extensive intraperitoneal adhesions will also prevent successful CAPD. Experience has shown that CAPD may be successfully employed in children with any of the following: polycystic kidney disease (with kidneys left *in situ* in most cases), vesicostomy, cutaneous ureterostomy, prune belly syndrome, bilateral Wilm's tumor, colostomy, recent abdominal surgery (if no draining wounds are present), concurrent cancer chemotherapy or corticosteroid therapy, and radiotherapy involving the peritoneum. Patient age, sex, prior ESRD therapy, primary renal disease and renal transplant status have no apparent influence on CAPD outcome, although these parameters have been examined only anecdotally [2, 44, 46, 89, 118].

Infants represent a patient group for whom CAPD/CCPD is the clear treatment of choice [2, 118]. Prior to the introduction of CAPD, pediatric ESRD treatment programs rarely accepted infants for treatment [119, 120]. As experience with the use of CAPD in infants has grown, it has become widely recognized that CAPD can be a practical and effective maintenance treatment in babies who develop ESRD as early as the first few days or weeks of life [105, 117, 121, 122, 123, 139].

The demonstrated success of this new treatment strategy for infants with ESRD raises complex social, ethical and legal issues which have recently become the subject of the bioethecist [124]. At issue is whether it is appropriate for any infant with ESRD to be denied renal replacement therapy, either by the medical team or by the parents. As with most such questions, there are no simple answers. Current policy in our center is to respect the wishes of the parents when they do not give us permission to treat their infant with CAPD. The availability of voluntary medical foster care has allowed three families who felt unable to care for their infants on CAPD to temporarily (1-2 yr) relinquish custody to the State. All 3 infants eventually returned to their natural parents after successful renal transplantation.

We believe that there are at least 3 major criteria which should be met before CAPD/CCPD can be recommended for any child.

1. *The child must be an eventual candidate for renal transplantation.* This is true for children accepted for treatment with any dialysis modality at the present time, since the quality of life on long term dialysis is not adequate for the child.

2. *The family should be motivated to learn and comply with the home dialysis program.* Motivation and ability to cope with the rigors of the home dialysis program may be the most important determinants of CAPD success [110]. No reliable criteria have been established by which family motivation and coping abilities can be predicted. Based on some surprisingly successful CAPD/CCPD families who have had low incomes or limited intelligence or nontraditional lifestyles, we now offer CAPD or CCPD to all families regardless of circumstances. Such a policy reflects the general bias of our program staff more than any other factor. Opas has recently noted the dramatic effect of a change in physician and nursing staff bias on patient selection for CAPD/CCPD at Childrens Hospital Los Angeles [104]. Between 1980 and 1982, 17 of 59 new dialysis patients 'chose' CAPD/CCPD. During the following 3 yr (1983-1985) 54 of 72 new patients were begun on CAPD/CCPD [104].

3. *The treating facility must be able to provide the necessary multidisciplinary support required by the child and family undergoing CAPD/CCPD.* CAPD for children is a team effort, usually requiring the active participation of pediatric nephrologists, pediatric urologists, pediatric surgeons, CAPD nurses, renal dieticians, renal social workers, child psychologists, child development specialists, and child life therapists. Children require a much greater investment

of time from each team member, with the primary CAPD nurse serving as the focal point for all aspects of the care of the child and family. We believe that one CAPD nurse can properly coordinate the care of no more than six pediatric patients; when the child/nurse ratio has exceeded 6:1 in our program the quality of care received by all patients has suffered and turnover within the nursing staff has increased.

5.5. Permanent peritoneal catheters for CAPD/CCPD

A reliable peritoneal catheter is the cornerstone of successful CAPD. The bulk of pediatric experience has been obtained with straight and curled Tenckhoff and Toronto Western Hospital catheters [125, 126, 127, 128, 129, 130]. All are available in an assortment of sizes from several manufacturers. No clearly superior pediatric catheter design has emerged, and controversy continues over the use of one or two cuffs, the optimum length of the subcutaneous tunnel and the optimum surgical placement procedure. The level of experience and committment of the surgical team is probably more important to the success of any given catheter than the choice of catheter type or placement technique.

The catheter placement procedure used in our center has been reported previously [125] and is depicted in Figure 1. Since 1982, we have used a modified, adult-size, curled, 1-cuff Tenckhoff catheter in all children weighing more than 5 kg. The cuff is glued by the manufacturer (Quinton Instrument Company, Seattle, Washington, 98121) at a point 5.0 cm above the onset of fenestrations in the curl. This short cuff-to-fenestration distance results in a catheter which begins curling almost immediately upon entry into the peritoneal cavity and which remains fixed to the anterior abdominal wall (see Figure 1a).

The catheter entry site and the course of the subcutaneous tunnel are chosen preoperatively, avoiding old surgical scars and attempting to keep the tunnel and exit site completely above the child's belt line. Infants with vesicostomies or colostomies should have an exit site located as far from the stoma as possible.

The operative procedure begins with a 2-4 cm incision made horizontally over the midportion of the rectus muscle near the level of the umbilicus. The anterior rectus sheath is incised and the rectus muscle separated bluntly. The peritoneum is exposed, fixed by two temporary sutures and then incised. Digital examination assures that no bowl is adherent to the peritoneum. The small patch of omental tissue which lies just below and is readily available through the incision is carefully exised, thus clearing a path for the catheter. This 'porthole' partial omentectomy need not remove more than about 10 square cm of omentum.

The curled catheter is soaked in saline to wet the dacron cuff and then threaded over a long, lubricated catheter guide. Care is taken to note the direction in which the catheter will begin to curl as it is pushed off of the guide. Catheter and guide are now introduced through the incision just beneath the anterior abdominal wall to a point in the midline several cm below the umbilicus. Holding the catheter guide in this position, the catheter is gently eased off of the guide until the cuff reaches the level of the peritoneal incision. As the catheter slides off of the guide

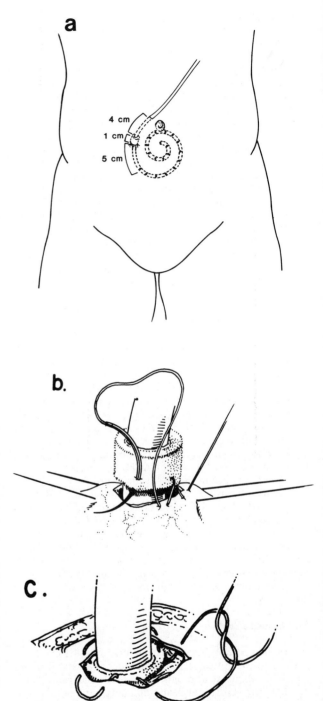

Figure 1. (a) Technique for placement of the short curled Tenckhoff catheter in a young child. A 4-cm subcutaneous tunnel is shown directed medially. Lateral direction of the tunnel is also acceptable (see Figure 2a). The 1-cm cuff is depicted sutured at the point of entry into the peritoneal cavity. Catheter fenestrations begin 5-cm below the cuff. (b) Attachment of the base of the cuff to the peritoneum with a nonabsorbable purse string suture. (c) Closure of the anterior rectus sheath incorporating the top of the cuff. Details of the surgical technique are given in the text. (Reprinted with permission from ref. 125).

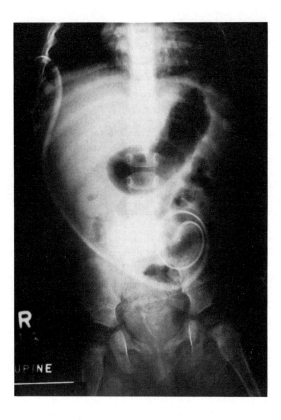

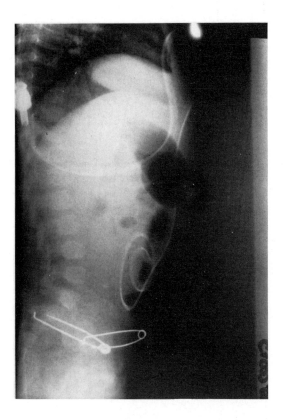

it will resume the curled configuration; care is taken to ensure that the curl lies flat beneath the abdominal wall in a plane which is anterior to the abdominal contents (see Figure 2b). When the curl is misdirected it can become entangled with omentum or loops of bowel as it slides off of the catheter guide.

The peritoneum is now closed around the catheter with a pursestring of nonabsorbable suture. The suture is passed through the substance of the cuff at its lowest point in several places (Figure 1b). When secured, this suture pulls a collar of peritoneum around the base of the cuff, creating a near-watertight seal and anchoring the catheter in position. A similar purse string suture is then used to close the anterior rectus sheath and fix it to the upper aspect of the cuff in a like manner (Figure 1c).

At this point, about 15 cc/kg of dialysate is infused and then drained immediately. If the closure is watertight and dialysate leaves the peritoneal cavity briskly, the catheter is felt to be in good functional position. If outflow is not brisk, the catheter is flushed; if dainage still is not improved, the catheter is removed and repositioned. Catheters which drain poorly in the operating room do not improve with use. Acceptance of anything less than excellent outflow at the time of catheter placement invites a second procedure.

When the catheter has been shown to infuse and drain freely, a short subcutaneous tunnel is created, with care taken that the skin exit aperture is small and fits snugly around the catheter. A 4 mm skin biopsy punch will create an ideal skin exit aperture for most Tenckhoff catheters. The direction of the tunnel may be either toward or away from the midline.

We next perform peritoneography in an effort to identify hernias which are a frequent complication of CAPD in children [131, 132]. Patients are placed in a reverse Trendelenberg position and peritoneography is performed by infusing 8/cc/kg of contrast material mixed with an equal volume of dialysate. An abdominal radiograph which includes the inguinal areas confirms correct positioning of the catheter and defines any inguinal hernias or patent *processus vaginalis* which might be present. If either is demonstrated, inguinal herniorrhaphy is performed. Umbilical and incisional defects are also closed at the time of catheter placement.

We usually continue dialysis following catheter placement, using frequent, low-volume exchanges (15cc/kg every 1-2 hr). For the first 48 hr after catheter placement, the child remains in bed except when the peritoneal cavity is empty. Exchange volume is increased slowly over the ensuing 5 to 7 days until the prescribed maintenance volume is reached (35-45 cc/kg). The dialysate contains 500 units of sodium heparin per liter and 125 mg of a first generation cephalosporin per liter for only the first 24 hr. Subsequent use of heparin is limited to those patients with obvious fibrin or blood in their dialysate and during episodes of peritonitis.

Between March, 1982 and December, 1986 we placed

Figure 2. (a) Supine abdominal radiograph showing a short curled Tenckhoff catheter in place in an 8 kg infant. The intraperitoneal catheter curl rides higher in the abdomen as a result of the lateral direction of the subcutaneous tunnel. (b) Lateral abdominal radiograph of the same infant showing the desired anterior position of the curled catheter, superficial to the peritoneal contents. (Reprinted with permission from ref. 125).

59 short curl catheters in Oregon children using the technique described above. Twenty-four of those catheters were eventually removed for reasons other than transplantation or patient death. Only 5 of 24 catheter failures were due to mechanical causes (leakage, 1; malposition, 2; breakage due to silastic rubber fatigue, 2). These results are listed in Tabel 4, and compared to mechanical catheter losses which have been reported by large pediatric CAPD/CCPD programs in Toronto [126] and Los Angeles [50]. The Toronto and UCLA programs employed a variety of catheters and used placement procedures which differed substantially from the technique used in Oregon [125, 126, 130].

Despite the encouraging disappearance of mechanical catheter failures from our program using the short curl technique (the last mechanical failure occurred in 1984), we continue to lose many catheters [19 of 24] to infectious complications (exit site/tunnel infections, complex peritonitis). Data from the National CAPD Registry show that, compared to adults, children tend to have a greater incidence of exit site and tunnel infections and are more likely to require catheter replacement during the first year of CAPD/CCPD [109].

5.6. The CAPD prescription

The current approach to CAPD mechanics in children has evolved empirically. Published guidelines from several different pediatric centers are strikingly similar despite diverse patient populations. Table 5 lists CAPD regimens used in three different pediatric CAPD programs [40, 41, 89] along with adult reference values [134]. In general, a CAPD regimen consisting of 4 or 5 exchanges, 35 to 45 cc/kg per exchange will provide adequate control of uremia. The 2.5% dextrose concentration is used most often in children, yielding an additional 35 to 50 cc/kg/day of net ultrafiltration (UF). Insensible and stool water losses in children usually amount to about 50 cc/100 kcal/day. With UF of 40 cc/kg/day in the anephric child, total fluid turnover in these children should be about 90 cc/100 kcal/day. Ad lib fluid intake in our young patients rarely exceeds this total. Anuric infants require aggressive fortification of formula feedings to achieve nutritional goals within these fluid limits [135].

Control of ultrafiltration must also be used to protect the infant or small child from dehydration. Ultrafiltration may not be diminished even in the face of up to 10% dehydration. Whenever there are increased body fluid losses as are seen with diarrhea, emesis, fever or decreased intake, the CAPD regimen must be adjusted to reduce daily UF.

5.7. Nutrition

Improved nutritional status has been documented in children who are begun on CAPD/CCPD, but normal nutritional status is uncommon in these children despite access

Table 4. Mechanical causes of catheter replacement in three pediatric programs

	Toronto [126]	*UCLA [50]*	*Oregon [125]*[a]
Total catheters at risk	78	167	59
Catheters replaced for mechanical causes			
Leakage	6	4	1
Obstruction	13	8	0
Malposition/migration	—	2	2
Cuff erosion	—	2	0
Breakage	—	1	2
Hernia	1	2	0
Total mechanical causes	20	19	5
Total catheters replaced[b]	26	74	24

[a] Short curled catheters only.
[b] Excludes catheters removed for renal transplantation or patient death.

Table 5. Representative pediatric CAPD regimens

Reference	*Prescribed exchange volume (ml/kg)*	*Mean total dialy urea clearance (ml/kg)1*	*Mean SUN (mg/dl)*	*Mean daily protein intake (g/kg)*
Saluksy *et al.* [41]	43	238	77	2.4[b]
Potter *et al.* [40]	35–50	164–224[a]	70	2.0[b]
Alexander *et al.* [89]	35–40	211	77	2.3[b]
Adult Guidelines [134]	25	238	89	1.4[c]

[a] Estimated.
[b] Estimated from dietary histories.
[c] Actual, from metabolic balance studies.

to an essentially unlimited diet [136]. Gains in nutritional status as reflected by increases in weight, muscle mass and/or skin fold thickness, have been reported most often in infants who were also receiving forced nutritional supplements or total diets via tube feedings [117, 137, 138, 139]. Guidelines for dietary management of infants and children receiving CAPD/CCPD have been published [121, 137, 140, 141]. These guidelines rely heavily on dietary recommendations developed for the general population of normal children; very little information is available from studies of dialyzed children fed controlled diets [143].

Current guidelines generally agree on the need to provide an energy intake of at least 100% of the Recommended Dietary Allowance (RDA) [142] for children of the same sex and height-age. Total energy intake will be augmented by an additional 8 to 20 kcal/kg/day derived from dialysate dextrose absorption [44].

There is less agreement on the optimum protein intake for children receiving CAPD/CCPD, reflecting the paucity of objective data on this subject. Precise nitrogen balance studies in stable adult males on CAPD have shown that when daily protein intake averages 1.4 g/kg, nitrogen balance is strongly positive [134]. Isolated measurements of nitrogen balance have been performed in a few children on CAPD [138], but available data are inadequate to determine the minimal protein (and energy) intake required to achieve positive nitrogen balance in pediatric CAPD patients of various ages. Dialysate protein losses are greater in children than in adults [51], and children often begin CAPD with evidence of protein wasting [136, 144], both factors which will increase protein requirements in children on CAPD.

Until better information becomes available it seems reasonable to ensure a minimum daily protein intake of 2.0 g/kg for children > 2 yr of age. This amount should be increased if dialysate protein losses are excessive, such as is seen during episodes of peritonitis and in smaller children and infants. Supplementation of dietary protein intake with intraperitoneally administered amino acids is currently under investigation [144].

Supplements of the water soluble vitamins should probably be provided all children receiving CAPD, but vitamins A, E and K are not recommended [121, 140]. Elevated levels of vitamin A have been reported in children receiving CAPD [145]. Specific recommentations for dietary supplements of vitamins and minerals have recently been published [140].

5.8. Growth

Poor growth has long been considered a consistent feature of children with ESRD, and those treated with chronic hemodialysis have been shown to grow poorly indeed [146, 147]. CAPD offers several theoretical advantages over hemodialysis which it was hoped would lead to improved growth, including essentially unrestricted diets, absorption of a regular carbohydrate energy boost from the dialysate and near steady-state biochemical control. Other features unique to CAPD could theoretically interfere with growth including anorexia caused by continuous dextrose absorption from the dialysate and excessive peritoneal losses of proteins and amino acids.

Despite nearly 10 years of experience with CAPD in children, a clear picture of the growth achievable by children on CAPD has only begun to emerge. Early controversies over how best to assess and report linear growth in children of different ages have not been fully resolved [148]. There is general agreement that only observation periods of 12 months or more can be reliably compared. Length, rather than height should be followed in infants until at least 24 months of age. Measurement techniques should closely follow established methods to minimize errors [149].

Controversy remains over the use of chronologic vs skeletal age as the standard for comparison. Chronologic age avoids the problems associated with differences in skeletal age determinations from center to center, while use of skeletal age allows comparison of growth rates among adolescents who may or may not have entered puberty [148]. Two methods for comparing observed growth to growth of normal children of the same sex and age (either chronologic or skeletal age) have become popular: the Standard Deviation Score (SDS or 'Z score') [150] and the Growth Velocity Index (GVI) [113].

Early observations by Kohaut suggested that the majority of children on CAPD grew at rates which were > 70% of expected (ie, GVI > 70%) [151, 152]. Fennell and associates compared growth among 58 children receiving various treatments for ESRD [114]. Nine were on CAPD, 15 were on hemodialysis, and 34 had received a renal transplant. Children receiving CAPD grew better than those treated by hemodialysis and almost as well as the transplanted children when all children up to 15.5 yr of age were considered. Average GVI in the CAPD and transplant groups was 77% and 80%, respectively. However, when children > 11 yr of age were excluded, a GVI of > 70% was observed in *no* hemodialysis patients, 33% of CAPD patients and 63% of transplant patients. This study illustrates the importance of similar age distributions among treatment groups when growth is to be compared.

Additional reports from single centers are consistent with the observation that growth rates of children on CAPD are about 80% to 90% of normal. Some children grow at 100% of normal rates, but true catch-up growth is rarely seen.

The National CAPD Registry recently compiled data on linear growth observed in 145 children during their first 12 months of treatment with CAPD/CCPD [153]. Growth was assessed by evaluating the observed change in Z score at initiation of CAPD/CCPD and following one year of therapy. Paired difference analysis demonstrated a widening of the gap between the children treated with CAPD/CCPD and normal children. Mean change in Z score for height after one yr of CAPD/CCPD was -0.31 for males and -0.28 for females. When patients were grouped by age, the mean change in Z score for height for males 0 to 4 yr of age was -0.89, which was significantly worse than older age groups.

These observations support concerns that infants and young children with ESRD, who are at highest risk for growth failure, do not experience normal growth when treated with CAPD/CCPD.

5.9. Special considerations in the treatment of infants with CAPD/CCPD

The additional problems encountered by infants treated with CAPD have been reviewed elsewhere [118, 154]. Experience with this age group is growing and recent reports have been generally favorable. Infants on CAPD/CCPD require aggressive nutritional support, often requiring forced feeding via nasogastric or gastrostomy tube when ad lib intake falls below recommended levels. Warady and associates recently reported the use of nasogastric tube feedings in 4 infants treated with CCPD, all of whom began dialysis during the first 4 weeks of life [117]. Mean energy and protein intakes were 105 ± 20 kcal/kg/day and 2.7 ± 0.7 gr/kg/day respectively. At one year, mean Z score for height was -1.33, which reflected a mean change in Z score of -0.7.

Recommendations for optimum energy and protein intake for infants < 2 yr of age treated with CAPD/CCPD are slowly evolving, but differences remain among published reports. Energy intake of 110 to 150 kcal/kg/day has been suggersted [140, 141, 138, 137, 121], with adjustments made for the individual infant should weight for height become excessive during growth. It seems reasonable to give at least 2.5 gr/kg/day of protein to these babies who rarely have problems with high BUN during vigorous growth. Higher protein intakes have also been recommended [137, 140].

5.10. Complications

5.10.1. Peritonitis
Data from the National CAPD Registry show that pediatric patients have a significantly greater peritonitis rate compared to adults (1.5 vs 1.3 episodes per patient yr), and a greater probability of experiencing an episode of peritonitis during the first year [109]. Peritonitis rates were also found to correlate with the pediatric experience of the treating center [153]. A reduced risk of developing first peritonitis was found for children treated at centers having a cumulative total of > 10 pediatric patients, with even better results obtained in centers treating > 20 pediatric patients. These data are consistent with earlier reports of dramatically lower peritonitis rates in some large pediatric centers [155].

5.10.2. Anemia
Recent reports have called attention to the improvement in anemia observed in children treated with CAPD. In one study, children on CAPD required 0.16 transfusions per month to maintain hematocrits at an average 21.9%, whereas children treated with hemodialysis required almost five times as many transfusions to maintain hematocrits at 19.6% [110]. In another large series of children on CAPD, transfusions were given to anephric children at a rate of one transfusion every 1.5 months, and about one half that rate to children with their own kidneys *in situ* [50].

5.10.3. Hypertension
Children on CAPD often experience improvement in control of hypertension. Among 10 children treated with both CAPD and hemodialysis, mean systolic blood pressure was significantly lower during CAPD (108 mm Hg vs 130 mm

HG) [110]. In another series, only one of 26 children on CAPD required antihypertensive medications [41].

5.10.4. Renal osteodystrophy
The majority of children receiving CAPD experience progression of renal osteodystrophy, despite treatment with various vitamin D preparations, calcium supplements and phosphate binders [156]. Salusky and associates have observed improved control of renal bone disease wth aggressive calcitriol therapy to maintain serum calcium levels 10.5 to 11.0 mg/dl [157]. The daily dose of calcitriol required to achieve these results in Salusky's patients ranged from 0.25 to 3.25 mcg/day. Calcium carbonate has been shown to be an effective phosphate binder in children and should replace aluminum-containing phosphate binders [158]. Frequent adjustments in calcitriol and calcium carbonate doses are often necessary to maintain serum calcium within the rather narrow target range of 10.5 to 11.0 mg/dl. Monitoring serum parathormone and alkaline phosphatase levels can also be helpful in assessing effectiveness of therapy. Aluminum-related bone disease should be suspected in patients who develop hypercalcemia which fails to resolve within a few days of withholding calcitriol therapy [157].

5.11. Survival

The probability of dying while on CAPD/CCPD at one year of therapy is substantially lower for pediatric patients when compared to adults (0.06 vs 0.17, respectively) [109]. However, infants and younger children may have a higher mortality risk than older pediatric patients. Mortality rates as high as 30% have been reported among small series of infants who began CAPD/CCPD during the first year of life, [105, 122]. The National CAPD Registry also found a substantially greater probability of dying on CAPD for this age group, but this difference was not statistically significant [109].

5.12. Termination of CAPD/CCPD

Data on termination of therapy is available from the National CAPD Registry; 204 children who terminated CAPD prior to September 1, 1986 were studied [153]. Two-thirds of these children left CAPD to receive a renal transplant. Of the 67 patients who were not transplanted, 14 died and 6 enjoyed return of renal function. Forty-one children were switched to another form of dialysis, primarily in-center hemodialysis. The most frequently cited reason for switching to another dialysis modality was excessive peritonitis. Membrane failure as evidenced by inadequate ultrafiltration or solute clearance was reported in 6 of the 204 children. Loss of ultrafiltration has been encountered with greater frequency in European children treated with CAPD [159, 160]. The reason for this geographic difference is unknown, but may relate to the prior use of acetate as a buffer in dialysate solutions available only in Europe [161].

5.13. Continuous cycling peritoneal dialysis (CCPD)

CCPD was developed in an attempt to combine the benefits of continuous peritoneal dialysis with the convenience of an automated delivery system. The use of CCPD in pediatric patients has been described in recent reports [50, 162, 163]. In general, results appear to be as good with CCPD as with CAPD. In one respect this is disappointing. A major theoretical advantage of CCPD over CAPD was a reduction in peritonitis rates. From somewhat limited available information it appears that in children there is no improvement in peritonitis rates with CCPD [164, 165]. Early data also suggest that children on CCPD have higher serum creatinine levels [162, 165], a finding which is difficult to interpret without more carefully controlled studies of dialysis mechanics in children treated with both CAPD and CCPD.

Reasons for choosing CCPD over CAPD will differ in the individual patient, and, as with the choice of CAPD over hemodialysis, will reflect the preferences and biases of the dialysis staff [166]. CCPD should be considered in patients with diminished ultrafiltration who might benefit from the use of frequent short exchanges. Children with hernias may also benefit from CCPD. If both parents work outside the home CCPD is obviously advantageous.

5.14. Quality of life of the child and family on CAPD/CCPD

There is little doubt that CAPD/CCPD offers children and their families a better quality of life than hemodialysis. Praise for the beneficial effects of CAPD on family life has been a consistent feature of published reports. The vast majority of older children who have experienced both modalities prefer CAPD over hemodialysis. Regular school attendance is a high priority in most pediatric CAPD programs; the ability to attend school every schoolday may be one of the most beneficial features of CAPD. We also encourage children to become active in sports and other normal childhood activities. Very few restrictions to physical exercise are necessary. We suggest avoidance of tackle football, wrestling and some forms of gymnastics which involve trauma to the abdomen (*e.g*, the uneven parallel bars). Swimming is readily accomplished by a variety of techniques [167, 168]. Family vacations are also encouraged and can be facilitated by the dialysate manufacturer who can usually arrange to have supplies shipped directly to the vacation site.

As with other home therapies for serious illnesses, the advantages derived from greater independence and self-reliance are not achieved without cost. Parent fatigue and 'burn-out' are commonly seen in the families of children on CAPD. Techniques for helping families deal with these problems have been described by Hall and associates [169]. Parents rarely spontaneously complain about the demands of the home dialysis regimen, although most are grateful for the opportunity to express their fatigue and frustration. Extensive involvement of the entire CAPD team in the emotional support of the family is essential. Regular telephone contact initiated by the CAPD nurses, social workers and dieticians has been helpful; more frequent clinic follow-up visits are also important during the first year on CAPD and whenever recurrent peritonitis or persistent exit site infections complicate therapy.

6. PERITONEAL DIALYSIS FOR INTOXICATIONS, INBORN ERRORS OF METABOLISM AND OTHER MISCELLANEOUS DISORDERS IN CHILDREN

6.1. Intoxications

Since the implementation of the Poison Prevention Packaging Act of 1970 there has been a dramatic decline in the incidence of accidental ingestions of regulated products by young children. Between 1974 and 1981 ingestions of aspirin, aspirin substitutes, oven cleaners and other lye-containing products, lighter fluids and anti-freeze by children under 5 yr of age decreased from 2.9 per 1000 children under 5 yr of age to less than 2.0 per 1000 [170]. Morbidity and mortality from accidental ingestions of aspirin and acetaminophen in this age group declined sharply during the same period. The death rate from accidental aspirin ingestion by young children decreased by 69% between 1970 and 1978 [171].

As gratifying as these statistics may be, the fact remains that many unintentional intoxications and deaths still occur each year among young children. In 1981 nearly 100 000 children under 5 yr of age were seen in emergency rooms in the United States because of accidental ingestion of hazardous substances [170].

Treatment of intoxications in small children remains an important if infrequently tested area of expertise for the nephrologist who is likely to be consulted regarding the advisability of dialysis in these situations. For many years peritoneal dialysis played an important role in the treatment of small children who had been poisoned with substances removable by dialysis [172]. The use of peritoneal dialysis in the treatment of poisoning is reviewed in detail in Chapter 12. For information regarding specific intoxications in children the reader in urgent need of this information is advised to contact the nearest Poison Control Center or to call the Rocky Mountain Poison Control Center in Denver, Colorado [303-629-1123].

In recent years the use of peritoneal dialysis to treat intoxications in children has almost disappeared in our center. Several factors seem to be responsible for this phenomenon. As noted above, the incidence of serious salicylate intoxication in young children has been steadily declining throughout the United States. In addition, a better understanding of the pathophysiology of salicylate intoxication has led to more successful use of forced diuresis and other supportive maneuvers in the child with intact renal function [173].

Improvements in acute hemodialysis techniques and equipment which have been specifically developed for use in small children have further reduced the use of peritoneal dialysis to treat intoxications [174]. Hemoperfusion techniques for pediatric patients have also been described [175]. Reliable percutaneous vascular access procedures and catheters designed for use in small children as well as single needle hemodialysis machinery have become widely available.

As a result of these and other developments, emergency hemodialysis is now available for infants and small children in pediatric dialysis centers throughout North America and Europe. Regardless of a patient's size, hemodialysis is many times more effective than peritoneal dialysis at removing dialyzable drugs and poisons [176, 177]. When a child has ingested a potentially lethal amount of a dialyzable poison, hemodialysis should be used whenever possible. Peritoneal dialysis is an acceptable alternative only for those children too small to receive hemodialysis at the facility in which they are being treated and too unstable to be safely transported to a pediatric dialysis center where hemodialysis could be performed expeditiously.

An exception to this preference for hemodialysis should be made for the child with impaired renal function who has iatrogenic NaCl poisoning. Peritoneal dialysis remains the treatment of choice for iatrogenic NaCl poisoning; corrective changes in osmolality may be brought about slowly and more safely with peritoneal dialysis than with hemodialysis [178, 179, 180].

6.2. Congenital hyperammonemia and other inborn errors of metabolism

Congenital urea cycle enzymopathies are characterized by a reduced capacity to synthesize urea, which leads to accumulation of ammonium and other nitrogenous urea percursors [181]. Severely affected neonates develop vomiting, lethargy, seizures and coma within the first few days of life. The central nervous system symptomatology is thought to be solely due to the effects of increased blood ammonium concentration. Emergency treatment is aimed at rapid and sustained removal of accumulated ammonium.

Peritoneal dialysis has emerged as the treatment of choice for infants with congenital hyperammonemic coma. The superiority of peritoneal dialysis over exchange transfusion in this setting has been demonstrated [182]. In studies performed in 53 episodes of hyperammonemic coma, ammonium was removed more rapidly with peritoneal dialysis than with exchange transfusion, and the rebound hyperammonemia which often follows treatment with exchange transfusion did not occur in babies treated with peritoneal dialysis. Hemodialysis is the most efficient method for removal of ammonium [183], but treatments with hemodialysis must be limited to several hours, whereas endogenous ammonium production in these babies is persistent

early in the course of treatment [182]. Peritoneal dialysis can be continued indefinitely, providing time during which the diagnosis of the specific urea cycle enzymopathy can be made and appropriate therapy instituted. Peritoneal dialysis removes ten times more nitrogen as glutamine than as ammonium; it has been suggested that the effectiveness of peritoneal dialysis in hyperammonemic infants may be due in part to the continuous removal of both ammonium and its precursors (glutamine, glutamate, and alanine) [182].

Peritoneal dialysis has also been useful in the acute management of several other congenital metabolic defects which do not always present with hyperammonemia. Successful treatment has been reported in cases of maple syrup urine disease [184], proprionic acidemia [185], and other congenital organic acidemias [186].

6.3. Miscellaneous pediatric disorders in which treatment with peritoneal dialysis has been attempted

Many of the serious afflictions of infants and children have been treated at one time or another with peritoneal dialysis. In 1966 Nora and associates demonstrated the effectiveness with which peritoneal dialysis removed fluid from children in intractable congestive heart failure [187]. Today such children would probably be as successfully treated wth one or more powerful diuretic agents unknown to Dr. Nora 20 yr ago.

Peritoneal dialysis has not been shown to be of sufficient benefit in the treatment of children with the following disorders to warrant continued use: hyaline membrane disease [188]; neonatal hyperbilirubinemia [189]; Reye's syndrome [190]; hepatic coma [191].

ACKNOWLEDGEMENTS

The author wishes to thank Edward S. Tank, M. D. for his assistance with descriptions of surgical procedures and Ms. Mary Blanchett and Ms. Janell McQuinn who prepared the manuscript.

REFERENCES

1. Popovich RP, Moncrief JW, Decherd JW *et al.*: The definition of a novel portable/wearable equilibrium peritoneal dialysis technique. Trans Am Soc Artif Intern Organs 5: 64, 1976.
2. Fine RN: Choosing a dialysis therapy for children with end-stage renal disease. Am J Kidney Dis 4: 249–252, 1984.
3. Stefanidis CJ, Balfe JW, Arbus GS *et al.*: Renal transplantation in children treated with continuous ambulatory peritoneal dialysis. Perit Dial Bull 3: 5–8, 1983.
4. Scharer K, Fine RN: Renal transplantation in children treated by CAPD: a report on a cooperative study. In: Fine RN, Scharer K, Mehls O (eds), CAPD in Children, Springer-Verlag, New York, pp 212–220, 1985.
5. Leichter HE, Salusky IB, Ettenger RB *et al.*: Experience with renal transplantation in children undergoing peritoneal dialysis (CAPD/CCPD). Am J Kidney Dis 8: 181–185, 1986.
6. Blackfan KD, Maxcy KF: The intraperitoneal injection of saline solution. Am J Dis Child 15: 19–28, 1918.
7. Bloxsum A, Powell N: The treatment of acute temporary dysfunction of the kidneys by peritoneal irrigation. Pediatrics

1: 52–57, 1948.
8. Swan H, Gordon HH: Peritoneal lavage in the treatment of anuria in children. Pediatrics 4: 586–595, 1949.
9. Odel HM, Ferris DO, Power MH: Peritoneal lavage as an effective means of extra-renal excretion. Am J Med 9: 63–77, 1950.
10. Fine J, Frank HA, Seligman AM: The treatment of acute renal failure by peritoneal irrigation. Ann Surg 124: 857–878, 1946.
11. Maxwell MH, Rockney RB, Kleeman CR *et al.*: Peritoneal dialysis: I. Technique and applications. JAMA 170: 917–924, 1959.
12. Segar WE, Gibson RK, Rhamy R: Peritoneal dialysis in infants and small children. Pediatrics 27: 603–613, 1961.
13. Etteldorf JN, Dobbins WT, Sweeney MJ *et al.*: Intermittent peritoneal dialysis in the management of acute renal failure in children. J Pediatr 60: 327–339, 1962.
14. Segar WE: Peritoneal dialysis in the treatment of boric acid poisoning. N Engl J Med 262: 798–800, 1960.
15. Etteldorf JN, Dobbins WT, Summitt RL *et al.*: Intermittent peritoneal dialysis using 5 per cent albumin in the treatment

of salicylate intoxication in children. J Pediatr 58: 226–236, 1961.

16. Lloyd-Still JD, Atwell JD: Renal failure in infancy, with special reference to the use of peritoneal dialysis. J Pediatr Surg 1: 466–475, 1966.

17. Manley GL, Collipp PJ: Renal failure in the newborn: treatment with peritoneal dialysis. Am J Dis Child 115: 107–110, 1968.

18. Lugo G, Ceballos R, Brown W *et al.*: Acute renal failure in the neonate managed by peritoneal dialysis. Am J Dis Child 118: 655–659, 1969.

19. Gianantonio CA, Vitacco M, Mendelbarzee J *et al.*: Acute renal failure in infancy and childhood. J Pediatr 61: 660–678, 1962.

20. Wiggelinkhuizen J: Peritoneal dialysis in children. S Afr Med J 45: 1047–1054, 1971.

21. Day RE, White RHR: Peritoneal dialysis in children: review of 8 years' experience. Arch Dis Child 52: 56–61, 1977.

22. Chan JCM: Peritoneal dialysis for renal failure in childhood. Clin Pediatr 17: 349–354, 1978.

23. Levin S, Winklestein JA: Diet and infrequent peritoneal dialysis in chronic anuric uremia. N Engl J Med 277: 619–624, 1967.

24. Feldman W, Baliah T, Drummond KN: Intermittent peritoneal dialysis in the management of chronic renal failure in children. Am J Dis Child 116: 30–36, 1968.

25. Palmer RA, Quinton WE, Gray J-F: Prolonged peritoneal dialysis for chronic renal failure. Lancet 1: 700–702, 1964.

26. Palmer RA, Newell JE, Gray J-F *et al.*: Treatment of chronic renal failure by prolonged peritoneal dialysis. New Engl J Med 274: 248–254, 1966.

27. Tenckhoff H, Schecter H: A bacteriologically safe peritoneal access device. Trans Am Soc Artif Intern Organs 14: 181–186, 1986.

28. Tenckhoff H, Meston B, Shilipetar G: A simplified automatic peritoneal dialysis system. Trans Am Soc Artif Intern Organs 18: 436–440, 1972.

29. Boen ST, Mion CM, Curtis FK *et al.*: Periodic peritoneal dialysis using the repeated puncture technique and an automatic cycling machine. Trans Am Soc Artif Intern Organs 10: 409–414, 1964.

30. Counts S, Hickman R, Garbaccio A, Tenckhoff H: Chronic home peritoneal dialysis in children. Trans Am Soc Artif Intern Organs 19: 157–167, 1973.

31. Hickman RO: Nine years' experience with chronic peritoneal dialysis in childhood. Dial Transplantation 7: 803, 1978.

32. Brouhard BH, Berger M, Cunningham RJ *et al.*: Home peritoneal dialysis in children. Trans Am Soc Artif Intern Organs 25: 90–94, 1979.

33. Baluarte HJ, Grossman MB, Polinsky MS *et al.*: Experience with intermittent home peritoneal dialysis (IHPD) in children (Abstract). Pediatr Res 14: 994, 1980.

34. Lorentz WB, Hamilton RW, Disher B *et al.*: Home peritoneal dialysis during infancy. Clin Nephrol 15: 194–197, 1981.

35. Potter DE, McDaid TK, Ramirez JA: Peritoneal dialysis in children. In: Atkins RC, Thomson NM, Farrell PC (eds), Peritoneal Dialysis, Churchill Linvingstone, New York, pp 356–361, 1981.

36. Oreopoulos DG, Katirtzoglou A, Arbus G, Cordy P: Dialysis and transplantation in young children (Letter). Brit Med J 1: 1628–1629, 1979.

37. Balfe JW, Irwin MA: Continuous ambulatory peritoneal dialysis in pediatrics. In: Legain M (ed), Continuous Ambulatory Peritoneal Dialysis, Excerpta Medica, Amsterdam, pp 131–136, 1980.

38. Alexander SR, Tseng CH, Maksym KA *et al.*: Clinical parameters in continuous ambulatory peritoneal dialysis for infants and young children. In: Moncrief JW, Popovich RP (eds), CAPD Update, Masson Publ USA, New York, pp 195–

209, 1981.

39. Kohaut EC: Continuous ambulatory peritoneal dialysis: a preliminary pediatric experience. Am J Dis Child 135: 270–271, 1981.

40. Potter DE, McDaid TK, McHenry K *et al.*: Continuous ambulatory peritoneal dialysis (CAPD) in children. Trans Am Soc Artif Intern Organs 27: 64–67, 1981.

41. Salusky IB, Lucullo L, Nelson P, Fine RN: Continuous ambulatory peritoneal dialysis in children. Pediatr Clin N Am 29: 1005–1012, 1982.

42. Guillot M, Clermont M-J, Gagnadoux M-F, Broyer M: Nineteen months' experience with continuous ambulatory peritoneal dialysis in children: main clinical and biological results. In: Gahl GM, Kessel M, Nolph KD (eds), Advances in Peritoneal Dialysis, Excerpta Medica, Amsterdam, pp 203–207, 1981.

43. Eastham EJ, Kirplani H, Francis D *et al.*: Pediatric continuous ambulatory peritoneal dialysis. Arch Dis Child 57: 677–680, 1982.

44. Balfe JW, Vigneaux A, Williamson J *et al.*: The use of CAPD in the treatment of children with end-stage renal disease. Perit Dial Bull 1: 35–38, 1981.

45. Schmerling J, Kohaut EC, Perry S: Cost and social benefits of CAPD in a pediatric population. In: Moncrief JW, Popovich RP (eds), CAPD Update, Masson Publ USA, New York, pp 189–193, 1981.

46. Alexander SR: Pediatric CAPD update – 1983. Perit Dial Bull (Suppl) 3: S15–S22, 1983.

47. Buoncristiani V, Cozarri M, Carobi C *et al.*: Semicontinuous semiambulatory peritoneal dialysis. Proc Eur Dial Transpl Assoc 17: 328, 1980.

48. Diaz-Buxo JA, Walker PJ, Farmer CD *et al.*: Continuous cyclic peritoneal dialysis. Trans Am Soc Artif Intern Organs 27: 51–53, 1981.

49. Price CG, Suki WN: Newer modifications of peritoneal dialysis: options in the treatment of patients with renal failure. Am J Nephrol 1: 97–104, 1981.

50. Von Lilien T, Salusky IB, Boechat I *et al.*: Five years' experience with continuous ambulatory or continuous cycling peritoneal dialysis in children. J Pediatr 111: 513–518, 1987.

51. Drachman R, Niaudet P, Dartois A-M, Broyer M: Protein losses during peritoneal dialysis in children. In: Fine RN, Scharer K, Mehls O (eds), CAPD in Children, Springer-Verlag, New York, pp 78–83, 1985.

52. Popovich RP, Personal communication. 1986.

53. Morgenstern BZ, Baluarte H: Peritoneal dialysis kinetics in children. In: Fine RN (ed), Chronic Ambulatory Peritoneal Dialysis (CAPD) and Chronic Cycling Peritoneal Dialysis (CCPD) in Children, Martinus Nijhoff, Boston, pp 47–62, 1987.

54. Putiloff PV: Materials for the study of the laws of growth of the human body in relation to the surface areas of different systems: the trial on Russian subjects of planigraphic anatomy as a means for exact anthropometry – one of the problems of anthropology. Report of Dr. PV Putiloff at the meeting of the Siberian Branch of the Russian Geographic Society, October 29, 1884, Omsk (summarized in ref. 56).

55. Wegner G: Chirurgische Bemerkungen uber die peritoneal Hohle, mit besonder Berucksichtigung der Ovariotomie. Arch Klin Chir 20: 51, 1887.

56. Esperanca MJ, Collins DL: Peritoneal dialysis efficiency in relation to body weight. J Pediatr Surg 1: 162–169, 1966.

57. DuBois D, DuBois EF: A formula to estimate the approximate surface area if height and weight be known. Arch Intern Med 17: 863–71, 1916.

58. Gruskin AB, Lerner GR, Fleischman LE: Developmental aspects of peritoneal dialysis kinetics. In: Fine RN (ed), Chronic Ambulatory Peritoneal Dialysis (CAPD) and Chronic Cycling Peritoneal Dialysis (CCPD) in Children, Martinus

Nijhoff, Boston, p. 37, 1987.

59. Driscoll JM, Heird WC: Maintenance fluid therapy during the neonatal period. In: Winters RW (ed), The Body Fluids in Pediatrics. Little, Brown, Boston, p 266, 1973.

60. Holiday MA: Metabolic rate and organ size during growth from infancy to maturity and during late gestation and early infancy. Pediatrics 47: 169–179, 1971.

61. McCance RA: The maintenance of chemical stability in the newborn in chemical exchange. Arch Dis Child 34: 361–370, 1959.

62. Nolph KD: Peritoneal anatomy and transport physiology. In: Drukker W, Parsons FM, Maher JF (eds), Replacement of Renal Function by Dialysis, 2nd Ed. Martinus Nijhoff, Boston, pp 440–456, 1983.

63. Mactier RA, Khanna R, Twardowski Z, Nolph KD: Role of peritoneal cavity lymphatic absorption in peritoneal dialysis. Kidney Int 32: 165–172, 1987.

63A. Khanna R, Mactier RA, Nolph KD and Groshong T: Why is ultrafiltration lower in children on CAPD? Abstracts, Amer Soc Neph 20: 100A, 1987.

64. Elzouki AY, Gruskin AB, Baluarte HJ *et al*.: Developmental aspects of peritoneal dialysis kinetics in dogs. Pediatr Res 15: 863–585, 1981.

65. Henderson LW: The problem of peritoneal membrane area and permeability. Kidney Int 3: 409–410, 1973.

66. Gruskin AB, Cote ML, Baluarte HJ: Peritoneal diffusion curves, peritoneal clearances, and scaling factors in children of differing age. Int J Pediatr Nephrol 3: 271–278, 1982.

67. Popovich RP, Pyle WK, Rosenthal DA *et al*.: Kinetics of peritoneal dialysis in children. In: Moncrief JW, Popovich RP (eds), CAPD Update, Masson Publ USA, New York, pp 227–242, 1981.

68. Morgenstern BZ, Pyle WK, Gruskin AB *et al*.: Transport characteristics of the pediatric peritoneal membrane (Abstract). Kidney Int 25: 259, 1984.

69. Morgenstern BZ, Pyle WK, Gruskin AB *et al*.: Convective characteristics of pediatric peritoneal dialysis. Perit Dial Bull 4: S155–158, 1984.

70. Kohaut EC, Alexander SR: Ultrafiltration in the young patient on CAPD. In: Moncrief JW, Popovich RP (eds), CAPD Update, Masson Publ USA, New York, pp 221–226, 1981.

71. Balfe JW, Hanning RM, Vigneaux A, Watson AR: A comparison of peritoneal water and solute movement in young and older children on CAPD. In: Fine RN, Scharer K, Mehls O (eds), CAPD in Children, Springer Verlag, New York, pp 14–19, 1985.

72. Kohaut EC: Effect of dialysate volume on ultrafiltration in young patients treatment with CAPD. Int J Pediatr Nephrol 7: 13–16, 1986.

73. Gordillo-Panigua G, Velasquez-Jones L: Acute renal failure. Pediatr Clin N Am 23: 817–828, 1976.

74. Dobrin RS, Kjellstrand C: The management of acute renal failure in pediatrics. In: Chapman A (ed), Acute Renal Failure. Churchill Livingstone, New York, pp 99–101, 1980.

75. Norman ME, Asadi FK: A prospective study of acute renal failure in the newborn infant. Pediatrics 63: 475–479, 1979.

76. Stapleton FB, Jones DP, Green RS: Acute renal failure in neonates: incidence, etiology and outcome. Pediatr Nephrol 1: 314–320, 1987.

77. Chesney RW, Kaplan BS, Freedom RM *et al*.: Acute renal failure: an important complication of cardiac surgery in infants. J Pediatr 87: 381–388, 1975.

78. Rigden SPA, Barratt TM, Dillon MJ *et al*.: Acute renal failure complicating cardiopulmonary bypass surgery. Arch Dis Child 57: 425–430, 1982.

79. Fong JSC, deChadraravian J-P, Kaplan BS: Hemolytic-uremic syndrome: current concepts and management. Pediatr Clin N Am 29: 835–856, 1982.

80. Gaudio KM, Siegel NJ: Pathogenesis and treatment of acute renal failure. Pediatr Clin N Am 34: 771–788, 1987.

81. Miller TR, Anderson RJ, Linas SL *et al*.: Urinary diagnostic indices in acute renal failure: a prospective study. Ann Intern Med 89: 47–50, 1978.

82. Ellis EN, Arnold WC: Use of urinary indices in renal failure in the newborn. Am J Dis Child 136: 615–617, 1982.

83. Mathew OP, Jones AS, Janes E *et al*.: Neonatal renal failure: usefulness of diagnostic indices. Pediatrics 65: 57–60, 1980.

84. Grylak L, Medani C, Hultzen C *et al*.: Nonoliguric acute renal failure in the newborn: a prospective evaluation of diagnostic indices. Am J Dis Child 136: 518–520, 1982.

85. Oh W: Renal function and clinical disorders in the neonate. Clin Perinatol 8: 215–223, 1981.

86. Arant BS Jr: Postnatal development of renal function during the first year of life. Pediatr Nephrol 1: 314–320, 1987.

87. Chan JCM: acute renal failure in children: Principles of management. Clin Pediatr 13: 686–695, 1974.

88. Groshong T; Dialysis in infants and children. In: Van Stone JC (ed), Dialysis in the Treatment of Renal Insufficiency. Grune & Stratton, New York, pp 234–236, 1983.

89. Alexander SR, Lubischer JT: Continuous ambulatory peritoneal dialysis in pediatrics: 3 years' experience at one center. Nefrologia (Madrid) 11: Suppl 2, 53–62, 1982.

90. Hodson EM, Kjellstrand CM, Mauer SM: Acute renal failure in infants and children: outcome of 53 patients requiring hemodialysis treatment. J Pediatr 93: 756–761, 1978.

91. Cannahan J, Cameron JS, Ogg CS *et al*.: Presentation, management, complications and outcome of acute renal failure in childhood: five years' experience. Br Med J 1: 599–602, 1977.

92. Book K, Ohgvist G, Bjork VO *et al*.: Peritoneal dialysis in infants and children after open heart surgery. Scand J Thorac Surg 16: 229–233, 1982.

93. Fine RN: Peritoneal dialysis update. J Pediatr 100: 1–7, 1982.

94. Leumann EP, Knecht B, Dangel P *et al*.: Peritoneal dialysis in newborns: technical improvements. In: Bulla M (ed), Renal Insufficiency in Children. Springer-Verlag, New York, pp 147–150, 1982.

95. Borzotta A, Harrison HL, Groff DB: Technique of peritoneal dialysis cannulation in neonates. Surg Gynecol Obstet 157: 73–74, 1983.

96. Shapiro RS: A homemade catheter for peritoneal dialysis in the neonate (Letter). J Pediatr 87: 160, 1976.

97. Steele BT, Vigneaux A, Blatz S *et al*.: Acute peritoneal dialysis in infants weighting <1500 grams. J Pediatr 110: 126–129, 1987.

98. Kanarek KS, Root E, Sidebottom RA, Williams PR: Succesful peritoneal dialysis in an infant weighting less than 800 grams. Clin Pediatr 21: 166–169, 1982.

99. Searle M, Lee HA: Peritoneal dialysis in infants (Letter). Br Med J 286: 1353, 1983.

100. Nash MA, Russo JC: Neonatal lactic acidosis and renal failure: the role of peritoneal dialysis. J Pediatr 91: 101–105, 1977.

101. Lorentz WB: Acute hydrothorax during peritoneal dialysis. J Pediatr 94: 417–419, 1979.

102. Posen GA, Luisello J: Continuous equilibration peritoneal dialysis in the treatment of acute renal failure. Perit Dial Bull 1: 6–7, 1980.

103. Abbad FCB, Ploos van Amstel SLB: Continuous ambulatory peritoneal dialysis in small children with acute renal failure. Proc EDTA 19: 607–613, 1982.

104. Opas LM: Technical aspects of CAPD/CCPD. In: Fine RN (ed), Chronic Ambulatory Peritoneal Dialysis (CAPD) and Chronic Cycling Peritoneal Dialysis in Children. Martinus Nijhoff, Boston, pp 87–110, 1987.

105. Kohaut EC, Alexander SR, Mehls O: The management of the infant on CAPD. In: Fine RN, Scharer K, Mehls O (eds), CAPD in Children. Springer-Verlag, New York, pp 97–105, 1985.

106. Popovich RP, Moncrief JW: Transport kinetics. In: Peritoneal Dialysis, Second Edition. Martinus Nijhoff, Boston, pp 115–158, 1985.
107. Rizzoni G, Broyer M, Brunner FP *et al.*: Combined report on regular dialysis and transplantation of children in Europe, 1985. Proc EDTA-ERA 23: 65–91, 1985.
108. National CAPD Registry Report #83–1, National Institutes of Health, April 15, pp 2–4, 1983.
109. Update on children who use CAPD/CCPD. Report of the National CAPD Registry of the National Institutes of Health, pp 6/1–6//10, January, 1987.
110. Baum M, Powell D, Calvin S *et al.*: Continuous ambulatory peritoneal dialysis in children: comparison with hemodialysis. N Engl J Med 307: 1537–1542, 1982.
111. Potter DE: Comparison of CAPD and hemodialysis in children. In: Fine RN (ed), Chronic Ambulatory Peritoneal dialysis (CAPD) and Chronic Cycling Peritoneal Dialysis (CCPD) in Children. Martinus Nijhoff, Boston, pp 297–306, 1987.
112. Brem AS, Toscano AM: Continuous cycling peritoneal dialysis for children: an alternative to hemodialysis treatment. Pediatrics 74: 254, 1984.
113. Stefanidis CJ, Hewitt IK, Balfe JW: Growth in children receiving continuous ambulatory peritoneal dialysis. J Pediatr 102: 681–685, 1983.
114. Fennell RS, Orak JK, Hudson T *et al.*: Growth in children with various therapies for end-stage renal disease. Am J Dis Child 138: 28–31, 1984.
115. Broyer M, Rizzoni G, Donckerwolcke R *et al.*: CAPD in children: data from the European Dialysis and Transplant Association (EDTA) Registry: In: Fine RN, Scharer K, Mehls O (eds), CAPD in Children. Springer-Verlag, New York, pp 30–40, 1985.
116. Gruskin AB, Alexander SR, Baluarte HJ *et al.*: Issues in pediatric dialysis. Am J Kidneys Dis 7: 306–311, 1986.
117. Waraday BA, Kriley M, Lovell H *et al.*: Growth and development of infants with end-stage renal disease receiving long-term peritoneal dialysis. J. Pediatr 112: 714–719, 1988.
118. Fine RN, Salusky IB, Ettenger RB: The therapeutic approach to the infant, child, and adolescent with end-stage renal disease. Pediatr Clin N Am 34: 789–801, 1987.
119. Potter DE, Holliday MA, Piel CF *et al.*: Treatment of end-stage renal disease in children: a 15-year experience. Kidney Int 18: 103, 1980.
120. Arbus GS, DeMaria JE, Galivanto J *et al.*: The first 10 years of the dialysis-transplantation program at The Hospital for Sick Children, Toronto. I: Predialysis and dialysis. Can Med Assoc J 120: 655, 1980.
121. Alexander, SR: CAPD in infants less than one year of age. In: Fine RN, Gruskin AB (eds), End Stage Renal Disease in Children. Saunders, Philadelphia, pp 149–171, 1984.
122. Kohaut EC, Whelchel J, Waldo DB, Diethelm AG: Aggressive therapy of infants with renal failure. Pediatr Nephrol 1: 150–153, 1987.
123. Salusky IB, von Lilien T, Anchondo M *et al.*: Experience with continuous cycling peritoneal dialysis during the first year of life. Pediatr Nephrol 1: 172–175, 1987.
124. Cohen C: Ethical and legal considerations in the care of the infant with end-stage renal disease whose parents elect conservative therapy. Pediatr Nephrol 1: 166–171, 1987.
125. Alexander SR, Tank ES, Corneil AT: Five years' experience with CAPD/CCPD catheters in infants and children. In: Fine RN, Scharer K, Mehls O (eds), CAPD in Children. Springer-Verlag, New York, pp 174–189, 1985.
126. Watson AR, Vigneux A, Hardy BE, Balfe JW: Six-year experience with CAPD catheters in children. Perit Dial Bull 5: 119–122, 1985.
127. Hogg RJ, Coln D, Chang J *et al.*: The Toronto Western Hospital catheter in a pediatric dialysis program. Am J Kidney

128. Alexander SR, Tank ES: Surgical aspects of continuous ambulatory peritoneal dialysis in infants, children and adolescents, J Urol 127: 501–504, 1982.
129. Hymes LC, Clowers B, MitchellC, Warshaw BL: Peritoneal catheter survival in children. Perit Dial Bull 6: 185–187, 1986.
130. Atkinson JB, Kenner K, Dzinovac J *et al.*: The surgeon's role in chronic peritoneal dialysis. J Pediatr Surg 18: 468, 1983.
131. Alexander SR, Tank ES: Technical considerations in the implantation of Tenckhoff catheters for continuous ambulatory peritoneal dialysis in children. Nefrologia (Madrid) 11: Suppl 2: 49–52, 1982.
132. Von Lilien T, Salusky IB, Yap HK *et al.*: Hernias: a frequent complication in children treated with continuous peritoneal dialysis. Am J Kidney Dis 10: 356–360, 1987.
133. Anderson RJ, Linas SL, Berns AS *et al.*: Nonoliguric acute renal failure. N Engl J Med 296: 1134–1138, 1977.
134. Blumenkrantz MJ, Koppel JD, Moran JK *et al.*: Nitrogen and urea metabolism during continuous ambulatory peritoneal dialysis. Kidney Int 20: 78–82, 1981.
135. Warren S, Conley SB: Nutritional considerations in infants on continuous peritoneal dialysis (CPD). Dial Transplant 12: 263–266, 1983.
136. Salusky IB, Fine RN, Nelson P *et al.*: Nutritional status of children undergoing continuous peritoneal dialysis. Am J Clin Nutr 38: 599, 1983.
137. Conley SB: Supplmental (NG) feedings of infants undergoing continuous peritoneal dialysis. In: Fine RN (ed), Chronic Ambulatory Peritoneal Dialysis (CAPD) and Chronic Cycling Peritoneal Dialysis (CCPD) in Children. Martinus Nijhoff, Boston, pp 263–269, 1987.
138. Wassner SJ, Abitbol C, Alexander SR *et al.*: Nutritional requirements for infants with renal failure. Am J Kidney Dis 7: 300–305, 1986.
139. Brewer ED, Holmes S, Tealey J: Initiation and maintenance of growth in infants with end-stage renal disease managed with chronic peritoneal dialysis and nasogastric tube feedings (Abstract). Kidney Int 29: 230, 1986.
140. Salusky IB: Nutritional recommendations for children treated with CAPD/CCPD. In: Fine RN (ed), Chronic Ambulatory Peritoneal Dialysis (CAPD) and Chronic Cycling Peritoneal Dialysis (CCPD) in Children. Martinus Nijhoff, Boston, pp 235–244, 1987.
141. Hellerstein S, Holliday MA, Grupe W *et al.*: Nutritional management of children with chronic renal failure. Summary of the task force on nutritional management of children with chronic renal failure. Pediatr Nephrol 1: 195–212, 1987.
142. Recommended Dietary Allowances, Ninth Revised Edition. Washington, DC: National Academy of Sciences, 1980.
143. Simmons JM, Wilson CJ, Potter DE *et al.*: Relation of calorie deficiency to growth failure in children on hemodialysis and the growth response to calorie supplementation. N Engl J Med 285: 653–656, 1971.
144. Hanning RM, Zlotkin SH, Balfe JW: Protein losses during CAPD in children: the role of dialysates containing amino acids. In: Fine RN (ed), Chronic Ambulatory Peritoneal Dialysis (CAPD) and Chronic Cycling Peritoneal Dialysis (CCPD) in Children. Martinus Nijhoff, Boston, pp 271–278, 1987.
145. Parrott KA, Stockberger R, Alexander SR *et al.*: Plasma vitamin A levels in children on CAPD. Perit Dial Bull 7: 90–92, 1987.
146. Kleinknecht C, Broyer M, Gagnadoux M-F *et al.*: Growth in children treated with long-term dialysis: a study of 76 patients. Adv Nephrol 9: 133–163, 1980.
147. Broyer M, Kleinknecht C, Lopirat C *et al.*: Growth in children treated with long-term hemodialysis. J Pediatr 84: 642–649, 1974.

Dis 3: 219–223, 1983.

148. Kohaut EC, Waldo FB: Growth in children on CAPD. In: Chronic Ambulatory Peritoneal Dialysis (CAPD) and Chronic Cycling Peritoneal Dialysis (CCPD) in Children. Martinus Nijhoff, Boston, pp 289–296, 1987.

149. Barratt TM, Broyer M, Chantler C et al.: Assessment of growth. Am J Kidney Dis 7: 340–346, 1986.

150. Potter DE, Broyer M, Chantler C et al.: Measurement of growth in children with renal insuffiency. Kidney Int. 14: 378–382, 1978.

151. Kohaut EC: Growth in children with end-stage renal disease treated with CAPD for at least one year. Perit Dial Bull 2: 159–160, 1982.

152. Kohaut EC: Growth in children treated with continuous ambulatory peritoneal dialysis. Int J Pediatr Nephrol 4: 93, 1983.

153. Pediatric population evaluation. Report of the National CAPD Registry of the National Institutes of Health, pp 9/1–9/9, January, 1987.

154. Alexander SR: Treatment of infants with ESRD. In: Fine RN, Gruskin Ab (eds), End Stage Renal Disease in Children. Saunders, Philadelphia, pp 17–29, 1984.

155. Fine RN, Salusky IB, Hall T et al.: Peritonitis in children undergoing continuous ambulatory peritoneal dialysis. Pediatrics 71: 806–809, 1983.

156. Hewitt RN, Salusky IB, Reilly BJ et al.: Renal osteodystrophy in children undergoing continuous ambulatory peritoneal dialysis. J Pedriatr 103: 729–734, 1983.

157. Salusky IB, Coburn JW, Brill J et al.: Bone disease in pediatric patients undergoing dialysis with CAPD or CCPD. Kidney Int 13: 975–982, 1988.

158. Salusky IB, Coburn JW, Foley J et al.: Effects of oral calcium carbonate on control of serum phosphorous and changes in plasma aluminum levels after discontinuation of aluminum-containing gels in children receiving dialysis. J Pediatr 108: 767–770, 1986.

159. Drachman R, Niaudet P, Gagnadoux M-F et al.: Modification of peritoneal ultrafiltration capacity in children undergoing peritoneal dialysis. Int J Pediatr Nephrol 6: 35, 1985.

160. Niaudet P: Loss of ultrafiltration and sclerosing encapsulating peritonitis in children undergoing CAPD/CCPD. In: Fine RN (ed), Chronic Ambulatory Peritoneal Dialysis (CAPD) and Chronic Cycling Peritoneal Dialysis (CCPD) in Children. Martinus Nijhoff, Boston, pp 201–219, 1987.

161. Faller B, Marechal JF, Brignon P: Ultrafiltration: acetate versus lactate in humans: a retrospective clinical longitudinal study. In: Khanna R, Nolph KD, Prowant P et al. (eds), Advances in Continuous Ambulatory Peritoneal Dialysis 1985, Perit Dial Bull, Toronto, p. 96, 1985.

162. Southwest Pediatric Nephrology Study Group: Continuous ambulatory and continuous cycling peritoneal dialysis in children. Kidney Int 27: 558–564, 1985.

163. Chormann ML, Staccone M, Edd P et al.: Experience with automated peritoneal dialysis (APD) in a pediatric population. In: Khanna R, Nolph KD, Prowant B et al. (eds), Advances in Continuous Ambulatory Peritoneal Dialysis, 1987. Perit Dial Bull, Toronto, pp 66–72, 1987.

164. Warady BA, Compoy SF, Gross Sp et al.: Pertonitis with continuous ambulatory peritoneal dialysis and continuous cycling peritoneal dialysis. J Pediatr 105: 726–730, 1984.

165. Alliapoulos JC, Salusky IB, Hall T et al.: Comparison of continuous cycling peritoneal dialysis with continuous ambulatory peritoneal dialysis in children. J Pediatr 105: 721–725, 1984.

166. Hogg RJ: Comparison of CAPD and CCPD in children. In Fine RN (ed), Chronic Ambulatory Peritoneal Dialysis (CAPD) and Chronic Cycling Peritoneal Dialysis (CCPD) in Children. Martinus Nijhoff, Boston, pp 307–315, 1987.

167. Vigneus A, Steele BT: CAPD is not a contraindication for swimming in children. Perit Dial Bull 2: 99, 1982.

168. Berzins Z: Stoma-adhesive allows safe swimming in CAPD patients. Perit Dial Bull 4:53, 1984.

169. Hall TL, Wilson M, Davidson D, Foley J: The importance of the CAPD nurse in dealing with patient/family burnout. In: Fine RN, Scharer K, Mehls O (eds), CAPD in Children. Springer-Verlag, New York, pp 207–211, 1984.

170. Unintentional poisoning among young children – United States. Morbidity and Mortality Weekly Report 32: 117–118, March 11, 1983.

171. Clarke A, Walton WW: Effect of safety packaging on aspirin ingestion in children. Pediatrics 63: 687–693, 1979.

172. Chan JCM, Campbell RA: Peritoneal dialysis in children: a survey of its indications and applications. Clin Pediatr 12: 131–139, 1973.

173. Temple AR: Acute and chronic effects of aspirin toxicity and their treatment. Arch Intern Med 141: 364–369, 1981.

174. Mauer SM: Pediatric renal dialysis. In: CM Edelmann Jr (ed), Pediatric Kidney Disease. Little Brown & Co, Boston, pp 493–502, 1978.

175. Papadopoulou ZL, Novello AC: The use of hemoperfusion in children, past, present, and future.- Pediatr Clin N Am 29: 1039–1052, 1982.

176. Van Stone JC: Hemodialysis. In: Gonick HC (ed), Current Nephrology, Vol 7. John Wiley & Sons, New York, pp 87–105, 1984.

177. Rubin J: Comments on dialysis solution composition, antibiotic transport, poisoning and novel uses of peritoneal dialysis. In Nolph KD (ed), Peritoneal Dialysis. Martinus Nijhoff, The Hague p 253 (Table), 1985.

178. El-Dahr S, Gomez RA, Campbell FG, Chevalier RL: Rapid correction of acute salt poisoning by peritoneal dialysis. Pediatr Nephrol 1: 602–604, 1987.

179. Miller NL, Finberg L: Peritoneal dialysis for salt poisoning. N Eng J Med 263: 1347, 1960.

180. Finberg L, Kinley J, Luttrell CN: Mass accidental salt poisoning in infancy. A study of a hospital disaster. JAMA 184: 187, 1963.

181. Shih VE: Congenital hyperammonemic syndromes. Clin Perinatol 3: 3–4, 1976.

182. Batshaw ML, Brusilow SW: Treatment of hyperammonemic coma caused by inborn errors of urea synthesis. J Pediatr 97: 893–900, 1980.

183. Donn SM, Swartz RD, Thoene JG: Comparison of exchange transfusion, peritoneal dialysis and hemodialysis for the treatment of hyperammonemia in an anuric newborn infant. J Pediatr 95: 67–70, 1979.

184. Sallan SE, Cottom D: Peritoneal dialysis in maple syrup urine disease. Lancet 2: 1423, 1969.

185. Russill G, Thom H, Tarlow MJ et al.: Reduction of plasma proprionate by peritoneal dialysis. Pediatrics 53: 281–283, 1974.

186. Mahoney MJ: Organic acidemias. Clin Perinatol 3: 61–78, 1976.

187. Nora JJ, Trygstad CW, Mangos JA: Peritoneal dialysis in the treatment of intractable congestive heart failure of infancy and childhood. J Pediatr 68: 693, 1966.

188. Boda D, Muranyi L, Altorjay I, Veress I: Peritoneal dialysis in the treatment of hyaline membrane disease in newborn premature infants. Acta Paediatr Scand 69: 90–92, 1971.

189. Hobolth N, Devantier M: Removal of indirect reacting bilirubin by albumin binding during intermittent peritoneal dialysis in the newborn. Acta Paediatr Scand 58: 171, 1969.

190. Pross DC, Bradford WD, Krueger RP: Reye's syndrome treated by peritoneal dialysis. Pediatrics 45: 845, 1970.

191. Krebs R, Flynn M: Treatment of hepatic coma with exchange transfusion and peritoneal dialysis. JAMA 199: 430, 1967.

18

PERITONEAL DIALYSIS IN DIABETICS

JACQUES ROTTEMBOURG

1. INTRODUCTION

Diabetes mellitus is the only growing cause of end stage renal disease (ESRD) in all of the industrialized countries [1, 2, 3]. Approximately one quarter of all diabetic patients suffer from renal failure and many of them die of ESRD [4]. Despite this large number, fifteen years ago only a few diabetic patients were accepted for dialysis in Europe and the United States with poor results [5]. Today every one agrees that exclusion of diabetic patients from renal replacement therapy is no longer acceptable when the socio economic environment is adequate and treatment facilities are available [6, 7, 8]. Diabetic patients should be offered all dialysis methods and renal or renal and pancreas transplantation within an integrated program [9, 10, 11]. In some parts of the United States, the number of diabetic patients in the dialysis-transplant programs reaches 25 to 30% [7] and in Europe around 12% with great differences between the latin countries and the nordic countries [12, 13]. Still today, despite the very encouraging results observed with renal transplantation [14] because of age and in some countries lack of either related or cadaver kidney donors, the majority of diabetic patients with ESRD are treated either exclusively or temporarily by dialysis methods [15, 16, 17, 18, 19]. Chronic peritoneal dialysis, as an alternative to haemodialysis for ESRD appeared in the mid-seventies with varying results [20, 21]. Recent developments mainly in relation to the continuous ambulatory peritoneal dialysis procedure (CAPD) have opened new therapeutic alternatives. From the experience gained in different countries since 1978, peritoneal dialysis is an appealing dialysis procedure in diabetic patients with both type I and type II diabetes [18, 19, 22, 23, 24, 25, 26]. CAPD has rapidly established itself as a viable alternative to haemodialysis [27, 28] and is now used extensively. In many centres, survival has been so encouraging that CAPD has become the preferred mode of therapy for diabetics [29, 30, 31].

2. CONTINUOUS AMBULATORY PERITONEAL DIALYSIS

Many papers have shown that an excellent control of both uremia and hypertension is possible using CAPD and reports by Flynn [32, 33] and different groups [18, 34, 35, 36, 37, 38] have shown that the intraperitoneal administration of insulin can restore the plasma glucose to near normal values without increased risk of peritonitis. Table 1 gives the choices of the first dialysis method offered since 1973 to 178 insulin dependent diabetic patients (IDD) with

Table 1. First choice of dialysis treatment in 178 diabetic patients treated at Hopital de la Pitié – Paris – France

	HD	IPD	CAPD	CCPD	TOTAL
1973–1974	9	–	–	–	9
1975–1976	13	1	–	–	14
1977–1978	16	2	1	–	19
1979–1980	19	–	13	–	32
1981–1982	9	–	18	4	31
1983–1984	10	–	17	3	30
1985–1986	9	2	16	–	27
1987	9	2	16	–	27
	91	6	73	8	178

ESRD in the Department of Nephrology of the Hospital de la Pitié in Paris. Results in such patients at four and five years of treatment are now becoming available and allow one to draw early conclusions [26, 27, 38].

2.1. The method – Blood glucose control

2.1.1. CAPD procedure

The CAPD procedure in diabetic patients is similar to the one used in non-diabetic patients. CAPD is conducted through an indwelling catheter: a double cuff Tenckhoff catheter with a preferential use of the curled type [39] or the new one with wings as a second subcutaneous cuff [40] or with the Toronto western Hospital catheter or the Swan neck catheter as proposed by the University of Missouri [41]. The average training period is around 20 days [42] even longer in blind diabetic patients [33]. Most patients perform four exchanges per day routinely using three 2 l bags with 1.5% dextrose concentration during the daytime and one 2 l bag with a 3.86% to 4.25% dextrose concentration overnight in order to effect adequate ultrafiltration. A 2.5% dextrose concentration can be occasionally used [25]. The exit site is protected during the first three months, but there are wide variations in the management of the exit site [43]. The patients are seen weekly during the first month after completion of training and monthly thereafter. Diabetic patients as others were recently trained to use the new disconnectable systems provided by various companies [44].

2.1.2. Insulin requirements

Insulin requirements of diabetic patients are influenced by uremia. Modifications of daily insulin doses when dialysis is started are unpredictable [45]. The intrapertioneal administration of insulin during CAPD in diabetic patients has been compared to treatment with an artificial pancreas and indeed there are certain similarities between physiological insulin secretion and the response to intra-peritoneal insulin administration [45, 47]. Intraperitoneally administered insulin closely mimics these physiological events. A large percentage of intraperitoneal insulin is absorbed into the portal vein [48]. The administered dose varies according to the glucose load. Peak insulin levels lag about 20–30 min behind the physiological peak and the duration of the peak achieved is longer [48, 49]. The reaction to insulin given as bolus injection is different from that produced when insulin is added to the dialysis solution prior to instillation [49]. Despite the lack of a clear understanding of the kinetics of insulin absorption across the peritoneum, the similarities observed between the physiological state of insulin secretion and intra-peritoneal insulin administration during CAPD encourage us to believe that this method will give better blood glucose control. Intra-peritoneal insulin administration requires higher daily insulin doses. These high insulin requirements may be due to such factors as: substantial binding and retention of insulin in the dialysis bag and tubing [50, 51], slow absorption from the peritoneal cavity with losses in the drained dialysate [49], degradation of insulin during transit to the systemic circulation, and altered effectiveness of insulin via the portal system.

2.1.3. Insulin injection sites

We investigated the advantages of different insulin injection sites in three different CAPD systems, in order to study insulin retention at the injection site, the amount of insulin contained in the first 50 ml of dialysate entering the peritoneal cavity and that in the remaining 1,950 ml of the dialysis solutiuon [52]. We suggested that for insulin injection sites into tubing, 99% of the insulin was contained in the first 50 ml as opposed to only 23% when the insulin was injected into bags [52]. Wide variations in the amount

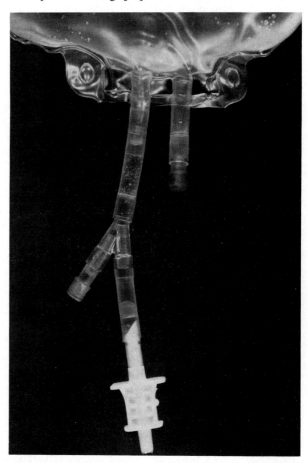

Figure 1. Injection port in the line of for CAPD (Baxter, Nivelles, Belgium).

of insulin absorbed to the PVC was found by various investigators. Amidon [53] and recently Wideroe [54] found large insulin binding to the bag, reaching 65% of the injected dose. Twardowski [55] showed minimal loss of insulin from adsorption onto PVC when it was injected into the dialysis bag. A special injection site was designed by many companies helping the patient in their insulin protocol administration (Figure 1).

2.1.4. Protocol for insulin administration and results
Patients on CAPD are taught to add generally regular insulin before the fluid is infused into the peritoneal cavity. The dose is adapted to the concentration of the glucose in the dialysate, to the carbohydrate intake from food, and the level of the previous measurement of blood glucose, Table 2 gives an estimation of the insulin requirements in insulin dependent diabetic patients treated by CAPD at the Hopital de la Pitié. During the period of assessment, because of occasional anorexia, nausea, vomiting and the diabetic lability, it is necessary to monitor the blood sugar level by the finger prick technique. The dose of insulin administered is either increased or decreased by 2 to 4 units. The aims of insulin requirements are to obtain fasting blood glucose levels around 7 mmol/l and to avoid 3 hr post prandial sugar levels of over 11 mmol/l. During the initial training period, the test is performed four times per day 5 to 10 min before draining the bag and occasionally 2 hr after meals. At home two such readings are performed daily, one during fasting and the second before supper. A series of seven readings during 24 hr are obtained once a month. Figure 2 give the results in 31 patients over a cumulative period of 131 months: all measurements are between 4 and 12 mmol/l without great variations. Many other centres have reported that intra-peritoneal insulin administration during CAPD achieves good blood glucose control [22, 26, 56, 57, 58]. In 37 CAPD patients at the Toronto Western Hospital, a similar protocol gave tight control of blood sugar: mean fasting blood glucose level were at 6.6 ± 2.7 mmol/l, mean one hour post breakfast were at 11.1 ± 3.3 mmol/l and mean one hour post lunch were at 9.9 ± 4.3 mmol/l. The correlation between the results given by the finger prick technique and the laboratory values seems to be good [59]. Some patients may be reluctant to perform numerous daily glucose measurements and one

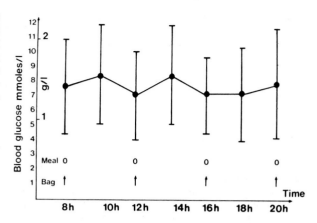

Figure 2. Blood glucose control at home in 31 diabetic patients over a 12 months period with seven daily readings once a month.

should be cautioned that the finger prick technique in some diabetics with severe vascular lesions can induce necrotic lesions [57].

2.1.5. Values of glycosylated hemoglobin (HbA₁C)
In recent years, it was asserted that mean blood sugar values do not provide a good indication of the clinical efficacy of any method of insulin administration. A better assessement in diabetic patients with normal renal function is given by the estimation of HbA_1C [60, 61]. Unknown uremic toxins, and impaired glucose metabolism in uremic patients interfere with the measurement of glycosylated hemoglobin [62]. Diabetics on CAPD always have a high HbA_1C. In our experience HbA_1C level was at $9.5 \pm 1.1\%$ at initiation and $8.2 + 0.6\%$ after two years of treatment [37]. In non-diabetic patients the level was $6.1 \pm 0.6\%$. In the Toronto Western Hospital Experience the mean HbA_1C level was at $9.1 \pm 1.0\%$ and higher than that of normal subjects at $6.2 + 0.9\%$ [26]. In CAPD diabetic patients the fructosamin test might be a better index of diabetic control.

2.1.6. Diet in CAPD diabetic patients
Considering a daily peritoneal absorption between 100 and 125 g of dextrose, and the daily loss of about 10 g of protein through the dialysate effluent, patients are asked to eat

Table 2. Estimation of insulin requirements and dialy carbohydrate intakes from food and dialysate in diabetics treated by CAPD. Hospital de la Pitie.

	Timing of bag exchange and meals				
	7 a.m.	12 a.m.	4 p.m.	8 p.m.	Total
Concentration of dextrose om 2 l bag (%)	1.5	1.5	1.5	4.0	
Routine dextrose absorption per 2 l bag (g)	25	20	20	60	125
Routine carbohydrate intake per meal (g)	30	70	20	40	160
Regular insulin injected (U)	18	26	14	30	88

a diet with a carbohydrate content ranging between 130 and 160 g/day and a protein content of about 1.5g/kg of body weight. Water and salt intakes are adjusted according to the residual renal function, the clinical status of hydration and the blood pressure values. Furosemide administration (250 to 500 mg/d) given orally can possibly contribute to the preservation of residual renal function [37].

2.1.7. CAPD in blind diabetics

Partial or total blindness constitutes a real handicap for using CAPD. However, Flynn and his colleagues have proved that when both patients and staff have enthusiasm blind diabetics can be trained to perform CAPD safely [31]. In some patients an Injecta Aid specially designed for the purpose of blind diabetics helps to inject insulin into the bag without contamination. In other cases a sighted person adds the insulin to all the bags used in the same day.

2.2. The clinical and biological status

The clinical status of a majority of diabetics, most of them insulin dependent, treated by CAPD can be judged as very good. After correction of predialysis overhydration, a steady weight gain can be observed during the first year of treatment requiring careful dietary control and adequate insulin management to avoid further increase in body weight. We recommend use of no more than one hypertonic exchange per day to minimize the effects of excessive glucose absorption.

Hypertension is easily controlled despite reduction or discontinuation of antihypertensive drugs over time. At the start of CAPD, 75 out of 81 patients received antihypertensive drugs, at one year 30 out of 62 patients and at two years 12 out of 32 patients. Unfortunately postural hypotension can be a major problem in some patients with major autonomic neurologic disorders, sometimes favored by an overuse of high dextrose concentration dialysate inducing hypovolemia.

The evolution of some major clinical and biological parameters is satisfactory as shown in various reports [18, 26, 42] and in Table 3 dealing exclusively with insulin dependent diabetics. Persistance of a relatively high hematocrit and hemoglobin level contributes to the well being of the patients. As in non-diabetics, serum albumin levels are in the lower normal range, creatinine is maintained in a steady state, and phosphorus levels are easily controlled without major doses of aluminium gels. The persistance of residual renal function, although slowly decreasing with time, is commonly but not always observed at least until the fourth year [37, 63]. Such a difference from what is routinely observed with either hemodialysis or intermittent peritoneal dialysis [64, 65] may be related to the stable high plasma osmolality, the absence of acute shifts with rapid reduction in extracellular volume and perhaps the routine administration of high doses of furosemide.

Permanent stable 24 hr peritoneal clearances were found in diabetics as in non diabetic patients on CAPD.

2.3. Technical complications

2.3.1. Acute peritonitis

Acute peritonitis remains the main complication with the method. This complication is in most cases benign and easily cured by local administration of antibiotics without lavage and hospitalization (see chapter on peritonitis). Whether the diabetic population is at lower or a greater risk of this complication is debated. With time, and the gradual introduction of various innovations the frequency of peritonitis has been reduced. Before the introduction of Y disconnectable systems [66], many centres reported the incidence of peritonitis in their diabetic population: Katirtzoglou and al. reported an incidence of one episode every

Table 3. Evolution of major clinical and blood parameters

Months	0-1	12	24	48
Patients (n)	81	62	32	9
Weight (kg)	62.8 ± 10.3	64.8 ± 10.2	63 ± 10	61.5 ± 8.2
Blood pressure				
Sys: mmHg	175 ± 25	144 ± 22	138 ± 30	135 ± 25
Diast: mmHg	95 ± 18	90 ± 14	88 ± 12	85 ± 12
S. albumin (G/L)	33.4 ± 4.8	33 ± 4	31 ± 5	30 ± 5
Creatinine (μmol/l)	910 ± 230	900 ± 170	890 ± 170	880 ± 120
P. bicarbonates (mmol/l)	21 ± 4	23 ± 4	24 ± 4	24 ± 3
Calcium (mmol/l)	2.2 ± 0.3	2.2 ± 0.3	2.3 ± 0.2	2.3 ± 0.2
Phosphorus (mmol/l)	1.7 ± 0.6	1.6 ± 0.4	1.5 ± 0.4	1.4 ± 0.4
Cholesterol (mmol/l)	5.6 ± 1.7	5.6 ± 1.8	5.5 ± 2.0	5.5 ± 1.7
Triglycerides (mmol/l)	2.2 ± 1.2	2.3 ± 1.3	2.6 ± 1.5	2.9 ± 1.9
Hemoglobin (g%)	8.6 ± 1.9	8.9 ± 2.1	9.8 ± 1.3	9.5 ± 1.5
Diuresis (ml/day)	980 ± 450	860 ± 330	800 ± 310	420 ± 250
Residual renal creat. clearance (ml/min)	4.4 ± 2.5	3.8 ± 2.1	3.6 ± 2.1	2.4 ± 1.6
Peritoneal creatinine clearance (ml/min)	4.6 ± 1.6	4.7 ± 1.8	4.8 ± 1.3	4.7 ± 1.2
Protein losses (g/day)	8.9 ± 2.9	9.8 ± 3.6	10 ± 4	10.5 ± 6

11.9 patient-months in nine insulin dependent diabetic patients [67]. At the Toronto Western Hospital the incidence of peritonitis among 37 diabetics was one episode every 20.3 patient-months [26]. Similarly in a larger group of 89 diabetic patients on CAPD in the area of metropolitan Toronto, the incidence of peritonitis was one episode every 10.9 patient-months [56]. At that time in our own unit, we obtained an incidence of peritonitis of one episode every 12.2 patient-months [36]. All these centres reported a similar, if not lower, incidence of peritonitis in diabetics compared to non-diabetics [68]. Furthermore, over the past few years the incidence of peritonitis in CAPD patients has been gradually decreasing. Over the last two years, 19 new diabetic patients were included in a prospective randomized trial, with 39 non-diabetic patients in order to study the incidence of peritonitis in relation to the type of connection used for bag exchanges comparing Y set disconnectable systems versus conventional systems [44]. Nine diabetic patients on disconnectable systems followed during 86 patient-months developed 4 peritonitis episodes while 10 diabetic patients on conventional systems followed during 106 patient-months developed 12 peritonitis episodes. The incidence in the group of diabetic patients on Y disconnectable systems was significantly lower than on conventional systems ($p<0.05$). Such results were not found in two Italian studies [69, 70] reporting a large discrepancy between diabetic patients and non-diabetic patients suggesting the possible contamination during insulin injection into the bags. Indeed the consequences of contaminating the bag cannot be prevented by the sterilization and the flushing effect on the connection site obtained with the Y connector.

Table 4 underlines the organisms responsible for the peritonitis. As in non diabetics, peritonitis in diabetics is predominantly caused by skin bacteria. More than 40% of the bacterial peritonitis is due to staphylococcus epidermidis. Other gram positive organisms include staphylococcus aureus, streptococcus viridans, acinetobacter, micrococcus and corynebacterium. In 20% of the bacterial peritonitis, a gram negative organism is found: escherichia coli, pseudomonas, klebsiella pneumoniae, or serratia. A very small fraction of 9% of the bacterial peritonitis is caused by fungi. In 17% of the cases, two or more organisms were found. One of the characteristics of the diabetic population is to develop aseptic peritonitis: thirty of those episodes were observed including 18 cases receiving antibiotics for

other reasons. Most peritonitis episodes, even in diabetic patients, are treated on an out-patient basis requiring 3 to 4 visits for each episode. But especially in diabetics, peritonitis may lead to fatal complications in relation to a perforated bowel, the organisms involved such as fungi, or frequent recurrence inducing severe malnutrition. Due to the enhanced and rapid absorption of glucose during peritonitis, hyperglycemia is frequently observed and insulin requirements increase. In parallel during the acute phase, the protein losses increase, the protein intakes decrease and the patient's nutrition must be watched closely; in some, parenteral nutrition should be considered. Generally the outcome of peritonitis treatment is good. Most patients continue on CAPD after the peritonitis is cured. A small percentage (2–5%) will dropout of the programme, either for recurrence of episodes or for the severity of the episode. Infections of the tunnel or at the exit site occur more frequently in the diabetic population [36].

2.3.2. Other abdominal complications

The other abdominal complications are not influenced by the diabetic status. Decreased ultrafiltration can be observed with or without a past history of recurrent peritonitis. Such a complication exposes the patient to chronic overhydration and requires transfer to hemodialysis or in some cases IPD, or CCPD [36, 71, 72]. It was mostly observed when dialysate with an acetate buffer was used [73]. Recovery of normal UF can be observed after a few weeks on an alternative procedure [72, 74]. Sclerosing peritonitis is a rare, but severe, complication of CAPD that can occur in diabetic as well as in non diabetic patients [74, 75]. Symptoms are nausea, vomiting, abdominal pain and intermittent subocclusion. A decrease in ultrafiltration rate is commonly observed. The real cause of such a severe complication remains unknown. The use of a dialysate with an acetate buffer instead of the lactate buffer commonly used may be a contributing although not exclusive risk factor for both decreasing ultrafiltration and sclerosing peritonitis [72, 74].

2.4. Metabolic and nutritional problems

2.4.1. Blood glucose control

In most patients an excellent control of blood glucose levels, the best among diabetics with ESRD, is made possible by using the intra-peritoneal route of insulin administration four times a day associated with frequent blood sugar monitoring [31, 37]. Clinical acute ketosis episodes never occured during the period under study. Hypoglycemia or hyperglycemia are seldom encountered except when patients develop malnutrition and/or peritoneal infection. Frequent blood sugar monitoring seems to be the best way to assess the blood glucose control, interpretation of glycosylated hemoglobin being difficult in uremic patients [62].

2.4.2. Lipid values

A marked increase in very low density lipoprotein (VLDL) bound triglyceride and decreased levels of high density lipoprotein (HDL) cholesterol concentrations are routinely observed in patients with ESRD dialyzed or not [76]. Serum triglycerides are frequently increased in diabetic patients treated by CAPD [26, 77, 78, 79] mainly during the first six months. The elevation remains moderate (Table 3) or

Table 4. Peritonitis during CAPD-CCPD in 8 diabetic-patients

140 Episodes		1 Episode per 14.2 pt-months	
Staph aureus	16	Escherichia Coli	9
Staph Epidermidis	41	Pseudomonas	10
Micrococcus	6	Serratia	4
Streptococcus	12	Klebs. Pneumoniae	7
Acinetobacter	14	Candida Albic.	6
Corynebacterium	6	Aspergillus	3
		Various	5

24 times 2 or more Organisms (17%)
30 times no Organism (21%)

even disappears if blood glucose levels are well controlled using the addition of insulin to the dialysate and if the daily use of dialysate with 4% dextrose concentration is restricted to one 2 l bag, although others have found such precautions ineffective [80]. The added potential risk of mild permanent hypertriglyceridemia among diabetic patient with ESRD remains debatable.

2.4.3. Malnutrition

Adequate nutrition is difficult to maintain in diabetic patients with gastroenteropathy leading to nausea, vomiting and diarrhea. In some cases, CAPD can exagerate gastrointestinal disorders requiring transfer to another method. The mean daily amino acid losses in the dialysate are around 2.25 g with 8–10 g of proteins [81]. These losses are small in comparison to the normal intake of 1.1–1.3 g protein/kg body weight/day. But during peritonitis the protein losses are excessive and in association with inadequate food intake due to poor appetite or inability to eat may induce malnutrition and produce severe hypoalbuminemia and hypoimmunoglobulinemia. Severe weight losses can be masked by a positive sodium balance and overhydration. Such a situation requires the administration of nutriment in large amounts. The oral route is often inadequate and intravenous administration, for example through a central catheter may be required. Larger caloric intakes will require adjustement of insulin doses and careful control of water and electrolyte balance is often difficult because of severe thirst. Hospitalization in an intensive care unit may be required.

During CAPD, various studies have shown that plasma levels of the essential aminoacids are low in CAPD patients [81, 82]. Of the non-essential aminoacids, tyrosine, and serine are low, whereas cystine, citrulline and 3 methylhistidine are high [81]. Compared to non diabetic patients, diabetics tend to have a less abnormal picture suggesting that intra-peritoneal administration of insulin may correct some metabolic abnormalities.

2.4.4. Replacement of glucose in the dialysate

To avoid some disadvantages of the use of glucose as the osmotic agent in peritoneal dialysis, including caloric load and hyperlipidemia, the search for alternative osmotic agents has justified active recent research [83, 84]. Diabetic patients could be the best candidates for such replacement. Replacement of glucose by xylitol, fructose, sorbitol, dextran aminoacid mixtures has been tested both in animals and in man [83]. Bazzato *et al* [85] have used xylitol in four diabetic patients treated by CAPD for six months [85]. Although xylitol can induce a lower need for insulin and a better control of hyperlipidemia, the administration of high doses of xylitol can induce an increase in plasma uric acid and lactic acid levels and deterioration of liver function. Dialysis with glycerol was initiated by De Paepe *et al.* [86] and prolonged by Matthys *et al.* [87, 88] in the same team, with a mean follow up of 18.2 months in 13 diabetic patients. Clinically this dialysate was well tolerated. Biochemical follow-up demonstrated a slight increase in hematocrit and a stable control of blood urea, creatinine, electrolytes and acid-base parameters. There were no signs of hemolysis and hepatotoxicity. Peritoneal ultrafiltration capacity and peritoneal creatinine clearances were well maintained over the whole follow-up period. There was no increase in the peritoneal protein loss with time. The daily blood glucose levels remained stable with a daily dose of intra-peritoneal insulin ranging from 50 to 67 units per day, which is comparable with dextrose dialysate (Table 2). But the use of glycerol containing dialysate causes some specific problems [89]; glycerol diffuses rapidly because of its lower molecular weight (90 daltons), and its ultrafiltration rate is lower than with glucose for equivalent caloric intakes [89]. Furthermore there is a risk of potential accumulation [88]; with the use of the 2,5% glycerol solution, the mean peak levels of glycerol increased up to 11.6 ± 2.3 mmol/l with peak values up to 49.6 mmol/l. Sometimes such high glycerol levels may induce a hyperosmolar syndrome, as it happened in the Belgian experience. There is also elevation of blood triglyceride levels.

Aminoacid solutions appear to be an attractive alternative to glucose. One and two per cent amino acid solutions were tested in malnourished patients [90, 91]. A 2% solution of aminoacid produced net ultrafiltration equivalent to a 4.25% glucose solution. In long term administration it appears to be beneficial only in malnourished patients. In patients with a normal total body nitrogen and an adequate protein intake, the possible loss of appetite associated with these solutions may neutralize the benefits of amino acid supplementation [91].

Many research groups have used glucose polymer solutions [84]. Mistry et al reported on the use of a high molecular-weight polymer (20 000 daltons), comparing a 5% glucose polymer with 1.36% glucose in non-diabetic patients [92]. There was an absorption of 14.4% of the glucose polymer.

2.5. Micro and macroangiopathy

2.5.1. Blood pressure

After six months on CAPD a large proportion of patients will remain normotensive without drugs [26, 36, 93]. Table 5 shows blood pressures in supine and orthostatic positions among 81 diabetic patients treated at Hospital de la Pitié, with the proportion of patients taking anti-hypertensive drugs and the mean number of tablets per patient and per day. If hypertension persists after one year, close attention to hydration status should be given, diabetics being very sensitive to over hydration and positive sodium balance. If anti-hypertensive drugs are required, over-dosage can lead to severe postural hypotension when hypovolemia is induced by using high dextrose concentration dialysates.

2.5.2. Visual status

To facilitate analysis, we grouped the results of tests of visual acuity into 5 categories: good vision from 20/20 to 20/60, impaired vision from 20/70 to 20/100, poor vision from 20/160 to 'count fingers', very poor vision with only light perception and totally blind. Status of visual acuity was available in 60 diabetic patients (120 eyes) treated at least one year by CAPD-CCPD (Table 6). Improvement was observed in 22% of the eyes, stabilization in 57% and deterioration in 21%. Most insulin dependent diabetics have irreversible retinal lesions before they start dialysis especially during the terminal phase of renal failure when hypertension tends to be severe [94]. Good control of blood

Table 5. Blood pressure in 81 diabetic-patients treated by CAPD-CCPD

Period, months	0-1	12	24	48
Patients (n)	81	62	32	9
Blood pressure				
mmHg Sup. Syst	175 ± 25	144 ± 22	138 ± 30	135 ± 25
Sup. Diast	95 ± 18	90 ± 14	88 ± 12	85 ± 12
Orthostatic Syst	160 ± 17	135 ± 16	130 ± 13	127 ± 17
Patients with antihypertensive drugs				
number	75	30	12	3
%	92	48	37	33
Mean number of tablets/day/patient	7.2 ± 3.1	3.5 ± 1.7	2.5 ± 1.7	2 ± 1

Table 6. Visual function in 60 diabetic-patients (120 eyes) treated at least one year by CAPD-CCPD

Stage	Acuity	Baseline number	%	Final number	%
1	20/20–20/60	38	32	48	40
2	20/70–20/100	40	33	39	32
3	20/160–Count Fingers	26	22	12	10
4	Light perception	10	8	12	10
5	Blind	6	5	9	8
		120	100	120	100

Table 7. Peripheral vascular complications during CAPD-CCPD in 81 diabetic-patients

24 patients required 44 amputations in the lower limbs
– 13 toes   13 forefeet
– 16 legs   2 tighs
10 patients died (mean age 67 yr)

34 patients presented destructive necrotic lesions
     toes and feet in   18 cases
     legs in   12 cases
     fingers in   4 cases

8 patients were operated
     6 reconstructive vascular bypass
     2 transluminal angioplasty

glucose and blood pressure, and also adequate specialized care are required to improve visual status when lesions are reversible. Vitreous surgery and pan-retinal photocoagulation can be highly beneficial and sight preserved even in dialyzed patients [93, 95, 96]. Those in whom deterioration was observed may already have far advanced proliferative retinopathy or other ophtalmological diseases.

2.5.3. Peripheral arteritis

Small vessel disease leading to ischaemic gangrene of the extremities is a common complication of type I diabetics. Severe peripheral vascular disease leading to gangrene and requiring amputations is still a too frequent complication observed in diabetics with ESRD. Such complications were observed in 24 patients with a high risk of sepsis and death (Table 7). A percentage of 29% of the patients have required amputations, a percentage close to the 25% observed among hemodialysis patients [19] and after successful renal transplantation [98]. CAPD has been considered a contributing factor to the acceleration of peripheral vascular disease [99]. Preexisting vascular disease might accelerate during CAPD in the presence of persistent hypotension [100]. In such patients it is wise to accept a lower standard of blood pressure control. A reduction of the amputation rate is certainly possible through adequate prevention including a foot care programme [7, 101, 102].

2.6. Neurological status

2.6.1. Peripheral neuropathy

Peripheral neuropathy is an almost constant finding in diabetic patients with ESRD induced by both diabetes and uremia. Abolition of peroneal nerve conduction velocity is present in about 25% of the patients and walking impairment, often mild, is present in 40 to 50% of cases. On CAPD progressive clinical improvement and stabilization are possible, but deterioration is also observed [26]. When measurable and despite so called 'adequate dialysis', low nerve conduction velocity values persists in most cases [19].

2.6.2. Autonomic nervous system dysfunction

Autonomic nervous dysfunction with clinical symptoms are encountered in about 10% of cases. Gastroparesis and the associated obstacles to nutrition with nausea, vomiting and diarrhea can contribute to severe malnutrition. Metoclopropamide facilitates gastric-emptying and may minimize gastric symptoms. Micturition disorders are in most cases asymptomatic but careful evaluation is required if the patient is a candidate for transplantation.

2.7. Hospitalization and rehabilitation

Duration of hospitalization and quality of rehabilitation will partly rely on selection criteria and the mean age of the patients considered. The overall hospitalization rate in recent published series [19, 26, 56] is between 30 and 40 days per patient per year including hospitalization for training, complications ·and social reasons. This is about twice the rate of hospitalization of non-diabetic patients of the same age. Peritonitis was the main cause of hospitalization until it was decided that simple acute peritonitis could be treated at home. The ambulatory treatment of peritonitis requires great care from the patient and the relatives and careful attention from the staff in charge. In our experience [19], the treatment of each peritonitis episode requires a mean of 4.2 ± 1.4 extra consultations and 3.5 ± 1.2 day-time hospitalizations in a specialized out-patient unit. The major cause of hospitalization is today the peripheral vascular disease with the various surgical procedures required: amputation, by-pass. At the Toronto Western Hospital, diabetics on CAPD spend 33 days per patient per year in a hospital which is almost twice as long as non-diabetic CAPD patients [26, 56].

Rehabilitation relies on many factors, not only medical. Only a minority of patients can resume their original occupation. In a series of 37 unselected diabetic patients trained for CAPD with a mean age of 49.8 yr (range 26 to 70) Khanna *et al* observed that 21 were able to carry out normal activity and seven of these were gainfully employed [26]. For retired persons, CAPD offers a unique means of home dialysis treatment avoiding tiring and costly travel to centers.

2.8. Causes of death, transfers – Survival

2.8.1. Causes of death

The main causes of death, increasing with age, are of vascular origin, including cerebrovascular accident, myocardial infarction, and also arteritis complicated by gangrene and sepsis often favored by malnutrition (Table 8). Peritonitis can be life threatening according to the pathogens involved, fungi for example, or some anatomical lesions, such as bowel perforation, as well as severe malnutrition induced by recurrent peritonitis episodes [36]. All series report some cases of cessation of treatment decided in agreement with the relatives when facing a situation where

Table 8. Outcome of 81 diabetic-patients treated by CAPD-CCPD at Hospital de la Pitié

Transfer to HD 19 pts		Death 29 pts	
Peritonitis	9	Lower limb amput. sepsis	10
Sclerozing peritonitis	4	Myocardial infarction	7
Loss of UF	1	Cerebro vasc Acc	4
Malnutrition	2	Peritonitis-perforation	2
Colon perforation	2	Cachexia	2
Access problem	1	Other causes	4

Transplantation 3 pts	Recovery of renal function 1 pt

Still on CAPD-CCPD 29 pts

multiple complications including dementia lead to permanent and definitive hospitalization.

2.8.2. Causes of transfer

Transfer mainly to hemodialysis, remains a frequent situation among diabetic patients treated by CAPD (Table 8). The main cause of transfer is alloted to severe abdominal complications including peritonitis, encapsulating sclerosing peritonitis, colic perforation and loss of ultrafiltration but also to permanent access problems and malnutrition [36, 103, 104]. In the juvenile population, a main cause of transfer should be transplantatiuon [26]. Unfortunately in most countries the lack of a donor, either living related or cadaveric is still a reality [16].

2.8.3. Survival

Actuarial survival rates on treatment by CAPD of diabetic patients during a period of 2 or 3 yr have been recently published [18, 26, 36, 56]. The number of patients treated remains small and long term follow-ups are not yet available. In all series, both actuarial survival rates, and technique success rates in diabetics are lower than in a non-diabetic population of the same age [7, 8, 9]. The actuarial technique success rates of all our insulin dependent diabetics treated between August 1978 and September 1987 by CAPD-CCPD with a mean age of 51.4 + 13.7 years (range 22–77) was 90%, 70% and 40% at 1, 2 and 4 yr respectively (Figure 3). In 31 patients under 50 years of age (mean age 38.8 years), the technique success rate at two years was 85%, but only 63% in 50 patients over 50 yr of age (mean 63 +P 8 yr). Such results are close to the most recent data published by Khanna *et al.* [56] dealing with 89 diabetic patients with a technique success rate of 35% at 3 yr and a patient actuarial survival of 58% at three years. In our population [27] as in the reports of Khanna [56] and Shapiro [28], survival on CAPD or hemodialysis seems to be comparable when age is the same. Similarly encouraging, 1 and 2 yr cumulative survivals for CAPD are given by several centres in North America, Australia and Europe [12, 104, 105].

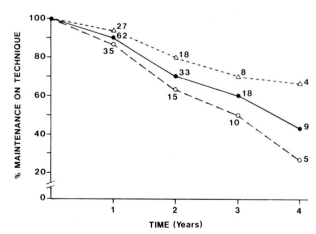

Figure 3. Actuarial technique survival rate: ———— in 81 diabetic patients treated by CAPD-CCPD and according to age in 31 patients less than 50 yr of age: - - - - - and – – – – in 50 patients aged more than 50 yr at start.

Despite the encouraging results observed with CAPD in diabetics type I or type II, such a method is not suitable to all patients. To offer to each patient the best, other forms, either continuous cyclic peritoneal dialysis (CCPD) or intermittent peritoneal dialysis (IPD) should be available.

3. OTHER FORMS OF PERITONEAL DIALYSIS

3.1. Continuous cyclic peritoneal dialysis

The multiple connections required during CAPD are the true limitations of the method. They are time consuming and increase the risk of peritonitis. Continuous cyclic peritoneal dialysis (CCPD) was designed by Diaz Buxo *et al.* [48] to avoid the several daily exchanges of CAPD while retaining the physiologic advantages of the method. Large series of diabetic patients treated by CCPD are not yet available. The American CAPD Registry reported 240 diabetic patients treated all over the country [107]. Early results including our own experience dealing with 8 patients during a 225 patient-months period are encouraging.

3.1.1. Method
An automatic peritoneal cycler is required. Commercial dialysates with different glucose concentrations are used. Selection of dialysate is made according to the patients need for ultrafiltration. Our routine schedule is four short nocturnal cycles using a 1.5% glucose solution. During the day time, the peritoneal cavity is filled with either a 4.2 or 4.5% glucose solution. Drainage is performed before the first nocturnal cycle.
Insulin can be administered to patients on CCPD, using the subcutaneous route. The peritoneal route is also possible and two methods have been proposed [108]. One schedule eliminates all subcutaneous insulin injections and initially uses an intraperitoneal dose of regular insulin that is equivalent to two times the previous 24 hour total subcutaneous dose. Fifty percent of the regular insulin is added to the diurnal bag (4.25% or 4.5% glucose concentrations) and the other 50 per cent is equally divided and injected into the bags used for the nocturnal exchanges. The total dose of insulin eventually required to obtain good blood glucose control is often close to three times the previous dose administered subcutaneously. The other schedule maintains a subcutaneous injection of 50 per cent of the previous subcutaneous insulin dose and adds 15 units of regular insulin to bags with 4.25% or 4.5% glucose concentrations and 10 units to bags with a 1.5% glucose concentration. Further gradual increments of intraperitoneal insulin doses with consequent reductions of subcutaneous insulin doses are made according to blood glucose concentrations routinely measured using the finger prick method.

3.1.2. Acceptance
Patient acceptance has been recorded as excellent with enjoyment of uninterrupted day activities and automated exchanges at night. CCPD allows connections under more aseptic conditions than CAPD with the consequent potential for a lower risk of infection. Indeed the rate of peritonitis

recorded by Diaz-Buxo was only one episode per 26 patient-months [109]. In our series, the rate was one episode per 39 patient-months [44]; 3 patients out of 8 were totally free of peritoneal infection. Other clinical and biological parameters are very similar to those observed among patients treated by CAPD, but the series are too small and the follow-up too short to authorize definite conclusions.

3.2. Intermittent peritoneal dialysis

Until 1977 intermittent peritoneal dialysis (IPD) was the only method of peritoneal dialysis available to treat insulin-dependent as well as non insulin dependent diabetics with ESRD, either at home or at the hospital. Very few patients were on treatment but early results were encouraging [65, 110]. Since 1978 the rapid development of CAPD as the preferential choice for many units to treat diabetics has restricted the indication for IPD. Nevertheless results recently published [111, 112] and new forms of IPD, such as nightly peritoneal dialysis or reciprocal peritoneal dialysis [113, 114] have clearly shown that IPD can be an adequate mode of therapy in high risk patients including diabetics.

3.2.1. Dialysis method and blood glucose control
The peritoneal access and the dialysis technique are similar to those used in a non-diabetic population. Two types of equipment to allow closed circuit delivery of the dialysis fluid are routinely used. The patients are treated either with an automatic cycler using commercially available dialysis solutions usually prepared in 5 or 10 l PVC containers or with a dialysis system using reverse osmosis treated water and concentrate solutions to prepare the adequate fluids required by different situations [64]. Standard dialysis schedules include 3 dialysis sessions of 10 to 14 hr duration per week. Large quantities of dialysis fluid, between 40 to 60 l per session, are required. Recently in patients with rapid transport shown by equilibrium tests, reciprocal (tidal) peritoneal dialysis or nightly peritoneal dialysis with lower volumes may be adequate [113, 114].
Most patients, at least at home, are dialyzed overnight. The composition of commercial dialysis solution routinely used is in mmol/l: Na 130–136, K 0–2, Cl 95, lactate 35, Ca 1.75, Mg 0.50, glucose 83 to 220.
Control of blood glucose requires careful monitoring using the 'finger prick' method. Most patients are on 2 to 3 daily subcutaneous injections of a mixture of regular and long acting insulin. Determination of the extra dose of insulin required on dialysis days is determined empirically and is a function of the dextrose concentration in the dialysis solution required to maintain an adequate water and electrolyte balance. Control of blood sugar can be achieved, either by supplementary subcutaneous injections or by addition of regular insulin to the dialysate [65].

3.2.2. Results
The largest series of diabetic patients treated by IPD recently reported by Mion *et al.* [64, 111] emphasizes the encouraging results which can be obtained in the long term in a high risk population. Actuarial survival rates and tech-

nique success rates differ according to the type of diabetes and age. Among type I diabetics with a mean age of 33.7 ± 5.5 y the patient survival rate was 95% at two years and 83% at 3 years which compares very favourably with the last results obtained in similar patients with hemodialysis [19, 28, 115]. Nevertheless, because of a high rate of transfer to CAPD or transplantation, the technique success rate was much lower respectively (65% at one year, 55% at 2 yr and 48% at 3 yr). Among type II diabetics with a mean age of 61.2 ± 7.9 IPD was almost the exclusive treatment and technique success rate and survival rate were almost identical with percentages of 79%, 68% and 41% at 1, 2 and 3 yr respectively. The main cause of death was vascular.

Because of repeated and important shifts in body fluids, good control of blood pressure among patients on IPD is often difficult requiring in most cases the use of anti-hypertensive drugs. Thirst, commonly observed among non-diabetic patients on IPD, in relation with hypernatremia occuring at the end of the session and/or immediately thereafter can be an important problem in diabetics leading to excessive water drinking and overweight. Rapid reduction in extracellular overload frequently encountered might explain the frequent decrease in residual renal function after starting dialysis [64], in contrast with what is observed among patients on CAPD. Because of high diet require-ments to avoid malnutrition and low peritoneal clearances, patients on IPD are at risk of inadequate dialysis. Decline of nerve conduction velocity on IPD has been reported [64]. Great attention should be paid to increase dialysis time up to 50 hr per week in patients with a large surface area.

Visual status can improve on treatment but deterioration has also been observed. As with any dialysis treatment, regular control of eye lesions is required leading in some cases to successfull surgery or retinal photocoagulation. The main advantage of IPD remains the very low rate of peritonitis observed also among diabetic patients. Eradi-cation of peritonitis was virtually obtained in both juvenile and type II diabetes treated at home. A rate as low as one episode per 12 patient-years has been observed in a group of 19 patients with a mean age of 33 y and a cumulative duration of treatment of 60 years [64]. Such results may be favored by the routine use of bacteriologic filters [116]. A higher rate of infection, although still very low, one episode per 5 patient-years, is observed in the non insulin dependent elderly group.

Severe abdominal complications are rarely observed on IPD. Nevertheless, sclerosing peritonitis has been reported in diabetics as in non-diabetics [75]. Among various po-tential risk factors, the role of an excessive use of hypertonic solution and/or use of an acetate buffered dialysate have been underlined [74, 75]. Such a complication can be associated with a progressive decrease of peritoneal ultra-filtration. Surprisingly patients on CAPD with a decreased transperitoneal ultrafiltration rate can recover completely after a few weeks of IPD as observed in two of our patients and by other groups [72].

Despite major handicaps, mainly cost and duration of dialysis, IPD can offer a safe and efficient home dialysis method to patients who for various reasons, including high vascular risk, recurrent peritonitis or loss of ultrafiltration, could not be treated by either home hemodialysis or CAPD.

4. PERITONEAL DIALYSIS VERSUS OTHER FORMS OF TREATMENT OF ESRD IN DIABETICS — THE BEST BUY

A valid comparison of results obtained in a diabetic population with the different treatments available remains difficult [7, 9, 15, 117, 118, 119, 120]. The series reported are often small with too short follow-ups. We have stressed how many factors such as age, type of diabetes and severity of vascular lesions can influence the prognosis. Social and economic factors play a significant role in the utilization of any mode of treatment. The choice of which renal replacement therapy should be used is largely influenced by the medical team's experience and preference as well as by the technical facilities available in a given country or even region. Negative and positive selection are a common consequence of such a reality. Nevertheless a rational approach to what should be the indications for peritoneal dialysis in a given patient is already possible.

To offer each patient the best buy, treatment of ESRD in diabetic patients requires an integrated program with all available transplantation and dialysis methods. The appropriate decision requires a careful medical psycholo-gical and social investigation including long and multiple conversations with the patient and his relatives.

Before deciding to put a diabetic patient on a peritoneal dialysis program, two main questions must be answered:
– Is the patient a candidate for transplantation?
– Should home dialysis be considered

4.1. Transplantation and peritoneal dialysis

Along with many, we consider that transplantation should be the first choice for juvenile diabetics less than 40 yr old [121]. Nevertheless, because of the shortage of cadaver donors, the frequent absence of living potential donors and the difficult ethical problems raised by transplantation between related persons, dialysis, at least in many European countries, will be required while the patient waits for a transplant [12, 16].

In such a group, if home dialysis is considered and the patient able to handle the technique himself, we propose CAPD as a first choice, which has many advantages. The CAPD technique does not require any machinery, offers full independance from relatives and allows by using the intraperitoneal route for insulin the best control of blood glucose level. CAPD does not jeopardize the chance of a successfull transplantation [15, 19, 26, 27, 122, 123]. The method can be used in the post-operative phase to control uremia in relation with acute tubular necrosis or early rejection.

If for some reason, mainly partial or total blindness, the patient cannot handle the CAPD technique, we believe that the daily exchange is difficult to impose on relatives and consider CCPD as the appropriate alternative. This tech-nique can offer adequate care without overtaxing the patient and family. With CAPD and CCPD the major risk remains peritonitis. Transplantation should not be performed within a short time following an episode of acute peritonitis. A delay of three to four weeks after treatment seems reas-onable although to our knowledge no controlled data on this topic are available.

If center dialysis must be considered while waiting for a transplant, hemodialysis, because of a shorter duration of dialysis, should be selected first, while intermittent peritoneal dialysis should be kept for patients who for various reasons, mainly vascular ones, cannot be hemo-dialyzed.

4.2. Hemodialysis versus peritoneal dialysis

Once again where to dialyse the patient remains the first question to answer before selecting the dialysis method.

If home dialysis is considered, CAPD can be the first choice for many diabetic patients of either type I or type II including the elderly. Recent reports [26, 27, 56] have underlined the high survival rate, the quality of life at least for many patients, the excellent control of blood glucose and an incidence of peritonitis almost equal and sometimes less than what is observed in a non-diabetic population. Nevertheless, the true shortcomings of CAPD should not be forgotten. Some patients will never be adequately trained and the help of a relative is not always available. The main drawbacks of CAPD remain the two different types of complications often found with the technique: malnutrition and recurrent peritonitis. Decreasing ultrafiltration rates and sclerosing peritonitis (although not specific for diabetic patients) raises the question of the long term function of the peritoneal membrane [74, 75, 124].

Intermittent and continuous cyclic peritoneal dialysis should be available to treat some diabetic patients at home either as a first choice or if transfer from CAPD is required [125]. Both techniques offer adequate control of uremia, allow home dialysis in diabetics with high vascular risk, diminish the risk of peritonitis compared to CAPD, reduce the technical burden either for the patient and/or the relatives and allow normal activities during the day, the machine or the cycler doing the dialysis during night.

Malnutrition present in some diabetic patients with gastro-enteropathy and uremia should be considered as a relative contrindication to starting peritoneal dialysis. In such patients high protein losses through the dialysate outflow can precipitate hypoalbuminemia and expose the patients to severe complications. Treatment by hemodialysis must sometimes temporarily precede therapy by various modes of peritoneal dialysis.

Results of peritoneal dialysis, sometimes excellent, but with many drawbacks, should not darken the regularly improving benefits offered to diabetics by hemodialysis mainly performed in centers, but also at home [17, 19, 27]. On a world basis hemodialysis remains the method most frequently used to treat insulin or non-insulin dependent diabetics with ESRD. An appropriate evaluation of all forms of treatment will require a few more years. To adapt to each case all methods should be available [7, 8, 19, 126]. Adequate facilities offering early transfer, when one method has failed, are part of an efficient end stage renal failure program for diabetics as well as for non-diabetics.

4.3. When to start peritoneal dialysis

In diabetics a high rate of vascular complications, mainly retinopathy and peripheral arteritis often jeopardize the otherwise excellent results obtained either with transplantation or dialysis methods. Uncontrolled high blood pressure is a frequent symptom of the terminal phase of end-stage renal failure leading to severe ocular lesions and to lethal cardiac or cerebral vascular complications. For such reasons diabetics could be considered as excellent candidates for early dialysis. However the true benefit of such a therapeutic approach versus the detriment to the patient and the community is hard to evaluate.

Criteria to start dialysis are similar for all dialysis methods. One advantage of peritoneal dialysis is the possibility of starting dialysis immediately after insertion of the catheter, while the AV fistula may not be used immediately requiring, if necessary, other temporary routes to vascular access.

For diabetic patients with easily controlled blood pressure and good nutritional status, starting dialysis when the creatinine clearance reaches 7 to 5 ml/min seems appropriate. Earlier dialysis can be considered only for patients who present refractory edema and/or severe hypertension despite high doses of antihypertensive drugs.

5. CONCLUSION

Peritoneal dialysis has proved to offer excellent treatment and a unique opportunity to treat insulin or non-insulin dependent diabetics at home. CAPD, as far as simplicity, control of blood glucose and cost are concerned, offers the best but should not rule out the other peritoneal dialysis techniques. IPD or CCPD are for some patients an excellent mode of treatment either permanent or transient. All forms of peritoneal dialysis should not be considered as the exclusive technique for the diabetic population but only an important part of an integrated program including hemodialysis and transplantation. Peritoneal dialysis is not the ultimate solution for obviously desperate situations.

ACKNOWLEDGEMENTS

The author wishes to express his gratitude to Marie-Laure Bertrand for her assistance in preparation of this manuscript.

REFERENCES

1. Avram MM: Diabetic renal failure Nephron 31: 285–290. 1982.
2. Friedman EA: Clinical imperatives in diabetic nephropathy. Kidney Int 23, (suppl) 14: S16–S19, 1982.
3. Friedman EA: Diabetic nephropathy. Strategies in prevention and managements. Kidney Int 21: 780–791, 1982.
4. Knowles HC: Magnitude of the renal failure problem in diabetic patients. Kidney Int 6. S1: 2–7, 1976.
5. Ghavanian M, Gutch CF, Kopp KF, Kolff WJ: The sad truth about hemodialysis in diabetic nephropathy. JAMA 222: 1386–1389, 1972.
6. Friedman EA: Overview of diabetic nephropathy. In: Keen H, Legrain M (eds), Prevention and Treatment of Diabetic Nephropathy. MTP, Lancaster,, pp. 3–19, 1983.

7. Friedman EA: Clinical strategy in diabetic nephropathy. In: E. Friedman et F. l'Esperance (eds), Diabetic Renal-Retinal Syndrome 3. Grune and Stratton, New York, 3: pp 331–337, 1986.

8. Legrain M: Diabetics with end stage renal disease: the best buy. Editorial. Diabetic Nephropathy 2: 1–3, 1983.

9. Legrain M, Gahl GM, Boudjemaa A, Rottembourg J: The case for dialysis in diabetics. Transplantation proceedings. 18, 6: 1693–1697, 1986.

10. Sutherland D, Fryd DS, Simmons RL, Ferguson RM, Najarian JS: Current status of kidney transplantation in uremic diabetics at the University of Minnesota. In: E. Friedman, F. l'Esperance. Diabetic Renal Retinal Syndrome 2 (eds), Grune and Stratton, New York, pp. 373–383, 1982.

11. Sutherland DER, Moudry K: Pancreas transplant registry report. Transplant Proc. 18, 6: 1747–1750, 1986.

12. Geerlings W, Broyer M, Brunner FP, Brynger H, Fassbinder W, Rizzoni G, Selwood HH, Tufveson G, Wing AJ: Combined report on regular dialysis and transplantation in Europe 1986. Nephr. Dial. Transpl. 2, 109–122, 1988.

13. Cameron JJ, Challah S: Treatment of end stage renal failure due to diabetes in the United Kingdom 1975–1984. Lancet 2: 962–966, 1986.

14. Belzer FO, Milper DT, Sollinger HW, Glass NR: Simplified kidney transplants in insulin dependant diabetics. In: Friedman E, l'Esperance F (eds), Diabetic Renal Retinal Syndrome 3. Grüne and Stratton, New York, pp 413–420, 1986.

15. Khauli RB, Steinmuller DR, Novick AC: A critical look at survival of diabetics with end stage renal disease: transplantation versus dialysis therapy. Transplantation 41: 598–601, 1986.

16. Jacobs C, Brunner F, Brynger H, Challah S, Kramer P, Selwood N, Wing A: The first five thousand diabetics treated by dialysis and transplantation in Europe. Diabetic Nephropathy 2: 11–16, 1983.

17. Kjellstrand C, Whitley K, Comty C, Shapiro F: Dialysis in patients with diabetes mellitus. Diabetic Nephropathy. 2:5–17, 1983.

18. Amair P, Khanna R, Leibel B, Pieratos A, Vas S, Meema E, Blair G, Chisholm L, Vas M, Zingg W, Dibenis G, Oreopoulos DG: Continuous ambulatory peritoneal dialysis in diabetics with end stage renal disease. N Eng J Med 306: 625–630, 1982.

19. Legrain M, Rottembourg J, Bentchikou A, Poignet JL, Issad B, Barthelemy A, Strippoli P: Dialysis treatment of insulin dependent diabetic patients. A ten years experience. Clinical Nephrology 21: 72–81, 1984.

20. Blumenkrantz M, Shapiro D, Mimura N, Oreopoulos DG: Maintenance peritoneal dialysis as an alternative in the patients with diabetes mellitus and end stage uremia. Kidney Int. 6 (Suppl 1): 108–114, 1974.

21. Rubin J, Oreopoulos DG, Blair RD, Chisholm LD, Meema HE, de Veber GA: Chronic peritoneal dialysis in the management of diabetics with terminal renal failure. Nephron 19: 265–270, 1977.

22. Lameire N, Dhaene M, Matthys E, de Paepe M, Vereerstraeten P, Dratwa M, Ringoir S: Experience with CAPD in diabetic patients. In: Keen H, Legrain M (eds), Prevention and Treatment of Diabetic Nephropathy. MTP Ltd. Lancaster, pp 289–297, 1983.

23. Polla-Imhoof B, Pirson Y, Lafontaine JJ, Vandenbroucke JM, Cosyns JP, Squifflet JP, Alexandre G, van Ypersele de Strihou C: Resultats de l'hémodialyse chronique et de la transplantation rénale dans le traitement de l'urémie terminale du diabétique. Néphrologie 3: 80–84, 1982.

24. Thomson NM, Simpson RW, Hooke D, Atkins RC: Peritoneal dialysis in the treatment of diabetic end stage renal failure. In: Atkins RC, Thomson NM, Farell PC. Peritoneal Dialysis (eds), Churchill Livingstone, New York, pp 345–355, 1981.

25. Khanna R, Wu G, Chisholm L, Oreopoulos D: Update: Further experience with CAPD in diabetics with end stage disease. Diabetic Nephropathy 2: 8–12, 1983.

26. Khanna R, Wu G, Prowant B, Jastrzebska J, Nolph KD, Oreopoulos DG: Continuous ambulatory peritoneal dialysis in diabetics with end stage renal disease: a combined experience of two North American centers. In: Friedman E, l'Esperance F (eds). Diabetic Renal Retinal Syndrome 3. Grüne and Stratton, New York, pp 363–381, 1986.

27. Rottembourg J: Le traitement de l'insuffisance rénale du diabétique. La Presse Med. 46: 437–440, 1987.

28. Shapiro FL: Haemodialysis in diabetic patients. In: H. Keen, M. Legrain (eds), Prevention and Treatment of Diabetic Nephropathy. MTP Ldt, Lancaster, pp 247–259, 1983.

29. Nolph KD, Cutler SJ, Steinberg SM, Novak JW: Continuous ambulatory peritoneal dialysis in the United States: A three year study. Kidney Int. 28: 198–205, 1985.

30. Zimmerman SW, Johnson CA, O'Brien M: Survival of diabetic patients on CAPD for over five years. Perit Dial Bull 7: 26–29, 1987.

31. Flynn CT: Long term continuous ambulatory peritoneal dialysis. Proc Europ Dial Transpl Ass 20: 700–704, 1983.

32. Flynn CT, Hibbard J, Dohrman B: Advantages of coninuous ambulatory peritoneal dialysis to the diabetic with renal failure. Proc Europ Dial Transpl Ass 16: 184–190, 1979.

33. Flynn CT: The diabetic on CAPD. In: Friedman E, L'Esperance F (eds), Diabetic Renal Retinal Syndrome 2, Grüne and Stratton, New York, pp 320–330, 1982.

34. Madden MA, Zimmerman S, Simpson DP: Continuous ambulatory peritoneal dialysis in diabetes mellitus. Amer J Nephrol 2: 133–139, 1982.

35. Legrain M, El Shahat Y, Rottembourg J, Balducci A, Jacobs C: Continuous ambulatory peritoneal dialysis versus other treatment modalities in end stage diabetic nephropathy. In G Jahl, M Kessel, K Nolph (eds). Advances in Peritoneal Dialysis. Excerpta Medica, Amsterdam, pp 365–368, 1981.

36. Rottembourg J, El Shahat Y, Agrafiotis A, Thuillier Y, de Groc F, Jacobs C, Legrain M: Continuous ambulatory peritoneal dialysis in insulin dependent diabetics: a 40 months experience. Kidney Int. 23: 40–45, 1983.

37. Rottembourg J, Issad B, Poignet JL, Strippoli P, Balducci A, Slama G, Gahl G: Residual renal function and control of blood glucose levels in insulin-dependent diabetics patients treated by CAPD. In: Keen H, Legrain M (eds), Prevention and Treatment of Diabetic Nephropathy. MTP Ltd, Lancaster, pp 339–352, 1983.

38. Rottembourg J, de Groc F, Issad B, Mehamha H, Souid M, Abada S, Gahl GM: Continuous ambulatory peritoneal dialysis in insulin dependent diabetics: advantages and Shortcomings. In: Mackowa M, Nolph KD, Kishimoto T, Moncrief JW (eds), Machine free Dialysis for Patient Convenience. ISAO Press. Cleveland: pp 75–80, 1984.

39. Rottembourg J, Jacq D, Vonlanthen M, Issad B, El Shahat Y: Straight or curled Tenckhoff peritoneal catheter for continuous ambulatory peritoneal dialysis. Perit Dial Bull 1: 123–124, 1981.

40. Rottembourg J, Quinton W, Durande JP, Brouard R: Wings as subcutaneous cuff in prevention of exit site infection in CAPD patients. Perit Dial Bull 7, S2: 63, 1987.

41. Twardowski ZJ, Khanna R, Nichols WK, Nolph KD, Prowant BF, Ryan LP, Russ J: Low complications rates with swan neck short tunnel Missouri peritoneal catheter. Perit Dial Bull 7, S2: 80, 1987.

42. Legrain M, Rottembourg J, Issad B, Cossette PY, Boudjemaa A: Continuous ambulatory peritoneal dialysis in diabetic patients. In IX Int. Congress of Nephrology. Los Angeles, Springer Verlag. New York, pp 1599–1610, 1984.

43. Oreopoulos DG, Baird-Helfrich G, Khanna R, Lum GM, Mathews R, Paulsen K, Twardowski ZJ, Vas SI: Peritoneal catheters and exit site. Pratices: current recommendations.

Perit Dial Bull 7: 130–137, 1987.

44. Rottembourg J, Brouard R, Issad B, Allouache M, Jacobs C: Prospective randomized study about Y connectors in CAPD patients. In: Khanna R, Nolph KD, Prowant B, Twardowski ZJ, Oreopoulos DG (eds), Advances in Continuous Ambulatory Peritoneal Dialysis. Perit Dial Bull Inc Toronto, 7: pp 107–113, 1987.

45. Avram MM, Paik SK, Okanya D, Rajpal K: The natural history of diabetic nephropathy: unpredictable insulin requirements. A further clue. Clin Nephrol 21: 36–38, 1984.

46. Porte DJ, Bagdade JD: Human insulin secretion: an integrated approach. Ann Rev Med 21: 219–240, 1970.

47. Graber AL: Chronic peritoneal dialysis in insulin dependent diabetes mellitus – diabetic clinical care-conference. J Tenn Med Ass 2: 74–78, 1981.

48. Schade DS, Eaton RP, Spencer W: The advantages of peritoneal route of insulin delivery. In: Irsigler K, Kunz KN, Owen DR, Regal H (eds), New Approaches to Insulin Therapy, MTP Press Lancaster, pp 31–39, 1981.

49. Balducci A, Slama G, Rottembourg J, Baumelou A, Delage A: Intraperitoneal insulin in uraemic diabetics undergoing continuous ambulatory peritoneal dialysis. Brit Med J 283: 1021–1023, 1981.

50. Twardowski ZJ, Nolph KD, Mac Gary TJ, Moore HL, Collin P, Ausman RK, Slimack WS: Insulin binding to plastic bag: a methodologic study. Am J Hosp Pharm 40: 575–579, 1983.

51. Johnson CA: Adsorption of insulin to the surface of peritoneal dialysis solution containers. Am J Kidney Dis 3: 224–228, 1983.

52. Rottembourg J, Carayon A, Benoliel D, Peluso F, Ozanne P: Critical evaluation of the injection site for insulin in CAPD for diabetic patients. In: JF Maher and JF Winchester (eds), Frontiers in Peritoneal Dialysis; Fields, Rich and Ass. New York, pp 283–287, 1986.

53. Amidon G, Reicher J, Curtis SM, Johnson A: Absorption of insulin to the surface of polyvinyl CAPD solution containers. Proc Dial Transplant Forum 10: 296–301, 1980.

54. Wideroe TE, Sineby LC, Berg KJ: Intraperitoneal (l 125) insulin absorption during intermittent and continuous peritoneal dialysis. Kidney Int 23: 22–28, 1983.

55. Twardowski ZJ: Insulin adsorption to peritoneal dialysis bags. Perit Dial Bull 3: 113–115, 1983.

56. Khanna R, Oreopoulos DG: CAPD in patients with diabetes mellitus. In: Gokal R. Editor. Continuous Ambulatory Peritoneal Dialysis. Churchill Livingstone – Edinburgh, pp 291–305, 1986.

57. Carta Q, Monge L, Triolo G, Dani F, Salomone M, Vercellone A, Vitelli A: Continuous insulin infusion in the management of uremic diabetic patients on dialysis: clinical experience with subcutaneous and intra peritoneal delivery. Diabetic Nephropathy 4: 83–87, 1985.

58. Groop LC, van Bonsdorff MC: Intra peritoneal insulin administration does not promote insulin antibody production in insulin dependent diabetes mellitus patients on dialysis. Diabetic Nephropathy 4: 80–82, 1985.

59. Friedman EA, Levits C, Hirsch S, Butt K: Feasibility of self blood glucose monotoring in uremic diabetics. In: Friedman E, L'Esperance F (eds), Diabetic Renal Retinal Syndrome 2. Grüne and Stratton, New York, pp 437–445, 1982.

60. Graft RJ, Porte JD: Glycosylated haemoglobin as an index of glycemia independent of plasma insulin in normal and diabetic subjects. Diabetes 27: 368–372, 1977.

61. Gabbay K: Glycohaemoglobin. A measure of glycaemic cruising altitude. In: Keen H, Legrain M (eds), Prevention and Treatment of Diabetic Nephropathy. Lancaster, MTP Ltd, pp 145–153, 1983.

62. Boer MJ, Miedema K, Casparie AF: Glycosylated haemoglobin in renal failure. Diabetologia 18: 437–440, 1980.

63. Rottembourg J, Issad B, Gallego JL, Degoulet P, Aime F,

Gueffaf B, Legrain M: Evolution of residual renal function in patients undergoing maintenance hemodialysis or continuous ambulatory peritoneal dialysis. Proc Europ Dial Transpl Ass 19: 397–401, 1982.

64. Mion C, Slingeneyer A, Canaud B, Oules R, Branger G, Chong G, Mourad G: Home intermittent peritoneal dialysis in the treatment of end-stage diabetic nephropathy. 1982 Update. In: Keen H and Legrain M (eds), Prevention and Treatment of Diabetic Nephropathy. Lancaster, MTP Ltd, pp 263–277, 1983.

65. Ahmads, Gallager N, Shen F: Intermittent peritoneal dialysis: Status reassessed. Trans Amer Soc Artif Intern Organs 25: 86–90, 1979.

66. Maiorca R, Cantaluppi A, Cancarini GC et al: Prospective controlled trial of a Y connector and disinfectant to prevent peritonitis in continuous ambulatory peritoneal dialysis. Lancet 2: 642–644, 1983.

67. Katirtzoglou A, Izatt S, Oreopoulos DG: Chronic peritoneal dialysis in diabetics with end stage renal failure. In: Friedman EA and L'Espereance F (eds), Diabetic Renal Retinal Syndrome 2. Grüne and Stratton, New York, pp 317–332, 1982.

68. Heaton A, Rodger ESC, Sellars L, Goodship THJ, Fletcher K, Nikolakakis N, Ward MK, Wilkinson R, Kerr DNS: Continuous ambulatory peritoneal dialysis after the honeymoon: review of experience in Newcastle 1979–1984. Br Med J 293: 938–941, 1986.

69. Maiorca R, Cancarini GC, Colombrita D: Further experience with Y system in continuous ambulatory peritoneal dialysis. In: Khanna R, Nolph KD, Prowant B, TWardowski ZT, Oreopoulos DG (eds), Advances in Continuous Ambulatory Peritoneal Dialysis 1986. Perit Dial Bull Inc Toronto, 6: pp 172–175, 1986.

70. Cantaluppi A, Scalamogna A, Castelnova C, Graziani G: Peritonitis prevention in CAPD. Long term efficacy of a Y connector and disinfectant. Perit Dial Bull 6: 58–61, 1986.

71. Faller B, Marichal JF: Loss of ultrafiltration in CAPD: clinical data. In: Gahl G, Kessel M, Nolph K (eds), Advances in Peritoneal Dialysis. Amsterdam, Excerpta Medica, 1981, pp 227–232.

72. Slingeneyer A, Canaud B, Mion C: Permanent loss of ultrafiltration capacity of the peritoneum in long term peritoneal dialysis: an epidemiological study. Nephron 33: 133–138, 1983.

73. Rottembourg J, Brouard R, Issad B, Allouache M, Ghali B, Boudjemaa A: Role of acetate in loss of ultrafiltration during CAPD. In: Berlyne GM, Giovannetti S (eds), Contribution to Nephrology. Karger-Basel 57: pp 197–206, 1987.

74. Rottembourg J, Gahl G, Poignet JL, Mertani E, Strippoli P, Langlois P, Tranbaloc P, Legrain M: Severe abdominal complications in patients undergoing continuous ambulatory peritoneal dialysis. Proc Europ Dial Transpl Ass 20: 236–242, 1983.

75. Slingeneyer A, Mion C, Mourad G, Canaud B, Faller B, Beraud JJ: Progressive sclerozing peritonitis: a late and severe complications of maintenance peritoneal dialysis. Trans Am Soc Art Int Organ 29: 633–640, 1983.

76. Norbeck H, Oro L, Carlson LA: Serum lipid and lipoprotein concentrations in chronic uremia. Act Med Scand 200: 487–495, 1976.

77. Gokal R, Ramos JM, McGurk JG, Ward MK, Kerr DNS: Hyperlipidaemia in patient on continuous ambulatory peritoneal dialysis. In: Gahl G, Kessel M, Nolph K (eds), Advances in Peritoneal Dialysis. Amsterdam, Excerpta Medica, pp 430–433, 1981.

78. Moncrief JW, Pyle WK, Simon P, Popovich RP: Hypertriglyceridemia, diabetes mellitus and insulin administration in patients undergoing continuous ambulatory peritoneal dialysis. In: Moncrief J, Popovich R (eds), CAPD Update. Masson, Yew York, pp 143–165, 1981.

79. Norbeck H: Lipid abnormalities in continuous ambulatory

peritoneal dialysis. In: Legrain M (eds), Continuous Ambulatory Peritoneal Dialysis. Excerpta Medica, Amsterdam. pp 298–301, 1979.

80. Beardsworth SF, Goldmith HJ, Stanbridge BR: Intraperitoneal insulin cannot correct the hyperlipidemia of CAPD. Perit Dial Bull 3: 126–128, 1983.

81. Dombros N, Oren A, Marliss EB, Anserson GH, Stern AN, Khanna R, Pehl J, Brades L, Roddella H, Labeil BS, Oreopoulos DG: Plasma amino acides profiles and amino acid losses in patients undergoing CAPD. Perit Dial Bull 2: 37–32, 1982.

82. Giordano C, De Santo NG, Capodicase G: Amino acid losses during CAPD. Clin Nephrol 14: 230–232, 1980.

83. Wu G: Osmotic agents for peritoneal dialysis solutions. Perit Dial Bull 2: 154–158, 1982.

84. Drouin JY, Jaudon MC, Guimont MC, Rottembourg J, Dubois M, Mollet M, Galli A, Legrain M: Le glucose doit-il et peut-il être remplacé dans les solutés utilisés pour la dialyse péritonéale? Thérapie 42: 209–217, 1984.

85. Bazzato G, Coli U, Landini S, Frascasso A, Morachiello P, Riguetto F, Scanferla F: Xylitol and low dosages of insulin: new perspectives for diabetic uraemic patients on CAPD. Perit Dial Bull 2: 161–165, 1982.

86. De Paepe M, Matthys E, Peluso F, Dokart R, Lameire N: Experience with glycerol as the osmotic agent in peritoneal dialysis in diabetic and non diabetic patients. In Prevention and treatment of diabetic nephropathy. Eds Keen H, Legrain M, Lancaster, PTP Ltd, pp 299–311, 1983.

87. Matthys E, Dolkart R, Lameire N: Extended use of a glycerol-containing dialysate in diabetic CAPD patients. Perit Dial Bull 7: 10–19, 1987.

88. Matthys E, Dolkart R, Lameire N: Potential hazards of glycerol dialysate in diabetic CAPD patients. Perit Dial Bull 7: 16–19, 1987.

89. Daniels FH, Leohnard EF, Cortell S: Glucose and gycerol compared as osmotic agents for peritoneal dialysis. Kidney Int. 25: 20–25, 1984.

90. Oren A, Wu G, Anderson G, Marliss E, Khanna R, Petit J, Mupas L, Rodella H, Brandes L, Roncari D, Kakis G, Harrison J, Mc Neil K, Oreopoulos DG: Effective use of amino-acid dialysate over four weeks in CAPD patients. Amer Soc Art Int Organs 29: 604–610, 1983.

91. Schilling H, Wu G, Petit J, Mitwalli A, Anderson GH, Ogilvie R, Oeropoulos DG: Effects of prolonged CAPD with amino acid containing solutions in three patients. In: Khanna R, Nolph KD, Prowant B, Twardowski ZJ, Oreopoulos DG (eds), Advances in Continuous Ambulatory Peritoneal Dialysis. Perit Dial Bull Inc Toronto 5: pp 49–55, 1985.

92. Mistry CD, Mallick NP, Gokal R: The use of large molecular weight glucose polyper (MW 20.000) as an osmotic agent in continuous ambulatory peritoneal dialysis. Khanna R, Nolph KD, Prowant B, Twardowski Z, Oreopoulos DG (eds), Advances in Continuous Ambulatory Peritoneal Dialysis. Perit Dial Bull Inc Toronto, 6: pp 7–11, 1986.

93. Rottembourg J, Bellio P, Maiga K, Remaoun M, Rousselie F, Legrain M: Visual function, blood pressure and blood glucose in diabetic patients undergoing continous ambulatory peritoneal dialysis. Proc Europ Dial Transpl Ass 21: 330–334, 1984.

94. Ramsay RC, Cantrill H, Knoblooch W, Comty CM, Najarian JS, Goetz FC: Visual status in diabetic patients following therapy for end stage nephropathy. In: Friedman E and l'Esperance F (eds), Diabetic Renal-Retinal Syndrome 3. Grüne and Stratton, New York, 3: 443–451, 1986.

95. Kohner E, Chahal P: Retinopathy in diabetic nephropathy. In prevention and treatment of diabetic nephropathy. Lancaster, MTP Ltd, pp. 191–196.

96. Diaz-Buxo JA, burgess WP, Greenman M, Chandler JT, Farmer CD, Walker PJ: Visual function in diabetic patients

undergoing dialysis: comparison of peritoneal and hemodialysis. Int. J. Artif. Organs. 7: 257–262, 1984.

97. Rottembourg J, Remaoun M, Maiga K, Bellio P, Issad B, Boudjemaa A, Cossette PY: Continuous ambulatory peritoneal dialysis in diabetic patients. The relationship of hypertension to retinopathy and cardiovascular complications. Hypertension (Suppl 2,) 7: 125–130, 1985.

98. Sutherland DE, Morrow CE, Fryd D, Ferguson R, Simmons R, Najarian JS: Improved patient and primary renal allograft survival in uremic diabetic recipients. Transplantation 34: 319–325, 1982.

99. Brown PM, Johnston KW, Fenton SSA, Cattran DC: Symptomatic exacerbation of peritoneal vascular disease with chronic ambulatory peritoneal dialysis. Clin Nephrol 16: 258–261, 1981.

100. Rottembourg J, Kahn JF, Mehamha H, Brouard R: Peripheral vascular disease in diabetic and non diabetic patients on CAPD. Perit Dial Bull S2, 65, 1986.

101. Rausher H, Levitz CS, Butt KMH, Friedman E: Podiatric contribution to limb preservation in diabetic renal transplant recipients. In: Friedman E, l'Esperance A (eds), Diabetic Renal Retinal Syndrome 2. New York, Grüne and Stratton, pp 419–426, 1982.

102. Ger R: Saving lost feet. In: Friedman E, l'Esperance F (eds), Diabetic Renal Retinal Syndrome 3. Grüne and Stratton, New York, 3: pp 119–130, 1986.

103. Abraham G, Zlotnik M, Ayiomamitis A, Oreopoulos DG: Drop out of diabetic patients from CAPD. In: Khanna R, Nolph KD, Prowant B, Twardowski Z, Oreopoulos DG (eds), Advances in Continuous Ambulatory Peritoneal Dialysis. Perit Dial Bull Inc Toronto, 7: pp 199–204, 1987.

104. Disney APS: Review of survival by treatment of diabetic nephropathy patients in Australia and New Zealand 1978–1984. Diabetic Nephropathy 4: 183–188, 1985.

105. Nolph KD, Steinberg S, Cutler SJ, Novak JW: Diabetic nephropathy and the CAPD registry. Diabetic Nephropathy 4: 161–162, 1983.

106. Diaz-Buxo JA, Walker PJ, CD, Chandler JT, Holt KL, Cox P: Continuous cyclic peritoneal dialysis. Trans Amer Soc Artif Int Organs 27: 51–53, 1981.

107. Nolph KD: Personal communication.

108. Diaz-Buxo J, Walker P, Farmer C, Chandler J, Burgess W, Holt K: Diabetic nephropathy experience with various dialytic therapies. Contemp Dialysis 4: 9–13, 1983.

109. Diaz-Buxo J, Chandler JT, Farmer CD, Walker P, Holt KL, Burgess WP, Orr SL: Long term observation of peritoneal clearances in patients undergoing peritoneal dialysis. ISAO Journal 6: 21–25, 1983.

110. Goldberg M, Baugham KB, Wombolt DG: Home intermittent peritoneal dialysis in high risk patients. In: Gahl G, Kessel M, Nolph K (eds), Advances in Peritoneal Dialysis. Amsterdam, Excerpta Medica. pp 138–143, 1981.

111. Mion C: Integration of peritoneal dialysis in a regional and stage renal disease programme: a French experience in Languedoc-Roussillon. In: Atkins C, Thomson N, Farell P (eds), Peritoneal Dialysis. Edinburgh, Churchill Livingstone, pp 395–403, 1981.

112. Mion C, Slingeneyer A, Canaud B, Mourad G: Optimized dialytic therapy for insulin dependent diabetics. In: Friedman EA and L'Esperance FA (eds), Diabetic Renal-Retinal Syndrome 3. Grüne and Stratton, pp 383–402, 1986.

113. Twardowski ZJ, Nolph KD, Khanna R, Gluck Z, Prowant BP, Ryan LP: Daily clearances with continuous ambulatory peritoneal dialysis and nightily peritoneal dialysis. Trans Am Soc Artif Intern Organs 32: 575–580, 1986.

114. Twardowski ZJ, Nolph KD, Khanna R, Prowant BF, Ryan LP, Moore HL, Nielsen MP: Peritoneal equilibration test. Perit Dial Bull 7: 138–147, 1987.

115. Farrell PC, Randerson DH: Comparison of CAPD with HD

and IPD. In: Gahl G, Kessel M, Nolph K (eds), Advances in Peritoneal Dialysis. Excerpta Medica, Amsterdam. pp 131–137, 1981.

116. Slingeneyer A, Mion C, Despaux E, Perez C, Duport J, Dansette AM: Use of a bacteriologic filter in the prevention of peritonitis associated with peritoneal dialysis: Long term clinical results in intermittent and continuous ambulatory peritoneal dialysis. In: Atkins RC, Thompson NP, Farrel PC (eds), Peritoneal Dialysis. Churchill Livingstone, Edinburgh, pp 301–312, 1981.

117. Jervell J, Brekke I, Fauchald P, Flatmark A: The management of uremia in diabetic nephropathy. Diabetic Nephropathy, 5: 52–54, 1986.

118. Legrain M, Rottembourg J, Bentchikou A, Strippoli P: The treatment of renal failure in diabetic patients. The best buy. In: Keen H, Legrain M (eds), Prevention and Treatment of Diabetic Nephropathy. MTP Ltd, Lancaster, pp 361–376, 1983.

119. Legrain M, Rottembourg J, Jacobs C: Traitement par dialyse et transplantation de l'insuffisance rénale chronique du diabétique. Diabete et métabolisme 11; 51–69, 1985.

120. Legrain M, Rottembourg J, Frantz Ph, Luciani J: Dialyse et transplantation chez le diabétique. La recherche du meilleur choix thérapeutique. In: Chatelain C, Legrain M (eds), Sé-minaires d'Uro Néphrologie Pitié-Salpétrière 11. Masson, Paris, pp 71–89, 1985.

121. Migliori RL, Simmons RL, Payne WD, Ascher NL, Sutherland DER, Najarian JS, Fryd D: Renal transplantation done safely without prior chronic dialysis therapy. Transplantation 43: 51–55, 1987.

122. Mousson C, Tanter Y, Chalopin JM, Rifle G: Programme dialyse péritonéale continue ambulatoire transplantation rénale chez la diabétique insulino-dependent au stade terminal de l'insuffisance rénale. Néphrologie 8: 205–210, 1987.

123. Najarian JS, Sutherland DER: Optimizing renal transplantation in diabetics. In: E. Friedman, L'Esperenace F (eds), Diabetic Renal Retinal Syndrome 3. Grüne and Stratton, New York, 1986, 3: pp 111–118.

124. Oreopoulos D: Peritoneal membrane: handle with care. Perit Dial bull 3: 111–113, 1983.

125. Diaz-Buxo JA: Clinical management of the diabetic patient: the role of continuous peritoneal dialysis. In: Khanna R, Nolph KD, Prowant B, Twardowski Z, Oreopoulos DG (eds), Advances in Continuous Ambulatory Peritoneal Dialysis, 6: pp 31–38, 1986.

126. Mejia G, Zimmerman SW: Comparison of continuous ambulatory peritoneal dialysis and hemodialysis for diabetics. Perit Dial Bull 5: 7–11, 1985.

19

THE STABILITY AND KINETICS OF PERITONEAL
MASS TRANSFER

MICHAEL D. HALLETT, REBECCA D. KUSH, MICHAEL J. LYSAGHT and PETER C. FARRELL

1. INTRODUCTION

Adequacy of peritoneal dialysis is dependent upon optimal solute and water transfer from the capillaries to peritoneal dialysate within the peritoneal cavity. Mass transfer is governed by the permeability of the capillary wall, the peritoneal interstitium and the mesothelial layer. Long-term exposure of these tissues to the processes and complications of CAPD may have an adverse effect on mass transfer, deleteriously affecting CAPD efficacy.

A number of studies have been performed to determine the long-term mass transfer stability of the peritoneal membrane. Some investigators have assessed long-term membrane permeability stability by sequential measurement of urea and creatinine clearances for mean periods ranging up to 19 months. Results are variable, some studies indicating no change in clearance with time [1–4], despite frequent bouts of peritonitis, while at least two other groups have found a significant reduction in small solute clearance with time [5–6]. Some investigators [7] have used consistency of serum solute concentrations as an indicator of peritoneal membrane function; little change was noted for periods up to 60 months using this technique. However, the latter is really a poor indicator of peritoneal membrane viability per se.

Loss of ultrafiltration capacity is another serious complication of long-term CAPD [8]. A number of factors have been generally implicated in loss of ultrafiltration capacity including the use of acetate buffer [9], patient gender and blood pressure [10]. Transient ultrafiltration reductions have been shown to occur during peritonitis [11–13] and are considered the result of a more open membrane. Ultrafiltration loss may occur 1 day before recognition of culture positive peritonitis [14]. There appears to be no relationship between the ultrafiltration capacity of the peritoneum and the number of peritonitis episodes [15, 16]. Huarte et al. [10] noted that ultrafiltration loss has been tentatively characterized as Type I or Type II. Type I is defined as a severe decrease in ultrafiltration capacity. Type II is a reduction in ultrafiltration capacity together with a fall in solute mass transfer. It is uncertain whether these categories are functionally independent, or which factors may lead to a predisposition toward one or the other problem. It may be hypothesized that decreases in the rate of solute transfer act to increase net ultrafiltration through slower loss of glucose osmotic gradient and vice versa. However, since stability of water transfer or ultrafiltration capacity is also dependent on membrane hydraulic permeability which may, logically, be expected to correlate with the membrane solute mass transfer coefficient, the net effect of reduction in both these factors becomes difficult to appreciate intuitively. The precise effect of simultaneous changes in mass transfer coefficient and hydraulic permeability on ultrafiltration can be estimated from theoretical models of ultrafiltration and mass transfer. (Techniques and their applications will be discussed in more detail in the section on ultrafiltration and measurement of hydraulic permeability).

Water and solute transfer are closely interconnected through the processes of simultaneous convection and diffusion. Thorough evaluation of membrane stability requires understanding and quantification of mass and water transfer characteristics of the peritoneum. Observation of the kinetics followed by appropriate mathematical model application may be used to quantify focussed measures of membrane permeability. Many studies have been satisfied with examining superficial indicators of permeability continuity. For example, clearance measurements which, although simple to perform, are multifactorial in nature, and variations may not necessarily reflect alterations in membrane morphology. Similarly, ultrafiltered volume, as an indirect measure of changes in membrane hydraulic permeability, may be affected by a number of other unrelated factors such as changes in lymphatic flow or initial dextrose or glucose concentration. The application of relatively simple kinetic models, particularly to solute transfer in CAPD, allows more direct measurement of membrane permeability, albeit as a lumped parameter, thereby overcoming dependence on otherwise independent parameters. The so-called mass transfer coefficient has been successfully used by us to evaluate the stability of peritoneal mass transfer.

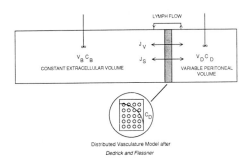

Figure 1. Compartmental model used to describe mass transfer in CAPD. Two well mixed compartments are separated by a membrane capable of bidirectional transport. The patient solute distribution volume, V_B, and concentration C_B are assumed constant. Dialysate volume and concentration are time dependent functions. (Inset refers to model by Dedrick and Flessner [28, 29, 30].

2. EVOLUTION OF CAPD SOLUTE KINETIC MODELS AND DEVELOPMENT OF THE MASS TRANSFER COEFFICIENT

All models can be described by the compartmental system shown in Figure 1. These models have recently been examined in a comparative fashion by Lysaght and Farrell [17] and Lysaght *et al.* [18] and are briefly summarized here.

In general Figure 1 describes a system in which it is assumed solutes and water transfer, in response to the additive contribution of convective and diffusive driving forces, across a dividing, homogeneous membrane; the latter is capable of bidirectional transfer, separating a constant solute extracellular distribution volume (V_B) and a variable peritoneal distribution volume (V_D). Differential and analytical equations can be developed to allow calculation of the membrane mass transfer coefficient from knowledge of the kinetics of peritoneal concentration and volume. Since V_B and C_B are assumed constant only the value of the constant blood concentration need be known from the blood compartment. The precise form of the equations is dependent upon simplifying assumptions involving inclusion of ultrafiltration and lymphatic flow and the degree of convective sieving. The mathematical development of these equations is as follows.

Mathematically, diffusive solute flux is represented by:

$$J_s = -D \frac{\partial C}{\partial x} . \quad [1]$$

For the special case of steady state, isothermal, diffusive transfer across a membrane of thickness δ, equation [1] becomes:

$$J_s = \frac{D_M}{\delta} . \Delta C = K_M \Delta C. \quad [2]$$

Convective transfer, on the other hand, results from solute drag in response to solvent movement across the membrane. In a system in which the solute species are able to diffuse across the membrane the transmembrane solvent flux is described by:

$$J_v = Lp(\Delta p - \sum \sigma_i \pi_i). \quad [3]$$

Total transmembrane convective solute flux is then given by:

$$J_{sc} = J_v.S.C. \quad [4]$$

Development beyond this point will depend upon the choice of simplifying assumptions. Nolph and Henderson [19] proposed a simplified model in which ultrafiltration and lymphatic flow are assumed negligible. Mass transfer is therefore assumed to occur exclusively via diffusion across a planar homogeneous membrane. The differential equation describing mass transfer from equation [2] without volume change becomes:

$$\frac{d(V_D C_D)}{dt} = V_D \frac{dC_D}{dt} = K_o A(C_B - C_D). \quad [5]$$

In this equation, $K_o A$ represents the membrane solute permeability term or mass transfer coefficient coupled with the membrane mass transfer area. Collectively this term is often referred to as the dialysance and abbreviated K_{BD} (units are typically ml/min) and is equivalent to the diffusive solute clearance at the beginning of an exchange or when the solute concentration within the peritoneum is negligible compared with the blood concentration. K_o represents the sum of the inverses of all the resistances to mass transfer between the plasma and the peritoneal dialysate. Equation [5] may be integrated and solved for K_{BD} ($K_o A$), assuming constant blood concentration, as shown below:

$$K_{BD} = \frac{V_D}{t} \ln \left[\frac{C_B - C_D^0}{C_B - C_D^t} \right] . \quad [6]$$

Equation [6] is adequate for large solutes (MW>10 000 daltons) which are completely sieved.

Example 1

The following β2-microglobulin data were collected from a patient undergoing chronic CAPD. Total dwell was 4.5 hr.

$C_B = 52.2$ mg/l
$C_D^t = 2.8$ mg/l (after a 2 hr dwell)
$C_D^0 = 2.2$ mg/l (after a 1 hr dwell)
$t = 60$ min
$V_D^0 = 1947$ ml
$V_D^t = 2038$ ml
average $V_D = 1993$ ml

Assuming negligible convective transport, as might be expected for large molecules such as β2-microglobulin, we can calculate the mass transfer coefficient from equation [6] assuming an average peritoneal volume.

$$K_{BD} = \frac{1993}{60} \ln \left[\frac{52.2 - 2.2}{52.2 - 2.8} \right] .$$

$$K_{BD} = \frac{1993}{60} 0.01$$

$$K_{BD} = 0.4 \text{ ml/min} .$$

More complex models [20, 21] include ultrafiltration and convection, assuming a nonselective membrane i.e S in equation [4] equals unity and that diffusive and convective transport are additive. The differential equation in this case is given by:

$$\frac{d(V_D C_D)}{dt} = K_{BD} (C_B - C_D) + C_B \frac{dV_D}{dt} \qquad [7]$$

and is integrated and solved for K_{BD} as follows:

$$K_{BD} = \frac{\overline{V}_D}{t} \ln \left[\frac{V_D^0 (\overline{C}_B - C_D^0)}{V_D^t (\overline{C}_B - C_D^t)} \right] \qquad [8]$$

Equation [8] is suitable for small solutes such as urea and creatinine which are not selectively sieved.

Example 2

Since the β2-m sieving coefficient is closer to zero than unity, equation [8] cannot be applied. This is illustrated as follows:

If the β2-m data obtained from the patient in example 1 were applied to equation [8] we obtain the following result.

$$K_{BD} = \frac{1993}{60} \ln \left[\frac{1947(52.2 - 2.2)}{2038(52.2 - 2.8)} \right] .$$

$$K_{BD} = -0.03 . \frac{1993}{60}$$

$$K_{BD} = -1.1 \text{ ml/min} .$$

The result is negative which, if peritoneal transfer is assumed a passive process, is physically impossible. However, such a value is theoretically predicted since the model must account for the excess material entering the peritoneum via the supposedly (by virtue of the assumptions used in developing equation [8]) non selective membrane. Clearly this assumption is invalid and equation [6] should be applied as previously shown.

In contrast, small molecules such as urea and creatinine are not selectively sieved i.e. $S \approx 1$. Urea data collected from the same patient are tabulated below.

$C_B = 27.0$ mmol/l
$C_D^t = 22.3$ mmol/l (after a 2 hr dwell)
$C_D^0 = 17.1$ mmol/l (after a 1 hr dwell)
$t = 60$ min
$V_D^0 = 1947$ ml
$V_D^t = 2038$ ml
average $V_D = 1993$ ml.

The mass transfer coefficient is calculated from equation [8] as follows:

$$K_{BD} = \frac{1993}{60} . \ln \left[\frac{1947(27.0 - 17.1)}{2038(27.0 - 22.3)} \right] .$$

$$K_{BD} = 33.2 . \ln [2.0]$$

$$K_{BD} = 23 \text{ ml/min} .$$

The analytical equations developed above are limited to cases where S either equals 0 or 1. Leypoldt *et al.* [24] have developed an analytical equation for cases where $S > 0$. Experimentally determined kinetic data are required to obtain the best fit values for K_{BD} and S. Alternatively, numerical methods may be applied to the solution of equation [7] for both K_{BD} and S. Computerised numerical methods, such as the well known Runge Kutta 4th order method, allow use of volume versus time profiles more closely approximating actual volume changes. This is in contrast to time-averaged values as used in analytical solutions described previously. Exponential [25] or, optimally, experimentally determined volume profiles may be used. However, while exponential profiles simplify computerised solution, they poorly represent experimental volumes after the first 100 min of dialysis, due to fluid loss from the peritoneum resulting from osmotic gradient reversal and/or lymphatic drainage. Net ultrafiltration is therefore highly dependent on these factors. The relevant importance of maintenance of positive osmotic gradient and lymphatic drainage on net ultrafiltration will be discussed in more detail in the section on ultrafiltration and measurement of hydraulic permeability.

Lymphatic drainage, as indicated in Figure 1, facilitates a non-selective outward solute flux from the peritoneal cavity to the extracellular volume. Thus far, the methods described to calculate the mass transfer coefficient have not considered the effect of peritoneal lymphatic drainage. The extent of lymphatic drainage from the peritoneal cavity has been studied by a number of investigators. Figures from the literature range from 11 ml/hr to 85 ml/hr [26]; this considerable variation is attributable to differences in experimental methodology. In view of the magnitude of this outward flow, Leypoldt *et al.* [27] developed equations to determine the effect of lymphatic drainage on the value of the mass transfer coefficient; they determined, using simplified models in which ultrafiltration was assumed negligible, that the error attributable to neglecting lymphatic flow is small. Typically a 5–10% error is evident for a lymphatic flow of 1 ml/min. Whether the calculated K_{BD} value over or underestimates the true value was found to be dependent more upon the method used to calculate the peritoneal volume than the magnitude of the lymphatic drainage. Lymphatic flow may be simply incorporated into equations [5] and [7], these equations integrated, and the values of K_{BD} compared with those calculated from equations [6] and [8]. Equation [5] for $S = 0$ and $Q_L > 0$ becomes

$$\frac{d(V_D C_D)}{dt} = K_{BD} (C_B - C_D) - Q_L C_D \qquad [9]$$

with an integrated solution given by

$$K_{BD} = (Q_F - Q_L) \frac{\ln \left[\dfrac{\overline{C}_B - (1 + \dfrac{Q_F}{K_{BD}}) C_{D1}}{\overline{C}_B - (1 + \dfrac{Q_F}{K_{BD}}) C_{D2}} \right]}{\ln \left[\dfrac{V_2}{V_1} \right]} - Q_F \quad [10]$$

Equation [7] for $S = 1$ and $Q_L > 0$ becomes

$$\frac{d(V_D C_D)}{dt} = K_{BD} (C_B - C_D) + \frac{dV_D}{dt} . C_B + Q_L C_B - Q_L C_D \qquad [11]$$

with an integrated solution given by

$$K_{BD} = (Q_F - Q_L) \frac{\ln\left[\dfrac{\overline{C}_B - C_{D1}}{\overline{C}_B - C_{D2}}\right]}{\ln\left[\dfrac{V_2}{V_1}\right]} - Q_F . \qquad [12]$$

Solutions for equations [9] and [11] assume that $dV_D/dt = Q_F - Q_L$.

We compared mass transfer coefficients for urea, creatinine and $\beta 2$-microglobulin in 5 patients assuming a range of lymphatic flow rates. Net ultrafiltration was determined from the difference in inlet bag volume and outlet drainage volume. For urea and creatinine, neglecting a lymphatic flow of 2 ml/min in equation [8] resulted in an overestimate in K_{BD} of 11%. An overestimate is expected since mass transfer due to unaccounted convection into the peritoneal cavity is considered, by the model, to be due to diffusion across a more permeable membrane. For $\beta 2$-microglobulin, K_{BD} was underestimated by 13% using equation [6]. This again is expected since, in this case, solute loss, through lymphatic removal, is not considered. Increasing lymphatic flow compounded the errors. While it is clear that neglecting lymphatic flow has only a small effect on the value of the mass transfer coefficient, the value of the true ultrafiltration rate is considerably underestimated by the value of the lymphatic drainage, if based on the observed volume change determined after a period of dialysis. Changes in ultrafiltered volume, therefore, may be related to changes in lymphatic drainage.

Dedrick and Flessner [28, 29, 30] attempted to model the peritoneum more closely with anatomical reality. The model proposes that the capillaries are uniformly distributed within a tissue matrix (see inset Figure 1). Since their principal interest was in peritoneal to blood solute transfer, equations were developed to describe mass transfer from the peritoneal fluid, through the tissue, across the capillaries and into the plasma; these equations apply just as easily to transfer in the opposite direction. The model attempts to overcome the limitations of the all-encompassing lumped sum parameter models, previously described, by mathematically describing the anatomical and physiological relationship between the various transfer resistances. Quantification of these resistances is therefore made theoretically possible. The complexity of numerical solution, however, precludes its routine practical application.

3. ULTRAFILTRATION AND MEASUREMENT OF HYDRAULIC PERMEABILITY

The mass transfer coefficient does not provide an independent measure of the membrane's ability to transfer or ultrafilter water in response to an osmotic gradient. This property is governed by the hydraulic permeability of the membrane as described in equation [3]. A model of ultrafiltration during CAPD has been recently developed by Jaffrin *et al.* [31] based on values for the membrane's hydraulic permeability and glucose mass transfer parameters (since osmotic gradient is dependent upon dialysate glucose concentration). In this model it is assumed that

net ultrafiltration equals the difference between total ultrafiltration and lymphatic flow and that the hydrostatic forces, Δp, shown in equation [3] are approximately in balance. Equations are derived to link peritoneal volume changes with the change in glucose concentration. The rate of change in the peritoneal volume is described below:

$$\frac{dV_D}{dt} = 19.3\, Lp\sigma(C_D - C_C)$$

where $C_c = 37 + Q_L/(19.3 . Lp\sigma)$ $\qquad [13]$

(C_D and C_C are in units of mOsmol/l).

Accurate solution of the unknowns requires simultaneous numerical integration of equations [11] (for $S \neq 1$) and [13]. However, for clinical purposes an estimate of $Lp\sigma$ may be obtained experimentally during the early phase of dialysis. The slope of the volume versus time curve may be calculated at $t = 0$ before appreciable change in the glucose concentration has occurred. The analysis is further complicated, however, since the value of C_C is theoretically dependent on permeability and lymphatic flow, neither of which are known; hence experimental rather than theoretical determination is required. A practical example is provided below.

Example 3
Volume data were obtained by Randerson and Farrell [25] from patients on a 2 l initial exchange volume (1.5% glucose = 75 mOsm/l). After the first 40 minutes dialysate volume from albumin dilution was found to be 2140 ml. If we assume that lymphatic drainage is equal to zero then $C_C = 37$ m Osm/l. From equation [13].

$Lp\sigma = 140/(19.3)(40)(75-37)$

$\qquad = 5 \; \mu l/min.mm \; Hg$

Jaffrin *et al.* [31] obtain a value of 6.5 $\mu l/min. mm$ Hg using numerical integration and curve fitting procedures. The value of $Lp\sigma$ obtained in this example could be improved by measuring C_D at the point where $dV_D/dt = 0$, thereby obtaining an estimate of C_C.

It becomes immediately evident from example 3 that accurate values for hydraulic permeability are difficult to obtain clinically. In view of these difficulties, changes in hydraulic permeability are most conveniently monitored indirectly through consistency of net ultrafiltered volume and osmotic gradient. Such methods are limited however, since, as we have seen, ultrafiltered volume is also dependent on factors independent of permeability, such as lymphatic drainage.

Although of limited clinical value, simultaneous numerical solution of equations [11] and [13] provides a mathematical method of determining the relationship between changes in glucose mass transfer coefficient (Gl K_{BD}), hydraulic permeability ($Lp\sigma$) and lymphatic flow (Q_L) and changes in ultrafiltration and the possible mechanism of ultrafiltration loss. Using a Runge Kutta 4th order numerical integration procedure, solutions for V_D may be determined for various values of Gl K_{BD}, $Lp\sigma$ and Q_L. Jaffrin *et al.* [31] quote typical figures for Gl K_{BD} and $Lp\sigma$ from the literature. They assume for the standard case a Gl K_{BD} of 10 ml/min and $Lp\sigma$ of 10 $\mu l/min.mm$ Hg. The value of the sieving coefficient, S, for glucose in equation [11] again from the literature may be taken as approximately equal to 0.7, although it can be shown that numerical solution is not strongly dependent on sieving coefficient. Figure 2 summarizes results from this analysis assuming a dwell time of 4 hr, an initial volume of 2 l (1.5% glucose solution) and a blood glucose osmolarity, $C_B = 7$ mOsmol/l.

Since the relationship between K_{BD} and $Lp\sigma$ is unknown it must be assumed that changes in one parameter will be equally reflected in the other since both parameters are dependant on membrane permeability or openness. It can be seen from Figure 2 that a linear dependence exists between ultrafiltration and lymphatic flow. The relationship between these parameters is essentially independent of the mass transfer coefficient and hydraulic permeability. To a degree this observation results from the assumption that mass transfer area is independent of small changes in peritoneal volume; this would appear to be a reasonable assumption [23].

Of particular interest is the changing relationship between ultrafiltered volume and glucose mass transfer coefficient and hydraulic permeability. If we assume values for Gl K_{BD} and $Lp\sigma$ equal to our standard case, ultrafiltration loss may be associated with either increases or decreases in these parameters due to the parabolic nature of the curves. Khanna and Oreopoulus [32] found that either increases or decreases in glucose, urea and creatinine mass transfer may be observed in patients with severe ultrafiltration loss. It would appear from this analysis, however, that proportionally greater reductions in mass transfer coefficient and permeability, for the standard case, are required to effect ultrafiltration losses equivalent to those which would result from increases in these factors. It might be expected, therefore, to see ultrafiltration loss associated more often with hyperpermeability than hypopermeability. Krediet *et al.* [33] found glucose and creatinine $K_{BD}S$ to be significantly higher in patients with poor ultrafiltration (defined as a maximal ultrafiltration capacity, MUC, using Dianeal 3.86%<1500 ml/24 hr/1.73 m²) than in patients with good ultrafiltration (MUC>3500 ml/24hr/1.73 m²). Our analysis also shows that changes in ultrafiltration capacity may occur independently of the mass transfer coefficient via changes in lymphatic drainage. The mechanisms or factors which contribute to permeability changes remain unclear.

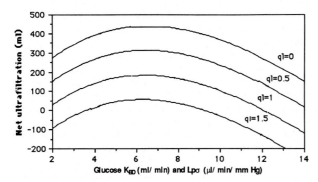

Figure 2. From mathematical modelling net ultrafiltration is linearly dependent on lymphatic drainage, ql (ml/min). A changing dependence on the mass transfer coefficient and hydraulic permeability is apparent.

4. THE MASS TRANSFER COEFFICIENT AND APPRAISAL OF PERITONEAL MEMBRANE STABILITY

As mentioned, clearance measurements have been readily used to plot long-term membrane stability. However, use of the mass transfer coefficient allows a focussed measure of membrane performance since its value is dependent only on membrane area and permeability. Hence, this approach allows the clinician to obtain more accurate measurement of membrane performance since changes in the mass transfer coefficient will reflect alterations in only these factors.

A number of studies have measured the mass transfer coefficient to investigate membrane stability with time on CAPD. Krediet [33] measured urea, creatinine and glucose $K_{BD}S$ in 38 patients on 75 occasions. No change was noted in any of these parameters for periods up to 24 months. Randerson and Farrell [22] measured mass transfer coefficients for urea, creatinine and B_{12} (using a two-pool model), using numerical methods together with an exponential ultrafiltration profile, to follow 15 patients over periods of up to two years. Three of these patients exhibited significant peritoneal permeability loss for the three solutes during the period of treatment. Although the remaining patients showed no significant change in urea and B_{12} mass transfer coefficients, a significant increase in pooled creatinine mass transfer coefficients was apparent.

An extention of this study by Spencer and Farrell [23] evaluated a further 8 patients for periods up to 30 months and obtained results indicating no change in membrane mass transfer coefficients for urea and creatinine. This study also provided a unique opportunity to compare the mass transfer coefficient variations in one patient over a five year period. No changes in mass transfer coefficients for urea and creatinine were apparent, even during such a prolonged period. In view of the importance of gaining representative and uniform estimates of K_{BD}, this study also examined the importance of intrapatient variability, dialysate volume (2 l vs. 1 l), and initial dialysate dextrose concentration on the measurement of K_{BD}. Results indicated that considerable intrapatient variation was present. It was suggested, given the asymptotic nature of the dialysate/plasma equilibration curve, that dialysate concentration data should only be included in the K_{BD} analysis if they were found to be less than 80-90% of corresponding plasma concentration values. While this method may reduce measurement error, such a technique will preclude measurement of high peritoneal membrane mass transfer coefficients and unduly bias results. A more effective method is to measure dialysate concentrations within the first 1 to 2 hr of a dialysis dwell.

Dialysate volume was also found to significantly affect the value of the mass transfer coefficient for urea ($K_{BD}S$ from 2 l exchanges were about 20% higher than those from 1 l exchanges) presumably due to a reduced membrane contact area. As would be expected, dextrose concentration was found to have no significant effect.

We have recently collected and reviewed mass transfer data from 145 patient observations at three centers in Japan (see acknowledgements). The mean time on CAPD was 24 ± 15 months. All patients were dialysed using 2 l of dialysate solution and were free of clinical peritonitis at time of evaluation. Peritonitis incidence averaged 1 episode per 20 patient months. Mass transfer coefficients for urea and creatinine were calculated from equation [8] in which the sieving coefficient is assumed equal to unity and

$$V_D^0 = \text{Initial volume of dialysate bag} + V_R \;(\cong 350 \text{ ml}) \quad [14]$$

$$V_D^F = \text{Final volume of dialysate bag (ml)} + V_R \quad [15]$$

$$C_D^0 = \text{Initial dialysate concentration (mg/l)}$$

$$\cong \frac{0.9 C_B V_R}{V_D^0} \quad [16]$$

$$\overline{V}_D = \frac{V_D^0 + V_D^t}{2} \quad [17]$$

$$t = \text{time on dialysis (min)} = 0.5\,t_I + t_d + 0.5 t_0 . \quad [18]$$

Initial dialysate volume included residual volume within the peritoneum resulting from incomplete drainage. The figure of 350 ml is based on the average value found by Spencer and Farrell [23] who measured residual volumes in 5 patients using dilution of residual RISA with a rinse volume. Initial dialysate concentration calculated in equation [16] accounts for solute within the residual volume. The concentration of urea and creatinine in this residual volume at the end of an exchange is assumed equal to 90% of blood levels. To minimize error resulting from the asymptotic nature of the C_D/C_B curve, bags in which the dialysate urea or creatinine concentration was greater than 90% of the plasma concentration at the end of an exchange were excluded. This technique will tend to exclude higher values of K_{BD} thereby lowering the average value for urea K_{BD} for this patient group. Generally, the K_{BD} was a 24 hr measurement, calculated from the average of the K_{BD} values from 3–4 exchanges on a given day. In addition to urea and creatinine mass transfer values, data on body weight, protein loss, dietary protein intake, ultrafiltered volume and grams glucose absorption were also collected. Dietary protein intake was calculated from the relationship derived by Randerson *et al.* [34]:

$$\text{DPI(gm/24hrs)} = 5.02(\text{Gu} + 3.12) . \quad [19]$$

Urea generation (Gu) is calculated from equation [20].

$$\text{Gu(mg/min)} =$$
$$\frac{1}{\Theta}\left[\sum_{i=1}^{n} V_{Di}^F C_{Di}^F + V_u C_u + V_s (C_B^F - C_B^0) \right] \quad [20]$$

where n represents the number of daily exchanges. For urea the solute distribution volume, V_s, may be assumed equal to 57% of body weight. Ultrafiltered volume, glucose absorption and protein loss were determined by calculating the difference in each quantity between the pre infusion and post drain dialysate. Values were summed over a 24 hr period. Averages and standard deviations for each parameter in this group are shown in Table 1.

Values for each parameter were plotted versus time on CAPD followed by simple linear regression analysis. Representative plots for urea and creatinine are shown in Figures 3 and 4.

This analysis suggested no significant correlation (based

Table 1 Average parameter values for patients from three centres in Japan. n<145 indicates data not recorded or excluded. Months on CAPD is equivalent for all parameters despite differences in n.

	n	mean ±SD
months on CAPD	145	24 ± 15
urea K_{BD}, ml/min	91	16 ± 6
creatinine K_{BD}, ml/min	142	9 ± 3
gms. glucose abs./24 hr	142	118 ± 37
weight, kg	145	58 ± 9
protein loss, g/24 hr	136	7 ± 3
dietary protein intake, g/24 hr/kg	99	1.1 ± 0.3

on a value of the β coefficient significantly different from zero) between any of the parameters listed in Table 1 and time on CAPD.

In addition we performed a more sensitive multiple linear regression analysis on data from nine patients from whom multiple follow up data had been obtained prospectively. All patients were male and had been assessed on 4 or more occasions.

Average time on CAPD at study onset for this group was 12 ± 12 months with a mean follow up duration of 21 ± 7 months. Peritonitis rate averaged 1 episode per 39 patient months over the period of study. Table 2 shows average values at study onset.

Multiple linear regression analysis [35] indicated a significant upward overall trend with time for creatinine K_{BD}

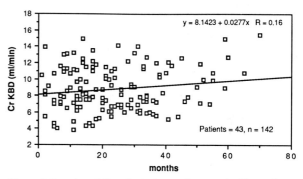

Figure 3. Based on 142 patient observations no significant change in creatinine K_{BD} is evident with time on CAPD. (The abscissa represents months on CAPD in Figures 3 and 4).

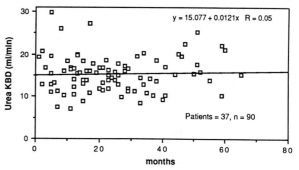

Figure 4. Based on 90 patient observations no significant change in urea K_{BD} is evident with time on CAPD.

Table 2 Average parameter values at study onset for 9 patients from whom follow data was obtained prospectively.

	n	mean ±SD
months on CAPD	9	12 ± 12
urea K_{BD}, ml/min	9	16 ± 3
creatinine K_{BD}, ml/min	9	7 ± 3
gms. glucose abs./24 hr	9	123 ± 41
weight, kg	9	61 ± 9
protein loss, mg/24hr	9	6 ± 3
dietary protein intake, g/24hr	9	1.1 ± 0.3

($F_{1,37}$=21.1, $p<0.01$). Significant individual changes with time were apparent within the group for glucose absorbed/24hr ($F_{9,29}$=3,4, $0.005<p<0.01$) and weight ($F_{9,31}$=11.5, $p<0.01$). Based on multiple linear regression, significant increases in weight were subsequently found for patients 4,6,7 ($p<0.01$) and 2($0.01<p<0.05$) and a significant fall for patient 8 ($p<0.01$). Significant increases in glucose absorbed/24 hr were found for patient 4 and 7 ($p<0.01$). However, no significant overall trend was indicated for these parameters. Creatinine K_{BD}, absorbed glucose and weight data for each patient are shown graphically in Figures 5–7.

No significant individual or overall trends were present for urea K_{BD}, protein loss, dietary protein intake, 24 hr ultrafiltration rate or volume ultrafiltered/gram glucose absorbed over the period of investigation. The absence of a significant rise in urea K_{BD} as demonstrated for creatinine may have been biased by exclusion of 24 hr dialysate collections with urea concentration in excess of 90% of the plasma concentration.

The results for creatinine K_{BD} are in general agreement with those of Randerson and Farrell [22] and may support a tendency toward hyperpermeability with increasing time on CAPD. While this result may suggest that ultrafiltration disorders associated with hyperpermeability are the main complication of long term CAPD, ultrafiltration loss was not found to be significant in this group.

5. CONCLUSIONS

Measurement of the mass transfer coefficient allows a convenient method of monitoring membrane solute transfer performance. It would appear from studies that have monitored the mass transfer coefficient over the longer term, that peritoneal permeability remains constant with time. However, our most recent study has indicated a possible

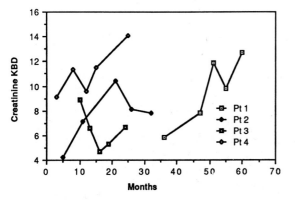
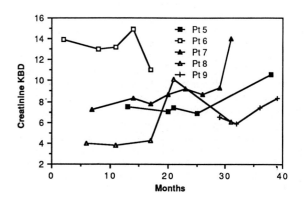

Figure 5. A significant overall upward trend in creatinine K_{BD} versus time on CAPD was apparent in 9 patients from whom follow up data were available.

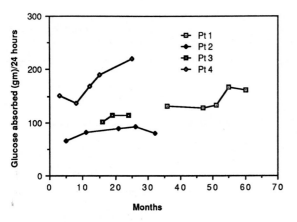
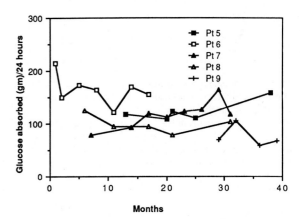

Figure 6. Although patients 4 and 7 ($p < 0.01$) exhibited significant increases in grams glucose absorbed per 24 hr versus time on CAPD, no significant overall trend was apparent in the 9 patient group.

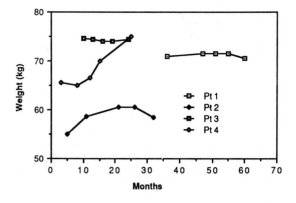
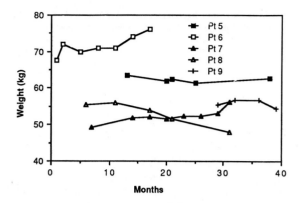

Figure 7. Patients 4, 6, 7 ($p < 0.01$) and patient 2 ($0.01 < p < 0.05$) exhibited significant rises in weight versus time on CAPD. Patient 8 ($p < 0.01$) showed a significant decrease in weight. However no significant overall trend was indicated in the 9 patient group.

increase in permeability for creatinine with long-term CAPD. Mathematical modelling of ultrafiltration indicates that a simultaneous increase or decrease in membrane solute and hydraulic permeability or membrane area may be associated with ultrafiltration loss. Stable mass transfer together with loss of ultrafiltration may be associated with increases in lymphatic drainage. In view of the propensity toward increases in the value of the creatinine mass transfer coefficient it may be that increased solute permeability is the more important cause of ultrafiltration loss in long-term CAPD; this possibility requires further confirmation. However even if this were confirmed there is widespread anecdotal evidence that resting the peritoneum would allow recovery of ultrafiltration capacity.

ACKNOWLEDGEMENTS

The combined data in Tables 1 and 2 and Figures 3 through 7 are based on studies conducted by Dr. R. Kush with the aid of Professor K. Ota, Tokyo Women's Medical College, Dr. K. Sakai of Kitazato University and Dr. Hidai of the Yokohama Clinic; these will be the subject of a more detailed future publication.

NOMENCLATURE

A = membrane area available for mass transfer, cm^2
C = solute concentration, mg/cm^3
CC = iso-osmotic glucose concentration, $mOsm/l$
D = solute diffusion coefficient, cm^2/min
δ = membrane thickness, cm
ΔC = solute concentration difference across the membrane, mg/cm^3
D_M = solute diffusion coefficient within the membrane, cm^2/min

Δp = hydraulic pressure difference, mmHg
$\Delta \pi$ = osmotic pressure difference, mmHg
Gu = urea generation, mg/min, averaged over time Θ
J_S = diffusive solute flux per unit area, mg/cm^2-min
J_{SC} = total convective solute flux, mg/min
J_V = volumetric flux, cm^3/min
K_{BD} = mass transfer coefficient invested with mass transfer area, ml/min
K_M = membrane permeability, cm/min
K_O = mass transfer coefficient, cm/min
Lp = hydraulic permeability, cm^3/min-mm Hg
Θ = urea data collection time, minutes
Q_F = peritoneal ultrafiltration, ml/min
Q_L = peritoneal lymphatic drainage, ml/min
S = solute sieving coefficient
σ = reflection coefficient
t = effective exchange time, min
t_D = dwell time, min
t_I = dialysate infuse time, min
t_O = dialysate drain time, min
V = solute distribution volume, cm^3
x = diffusion distance, cm

Subscripts

B = blood
D = dialysate
i = species i
R = residual
u = urine

Superscripts

O = value at time=0
F = final
t = value at time=t

Diacritical bar denotes average value.

REFERENCES

1. Rubin J, Nolph K, Arfania D, Brown P, Prowant B: Follow up of peritoneal clearances in patients undergoing CAPD. Kidney Int 16: 619–623, 1979.
2. Rodger RSC, Goodship THJ, Nikolakakis N, Ashcroft R, Wilkinson R, Ward M: Sequential measurements of ultrafil-tration capacity and peritoneal clearance show no loss of membrane function in patients treated by CAPD. Kidney Int 28(2): 311, 1985.
3. De Santo NG, Capodisaca G, Senatore T, Cicchetti D, Cirillo D, Damiano M, Giordano C: Stability of peritoneal urea clearances in continuous ambulatory peritoneal dialysis. Int J of Art Organs 2: 193–196, 1979.
4. Von Lillien T, Salusky IB, Alliapoulos JC, Leichter HE, Wilson

M, Hall TL, Fine RN: The effect of chronic CAPD/CCPD treatment and peritonitis on peritoneal clearances in paediatric patients. Paediatric Research 19(4) pt 2: 385(A), 1985.

5. Sang Yong Ahn, dong Cheol Han, Seung Duk Hwang, Hi Bahl Lee: Changes in peritoneal solute transport during long-term continuous ambulatory peritoneal dialysis. Kidney Int 31(1): 248, 1987.

6. Finkelstein FO, Kliger AS, Bastl C, Yap P: Sequential clearance and dialysance measurements in chronic peritoneal dialysis patients. Nephron 18: 342–347, 1977.

7. Gilmour J, Wu G, Khanna R, Schilling H, Mitwalli A, Oreopoulos D: Long term continuous ambularoty peritoneal dialysis. PD Bulletin: april-june 1985.

8. Slingeneyer A, Canaud B, Mion C: Permanent loss of ultrafiltration capacity of the peritoneum in long term peritoneal dialysis: an epidemiological study. Nepron 33: 133–138, 1983.

9. Rottembourg J, Issad B, Mehamha H, Legrain M: Evolution of the ultrafiltration rate during CAPD: role of acetate and lactate buffers. Kidney Int 28(2): 311, 1985.

10. Huarte E, Sepas R, Carmona AR, Fontan MP, Ortega O, Martinez ME, Miguel JL, Socilia LS: Peritoneal membrane failure (PF) as a determinant of the CAPD future (an epidemiologically, functional and pathological study). Kidney Int 28(2): 307, 1985.

11. Raja RM, Kramer MS, Rosenbaum JL, Bolisay C and Krug M: Contrasting changes in solute transport and ultrafiltration with peritonitis in CAPD patients. Trans Am Soc Artif Internal Organs 27: 68–70, 1981.

12. Rubin J, Ray R, Barnes T, Bower J: Peritoneal abnormalities during infectious episodes of continuous ambulatory peritoneal dialysis. Nephron 29: 124–127, 1981.

13. Krediet R, Zuyderhoudt FMJ, Boeschoten EW, Arisz L: Alterations in peritoneal transport of water and solutes during peritonitis in continuous ambulatory peritoneal dialysis patients. Eur J Clin Invest (UK) 17(1): 43–52, 1987.

14. Wideroe T, Smeby LC, Mjaland S, Dahl K, Berg KJ, Aas TW: Long term changes in transperitoneal water transport during CAPD. Nephron 38: 238–247, 1984.

15. Slingeneyer A, Canaud B, Mion C: Permanent loss of ultrafiltration capacity of the peritoneum in long term peritoneal dialysis: an epidemiological study. Nephron 33: 133–138, 1983.

16. Cole CH, Roy D, Prichard S: Ultrafiltration capacity of the peritoneum as a function of peritonitis in patients on CAPD. Kidney Int 25(6): 997, 1984.

17. Lysaght MJ, Farrell PC: Membrane phenomena and mass transfer kinetics in peritoneal dialysis. J Mem Sci (in press).

18. Lysaght MJ, Hallett MD, Farrell PC: Evolution of transport theory in CAPD. Clinical Nephrology (in press).

19. Henderson LW, Nolph KD: Altered permeability of the pe-ritoneal membrane after using hypertonic peritoneal dialysis fluid. J Clin Invest 48: 992–1001, 1969.

20. Babb AL, Johansen MJ, Strand H, Tenckhoff H, Scribner BH: Bi-directional permeability of the human peritoneum to middle molecules. Proc Eur Dial Transplant Assoc 10: 247–262, 1973.

21. Garred L, Canaud B, Farrell PC: A simple kinetic model for assessing peritoneal mass transfer in CAPD. ASAIO J 6(3): 131–137, 1983.

22. Randerson DH, Farrell PC: Long term peritoneal clearance in CAPD. In: Atkins RC, Thomson N, Farrell PC (eds), Peritoneal Dialysis. Churchill Livingstone: pp 22–29, 1981.

23. Spencer P, Farrell PC: Solute and water transfer kinetics in CAPD. In: Gokal (ed), Continuous Ambulatory Peritoneal Dialysis. Churchill Livingstone, Edinburgh: pp 38–55, 1986.

24. Leypoldt JK, Parker HR, Frigon RP, Henderson LW: Molecular size dependence of peritoneal transport. J Lab Clin Med 110(2): 207–216, 1987.

25. Randerson DH, Farrell PC: Mass transfer properties of the human peritoneum. ASAIO J 3: 140–25, 1980.

26. Mactier RA, Khanna R, Twardowski ZJ, Nolph DK: Role of peritoneal cavity lymphatic absorption in peritoneal dialysis. Kidney Int 32: 165–172, 1987.

27. Leypoldt JK, Pust AH, Frigon RP, Henderson LW: Dialysate volume measurements required for determining peritoneal solute transport. Kidney Int: 1987 in review.

28. Dedrick RL, Flessner MF, Collins JM, Schultz JS: Is the peritoneum a membrane? ASAIO J 5(1): 1–8, 1982.

29. Flessner MF, Dedrick RL, Schulz JS: A distributed Model of peritoneal plasma transport: theoretical considerations. AM J Physio 246: 597–607, 1984.

30. Flessner MF, Dedrick RL, Schulz JS: A distributed model of peritoneal-plasma transport: analysis of experimental data in the rat. Am J Physiol 248: 413–424, 1985.

31. Jaffrin MY, Odell RA, Farrell PC: A model of ultrafiltration and glucose mass transfer kinetics in peritoneal dialysis. Artificial Organs 11(3): 198–207, 1987.

32. Khanna R, Oreopoulos D: Complications of peritoneal dialysis other than peritonitis. In: Nolph KD (ed), Peritoneal dialysis. Nijhof: pp 441–524, 1985.

33. Krediet RT, Boeschoten EW, Zuyderhoudt FMJ, Arisz L: Peritoneal transport characteristics of water, low-molecular weight solutes and proteins during long-term CAPD. Peritoneal Dialysis Bulletin 6(2): pp 61–65, 1986.

34. Randerson DH, Chapman GV, Farrell PC: Amino acid and dietary status in CAPD patients. In: Atkins RC, Thompson NM, Farrell PC (eds). Peritoneal dialysis. Churchill Livingstone: pp 179–191, 1981.

35. Weisberg S: Applied linear regression. John Wiley (pub): New York, 1982.

20

THE USA CAPD REGISTRY

CHARACTERISTICS OF PARTICIPANTS AND SELECTED OUTCOME MEASURES FOR THE PERIOD JANUARY 1, 1981, THROUGH AUGUST 31, 1987

ANNE S. LINDBLAD, JOEL W. NOVAK and KARL D. NOLPH

PREFACE

The National Institutes of Health have supported a CAPD Registry since 1981. Since there has been no USA Registry for patients undergoing all forms of chronic dialysis therapy, the USA CAPD Registry was created to monitor certain outcome measures during the rapid growth and development of this relatively newer form of therapy. A portion of the 1988 Registry Report is included in this book for several reasons. First, the report represents the status of the Registry at the time this book was prepared. This may clarify to some extent the state of affairs impacting on the thinking of respetive authors. Secondly, the Report includes cumulative data over the life span of the Registry since 1981 and portrays much of what has happened to CAPD and CCPD over the time period from the first to the third edition of the book.

We are pleased to have this example of the Registry report included in this book.

Gladys Hirschman, M.D.
Director, Chronic Renal Disease Program,
National Institute of Arthritis, Diabetes
      and Digestive and Kidney Diseases,
National Institutes of Health,
Bethesda, Maryland   USA

Karl D. Nolph, M.D.
Director, Division of Nephrology,
Professor of Medicine,
Department of Medicine,
University of Missouri Health Sciences Center,
VA Hospital and Dalton Research Center,
Clinical Coordinator of the CAPD Registry,
Columbia, Missouri   USA

1. INTRODUCTION

1.1. The National CAPD Registry and the Registry Report

The National CAPD Registry, sponsored by the National Institute of Diabetes and Digestive and Kidney Diseases (NIDDK), is responsible for developing information regarding the number of patients receiving CAPD and/or CCPD therapy, their characteristics, the extent of some of the more important treatment-related complications and selected outcomes to the therapy.

Registry operations are conducted through a Clinical Coordinating Center (CCC) at the University of Missouri, under the direction of Karl D. Nolph, M.D., and a Data Coordinating center (DCC) located at The EMMES Corporation in Potomac, Maryland. Joel W. Novak, M.S. serves as principal director of the DCC and Anne S. Lindblad, M.S. serves as project director. The Clinical Coordinating Center acts as liaison between the Registry and the medical community, and specifically assists in information dissemination. The primary responsibility of the Data Coordinating Center is to operate the data collection and processing system, provide epidemiological and biostatistical support, and produce technical reports such as this, in collaboration with Dr. Nolph and his staff at the University of Missouri. Staff of the Kidney-Urology Branch (DKUHD), NIDDK, are collaborators in the project as are members of the Executive Advisory Committee (see Appendix I).

The Registry began operations on a pilot basis in January, 1981 with the participation of 15 centers; and, it became fully operational in October, 1981, with a roster of 184 participating centers. At this writing, 493 clinical centers in the United States participate in the Registry program. The CAPD Registry is scheduled to be discontinued in the Summer of 1988, but will be replaced by a total ESRD Registry which will monitor experiences with all types of therapies in ESRD patients.

This report summarizes data on 24 932 patients received by the Data Coordinating Center from the 493 participating centers as of August 31, 1987. Section 2 describes the size of the Registry and documents its growth. Further, it defines the patient cohorts that are available for analysis. In Sections 3, 4 and 5 we describe the characteristics of the patients who have been registered, the complications of treatment that they have experienced and outcomes of their treatment e.g. death, transfer to another modality and transplantation.

2. REGISTRY PATIENT POPULATION

As of August 31, 1987 when the Registry's files were closed for the current analysis, 24 932 patients had been registered with the National CAPD Registry. The majority of the patients, 92% (23 043), initially received CAPD; 1672 (7%) initially received CCPD. An additional 217 patients were reported to have initially received combination therapy with both CAPD and CCPD.

2.1. Classification of patients

As might be expected, patients participating in the Registry vary widely. Two characteristics of unusual significance when analyzing patient responses to treatment are: experience on CAPD or CCPD prior to being registered and experience with an alternate ESRD therapy, prior to registration. Patients who received CAPD or CCPD prior to registration must be regarded as the survivors of a larger group of patients, who should not be grouped with newly treated patients when analyzing outcomes of CAPD or CCPD therapy. Similarly, patients who are known to have received (and likely failed) an alternate form of replacement therapy prior to commencing CAPD/CCPD should also be considered separately from previously untreated patients in analyses of outcomes since they may have very different prognoses.

To facilitate a discussion of the patient subgroups represented in the Registry, patients are classified with respect to prior CAPD, CCPD or other ESRD therapy. The classification scheme identifies four subgroups of particular interest:

1A – No replacement therapy for ESRD prior to registration.

1B – No CAPD/CCPD prior to registration but prior experience with alternative forms of replacement therapy.

2A – Experience with CAPD/CCPD prior to registration.

2B – Experience with both CAPD/CCPD and an alternative form of replacement therapy prior to registration.

Reference is made in all of our reports to these categories when describing the group(s) that are analyzed and the experiences reported.

2.2. Registration by class

Of the 24 932 patients ever registered, 17 845 (72%) were registered at the time that CAPD or CCPD therapy was initiated (viz. Classes 1A (8373) and 1B (9472) as defined above). The remaining 7087 patients (Class 2A and 2B) had been diagnosed earlier and treated with some other form of ESRD therapy (see Exhibit 2–1).

2.3. Registration by class and year

Exhibit 2–2 details the yearly accrual of patients receiving CAPD and CCPD from the time of the Registry's activation. As of August 31, 1987, a total of 23 043 patients had been registered on CAPD. Note that this number reflects a 318% overall increase in the number of registrants over the 1981–1982 figure of 5509. The yearly increases of approximately 20–30% which have been seen are thought to be the result of increases in the number of participating centers, the total number of ESRD patients and the fraction of ESRD patients being offered CAPD therapy. CCPD registrations have also been rising; more CCPD patients were registered in 1986 than in any previous year.

2.4. Patient follow-up and data currency

Eighty-eight percent of the 24 932 registered patients (22 040) have follow-up information available and consequently are available for analysis in this report. Of those with follow-up, 14 967 received CAPD therapy (6945 Class 1A and 8022 Class 1B) and 1013 received CCPD therapy (515 Class 1A and 498 Class 1B) as the initial treatment for end stage renal disease (see Exhibit 2–3).

Exhibit 2–4 summarizes the status of patients reported to be on CAPD/CCPD at the time of last reported contact. As of August 31, 1987, 82% of participating centers (405/ 493) had submitted follow-up reports regarding patient contacts during 1987; those centers are considered to be fully active. Eighty-eight centers had not submitted follow-up reports in 1987 for any of their patients and are considered to be 'provisionally inactive'. Among the 405 actively participating centers, 93% of patients (8990/9711) last reported to be on CAPD/CCPD have data reflecting their status at some time during the preceding 12 month period (September 1, 1986 – August 31, 1987). Over three-quarters of the patients 666/876) with last contact prior to September 1, 1986 were patients who transferred to another center. Note that if the patient's new center is not a Registry participant, further follow-up is considered unlikely. An additional 1204 patients last reported as continuing on CAPD/CCPD are no longer being followed as the participating center is no longer an active Registry participant.

Exhibit 2–5 graphically illustrates the number of patients registered versus the number of patients with current follow-up by class of patient as defined earlier. The latter group includes patients continuing CAPD/CCPD and for whom information was received in the last 12 months, as well as patients who discontinued CAPD/CCPD as of the last report. For Class 1A and 1B patients data currency is in excess of 94%; for all classes of patients data currency exceeds 88%.

2.5. Registry coverage

While, the true number of patients receiving CAPD in the United States is not known, reports of the Health Care Financing Administration (HCFA) are available which indicate the number of patients reimbursed for CAPD as of December 31st of each year. Assuming HCFA's reports provide a reasonable estimate of the true size of the CAPD population, we have estimated the Registry's coverage by comparting such data to the number of currently active patients reported by the Registry. Note that information provided by the HCFA does not report on CCPD patients prior to 1984. Exhibit 2–6 presents data on the number of patients receiving CAPD and CCPD; as of December 31st of each year, as reported by HCFA and estimated by the National CAPD Registry. Note that the data suggest that the National CAPD Registry has enrolled and followed approximately half of the CAPD population in the United States, through 1986.

2.6. Census and flow of CAPD patients

The National CAPD Registry has undergone constant change and growth since its inauguration in 1981. Every year an increasing number of patients receiving CAPD are registered. Notwithstanding the fact that patients routinely leave the Registry when they receive a kidney transplant, transfer to an alternate replacement therapy or die, the number of patients under follow-up at the end of each year has increased such that there has been an estimated four-fold increase since 1981. Figure 2–7 illustrates the yearly census and flow of CAPD Registry patients. For the purposes of Figure 2–7, patients who leave the Registry but return to CAPD/CCPD within 8 months are counted as continuing on CAPD/CCPD. Note that for later analysis regarding transfers off of CAPD/CCPD, patients who have discontinued CAPD/CCPD for more than 30 days are considered to have permanently transferred.

When the Registry began in 1981, a bolus of patients was entered as newly recruited centers registered patients already receiving CAPD. In 1983, a decrease in absolute numbers of new registrants was observed, as the influx of new centers stabilized. However, since 1983 a steady increase in registrations has been observed, as new centerss continue to join the Registry, with the result that in 1986 newly registered patients increased markedly to 5181. Note that new registrations exceed patient losses in every year.

Exhibit 2–1. Number of patients registered by class and type of dialysis

Type of dialysis	Class of patient				
	1A	1B	2A	2B	Total
CAPD	7695	8822	2557	3969	23 043
CCPD	592	569	249	262	1 672
CAPD and CCPD	86	81	26	24	217
Total	8373	9472	2832	4255	24 932

Exhibit 2–2. Number of patients registered and year of registration by class

Class	1981-1982	1983	1984	1985	1986	1987*	Total
CAPD							
1A	921	888	1353	1639	1823	1071	7 695
1B	1999	1352	1375	1508	1617	971	8 822
2A	658	153	242	446	596	462	2 557
2B	1931	304	401	403	573	357	3 969
Total	5509	2697	3371	3996	4609	2861	23 043
CCPD							
1A	33	42	83	95	175	164	592
1B	68	72	96	75	146	112	569
2A	13	23	15	17	101	80	249
2B	53	30	31	28	71	49	262
Total	167	167	225	215	493	405	1672

* Includes information received through August 31, 1987.
Note: Table excludes the 217 patients treated by a combination of CAPD and CCPD

Exhibit 2–3. Number of patients with follow-up by class and type of dialysis

Type of dialysis	Class of patient				
	1A	1B	2A	2B	Total
CAPD	6945	8022	2136	3304	20 407
CCPD	514	498	219	221	1 453
CAPD and CCPD	68	67	23	22	180
Total	7528	8587	2378	3547	22 040

Exhibit 2–4. Last contact and status according to activity classification of center for patients last reported to be on CAPD/CCPD

Date of last reported contact	Status at last contact		
	On CAPD/CCPD with follow-up data	Transferred to another center	Registered only
Active centers (405)			
1981–1983	1	203	98
1984	0	151	9
1985 (Jan – April)	1	46	22
1985 (May – Aug)	1	60	9
1985 (Sept – Dec)	24	64	14
1986 (Jan – April)	13	72	11
1986 (May – Aug)	1	70	6
1986 (Sept – Dec)	93	109	32
1987 (Jan – April)	504	34	0
1987 (May – Aug)	7018	31	1169
Total	7656	860	1370
Provisionally inactive centers (88)			
1981–1983	262	22	249
1984	96	20	18
1985 (Jan – April)	23	7	2
1985 (May – Aug)	81	13	29

Exhibit 2–4. Continued

Date of last reported contact	Status at last contact		
	On CAPD/CCPD with follow-up data	Transferred to another center	Registered only
1985 (Sept – Dec)	55	5	18
1986 (Jan – April)	96	2	54
1986 (May – Aug)	67	1	32
1986 (Sept – Dec)	32	0	20
1987 (Jan – April)	0	0	0
1987 (May – Aug)	0	0	0
Total	712	70	422

Exhibit 2–5. Currency of data by class of case

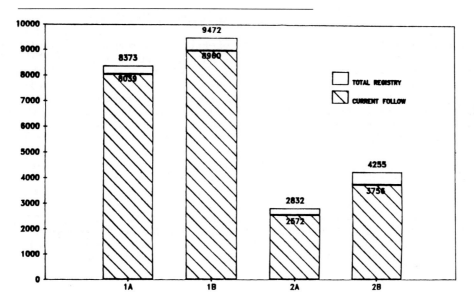

Exhibit 2–6. Number of patients receiving CAPD/CCPD at year end

CAPD/CCPD	1981	1982	1983	1984	1985	1986	1987*
HCFA**	4347	6523	8532	10 854	12 189	13 220	N.A.
Registry	1949	3554	4070	5 003	6 122	7 184	7600
% Registry coverage	45	54	48	46	50	54	N.A.

  * On CAPD or CCPD as of August 31, 1987.
** Includes patients reported to be on CCPD in 1984, 1985, and 1986.

Exhibit 2–7. Census and flow of the national CAPD registry by year* 1981–1987**

	1981	1982	1983	1984	1985	1986	1987
Newly registered patients	2276	3411	2871	3622	4261	5181	3310
Transplants	31	164	265	361	476	694	341
Transfers	152	627	737	767	971	1136	585
Deaths	106	428	630	840	1028	1346	715
On CAPD/CCPD as of December 31st of each year	1949	3554	4070	5003	6122	7184	7600

* Totals as of December 31st of each year.
** Reflects the last reported status of all Registry patients received by the Data Coordinating Center as of August 31, 1987.

3. PATIENT CHARACTERISTICS

This section details the characteristics of the 22 040 patients for whom outcome information is available, and who form the basis of the analyses that follow. At the time of registration 20 319 of those patients were receiving CAPD; 1443 were receiving CCPD. As not all demographic data are available for all patients, patient totals on which percentages are based may vary slightly from characteristic to characteristic. Patients who reported using a combination of CAPD and CCPD are not reflected in this summary or in the outcome evaluations that follow.

Sex, age, race and primary renal disease type are summarized in Exhibit 3–1 for all CAPD and CCPD patients, irrespective of therapy received prior to registration. Overall, male patients outnumber female patients in the Registry; and, white patients outnumber blacks and those of 'other' races. The median age of Registry patients is 52 yrs, and diabetic glomerulosclerosis, reported in 26% of patients, is the most frequently cited type of primary renal disease.

Exhibit 3–1 compares the distribution of patient characteristics of all persons with end-stage renal disease (ESRD) as reported by the Health Care Financing Administration [1]. Several differences in these populations are noteworthy. Whereas diabetic glomerulosclerosis is the most frequently cited primary renal disease type in the CAPD Registry, accounting for 26% of Registry patients, only 18% of the total ESRD population are so diagnosed. Chronic glomerulonephritis and hypertensive renal disease are more commonly reported in the ESRD population, occurring in 23% and 22% of this cohort. These two disease types account for only 17% and 15% of Registry patients respectively. The Registry population appears to be younger with a higher percentage of white patients. Sixty-nine percent of Registry patients are under 40 yrs of age compared to 53% of all ESRD patients, and approximately three-quarters (76%) of Registry patients are white, whereas only 64% of all ESRD patients are white. The distribution of sex appears to be similar between the Registry and the ESRD cohorts, with males accounting for more than half of both populations.

3.1. Sex and age distributions

Distributions of age by sex are provided separately for patients whose initial therapy was CAPD and CCPD (see Exhibits 3–2 and 3–3). Males and females are evenly distributed on CCPD therapy while a higher proportion of males (55%) are reported for CAPD. CCPD patients tend to be younger then CAPD patients, with 17% of CCPD patients being under the age of 20 yrs. In contrast only 5% of the CAPD population is under the age of 20 yrs. From data presented in Exhibit 3–2, it is evident that males and females on CAPD are similarly distributed among age groups. Age distribution on CCPD is also similar for males and females with only minor differences observed in the < 5 yr of age category and 20–29 yr-olds. Five percent of males are less than 5 yrs of age, while 2% of females fall into this group. Twelve percent of the females receiving CCPD are between the age 20–29, while 7% of males are in their 20's. The median age for males and females on CCPD is 47 yrs and 48 yrs, respectively.

3.2. Race and age distribution

Distributions of race by age are also provided separately for CAPD (Exhibit 3–4) and CCPD (Exhibit 3–5) patients. Race categories are similarly distributed among patients using CAPD and CCPD, with three-quarters of patients reported as white. As noted in earlier Registry reports, white patients tend to be older with 36% being 60 yrs of age or older, while 23% of blacks and 'other' races fall into this age group. Patients classified in the 'other' race category tend to be younger; 19% of patients were under 30 yrs of age compared to 14% of white and blacks.

3.3. Primary renal disease — CAPD

The Registry collects frequency information on 16 primary renal disease diagnoses. Patients, whose primary renal disease diagnoses do not fall into one of these categories, are classified as 'other'. As indicated in Exhibit 3–6, five categories of renal disease account for 73% of all patients on CAPD: diabetic glomerulosclerosis (26%), chronic glomerulonephritis (17%), hypertensive renal disease (15%), interstitial nephritis/chronic pyelonephritis (8%), and polycystic kidney(s) (6%). The remaining 27% of patients are distributed among 11 diagnostic categories, no one of which accounts for more than 4% of all patients.* Note that 11% of patients could not be classified into any one of the 16 disease types used; and, 6% of patients are coded as disease type unknown.

The distributions by primary renal disease of patients with follow-up information who were registered in 1981–82, 1983, 1984, 1985 and 1986 are given in Exhibit 3–6. Note that only 64% (1,830/2,861) of CAPD patients re-gistered in the first 8 months of 1987 are reported, as follow-up information has not been received for many of the newly registered patients. As can be seen, there continues to be an increase in the proportion of patients with diabetic glomerulosclerosis who enter the Registry each year. In 1981–83, 21.4% of the patients entered were diagnosed with diabetic glomerulosclerosis increasing to 30.9% in the first eight months of 1986. Corresponding decreases are observed in patients with chronic glomerulonephritis and polycystic kidney(s). A noticeable increase in the percentage of patients entering the Registry after 1984 with interstitial nephritis/chronic pyelonephritis is also observed. These results are essentially identical for all registered patients irrespective of follow-up information status.

Exhibit 3–1. Percent of patients with selected characteristics by type of therapy

| Selected characteristic | Therapy type | | Total (n=21 860) | Total ESRD [1] (n=90 621) |
	CAPD (n=20 407)	CCPD (n=1 453)		
Sex				
Male	55	51	55	53
Female	45	49	45	47
Race				
White	76	74	76	64
Black	17	20	17	31
Other	7	6	7	4
Primary renal disease type				
Diabetic glomerulosclerosis	26	27	26	18
Chronic glomerulonephritis	17	15	17	23
Hypertensive renal disease	15	11	15	22
Interstitial nephritis/chronic pyelonephritis	8	8	8	*
Polycystic kidney(s)	6	5	6	*
All other types	28	33	28	*
Age (yr)				
<5	1	4	1	<1
5–9	1	4	1	<1
10–19	3	9	4	1
20–39	25	24	25	18
40–59	38	30	38	34
>60	33	30	33	47
Median age	53	47	52	*

1 End-Stage Renal Disease Patient Profile Tables – 1985. Contemporary Dialysis and Nephrology. March 1987, p. 34–40.
* Not provided.

---

* The reader should note that the diagnoses reported are the clinical impressions given by the attending physician and do not conform to uniform definitions.

Exhibit 3–2. CAPD: Age* distribution by sex

Age group in years	Total patients		Sex	
	N	(%)	Male %	Female (%)
<1	75	0.4	0.3	0.4
1–4	105	0.5	0.6	0.5
5–9	166	0.8	0.9	0.8
10–14	257	1.3	1.2	1.3
15–19	335	1.7	1.4	2.0
20–29	1843	9.1	7.9	10.6
30–39	3111	15.4	15.8	14.9
40–49	3203	15.8	16.0	15.6
50–59	4449	22.0	21.2	23.0
60–69	4465	22.0	22.9	21.0
70–79	1942	9.6	10.2	8.8
80–89	287	1.4	1.6	1.2
≥90	8	<0.1	<0.01	<0.01
Total patients	20 246		11 189	9056
Percent patients	(100)		(55)	(45)

* Age at time of registration.

Exhibit 3–3. CCPD: Age* distribution by sex

Age group in years	Total patients		Sex	
	N	(%)	Male %	Female (%)
<1	17	1.2	1.6	0.7
1–4	33	2.3	3.3	1.3
5–9	50	3.5	2.9	4.1
10–14	69	4.8	5.2	4.4
15–19	59	4.1	4.1	4.1
20–29	133	9.2	6.9	11.7
30–39	219	15.2	15.8	14.6
40–49	184	12.8	14.0	11.5
50–59	246	17.1	16.9	17.3
60–69	280	19.5	19.9	19.0
70–79	121	8.4	8.2	8.7
80–89	26	1.8	1.4	2.3
≥90	2	0.1	0	0.3
Total patients	1439		735	704
Percent patients	(100)		(51)	(49)

* Age at time of registration.

Exhibit 3–4. CAPD: Age* distribution by race

Age group in years	Total patients N	Total patients (%)	White (%)	Black (%)	Other (%)
<1	75	0.4	0.4	0.3	0.4
1–4	105	0.5	0.5	0.4	1.0
5–9	166	0.8	0.8	0.6	1.4
10–14	257	1.3	1.2	1.0	2.9
15–19	335	1.7	1.6	1.8	2.2
20–29	1840	9.1	9.0	8.9	10.8
30–39	3110	15.4	14.8	17.8	15.2
40–49	3194	15.8	14.3	20.8	19.8
50–59	4449	22.0	21.2	25.1	22.8
60–69	4465	22.1	23.5	17.8	16.5
70–79	1938	9.6	11.0	4.8	6.1
80–89	287	1.4	1.6	0.6	0.9
≥90	8	<0.1	<0.1	<0.1	0
Total patients	20 229		15 423	3536	1270
Percent of patients	(100)		(76)	(17)	(6)

* Age at time of registration.

Exhibit 3–5. CCPD: Age* distribution by race

Age group in years	Total patients N	Total patients (%)	White (%)	Black (%)	Other (%)
<1	17	1.2	0.9	1.4	3.4
1–4	33	2.3	2.2	1.0	6.8
5–9	50	3.5	3.3	2.5	9.1
10–14	69	4.8	5.0	4.2	4.6
15–19	60	4.2	3.6	5.3	8.0
20–29	133	9.2	9.4	8.8	9.1
30–39	219	15.2	15.1	17.9	8.0
40–49	183	12.7	11.9	15.4	13.6
50–59	246	17.1	17.3	17.2	14.8
60–69	280	19.5	20.1	17.2	19.3
70–79	121	8.4	9.4	6.3	3.4
80–89	26	1.8	1.8	2.5	0
≥90	2	0.1	0.1	0.4	0
Total patients	1439		1066	285	88
Percent of patients	(100)		(74)	(20)	(6)

* Age at time of registration.

Exhibit 3–6. CAPD: Distribution of patients by primary renal disease type according to year of registration

Renal disease type	Total patients N	(%)	1981–1983 (%)	1984 (%)	1985 (%)	1986 (%)	1987* (%)
Diabetic glomerulosclerosis	5092	(25.9)	21.4	25.6	28.0	29.7	30.9
Chronic glomerulonephritis	3377	(17.2)	21.3	17.0	14.4	14.3	13.6
Hypertensive Renal Disease	3024	(15.4)	16.0	14.2	14.5	15.7	16.1
Polycystic kidney(s)	1247	(6.4)	7.5	6.3	5.6	5.5	5.3
Interstitial nephritis/ chronic pyelonephritis	1522	(7.8)	6.6	8.7	8.7	8.3	7.9
Systemic immunological disease with renal involvement	569	(2.9)	3.1	3.1	3.1	2.5	2.4
Rapidly progressing glomerulonephritis	440	(2.2)	2.3	2.2	2.2	2.3	2.0
Obstructive uropathy	392	(2.0)	2.4	1.6	1.9	1.9	1.6
Familial nephritis	187	(1.0)	1.3	0.8	0.6	0.7	0.9
Amyloidosis with renal involvement	106	(0.5)	0.6	0.4	0.6	0.5	0.5
Renal infarct, 2nd to vascular occlusion	110	(0.6)	0.5	0.6	0.6	0.5	0.8
Aplastic-hypoplastic kidney(s)	93	(0.5)	0.6	0.4	0.5	0.2	0.6
Stone forming renal disease	82	(0.4)	0.6	0.4	0.4	0.4	0.1
Nephrectomy, 2nd to cancer	80	(0.4)	0.4	0.4	0.4	0.4	0.4
Gouty nephropathy	37	(0.2)	0.2	0.3	0.1	0.2	0.1
Bilateral cortical necrosis	23	(0.1)	0.1	0.1	0.2	0.2	0.1
Other	2049	(10.6)	8.9	11.6	12.0	10.4	11.4
Unknown	1219	(6.2)	6.3	6.3	6.2	6.3	5.6
Number of patients	19 649		7103	2821	3662	4233	1830
Percent of patients	100		36	14	19	22	9

* Follow-up information received as of August 31, 1987.

4. COMPLICATIONS OF TREATMENT

The National CAPD Registry routinely collects information on major complications associated with continuous peritoneal dialysis: peritonitis, exit site and tunnel infections and catheter replacements. Complications occurring in Class 1 and Class 2 patients are considered separately as the Registry has no knowledge of the problems experienced by Class 2 patients prior to registration. Note that the available data may overstate the number of episodes experienced by some patients as there are no clear criteria for differentiating between a new, distinct episode and the persistence of a previously reported complication.

Exhibits 4–1 through 4–9 detail complication rates and probability distributions for the time to first episode of selected complications. Rates are based on patient yrs of observation [2]. Class 1 patient yrs are calculated from the day CAPD/CCPD therapy was initiated to the last reported contact date or date of CAPD/CCPD termination. Observation times for Class 2 patients are calculated from the date of entry on the Registry to the date of last contact or CAPD/CCPD termination.

Rates per patient yr are calculated as follows:

Rate per patient year =

$$= \frac{\text{Total \# of Episodes Reported by the Cohort}}{\text{Total Years Cohort Under Observation}}$$

The probability distributions which reflect the time of first episode of an event were estimated using the methods

of Kaplan-Meier [3]. Distributions of first complications were calculated for Class 1 patients only, as Class 2 patients may have had a first event prior to being followed by the Registry.

Probability distributions have also been calculated separately by year of registration to assess possible time trends. As dates of complications were not reported prior to 1984 and are no longer reported as of October 31, 1986, times to first episode were estimated using the median of the interval in which the event was reported as the date of event.

4.1. Peritonitis — CAPD

The National CAPD Registry defines peritonitis as turbid dialysate with white blood count greater than 100 cells per cubic millimeter. Abdominal symptoms and/or positive culture are not required for diagnosis of peritonitis. Overall the peritonitis rate per patient yr (ppy) for CAPD patients is 1.4 events. Class 1 patients experienced 1.3 peritonitis episodes ppy (Exhibit 4–1). The probability of Class 1 patients experiencing at least one episode of peritonitis is found to be 40% by the end of the sixth month of therapy; at the end of 24 months of therapy, the chances that a patient will have experienced at least one episode of peritonitis doubles to 79% (Exhibit 4–2). The median time to first peritonitis is estimated to be 8.4 months.

An increase in reported peritonitis episodes has been observed among patients registered in the first 8 months of 1987. The estimated peritonitis rate per patient yr for

Class 1A patients in this cohort is 1.4 events, compared with 1.2 and 1.3 episodes ppy for patients registered in 1986 and 1985 respectively (Exhibit 4–3). The reason for this apparent increase is not clear, although the introduction by the Registry of new data collection forms, which require less rigorous documentation of peritonitis episodes, may have influenced reporting practices. Note also that the cumulative rates among calender cohorts are not strictly comparable, as earlier cohorts have had more time for the development of repetitive complications.

The probability that a Class 1 CAPD patient who entered the Registry prior to 1984 experienced the first episode of peritonitis in the first 6 months on therapy is 43%; for the cohort registered after 1983 it is 38%. This observed decline in the probability of first peritonitis is maintained at 12 months, but disappears at 18 months (Exhibit 4–4). Note that estimates beyond 18 months are not considered reliable, as follow-up data for patients in the later cohort is not sufficiently mature.

4.2. Exit site tunnel infections — CAPD

Differentiation between exit site and tunnel infections is difficult to determine in the usual clinical setting. Accordingly, the Registry classifies these events as one complication. The rate per patient year of observation for exit site/tunnel infections was 0.6 regardless of patient classification (Exhibit 4–1). Note that less than one quarter of the patients experience the first episode in the first 6 months of therapy and the probability that a patient has experienced at least one event by the end of the second year is less than 50% (Exhibit 4–5). The median time to first episode of exit site/tunnel infection is estimated to be 26.7 months.

The possibility of a small decrease in the number of exit site/tunnel infections reported for Class 1A patients is suggested, as a rate of 0.6 was observed for 1981-1982 and ppy rates of 0.5 or less were observed in successive yrs through 1985. A similar observation is reported for Class 1B patients (Exhibit 4–3). An increase in the number of exit site tunnel infections reported has been observed for both the 1986 and the 1987 cohorts. However, a decrease in the probability of experiencing a first episode of exit site/tunnel infection continues to be noted for patients registered after 1983 compared to patients registered in 1981–1983. At one year, the probability of experiencing a first episode of exit site/tunnel infection is 37% for patients registered in 1981–1983; for patients registered after 1983, it is 30%. Note that confidence intervals are non-overlapping throughout the 18 month period.

4.3. Catheter replacements — CAPD

Participating clinical centers are asked to report on the frequency of catheter replacements for those patients continuing with CAPD. Note that catheters that are removed due to failure and not replaced are not reported, nor is it likely that early catheter failures, i.e. prior to the first successful exchange are reported to the Registry. For these reasons, the catheter replacement rates reported by the Registry are considered to be underestimates of the true rate of catheter failure.

Overall catheter replacement rates for Class 1 patients

were observed to be 0.2 events ppy; for Class 2 patients the observed rate is 0.3 events ppy (Exhibit 4–1). The probability of having at least one catheter replaced by end of two yrs of therapy was 32% (Exhibit 4–6). Unlike peritonitis and exit site/tunnel infections, catheter replacement rates and probabilities of the first replacement occurring do not appear to vary by yr of registration (Exhibits 4–3 and 4–4). However the probability of a first catheter replacement within six months was 12 percent for patients registered in 1981–1983 compared to 9 percent for patients registered in 1984–1986.

4.4. Any complications — CAPD

Exhibit 4–7 illustrates the probability distribution estimate of the time to a first episode of peritonitis, exit site/tunnel infection or catheter replacement. Note that the chance that a CAPD patient will experience at least one of these three complications is 53% at 6 months. By the end of the second yr of therapy, 88% of patients are expected to have experienced at least one of these three types of complications.

4.5. CCPD complications

Similar data summaries have been prepared for patients receiving CCPD. Complication rates and probability distribution estimates of the time to first complication are presented in Exhibits 4–8 and 4–9. As patients are not randomly allocated to treatment with CAPD or CCPD, comparisons of the two modalties are subject to selection biases; and hence, caution should be used when evaluating differences in complication rates and probability distributions for the two modalities.

As illustrated in Exhibit 4–8, complication rates per patient yr across all categories were lower for Class 1 CCPD patients than for Class 2 CCPD patients. As in CAPD, peritonitis is the most frequently encountered complication among CCPD patients; and, approximately half (54%) of all Class 1 CCPD patients are expected to have experienced at least one episode of peritonitis by the end of their first yr of therapy (Exhibit 4–9). First catheter replacements are expected to occur in 21% of CCPD patients by the end of one yr of therapy; 29% of CCPD patients will have had a catheter replacement by the end of two yrs of therapy. Nearly half of all CCPD patients will have had a first exit site/tunnel infection by the end of two yrs.

4.6. Hospitalizations — CAPD/CCPD

Due to the restructuring of the data collection procedures of the National CAPD Registry, requests for detailed information on days hospitalized for CAPD/CCPD patients were terminated after October 31, 1986. Exhibit 4–10 presents a summary of mean days hospitalized per patient yr based only on information received through October 31, 1986.

CAPD and CCPD patients are reported to be hospitalized for 19 and 20.8 days ppy respectively for all causes, of which 8 days (42%) are directly attributed to CAPD related complications such as peritonitis, exit site/tunnel infections, catheter replacements, etc. Patients with CAPD or CCPD experience prior to entering the Registry (Class 2) are reported to have at least an additional day ppy of hospitalization for CAPD or CCPD related causes (Exhibit 4–10).

Exhibit 4–1. CAPD: Occurrence* of selected complications by class of patients

Complication	Total	1A	1B	2A	2B
*Rates**					
Peritonitis	1.4	1.3	1.3	1.6	1.6
Exit site/ tunnel infections	0.6	0.6	0.6	0.6	0.6
Catheter replacement	0.2	0.2	0.2	0.3	0.3
Based on					
Patient	20 265	6925	7985	2113	3242
Patient-years	24 292	7924	9848	2153	4366

* Number of episodes per patient-years of observation.

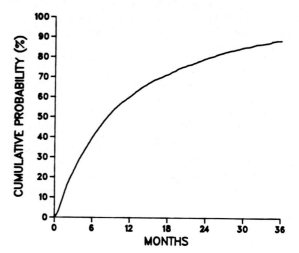

Exhibit 4–2. CAPD: Cumulative probability of experiencing first episode of peritonitis (class 1 patients only)

Cumulative probabilities and 95% Confidence Intervals (C.I.) for Exhibit 4–2.

	Months on CAPD					
	6	12	18	24	30	36
Cumulative Prob.	40	60	71	79	85	88
95% C.I.	(39, 41)	(59, 61)	(70, 73)	(78, 81)	(83, 86)	(87, 90)

Exhibit 4–3. CAPD: Complication rates* by year of registration

	1981	1982	1983	1984	1985	1986	1987**
Class 1A patients							
Peritonitis	1.3	1.4	1.3	1.3	1.3	1.2	1.4
Exit site/tunnel inf.	0.6	0.6	0.5	0.5	0.5	0.6	0.9
Catheter replacement	0.2	0.3	0.3	0.2	0.2	0.2	0.3
Patients	177	679	851	1309	1554	1696	663
Patient years	338	1188	1295	1834	1806	1296	165
Class 1B patients							
Peritonitis	1.3	1.4	1.3	1.3	1.3	1.3	1.5
Exit site/tunnel inf.	0.6	0.6	0.6	0.5	0.5	0.6	0.7
Catheter replacement	0.2	0.2	0.2	0.2	0.2	0.2	0.3
Patients	424	1405	1313	1399	1423	1512	586
Patient years	864	2249	2106	1805	1582	1103	141

* Number of episodes per patient year.
** Reflects information received through August 31, 1987.

Exhibit 4-4. CAPD: Cumulative probabilities and 95% Confidence Intervals (C.I.) of experiencing selected events for the first time by year registered

	Months from initiation of CAPD					
	6		12		18	
Events and year of registration	Prob.	95% C.I.	Prob.	95% C.I.	Prob.	95% C.I.
Peritonitis						
1981–1983	43	(42, 45)	63	(61, 64)	72	(71, 74)
1984–1987*	38	(37, 39)	59	(57, 60)	71	(69, 73)
Exit site/tunnel inf.						
1981–1983	26	(25, 28)	37	(35, 39)	45	(43, 47)
1984–1987*	19	(18, 20)	30	(29, 32)	38	(36, 40)
Catheter Replacement						
1981–1983	12	(11, 13)	19	(18, 21)	26	(24, 28)
1984–1987*	9	(8, 9)	17	(16, 18)	24	(23, 26)
Any of above						
1981–1983	59	(57, 60)	74	(73, 76)	84	(83, 85)
1984–1987*	51	(49, 52)	71	(70, 72)	81	(80, 83)

* As of August 31, 1987

Exhibit 4-5. CAPD: Cumulative probability of experiencing first exit site/tunnel infection (class 1 patients only)

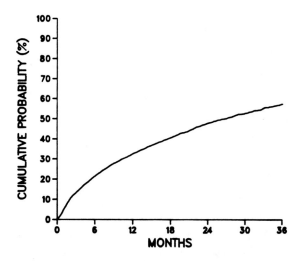

Cumulative probabilities and 95% Confidence Intervals (C.I.) for Exhibit 4-5.

	Months on CAPD					
	6	12	18	24	30	36
Cumulative Prob.	21	32	40	48	53	57
95% C.I.	(21, 22)	(31, 34)	(39, 42)	(46, 50)	(50, 55)	(55, 60)

Exhibit 4-6. CAPD: Cumulative probability of experiencing first catheter replacement (class 1 patients only)

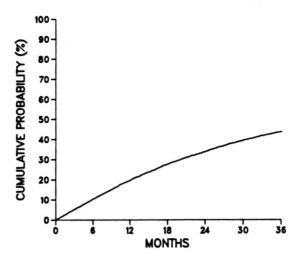

Cumulative probabilities and 95% Confidence Intervals (C.I.) for Exhibit 4–6.

	Months on CAPD					
	6	*12*	*18*	*24*	*30*	*36*
Cumulative Prob.	10	18	25	32	37	42
95% C.I.	(9, 10)	(17, 18)	(23, 26)	(30, 33)	(35, 39)	(40, 45)

Exhibit 4-7. CAPD: Cumulative probability of experiencing first complication (class 1 patients only)

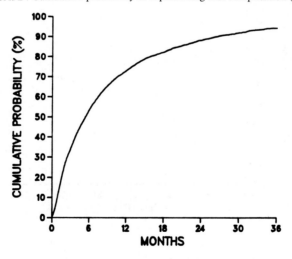

Cumulative probabilities and 95% Confidence Intervals (C.I.) for Exhibit 4–7.

	Months on CAPD					
	6	*12*	*18*	*24*	*30*	*36*
Cumulative Prob.	53	73	82	88	92	94
95% C.I.	(52, 54)	(72, 74)	(81, 83)	(87, 89)	(91, 93)	(93, 95)

* Peritonitis, exit site/tunnel infection, catheter replacement.

Exhibit 4–8. CCPD: Occurrence* of selected complications by class of patients (class 1 patients only)

Complication	Total	Class of patient			
		1A	*1B*	*2A*	*2B*
*Rates**					
Peritonitis	1.3	1.1	1.2	1.5	1.6
Exit site/ tunnel infections	0.6	0.5	0.6	0.7	0.6
Catheter replacement	0.3	0.2	0.3	0.5	0.3
Based on					
Patient	1446	515	496	217	218
Patient-years	1248	401	504	131	213

* Number of episodes per patient-years of observation.

Exhibit 4–9. CCPD: Cumulative probabilities and 95% Confidence Intervals (c.i.) of experiencing selected events for the first time by number of months on CCPD (class 1 patients only)

Number of months from initiation of CCPD	Event type							
	Peritonitis		*Exit site/tunnel infection*		*Catheter replacement*		*Any complication*	
	Prob.	*95% C.I.*	*Prob.*	*95% C.I.*	*Prob.*	*95% C.I.*	*Prob.*	*95% C.I.*
6	35	(31, 38)	20	(16, 23)	11	(8, 13)	49	(45, 52)
12	54	(49, 60)	29	(24, 34)	21	(17, 26)	69	(64, 73)
18	64	(57, 70)	40	(33, 47)	26	(20, 34)	78	(72, 83)
24	75	(67, 82)	48	(39, 56)	29	(22, 38)	87	(80, 91)

Exhibit 4–10. Mean days hospitalized per patient year of observation

Class	*CAPD*		*CCPD*	
	All causes	*CAPD Complications*	*All causes*	*CCPD complications*
1A	19.4	7.0	19.8	7.4
1B	18.8	7.3	21.1	7.8
2A	21.2	8.5	24.2	11.9
2B	19.8	9.0	20.0	9.2
Total	19.4	7.7	20.8	8.3

5. TERMINATION OF CONTINUOUS PERITONEAL DIALYSIS

For the most part, patients terminate CAPD or CCPD therapy for one of three reasons:
- Transfer to another type of dialysis.
- Transplantation.
- Death.

On rare occasions CAPD/CCPD may be terminated because of a return of kidney function or because a patient refuses further therapy for end stage renal disease with no return of kidney function.

Patient transfers are considered to have occurred when a change to another dialysis modality is made with no intention to return to peritoneal dialysis or when a transfer of at least a four week duration is reported. Transfer to another replacement therapy often represents CAPD/CCPD failure – while the same cannot be said for transplants that are performed. Transplantation and transfer are routinely reported for patients followed by the Registry. Patient death is reported to the Registry only if it occurs while the patient is still receiving CAPD or CCPD – or if it occurs within two weeks of transfer to another therapy.

Probability distributions portraying the cumulative probability over time of transfer to another replacement therapy, transplantation, and death are estimated using the methods of Kaplan-Meier [3]. It is important to note that these probability distributions are not additive, in part due to the reporting of multiple events on a single patient. For example, patients who transfer to another modality and die within two weeks of that transfer will count as an event in both the transfer distribution and the death distribution. The results which follow reflect data submitted for Class 1 CAPD or CCPD patients only. Summaries for Class 2 patients are not provided as true time on peritoneal therapy cannot be estimated in previously treated patients.

5.1. Probability of transferring to an alternate dialysis modality — CAPD

Patients who have received CAPD for varying lengths of time may decide to discontinue CAPD in favor of hemodialysis, IPD or terminate all dialysis with no return of kidney function. Such patients are considered to be CAPD transfers for this analysis. Patients who die while on CAPD, transfer to another center and subsequently are lost to follow-up, receive a kidney transplant, discontinue dialysis due to a return in kidney function, or change to CCPD are not considered transfers. Such patients contribute information only for the time they are known to be receiving continuous peritoneal dialysis and are censored in the analyses that have been performed.

The estimated probability distribution for transferring off of CAPD is illustrated in Exhibit 5-1. Note that the probability of transferring to another modality doubles from 10% at 6 months to 20% at one year. After 18 months the probability of a transfer increases by approximately 6% every 6 months. By three years, 44% of patients have discontinued CAPD in favor of an alternate dialysis modality.

5.2. Probability of transplantation — CAPD

An alternative to dialysis for the end stage renal disease patient is transplantation. The availability of a suitable kidney, patient preference and medical considerations are all factors which influence the decision to transplant. For analysis purposes, patients receiving a transplant are counted as having experienced the event, all other patients, regardless of status (i.e., continuing CAPD, death, transfer, etc.) are censored as of the last day known to be on CAPD.

From Exhibit 5-2 it is evident that the majority of CAPD patients do not receive a transplant. Twenty percent of patients are reported to have received a transplant by the end of year two; and the cumulative probability of a transplant occurring increases to only 25% by the end of year three.

As children are more likely to receive a transplant than adults, Exhibit 5-3 displays the probability separately for three groups of patients: age < 20 yrs, nondiabetics age 20–59 yrs (standard), diabetics or patients 60 yrs of age or older. For the purposes of this analysis all Class 1 patients are considered regardless of therapy (i.e., CAPD or CCPD). The two year probability of a transplant is 25% for the 'standard' population, 50% greater than the 12% transplant probability observed for diabetics or patients 60 yrs of age or greater. Children experience the greatest transplantation rate with 51% expected to receive a kidney transplant at two years; more than double the probability for the 'standard' group.

5.3. Probability of death while on CAPD

As previously indicated, deaths are reported to the Registry only if they occur while the patient is receiving CAPD or within two weeks of transfer to an alternative modality such as hemodialysis, IPD, or transplantation. Therefore, all patients not reported as dead provide information only for as long as they remain on CAPD. It should be understood, that those patients who subsequently die are not reflected in the Registry data base.

The probability distribution estimate of death while on CAPD, given in Exhibit 5-4, reveals a fairly constant increase in the cumulative probability of death with time. After six months on CAPD, deaths are observed to have occurred in 8% of patients, while the cumulative probability of death is 16% for patients who have been on treatment for twelve months. Increases of similar magnitude are observed at 18 months and 24 months. After 30 months on therapy, 36% of patients are reported as having died.

5.4. Probability of discontinuing CAPD for any reason

As suggested earlier, patients who use CAPD as a replacement therapy for end stage renal disease can be expected to discontinue this treatment modality due to a variety of reasons: transfer to hemodialysis, IPD, discontinuation of all dialysis with or without return of kidney function, death or transplantation. Considering terminations for any reason as an event yields the probability distribution displayed in Exhibit 5-5. For patients coming to CAPD for the first time, over half (54%) may be expected to leave CAPD within 18 months; and after three years on therapy, three-quarters of the patients will have terminated CAPD. Of potential clinical significance, twenty-five percent of patients may be considered as 'long term' CAPD users.

5.5. Probability of discontinuing CCPD

Probability distributions corresponding to patients beginning peritoneal dialysis with CCPD were estimated in a similar manner to those for CAPD patients. Patients changing from CCPD to CAPD were not considered transfers. Note that the estimates based on the CCPD patient population are subject to change when more follow-up on CCPD patients becomes available, as confidence bands at two years are rather sizeable.

The probability of transferring from CCPD to hemodialysis or IPD, or discontinuing all dialysis with no return of kidney function, as shown in Exhibit 5–6, indicates that more than one-third of patients (37%) leave CCPD by two years in favor of an alternative dialysis modality. Transplants occur less frequently than transfers with approximately twenty-eight percent of the patients receiving a transplant within the first two years of therapy. However, a tripling of the probability of being transplanted was observed between the 0–6 month period (5%) and 6–12 month period (16%) (Exhibit 5–7). Similarly, the cumulative probability of death doubles the first six months (11%) to the second six months (22%); and, by 18 months approximately one-third of patients (31%) are reported as having died while on CCPD (Exhibit 5–8). The cumulative probability of discontinuing CCPD for any reason as illustrated in Exhibit 5–9 is estimated to be 49% at 1 yr and 72% at 2 yrs.

5.6. Follow-up of transfers to hemodialysis — CAPD/CCPD

Although reasons for discontinuing CAPD/CCPD have previously been reported, a new follow-up form was instituted by the Registry in November, 1986 which provides more detailed information on this very important topic. Centers were requested to prospectively complete this form for all patients transferring to hemodialysis in the period July 1, 1986 to present. Information has been received on 1030 patients and is summarized in Exhibit 5–10. Most patients transferring to hemodialysis receive in-center dialysis with only 2% of transferred patients utilizing home hemodialysis. Twenty-six percent of the patients were reported to have discontinued CAPD/CCPD primarily due to excessive peritonitis, 14% due to patient or family choice or inability to cope, and 11% due to exit site/tunnel infections. In all, almost half of all patients' (48%) primary reason for transferring to hemodialysis was due to a CAPD/CCPD related complication (peritonitis, exit site/tunnel infection, CAPD related hospitalization, catheter leak, malfunction or failure, or hernia). An additional 9% transferred because peritoneal dialysis could not meet biochemical or fluid standards.

Fifty-one of the 1030 patients (5%) who were reported to have transferred to hemodialysis since July 1, 1986, have subsequently returned to CAPD/CCPD as of August 31, 1987. Median time to return was 70 days with minimum and maximum time to return of 28 and 330 days respectively. The primary reasons these patients discontinued CAPD/CCPD are listed in Exhibit 5–11. Sixty percent (31/51) of patients had left CAPD/CCPD due to complications of peritoneal dialysis (peritonitis, exit site/tunnel infections, catheter leak or malfunction, or hernia). Of the 110 patients who discontinued CAPD/CCPD due to exit site/tunnel infections, 14% (15/110) have returned to CAPD/CCPD. Only 5% (14/268) of patients transferring to hemodialysis due to excessive peritonitis while on CAPD/CCPD have returned to CAPD/CCPD. As the maximum follow-up time of this cohort is only 1 year, continued follow-up may provide further insight as to why patients leave CAPD/CCPD in favor of hemodialysis and, if these transfers are permanent.

5.7. Follow-up of kidney transplants — CAPD/CCPD

In the period beginning July 1, 1986 through August 31, 1987, 764 reports have been received which summarizes information concerning kidney transplants. From these reports, it is estimated that 19% of patients (144/764) received a kidney from a living related donor (Exhibit 5–12). Four percent of patients received hemodialysis immediately prior to the transplant and, sixty-eight percent of patients required no form of dialysis in the 2 week post-operative period. Of the 229 patients who required dialysis, the majority (73%) used peritoneal dialysis.

5.8. Follow-up of patient deaths — CAPD/CCPD

Registry participants were requested to prospectively provide information with regard to events preceding a patient's death, as well as the probable cause of death for all deaths reported from July 1, 1986 to present. Forms summarizing these items have been received for 1295 patients, and the results are detailed in Exhibit 5–13. Eighty-three percent of the patients were reported to have used peritoneal dialysis up until the time of death. Only 14% reported to have received maintenance hemodialysis between the last peritoneal dialysis exchange and date of death. Only 13 patients (1%) received a transplanted kidney within two weeks of death. Ten percent of patients were reported to have had a complication of peritoneal dialysis as a contributing factor in the patient's demise. An additional 10% had a complication present at the time of death, but it was not considered to have contributed to the patient's death. The majority of patients (73%) were claimed to have died from causes unrelated to renal disease or peritoneal dialysis. Thirteen percent died as a consequence of renal disease and 5% succumbed due to both renal disease and causes unrelated to renal disease or peritoneal dialysis.

Exhibit 5–1. CAPD: Cumulative probability of transfer* (class 1 patients only)

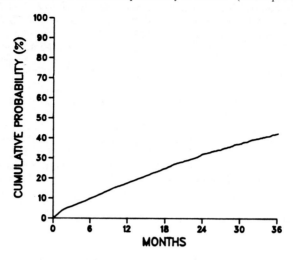

Cumulative probabilities and 95% Confidence Intervals (C.I.) for Exhibit 5–1.

	Months on CAPD					
	6	12	18	24	30	36
Cumulative Prob.	10	20	28	34	39	44
95% C.I.	(10, 11)	(19, 20)	(26, 29)	(32, 35)	(37, 41)	(42, 46)

* Transfer to hemodialysis, IPD, or off dialysis with no return of kidney function

Exhibit 5–2. CAPD: Cumulative probability of receiving a kidney transplant (class 1 patients only)

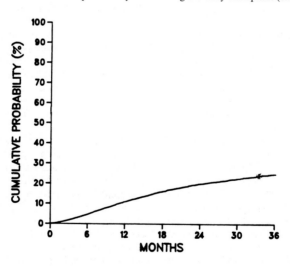

Cumulative probabilities and 95% Confidence Intervals (C.I.) for Exhibit 5–2.

	Months on CAPD					
	6	12	18	24	30	36
Cumulative Prob.	4	11	16	20	22	25
95% C.I.	(4, 5)	(10, 12)	(15, 17)	(18, 21)	(21, 24)	(23, 27)

Exhibit 5-3. CAPD or CCPD: Cumulative probability of transplantation: pediatrics vs standard vs other (class 1 patients only)

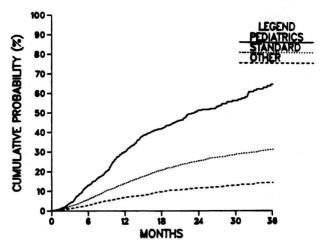

Cumulative probabilities and 95% Confidence Intervals (C.I.) for Exhibit 5-3.

	Months on CAPD					
	6	12	18	24	30	36
Pediatrics*						
Cumulative Prob.	13	30	42	51	56	64
95% C.I.	(10, 16)	(26, 35)	(37, 47)	(45, 57)	(48, 64)	(56, 72)
Standard**						
Cumulative Prob.	6	14	21	25	29	31
95% C.I.	(5, 6)	(13, 15)	(19, 22)	(23, 28)	(26, 31)	(28, 34)
Other***						
Cumulative Prob.	3	7	10	12	13	14
95% C.I.	(2, 3)	(6, 8)	(9, 11)	(10, 14)	(11, 15)	(12, 17)

* Patients under 20 yrs of age.
** Patients between the age of 20–59 yrs of age not diagnosed with diabetic glomerulosclerosis.
*** Patients >59 yrs of age or patients diagnosed with diabetic glomerulosclerosis.

Exhibit 5-4. CAPD: Cumulative probability of death* (class 1 patients only)

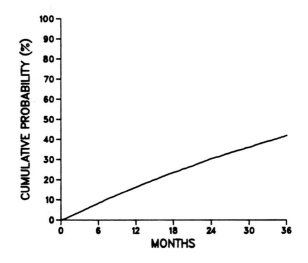

Cumulative probabilities and 95% Confidence Intervals (C.I.) for Exhibit 5–4.

	Months on CAPD					
	6	*12*	*18*	*24*	*30*	*36*
Cumulative Prob.	8	16	23	30	36	42
95% C.I.	(8, 9)	(15, 17)	(22, 25)	(29, 32)	(34, 38)	(40, 44)

* While on CAPD or within two weeks of CAPD termination.

Exhibit 5–5. CAPD: Cumulative probability of discontinuing CAPD therapy for any reason*   (class 1 patients only)

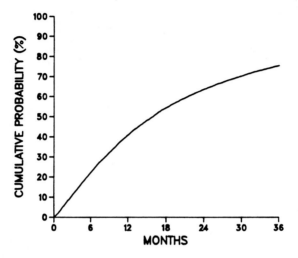

Cumulative probabilities and 95% Confidence Intervals (C.I.) for Exhibit 5–5.

	Months on CAPD					
	6	*12*	*18*	*24*	*30*	*36*
Cumulative Prob.	22	41	54	63	70	75
95% C.I.	(21, 23)	(40, 42)	(53, 55)	(62, 65)	(69, 71)	(74, 76)

* Transfer to hemodialysis or IPD, transplantation, discontinuing dialysis with or without return of kidney function, death.

Exhibit 5–6. CCPD: Cumulative probability of transfer* (class 1 patients only)

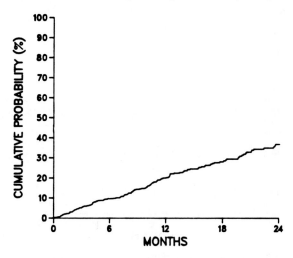

Cumulative probabilities and 95% Confidence Intervals (C.I.) for Exhibit 5–6.

	Months on CAPD			
	6	*12*	*18*	*24*
Cumulative Prob.	10	20	28	37
95% C.I.	(8, 12)	(14, 24)	(23, 34)	(30, 44)

* Transfer to hemodialysis, IPD, or off dialysis with no return of kidney function.

Exhibit 5–7. CCPD: Cumulative probability of receiving a kidney transplant (class 1 patients only)

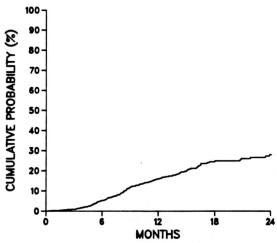

Cumulative probabilities and 95% Confidence Intervals (C.I.) for Exhibit 5–7.

	Months on CAPD			
	6	*12*	*18*	*24*
Cumulative Prob.	5	16	24	28
95% C.I.	(4, 7)	(13, 20)	(19, 30)	(21, 36)

Exhibit 5-8. CCPD: Cumulative probability of death* (class 1 patients only)

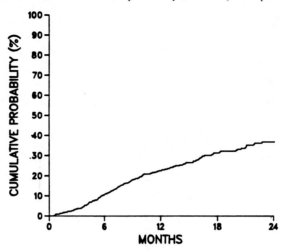

Cumulative probabilities and 95% Confidence Intervals (C.I.) for Exhibit 5-8.

	Months on CAPD			
	6	*12*	*18*	*24*
Cumulative Prob.	11	22	31	37
95% C.I.	(8, 13)	(19, 27)	(26, 37)	(30, 44)

* While on CCPD or within two weeks of CCPD termination.

Exhibit 5-9. CCPD: Cumulative probability of discontinuing CCPD for any reason* (class 1 patients only)

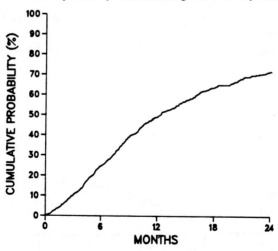

Cumulative probabilities and 95% Confidence Intervals (C.I.) for Exhibit 5-9.

	Months on CAPD			
	6	*12*	*18*	*24*
Cumulative Prob.	25	49	64	72
95% C.I.	(22, 28)	(45, 53)	(59, 68)	(67, 76)

* Transfer to hemodialysis, IPD, transplantation, discontinuing dialysis with or without return of kidney function, death.

Exhibit 5–10. Follow-up of transfers to hemodialysis summary

	Frequency	Percent (n=1,030)
Type of hemodialysis		
In-center	991	96
Home	20	2
Unknown	19	2
Primary reason discontinuing PD		
Peritoneal dialysis unable to meet fluid standard	45	4
Peritoneal dialysis unable to meet biochemical standard	48	5
Visual/manual impairment	13	1
Excessive peritonitis	268	26
Exit site/tunnel infection	110	11
Hospitalization for CAPD-related complications	18	2
Hospitalization for other than CAPD-related complications	10	1
Catheter leaks and malfunctions	41	4
Catheter failure	26	3
Hernia	21	2
Other medical reasons	159	15
Patient/family choice/inability to cope	148	14
Desire for change	27	3
Socioeconomic reasons	3	<1
Other	90	9
Unknown	3	<1

Exhibit 5–11. Primary reason for leaving CAPD in patients who transferred from CAPD to hemodialysis and subsequently returned to CAPD

Primary reason	Frequency	Percent (n=51)
Excessive peritonitis	14	27
Exit site/tunnel infection	15	29
Catheter leak/malfunction	1	2
Hernia	1	2
Other medical reason	8	16
Patient/family choice/inability to cope	2	4
Desire for change	1	2
Other reason	4	8
Not stated	4	8

Exhibit 5–12. Follow-up of kidney transplant summary

	Frequency	Percent (n=764)
Transplanted kidney – living related donor		
No	618	81
Yes	144	19
Unknown	2	<1
Last dialysis prior to transplant		
Peritoneal dialysis	730	96
Hemodialysis	29	4
Unknown	5	<1
Dialysis type in 2-week post-op period		
None	522	68
Peritoneal dialysis	168	22
Hemodialysis	61	8
Unknown	13	2

Exhibit 5–13. Death summary

	Frequency	Percent (n=1,295)
Last dialysis type prior to death		
Peritoneal dialysis	1079	83
Hemodialysis	184	14
Unknown	32	2
Received kidney transplant within 2 weeks prior to death		
No	1281	99
Yes	13	1
Unknown	1	<1
Complication of peritoneal dialysis present at death		
No	1032	80
Yes, not contributing factor in patient's demise	124	10
Yes, minor contributing factor in patient's demise	64	5
Yes, major contributing factor in patient's demise	67	5
Unknown	8	1
Cause of death		
Renal disease	163	13
Unrelated to renal disease or peritoneal dialysis	947	73
Both renal disease and unrelated causes	60	5
Unknown	125	10

ACKNOWLEDGEMENTS

The authors wish to thank all participating centers for providing the data on which this report is based.

We gratefully acknowledge the assistance of the following staffs of The EMMES Corporation and the University of Missouri, without whom the report could not have been completed:

Joanne Damours
Marsha Denekas
Cecily Fritz
Jag Gill
Jeanette Leroux
Warren Pendleton
Kelly Raygor
Phyllis Scholl
Carol Smith
Tamara Voss

Questions regarding this report and requests for additional copies should be addressed to:

National CAPD Registry,
Data Coordinating Center,
The EMMES Corporation,
11325 Seven Locks Road, Suite 214,
Potomac, MD 20854, USA.
800–638–2578; in Maryland, 301–299–8655

For other information about the Registry project, contact:
Karl D. Nolph, M.D., or Mr. Jag Gill,
Division of Nephrology (MA436),
University of Missouri Health Sciences Center,
Columbia, MO 65212, USA.
314–882–7991

REFERENCES

1. End-Stage Renal Disease Patient Profile Tables – 1985. Contemporary Dialysis and Nephrology. p. 34–40: March, 1987.
2. Kahn HA: *An Introduction to Epidemiologic Methods.* Oxford University Press: New York, 1983.
3. Kaplan E, Meier P: Nonparametric estimates from incomplete observations. J. Am Stat Assoc 53: 457–458, 1958.

APPENDIX 1
NIH Project Officer

Gladys Hirschman, M.D.
Chronic Renal Disease Program
Kidney-Urology Branch (DKUHD)
NIDDK
Bethesda, Maryland

Executive Advisory Committee Members of the National CAPD Registry

Steven Alexander, M.D.
University of Texas Health Center at Dallas
Dallas, TX

Christopher R. Blagg, M.D.
Northwest Kidney Center,
Seattle, WA

John A. Goffinet, M.D.
VA Hospital
West Haven, CT

Richard Hamburger, M.D.
Indiana University Medical Center
Indianapolis, IN

Robert Hamilton, M.D.
Bowman Gray School of Medicine
Winston-Salem, NC

Joanne Hoover, M.D., MPH
University of Washington,
Seattle, WA

John F. Maher, M.D.
Uniform Services University of Health Sciences
Bethesda, MD

George W. Williams, Ph.D.
Cleveland Clinic Foundation
Cleveland, OH

21

PERITONEAL DIALYSIS RESULTS IN THE EDTA REGISTRY

THOMAS A. GOLPER, WILLEM GEERLINGS, NEVILLE H. SELWOOD, FELIX P. BRUNNER
and ANTONY J. WING

1. EDTA REGISTRY QUESTIONNAIRES

Directors of renal units in thirty-four European countries with a base population in 1985 of 582 million people (WHO Statistics Annual) submitted data to the Registry of the European Dialysis and Transplant Association – European Renal Association (EDTA Registry). The Registry maintained a computerised data base of 111 378 patients who were alive on dialysis or with a functioning transplant on 31 December 1985 [1]. This represents a 9% increase in the size of the data base since 31 December 1984 [2] and a 42% increase since the end of 1982 [3]. Information has been provided by an uninterrupted sequence of annual returns which commenced in 1965, and it is currently held on the dedicated VAX 11/750 computer at St Thomas' Hospital in London.

Data have been recorded on two types of questionnaires. The centre questionnaire provides a summary of the activities in each unit, and the contents vary slightly from year to year. An individual patient questionaire is completed for every subject accepted for renal replacement therapy (RRT). The information requested includes patient identification facts with date of birth, a coded entry for the primary renal disease (PRD) leading to end stage renal failure (ESRF), graft and dialysis details where appropriate, malignancies, date and cause of death. The treatment sequence for each patient is described by a number code for the modality and a date for the start of each treatment. This date sequence is used for incidence and prevalence statistics and for calculation of patient and technique survival rates. In most analyses described in this chapter, the data base from the individual patient questionnaires has been used. When the centre questionnaire is used, it will be mentioned. The Registry publishes figures from both questionnaires and there may be differences due to either incomplete or double reporting or from the retrospective correction of data from previous years. Questionnaires were received from 85% of all the European centres, and returns were complete for some countries [1–7].

In the 1981 patient questionnaire, special questions were asked regarding why continuous ambulatory peritoneal dialysis (CAPD) was used, how many days of hospitalisation were needed while on CAPD, and, if appropriate, why CAPD was abandoned during 1981. In 1982, the number of catheter insertions, days of hospitalisation, and reason for abandonment of CAPD were requested. In 1983 and 1984 the reason for abandonment was requested. In every year the number of episodes of peritonitis was requested. Because certain information is available only in a particular year or years, we have elected to follow the CAPD cohorts of the particular year in which the specific question was requested.

2. STATISTICAL METHODOLOGY

Overall survival on renal replacement therapy (RRT) was calculated by the Selwood method [8] because it provides insights relevant to the contribution of each method of treatment (MOT) to overall survival. In Selwood's computation each patient is entered from the date of first treatment and the only exit is death. Patients are not censored when they change MOT but are retained in the overall survival calculation, joining the other patients on the new therapy from the date of their change. Actuarial convention is followed and if the patient is on therapy for less than a full interval, it counts as 0.5 of an interval. The analysis gives the numbers of patients on each therapy separately at definable intervals after the first treatment. In other words, this method describes the proportional contribution of each therapy at a specified time after commencement of RRT. The cohort of patients entering a Selwood analysis must be defined clearly. If treatment policies are undergoing change, then the cohort should be selected over an appropriate period of entry. Policies were changing during the periods covered in the analysis described in this chapter. Therefore, we have specifically chosen certain cohorts which will be mentioned as their results are displayed. In addition, the unique nature of the questions asked in certain years contributes to the selection of certain cohorts for in-depth analyses.

Interval mortality on RRT is the resultant of the interval

mortalities of all MOTs taking into account the proportions of patients on each MOT. The Selwood method would cause confusion if it were used to express cumulative survival on the MOTs separately, and it certainly cannot be used to compare the results of different MOTs, only their relative contributions to treatment and survival. The reason can be exemplefied: if a patient changes to CAPD for the first time during his/her second year of RRT, then the patient's survival on CAPD counts during his/her second year of RRT and amongst other patients who were on CAPD during their second year of replacement therapy. Only a proportion of these will have started replacement therapy on CAPD and be in their second year of CAPD.

An advantage of the Selwood method is that it does not ignore antecedent histories. Conventional survival calculation on any MOT views the MOT in isolation with the survival clock reset at zero time for each patient as he/she commences the MOT being evaluated. It may become policy in certain countries to utilise a specific MOT for patients who have failed other MOTs and, in doing so, have suffered complications which heighten their risk for untoward consequences. The Selwood approach does not obscure this situation.

In addition to the Selwood approach we will also give survival data utilising the traditional actuarial approach. In these analyses, the clock starts when the MOT starts and a change in MOT censors a patient at the date of change. When this approach is used we will attempt to make it clear why we elected to use it for the point we are emphasising, and we will specify the conditions applied to the analysis. When referring to patient survival, survival 'on' CAPD means that actuarial survival starts when CAPD starts and transplantation or switching to another form of dialysis causes censoring. Survival 'after' CAPD means the clock starts when CAPD commences and that only the patient's death serves as the end-point, without censoring for shifts of MOTs.

3. GENERAL RESULTS

At the close of 1985, 7.5% of European ESRF patients were being treated by peritoneal dialysis with 88% of those being on continuous peritoneal dialysis (CPD) (Table 1, Figure 1). A very small fraction of this CPD population

Table 1. Methods of treatment of live registered patients on 31 December 1985.
A small fraction of the CAPD population was actually undergoing CCPD.

Method of treatment	*All patients*			
	n	*%*	*PMP*	*Mean age*
CAPD	7 377	6.6.	12.7	53.2
IPD	942	0.9	1.6	57.7
Hospital haemodialysis	69 991	62.8	120.2	51.9
Home haemodialysis	7 054	6.3	12.1	46.8
Transplant	26 014	23.4	44.7	39.7
Total registry	111 378	100.0	191.3	48.8

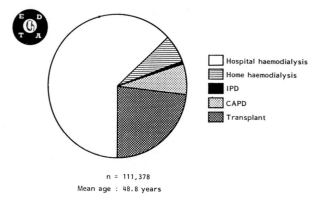

n = 111,378
Mean age : 48.8 years

Figure 1. Proportions of live patients recorded by the Registry on each MOT on 31 December 1985. A very small fraction of the CAPD population was actually undergoing CCPD.

was undergoing CCPD, hence the general descriptive term CPD instead of CAPD. The CPD patients had a mean age of 53.2 years and the IPD patients were slightly older. Home haemodialysis patients and patients with a functioning graft were younger than the peritoneal dialysis patients (Table 1). There were 12.7 CPD patients per million population (pmp), ranking third after hospital haemodialysis and transplantation. Ten and a half per cent of all ESRF patients in Europe were >65 yr old (Table 2), compared to 8% at the end of 1982 [3]. Thirteen per cent of these elderly patients received CPD and only 1% had a functioning graft. Children who commenced treatment under the age of 15 yr accounted for just over 3% of the total patients, similar to the proportion observed in 1982. However, unlike 1982, 7.8% of children were treated by CPD, an increase of 50%. This increase had been a progressive rise over the intervening years (data not shown). Furthermore, the mean age of the children treated by CPD was considerably lower than for children receiving haemodialysis or with a functioning graft (Table 2). Therefore, it can be seen that CAPD has made a significant contribution to the treatment of ESRF in Europe, especially at the extremes of age.

The extent of the contribution varied widely between countries (Table 3).

The number of ESRF patients on an MOT in the total Registry rose from 135 pmp in 1982 to 191 pmp in 1985. In many countries, expansion of haemodialysis facilities has been limited (eg United Kingdom), hence the dependence on CAPD. The percentage of centres performing CAPD in selected countries is shown over a five year time span in Figure 2 (see Section 4).

In the mid-1970s intermittent peritoneal dialysis (IPD) began to make a small contribution to the dialysis programme and was promptly overtaken by the soaring growth of CAPD. Subsequently there was a major decline in the fraction of patients treated by haemodialysis and IPD, while there was an increase of both CAPD and transplantation (Figure 3). From 1978 to 1980 in the UK, Sweden, Italy, France and Belgium there was a rapid growth in the proportion of patients on CAPD (Figure 4). In Sweden, Italy, France and Belgium this growth plateaued while in the UK it persisted. Since 1982 there was a parallel rise

Table 2. Methods of treatment of live elderly patients (aged over 65 years at first treatment) and of children (aged under 15 years at first treatment) on 31 December 1985. A very small fraction of the CAPD population was actually undergoing CCPD.

	Age at start of treatment							
	Less than 15 yr				More than 65 yr			
Method of treatment	n	%	PMP	Mean age	n	%	PMP	Mean age
CAPD	279	7.8	0.4	11.0	1 532	13.0	2.6	72.2
IP	22	0.6	0.03	8.1	324	2.8	0.6	73.8
Hospital haemodialysis	1309	36.8	1.8	15.3	9 618	82.1	16.5	72.9
Home haemodialysis	119	3.3	0.2	19.4	121	1.0	0.2	72.5
Transplant	1833	51.5	2.6	16.4	116	1.1	0.2	70.8
Total registry	3562	100.0	5.0	15.6	11 711	100.0	20.1	72.8

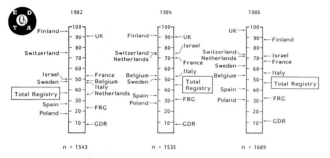

Figure 2. Per cent of centres which performed CAPD on 31 December 1982, 1984 and 1986 in selected countries.

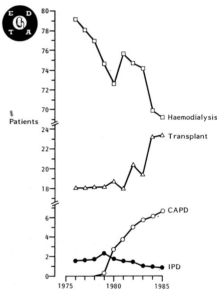

Figure 3. Per cent of patients alive on different MOTs at the end of each year. Note the twice interrupted scale.

in the Netherlands. Only 1% of the large number of patients on therapy in the Federal Republic of Germany (FRG) were on CAPD. Eastern European countries commenced CAPD later and there has been growth in CAPD commensurate with the increase in ESRF patients treated pmp (Figure 4, Table 3).

4. CAPD CENTRES

Figure 2 covers a five year time span and shows the per cent of centres performing CAPD in 13 selected EDTA countries and for the total Registry. These data were compiled from centre questionnaires. Over this 5 yr span the overall number of centres responding increased about 9% but for the countries with the greatest number of centres (e.g. FRG, Italy, France and Spain), there was no substantial increase. In most countries the per cent of centres performing CAPD increased, notably in Poland, Spain, Israel and the Netherlands. Other countries appeared to have a broad commitment to CAPD from 1982 which persisted (e.g. Finland, UK and Switzerland). The FRG and GDR have persistently demonstrated little interest in CAPD.

The rapid expansion of CAPD led to a peak in 1980 of centres performing their first CAPD training (Figure 5). There was a subsequent decline after 1980. This decline is also noted in the number of centres which commenced haemodialysis or transplantation for the first time in each year shown in Figure 5. This indicates that expansion of

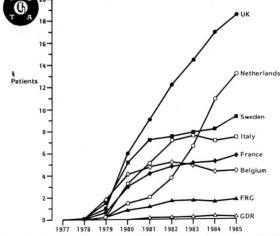

Figure 4. Per cent of all living ESRF patients treated by CAPD in eight selected countries from 1977 to 1985.

Table 3. Registered patients known to be alive on 31 December 1985, in 34 countries. A small fraction of the CAPD population was actually undergoing CCPD.

Country	IPD	CAPD	Haemodialysis or Haemofiltration				% home of total	With functioning grafts	Total	PMP
			Hospital	Home	Total					
Algeria	0	26	211	2	213	0.9	23	262	14.3
Austria	1	17	1301	45	1346	3.3	515	1879	250.5
Belgium	3	159	2187	100	2287	4.4	1148	3597	367.0
Bulgaria	0	3	877	16	893	1.8	23	919	102.1
Cyprus	0	0	119	0	119	0	46	165	275.0
Czechoslovakia	5	0	915	2	917	0.2	299	1221	80.3
Denmark	34	167	385	43	428	10.0	514	1143	224.1
Egypt	34	8	992	1	993	0.1	121	1156	29.7
Fed Rep Germany	217	363	14 849	1241	16 090	7.7	3160	19 830	324.0
Finland	6	170	247	2	249	0.8	628	1053	219.4
France	165	949	9832	2128	11 960	17.8	3383	16 457	308.2
German Dem Rep	6	4	1515	0	1515	0	532	2057	122.4
Greece	2	196	1179	3	1182	0.2	229	1609	173.0
Hungary	34	5	460	1	461	0.2	157	657	61.4
Iceland	0	5	10	0	10	0	14	29	145.0
Ireland	3	60	216	23	239	9.6	309	611	185.2
Israel	52	225	887	44	931	4.7	325	1533	403.4
Italy	127	1279	12 780	806	13 586	5.9	2191	17 183	302.5
Lebanon	0	0	16	0	16	0	1	17	6.3
Libya	0	0	83	0	83	0	12	95	32.8
Luxembourg	0	0	81	5	86	5.8	14	100	250.0
Morocco	0	0	102	0	102	0	6	108	4.9
Netherlands	1	298	1482	146	1628	9.0	354	2281	162.9
Norway	6	25	184	3	187	1.6	706	924	225.4
Poland	47	13	1010	0	1010	0	349	1419	40.1
Portugal	1	17	2181	0	2181	0	188	2387	243.6
Spain	71	656	8511	302	8813	3.4	2437	11 977	323.7
Sweden	22	233	795	90	885	10.2	1373	2513	302.8
Switzerland	4	263	985	169	1154	14.6	900	2321	357.1
Syria	0	0	0	0	0	0	1	1	0.1
Tunisia	1	15	327	0	327	0	8	351	56.6
Turkey	13	15	573	2	575	0.3	128	731	16.5
United Kingdom	58	2141	1872	1839	3711	49.6	5684	11 594	207.4
Yugoslavia	29	65	2827	41	2868	1.4	236	3198	144.7
Total registry	942	7377	69 991	7054	77 045	9.2	26 014	111 378	191.3

populations depended in recent years on the development of existing centres rather than the opening of new ones. Figure 2 data would corroborate this interpretation. A further breakdown of these data is seen in Figure 6 which details four selected countries. In Belgium, FRG and the UK, the pattern was similar to the total Registry as shown in Figure 5, while for the GDR there appeared to be a pattern of limited expansion. Again from Figure 2 it can be noted that the GDR policies towards CAPD have not changed much over time.

5. DEMOGRAPHY: CAPD PATIENTS

Graphing the numbers of patients alive on each MOT demonstrates the relationship of peritoneal dialysis to haemodialysis and transplantation (Figure 7). The rates of increase of all three MOT appear to be equal. The different

patterns in growth of numbers of patients alive pmp on each MOT in a selection of European countries are shown in Figure 8. In all countries except the UK and perhaps Sweden, the numbers on haemodialysis or with a transplant have grown at the same or at a greater rate than those on CAPD. In the UK limited hospital haemodialysis facilities have forced physicians to expand CAPD. Gokal et al have expressed concerns that CAPD expansion in the absence of an expansion in back-up haemodialysis stations will stress the existing haemodialysis facilities [9, 10]. However, in general, the proportion of live ESRF patients on CAPD correlated in each country with the number of patients pmp on CAPD (Figure 9). Thus expansion of CAPD has generally accompanied an expansion of all ESRF services.

The rate of acceptance for CAPD in different countries in 1985 is shown in Figures 10–12, expressed pmp. Israel, Finland and the UK accepted the most patients pmp on

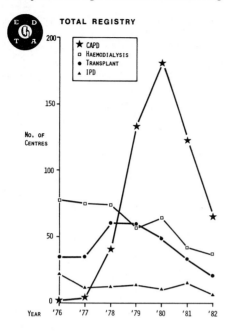

Figure 5. Commencement of MOTs in Europe, 1976-82. Numbers of centres are plotted according to the year in which they claimed to have treated their first patient on ech MOT.

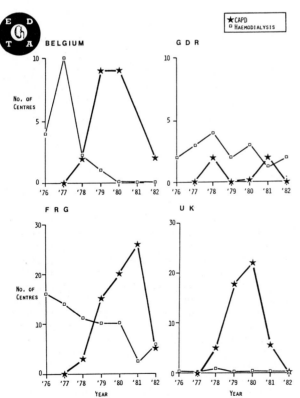

Figure 6. Commencement of CAPD and haemodialysis in four European countries, 1976-82. Numbers of centres are plotted according to the year in which they claimed to have treated their first patient on each therapy.

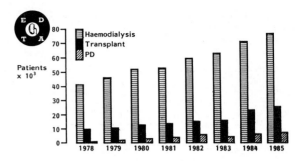

Figure 7. Numbers of total Registry patients alive on haemodialysis, with a functioning transplant or on peritoneal dialysis at the end of each year 1978–85.

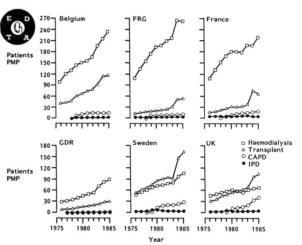

Figure 8. Numbers of patients alive per million population (pmp) at the end of each year 1976–85, according to MOT, in six selected countries.

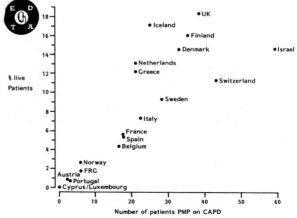

Figure 9. Contribution of CAPD to national programmes on 31 December 1985, showing the correlation between per cent of all living ESRF patients on CAPD and the number of CAPD patients pmp.

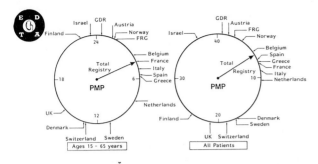

Figure 10. Rate of acceptance into CAPD per million population for the age group 15–65 yr and for all CAPD patients in selected countries during 1985.

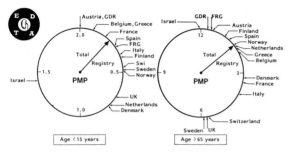

Figure 11. Rate of acceptance into CAPD per million population for the young and the elderly during 1985.

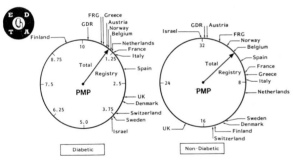

Figure 12. Rate of acceptance into CAPD per million population for diabetics and non-diabetics during 1985.

to CAPD. Israel consistently led all categories (all patients, aged <15 yr, 15–65, >65 yr) and was second only to Finland for diabetics. In fact, the policy in Finland of offering CAPD to the many diabetics treated in their country was responsible for its high rate of CAPD and indicated an approach which was different to that of Sweden, Denmark and Norway – other Nordic countries with a high incidence of diabetic nephropathy. Brunner et al recently reported an in-depth analysis of RRT in European diabetics [11]. Finland's non-diabetic acceptance rate was ranked fourth. Eastern European countries accepted fewest patients for CAPD (Figure 12).

When rate of acceptance according to age was considered, Israel, Denmark, the Netherlands and the UK accepted the most children. Israel, Sweden, the UK and Switzerland accepted the most patients over 65 yr old (Figure 11). In Table 4, we have ranked countries by their CAPD acceptance rate pmp (column 1). The CAPD acceptance rate did not necessarily correlate with the country's rank of total ESRF patients acceptance rate (column 2), or with the per cent of ESRF patients (column 3) or all dialysis patients on CAPD (column 4). On the other hand, with the exception of Italy, these countries had a higher percentage of dialysis patients on CAPD than did the total Registry (column 4).

Table 5 is an analysis of 1985 data from countries selected for having an emphasis on home haemodialysis (column 1). We attempted to evaluate the attitudes or policies in these countries towards the therapies which make patients less dependent on dialysis centres, i.e. transplantation, home haemodialysis and CAPD. With the exception of France, these countries appeared to be committed to all three therapies. France was committed to home haemodialysis but less so to CAPD or transplantation.

The data displayed in Table 6 are a breakdown of the data from Figure 12, accentuating the CAPD acceptance rate pmp by age ranges and presence or absence of diabetes. Again, the high acceptance rate of diabetes aged 15–65 yr in the Nordic countries exceeded that elsewhere in Europe. For the total Registry, ages 15–65 yr, the diabetic acceptance rate was about one-quarter of the non-diabetic rate. However, for the elderly (aged over 65), the diabetic acceptance rate was about one-quarter of the non-diabetic rate. However, for the elderly (aged over 65), the diabetic acceptance is not known. The overall CAPD acceptance rate pmp in

Table 4. All countries with a CAPD acceptance rate >20 patients pmp. In column 2 is the rank from 1 to 34 of countries in the Registry by ESRF patients pmp.

Country	CAPD patients alive, PMP	ESRF patients alive, PMP ranking	% of ESRF patients on CAPD	% of dialysis patients on CAPD
Israel	59.2	1	14.7	18.6
Switzerland	40.5	3	11.3	18.5
United Kingdom	38.3	16	18.5	36.2
Finland	35.4	15	16.1	40.0
Denmark	32.7	14	14.6	26.6
Sweden	28.1	7	9.3	20.4
Iceland	25.0	20	17.2	33.3
Italy	22.5	8	7.4	8.5
Netherlands	21.3	19	13.1	15.5
Greece	21.1	18	12.2	14.2
Total registry	12.7		6.6	8.6

Table 5. Countries with at least 10% of all haemodialysis patients on home haemodialysis.

Country	% of all haemodialysis at home	% of total dialysis on home haemodialysis	% of total dialysis on CAPD	% total of ESRF population transplanted	ESRF patients PMP
United Kingdom	49.6	31.1	36.2	49.0	207.4
France	17.8	16.3	7.3	20.6	308.2
Switzerland	14.6	11.9	18.5	38.8	357.1
Sweden	10.2	7.9	20.4	54.6	302.8
Denmark	10.0	6.8	26.6	45.0	224.1
Total registry	9.2	8.2	8.6	23.4	191.3

Table 6. Rate of acceptance into CAPD during 1985 (PMP)

| Country | Age <15 yr | | Age 15–65 yr | | Age >65 yr | |
	Diabetic	Non-diabetic	Diabetic	Non-diabetic	Diabetic	Non-diabetic
Austria	0	0.0	0.93	0.53	0.0	0.53
Belgium	0	0.10	0.81	3.04	0.0	2.03
Denmark	0	0.78	2.54	10.76	0.59	2.54
Finland	0	0.41	9.18	13.47	0.20	1.02
France	0	0.20	1.13	3.38	0.02	3.09
Fed Rep Germany	0	0.31	0.57	1.18	0.08	0.38
German Dem Rep	0	0.0	0.17	0.30	0.0	0.28
Greece	0	0.10	0.51	5.26	0.20	1.72
Israel	0	1.44	3.12	20.38	0.96	11.03
Italy	0	0.37	0.72	4.38	0.60	3.19
Netherlands	0	0.76	0.97	7.01	0.28	1.46
Norway	0	0.48	0.72	0.96	0.24	1.45
Spain	0	0.29	1.71	4.05	0.23	1.14
Sweden	0	0.48	3.48	7.43	0.48	5.40
Switzerland	0	0.46	3.50	9.59	0.30	5.02
United Kingdom	0	0.68	2.66	12.53	0.28	5.06
Total registry	0	0.26	0.90	3.47	0.17	1.60

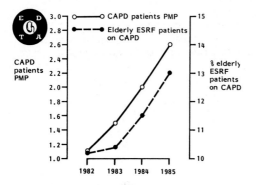

Figure 13. CAPD is growing in popularity as a MOT for elderly patients.

1985, for both diabetics and non-diabetics, was twice what it was in 1982 (3).

It appears that peritoneal dialysis has been a major contributor to the increased acceptance rate of elderly patients for RRT. In 1985, CAPD (13.0%) and IPD (2.8%) together supported 15.8% of all patients over 65 yr of age. In 1982, 14.5% were on these MOT. However, the number of elderly patients on RRT increased from 6,544 in 1982 to 11,711 in 1985, and therefore the acceptance of elderly patients for CAPD rose dramatically (Figure 13). This phenomenon has been well described in the UK by several observers (9, 10, 12, 13, 14).

These demographic data show that although CAPD has been deployed speedily during recent years in Europe, it was used for only a small proportion of patients overall. Furthermore, its recent popularity has not been achieved by reduction in numbers of patients on haemodialysis (although the proportion of patients on haemodialysis decreased), nor has the popularity of CAPD caused a reduction in the rate of increase in the haemodialysis population (Figure 7). The rate of acceptance of new patients for RRT has increased and that is where the contribution of CAPD was manifested.

6. SELECTION OF PATIENTS FOR CAPD

In Figures 3 and 7 the per cent and absolute numbers, respectively, of patients alive on each MOT are displayed. Analysis of antecedent treatment showed that most patients who commenced CAPD in the years 1982–1985 did so as new patients to ESRF therapy (Figure 14). Nonetheless, a substantial proportion of CAPD patients came from other forms of dialysis and a small fraction came from failed transplants. No trends over the years were apparent. Of the non-diabetics commencing CAPD, over 20% came from haemodialysis while 55% were new to ESRF therapy. For diabetics 15% came from haemodialysis and 67% were new to ESRF therapy. These data suggest that CAPD was preferred for diabetic patients, a finding noted in several other investigations [3, 9, 10, 11, 12, 15, 16].

However, this was only one aspect of the MOT selection bias for diabetics. From Figures 15 and 16, the roles of the different MOTs in different regions of Europe are displayed for diabetic patients in the transplantable age range. In Latin countries (France, Italy, Portugal and Spain, Figure 15) very few diabetics were grafted and CAPD was employed for 25% of the cases. In Nordic countries (Denmark, Finland, Iceland, Norway and Sweden, Figure 16) many diabetics started therapy with transplantation, and subsequent transplantation appeared to draw patients from the other MOTs with equal proportions. Nonetheless, about 25% of all diabetics commencing ESRF therapy in the Nordic countries were initially treated by CAPD.

The role of age in the selection of patients for a MOT has been described previously in Tables 1, 2 and 6 and Figures 10, 11 and 13. There appeared to be a selection bias for CAPD in the elderly. As discussed above, there also appeared to be a selection bias for CAPD as the MOT in diabetics. Of diabetics who started RRT, 85% of type I patients and 65% of type II patients did so before the

age of 65 yr [11, 17]. The age distribution and median age of diabetic patients (both types) at the start of RRT in 1983–85 are shown in Figure 17. If one looks at the primary renal disease of patients maintained by dialysis throughout the years of Registry activity (Figure 18), only diabetes stands out as showing bias for peritoneal dialysis over haemodialysis. Patients with cystic disease were more often treated preferentially with haemodialysis, presumably for mechanical/technical reasons related to large cysts. The slight increase of renal-vascular patients treated by CAPD may reflect the tendency for patients with this disorder to be older. An analysis of recent years confirmed this general pattern of selecting CAPD as first MOT for diabetics [11].

Because the patient questionnaires asked different questions in certain years, we could not address the same question each year. We have selected the 1981 patient questionnaire as an example. Reasons for choice for CAPD were recorded that year by numeric code. In this and subsequent sections we will describe the findings of that 1981 cohort of CAPD patients. Previous MOT, age, sex and primary renal disease were responses present each year on the patient questionnaire.

The reasons for choice of CAPD were separated into three categories; those patients for whom CAPD was regarded as 'temporary', 'enforced' or as 'first choice' treatment. CAPD was considered 'first choice' treatment for over 50% of all age groups and both sexes (Figure 19). There was a tendency for its preference as 'first choice' treatment to increase with age, and also in males. CAPD

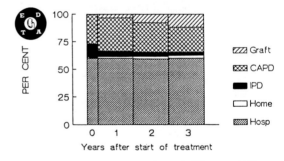

Figure 15. Proportional contribution of different MOTs to the treatment of diabetics who started RRT between 1980–85, aged 15–54 yr. (Latin = France, Italy, Portugal, Spain).

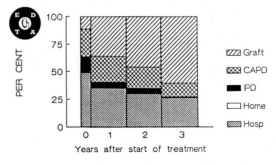

Figure 16. Proportional contribution of different MOTs to the treatment of diabetics who started RRT between 1980–85, aged 15–54 yr. (Nordic = Denmark, Finland, Iceland, Norway, Sweden).

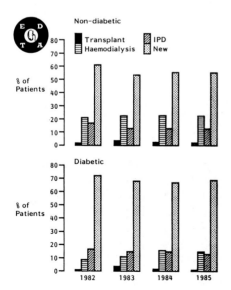

Figure 14. Previous treatment in non-diabetic and diabetic patients who commenced CAPD in the years 1982–85. 'New' patients are those for whom CAPD was the first recorded MOT.

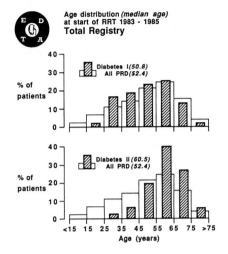

Figure 17. Age distribution and median age at start of RRT in 1983-85 for all patients (all PRD, open bars) and for patients with nephropathy due to insulin dependent (type I) diabetes (upper panel, slashed bars) and non-insulin dependent (type II) diabetes (lower panel, slashed bars).

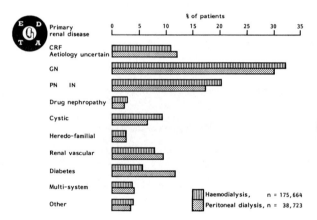

Figure 18. Primary renal disease in patients treated by CAPD and haemodialysis, since the start of the Registry. (PN IN = pyelo/interstitial nephritis).

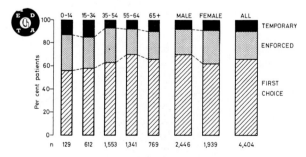

Figure 19. Reason for choice of CAPD according to age and sex in 1981. ('temporary' indicates that CAPD was carried out whilst waiting for transfer to haemodialysis or transplantation; 'enforced' indicates that CAPD was necessary because haemodialysis and transplantation were technically or medically impossible or had failed).

was more likely to be used as a 'temporary' measure in younger patients awaiting transfer to haemodialysis or transplantation. The proportion of patients for whom CAPD was said to be 'enforced' treatment (because of non-availability or failure of alternative therapy, or medical and technical contra-indicatios) was consistent throughout the age groups, but was larger in females than in males.

The percentage for whom CAPD was considered to be 'enforced' in the Federal republic of Germany was strikingly larger than most other countries (Figure 20). Sweden and the UK considered CAPD the 'first choice' treatment in over 70% of patients for whom it was used. CAPD was more often considered treatment of 'first choice' in diabetic patients than non-diabetics, and was less often considered an 'enforced' treatment (Figure 21). The proportions thus varied between countries with replies from the Federal Republic of Germany reflecting different physician attitudes in that country. In almost 90% of diabetic patients on CAPD in the United Kingdom, CAPD was considered the treatment of 'first choice'.

It is clear from the above data that the CAPD population in Europe differed in many important respects from the haemodialysis and transplant populations. These differences resulted from variation in clinical policy and practice and from contrasting attitudes to the role of CAPD in the different countries. Results of treatment by the different MOTs can only be compared when these selection biases are considered. Recently several investigations have attempted this [9, 10, 12, 16]. It is important to emphasise that patients have been selected, not randomly assgned to MOTs.

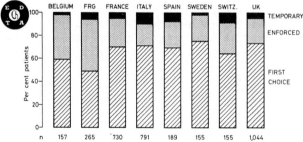

Figure 20. Reason for choice of CAPD acording to country in 1981. For meaning of 'temporary' and 'enforced', see Figure 19.

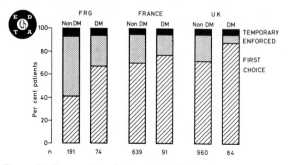

Figure 21. Reason for choice of CAPD in diabetics and non-diabetics in 1981. For meaning of 'temporary' and 'enforced', see Figure 19.

7. MANAGEMENT OF PATIENTS ON CAPD

In 1982 the patient questionnaire inquired specifically about catheter insertions. These results were detailed in the Second Edition of this text (3) and will only be summarised here. Neither age nor sex played a role in determining how many catheters were placed in an individual patient. Over 70% of patients did not require more than one catheter. More catheter insertions were required in those patients who had more frequent episodes of peritonitis.

In 1981 and 1982 the patient questionnaire inquired specifically about hospitalisation related to peritonitis while receiving CAPD. These data were also presented in the Second Edition [3] and are summarised here. Thirty per cent of diabetic patients spent 2–6 weeks hospitalised compared to 20% of non-diabetics. Over 40% of each group were not hospitalised for peritonitis. As the length of time on CAPD increased, so did the likelihood of hospitalisation for peritonitis. Age did not contribute to hospitalisation for peritonitis.

The reason for abandonment of CAPD (death and transplantation are excluded as reasons) were recorded from 1981 through 1984. Because of the nature of the questions and responses, we chose the latter two years only for analysis. Table 7 includes a variety of categories including age and duration on CAPD. What is not displayed is that the results in 1983 were very similar to those in 1984, diabetics were the same as non-diabetics, and males abandoned CAPD proportionally for the same reasons as did females. However, although males and females abandoned CAPD for the same reasons in 1983 and 1984, they did not do so with an equal frequency. During these two years 55% of all CAPD patients were male. However, 64% of all patients who abandoned CAPD were male. Therefore during this interval females had a lower abandonment rate than their male counterparts. Table 7 then addresses where differences were observed. Older patients abandoned CAPD for peritonitis less frequently than their younger counterparts but more often for inability to cope with the task of performing the procedure. As one would expect, patients who abandoned CAPD in less than three months usually did so for reasons other than peritonitis. Patients who

abandoned CAPD after three months demonstrated a higher likelihood of abandoning CAPD because of peritonitis the longer they were on CAPD. Similarly, being unable to cope with the procedure was less likely to cause abandonment the longer one stayed on this MOT.

We next lumped together all reasons for abandonment (again excluding death and transplantation) to plot actuarial technique survival curves for the 1981 cohort whose reason for using CAPD was known. The Registry has followed these patients for five years. If the number entering an at risk interval was < 30 patients, the plot ceases. Figure 22 shows the technique survival of this 1981 cohort by age and reason ('temporary', 'enforced', 'first choice') for CAPD. The patients > 65 yr of age in whom CAPD was 'enforced' had a high rate of technique survival. This is possibly a consequence of low patient survival (see Section 8 below). These patients died on CAPD with functioning technique. The 'temporary', age 15 to 64, were preordained to have a low technique survival. Their overall patient survival was high (see Section 8 below) probably reflecting effective individualised therapy after 'temporary' CAPD. For those patients for whom CAPD was their 'first choice' MOT, the >65 age group had the best technique survival. As one will see below (Section 8), this group had a low patient survival, again implying that these patients were retained on CAPD until their death. Figure 23 plots the actuarial technique survival in diabetic and non-diabetic

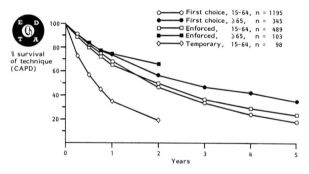

Figure 22. CAPD technique survival in the 1981 cohort for whom the reason for choice of CAPD was known.

Table 7. Reasons for CAPD abandonment, 1983 and 1984

Specific categories (n)	Peritonitis (%)	Other abdominal complications (%)	Inadequate dialysis/UF (%)	Pt. unable to cope with CAPD (%)	Patient request (%)	Family request (%)	Other complications related to CAPD (%)	Other (%)
Over 65 yr old (323)	48	11	12	11	5	2	10	1
Under 65 yr old (1342)	53	12	15	5	6	1	8	0
On CAPD <3 mo (270)	33	16	16	10	10	1	14	0
On CAPD 3–12 mo (577)	55	11	10	9	5	2	8	0
On CAPD >12 mo (818)	57	11	17	3	5	0	6	1
All patients (1665)	52	12	14	6	6	1	8	1

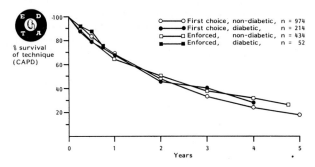

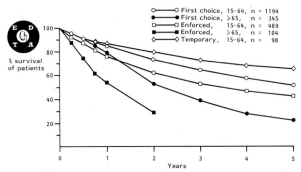

Figure 23. CAPD technique survival in the 1981 cohort for whom the reason for choosing CAPD was known. Diabetics are compared to non-diabetics. The number of 'temporary' diabetics was too small to include.

Figure 24. 1981 CAPD cohort patient survival rate 'on' and 'after' CAPD. The time clock began when CAPD began and switching MOT did not censor the patient.

CAPD patients in this 1981 cohort. There was no difference in technique survival for these diabetic regardless of the reason for choosing CAPD.

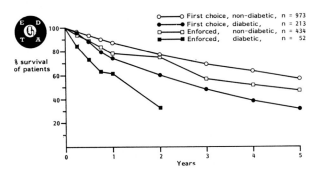

8. PATIENT SURVIVAL ON CAPD

We were particularly interested in following the 1981 cohort for whom the reason for choosing CAPD was known. Patient survival was calculated using traditional actuarial methodology. The survival time clock began at date of commencement of CAPD in 1981 and followed patient survival from that date on, irrespective of changes in MOT. Figure 24 is the actuarial plot of patient survival by age and reason for using CAPD. The 'temporary' patients had a survival rate superior to that of the other groups and the elderly 'enforced' group had the worst patient survival rate. The younger 'first choice' patient survival rate was superior to the elderly 'first choice' patient survival rate. We think that the survival of the 'temporary' group reflected the individualisation of therapy that occurred after CAPD terminated. This group demonstrated the worst technique survival (Figure 22), which supports this interpretation. The final analysis of this 1981 cohort is plotted in Figure 25 comparing diabetics and non-diabetics. The survival of the non-diabetrics was greater, regardless of reason for choosing CAPD. The 'first choice' groups did better than the 'enforced' groups.

We were interested in the effect of antecedent RRT on the outcome of CAPD. We elected to follow CAPD patients who had previously been haemodialysed. The actuarial survival of patients while 'on' CAPD from 1983 to 1986, categorised by being diabetic or not, and whether their MOT immediately preceding CAPD was haemodialysis or not is plotted in Figure 26. As expected, the non-diabetics demonstrated greater survival ratres. Within the disease categories survival rate was greater if the patients were switched from haemodialysis to CAPD compared to those patients entering CAPD who had not previously experienced haemodialysis. For these same patients we evaluated CAPD technique survival wth death being the only censoring criterion. Thus any switch to another RRT after CAPD counted as a technique 'death' for CAPD. These curves plotted in Figure 27 yielded the

Figure 25. 1981 CAPD cohort patient survival rate 'on' and 'after' CAPD, diabetics compared to non-diabetics. The time clock began when CAPD was begun and switching MOT did not censor the patient.

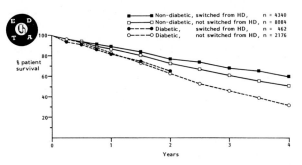

Figure 26. Actuarial patient survival 'on' CAPD from 1983-86, diabetic versus non-diabetic, and whether the immediately preceding MOT was haemodialysis or not. 'N' refers to the number entering the first at risk interval. The curves cease when the number entering that interval is <30.

opposite results of those seen for patient survival. Patients switched to CAPD from haemodialysis had the worst CAPD technique survival, independent of diabetes. Therefore, it appears that haemodialysis antecedent to CAPD had an effect on subsequent outcome and was associated with greater patient and worse technique survival. It also appears that survival on haemodialysis and transfer to CAPD (the selection criteria), and then subsequent transfer from CAPD (worst technique survival) resulted in the best patient survival. However, in all

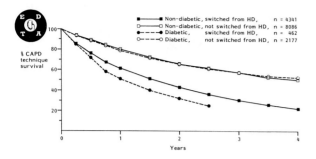

Figure 27. Actuarial CAPD technique survival, diabetics versus non-diabetics, from 1983–86, whether the MOT immediately preciding CAPD was haemodialysis or not. 'N' refers to the number entering the first at risk interval. The curves cease when the number entering that interval is <30.

probability it was the fittest patients who changed therapies in the process of selecting the best treatment for each individual.

To evaluate the role of each MOT in overall patient survival, the Selwood computation, as described in Section 2, was applied. Figure 28 is a Selwood computation comparing the contribution to survival of the different MOTs for patients beginning RRT in 1979 and 1983. CAPD was used as first treatment for 3% of the 1979 cohort and for over 10% of the 1983 cohort.

Transplantation made a growing contribution with time for both cohorts, consistent with the data in Figure 3. The late introduction of transplantation emphasis that the patients who received grafts are those who have survived the early months of dialysis. Figures 22-27 should be interpreted in this light. Home haemodialysis made a smaller contribution in 1983 than in 1979 and it appears that home haemodialysis was being progressively eclipsed by CAPD for patients who could cope with independent dialysis.

Despite a progressive increase in the average age of new patients commencing RRT year by year (Table 1) [2, 3, 18, 19], the overall survival on RRT improved from 87.4% at one year and 77.4% at two years for the 1979 cohort to 88.6% and 79.2%, respectively, for the 1983 cohort. Tabless 8–10 record a summary of results from Selwood analyses for European patients whose first treatment was

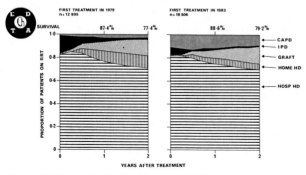

Figure 28. Proportional contributions of different MOTs for patients commencing RRT in 1979 and 1983. Since CAPçD was not yet a treatment code in 1979, the 1979 CAPD data were indirectly derived from other codes and mini-questionnaires.

Table 8. Proportions of patients on different modes of therapy at start of first treatment of 7664 patients in 1983 and at the first and second anniversaries with overall cumulative survival. Age 15–55 and 'standard' primary renal disease (excludes multisystem and hereditary disease, but includes cystic diseases).

Age 15–55, standard PRD

Method of therapy	Proportion of patients on RRT		
	Start	1 yr	2 yr
CAPD	0.07	0.07	0.06
IPD	0.06	0.01	0.01
Graft	0.01	0.09	0.19
Home HD	<0.01	0.07	0.08
Hosp. HD	0.87	0.79	0.72
Overall survival %		94.0	88.3

Table 9. Proportions of patients on different methods of therapy at start of first treatment of 2150 patients in 1983 and at first and second anniversaries with overall cumulative survival. Age over 65 and 'standard' primary renal disease (excludes multisystem and hereditary disease, but includes cystic diseases).

Age >65, standard PRD

Method of therapy	Proportion of patients on RRT		
	Start	1 yr	2 yr
CAPD	0.12	0.14	0.14
IPD	0.08	0.04	0.04
Graft	0	<0.01	0.01
Home HD	<0.01	0.01	0.01
Hosp. HD	0.80	0.82	0.82
Overall survival %		82.4	66.7

in 1983. Comparison of Table 8 and Table 9 shows the influence of the age of patients at date of first treatment on the contribution of different MOTs. These two tables include only patients with standard primary renal diseases (see caption table 8). CAPD has made a particularly noticeable contribution to the treatment of patients aged over 65, rising from 0.12 at start of RRT to 0.14 at the end of two yr. Among adults aged 15–55 the contribution was half as great (0.06–0.07).

Neither renal transplantation nor home haemodialysis contributed much to the treatment of patients aged over 65 who commenced RRT in 1983. The proportion of adults aged 15–55 who were dependent on hospital haemodialysis decreased progressively with time on RRT but there was no such reduction in the proportion of over 65's who relied on this therapy in the pooled European results. Overall survival after two years on RRT was 88.3% for patients aged 15–55; it was 66.7% for those aged over 65.

Table 10 shows how CAPD has been used preferentially for the treatment of patients with diabetic nephropathy, around one-quarter of whom were on CAPD at any time after commencement of RRT. Overall survival for patients

Table 10. Proportions of patients on different methods of therapy at start of first treatment of 1664 patients in 1983 and at first and second anniversaries with overall cumulative survival. All ages and diabetic nephropathy.

All ages, diabetic nephropathy

Methods of therapy	Proportion of patients on RRT		
	Start	*1 yr*	*2 yr*
CAPD	0.24	0.27	0.25
IPD	0.12	0.06	0.04
Graft	0.01	0.08	0.14
Home HD	0	0.01	0.01
Hosp. HD	0.63	0.61	0.61
Overall survival %		78.7	60.7

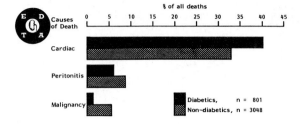

Figurie 30. Causes of death in diabetic and non-diabetic CAPD patients between 1983–86. Sixty CAPD patients who died in this period could not be classified as either diabetic or non-diabetic, explaining the different 'n' in Figures 29 and 30.

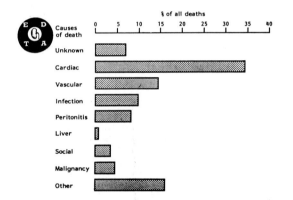

Figure 29. Causes of death in 3909 CAPD patients between 1983-86.

with diabetic nephropathy of all ages combined was inferior to that of the over 65 year-olds with standard primary renal diseases.

The causes of death for CAPD patients between 1983 and 1986 are graphed in Figures 29 and 30. 3909 CAPD patients died during this interval. We looked at the causes of death in relation to the duration of CAPD (<12 months or >12 months) and found no significant differences. Cardiac causes accounted for 33% of all deaths on CAPD from 1983 to 1986. For all the causes of death cited in Figure 29, we compared diabetics to non-diabetics. Figure 30 shows only those categories where diabetics and non-diabetics differed in the frequency of recorded causes of death. Diabetics were more likely to die of cardiac events as noted by others [11, 20] and non-diabetics were more likely to die from peritonitis or malignancies.

9. PERITONITIS

The patient questionnaire has evolved simultaneously with CAPD and certain questions or analyses addressing peritonitis were performed only in particular years. The findings of Wing et al described in the 2nd Edition of this text should be reiterated [3]. From the unique questions

in 1982, they noted that of the patients who did not experience peritonitis, 89% required only one catheter. Of those patients who experienced four or more episodes or peritonitis, 32% required new catheters. Furthermore, diabetics did not experience more frequent peritonitis than non-diabetics. However, diabetics did spend more time in hospital for peritonitis than non-diabetics. Almost 30% of diabetics spent 2 to 6 weeks hospitalised compared to 20% of the non-diabetics. For all patients the longer the duration of CAPD, the greater the likelihood of hospitalisation for peritonitis. The pattern of hospitalisation was not different between the middle-aged and the elderly. These 1982 data from the EDTA Registry have been confirmed by other investigators who have not found an increased hospitalisation rate in CAPD populations, which tend to be older than the haemodialysis population [9, 10]. Fifty per cent of the 1982 CAPD cohort was free of peritonitis while 7% had four or more episodes. The frequency of peritonitis increased the longer a patient was on CAPD. Of those patients on CAPD for 6–12 months, 40% had had at least two episodes of peritonitis.

Of the 1981 cohort for whom the reason for choosing CAPD was known prospectively, 38.6% of the 'first choice' (see Section 6 for details of these choices) patients were peritonitis-free during that year. Of the patients for whom CAPD was not the 'first choice' 47.6% remained free of peritonitis for 1981.

We determined peritonitis rates in patients on CAPD at some time in 1984 or 1985 by totalling episodes and dividing by the patient-years of CAPD which were calculated from each individual's dated treatment sequence. Table 11 shows the peritonitis rates in 14 selected countries and for the entire Registry in both years of the analysis. Observed differences could be related to national policies toward CAPD, for example, wider usage in the UK compared to the FRG, or to unique regional practices, such as the use of the Y-set in Italy, France, and Belgium. However, it is not possible to separate the effect of these influences from those of other variables.

We next evaluated peritonitis rates according to age (<15 yr, 15–64.9 yr, and >65 yr),duration of CAPD therapy (<3 months, 3–5.9 months, and >6 months), and the presence or absence of diabetes. Patients with no primary renal disease code were censored from Table 12 but were eligible for Table 11. Table 12 shows the peritonitis rates for these various categories. Infection rate in diabetics was not different from that of the non-diabetics, an observation

Table 11. Peritonitis rates in selected European countries

| Country | Episodes/yr | |
	1984	1985
Belgium	0.77	0.69
Denmark	1.79	0.94
Finland	1.96	0.94
France	1.29	0.77
Federal Republic of Germany	1.00	0.60
Greece	1.12	0.52
Israel	2.71	1.50
Italy	1.05	0.63
Netherlands	1.47	—
Spain	1.27	0.81
Sweden	1.16	0.53
Switzerland	0.98	0.83
United Kingdom	1.53	3.29
Yugoslavia	1.70	1.51
Total registry	1.34	1.44

Table 12. Combined 1984–85 CAPD peritonitis rates by age, duration of CAPD and diabetic status

Age (yr)	Duration of CAPD (months)	Diabetics	Non-diabetics
<15	<3	0 *	3.00
	3–5.9	0 *	1.42
	>6	2.84 *	1.13
	Total	2.51 *	1.23
15–64.9	<3	3.98	3.48
	3–5.9	1.71	2.31
	>6	1.33	1.29
	Total	1.44	1.40
65+	<3	3.96	3.75
	3–5.9	1.71	2.44
	>6	1.17	1.27
	Total	1.36	1.44
All ages	<3	3.98	3.52
	3–5.9	1.71	2.29
	>6	1.31	1.28
	Total	1.44	1.40

* Very small data base used to derive these values.

noted previously [21–23]. Infection rate was highest in those patients on CAPD for less than 3 months, and was lowest in those patients on CAPD for 6 months or greater, irrespective of age or primary renal disease. This probably reflects cumulative patient selection by which individuals with high infection rates either died or were changed to other therapy.

10. SUMMARY/CONCLUSIONS

CAPD has made a substantial contribution to the treatment of ESRF in many European countries. National policies differed markedly within the EDTA member countries.

ACKNOWLEDGEMENTS

The authors gratefully acknowledge the assistance of the Registry personnel and the Registration Committee, and the collaboration of the Directors of the European centres who have contributed data to the Registry. The Registry is funded in part by the parent Association, by European Governments, and by commercial companies. Dr Golper was on sabbatical leave from The Oregon Health Sciences University and the Portland Veterans Administration Medical Centre.

REFERENCES

1. EDTA Registration Committee EDTA Registry centre survey, 1985. Nephrol Dial Transpl: 1987 (in press).
2. EDTA Registration Committee: Demography of dialysis and transplantation in Europe, 1984. Nephrol Dial Transpl 1: 1–8, 1986.
3. Wing AJ, Moore R, Brunner FP *et al.*: Peritoneal dialysis results in the EDTA Registry. In: Peritoneal Dialysis, Second Edition. Nolph K (ed), Martinus Nijhoff Pub, Boston: pp 637–665, 1985.
4. Brunner FP, Broyer M, Brynger H *et al.*: Combined report on regular dialysis and transplantation in Europe, XV, 1984. Proc EDTA – ERA, 22nd Congress, Brussels, 22: 3–54, 1985.
5. Kramer P, Broyer M, Brunner FP *et al.*: Combined report on regular dialysis and transplantation in Europe, XIV, 1983. Proc EDTA-ERA, 21st Congress, Florence, 21: 2–68, 1985.
6. Wing AJ, Broyer M, Brunner FP *et al.*: Combined report on regular dialysis and transplantation in Europe, XIII, 1982. Proc EDTA-ERA, 20th Congress, London, 20: 2–75, 1983.
7. Broyer M, Brunner FP, Brynger H *et al.*: Combined Report on regular dialysis and transplantation in Europe, XII, 1981. Proc EDTA-ERA, 19th Congress, Madrid, 19: 2–59, 1983.
8. Geerlings W, Selwood NH, Brunner FP *et al.*: The contribution

of CAPD to overall survival on renal replacement therapy in Europe. Proc Xth Congress of the Intern Soc Nephrology: 1987 (in press).
9. Gokal R, King J, Boyle S *et al.*: Outcome in patients on continuous ambulatory peritoneal dialysis and haemodialysis: 4-yr analysis of a prospective multicentre study. Lancet 2: 1105–1109, 1987.
10. Gokal R, Baillod R, Boyle S *et al.*: Multicentre study on outcome of treatments in patients on continuous ambulatory peritoneal dialysis and haemodialysis. Nephrol Dial Transpl 2: 172–178, 1987.
11. Brunner FP, Brynger H, Challah S *et al.*: Renal replacement therapy in patients with diabetic nephropathy 1980–85. Data from the EDTA Registry. (manuscript submitted)
12. Burton PR, Walls J: Selection adjusted comparison of life expectancy of patients on continuous ambulatory peritoneal dialysis, haemodialysis and renal transplantation. Lancet 1: 1115–1119, 1987.
13. Wing AJ, Broyer M, Brunner FP *et al.*: The contribution of continuous ambulatory peritoneal dialysis in Europe. ASAIO 6: 214–219, 1983.
14. Editorial: CAPD – the white knight? Lancet 2: 1127–8, 1987.
15. Zimmerman SW, Johnson CA, O'Brien M: Long-term survivors

on peritoneal dialysis. Am J Kid Dis 10: 214–249, 1987.

16. Capelli JP, Camiscioli TC, Vallorini RD: Comparative analysis of survival on home haemodialysis, in-center hemodialysis and chronic peritoneal dialysis (CAPD-IPD) therapies. Dial and Transpl 14: 38–52, 1985.

17. EDTA Registration Committee. Combined report on regular dialysis and transplantation in Europe, XVII, 1986. Presented by W Geerlings: West Berlin, October 1987.

18. Nicholls AJ, Waldek S, Moorehead PJ *et al.*: Impact of continuous ambulatory peritoneal dialysis on treatment of renal failure in patients over 60. Br Med J 288: 18–19, 1984.

19. Taube DA, Winder EH, Ogg CS: Successful treatment of middle-aged and elderly patients with end-stage renal disease. Br Med J 286: 2018–2020, 1983.

20. Abraham G, Zlotnik M, Ayiomamitis A *et al.*: Drop-out of diabetic patients from CAPD. In: Advances in Continuous Ambulatory Peritoneal Dialysis. Ed. Khanna R, Nolph KD, Browant B, Twardowski ZJ, Oreopoulos DG: Peritoneal Dialysis Bulletin Inc. Univ of Toronto Press: Toronto, 1987.

21. Williams C, Belvedere D, Cattran D *et al.*: Experience with CAPD in diabetic patients in Toronto. Perit Dial Bull 2 (suppl): S12–S14, 1982.

22. Steinberg SM, Cutler SJ, Novak JW, Nolph KD: The USA CAPD Registry. Nolph KD (ed). In: Peritoneal Dialysis 2nd Edition. Martinus Nijhoff Publishing: Boston, 1985.

23. Khanna R, Oreopoulos DG: CAPD in patients with diabetes mellitus. Gokal R (ed). In: Continuous Ambulatory Peritoneal Dialysis. Churchill Livingstone: Edinburgh, 1986.

22

QUALITY OF LIFE IN PERITONEAL DIALYSIS PATIENTS: INSTRUMENTS AND APPLICATION

HOWARD J. BURTON, ROBERT M. LINDSAY, STEPHEN A. KLINE, and PAUL A. HEIDENHEIM

1. INTRODUCTION

For the past 25 years, dialysis has been advocated as an artificial replacement therapy for the functional loss of kidneys. Thousands of patients with chronic renal failure have been kept alive who otherwise would·have died. At present, in excess of 80 000 persons in the United States are on dialysis, a dramatic increase from the 2398 of 15 years ago [1]. This increase, in large measure, is due to the technological and treatment advances in renal replacement therapy. However, technologies such as automated dialysis systems [2, 3], bacteriologically safe catheters [4], and modified peritoneal dialysis procedures such as CAPD [5] or its automated nocturnal form, 'prolonged dwell' peritoneal dialysis [6], do more than sustain life. They enhance patients' physical status and tolerance for home treatment [7] and free them from the constraints of extracorporeal hemodialysis [8], thus contributing to overall improvement in patients' cognitive acuity and psychosocial functioning [9–12].

Nonetheless, these innovations in technique and care can have negative effects. They foster case mix and treatment approaches which in some respects mitigate against patient adjustment, thus diminishing quality of life [13]. They accelerate the assignment of patients to alternative treatment settings, often inappropriately, with subsequent negative outcomes for both the patient and family [14]. When the total treatment process is further complicated, preexisting patient/family system irritants are exacerbated and in many instances evolve into major psychosocial problems, which if untreated, can be detrimental to the very survival of the patient [15].

Evidence that psychosocial variables may be more important than physiological ones in determining success, failure, and ultimately survival of the patient on home

dialysis [16, 17] has major implications. Obviously, if survival rates are to continue to improve, factors negatively affecting individual patient well being must be identified. Corrective steps should be taken to minimize their impact and measures implemented to prevent their recurrence. These actions are especially important for those CAPD patients who have an estimated 50% chance of home failure after their initial two year treatment period, and a 80% chance of failure after 48 months [18].

Corrective actions can also benefit those patients who are part of the natural shift from centre dialysis to home treatment, and whose numbers are steadily increasing. For example, there was an approximately 114 percent increase of new CAPD and home hemodialysis patients in the last fifteen years in the United States. Interestingly, there was a rapid increase in the CAPD population from 7.8% of the home dialysis population in 1975 to 62.5% of the population in 1983 [1]. This trend has been similarly noted in Canada where currently 41% of new patients are being treated by CAPD and 35% of all patients on dialysis are being treated by it [19]. Current rates of organ transplantation indicate that this picture is unlikely to change. For these home dialysis patients, failure usually means a return to (high cost) in-hospital hemodialysis units.

The introduction of quality of life issues into regional home dialysis centres has sensitized renal team members to the importance of psychosocial parameters in reducing patient mortality and morbidity. As a consequence, the staff require more precision, clarity, and utility in their measurement. We have responded to this need by developing a dialysis related quality of life test battery that forgoes the traditional use of indices of health which rely on measures of the presence or absence of disease, life tables, and mortality rates. This latter approach, as exemplified by the article entitled 'Mortality, Morbidity, and Life Satisfaction in the Very Old Dialysis Patient' [20], illustrates the narrow medical-reductionist practice of utilizing well being indicators [21] that are easily quantifiable. We also rejected single summary statistics like the time trade-off method [22–25] and composite scores of quality of life, which capture the global characteristics of life satisfaction, happiness, sense of well being or similar constructs [26, 27] because they may provide incomplete or misleading pictures of life conditions [28]. They are not sensitive to many relevant factors, and as relative gross measures of health they are at variance with the present need by renal units for a health assessment that captures specific domains of quality of life.

This chapter addresses these issues of measurement, application and identification of critical quality of life indices. It provides an overview of psychosocial characteristics considered important for the successful adaptation of peritoneal patients, especially those on home treatment. It describes a multi-method approach to the measurement of quality of life that is reliable, valid and useful for estimating patients' perception of their well being. Lastly, it offers pragmatically useful information regarding the determinants of success in long-term CAPD patients together with predictive models and suggestions as to how to choose a dialysis therapy for a given patient. In large measure, it will draw from our ongoing research which over the last ten years has been directed to the task of identifying factors influencing both outcome and quality of life for a substantial sample of patients on home, center and self-care dialysis [29–31].

2. A QUALITY OF LIFE PERSPECTIVE OF ESRD

Because kidney disease inflicts upon both patients and their families a multitude of problems of a psychosocial nature, renal team members are frequently confronted with concerns about quality of life. They realize that renal replacement therapy generally requires modifications of the patients' extra-familiar social activities and intra-familiar social interactions [32–35]. Prescribed social roles are altered [36]; individual work patterns changed; career advancements blocked [37, 38]; and unemployment or early retirement more likely [39–43]. Patients report a reduction in the frequency of sexual intercourse, an inability to maintain a penile erection, and a general loss of sexual interest and arousal [44–48]. There is a change in intrapsychic coping as patients manifest signs of depression, anxiety, and social withdrawal, and express feelings of worthlessness and hopelessness. Mood and affect fluctuate. Intellectual processes decrease, and patients complain of memory loss and disturbances in their patterns of sleep [49–51]. Staff recognize that when unabated, the dependence on artificial life support devices, adherence to a strict medical regimen, greater financial hardships and a decrease in physical and social functioning, singularly or collectively, can cause major life style disruptions and require considerable psychological and social accommodation.

2.1. Living and dying

The dilemma for the renal patient is a difficult one. It is a dilemma that concerns itself as much with living as with dying. On the one hand, the patient fears life will be shortened by premature death. On the other hand, he is fearful that if he continues to live by artificial means, life may not be acceptable to himself or his family. He also fears that his physical health and his level of activity will decline and that his daily existence will be plagued by the constant threat of death and its accompanying stress. Peritoneal dialysis, he knows, will prolong his life but it is hard for him to accept that it will not return him to his former level of functioning.

For most patients, the conflicts of living and dying are resolved through positive adjustments. For others, the conflict is solved by suicide. Resolution by suicide is not surprising if one accepts the premise that all people have self destructive mechanisms [52]. Everyone controls these mechanisms until the environment invites one to stop living, an invitation that usually takes the form of a subtle message questioning the meaning and value of one's very being. It is theoretically simple for ESRD patients to end their lives because of the intrinsic nature of their disease and their potential control over their immediate environment; what is remarkable is that so few choose to terminate life.

Nonetheless, suicidal ideation and behavior are serious problems among dialysis patients [53]. Self destruction can be a preoccupation with patients, typically with difficulty facing the implications of their illness and struggling for a minimal existence.

The notion that patients often think about taking their life is generally accepted by the treatment team. However, they are in less agreement as to the number who actually do. Estimates of reported suicides range from four to 400 times that of the general population [54, 55]. To a large degree, rate discrepancies are based on differing opinions as to what constitutes genuine suicidal behaviour. Diet violations, for example, often are seen as the primary means of self destruction, but there is some question as to whether they should be evaluated from a suicidal framework.

Regardless of the interpretation of treatment abuses, significant numbers of patients find being chronically ill and in need of constant medical care almost as intolerable as the fear of imminent death. Paradoxically, their simple, almost fatalistic, attitude seems to act as an adequate psychological defense against lethal self destructive behaviour [56].

2.2. Compliance vs noncompliance

Nephrologists and dialysis nurses have major concerns about nonadherence to prescribed medical regimens. They know that noncompliance, especially to nutritional requirements is one of the most significant medical complications attendant on long term dialysis patients. They also acknowledge that for many, it becomes the vehicle for acting out conflicting feelings towards treatment. Carried to extremes, it can jeopardize the patient's life. This is equally true for both peritoneal and hemodialysis. Granted that CAPD may be less complex and the dietary and fluid restrictions less limiting, but it still requires major changes in the patient's lifestyle and coping strategies.

Reasons for noncompliance are complex and individualized but are understandable, given that dietary restrictions block the accustomed stress outlets such as eating, alcohol consumption or smoking excessively, and require a major readjustment from previous habits of consumption. Health belief motivators, the high value patients place on their health, and educational programs geared to diet management all fail to predict compliance and have no significant long-term effects on compliant behaviour [57, 58]. On the other hand, compliance is known to be positively associated with the measured internal locus of control [57], social support, knowledge of disease or therapy, stresses and strains, patient motives and perceived utility, and with age, education, social class, income and occupational status [59].

Additionally, how the patients feel about their illness can influence their degree of compliance [60]. For instance, statements of acceptance of the illness; not blaming others for their condition; acceptance of responsibility for their care; ability to control their anxiety concerning their illness; and recognition of gains in some instances from their illness, all indicate a positive feeling and tend to predict compliance with the medical regimen. Noncompliers look on their illness as an enemy or burden which renders them defenceless and powerless. Their illness is seen as being unjust. They accept dependency, become preoccupied with their illness, like to talk about it but will not become involved in their care. Negative feelings such as these tend to predict non-compliant behaviour.

According to Czaczkes and DeNour [61], compliance is important to physical well being and survival. Our data assessing outcomes (success, failure, death) on 117 patients at 17 months home treatment supports the former premise but not the latter [62]. Compliers over the first two years consistently had better physiological functioning than non-compliers and, indeed, the tendency of the non-compliers was to worsen their physiological status with time. Of notable interest is that hemodialysis non-compliers had a very high incidence of treatment related stress, whereas, there was no difference between compliers and non-compliers treated by CAPD.

Dialysis patients generally have problems complying. At some time, they cheat by not adhering to nutritional requirements or by altering their dialysis procedures. In part, variability in willingness to comply can be attributed to personality facctors. Low frustration tolerance and primary and secondary gains from the 'sick role' are commonly associated with noncompliance [63]. Physicians can use personality features to assure successful outcomes for CAPD patients. Meticulous, even obsessive-compulsive patients, for example, do well with their regular charting of exchanges, blood pressure and drugs, as well as with thorough care of the catheter [64]. Case studies have reported that patients who are compulsive and compliant and who manage their treatment accordingly, do extremely well on CAPD [65].

3. LOSS AND THREAT OF LOSS

3.1. Employment

The degree of rehabilitation is a major criteria used to establish a patient's adaptation to treatment. Conclusions as to the vocational rehabilitation of peritoneal patients are difficult to draw, since most studies pertinent to this area relate only to hemodialysis [66–72]. Yet it is plausible to expect that the working status of PD patients would depend on the same relevant characteristics as that of hemodialysis patients, namely, medical and psychological status [38] and social environment [73]. Participation in non-vocational activities and constructive interpersonal relationships which are positively associated with vocational rehabilitation [74, 75], and psychological manifestations like denial, displacement and projections which are negatively associated with poor rehabilitation [76] should similarly apply.

Full employment has been and still is, the ideal goal of most dialysis patients. For the group as a whole, it is unfortunately seldom attained. Research in 1977 by Hagarty and Hagarty [77] of centre and home peritoneal patients showed only 40% were employed. Of those employed, 64% were white collar workers; 36% were unskilled labourers. In 1980, we reported that 47% of home dialysis patients were employed of which 75% were married, and fifty percent were both males and under 40 years of age. This data suggests that many peritoneal dialysis patients are unemployed due to the disease and treatment, and not by choice [29]. Of the PD patients on CAPD, only eight percent remained at the same premorbid job; 20% moved to a different job and 72% left their employment because of their chronic illness. Almost three quarters of those employed worked less than a 40 hr week. Compared to employed hemodialysis patients, those CAPD patients who were working reported more problems in obtaining salary increases, and in receiving and accepting promotions. But they experienced fewer problems with their employers and fellow workers, and were less likely to transfer to a new job. In terms of continuity of employment (pre/post chronic renal insufficiency), hemodialysis patients had greater job stability than those on CAPD. This was equally true of housewives, who were more likely to resume their household duties [78, 79]. These findings have since been replicated [80, 81].

Comparisons of our most recent findings about vocational rehabilitation with that of others is difficult. Whereas some researchers speak about only two categories – complete vocational rehabilitation (full time employment) and no rehabilitation at all, we include in our definition employment status, absenteeism from work and interference wth household and work activities. Additionally, our findings are based on a home dialysis population comprising 28% hemodialysis, 5% IPD and 67% CAPD. Still, the percentage we found to be gainfully employed at the start of their home training program [48.5%] and at the end of a two year experience [42.9%] are similar to the 52% reported by Czaczkes and DeNour [61], higher than the 31.6% reported by Cadnapaphornchai *et al.* [82], but much lower than those reported by Cameron *et al.* [83], Pendras and Pollard [84], Disney and Row [85], and Brunner *et al.* [86], each of whom report in excess of 70%. Differences in the reported percentages which range from 32% to 92% may be due to differences in patient populations or differences in dialysis hours or schedules. For instance, Tews [71] notes that patients with full-time employment tend to be dialyzed in evening or night shifts, and that patients with high overall stress including medical problems, adaptation to dialysis and problems of a personal or family nature are more likely to be out of work than patients with low overall stress.

Dialysis is particularly problematic for those patients working at the onset of their chronic condition. The necessity for physical restrictions makes previous employment involving manual activity prohibitive, while the illness-related absences from work diminishes job responsibilities. The almost a week per month rate of absenteeism of our study patients, pre-home treatment, confirms the observations of others. However, within 17 months, absenteeism was reduced dramatically to that of less than half a day a month on average [30]. This probably reflects the flexibility in dialysis scheduling of home treatment which is known to enhance patient rehabilitation in terms of full time employment [61].

While the level of vocational rehabilitation is used by medical teams as an index of improved quality of life, very little is known about how patients feel and think about their work. Some researchers found that 95% of their patients believe they work as efficiently as they did before dialysis. Others report that many patients complain of decreased work efficiency [87]. We found that home dialysis posed little interference for work. Similarly, there was much less interference with household chores as one proceeds with home dialysis [88].

From reported findings it is evident that threat of loss of job is always present for ESRD patients, but actual loss of employment varies from patient to patient. For the majority of patients, a reduction in occupational status within their community is a common occurrence, and a disproportionate number are forced to either alter their job responsibilities, or leave or change their employment. For those engaged in occupations less physically demanding and/or amenable to flexibility, it is easier to maintain employment [66]. In certain occupations, the necessity for regular bag changes creates a problem for those on CAPD [67].

From our clinical observations, it is apparent that rehabilitation usually includes plans by the renal staff and the patient for their return to full time employment. This goal reflects the North American value that work is an important indicator of well being and, therefore, is viewed as a worthwhile treatment objective. Unfortunately, disincentives to work, such as eligibility for benefits, are counterproductive and frequently undermine the efforts of vocational rehabilitation. A case in point are those individuals who, in the initital stages of treatment and while adjusting to their condition, choose to receive municipal, state or federal assistance or long term disability benefits. At some time in the future, if they seek out part time work as an initial step to full employment, they and their families can face major financial difficulties. Many governmental programs are inflexible and fail to consider earnings from part time work. Benefits like medication and transportation may have to be assumed by the patient when he becomes employed. These bureaucratic disincentives, when compounded by the time requirements of dialysis and the possibility that a bag change may need to occur on the job, often create problems for the patient that far outweigh the advantages of being employed.

3.2. Body image, self image and self esteen

Body image is the central and personal representation of body parts and of the body as a whole. It influences what a person does and does not do, attitudes and opinions, even more so than does the realistic image of the body [89]. Perceptions of distorted body image tend to arouse great emotional tension, to disrupt habitual patterns of daily behaviour, to reduce mental efficiency and produce painfully unpleasant effects [90].

According to Deutsch [91], the stress associated with fear of loss of bodily parts is rarely, if ever, definitively solved. For patients with chronic renal failure, these fears are particularly common. Loss of body function or part of the body has been recorded as a major cause of stress by Cummings [92], DeNour and Czaczkes [93], and Wright and colleagues [94]. Abram [95], Kestenbaum [96], Shea and co-workers [97], and Kemph [98] have also given special attention to the unpleasant effects that follow disturbance in body image.

Patient-machine relationships and their influence on body image received much attention in the late 1960s and early 1970s as did concern with the arteriovenous shunts and their effects on general appearance [93]. Problems related to body image still occur but do so less frequently and with less severity as in the earlier days of dialysis. Changes in body image, however, remain a major source of stress for those who are attached to artificial devices or have their kidneys removed [61]. Diminution of body image is also evident for those on CAPD. It occurs as a frequent reaction to the presence of a permanent catheter, the wearing of an empty CAPD bag [67], the noises produced by the fluid and the sensation of feeling full [64].

Distortions of self image are quite common in dialysis patients. Their perceptions of self in relation to their environment is a major determinant. This is especially true as it relates to shifts in social roles, patient-staff interactions, and the physical changes related to renal failure. Perceptive clinicians are cognizant that increased dependency on family and staff and perceived loss of stature are particularly difficult for those patients who put a high premium on self sufficiency and independence. Loss of self image is especially a problem felt by previously independent males [99]. Self image is negatively correlated with an ability to adequately perform employment or household tasks, economic status, aspirations for the future, physical appearance, and the feeling of attractiveness [92].

As for loss of esteem, a number of events are contributing factors. Some people associate it with the loss of intellectual functioning secondary to uremic toxins, with feelings of estrangement and loneliness and with the loss of interest in the immediate environment [92, 100, 101]. Others maintain self esteem is seriously affected by loss of membership in social groups, failures of plans or ventures, decrease in financial and occupational status, frustration of drives, and by the role reversal which frequently occurs as a consequence of inactivity [94, 95]. Shame and feelings of failure and weakness are also concomitant with feeling of loss of self esteem [102].

In summary, peritoneal dialysis patients behave similarly to those on hemodialysis and to others with chronic illness. Each patient handles the threat of loss, or actual loss, of body image, self image and self esteem as an outgrowth of previously existing personality development, of the ways of coping with previous conflicts and anxieties, and of the meaning attached to the current illness [103].

3.3. Sexual relations

Information regarding patients' sexual relations was sparse in the early years of dialysis. More recently, a wealth of data on this subject has been published and a clearer picture of that aspect of adjustment emerges. The most frequently cited observation is the deterioration of sexual function in both sexes after dialysis, despite improvement in general physical condition and in hormonal balances [104]. Men and women both report a decrease in libido and a marked reduction in frequency of intercourse [105]. Significant correlations have been reported between the problems of potency and libido, and those of vocational rehabilitation, depression, self image, sick role, dominance, and age at the time of diagnosis [76, 106, 107].

Our experience is that both CAPD and hemodialysis patients complain frequently about marital and sexual concerns [108]. Hemodialysis patients, however, experience significantly more problems with sexual dysfunction than those on CAPD. They are more concerned by their loss of libido, and avoid sexual activity out of fear of damage to their blood access devices. This appears especially true of females. Compared with CAPD patients, those on hemodialysis also complain more often of loss of sexual identity and attractiveness. Even those between 60 and 79 years of age on hemodialysis indicate greater changes in sexual activity and loss of sexual attractiveness than their counterparts on CAPD.

These findings should not minimize the unique sexual problems faced by patients on CAPD. Sexual difficulties do arise from the belief that the 'bag' is ugly and undesirable [60]. Individuals partake of sexual activities less often. We noted a 30% increase in those who no longer engaged in intercourse after having commenced CAPD and there was a fourfold increase of men who reported difficulty maintaining an erection [109].

'Unfortunately, sexual functioning is an area of the patient's life that the nurse often feels most uncomfortable or incapable of helping the patient express [110]'. It need not be. At the outset, the nurse should accept the fact and impart to the patient with conviction that sexual functioning of dialysis patients can be normal when those factors that interact and influence with it are also normal. Sexual activities will continue only if the patient is physically sound, his or her marital relations are satisfactory and if psychiatric complications, especially depression, are minimized.

This requires that the staff obtain an adequate assessment of sexual functioning and explore with the patient and sexual partner the meaning of sexuality. As a useful first approach, Lancaster [111] suggests that the history taking enterprise elicit answers to five basic questions:

1. How does the patient express his needs for dependency, independency, intimacy, or isolation?
2. How is the loss of sexual potency related to other areas of functioning such as job, sports, or hobbies?
3. How does one define himself or herself in light of a changing body image?
4. Does one's view of masculine or feminine roles undergo changes?
5. Is there enough trust, sharing, and communication between the partners and staff to deal with these personal issues?

This process of sharing problems with a careful listener, according to Lancaster, frequently results in the couple finding they can work out many of their own difficulties. He recommends that the nurse center the therapeutic encounter around 'being' rather than 'performing'. This should help the couple recognize the human needs of touch, tenderness and respect, above but not independent of, the masculine or feminine role. And by setting aside personal values, the couple's personal style of giving and sharing affection is legitimized.

3.4. Social/leisure activities

Social participation and deployment of leisure time are non-work activities known to be strongly related to a sense of well being [112]. This is a belief held widely by renal staff. Those dialysis patients and families who pursue outside interests are seen as better adjusted emotionally. The staff believe outside interests provide the opportunity for those on dialysis to become absorbed in an activity which distracts from self preoccupation and excessive introspection. Keeping personal concerns at a distance, they argue, appears to recharge the patient's emotional and intellectual apparatus to deal more effectively and objectively with his/her personal problems.

Research indicates that the dialysis regimen interferes with both social interaction and recreation thereby posing one of the greatest threats to patients' sense of well being [113, 114]. The magnitude of change varies according to age, modality and setting. Older patients experience a marked reduction in their leisure activities [115]. Compared to younger and middle age home patients, the elderly participate less often in physical and social activities. They also have a tendency to engage in fewer sedentary and community pursuits [116]. This is not to discount the fact that older dialysis patients perceive their life quality to be better than do younger dialysants [28]. They utilize social support as well as, and in some instances, better than their younger cohorts, and as a group evidence less psychological dysfunction and a greater capacity to handle a variety of important stressors [116].

Hemodialysis with its complex treatment regimen limits life style and restricts extra-familiar social activity [74, 117]. Even the simpler process of CAPD can diminish physical activities, but less so than hemodialysis [118]. Comparatively, those on CAPD spend significantly less time on sedentary activities, whereas home hemodialysis patients increase their passive activities over time. As for home and in-centre dialysis patients, both report a significant decrease in social functioning [119].

All available data support the hypothesis that social

activities for those with chronic kidney disease are limited. The majority continue with passive recreation – listening to the radio, reading newspapers or watching television [120]. Roughly 50% of patients are involved in sports, or active recreation including swimming, golf, hunting and fishing [77]. Approximately sixty percent of patients report that their leisure activities decrease somewhat. Eighteen percent had a significant decrease [121]. DeNour [115] reported that nearly 50% of her sample hardly participated in social leisure activities. She suggests that failure to participate in certain activities may reflect lack of interest. Although nearly 60% of her patients reported maintained interest in individual leisure activities, a much smaller number reported maintained interest in family leisure activities [38%] and in social leisure activities [33%]. This data is supported by others who report few dialysis patients are inclined to socialize out of the house [29], and that their participation in clubs and associations is almost nonexistent [118]. While the overall benefits of socialization are welcomed, not all outcomes are desired. Avoidance of personal involvement with fellow patients has been linked to survival in both men and women [122].

Despite this gloomy picture, there is a ray of hope. More encouraging figures suggest that we can expect 25% of chronic renal failure patients to have some decrease in social activities, but only 20 percent to have a marked decrease. Rates of participation will increase with input from renal team members. By insisting that patients participate in exercise programs, not only will their activity be increased and interpersonal functioning improved significantly, but they will also experience less anxiety and depression [123]. More importantly, these beneficial effects can be long lasting [124]. Additionally, staff efforts directed at keeping the patient working will be rewarded. Those who remain in their occupation also continue their leisure activities without a great change [121, 61].

4. COPING WITH ILLNESS

Anxiety and depression

Anxiety, a frequently observed reaction [38, 125], manifests high levels in all ESRD patients. As a group, they show significantly higher levels than normal individuals [40]. Much of the anxiety is related to the fear of dying and of peritonitis, psychological stresses, financial worries, changes in lifestyle, and the perceived loss of support from the hospital staff [126]. Anxiety is particularly evident during the first three to six months of dialysis, when the majority of patients experience intense awareness of, and vulnerability to, the stresses inherent in their situation [95–98].

Sex differences are clearly evident. Women are more likely to be anxious than are men, irrespective of mode of treatment [118]. However, females on CAPD are significantly less anxious than those on hemodialysis, and show a marginal decrease in their anxiety during the initial home experience. This is in contrast to the marked increase in anxiety for females on hemodialysis [108]. In selecting patients for a home program, these differences should be considered.

With CAPD, age has little influence on how a patient group experiences anxiety. Anxiety in patients over 65 is similar to that of younger individuals. However, there is a trend for those in the middle years (age 45–64) to experience greater anxiety than those older and younger [116]. The young and old patients show marginal differences. Despite the minimal differences in expressed anxiety, the renal team should be aware that elderly dialysis patients experience anxiety states with greater frequency than the elderly in the general population. These attacks usually are transient and commonly occur in response to sudden changes in the environment or in health status.

Patients who are stressed and anxious usually are depressed. Depression, in fact, has been called the most common complication of dialysis [127, 128]. It may be manifested by a 'giving up' syndrome in which patients no longer actively participate in their own care, and disregard their medical instructions [129]. In these circumstances, severe complications and death frequently occur. Depression as the primary problem of dialysis has been questioned [130]. A number of studies have failed to find elevated levels of depression in their dialysis subjects [131–137]. Because these levels vary considerably, this may reflect a peculiarity in sample selection. It could also reflect the preference of the researcher to focus solely on clinical depression.

There is also disagreement as to the reasons for the existence of depression. Some argue, it is a function of patients' realization of the complex responsibilities in their 'new life' [138]. Others state it is a gradually developing entity, evolving from dialysis patients' continuous struggle to cope with day-to-day stresses [139]. It is speculated that depression originates from guilt over regime violations; shame related to physical appearance; difficulties caused to others; and to the nature of the illness [140].

Regardless of etiology, depression in ESRD patients is significantly deeper than in the general population [94, 140, 141]. We know that patients may suffer severe depressive reactions, even after they have been stabilized medically through dialysis [129, 139]. These reactions often are accompanied by apathy and suicidal ideation, and can be sufficiently severe to impede the patient's cooperation in self care and adherence to dietary restrictions.

We also know that the incidence and prevalence of depression are highest in those dialysis patients age 55 to 70 [142]. Their clinical picture of depression is similar to that of elderly individuals in general. Like their counterparts, they are less likely than young persons to admit to the symptoms of depression itself. They are more likely to complain of the symptoms of anxiety, somatization, hypochondriasis, or to a loss of concentration and memory deficit [143]. The elderly dialysis patient may manifest an atypical picture of masked depression. Here, the clinical presentation may be one of apathy, withdrawal, somatic complaints and functional slowness [144]. Interestingly, CAPD patients over 65 are significantly less depressed than those in the middle years. Their depression scores compare favorably to those CAPD patients under age 45 [116].

Renal team members need be cognizant of the fact that amog all the psychosocial parameters we examined, depression distinguishes more clearly those who failed, succeeded or died while on a home program [15, 16]. Additionally, the severity and type of depression is of particular importance to outcome [145]. The depressive profile (Type 1) of those patients who succeed on home dialysis is one of profound anxiety, with elevated levels of self-depreciation, social introverson, and hypochondriasis. The profile of those at risk to die (Type II) is one of a tendency toward pre-occupation with complaints, degradation of self as being worthless, unpleasant, and undeserving, and an inclination to be downhearted, despondent, and pessimistic.

In the presence of a Type I profile, patients are likely to manage well on a home dialysis program. A clinical and psychological profile associated with failure to survive (Type II) warrants emergency intervention by the dialysis team. The minimum response would include a clinical psychological assessment with immediate institution of necessary supportive measures. Identification of key determinants that may impede survival may help to minimize unnecessary mortality and morbidity by early appropriate intervention and will likely improve patients' adaptation to this illness, thus influencing their quality of life.

Unfortunately, it is not unusual for depressed ESRD patients to remain untreated. Because the symptoms of depression and uremia often overlap, the former can be mistakenly attributed to the disease process itself. An imbalance in biochemical structure (i.e. elevated BUN levels, acidemia, electrolyte disturbances, and disordered calcium metabolism) may cause the patient to exhibit a depressed affect [146]. Thus in assessing dysphoric symptoms, consideration should be given to the possibility of chemical imbalance [147]. This is less likely to occur in those patients dialyzing by innovative peritoneal procedures, since these procedures purport to have the advantage over hemodialysis in maintenance of a steady biochemical state in the blood [148]. Consideration should also be given to the possibility of a depression being induced by antihypertensive medications, steroids, barbiturates, cimetidine, and benzodiazepines [146].

It is apparent that untreated depression creates management problems of great magnitude. If not resolved, it may endanger patients' lives. The severely depressed grow chronically more preoccupied with feelings of unworthiness, failure or hopelessness. They lose initiative and interest and lapse into repetitive expressions of futility with their situation. Where the patient is more obtunded clinically or where there is suicidal risk, antidepressants may have a role.

4.2. Adaptive vs maladaptive denial

Denial is a frequently used mechanism employed by dialysis patients to cope, especially with depression [95, 113, 149, 150]. It is a necessary tool for dealing with uncertainties and unfortunate realities in their lives, and a useful, effective means of helping them handle their continuing unsatisfactory physical condition [151].

The use of denial to cope with chronic renal failure can be a blessing for the patient, and no attempt should be made to substitute a more realistic attitude [117]. Used up to a point, denial permits the patient to live with his illness. It is a characteristic reaction to stress and in fact is used more by dialysis patients than any other group of chronically ill [152]. Denial should be viewed as a constant

mechanism which protects the patient from experiencing intensive feelings of helplessness when they are depressed. It reduces the appreciation of stresses and concerns and, indeed, has been found to positively correlate with success on home hemodialysis in males over the age of 45 [16].

However, as Yanagida and associates point out [152] patients with low levels of denial may be more difficult for staff to treat. They are more likely to experience negative effects, and yet compliance may not be better. In some cases, massive denial can disrupt basic reality. It can cause a patient to view any sort of psychiatric intervention with suspicion, negativity and indifference. Excessive denial is a potential killer when the individual refuses to accept the demands and limitations of his disease. There are case studies that suggest massive denial may be of delusional proportions [153]. Denial may prevent the patient from hearing instructions and information, from recognizing emotional conflicts and difficulties, and may cause the patient to ignore necessary medical procedures.

Denial appears to be employed differently across dialysis age groups but in a consistent way. For instance, in our CAPD population, we found that it significantly increases with age but has no relationship to gender, mode of dialysis or length of time on a home program [118]. Clinically speaking, we found that there is an intermediate range of defensive strength in the use of denial which allows optimal coping, while extreme deviations on either side have adverse effects. In the absence of denial, stress prevails. If it dominates the patient's function, it seriously restricts the ability to concentrate on external or internal threats and to deal with them effectively. This delicate dilemma seems to have been solved most successfully by the elderly, who experience much less stress than do younger people and are better able to handle a variety of problems [116].

4.3. Stresses and concerns

Of the causes of stress for ESRD patients, twelve are usually cited: frequent and/or prolonged hospitalization, loss or threat of loss, frustration of basic drives, role changes, restrictions, dependency, an increase in aggression, threat of death, changes in body image and self image, activities of daily living and the stresses associated with the illness per se and the treatment process.

While the sources of stress are similar for both CAPD and hemodialysis patients [154, 155], the frequency with which they occur and the extent of discomfort differ. Overall CAPD patients experience significantly fewer episodes of stress and the severity is less [8, 156]. Both groups report physical weakness as the most common stressor. The stress associated with fluid restrictions, sleep disturbances, headaches, and decreased sexual functioning is significantly lower for CAPD patients than for hemodialysis subjects [156]. Females on hemodialysis report much more stress and concern than those on CAPD. Males did not differ in the frequency of experienced stress, but men on CAPD did indicate less concern [78, 79].

The most stressful items identified by the CAPD patients in a study by Eichel [154] were fatigue and limitations in activity. We found CAPD patients to be concerned more about having to alter or cancel vacation plans than their feelings of dependence on others, the financial problems they face or their decrease in sexual ability. They are least concerned about marriage strain, loss of family roles and care of children [29]. CAPD and IPD home patients have a great fear of infection, followed closely by feelings of being physically weak, fear of death, cramps and an inability to sleep. They are rarely affected by the stresses associated with headaches, itchiness, fear of blood clotting, pain during dialysis, dietary restriction and fear of losing dialysis sites [29, 30].

Coping capabilities of dialysis patients varies with age. We discovered that at the start of a home training program, the stress associated with life crises in those under age 40 is proportionately higher than those 60 and over, or those in their middle years. This finding held true after three months of home therapy, even with an overall increase among all patients [118]. This increase was especially evident with respect to changes in personal, recreational and sleeping habits, living conditions, spouses beginning or stopping work, trouble with in-laws, arguments with spouses, death of a close friend, major financial changes, sexual difficulties, changes in health of other family members and stress related to personal injury or illness. These findings confirm those of others [97, 157, 158].

Besides major life crises, home dialysis patients over 60 also experience the least stress associated with activities of daily living [116], a pattern that holds true of CAPD as well [156]. Elderly patients likewise report less stress from their dialysis treatment. Compared to those younger, older CAPD patients ($>$ 65) are significantly less concerned by cramps, pain or discomfort during dialysis, headaches, fear of death, fear of blood clotting, fear of loss of dialysis sites, being physically weak and up and down health [156].

4.4. Dependency vs independency

Dependence on dialysis, on the medical team and on family members is a major source of stress and a likely encumbrance to successful adaptation to renal failure. All dialysis patients are reliant on someone or something for assistance and emotional support. Contingent on the degree and nature of his physical and emotional impairment, the patient may be unable to take care of many of his medical needs and become dependent. Most patients handle this situation well. While some react through passive dependence, others deny the realities of the situation.

Those who adopt the dependent role obtain gratification in being cared for, and resist learning to care for themselves. In extreme cases, patients become almost parasitic and find themselves in a role at odds with the strongly valued attribute of 'self reliance'.

In attempts to develop self reliance, dialysis patients should be reminded that much of their overall physical and mental adjustment depends upon how well they accept responsibility of their own treatment. Home peritoneal dialysis self-care programs directed to this end (i.e. bringing about patient independence) have not been that successful [159]. Patients will modify the self care approach by involving a partner in some significant part of their training and treatment, usually, prior to completion of the training course. This has certainly been our experience with CAPD which purports to offer total patient independence. Large numbers of patients on this modality have dialysis assistants

and complain of being dependent on others [29]. It has been suggested that a home peritoneal patient's need for social interaction may supersede the need for independence of self treatment [159]. There is no argument on our part as to the important influence that social interaction and social support have in influencing outcome in ESRD [160].

4.5. Family and marital relationship

Families are invariably affected by the illness of the dialysis patient, and must learn to cope with the latter's fluctuating health, physical weakness and threat of death. They may also face loss of income and have to alter or forego vacations. Families often deny or refuse to accept the realities of the illness [158].

For families in stress, adjustment for the spouse is particularly difficult [161]. Many are troubled by depression and grief, and some feel hostility because of the patient's increased dependency [162]. When multiple roles are assumed, including those of the patient, the spouse may become even more exhausted and deeply depressed [162].

Fortunately, the majority of families are able to cope. A comprehensive study of centre and home dialysis showed that nearly 50% of the patients felt the quality of their marriage had not been affected by dialysis. Indeed, approximately 40% thought the illness had strengthened their marriage. Only six percent reported that the illness was responsible for their separation [31]. We found that CAPD patients indicated more support from their household members and greater satisfaction with interspousal relationships than did their counterparts on home hemodialysis. Yet they were as equally dependent on their spouses [163, 164].

5. MULTI-METHOD ASSESSMENT OF CHRONIC RENAL FAILURE

Because the concept of quality of life is generally subjective, its empirical assessment is difficult. People's perceptions of it differ depending on personal expectations, experience, attitudes, values, or philosophy. Definitions often remain implicit or vaguely described [165–169]. Included in its many descriptions are a person's ability to perform the ordinary activities of daily life, the ability to realize life plans, or alternatively, an objective measures of one's environment [170]. To further compound the problem, indices of quality of life often include, in its formulation, overlapping and unspecified concepts [171]. This leads to inconsistencies in the interpretation of what actually constitutes the concept under consideration [27]. Nonetheless, quality of life has become a popular phrase indicating a state of well being against which comparison can be made with the processes and outcomes of health care.

A review of the literature indicates that well being measures have a wide range of applications prescribed in part by the purpose of the particular research [112, 165, 173]. Social adjustment scales have been applied to psychiatry since the 1950's and were extensively reviewed by Weissman [171, 174]. To address the nonpsychiatric patient population, a number of disease-specific instruments have also been developed [175]. Quality of life estimates apply to patients with cardiovascular problems [176], diabetes

[177], joint diseases [178], chronic lung disease [179], and rheumatoid arthritis [180], to name but a few. Instruments have assessed functional ability [181, 182], recorded health status [183–185], or focused on one aspect of illness such as daily life skills [186], adjustment to illness [187], meaning of illness [188], or illness behaviour [189].

Churchill, in his review of tools used to estimate quality of life in end-stage renal disease, suggests that they can be conceptually divided into those that provide a global assessment of well being and those that attempt to 'identify the components which contribute to perceived quality of life' [22]. He reports studies by Levy and Wynbrandt [190], Brown *et al.* [191]. Bergsten *et al.* [192], DeNour and Shannon [193], and Laborde and Powers [26] as exemplifying global assessments. Representative studies of quality of life directed to more specific constructs are not reported, but have been extensively documented by Ferrans and Powers [27]. They note that there is an infinite number of aspects of life which should be included in quality of life measurement of which the following are of special merit: subject assessment of life satisfaction [194], socioeconomic status [195], physical health [196], affect [197], perceived stress [198], friendship [199], family [200], marriage [201], life goals [202], housing and neighborhood [203], self-esteem [204], depression [195], psychological defense mechanisms [193], and coping [190].

We conclude from these studies that quality of life measurement is still in a state of flux. There is no consensus as to the preference for single or multi-dimensional indicators or the appropriateness of subjective rather than objective measures. Nor is there consensus as to the framework by which quality of life concepts should be measured [205]. However, there is general agreement as to the need for a scale with proven psychometric properties that provides a simple, systematic method to assess the effects of disabling illness, to monitor its progress and to predict its course.

Over the past ten years, the authors have directed their research endeavours to the realization of this task. The degree to which we have succeeded is reflected in the use of our quality of life questionnaire in research studies in both North America and Europe. Our scales have demonstrated that they are capable of revealing, patients' hopes, fears, successes, disappointments and problems. As such, the questionnaire has import as a screening tool to identify the at risk patient. In clinical trials, the instrument has shown good monitoring capabilities and predictive power. These characteristics should be of value to psychiatrists, psychologists and social workers, whose professional roles involve therapeutic interventions aimed at improving the quality of life of their patients. Augmenting their clinical impressions with empirical data should be of benefit to them in both tailoring specific aspects of treatment delivery to suit patients' individual lifestyles, and in maximizing the effectiveness of treatment.

5.1. Renal disease test battery of biopsychosocial functioning

The test battery was developed from data obtained over the last ten years on approximately 1000 ESRD patients from hospital, home or satellite care centres in North America and Europe. The data was used to create a multidimensional instrument that captures specific domains of quality of life. This approach acknowledges the multifaceted nature of the concept, the variability of importance that people attach to each dimension, and the fact that domains impact differently on well being [200, 206]. Employing varying health indices as opposed to a single measure allows an examination of the interrelationships between indicators, and for a more precise specification as to which aspects of adjustment are predictive. It also allows for the utilization of both subjective and objective measures, a strategy preferred by George and Bearon [207], for assessing quality of life and tapping patients' subjective experiences.

This self-report, pencil and paper questionnaire incorporates life domains important to persons with renal disease: social/leisure time activities, biophysical stress, social/emotional support, psychological coping mechanisms, physiological status, fatigue and sleep disturbances, household management and work performance. The domains have a crucial element in common. All reflect variations in personal resources. In this respect, they parallel the three clusters of psychosocial indicators of Zill's [208] conceptual framework of 'effective life management':
a) indicators of environmental stress:
b) indicators of social functioning; and
c) indicators of 'coping resources' available.
The test battery is designed within this framework. As a model, it assumes that patients have a greater or lesser command of their personal resources which will determine variations in effective life management. It further presumes that the various domains of life experience vary widely with differing modalities, settings and equipment. Item selection, scale construction and field testing were carried out in accordance with the guidelines for measuring quality of life as suggested by Guyatt *et al.* [175].

The instrument has been used as a descriptive, predictive and evaluative index of quality of life. Used descriptively, it has distinguished between groups of dialysis patients selected on the basis of age, sex, and treatment modality [29–31]. As a predictive index of health outcome it has foretold survival on home dialysis [15] and adaptation to home hemodialysis [16]. We used selected domains from the battery in applied research to evaluate new dialysis procedures [209] and equipment [210]. Under all three applications, the instrument proved to be valid, reliable and sensitive to individual change and subgroup differences. Since the scales are short and easy to complete, and can be used individually or in combination, they are suitable for clinical use in the routine monitoring and assessment of renal patients.

5.2. Assessing personality dysfunction

Most of the current research by psychonephrologists is directed to establishing the relationship between personality and adaptation [211]; predicting emotional adjustment and survival [15, 212] or assessing personality traits [213]. Preference is usually given to the use of assessment tools oriented to the measurement of psychopathology (eg. MMPI). Inevitably, the reliability and validity of these devices have not been established on an ESRD population.

In some respects, this relates to the problems that this medical condition poses for traditional psychological test batteries [214].

The assessment tool we selected (Basic Personality Inventory – BPI) emphasizes symptom formation rather than psychopathology and has proven psychometric properties [214, 215] which are not diluted with use with an ESRD population [29, 30]. By establishing suitability prior to use we adhered to the admonition of Osberg *et al.* [10] not to use psychological tools validated only in normal populations but rather to validate the instrument on the population for which their use is intended.

The BPI, developed out of the work of Hoffman, Jackson and Skinner [216] is a 12-scale, 240-item, true/false inventory based on modern principles of test construction for item writing and selection procedures [217, 218]. The scales represent relatively independent aspects of traditional dimensions of psychological dysfunction. The reliabilities for the six subscales used in our ESRD studies (i.e. hypochondriasis, depression, denial, anxiety, social introversion, self depreciation) range from a high of 0.84 to a low of 0.63 (Table 1). The overall Cronbach's alpha, which is a conservative estimate of internal consistency, was 0.76. The remaining scales were not utilized because the dimensions measured were considered less appropriate to the medical condition under investigation.

5.3. Assessing dialysis stress

The quality of life of ESRD patients can be altered by the presence and severity of the symptoms of the disease and the symptoms induced by treatment. We found [219], as have others [220], that dialysis stress related symptoms not alleviated by medication or diminished by psychotherapeutic intervention increases the likelihood of an unfavourable prognosis.

Our dialysis stress scale (DSS) is the precursor of instruments developed by Baldree *et al.* in 1982 [221] and modified for a CAPD population by Eichel [220] in 1986. The DSS consists of two 7-item subscales that captures patient stress related to the symptoms of chronic uremia (Disease Related Stress – DRS) and those stress symptoms that stem from the problems and discomforts of dialysis and other therapeutic demands (Treatment Related Stress – TRS).

Items on the Disease Related Scale reflect fears and concerns generally related to chronic renal failure and include: being physically weak, fear of death, fear of blood clotting, up and down health, itching, inability to sleep, sexual functioning. The scale scores provide an estimate of incidence, total and mean per item stress. Reliabilities, as reported in Table 1, are quite acceptable.

Items specific to the Treatment Related Stress Scale (TRS) include: cramps, pain or discomfort during dialysis, fear of access site problems, infections, dietary and liquid restrictions. Scoring is identical to that of the Disease Related Stress Scale. Scale reliability is noted in Table 1. Evidence of content and construct validity for the disease and treatment stress scales is reported elsewhere [29, 30, 209].

For use as an evaluative index, the Dialysis Stress Scale has been revised. In the first revision, nine items were selected that reflected only somatic symptoms (e.g. nausea, vomiting, headache, dizziness, back and chest pain, hypotension, muscle cramps and smarting of extremities). This new scale (Somatic Symptoms Distress Scale – SSDS) performed well in an evaluative randomized pilot study comparing the adequacy of dialysis of an in-center hemodialysis sample utilizing different dialyzers [210]. An expanded version of the Somatic Symptom Distress Scale is currently being field tested in a number of European dialysis centers. Preliminary data indicates it is both reliable and valid across cultures [222].

A 53-item Treatment Related Stress Scale was developed for use with a CAPD patient population. Field tests in a pilot study [211] of a stratified random sample of 50 CAPD patients from seven American dialysis centres established excellent psychometric properties (Table 1). Confirmatory evidence of reliability and validity was reported by Schreiber *et al.*, in an evaluative clinical trial of dialyzer use with 103 CAPD patients from seven American and three Canadian hospitals [210].

5.4. Assessing stresses of daily living

Empirical referents for quality of life include mobility, performance of social roles and the ability and energy to perform necessary daily activities. These elements are significantly influenced by the patient's overall functional capacity. If the patient's capacity to carry out the usual activities of day-today life are seriously impaired by uremic symptoms and psychological dysfunctioning, stress results.

The Psychosocial Stress Scale (PSS), as originally designed, was an eight-item scale which records stress related to financial problems, marriage strain, loss of family role, the need for changing one's vacation plans, altered body image, child care problems, sexual functioning and dependency needs. Scale reliability is reported in Table 1. By adding items (e.g. work, intimacy, recreation, isolation), the psychometric properties of the revised 211-item scale have been enhanced (Table 1). Based on studies of hemodialysis and peritoneal patients, there is evidence for both content and construct validity [209, 210, 223, 224].

5.5. Assessing social support

Social support is defined as information received by the respondent that he is loved, wanted, respected, valued, and a part of a context he can count on should the need arise. The Social Support Scale (SSS) is comprised of seven sets of vignettes from the original 16 developed by Kaplan and modified by Turner using a story identification technique [225–227]. Evidence suggests social-support mechanisms function as moderators of stress and as independent variables in determining health status [225, 226]. Scale reliability based on a ESRD (Table 1) and non-renal failure population is above average [227]. Validity has been documented by the authors of the scale.

5.6. Assessing primary group support

Primary groups may include one's family, friends, fellow workers, and neighbors. Primary group support is assessed by a Dialysis Interpersonal Relationship Index (DIPI). The

Table 1. Description of scales

	Range	Number of items	Home dialysis patients	
			N	*
Dialysis stress				
Global	0–6	14	162	0.81
Disease Process	0–6	7	267	0.65
Treatment Related	0–6	7	166	0.67
Somatic Symptoms	0–5	9	50	0.74
Treatment Related Stress (CAPD)	0–5	53	50	0.92
Psychosocial stress				
PSS (Original)	0–6	8	99	0.68
PSS (Revised)	0–6	21	50	0.88
Dialysis interpersonal relationship				
Global	0–5	26	87	0.88
Spouse	0–5	6	216	0.85
Household	0–5	6	143	0.67
Extended Family	0–5	6	242	0.82
Friends	0–5	6	262	0.84
Social Support	9–45	7 sets	247	0.78
Marriage dyad				
Dyadic Consensus	0–5	13	150	0.90
Dyadic Cohension	0–5	5	179	0.70
Basic Personality Inventory				
Depression	0–1	20	226	0.84
Denial	0–1	20	233	0.72
Anxiety	0–1	20	229	0.79
Self Depreciation	0–1	20	215	0.63
Social Introversion	0–1	20	236	0.79
Hypochondriasis	0–1	20	226	0.75
Patient self assessment	0–4	7	226	0.78
Locus of control	0–4	6	137	0.65
Personal Locus Control	0–4	2	90	0.70
Ideological Locus Control	0–4	4	90	0.61

* = Cronbach's Reliability Alpha

index requires the respondent to assess the amount of mutual understanding, perceived support, closeness and level of satisfaction with the relationship. The Global Index comprises four subscales (spouse, family at home, extended family, friends) each containing four items. Global and subscale reliabilities [29] are within an acceptable range (Table 1).

DIPI items are not representative of a particular universe of items, and thus content validity is not at issue. Construct and discriminant validity was established by correlating the scale with the Social Support Scale. Discriminant validity of the Spouse subscale, was determined by correlating it with Spanier's Marriage Dyad Cohesion and Consensus scales [228].

5.7. Assessing leisure and recreational activity

Viewed as a social indicator, social/leisure time activity is an objective measure. As a concept, it is relevant to social norms and is a common index of the well being of a society or a population stratum within society. Spare time (non-work) activities are most strongly related to a global index of well being [112]. Despite its importance as a measure of well being, there is little information about leisure pursuits of ESRD patients. The conflicting picture presented by those few studies undertaken [50, 121, 115] underscore the fact that it is more difficult to assess change in this area than to assess rehabilitation or compliance.

The Social Leisure Activities Inventory (SLAI) establishes the degree to which patients participate in various activities – physical, sedentary, social and community-based, in a typical month. Items represent a cross section of active and passive activities which the patient can engage in alone or with others. There is no overall score. Scores represent a computed average of the ratings of the scale items.

Because the SLAI is an inventory of separate activities

rather than as a unified scale where all items measure the same underlying concept, there is no reason to expect that persons who engage in one activity would necessarily engage in another similar activity. Consequently, the degree of intercorrelation among items is expected to be low, and the issue of internal consistency is not really relevant. Since the items selected are similar to those used by a national study of 'The Use of Time in American Society' [229], there is no question as to content validity. Use of the SLAI with a dialysis population supports this assumption. Most items are relevant to a sizeable number of respondents, and even the least popular activities are engaged in by over 10% of the samples most of the time.

5.8. Patient self-assessement

Credence should be given to patients' perception as to how they are coping. In contrast to functional capacity, which can be determined objectively by a variety of tests (e.g. BPI), the patients' opinion as to their health status is entirely subjective. Evidence supports the use of self-evaluative reports as accurately reflecting individual well being [230].

Our Dialysis Self-rating Scale requires a subjective estimate of performance in six key areas of functioning and an overall assessment of how well they are doing. A global score is calculated by taking the mean of the seven ratings. Table 1 records the reliability estimates. Validity is presently being established.

5.9. Assessing feelings of helplessness

Recently, much attention has been accorded to dialysis patients' locus of control. This concept refers to an individual's feelings that major life occurrences are either contingent upon personal behaviour and effort (internal locus of control) or upon forces that are beyond personal influence (external locus of control). Health related research of locus of control is certainly not capricious, since the construct compliments the philosophy of renal units that improvements in health status relate to individuals taking charge of their own health behaviour.

Locus of control has played an important role in nephrological research. Fish and Karabenick [231] found a significant association between those patients with internal control and high self esteem. Snyder [232] reports that externals perceived both little social support and high stress from the treatment. Galaz [233] noted that individuals who adjusted better to hemodialysis are internal, while those making a poorer adjustment tend to be external. Goldstein and Rezikoff [234] report that dialysis patients at the external end of the locus of control continuum are more likely to reject a real commitment to treatment. This is disturbing given that most dialysis patients have an external locus of control [235–236]. There is a ray of hope however, in the finding that continuance in dialysis over the long period corresponds to an increase in feelings of personal control by the patient [236].

Our six item measure [29] was developed from a previously abridged 11-item I-E Scale [237]. These shorter versions were intended to improve on the original 29-item index [238] by being relevant to the population being studied. Through the use of a more differentiated response

to individual items they also enhanced the scales' reliability (Table 1). Based on a pretest of 137 dialysis patients we were able to distinguishes between two levels of I-E, namely personal and ideological. These two factors have been noted by other researchers [239, 240].

6. ADAPTING SUCCESSFULLY TO CAPD

Nephrology staff invariably ask 'What factors distinguish patients who succeed at CAPD and those who fail, be it by death or return to centre?' In an attempt to answer this question, we collected physiological and psychosocial data on 150 patients over the first three months of CAPD therapy. At the end of this period, we found 27 percent of the patients continued with their original treatment and believed themselves to be 'successfully adapted' (i.e. feeling very well physically, socially and emotionally). Twenty one percent were still on CAPD but considered themselves to be 'qualified adapters' (i.e. doing fairly well). Seventy-nine patients (52%) either died or returned to in-centre dialysis.

Analysis, excluding qualified adapters showed gender differences between successful adapters. Thirty-eight percent of the total female population were successful as opposed to 26 percent of the males. However, age was of no influence. Adapters were significantly less depressed and less anxious than failures.

CAPD patients who adapted well at home also adapted well in their marriages and family relationships. Compared to those who failed, their marriages were more intact (i.e. marital cohesion); their interpersonal relationships with household family members, usually children, were more intense. However, this was not true of relationships involving extended family or friends. Adapters were less involved in community activities; were more socially introverted, and scored more internally than failures.

They were also physiologically better as judged by routine clinical hematological and biochemical examinations, and they had less morbidity as defined by hospital admissions. Adapted patients had 0.09 hospital admissions/patient/ month whereas those who returned to in-center hemodialysis or died showed, respectively, 0.29 and 0.25 admissions per patient month ($p < 0.008$).

More recently, we looked at long term adjustment to home dialysis. Analysis was based on 308 patients, the majority (72%) of which were on peritoneal procedures. The logistic regression models that predict both survival and successful adaptation are interesting in that they support our belief that differing variables influence ESRD outcomes. For instance, the regression equation predicting survival at 17 months, from independent variables collected at the start of the home training program, relates age and the initial renal diagnosis. On further examination, this indicates the poor prognosis of that group of patients who have diabetic nephropathy. On the other hand, the model to predict successful adaptation is more influenced by psychosocial factors such as the level of social introversion and the degree of stress that the patient experiences from his treatment regimen. We expect that predictive models will generate dissimilar profiles dependent upon the duration of home treatment. This would also apply to regression models for patients on CAPD, home hemodialysis and self-care hemodialysis.

These results indicate that information obtained from psychosocial profiling at the patient's initial presentation will augment pathophysiological information in helping the physician select the most beneficial treatment for the patient. Modelling could indicate whether or not it is worthwhile training a patient for a home dialysis program. Besides, it will identify those factors which might be important in possible failures and, thus, allow appropriate intervention to be instituted at an early stage. In the long run, we hope it will lead to a selective choice of treatment model for a given patient.

7. THE CHOICE OF A TREATMENT MODALITY FOR HOME DIALYSIS

It appears that the stresses of home dialysis are not a uniform problem and they may be influenced by the type of dialysis therapy in selected groups of patients. Review of data indicates that the frequency and degree of stresses and concerns are more relevant to those patients treated by hemodialysis, especially in the younger age groups. Furthermore, irrespective of modality, they are directly related to the degree of depression and anxiety that the individual has as part of his/her basic personality traits. Thus, it can be assumed that patients who demonstrate high levels of depression or anxiety will find home hemodialysis a stressful form of therapy; a dialysis patient who is not unduly depressed

and who has a 'healthy' level of denial may more readily cope with that treatment mode.

On the other hand, CAPD appears to interfere with employment and household work, and is likely to hamper an individual's return to employment especially if the patient is male and of the older age group. Thus, males who are strongly motivated to continue working, particularly if over 45 years of age, might best be treated by hemodialysis. However, the young female patient who is not employed will likely prefer CAPD, a treatment modality associated with less stress and concern. The preference would be enhanced if her personality profile showed elevated levels of depression, anxiety, self depreciation or social introversion.

The management of patients with ESRD is obviously not the sole domain of any particular treatment modality. Consequently, a flexible attitude should be adopted by renal units, and patients should be guided towards the type of dialysis therapy that best suits them. It is obvious that every geographic region should have all forms of peritoneal and hemodialysis modalities at its disposal. This is becoming more important as financial pressures force renal teams to maintain as large a percentage of patients outside the hospital setting as possible.

Thus, it is imperative to be cognizant of non-physiological parameters which may influence patient survival and probabilities of success of a given treatment modality. Identification of these key determinants should help minimize unnecessary mortality and morbidity by stimulating early intervention, thereby improving patients' adaptation to their illness and ultimately their quality of life.

REFERENCES

1. Rosansky S, Eggers P: Trends in the US end-stage disease population: 1973–1983. Am J Kidney Disease 9(2): 91–97, 1987.
2. Lasker N, McCauley EP, Possarotti CT: Chronic peritoneal dialysis. Trans Am Soc Artif Internal Organs 12: 94–97, 1966.
3. Tenckhoff H, Weston B, Shilipetar G: A simplified automatic peritoneal dialysis system. Trans Am Soc Artif Internal Organs, 18: 436–440, 1972.
4. Tenckhoff H, Schecter H: A bacteriologically safe peritoneal access devise. Trans Am Soc Artif Internal Organs 14: 181–186, 1968.
5. Moncrief JW et al.: Continuous ambulatory peritoneal dialysis best treatment for end-stage renal disease. Kidney Int 17: S23–5, 1985.
6. Price CG, Suki WN: Newer modifications of peritoneal dialysis: Options in the treatment of patients with renal failure. Am J Nephrol. 1: 97–104, 1981.
7. Oreopoulos DG: Chronic peritoneal dialysis. Clin Neph. 9: 165–173, 1978.
8. Lindsay RM: Adaptation to home dialysis: The use of hemodialysis and peritoneal dialysis. AANNT Journal, 9(4): 49–52, 1982.
9. Teschan PE, Ginn HE, Bourne Jr, et al.: Quantitative indices of clinical uremia. Kidney Int 15: 676–697, 1979.
10. Osberg JW, Meares GJ, McKee DC: Intellectual functioning renal failure and chronic dialysis. J of Chronic Dis, 35(6): 445–456, 1982.
11. Burton HJ, DeNour AK, Conley JA et al.: Comparison of psychological adjustment to continuous ambulatory peritoneal dialysis and home hemodialysis. Peritoneal Dialysis Bulletin 2(2): 76–78, 1982.

12. Burton HJ, Lindsay RM, Kline SA: Social Support as a mediator of psychological dysfunctioning and a determinant of renal failure outcomes. Clinical and Experimental Dialysis and Apheresis, 7(4): 371–389, 1983.
13. Evans RW, Manninen D, Garrison L et al.: The quality of life of patients with end-stage renal disease. N Eng J Med, 312(9): 553–559, 1985.
14. Evans DH. The treatment of kidney disease: an analysis of medical care process, medical care structure and patient outcomes. Unpublished doctoral dissertation. Duke University, 1979.
15. Wai L, Richmond J, Burton HJ, et al.: Influence of psychosocial factors on survival of home dialysis patients. Lancet 2: 1155–1156, 1981.
16. Richmond JM, Lindsay RM, Burton HJ: Psychological and physiological factors predicting the outcome on home hemodialysis. Clinical Nephrology 17(3): 109–113, 1982.
17. Burton HJ, Kline SA, Lindsay RM, et al.: Relationship of depression to survival in chronic renal failure. Psychosomatic Medicine 48 (3/4): 261–269, 1986.
18. Lindsay RM, Burton HJ, Kline SA: Quality of life and psychosocial aspects of chronic peritoneal dialysis. In: KD Nolph, Peritoneal Dialysis (2nd ed.) Boston: Martinus Nijhoff Publishers, pp. 668–684, 1985.
19. Posen G, Arbus G, Hutchinson T, et al.: Survival comparison of adult non-diabetic patients treated with either hemodialysis or CAPD for End-stage renal failure. Peritoneal Dialysis Bulletin 7(2): 78–79, 1987.
20. Westlie L, Umen A, Nestrud S, et al.: Mortality, morbidity, and life satisfaction in the very old dialysis patient. Trans Am Soc Intern Organ 30: 21–30, 1984.
21. Berg O: Health and quality of life. Acta Sociologica 18(1): 3–22, 1975.

22. Churchill DN, Torrance GW, Taylor DW, *et al.*: Measurement of quality of life in end-stage renal disease; the time trade-off approach, Clin Invest Med. 10(1): 14–20, 1987.

23. Churchill DN, Morgan J, Torrance G: Quality of life in end stage renal disease. Peritoneal Dialysis Bull. 4: 20–23, 1984.

24. Torrance GW, Thomas WH, Sackett DL: A utility maximization model for evaluation of health care programs. Hlth Services Rs 7: 118–33, 1972.

25. Sackett DL, Torrnace GW: The utility of different health states as perceived by the general public. J Chron Dis 31: 697–704, 1978.

26. Laborde JM, Powers MJ: Satisfaction with life for patients undergoing hemodialysis and patients suffering from osteoarthritis. Research in Nursing & Health 3: 1924, 1980.

27. Ferrans GE, Powers MJ: Quality of life index: development and psychometric properties. Advances in Nursing Science, 8(1): 15–24, 1985.

28. Chubon RA: Quality of life and persons with end-stage renal disease. Dialysis & Transplantation, 15(8): 450–452, 1986.

29. Burton HJ, Canzona L, Lindsay RM, *et al.*: Adaptation to Home Dialysis: The Health Care Research Unit Report. University of Western Ontario (London), 1–387, 1980.

30. Burton HJ, Lindsay RM, Canzona L, *et al.*: Adapting to a home dialysis program – The Ontario experience. Ontario Ministry of Health (DM 338): 1–33, 1985.

31. Burton HJ, Lindsay RM, Akhtar M.: Factors Influencing Outcome of Home and Satellite Care Patients. Department Psychiatry, Toronto Western Hosptial, 1–65, 1986.

32. O'Brien ME: Effective social environment and hemodialysis adaptation: A panel analysis. J of Hlth and Soc Beh, 21 (Dec): 360–370, 1980.

33. Beard MP: Changing family relationships. Dialysis and Transplantation, 4: 35, 1975.

34. Roper E, Raulson A, Cramer D.: Attitudinal barriers in dialysis communication. AANNT Journal 4(4): 179–98, 1977.

35. Sorensen E: Group therapy in a community hospital dialysis unit. J Am Med Assoc. 221(8): 899–901, 1972.

36. Kossoris P: Family therapy as an adjunct to hemodialysis and transplantation. Am J Nur 70: 1730–33, 1970.

37. DeNour AK: Medical staffs' attitudes and patients' rehabilitation. Proc Eur Dial Transpl Assoc 17: 520–523, 1980.

38. Decker RS: Vocational placement services for the renal disease client. Dial & Transp., 7(6): 561–66, 1978.

39. Ford JF: Rehabilitation – what does it mean and who is repsonsible. In: GE Schreiner (ed.), Controversies in Nephrology, Vol 1. Georgetown, University, 1979, pp. 181–190.

40. Lindsay RM, Oreopoulos DG, Burton HJ: A comparison of CAPD and Hemodialasis in adaptation to home dialysis. In: JW Moncrief and RP Popovich (eds.), CAPD Update, Masson Publishing, 1981. pp. 171–179.

41. Palmer S, Canzona L, Conley J, *et al.*: Vocational adaptation of patients on home dialysis: its relationship to personality, activities and support received. J Psychosom Res 27(3): 201–207, 1983.

42. Kawaguchi Y, Ota K: Continuous ambulatory peritoneal dialysis: One year's experience of cooperative study in Japan. In: Gahl GM, Kessel M, Nolph KD (eds), Advances in Peritoneal Dialysis, Excerpta Medica, Princeton, 1981, 233–239.

43. Gutman RA, *et al.*: Physical activity and employment status of patients on maintenance dialysis. N Eng J Med 304: 309, 1981.

44. Procci WR: The study of sexual dysfunction in uremic males: Problems for patients and investigators. Clinical and Experimental Dialysis and Apheresis 7(4): 289–302, 1983.

45. Davenport U, Strawgate-Kanefsky L: A CAPD patient group on sexuality – A critical view. Clinical and Experimental Dialysis and Apheresis, 7(4): 303–312, 1983.

46. Levy NB: Sexual dysfunctions of hemodialysis patients. Clinical and Experimental Dialysis and Apheresis, 7(4): 275–288, 1983.

47. Stout J, Auer J, Kincey J, *et al.*: Sexual and marital relationships and dialysis, – The patients' viewpoint. Peritoneal Dialysis Bull. 7(2) April–June: 97–101, 1987.

48. Degen K, Strain J, Zumoff B: Biopsychosocial evaluation of sexual functioning in end-stage renal disease. In: Levy N (ed), Psychonephrology 2, Psychological Problems in Kidney Failure and Their Treatment. Plenum Publ. New York, pp 223–234, 1983.

49. Gilli P, Bastiani P, Rosati R, *et al.*: Impairment of the mental status of patients on regular dialysis treatment. Proc Eur Dial Transp Assoc. 17: 306–311, 1980.

50. Freidman EA, Goodwin NJ, Chaudhry L: Psychosocial adjustment to maintenance hemodialysis. 1. NY J Med 70: 629–637, 1970.

51. Anger D: The psychologic stress of chronic renal failure and long-term hemodialysis. Nurs Clin North Am., 10: 449–460, 1975.

52. Jourard SM: The invitation to die. In: Schneidman ES (ed). On the Nature of Suicide. Jossey-Bass. New York, 1969.

53. Gelfman M, Wilson EJ. Emotional reactions in a renal unit. Comp Psych 13: 283, 1972.

54. Abram HS, Moore GL, Westervelt FBB, Jr. Suicidal behaviour in chronic dialysis patients. Am J Psychiatry 127: 1199, 1971.

55. Haenel T, Brunner F, Battegay R. Renal dialysis and suicide: occurrence in Switzerland and in Europe. Comp Psychiatry 1: 140, 1980.

56. Norton CE. Attitudes toward living and dying in patients on chronic hemodialysis. Ann NY Acad Sci 164: 720, 1969.

57. Bollin BW, Hart LK: The relationship of health belief motivations, health locus of control and health valuing to dietary compliance of hemodialysis patients. AANNT Journal, October: 41–47, 1982.

58. Kutner NG, Brogan D, Kutner MH: End-stage renal disease treatment modality and patients' quality of life. Am J. Nephrol. 6: 396–402, 1986.

59. Haynes RB, Sackett DL. A Workshop Symposium: Compliance with Therapeutic Regimens, Annotated Bibliography. McMaster University Medical Centre, Hamilton, Ontario, 1974.

60. Cheek JN, Patient feeling about illness: Do they affect compliance with the therapeutic regimen. AANNT Journal, October: 17–20, 1982.

61. Czaczkes, JW, Kaplan DeNour. Chronic Hemodialysis as a Way of Life. New York: Brunner/Mazel Publishers, p. 81. 1978.

62. Lindsay RM, Burton HJ, Heidenheim P: Compliance, denial and dialysis success. In: Levy N (ed), Psychonephrology IV, Plenum Publ, New York, (In press).

63. DeNour AK, Czaczkes AW: Personality factores in chronic hemodialysis patients causing noncompliance with the medical regime. Psychosom Med 34: 333, 1972.

64. Gonsalves-Ebrahim L, Gulledge AD, Miga D: Continuous ambulatory peritoneal dialysis: psychological factors. Psychosomatics 23: 944, 1982.

65. Blagg C: Continuous ambulatory peritoneal dialysis. Am J Kidney Dis 3: 378, 1982.

66. Kutner NG, Cardenas DD: Rehabilitation status of chronic renal disease patients undergoing dialysis: variations by age category. Arch Phys Med Rehabil 62: 626, 1981.

67. Oreopoulos DG, Khanna R: The present and future role of continuous ambulatory peritoneal dialysis (CAPD). Am J Kidney Dis 11: 381, 1982.

68. Calsyn DA, Sherrard DJ, Hyerstay BJ, *et al.*: Vocation adjustment and survival on chronic hemodialysis. Arch Phys Med Rehabil 32: 483, 1981.

69. Gutman RA, Stead UW, Robinson RR. Physical activity and

employment status of patients on maintenance dialysis. N Engl J Med 304: 309–313, 1981.

70. Rosenbaum I, Atcherson E, Corry RJ: Rehabilitation and the transplant patient. Dialysis and Transplant 10: 136, 1981.

71. Tews HP, Schreiber WR, Huber W, *et al.*: Vocational rehabilitation and dialyzed patients: a cross sectional study. Nephron 26: 130, 1980.

72. Palmer S, Canzona L, Conley J, *et al.*: Vocational adaptation of patients on home dialysis -its relationshipo to personality, activities and support received. J Psychosomatic Res 27: 201, 1983.

73. Shapiro FL, Schwalbach A: Rehabilitation: its implementation and effectiveness in a dialysis setting. J Chron Dis 26: 613–616, 1973.

74. Goldberg RT: Rehabilitation of patients on chronic hemodialysis and after renal transplantation: a comparative study. Scand J Rehabil Med 6: 65, 1974.

75. Malmquist AA: A prospective study of patients in chronic hemodialysis – II Predicting factors regarding rehabilitation. J of Psychosom. Res 12: 339, 1973.

76. DeNour KA, Czaczkes JW: Personality factors influencing vocational rehabilitation. Arch General Psychiatry 32: 573, 1975.

77. Hagarty SF, Hagarty LM: Beyond survival: a study of the rehabilitation of kidney dialysis and transplant patients. Laidlaw Foundation, Toronto, Canada, 1977.

78. Lindsay RM, Oreopoulos DG, Burton HJ, *et al.*: Adaptation to home dialysis: a comparison of continuous ambulatory peritoneal dialysis and hemodialysis. In: M Legrain (ed), Continuous Ambulatory Peritoneal Dialysis, Excerpta Medica, Amsterdam, 1980, 120–130.

79. Lindsay RM, Oreopoulos DG, Burton HJ, *et al.*: The effect of treatment modality (CAPD vs hemodialysis) in adaptation to home dialysis in Canada. In: RC Atkins, NM Thomson, PC Farrell (eds), Peritoneal Dialysis, Churchill, Livingstone, Edinburgh, 1981, pp 385–394.

80. Lindsay RM, Burton HJ, Heidenheim P: Is CAPD for everyone? In: N. Levy (ed), Psychonephrology IV. Plenum Publ, New York. (In press).

81. Wiltshire S. The Quality of Life of Patients on Self-Care Hemodialysis and Continuous Ambulatory Peritoneal Dialysis. PhD Dissertation, School of Professional Psychology, UCLA Berkeley, 1982.

82. Cadnapaphornchai P, Chakko K, Holmes J, *et al.*: Analysis of 5 year experience of home dialysis as a treatment modality for patients with end-stage renal failure. Am J of Med. 57: 789, 1974.

83. Cameron JS, Ellis FG, Ogg CS, *et al.*: A comparison of mortality and rehabilitation in regular dialysis and transplantation. Proc Eur Dial Transplant Assoc. London: Pitman Medical. Vol 7: 25, 1970.

84. Pendras JP, Pollard TL: Eight years' experience with a community dialysis centre. The Northwest Kidney Center. Trans Am Soc Art Inter Organs 16: 72, 1970.

85. Disney A, Row P: Australian maintenance dialysis survey. Medical Journal of Australia. 2: 651–1974.

86. Brunner PP, Giesecke B, Garland HJ, *et al.*: Combined report on regular dialysis and transplantation in Europe. V, 1974. Pro Eur Dial Trans Assoc. London: Pitman Medical, Vol 12: 3, 1976.

87. Baillod RA, Crockett RE, Ross A: Social and psychological aspects of regular haemodialysis treatment. Pro Eur Dial and Transplant Assoc. Excerpta Medica Foundation. Amsterdam, Vol V, 97, 1969.

88. Huber W, Strauch-Rahauser G, Werner J, *et al.*: Factors influencing rehabilitation in regular haemodialysis – A standardized questionnaire in 222 patients. Pro Eur Dialy Transplant Assoc. Bath: Pittman Press, Vol 9, 257, 1972.

89. Fisher S, Cleveland SE: Body Image and Personality, Von Nostrund, New York, 1958.

90. Cameron N: Personality Development and Psychopathology. Houghton Mifflin Company, Boston, 1963.

91. Deutsche H: Some psychoanalytic observations in surgery. Psychosomatic Med 4: 10, 1942.

92. Cummings J: Hemodialysis; the pressures and how patients respond. Am J Nursing 70, 1970.

93. DeNour AK, Czaczkes SW: Psychological and psychiatric observations in patients in chronic haemodialysis. Proc Eur Dialysis Transplant Assoc 5: 67, 1969.

94. Wright RD, Sand P, Livingston G: Psychological stress during hemodialysis for chronic renal failure. Ann Intern Med 64: 611, 1966.

95. Abram HS: The psychiatrist, the treatment of chronic renal failure and the prolongation of life: II. American Journal of Psychiatry, 126: 157, 1969.

96. Kestenbaum JM: Psychological adjustment to hemodialysis. Paper presented at the American Psychological Association, Chicago, Illinois, 1975.

97. Shea EJ, Bogdan A, Freeman RB, *et al.*: Hemodialysis for chronic renal failure IV: Psychological considerations. Ann Intern Med 62: 558, 1965.

98. Kemph JP: Renal failure, artificial kidney and kidney transplants. American Journal of Psychiatry 122: 1270, 1966.

99. Schreiner GE: The Artificial Kidney, 8: 42–45, 1959.

100. Menzies IG, Stewart WK: Psychiatric observations on patients receiving regular dialysis treatment. Br. Med J 1: 544, 1968.

101. McKegney FP, Lange D: The decision to no longer live on chronic hemodialysis. Am J Psychiatry 128: 267, 1971.

102. Wittkower E: Psychological aspects of physical illness. Can Med Assoc J 66: 220, 1952.

103. Ballak L: Psychology of Physical Illness. Grune and Stratton. New York, 1952.

104. Levy NB. Psychological reactions to machine dependency. Psychiat Clin North Am 4: 351, 1981.

105. Larsen NA. Sexual problem of patients on RDT and after transplantation. Proc Eur Dialysis and Transplant Assoc. The Pitman Press, Bath, 9: 271, 1972.

106. Abram HS, Hester LR, Sheridan WF, *et al.*: Sexual functioning in patients with chronic renal failure. J Nervous Mental Dis 160: 220, 1975.

107. Holcomb JL, MacDonald RW: Social functioning of artificial kidney patients. Social & Sci Med: 109, 1973.

108. Burton HJ, Klatt H, Conley JA, *et al.*: Stresses associated with sexual adjustment of end stage renal disease patients commencing home dialysis: a comparison between hemodialysis and CAPD. Contemporary Dialysis, 25, 1981.

109. Kline SA, Burton HJ, Lindsay RM: Sexual problems of patients on Continuous Ambulatory Peritoneal Dialysis. Unpublished data.

110. Lancaster L: The Patient with End-stage Renal Disease. New York: John Wiley & Sons, 1979.

111. Lancaster L: Home study Program Renal failure: Pathophysiology, assessment and intervention. Critical Care Nurse. Jan/Feb.: 40–55, 1982.

112. Campbell DT, Converse P, Rogers W: The Quality of American Life. Russell Sage Foundation, New York, 1976.

113. Short MJ, Alexander RJ: Roles of denial in chronic hemodialysis. Arch General Psychiatry 20: 433, 1969.

114. Freidman EA, Goodwin NJ, Chaudhry L: Psychosocial adjustment to maintenance hemodialysis: II NY State J Med 70: 767, 1970.

115. DeNour AK: Social adjustment of chronic dialysis patients. Am J Psych 139(1): 97–100, 1982.

116. Kline SA, Burton HJ: The elderly patient on dialysis – psychosocial considerations. Psychosocial Aspects of Elderly Patients on Dialysis. In: Geriatric Nephrology, (ed) DG Oreopoulos, Martinus Nijhoff Publishers, Boston, Mass., 183–202, 1986.

117. Glassman RM, Siegel A: Personality correlates of survival

in a long-term hemodialysis program. Arch General Psychiatry 22: 566, 1970.

118. Burton HJ: Survival without the machine: a comparison of the psychosocial effectiveness of continous ambulatory peritoneal dialysis (CAPD) and home hemodialysis. Dr. P.H. Dissertation, University of Pittsburgh, 1981.

119. Mock LA: Psychosocial aspects of home and in centre dialysis. Ph.D. Dissertation, University of Houston, 1975.

120. Strauch M, Huber W, Rahauser G, et al.: Rehabilitation in patients undergoing maintenance haemodialysis: Results of a questionnaire in 15 dialysis centres. Pro Eur Dial Transplant Assoc. London: Pitman Medical, Vol 8, 28, 1971.

121. Shulman R, Pacey I, Diewold P: The quality of life on home hemodialysis. Presented at the European Conference on Psychosomatic Research, Edinburgh, 1974.

122. Foster FC, Cohn GL, McKegney FD: Psychobiologic factors and individual survival on chronic renal hemodialysis. A two-year followup: I, Psychosom Med. 35(1): 64–87, 1973.

123. Carney RM, McKevitt PM, Goldberg AP, et al.: Psychological effects of exercise training in hemodialysis patients. Nephron 33: 179–181, 1983.

124. Carney RM, Templeton B, Hong BA, Harter HR, et al.: Exercise training reduces depression and increases the performance of pleasant activities in hemodialysis patients. Nephron 47: 194–198, 1987.

125. Eschbach JN Jr. Barnett BM, Daly S, et al.: Hemodialysis in the home. Annals of Internal Medicine 67: 1149, 1967.

126. Brand L, Komorita NJ: Adapting to long term hemodialysis. Am J Nursing 66: 1178, 1966.

127. DeNour AK, Shaltield J, et al.: Emotional reactions of patients on chronic hemodialysis. Psychosomatic Med 30: 521, 1968.

128. Wing AJ, Broyer M. Brunner FP, et al.: Combined report on regular dialysis and transplantation in Europe, I4XIII, 1982. In: AM Davison, PJ Guillou (eds), Proceedings of the Europeean Dialysis and Transplant Association – European Renal Association, Vol. 20, Pitman Publ, London, England, 1983, pp 2–75.

129. Lefebvre P, Nobert A, Crombez JC: Psychological and psychopathological reactions in relation to chronic hemodialysis. Can Psychiatric Assoc J 17: 55, 1972.

130. Binik Y: Coping with chronic life threatening illness: Psychosocial perspectives on end-stage renal disease. Can J Behav Sci Comp 15: 373, 1983.

131. Burke HR: Renal patients and their MMPI profiles. J Psychol 101: 229, 1979.

132. Trieschmann RB, Sand PL: WAIS and MMPI correlates of increasing renal failure in adult medical patients. Psychol Rep 2: 1251, 1971.

133. Devins GM, Binik YM, Gorman P, et al.: Perceived self-efficacy outcome, expectancies and negative mood states in end stage renal disease. J Abnormal Psychol 91: 241, 1982.

134. Devins GM, Binik YM, Hollomby B, et al.: Helplessness and depression in end stage renal diseas. J Abnormal Psychol 90: 531, 1981.

135. Livesley WJ. Psychiatric disturbances and chronic hemodialysis. Br Med J 2: 306, 1979.

136. Livesley WJ. Factors associated with psychiatric symptoms in patients undergoing chronic hemodialysis. Can J Psychiatry 26: 562, 1981.

137. Lowry MR. Frequency depressive disorder in patients entering home hemodialysis. J Nervous Mental Dis 167: 199, 1979.

138. Abram HS, Wadlington W. Selection of patients for artificial and transplanted organs. Ann Intern Med 69: 615, 1968.

139. Cramond WA, Knight PR, Lawrence JR: The psychiatric contribution to a renal unit undertaking chronic hemodialysis and renal hemo transplantation. Br J Psychiatry 113: 1201, 1967.

140. Reichsman F, Levy NB: Problems in adaptation to main-

tenance hemodialysis. Arch Intern Med 130: 859, 1972.

141. Lindsay RM: Adaptation to home dialysis: The use of hemodialysis and Peritoneal Dialysis. AANNT Journal, Aug: 49–51, 74, 1982.

142. Levy NB: Coping with maintenance hemodialysis – Psychological considerations in the care of patients. In: Clinical Aspects of Uremia and Hemodialysis (ed), SC Massry and AL Sellers. Springfield: CC Thomas, 1976.

143. Liptzin B: Psychiatric aspects of aging. In: Rowe JW, Besdine RW (eds) Health and Disease in Old Age. Boston: Little, Brown and Company. 85–96, 1982.

144. Epstein L: Symposium on age differentiation in depressive illness – Depression in the elderly. J of Geront. 31: 278–282, 1976.

145. Burton HJ, Kline SA, Lindsay RM, et al.: The relationship of depression to survival in chronic renal failure. Psychosom. Med. 48(3,4): 261–269, 1986.

146. Rakin PL: Psychiatric aspects of end-stage renal disease: Diagnosis and management. In: WJ Stone and PL Rabin (eds) End-stage renal disease: An Integrated Approach. New York: Academic, 1983.

147. Yanagida E, Streltzer J: Limitations of psychological tests in a dialysis population. Psychosom Med. 41: 557–567, 1979.

148. McRae C: Cognitive-behavioral mediators of depression in chronic illness: An investigation of the links between symptoms of disease and depression in patients on home kidney dialysis. PhD dissertation, University of Iowa, 1987.

149. Beard BH: Fear of death and fear of life. Arch General Psych 21: 373, 1969.

150. Freyberger H: Six years' experience as a psychosomaticist in a hemodialysis unit. Psychotherapy and Psychosomatic 22: 226, 1973.

151. MacNamara M: Psychosocial problems in a renal unit. Br J Psych 113: 1231, 1967.

152. Yanagida EH, Streltzer J, Siemsen A: Denial in dialysis patients: Relationship to compliance and other variables. Psychosomatic Medicine 43(3): 271–280, 1981.

153. Coogan JP: Psychiatry for the slowly dying. Report on a program at Los Angeles County Hospital, SK and F Psychiatric Reporter. 45: 4, 1969.

154. Eichel CJ: Stress and coping in patients on CAPD compared to hemodialysis patients. ANNA Journal 13(1): 9–13, 1986.

155. Sorrels A, Blackson C, Moncrief J: Getting back to reality: Psychosocial adjustments in CAPD. Nephrology Nurse, 4(3): 22–23, 1982.

156. Kline SA, Burton HJ, DeNour AK, et al.: Patient's self assessment of stressors and adjustment to home hemodialysis and CAPD. Peritoneal Dialysis Bull 5(1): 36–39, 1985.

157. Lindsay RM, Burton HJ: Psychosocial Factors. In: Fenton S, Kaye M, Price J (eds). The Treatment of End-Stage Renal Disease by Peritoneal Dialysis. Princeton Junction, New Jersey. Communications Media for Education, 139–149, 1982.

158. Shambaugh PW, Kanter SS: Spouses under stress. Group meetings with spouses of patients on hemodialysis. Am J Psychiatry 126: 928, 1969.

159. Snavely CA: Patient independence in home peritoneal dialysis: One center's experience with self care. Dialysis & Trans 9(11): 1052–1054, 1980.

160. Burton HJ, Lindsay RM, Kline SA: Social support as a mediator of psychological dysfunctioning and a determinant of renal failure outcomes. Clin. Exper Dialysis and Aphesesis 7(4): 371–390, 1983.

161. Molumphy SD, Sporakowski MJ: The family stress of hemodialysis. Family Relations, 33: 33–39, 1984.

162. Shambaugh PW, Hampers CL, Bailey G, et al.: Hemodialysis in the home – emotional impact on the spouse. Trans Am Soc Artif Intern Organs 13: 41, 1967.

163. Conley J, Burton HJ, DeNour AK: Support systems for patients and spouses on home dialysis. International Journal

of Family Psychiatry, 2(1/2): 45–54, 1981.

164. Palmer SE, Canzona L, Wai L: Helping families respond effectively to chronic illness. In: Coping With Physical Illness: New Perspectives (ed.) Rudolf H. Moss. Plenum Pub: New York: 1984, 283–294.

165. Najman JM, Levine S: Evaluating the quality of life: current state of the art. Archives of Physical Medicine Rehabilitation 63: Feb, 1982.

166. Flanagan JC: Measurement of the quality of life. Archives of Physical Medicine & Rehabilitation, 63, 1982.

167. Freed MM: Quality of life: the physician's dilemma. Archives of Physical Medicine Rehabilitation 65: 3, 1984.

168. van Dam FS, Somers R, von Beek-Couzijn AL: Quality of life: some theoretical issues. Journal of Clinical Pharmacology 21, 1981.

169. Andrews FM, McKinnell AC: Measures of self reported well being: their affective, cognitive and other components. Social Indicators Research 8, 1980.

170. Zautra A, Goodhart D: Quality of life indicators: A review of the literature. Community Mentl Health Rev, 4(1): 1–10, 1979.

171. Weissman M, Sholomskas D, Karen J: The assessment of social adjustment. Arch Gen Psychiatry, 38: 1250–1258, 1981.

172. Ferrans GE, Powers MJ: Quality of life index: development and psychometric properties. Advances in Nursing Science, 8(1): 15–24, 1985.

173. Baker F, Intagliata J: Quality of life in the evaluation of community support systems. Eval Program Planning 5: 69–79, 1982.

174. Weissman MM: The assessment of social adjustment: A review of techniques. Arch Gen Psychiatry. 32: 357–365, 1975.

175. Guyatt GH, Bombardier C, Tugwell PX: Measuring disease-specific quality of life in clinical trials. CMAJ, 134: 889–895, 1986.

176. Goldman L, Hashimoto D, Cook EF: Comparative reproducibility and validity of systems for assessing cardio-vascular functional class: advantages of a new specific activity scale. Circulation, 64: 1227–1234, 1981.

177. Peyrot M, McMurry J: Psychosocial factors in diabetes control: Adjustment of insulin-treated adults. Psychosom Med 47(6): 542–557, 1985.

178. Tugwell P, Bombardier C, Buchannan W, et al.: The ability of the McMaster disability questionnaire to detect sensitivity to change in rheumatoid arthritis [abstr]. Clin Res 31: 239, 1983.

179. Mahler DA, Weinberg DH, Wells CK, et al.: Measurement of dyspnea: description of two new indices, inter-observer agreement and physiological correlations. Am Rev Respir Dis 24(suppl 1): 138, 1982.

180. Fries JF, Spitz PW, Young DY: The dimensions of health outcomes: the health assessment questionnaire, disability and pain scales. J Rheumatol, 5: 789–793, 1982.

181. Jette AM: Functional Status Instrument: Reliability of a chronic disease evaluation instrument. Arch Phys Med Rehabil, 61: 395–401, 1980.

182. Helewa A, Goldsmith CH, Smyth HA: Independent measurement of functional index in rheumatoid arthritis. Scand J Rheumatol, 2: 71–77, 1973.

183. Meenan RF: The AIMS approach to health status measurement: Conceptual background and measurement properties. J Rheumatol, 9: 785–788, 1982.

184. Brook RH, Ware JE, Davied-Avery R, et al.: Overview of adult health status measures fielded in RAND's health insurance study. Med. Care, 17 (suppl.): 1–131, 1979.

185. Grieco A, Long CL: Investigation of the Karnofsky performance status as a measure of quality of life. Health Psychol 3: 129–142, 1984.

186. Berger M, Babbitt RA, Pollard WE, et al.: The Sickness Impact Profile: Validation of a health status measure. Med. Care, 14: 57–67.

187. Derogatis LR: The psychosocial adjustment to illness scale (PAIS). J Psychosomatic Res 30(1): 77–91, 1986.

188. Pritchard M: Measurement of illness behaviour in patients on haemodialysis and awaiting cardiac surgery. J Psychosomatic Res. 23: 117–130, 1979.

189. Goldsmith C: Illnss behavior of dialysis patients, staff response, and coping measures. AANNT Journal, Dec: 38–41, 1982.

190. Levy N, Wynbrandt G: The quality of life on maintenance hemodialysis. Lancet, Part 1: 1328–1330, 1975.

191. Brown DJ, Craick CC, Davies SE, et al.:: Physical, emotional and social adjustments to home dialysis. Med J Aust, 1: 245–247, 1978.

192. Bergsten E, Asaba H, Berstrom J: A study of patients on chronic hemodialysis. Scan J Soc Med Suppl II, 1977.

193. DeNour AK, Shannon J. Quality of life of dialysis and transplant patients. Nephron, 25: 117–120, 1980.

194. Campbell A: Subjective measures of well-being. Am Psychol, 31: 117–124, 1976.

195. Bonney S, Finkelstein F, Lytton B, et al.: Treatment of end-stage renal failure in a defined geographic area. Arch Intern Med 138: 1510–1513, 1978.

196. Johnson J, McCauley C, Copley J: The quality of life of hemodialysis and transplant patients. Kidney Int, 22: 286–291, 1982.

197. Keon T, McDonald B: Job satisfaction and life satisfaction: An empirical evaluation of their inter-relationship. Hum Relations, 35: 167–180, 1982.

198. Tietze M: Maintenance hemodialysis stressors, hierarchy of human needs, and nursing interventions: A patient perspective. AANNT Journal 11(1): 13–17, 1984.

199. Burton HJ, Kline SA, Lindsay RM et al.: The role of support in influencing outcome of ESRD. General Hospital Psychiatry 10: 4, 260–266, July 1988.

200. Campbell A: The Sense of Well-Being in America. New York, McGraw-Hill, 1981.

201. Mass M. DeNour AK: Reactions of families to chronic hemodialysis. Psychotherapy and Psychosomatics,, 26: 20, 1975.

202. Neugarten G, Havinghurst R, Tobin S: The measure of life satisfaction. J Gerontol, 16: 134–143, 1961.

203. Campbell A, Converse P: Human Meaning of Social Change. New York, Russell Sage Foundation, 1976.

204. Conte V, Salamon M: An objective approach to the measurement and use of life satisfaction with older persons. Measure Eval Guidance, 15: 194–200, 1981.

205. Liang MH, Cullen KE, Larson MG: In search of a more perfect mousetrap: (Health status or quality of life instrument). J Rheumatol, 9: 775–779, 1982.

206. Campbell A, Converse P, Rogers W: The Quality of American Life. New York, Russell Sage Foundation, 1976.

207. George LK, Bearon LB: Quality of Life in Older Persons. New York, Human Sciences Press, 1980, 1–14.

208. Zill N: Developing indicators of effective life management. Paper delivered at the Urban Regional Information System Association Meeting, Aug 19–31, 1973, Atlantic City, New Jersey.

209. Lindsay RM, Burton HJ: An evaluation of the Hospal Dialysis System and of its role in safely reducing dialysis time. Victoria Hospital Renal Unit, London, Canada. 1987.

210. Schreiber MJ, Burton HJ, Lindsay RM, Kline SA. An Evaluation of the Sterile Connection Device and its Role in Improving Quality of Life for CAPD Patients. Dept. Psychosocial Medicine, Toronto Western Hospital, 1–89. 1987.

211. Greenberg M: Personality and adjustment in hemodialysis patients. Dial & Trans Nov: 9–13, 89, 1977.

212. Fishman DB, Schneider CJ: Predicting emotional adjustment in home dialysis patients and their relatives. Journal of Chronic Diseases 25: 99–109, 1972.

213. DeNour AK, Czaczkes JW: Psychological and psychiatric

observations on patients on chronic hemodialysis. Pro Eur Dial & Trans Assoc 5: 67–70, 1968.

214. Holden RR, Reddon JR, Jackson DN *et al.*: The construct heuristic applied to the measurement of psychopathology. Multivariate Behavioural Research, 18: 37–46, 1983.
215. Holden RR: Item subtlety, face validity and the structured assessment of psychopathology. Ph.D. Dissertation, University of Western Ontario, 1982.
216. Hoffman H, Jackson DN, Skinner H: Dimensions of psychopathology among alcoholic patients. Journal of Studies on Alcohol 36: 825–837, 1975.
217. Jackson DN: A sequential system for personality scale development. In: C. Spielberger (ed.), Clinical and Community Psychology, Vol. 2, Academic Press, New York, 1970.
218. Jackson DN: Orthogonal components of psychopathology: a fresh approach to measuring the constructs underlying MMPI clinical scales. Presented at Society of Multivariate Experimental Psychology, Oregon, November, 1975.
219. Kline SA, Burton HJ, DeNour AK, *et al.*: Patient's self assessment of stressors and adjustment to home hemodialysis and CAPD. Peritoneal Dialysis Bulletin 5(1): 36–38, 1985.
220. Eichel CJ: Stress and coping in patients on CAPD compared to hemodialysis patients. ANNA Journal 13(1): 9–13, 1986.
221. Baldree K, Murphy S, Powers M: Stress identification and coping patterns in patients on hemodialysis. Nursing Research 31(2): 107–112, 1982.
222. Burton HJ, Lindsay RM, Heidenheim P: Quality of Life: Measurement and Application, The Gambro Clinical Trials Workshop, Copenhagen, Denmark, February, 1988.
223. Manuel A, Saiphoo C, Burton HJ, *et al.*: Adequacy of dialysis: a pilot study comparing the effect of dialysis with the Disscap 160 and Biospal 3000S dialyzers on urea kinetics and well being questionnaire. In: Blood Purification in Perspective: New Insights and Future Trends. ISAO Press, 170–175, 1987.
224. Burton HJ, Lindsay RM, Kline SA: du Pont Sterile Connection Device: A Field Trial. Dept. Psychosocial Medicine, Toronto Western Hospital, 1–51, 1985.
225. Cobb S: Social support as a moderator of life stress. Psychosom Med 38(5): 300, 1976.
226. Kaplan A: Social support: the construct and its measurement. Bachelor's Thesis. Brown University, 1977.
227. Turner RJ, Frankel BG, Levin D, *et al.*: Social support: conceptualization, measurement and implications for mental health. In: Greenley JR (ed), Research in community and mental health. Vol. III. Jai Press, Greenwich, 1985.
228. Spanier G: Measuring dyadic adjustment: new scales for assessing the quality of marriage and similar dyads. J Marriage and Fam 2: 15, 1976.
229. Robinson JP, Shaver PR: Measures of social psychological attitudes. Ann Arbor, Michigan: Institute for Social Research, University of Michigan, 1973.
230. Froberg DG: Consistency of self-ratings across measurement conditions and test administrations. Evaluation & The Health Professions, 7(4): 471–484, 1984.
231. Fish B, Karabenick S: Relationship between self-esteem and locus of control. Psychological Reports, 29: 789, 1971.
232. Snyder W: Factors affecting adherence to diet and medication orders by hemodialysis patients. MSc. Dissertation, The University of Michigan, 1977.
233. Galaz A: Psychological aspects related to the adjustment of hemodialysis patients. PhD dissertation. The University of Oklahoma, 1972.
234. Goldstein AM, Reznikoff M: Suicide in chronic hemodialysis patients from an external locus of control framework. Am J Psych 127:1204, 1973.
235. Gentry M, Davis GC: Cross-sectional analysis of psychological adaptation to chronic hemodialysis. J of Chronic Dis. 25: 545, 1972.
236. Mlott SR, Allain A: Personality correlates of renal dialysis patients and their spouses. Southern Medical Journal 67(81): 941–944, 1974.
237. Valecha GK: Construct validation of internal-external locus of control. PhD Dissertation. Ohio State University, 1972.
238. Rotter JB: Generalized expectancies for internal versus external control of reinforcement. Psychological Mono 80(1)609, 1966.
239. Gurin P, Gurin G, Lao RC, *et al.*: Internal-external control in the motivational dynamics of negro youth. Journal of Social Issues 25: 29–53, 1969.
240. Mirels HL: Dimensions of internal versus external control. J of Consult and Clin Psycho, 34: 226–221, 1970.

INDEX OF SUBJECTS

450

452